# PRONUNCIATION

You can use this dictionary to learn how to pronounce medical terms. The pronunciation appears in parentheses between the term and the beginning of its definition. The pronunciation of terms defined in this dictionary is indicated with letters of the English alphabet rather than with phonetic symbols. The following key shows the sounds represented by these letters.

## VOWELS

ā   day, care, trait, gauge
a   mat, damage, far
ă   about, hepatitis, data, tartar
ah  father, what
aw  raw, fall, cause
ē   ego, here, bead, beet, artery
e   bed, head, therapy, teratoma

ĕ   erythrocyte, genesis, system, lower
ī   isle, lie, pyre, bacilli
i   igloo, hip, irritate
ĭ   pencil, circus
ō   oval, form, go
o   got, bought
ŏ   oven, bottom, motor
ow  cow, hour
oy  boy, oil

ū   prune, fruit, genu, food
yū  cube, urine, beauty, value
u   put, wool
ŭ   upset, putt, murmur, tough

## CONSONANTS

b   bad, tab
ch  child, itch
d   dog, bad
dh  this, smooth (cf. th)
f   fit, defect; phase, hyphen; tough
g   got, bag
h   hit, behold
[h] Denotes an approximation of a tone used in French words whereby the sound is pulled to the back of the tongue. The closest equivalent in English is found in the

word 'zone' wherein the ending of that word is pronounced as if swallowed.
j   jade; gender, rigid, edge (cf. g)
k   cut, tic; tachycardia (cf. ch)
ks  extra, tax
kw  quick, aqua
l   law, kill
m   me, timid, bum
n   no, tender, run
ng  ring

p   pan, upset, top
r   rot, atropy, tar
s   so, distill, mess (cf z); center, council (cf k)
sh  show, wish; social
t   ten, batter, put
th  thin, with (cf dh)
v   vote, oven, nerve
w   we, awake, tow
y   yes, payload
z   zero; disease, faces (cf s); xiphoid (cf ks)
zh  azure, vision, measure

# BUILDING BLOCKS OF MEDICAL LANGUAGE

The most common medical word parts can be found in the appendix section of this dictionary. These are prefixes, suffixes, and combining forms that make up 90 to 95 percent of medical vocabulary.

Throughout the A–Z section these terms are marked with the ♻ symbol.

♻ **ab-** from, away from, off
♻ **abs-** from, away from
♻ **acantho-** thorn
♻ **ad-** increase, adherence, motion toward, very
♻ **adeno-** gland
♻ **alge-** pain
♻ **ambi-** around, on (both) sides, on all sides, both

♻ **anti- 1** against, opposing, **2** curative, **3** antibody
♻ **cheilo-** lip
♻ **derm-** skin
♻ **dermato-** skin
♻ **gingivo-** gums
♻ **glosso-** tongue
♻ **histio-** tissue
♻ **histo-** tissue

♻ **hydro-** water, hydrogen
♻ **hyper-** excessive, above normal
♻ **hypo-** beneath, diminution, deficiency, the lowest
♻ **intra-** within
♻ **karyo-** nucleus
♻ **kerato-** cornea
♻ **kilo-** one thousand ($10^3$)

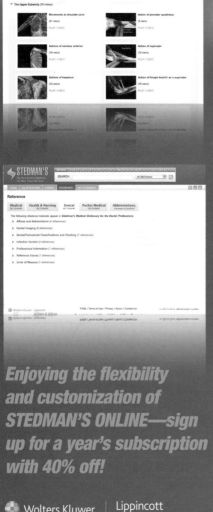
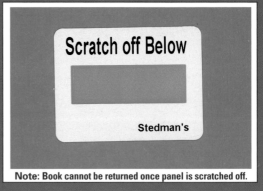

# Stedman's
# Dental Dictionary

## ILLUSTRATED
### SECOND EDITION

Wolters Kluwer | Lippincott Williams & Wilkins
Health

Philadelphia · Baltimore · New York · London
Buenos Aires · Hong Kong · Sydney · Tokyo

*Senior Publisher:* Julie K. Stegman
*Brand Manager:* Jennifer Feldman
*Product Director:* Eric Branger
*Product Manager:* Tiffany Piper, Amy Burroughs
*Chief Copyeditor:* Raymond Lukens
*Copyeditor & Pronunciations:* Kristi Lukens
*Typographic Design:* Parkton Art Studio, Inc.
*Compositor:* Absolute Service, Inc.
*Manufacturing Coordinator:* Margie Orzech-Zeranko

**DISCLAIMER**
Care has been taken to confirm the accuracy of the information present and to describe generally accepted practices. However, the authors, editors, and publisher are not responsible for errors or omissions or for any consequences from application of the information in this book and make no warranty, expressed or implied, with respect to the currency, completeness, or accuracy of the contents of the publication. Application of this information in a particular situation remains the professional responsibility of the practitioner; the clinical treatments described and recommended may not be considered absolute and universal recommendations.

The authors, editors, and publishers have exerted every effort to ensure that drug selection and dosage set forth in this text are in accordance with current recommendations and practice at the time of publication. However, in view of ongoing research, changes in government regulations, and the constant flow of information relating to drug therapy and drug reactions, the reader is urged to check the package insert for each drug for any change in indications and dosage and for added warnings and precautions. This is particularly important when the recommended agent is a new or infrequently employed drug.

Some drugs and medical devices presented in this publication have Food and Drug Administration (FDA) clearance for limited use in restricted research settings. It is the responsibility of the health care provider to ascertain the FDA status of each drug or device planned for use in their clinical practice.

**Library of Congress Cataloging-in-Publication Data**

CIP information available upon request.

# Contents

How to Use this Dictionary ........................................................... inside cover

A Message from the Publisher ................................................................ iv

Consultants in the Dental Professions ........................................................ vii

Consultants to the Stedman's Dictionaries ................................................... ix

Illustrations Index ......................................................................... xviii

Illustrations Sources ....................................................................... xxiv

Artwork Credits ............................................................................ xxxi

A-Z Vocabulary ................................................................................ 1

Image Insert: Oral Conditions and Disorders ............................................... A1

Contents to the Appendices ............................................................... APP 1

# A Message from the Publisher

S tedman's, first produced as Dunglison's *New Dictionary of Medical Science and Literature* in 1833, has a long-standing tradition of excellence. With this new edition of *Stedman's Medical Dictionary for the Dental Professions,* we strove to continue this reputation of excellence, providing our readers with our most comprehensive dictionary devoted to the dental professions, delivered in print and now online as well.

Featuring more than 16,000 entries and 600 illustrations, *Stedman's Medical Dictionary for the Dental Professions, 2nd Edition*, provides students, educators, and practitioners access to the core language for the dental professions, including dentists, dental hygienists, dental assistants, dental lab technicians, and dental office employees.

## Features of Stedman's Dental Dictionary

Accuracy, timeliness and comprehensive content are the hallmarks of any Stedman's Dictionary and every dictionary produced undergoes a rigorous content review. With this new edition, every term and definition was reviewed by leading experts in the dental professions. Each entry was reviewed for accuracy, currency, and application to the dental professions.

- **Art Program** Each of the more than 600 images in this edition were reviewed by our content experts to ensure the images were of the highest quality to increase the reader's understanding of illustrated terms. You also will notice a color insert that includes images covering common oral diseases.

- **Pronunciations** A written pronunciation has been provided for nearly every entry in the dictionary to aid in the reader's understanding of the terminology. A pronunciation key is provided on the "How to Use This Dictionary" page on the inside cover of the dictionary.

- **Cross-References in Blue** Some entries do not have definitions; they are synonyms that point the reader to the preferred main term where the definition appears. All such synonyms are printed in blue, signaling readers to look up the preferred term to find the definition.

- **Building Blocks** Greek and Latin word parts account for about 90 percent of medical language, so identifying and learning these word parts is an integral part of understanding medical language. A recycle symbol icon (♻) is used to identify these prefixes, suffixes, and combining forms in the margins of the A-Z section.

- **Terminologia Anatomica** All the Gross Anatomy terms in this edition reflect the most recent anatomical nomenclature (*Terminologia Anatomica*) approved by the Federative Committee on Anatomical Terminology. All the Latin anatomical terms and their English translations are identified with a [TA] within the text of the dictionary.

- **Etymologies** The origins of word parts are included in angle brackets for select terms to aid in the reader's learning and understanding of dental terminology.

- **Appendices** Twenty-four quick-reference appendices have been added as a resource for readers, including Common Medical/Dental Abbreviations and Acronyms, Classifications of Periodontal Diseases and Conditions, Dental and Periodontal Charting, Guidelines for Infection Control in Dental Health Care Settings, and Dental Imaging Errors.

- **Free bonus online subscription!** Included with your dictionary, you will find an access code that provides a free subscription to the Dental Dictionary content on stedmansonline.com. This subscription includes all the content from the dictionary in an easy-to-navigate online interface. In addition, you will find audio pronunciation, so that readers can not only read the written pronunciation, they can hear words pronounced. Terms also are supported by illustrations, animations, and videos. Users also can customize online content by creating notes about specific terms, adding terms, and saving search results and images in MyStedman's.

## Acknowledgments

We at Lippincott Williams & Wilkins are grateful to our consultants from the dental professions for their help in reviewing, writing, and revising the thousands of entries in this dictionary. Without them, none of the terminology presented here would be relevant or useful. We are also indebted to the many reviewers who assisted us in making critical decisions about the presentation of the dictionary, the dictionary entries themselves, and the content presented in this new edition.

As with other Stedman's dictionaries, the development of this new edition, *Stedman's Medical Dictionary for the Dental Professions,* has greatly benefited from the experience and expertise of Ray Lukens, Chief Copyeditor, whose patience, dedication, and hard work have given this edition an unparallel level of quality. We continue to thank him for supporting our efforts to produce the most accurate, comprehensive, and timely resource for you.

## Your Medical Word Resource Publisher

We strive to provide our readers, including students, educators, and practitioners, with the most up-to-date and accurate medical language references. We, as always, welcome any suggestions you may have for improvements, changes, corrections, and additions—whatever makes it possible for this Stedman's product to serve you better.

| | | |
|---|---|---|
| Julie K. Stegman | Eric Branger | Jennifer Feldman |
| Senior Publisher | Product Director | Brand Manager |

*Stedman's Dental Dictionary, Illustrated, 2nd Edition*
Lippincott Williams & Wilkins
Baltimore, Maryland

# Consultants in the Dental Professions

**Bonnie Blank, RDH, BSc, MA**                           Dental Hygiene
Dental Hygiene Faculty, Camosun College, Victoria, BC, Canada

**Jason William Clark**                                   Dental Hygiene
Burlington, ON, Canada

**Bertha C. Escobar-Poni, MD**                            Dental
Associate Professor, Pathology and Human Anatomy, Loma Linda
University, Loma Linda, CA, USA

**Robyn Hyatt, RDH, PhD**                                 Dental Hygiene
Dental Hygiene Program Director, Dental Hygiene, Fortis College, Salt
Lake City, UT, USA

**Sylvia Ieraci, RDH, BSc, Med**                          Dental Hygiene
Dental Hygiene Program Director, Canadian Business College, Toronto,
ON, Canada

**Carolyn Ray, RDH, Med**                                 Dental Hygiene
Professor, Dental Hygiene, University of Oklahoma Health Sciences
Center, Oklahoma City, OK, USA

**George S. Schuster, DDS, MS, PhD**                      General Editor,
Ione and Arthur Merritt Professor, Emeritus, Medical College of        Dental
Georgia, School of Dentistry, Augusta, GA, USA

**Cheryl M. Westphal, RDH, MS**                           Dental Hygiene
Assistant Dean for Allied Health Programs, Director, Dental Hygiene
Program, New York University, New York, NY, USA

**Karen Sue Williams, RDH, MS**                           Dental Hygiene
Assistant Professor, Fones School of Dental Hygiene, University of
Bridgeport, Bridgeport, CT, USA

# Consultants to the Stedman's Dictionaries

**Naomi Adams, RN, BN, CLNC**  
CEO, Adams Medical-Legal Consulting, Woodbridge, VA, USA;  
Instructor, Practical Nursing Program MCI@ECPI College of  
Technology, Manassas, VA, USA

ESL

**Steven Ades, MD, FRCPC**  
Associate Professor of Medicine and Oncology, McGill University  
Health Center, Montreal, Quebec, Canada

Oncology

**Amy S. Alfriend, RN, MPH, COHN-S/CM**  
Assistant Director, Division of Occupational and Environmental  
Medicine, Johns Hopkins University School of Medicine, Baltimore,  
MD, USA

Nursing

**R. Donald Allison, PhD**  
Associate Scientist, Department of Biochemistry and Molecular Biology,  
University of Florida College of Medicine, Gainesville, FL, USA

Biochemistry

**Debra Kay Arver, RDH, BSDH, Masters Candidate**  
Dental Hygiene Instructor, Argosy University Health Sciences,  
Department of Dental Hygiene, Eagan, MN, USA

Dental Hygiene

**Tricia Berry, OTR/L, MATL**  
Director of Clinical Placement, Kaplan University, Johnston, IA, USA

Medical  
Assisting

**Dolores Bertoti, MS, PT**  
Associate Professor and Department Chair, Alvernia College, Reading,  
PA, USA

Physical  
Therapy

**David A. Bloom, MD**  
The Jack Lapides Professor of Urology, University of Michigan, Ann  
Arbor, MI, USA

Genitourinary  
Surgery

**Jane Bruner, PhD**  
Chair, Department of Biological Sciences, California State University,  
Stanislaus, Turlock, CA, USA

Bacteriology

**Mary Ellen Camire, PhD**  
Professor, Department of Food Science and Human Nutrition, University  
of Maine, Orono, ME, USA

Nutrition

**Kathleen E. Cavanagh, BSC, DVM**  
Fonthill, ON, Canada

Veterinary  
Medicine

**Mitchell Charap, MD, FACP**                              Internal
The Abraham Sunshine Associate Professor of Clinical Medicine,          Medicine
Associate Chair for Postgraduate Programs, Program Director,
Department of Medicine, NYU School of Medicine, New York, NY,
USA

**George P. Chrousos, MD, FAAP, MACP, MACE**                Endocrinology
Professor and Chairman, First Department of Pediatrics, Athens
University Medical School, Aghia Sophia Children's Hospital, Athens,
Greece

**Mark B. Constantian, MD**                                 Plastic/
St. Joseph Hospital, Southern New Hampshire Medical Center, Nashua,     Reconstructive
NH, USA                                                    Surgery

**Arthur F. Dalley, II, PhD**                               Gross Anatomy
Professor of Cell and Developmental Biology and Director, Gross
Anatomy Program, Department of Cell and Developmental Biology,
Vanderbilt University School of Medicine, Nashville, TN, USA; Adjunct
Professor for Anatomy, Belmont University School of Physical Therapy,
Nashville, TN, USA

**Ivan Damjanov, MD, PhD**                                  Pathology/
Professor of Pathology, University of Kansas School of Medicine,        Anatomy
Kansas City, KS, USA

**John A. Day, Jr., MD, FCCP**                              Pulmonary
Assistant Professor of Medicine, University of Massachusetts Medical    Diseases
School, Worcester, MA, USA

**John H. Dirckx, MD**                                      Etymologies
Dayton, Ohio, USA                                          and High
                                                           Profile Terms

**Philip Docking, EdD, MSc, Cert Ed, RN MFPHC**            Nursing
Associate Director, Education and Development, HMI Institute of Health
Sciences, Singapore

**Mark Drnach, PT, DPT, MBA, PCS**                          Physical
Clinical Associate Professor, Department of Physical Therapy, Wheeling  Therapy
Jesuit University, Wheeling, WV, USA

**Michelle R. Easton, PharmD**                                    **Pharmacy**
Assistant Dean, Professional and Student Affairs and Associate
Professor, School of Pharmacy, University of Charleston, Charleston,
WV, USA

**Nancy L. Evans, RN, MS**                                    **Nursing**
Professor of Nursing, Bristol Community College, Fall River, MA, USA

**Thomas W. Filardo, MD**                                    **Chief**
Physician-Consultant, Evendale, OH, USA                       **Lexicographer**
                                                              **and New Terms**
                                                              **Editor**

**Benjamin K. Fisher, MD, FRCP(C)**                           **Dermatology**
Professor Emeritus, University of Toronto Medical School, Toronto,
Ontario, Canada

**Lee A. Fleisher, MD**                                       **Anesthesiology**
Robert D. Dripps Professor and Chair of Anesthesiology and Critical
Care, Professor of Medicine, University of Pennsylvania School of
Medicine, Philadelphia, PA, USA

**Robert J. Fontana, MD**                                     **Gastroenterology**
Associate Professor of Medicine, University of Michigan, Ann Arbor,
MI, USA

**Paul J. Friedman, MD**                                      **Radiology**
Professor Emeritus, Department of Radiology, University of California,
San Diego, CA, USA

**Leslie P. Gartner, PhD**                                    **Histology**
Professor of Anatomy, Department of Biomedical Sciences, Dental
School, University of Maryland at Baltimore, Baltimore, MD, USA

**Douglas J. Gould, PhD**                                     **Gross Anatomy**
Associate Professor, University of Kentucky College of Medicine,
Lexington, KY, USA

**Mary Kaye Griffin, BSH RT (R) (M)**                         **Radiology**
Radiology Program Director, Spencerian College, Louisville, KY, USA   **Technology**

**Joyce P. Griffin-Sobel, PhD, RN, AOCN, APRN.BC, CNE**       **Nursing**
Director, Undergraduate Programs, Bellevue School of Nursing, Hunter   **Oncology**
College, New York, NY, USA

**Steven Gutman, MD, MBA**                                **Stains/**
Director, Office of In Vitro Diagnostics, Center for Devices and    **Procedures**
Radiological Health, Food and Drug Administration, Rockville, MD,
USA

**Duane E. Haines, PhD**                                  **Neuroanatomy**
Professor and Chairman of Anatomy, Professor of Neurosurgery and of
Neurology, University of Mississippi Medical Center, Jackson, MS, USA

**Kerri Hines, RN, BSN**                                  **Nursing**
San Jacinto College, Houston, TX, USA

**Nicholas M. Hipskind, PhD, CCC-A**                      **Audiology**
Professor Emeritus, Department of Speech and Hearing Sciences,
Indiana University, Bloomington, IN, USA

**Nancy Hislop, RN, BSN**                                 **Medical**
Online Instructor, Globe University/Minnesota School of Business,   **Terminology**
Richfield, MN, USA

**Nicola C. Y. Ho, MD**                                   **Genetics**
Assistant Professor of Pediatrics and Active Staff of Johns Hopkins
Medical Institutions, Baltimore, MD, USA

**Iain H. Kalfas MD, FACS**                               **Neurosurgery**
Chairman, Department of Neurosurgery, Cleveland Clinic Foundation,
Cleveland, OH, USA

**John B. Kerrison, MD**                                  **Ophthalmology**
Assistant Professor of Ophthalmology, Neurology, and Neurosurgery,
Wilmer Eye Institute, Johns Hopkins Hospital, Baltimore, MD, USA

**Jeffrey L. Kishiyama**                                  **Immunology**
Associate Clinical Professor of Medicine, University of California, San
Francisco, CA, USA

**Marian Kovatchitch, MS, RN**                            **Nursing**
Dean of Academic Affairs, St. Elizabeth College of Nursing, Utica, NY,
USA

**John M. Last, MD, FRACP, FRCPC, FFPH(UK)**              **Medical**
Professor Emeritus, Department of Epidemiology and Community        **Statistics/**
Medicine, University of Ottawa, Ottawa, Ontario, Canada            **Epidemiology**

**James L. Lear, MD**
Founder, Scientific Imaging, Inc., Larkspur, CO, USA; Professor and
Director, Division of Nuclear Medicine, University of Colorado Health
Sciences Center, Denver, CO, USA

**Nuclear
Medicine**

**Joseph LoCicero, III, MD**
Professor and Chair, Department of Surgery, University of South
Alabama, Mobile, AL, USA

**Thoracic
Surgery**

**Kathy A. Locke, BA, CMA, RMA**
Program Coordinator, School of Health Science, Northwestern Business
College, Bridgeview, IL, USA

**Medical
Assisting**

**James M. Madsen, MD, MPH, FCAP, FACOEM COL, MC-FS,
USA**
Scientific Advisor, Chemical Casualty Care Division, U.S. Army Medical
Research Institute of Chemical Defense (USAMRICD), APG-EA, MD;
Associate Professor of Preventive Medicine and Biometrics; Assistant
Professor of Pathology; Assistant Professor of Military and Emergency
Medicine; Assistant Professor of Emerging Infectious Diseases, Uniformed
Services University of the Health Sciences, Bethesda, MD, USA

**Weapons of
Mass
Destruction/
Bioterrorism**

**Connie R. Mahon, MS, CLS**
Microbiologist, Center for Drug Evaluation and Research, U.S. Food and
Drug Administration, Rockville, MD, USA

**Clinical Lab
Sciences,
Bacteriology
and Mycology**

**Lisa Marcucci, MD**
Fellow, Division of Critical Care, Department of Surgery, Johns Hopkins
University, Baltimore, MD, USA

**Biography/
Eponyms**

**Gail Metzger, MS, OTR/L**
Assistant Professor, Department of Occupational Therapy, Alvernia
College, Reading, PA, USA

**Occupational
Therapy**

**Laurie A. Milliken, PhD**
Associate Professor, Department of Exercise and Health Sciences,
University of Massachusetts Boston, Boston, MA, USA

**Exercise
Science**

**Keith L. Moore, MSc, PhD, FIAC, FRSM**
Professor Emeritus, Division of Anatomy, Department of Surgery,
Faculty of Medicine, University of Toronto, Toronto, Ontario, Canada;
Recipient of the 2007 Henry Gray/Elsevier Distinguished Educator
Award, awarded by the American Association of Anatomists

**Embryology
and British
Medical
Terminology**

**Marianna M. Newkirk, MSc, PhD**                                 Rheumatology
Associated Professor of Medicine, Physiology, Microbiology and
Immunology, McGill University, Montreal, Quebec, Canada

**Marilyn H. Oermann, PhD, RN, FAAN**                             Nursing
Professor and Division Chair, School of Nursing; Editor, Journal of
Nursing Care Quality; The University of North Carolina at Chapel Hill,
Chapel Hill, NC, USA

**J. Patrick O'Leary, MD**                                        General
Associate Dean for Clinical Affairs, The Isidore Cohn, Jr. Professor and   Surgery
Chairman of Surgery, LSU Health Sciences Center, New Orleans, LA,
USA

**Kathleen M. O'Malley, CPhT**                                    Pharm Tech
American Medical Careers, Flint, MI, USA

**Stephen J. Peroutka, MD, PhD**                                  Biotechnology
Consultant, Hillsborough, CA, USA

**Sharon T. Phelan, MD, FACOG**                                   Obstetrics/
Professor, Department of Obstetrics and Gynecology, University of New      Gynecology
Mexico, Albuquerque, NM, USA

**Wanda Pierson, RN, MSN, PhD**                                   Nursing
Chair, Nursing Department, Langara College, Vancouver, BC, Canada

**Susan Polasek, MA, RD, LD**                                     Nutrition
Austin, TX, USA

**Richard A. Prayson, MD**                                        Neuropathology
Section Head of Neuropathology, Department of Anatomic Pathology,
Cleveland Clinic Foundation, Cleveland, OH, USA

**Lisa Radak, RT(R)(T)(CT)**                                      Radiation
Academic Clinical Coordinator, Radiation Therapy Program, Baker           Therapy
College of Jackson, Jackson, MI, USA

**Deneen Raysor, BS, CPT**                                        Physiology
Exercise Physiologist, Aquatic and Fitness Center, Philadelphia, PA,
USA

**William Reichel, MD**                                           Geriatrics
Affiliated Scholar, Center for Clinical Bioethics, Georgetown University,
School of Medicine, Washington, DC, USA

**Jo Ann Runewicz, RN, C, MSN, EdD**                    **Nursing**
Drexel University, Philadelphia, PA, USA


**Georgina Sampson, RHIA**                             **Health Information**
Professor, Rasmussen College, Brooklyn Park, MN, USA   **Technology**


**George S. Schuster, DDS, MS, PhD**                   **Dentistry**
Ione and Arthur Merritt Professor, Emeritus, Medical College of
Georgia, School of Dentistry, Augusta, GA, USA


**Linda N. Sevier, MD**                                **Pediatrics**
Pediatric Faculty, The Children's Hospital at Sinai, Baltimore, MD,
USA


**Susan Slajus, MBA, RHIA**                            **Health Information**
Davenport University, Grand Rapids, MI, USA            **Technology**


**James B. Snow, Jr., MD, FACS**                       **Otorhinolaryngology**
Former Director, National Institute on Deafness and Other
Communication Disorders, National Institutes of Health, Bethesda,
MD, USA; Professor Emeritus of Otorhinolaryngology, University
of Pennsylvania, Philadelphia, PA, USA


**Carlotta South, AAS, ADN, RN**                       **Nursing**
San Jacinto College North, Houston, TX, USA


**Linda Spang, EMT-P, RMA, JD**                        **Emergency**
Department Coordinator Allied Health, MA Program Director,   **Medical Services**
Davenport University, Lansing, MI, USA


**Margaret M. Spieth, MAEd, CMT**                      **Medical**
Faculty, Medical Transcription Program, Moraine Park Technical   **Transcription**
College, West Bend, WI, USA


**Scott Stanley, EdD, RRT, FAARC**                     **Respiration**
Assistant Dean for Undergraduate Affairs, Health and Liberal Arts   **Therapy**
Director of the Respiratory Care Programs, School of Professional
and Continuing Studies, Northeastern University, Boston, MA, USA


**Erin K. Stauder, M.S. CCC/SLP**                      **Speech-Language**
Speech-Language Pathologist, Loyola College in Maryland,   **Pathology**
Baltimore, MD, USA

**Nona K. Stinemetz, LPN**
Vatterott College, Des Moines, IA, USA

Medical
Terminology

**Roger M. Stone, MD, MS, FAAEM, FACEP**
Clinical Assistant Professor, Emergency Medicine Residency, University
of Maryland School of Medicine, Baltimore, MD, USA; EMS Medical
Director, Montgomery and Caroline Counties, MD, USA

Emergency
Medicine

**Janet L. Stringer, MD, PhD**
Associate Professor of Pharmacology and Neuroscience, Baylor College
of Medicine, Houston, TX, USA

Pharmacology/
Toxicology

**Deanna A. Sutton, PhD, MT, SM(ASCP), RM, SM(NRM)**
Assistant Professor, Department of Pathology, Administrative Director,
Fungus Testing Laboratory, University of Texas Health Science Center
at San Antonio, San Antonio, TX, USA

Medical
Mycology

**Robin Sylvis, RDH, MS**
Director, International Business Development, The CoreMedical Group,
Salem, NH, USA

Dental Hygiene

**Geoffrey Tabin, MD**
Professor of Ophthalmology and Visual Sciences, Moran Eye Center,
University of Utah, Salt Lake City, UT, USA

Ophthalmology
and Optometry

**Nina Thierer, CMA (AAMA), BS, CPC, CCAT**
Ivy Tech Community College Northeast, Fort Wayne, IN, USA

Medical
Assisting

**Walter R. Thompson, PhD, FACSM, FAACVPR**
Professor, Department of Kinesiology and Health, College of Education;
Professor, Division of Nutrition, School of Health Professions, College
of Health and Human Sciences, Georgia State University, Atlanta, GA,
USA

Exercise
Science

**Kelly S. Ullmer, ND, LDHS, OTR**
Sheboygan, WI, USA

Alternative/
Holistic
Medicine

**Alexandra Valsamakis, MD, PhD**
Assistant Professor of Pathology, Johns Hopkins School of Medicine,
Baltimore, MD, USA

Virology

**Amy Carson VonKadich, MEd, RTT**
Radiation Therapy Program Director, New Hampshire Technical
Institute, Concord, NH, USA

Radiology
Technology

**Galen S. Wagner, MD**                                    Cardiology
Duke University Medical Center, Durham, NC, USA

**Bruce J. Walz, PhD**                                    Emergency
Professor and Chair, Department of Emergency Health Services,    Medical
University of Maryland, Baltimore County, Baltimore, MD, USA    Services

**Marsha Wamsley, RN, MS**                                Nursing
Professor of Nursing, Sinclair Community College, Dayton, OH, USA

**Dr. Brian J. Ward**                                     Parasitology/
Chief, McGill University Division of Infectious Diseases, Departments    Tropical
of Medicine & Microbiology, McGill University, Montreal, Quebec,    Medicine
Canada

**Ruth Werner, LMP, NCTMB**                               Massage
Faculty, Myotherapy College of Utah, Layton, UT, USA      Therapy

**Barry M. Westling, MS, RRT-NPS, RPFT**                  Respiratory
Program Director, Respiratory Therapy, San Joaquin Valley College,    Therapy
Visalia, CA, USA

**Asa J. Wilbourn, MD**                                   Neurology
Director, EMG Laboratory, Cleveland Clinic; Clinical Professor of
Neurology, Case University School of Medicine, Cleveland, OH, USA

**Helaine R. Wolpert, MD**                                Clinical
Anatomic and Clinical Pathologist, Newton, MA, USA        Pathology/
                                                          Hematology/
                                                          Laboratory
                                                          Medicine

**Douglas B. Woodruff, MD**                               Psychiatry/
Private Practice, Baltimore, MD, USA                      Psychology

**David B. Young, PhD**                                   Physiology
Professor, Physiology and Biophysics, University of Mississippi Medical
Center, Jackson, MS, USA

**Joseph D. Zuckerman, MD**                               Orthopaedics
Professor & Chairman, Department of Orthopaedic Surgery, NYU –
Hospital for Joint Diseases, New York, NY, USA

# Illustrations Index

The Illustrations Index provides a quick way to find any image in Stedman's Dental Dictionary. The page number accompanying each term listed below tells you where an illustration of that term is found. A page number preceded by the letter A indicates the image can be found in the color insert, a 16-page section dedicated to oral conditions and disorders. When you look up a word in the A to Z section, you can tell if it is illustrated—either at the word itself or in the insert or appendices—if it is accompanied by this symbol: ⬛.

abfraction  **198**

abrasion  **A4**

abscess  **A2**

abutment  **4**

accessory cusp  **6**

acid etching process for enamel  **9**

acquired hypodontia  **10**

acrylic teeth for maxillary and mandibular dentures  **12**

actinic cheilosis  **A8**

actinomycotic gingivitis  **A11**

acute atrophic candidiasis  **A11**

acute pseudomembranous candidiasis  **A11**

Addison disease  **A14**

adenoid cystic carcinoma  **16**

adenomatoid odontogenic tumor  **A16**

alginate impression material, loading maxillary tray with  **27**

alveolar abscess  **31**

amalgam alloy, forms of  **33**

amalgam fillings in teeth  **230**

amalgam overhang  **424**

amalgam restorations and fixed bridge  **233**

amalgam tattoo  **33**

ameloblastic fibro-odontoma  **A16**

ameloblastoma  **A16**

amelogenesis imperfecta  **35, A3**

anesthesia, dental injections  **40**

angioedema  **41**

angioedema: latex allergy  **336**

Angle classification of malocclusion  **42**

angular cheilitis  **A8**

ankyloglossia  **44**

ankylosis  **44**

aphthae  **54**

aphthous stomatitis  **A7**

aphthous ulcer  **54**

apical periodontitis  **55**

arcs, maxillary and mandibular  **57**

articulator  **61**

aspects, facial and lingual  **219**

atlantoaxial joint  **65**

attached gingiva  **66**

attrition  **67, A4**

baby bottle tooth decay (nursing bottle caries)  **74**

Barton bandage  **78**

beading or periphery wax  **597**

Bell palsy  **82**

bifid uvula  **84**

bitewing radiograph showing brackets, wires, and stainless-steel ligatures  **94**

blade implant  **88**

blue nevus  **90**

bonded abrasion instruments  **2**

bone loss, generalized  **91**

bridge  **95**

brown hairy tongue  **A7**

buccal mucosa and caliculus angularis  **104**

buccal space infection  **97**

buccal tube  **98**

bulla  **100**

burnished calculus  **101**

calculus  **103**

calculus bridge  **103**

calculus removal  **43**

canalicular adenoma   17

candidal cheilitis   **A8**

candidiasis   **105**

candidiasis, chronic atrophic   **A11**

candidiasis, chronic hyperplastic   **A11**

carcinoma appearing as erythroplakia   **A9**

caries   **108, A1**

caries and chronic periapical
    inflammation   **A2**

caries associated with xerostomia   **602**

caries, recurrent   **487**

caries, restoration of   **494**

caries, root   **501**

cell-mediated hypersensitivity   **A14**

ceramomental crown, layers in construction
    of   **588**

cervical vertebrae   **118**

cheilitis glandularis   **A8**

cheilitis granulomatosa   **A8**

cicatricial pemphigoid   **A11**

cigarette keratosis   **A10**

cleft lip and cleft palate   **127**

cleidocranial dysostosis   **127**

clinical attachment loss, measurements
    for   **128**

complete denture prosthesis   **133**

completed endodontic treatment, radiograph
    of   **200**

concavity on mesial surface of maxillary
    premolar tooth   **135**

concrescence **136**

condensing and carving procedures   **136**

condensing osteitis   **A6**

condyloma acuminata   **A13**

cone-cut   **138**

congenital epulis of newborn   **138**

Coxsackievirus hand-foot-and-mouth
    disease   **268**

curette   **152**

cyclic neutropenia   **A5**

cyst, Blandin-Nuhn   **A5**

cyst, botryoid lateral periodontal   **A6**

cyst, buccal bifurcation   **97**

cyst, dentigerous   **167**

cyst, dermoid   **A5**

cyst, epidermal   **203**

cyst, eruption   **207**

cyst, lateral periodontal   **335**

cyst, nasoalveolar   **393**

cyst, oral lymphoepithelial   **351, A5**

cyst, salivary duct   **520**

cyst, traumatic bone   **91**

cystic hygroma   **154**

debanding and debonding
    armamentarium   **157**

decay, recurrent   **487**

defect, circumferential (moat)   **A2**

defect, three-wall bone   **A2**

defect, two-wall cratering   **A2**

defect, vertical one-wall   **158**

defects due to poor carving   **234**

dehiscences and fenestrations   **227**

dens   **161**

dens invaginatus   **161**

dental casting equipment   **110**

dental cement in pulpal protection   **114**

dental curing lights   **341**

dental dam clamps   **163**

dental film techniques   **231**

dental handpiece with disposable prophylaxis
    angle   **471**

dental implant, radiographic image of   **164**

dental instruments for manual cutting
    procedures   **269**

dental waxes   **93**

dentin dysplasia   **169**

dentin tubules and pulpal nerve endings   **397**

dentinal tubules   **168**

dentinogenesis imperfecta   **169, A4**

dentist-retrievable prosthesis   **166**

dentition, deciduous and permanent   **170**

dermoid cyst   **173**

desmoplastic fibroma   **A15**

development of teeth and odontogenic
   tumors   **34**

diastema   **176**

dilaceration of third molar   **178**

direct digital imaging system   **178**

discoid lupus erythematosus   **180**

distal drift of mandibular premolars and
   canine   **185**

ecchymosis   **189**

ectopic enamel   **190**

ectopic eruption   **191**

enamel formation in teeth   **197**

enamel hypoplasia   **197**

enameloma   **198**

endosseous dental implant   **201**

endosseous single-tooth implant restored with
   crown   **165**

endosteal implants   **201**

Epstein pearl   **205**

epulis fissuratum   **A15**

erosion   **100, 206, 340, A4**

erythema multiforme   **A5**

erythroleukoplakia   **A9**

erythroplakia   **208**

Ewing tumor   **212**

exfoliating tooth   **213**

exfoliative cheilitis   **A8**

exostoses, maxillary and mandibular   **214**

explorers   **215**

extrinsic staining   **218**

fabrication of dental cast   **163**

face masks   **359**

facial muscles   **220**

facial nerve [CN VII]   **221**

facial palsy   **222**

fascia of head and neck   **225**

fiber groups of the periodontium   **228**

figure 8 mixing technique for dental
   cements   **113**

fimbriated fold   **231**

fissure sealant   **232**

fissured tongue   **232**

fistula   **233**

fixed appliance system   **233**

floor of mouth and vestibule of oral
   cavity   **383**

focal argyrosis   **237**

focal epithelial hyperplasia   **237**

focal eruption gingivitis   **254**

foliate papilla   **238**

Fordyce spots   **239**

frictional keratosis   **327**

full mouth survey   **550**

fusion   **245**

Gardner syndrome   **A6**

gel etchant   **249**

gemination   **320**

gemination, variants of   **249**

gemination: twinning, fusion, and
   concrescence   **580**

geographic stomatitis   **A8**

geographic tongue   **250, A7**

giant cell fibroma   **A15**

Gillmore needles   **252**

gingiva   **252**

gingival abscess   **252**

gingival avulsion   **71**

gingival edema due to hypothyroidism   **297**

gingival fibromatosis   **253**

gingival overgrowth   **A10**

gingival recession due to frenal pull   **254**

gingivitis   **3**

glass ionomer cement   **255**

gloves   **257**

gold crown   **150**

Gracey curette series   **260**

hairy leukoplakia   **267, A10**

hard palate   **269**

Hawley retainer   **269**

hemangioma   **272**

hematoma   **272**

hereditary hemorrhagic
   telangiectasia   **277, A9**

herpes zoster   **A12**

hormonal gingivitis   **282**

Hutchinson incisors   **284**

hybrid composite resin   **285**

hypercementosis   **287**

hyperdontia   **288**

hyperplastic pulpitis   **290**

hypodontia   **294**

hypohidrotic extodermal dysplasia   **A4**

idopathic osteosclerosis   **A6**

immediate hypersensitivity   **A14**

impacted mandibular third molar   **301**

implant superstructure   **302**

implant-supported prosthesis   **302**

impression taken using triple tray   **303**

impression trays   **303**

indirect vision   **306**

infection routes, intracranial cavity   **318**

infectious mononucleosis   **307**

inflammatory fibrous hyperplasia   **290**

inlays and amalgams   **310**

innervation of teeth   **311**

intrinsic staining   **236, 319, A4**

irritation fibroma   **322**

labial lymphangioma   **350**

labial mucosa   **330**

lateral incisor   **335**

Le Fort classification of facial fractures   **337**

lead line   **337**

leukoedema   **340**

leukoplakia   **340, A10**

lichen planus   **A9**

lichenoid drug eruption   **A13**

lichenoid mucositis   **A13**

light-cure dental resin kit   **341**

line angle   **342**

linea alba buccalis   **98**

lingual tonsil   **344**

lip pits   **346**

lipoma   **346**

lower gingiva (gums)   **264**

Ludwig angina   **349**

lupus-like drug eruption   **A13**

lymph nodes of head and neck   **350**

lymphangiomas causing macroglossia   **A15**

macrodontia   **352**

macroglossia   **352**

magnetostrictive ultrasonic device   **353**

major aphthous ulcer   **A6, A7**

mandible   **355, 356, 552**

mandible fractures, sites and incidence
   of   **241**

mandibular first, second, and third molars
   (radiograph)   **380**

mandibular molar area   **355**

mandibular molars and premolars   **441**

mandibular osteoma   **422**

mandibular tori   **357**

marginal gingiva and gingival groove   **253**

marginal gingivitis   **358**

masseteric space infection   **307**

maxilla   **362**

maxillary artery and branches   **363**

maxillary teeth and palate   **428**

median rhomboid glossitis   **A7**

melanoma   **367**

melanoplakia with attached gingiva   **368**

melanotic macula, oral (labial)   **353**

mesial furcation   **245**

mesioangular impaction   **164**

microdontia   **375**

microleakage and effects of alteration of
   temperature   **376**

migration of second premolar and partial
   eruption   **377**

mixing process for zinc-phosphate
   cement   **605**

modified pen grasp   **379**

morsicatio buccarum   **382**

mouth breathing   **383**

mouth guard   384

mouth mirror   384

mouth mirror, parts of   312

mucocele   384

mucogingival junction   385

muscles of mastication   360

natal tooth   394

necrotizing ulcerative gingivitis   395, A11

necrotizing ulcerative periodontitis   395

nerves, teeth and skull   396

nerves, temporomandibular region   558

neurofibromatosis   398

nicotine stomatitis   A10

nicotine stomatopathy   536

nodule   402

oculoauriculovertebral occlusion (Goldenhar
   syndrome)   259

odontoameloblastoma   A16

odontoblastic processes   411

odontogenic keratocyst   412

odontoma, complex   A16

odontoma, compound   A16

open contact, poor restoration contour   141

oral cavity   417, 543

oral trauma   331

orofacial granulomatosis   A7

oropharynx and tonsillar pillars   419

orthodontic appliance   420

orthodontic fixed lingual retainer   494

overjet   424

palate   427

panoramic radiograph   430

papillae of tongue, filiform and
   fungiform   230

papilloma   431

papule   431

paranasal sinuses   433

parotid gland   435

parotid papilla   431

parulis   436, A15

pemphigus vulgaris   A11

periapical abscess   440

periapical cemento-osseous dysplasia   A16

periapical inflammation   A2

pericoronitis   441

periodontal abscess   442

periodontal abscess, fluctuant and
   pointing   458

periodontal attachment system   443

periodontal disease   443

periodontal dressings, mixture and placement
   of   444

periodontal file   444

periodontal probes   445

periodontitis   445, A2, A3

periodontium, healthy   446

permanent secondary dentition   510

permanent teeth with approximate age of
   eruption   447

petechiae   448

Peutz-Jeghers syndrome   A14

plaque   166

pleomorphic adenoma   456

porcelain fused to metal crown   460

pregnancy tumor   A15

primary herpetic gingivitis   A12

primary herpetic gingivostomatitis   A12

primary lymphoma of palate   557

primary teeth with approximate age of
   eruption   467

probing depth   468

proliferative verrucous leukoplakia   A9

protective eyewear   472

pseudoaphthae   149

pustule   478

pyogenic granuloma   479, A15

radiolucent area   484

ranula   485, A5

recession   486

recurrent herpes simplex   A12

regional adontodysplasia   412

removable partial denture   490

restoration **151**

retraction **495**

retrocuspid papilla **496**

root canal filling **501**

root canal therapy **501**

rubber cup and polishing agent **143**

salivary glands: parotid, submandibular,
   sublingual **505**

scalloped tongue showing impressions of
   teeth **A7**

scar **507**

secondary palate development **511**

shovel-shaped incisors **519**

sialolithiasis **520**

sickle scalers **521**

sinus tracts **523**

smoker's melanosis **A13**

snuff dippers patch **436**

socket sclerosis **A6**

soft palate **240**

squamous cell carcinoma **532, A9**

Stevens-Johnson syndrome **A5**

Sturge-Weber angiomatosis **539**

subgingival scaling and root planing **502**

succedaneous dentition development **544**

supereruption **546**

supernumerary root **547**

supragingival calculus deposits, detection
   of **548**

sutures, types of **551**

systemic fluoride **236**

systemic lupus erythematosus **A4**

talon cusps **555**

taurodontism **556**

teeth types **304**

teeth, longitudinal sections **55**

temporomandibular joint **559**

temporomandibular joint, dislocation of **180**

tongue **568**

tooth anatomy **39**

tooth formation **570**

tooth, antenatal and after eruption **570**

toothbrush abrasion and abfraction **2**

torus palatinus **571**

transillumination **574**

trauma, lip **575**

traumatic ulcer **582, A6**

unerupted 3rd molar **583**

unicystic ameloblastoma **A16**

varicella **A12**

veneers **588**

verruca vulgaris **589**

vesicle **590**

viral hepatitis antigens and antibodies,
   nomenclature of **276**

vital tooth whitening **598**

wheel brush used in polishing **459**

white hairy tongue **A7**

white sponge nevus **598, A10**

working ends, unpaired and paired **599**

Z-tract injection technique **605**

# Illustration Sources

Courtesy of Dr. Kenneth Abramovitch. From Langlais RP, Miller CS, Nield-Gehrig JS. *Color Atlas of Common Oral Diseases*. 4th ed. Baltimore, MD: Lippincott Williams & Wilkins; 2009 (macroglossia).

From Agur AM, Dalley AF. *Grant's Atlas of Anatomy*. 11th ed. Baltimore, MD: Lippincott Williams & Wilkins; 2004 (atlantoaxial joint).

Courtesy of Ralph Arnold. From Langlais RP, Miller CS, Nield-Gehrig JS. *Color Atlas of Common Oral Diseases*. 4th ed. Baltimore, MD: Lippincott Williams & Wilkins; 2009 (acute necrotizing ulcerative gingivitis, class V caries: maxillary anteriors).

From Bickley LS, Szilagyi P. *Bates' Guide to Physical Examination and History Taking*. 8th ed. Philadelphia, PA: Lippincott Williams & Wilkins; 2003 (patient with Bell palsy, torus palatinus).

From Blackbourne LH MD. *Advanced Surgical Recall*. 2nd ed. Baltimore, MD: Lippincott Williams & Wilkins; 2004 (regions of the mandible).

Courtesy of Cavallucci D, CDA, EFDA, RDH. Harcum College, Bryn Mawr, PA (dental film techniques: occlusal, bitewing, periapical).

Courtesy of Dr. Israel Chilvarquer. From Langlais RP, Miller CS, Nield-Gehrig JS. *Color Atlas of Common Oral Diseases*. 4th ed. Baltimore, MD: Lippincott Williams & Wilkins; 2009 (compound odontoma).

Courtesy of Dr. Walter Colon. Langlais RP, Miller CS, Nield-Gehrig JS. *Color Atlas of Common Oral Diseases*. 4th ed. Baltimore, MD: Lippincott Williams & Wilkins; 2009 (necrotizing ulcerative periodontitis: photograph).

From Fleisher GR MD, Ludwig S MD, Baskin MN MD. *Atlas of Pediatric Emergency Medicine*. Philadelphia, PA: Lippincott Williams & Wilkins; 2004 (alveolar abscess, baby bottle tooth decay, cervical vertebrae, Coxsackievirus hand-foot-and-mouth disease, exfoliating tooth, fistula, gingival avulsion, gingivitis, natal tooth, patient with facial palsy).

Courtesy of Dr. Franklin Garcia-Godoy. From Langlais RP, Miller CS, Nield-Gehrig JS. *Color Atlas of Common Oral Diseases*. 4th ed. Baltimore, MD: Lippincott Williams & Wilkins; 2009 (eruption cyst).

From Gladwin M, Bagby M. *Clinical Aspects of Dental Materials: Theory, Practice, and Cases*. 2nd ed. Baltimore, MD: Lippincott Williams & Wilkins; 2004 (acid etching process, acrylic teeth, amalgam overhang, anterior vertical bitewing radiograph showing brackets, wires, and stainless-steel ligatures, articulator, beading or periphery wax, bonded abrasion instruments, buccal tube, caries: restoration, cement: mixing process for zinc-phosphate type, condensing and carving procedures, defects due to poor carving, dental casting equipment, dental cement in pulpal protection, dental dam clamps, dental instruments for manual cutting procedures, dental waxes, fabrication of dental cast by pouring dental stone into impression, face masks, figure 8 mixing technique, forms of amalgam alloy, gel etchant, Gillmore needles, glass ionomer cement, gloves, impression taken using triple tray, impression trays, inlays and amalgams, layers in construction of ceramomental crown, light-cure dental resin kit, loading maxillary tray with alginate impression materials, microleakage and effects of alteration of temperature, mixture and placement of periodontal dressings, mouth guard, office-applied vital tooth whitening, orthodontic appliance, orthodontic fixed lingual retainer, protective eyewear, root canal therapy: radiographs, wheel brush used in polishing).

From Gladwin M, Bagby M. *Clinical Aspects of Dental Materials: Theory, Practice, and Cases.* 3rd ed. Baltimore, MD: Lippincott Williams & Wilkins; 2009 (complete denture prosthesis, dental curing lights, fissure sealant, hybrid composite resin, porcelain fused to metal crown, removable partial denture, restoration).

From Gold DH MD, Weingeist TA MD PhD. *Color Atlas of the Eye in Systemic Disease.* Baltimore, MD: Lippincott Williams & Wilkins; 2001 (oculoauriculovertebral occlusion: Goldenhar syndrome).

From Goodheart HP MD. *Goodheart's Photoguide of Common Skin Disorders.* 2nd ed. Philadelphia, PA: Lippincott Williams & Wilkins; 2003 (hairy leukoplakia, pyogenic granuloma, systemic lupus erythematosus).

From Harwood-Nuss A MD FACEP, Wolfson AB MD FACEP FACP, et al. *The Clinical Practice of Emergency Medicine.* 3rd ed. Philadelphia, PA: Lippincott Williams & Wilkins; 2001 (Barton bandage, fascial planes of head and neck, mandible: posteroanterior radiograph, mandible: sites and incidence of fractures, parotid gland).

Courtesy of Dr. Sheryl Hunter. From Langlais RP, Miller CS, Nield-Gehrig JS. *Color Atlas of Common Oral Diseases.* 4th ed. Baltimore, MD: Lippincott Williams & Wilkins; 2009 (congenital epulis of newborn).

Courtesy of Dr. Tom Kluemper. From Langlais RP, Miller CS, Nield-Gehrig JS. *Color Atlas of Common Oral Diseases.* 4th ed. Baltimore, MD: Lippincott Williams & Wilkins; 2009 (Angle classification of malocclusion: class II division 1, left; class III, right; class III, center).

From Langlais RP, Miller CS. *Color Atlas of Common Oral Diseases.* 3rd ed. Baltimore, MD: Lippincott Williams & Wilkins; 2003 (accessory cusp, acquired hypodontia, adenoid cystic carcinoma, amalgam fillings in teeth, amalgam tattoo caused by retrograde amalgam, amelogenesis imperfecta, angioedema, angioedema: latex allergy, ankyloglossia, ankylosis, aphthae, aphthous ulcer, apical periodontitis, attached gingiva, attrition along incisal surfaces, bifid uvula, buccal bifurcation cyst, buccal mucosa and caliculus angularis, buccal space infection, bulla, calculus, calculus bridge, canalicular adenoma, cleft lip and cleft palate, cleidocranial dysostosis, concrescence, cystic hygroma, dehiscences and fenestrations, dens invaginatus, dental lamina cysts and Epstein pearl, dentigerous cyst, dentin dysplasia, dermoid cyst, dilaceration of third molar, discoid lupus erythematosus, distal drift of mandibular premolars and canine, ecchymosis, ectopic eruption, enamel formation in teeth, enamel hypoplasia, enameloma, epidermal cyst, erosion: due to chronic induced vomiting, erosion: due to lemon sucking, erosion: lichen planus, erythroplakia, Ewing tumor, extrinsic staining, filiform and fungiform papillae of tongue, fimbriated fold, fissured tongue, fluctuant and pointing periodontal abscess, focal argyrosis, focal epithelial hyperplasia, focal eruption gingivitis, foliate papilla, Fordyce spots, frictional keratosis, gemination, twinning, fusion, and concrescence, generalized bone loss, geographic tongue, gingival abscess, gingival edema due to hypothyroidism, gingival fibromatosis, gingival recession due to frenal pull, gold crown, hard palate, healthy periodontium, hemangioma, hematoma, hereditary hemorrhagic telangiectasia, hormonal gingivitis, hypercementosis, hyperdontia, hyperplastic pulpitis, hypodontia, inflammatory fibrous hyperplasia, intrinsic staining: fluorosis, intrinsic staining: nonvital right central incisor, irritation fibroma, labial lymphangioma, labial mucosa, lateral periodontal cyst, lead line, leukoedema: buccal mucosa, leukoplakia, linea alba buccalis, lingual tonsil, lipoma, Ludwig angina, macrodontia, mandibular first, second, and third molars (radiograph), mandibular molar area (radiograph), mandibular molars and premolars (periapical radiograph), mandibular osteoma, mandibular tori, marginal gingiva and gingival groove, marginal gingivitis, masseteric space infection, maxilla: lateral incisor (radiograph), maxillary and mandibular exostoses, melanoplakia with attached gingiva, microdontia, migration of second premolar and partial eruption buccal to first molar, moderate periodontitis, morsicatio buccarum, mouth breathing, mucocele, mucogingival junction, nasoalveolar cyst, neurofibromatosis, nicotine stomatopathy, nodule, odontogenic keratocyst, open contact, oral melanotic macula, oral lymphoepithelial cyst, papilloma, papule, parotid papilla, parulis, periapical abscess, pericoronitis, periodontal abscess, petechiae, plaque, pleomorphic adenoma, primary lymphoma of palate: telangiectasia, pseudoaphthae, pustule, rampant caries associated with xerostomia, ranula, recurrent caries, regional adontodysplasia, retrocuspid papilla, root caries, salivary duct cyst, scar, shovel-shaped incisors, sialolithiasis, sinus tracts, snuff dipper's patch, soft palate, squamous cell carcinoma, Sturge-Weber angiomatosis, supereruption, supernumerary root, talon cusps, taurodontism, toothbrush abrasion and abfraction, trauma: swollen ulcerated upper lip, traumatic bone cyst, traumatic ulcer, variants of gemination, verruca vulgaris, vertical one-wall defect, vesicle, white sponge nevus, abrasion: worn by friction against porcelain, abscess, actinic cheilosis: everted, actinic cheilosis: vermilion border lost, actinomycotic gingivitis, acute atrophic candidiasis, Addison disease: hypermelanosis, Addison disease: pigmentation of lips, adenomatoid odontogenic tumor, ameloblastic fibro-odontoma, ameloblastoma: soap-bubble locules, amelogenesis imperfecta type II-C, angular cheilitis, aphthous stomatitis, botryoid lateral periodontal cyst, brown hairy tongue, candidal cheilitis, carcinoma appearing as erythroplakia, caries and chronic periapical inflammation, caries: class III lateral incisor, caries: class IV involving lateral incisor and class III involving central incisor, cell-mediated hypersensitivity:

alloy contact, cell-mediated hypersensitivity: benzocaine, cell-mediated hypersensitivity: thiazide, cheilitis glandularis, cheilitis granulomatosa, chronic atrophic candidiasis, chronic hyperplastic candidiasis, cicatricial pemphigoid, circumferential defect and nonvital tooth, class I caries: before and after preparation, class I caries: below occlusal enamel first molar, class VI caries: premolar cusp tip, condensing osteitis, condyloma acuminata, cyclic neutropenia, cyclic neutropenia: floating teeth and gingival erythema, cyst of Blandin-Nuhn, dentiogenesis imperfecta, dermoid cyst, desmoplastic fibroma, epulis fissuratum, erosion: carbonated beverages, erosive lichen planus, erythema multiforme, erythroleukoplakia, exfoliative cheilitis, Gardner syndrome, geographic stomatitis, geographic tongue, giant cell fibroma, hereditary hemorrhagic telangiectasia, herpes zoster, HIV-associated condyloma acuminata, HIV-associated hairy leukoplakia, HIV-associated necrotizing ulcerative gingivitis, hypohidrotic extodermal dysplasia, idopathic osteosclerosis, immediate hypersensitivity, intrinsic staining: pink tooth of Mummery, intrinsic staining: tetracycline staining, leukoplakia: hyperkeratosis of soft palate, lichen planus: plaque form, lichenoid drug eruption: drug withdrawal, lichenoid drug eruption: lateral tongue, lichenoid mucositis, lupus-like drug eruption, lymphangiomas causing macroglossia, major aphthous ulcer: soft palate, major aphthous: gingival ulcers, major aphthous: tongue ulcers, median rhomboid glossitis, nicotine stomatitis, nifedipine-induced gingival overgrowth: palate and side, odontoameloblastoma, oral lymphoepithelial cyst, parulis, pemphigus vulgaris, periapical cemento-osseous dysplasia, periapical inflammation, periapical inflammation, periapical inflammation, Peutz-Jeghers syndrome: buccal mucosa and lips, phenytoin-induced gingival overgrowth, pregnancy tumor, primary herpetic gingivitis, primary herpetic gingivostomatitis: lesions around teeth and multiple areas of gingivitis, proliferative verrucous leukoplakia, pyogenic granuloma, radiographic evidence of class II caries, ranula, recurrent herpes simplex: in patient with HIV, recurrent herpes simplex: multiple gingival ulcers, recurrent herpes simplex: on hard palate, smoker's melanosis: buccal mucosa and soft palate, socket sclerosis, squamous cell carcinoma: floor of mouth and ventral tongue, Stevens-Johnson syndrome, three-wall bone defect, traumatic ulcer, two-wall cratering defect, unicystic ameloblastoma, varicella, white hairy tongue, white sponge nevus).

From Langlais RP, Miller CS, Nield-Gehrig JS. *Color Atlas of Common Oral Diseases*. 4th ed. Baltimore, MD: Lippincott Williams & Wilkins; 2009 (dentinogenesis imperfecta, enamel pearls, lip pits, necrotizing ulcerative periodontitis: radiograph, advanced periodontitis: class III furcation, attrition: polished incisials abrasion, cigarette keratosis, mild periodontitis, moderate periodontitis, moderate to severe periodontitis: 4-mm moat defect, orofacial granulomatosis, periapical inflammation, scalloped tongue showing impressions of teeth).

From Langland OE, Langlais RP, Preece JW. *Principles of Dental Imaging*. 2nd ed. Baltimore, MD: Lippincott Williams & Wilkins; 2002 (cone-cut, full mouth survey).

Courtesy of Dr. Roger A. Lawton and Nobel Biocare. From Gladwin M, Bagby M. *Clinical Aspects of Dental Materials: Theory, Practice, and Cases*. 3rd ed. Baltimore, MD: Lippincott Williams & Wilkins; 2009 (endosseous single-tooth implant restored with crown).

Courtesy of Dr. Nancy Mantich. From Langlais RP, Miller CS, Nield-Gehrig JS. *Color Atlas of Common Oral Diseases*. 4th ed. Baltimore, MD: Lippincott Williams & Wilkins; 2009 (blue nevus).

From Melfi RC. *Permar's Oral Embryology and Microscopic Anatomy*. 10th ed. Philadelphia, PA: Lippincott Williams & Wilkins; 2000 (dentinal tubules: electron micrograph).

From Moore KL, Agur A. *Essential Clinical Anatomy*. 2nd ed. Philadelphia, PA: Lippincott Williams & Wilkins; 2002 (osseous structures of palate, tongue: A & C).

From Moore KL PhD FRSM FIAC, Dalley AF II PhD. *Clinical Oriented Anatomy*. 4th ed. Baltimore, MD: Lippincott Williams & Wilkins; 1999 (dens, dislocation of temporomandibular joint, distribution of facial nerve, floor of mouth and vestibule of oral cavity, innervation of teeth, longitudinal sections of teeth, maxillary artery and branches, maxillary teeth and palate, salivary glands: parotid, submandibular, and sublingual, temporomandibular joint, tongue: B).

Courtesy of Dr. Rick Myers. From Langlais RP, Miller CS, Nield-Gehrig JS. *Color Atlas of Common Oral Diseases*. 4th ed. Baltimore, MD: Lippincott Williams & Wilkins; 2009 (fusion).

From Nield-Gehrig JS, Willmann DE. *Foundations of Periodontics for the Dental Hygienist*. 2nd ed. Baltimore, MD: Lippincott Williams & Wilkins; 2007 (palatal gingiva of patient with chronic periodontitis, chronic periodontitis: probe inserted in pocket, aggressive periodontitis).

From Nield-Gehrig JS. *Fundamentals of Periodontal Instrumentation & Advanced Root Instrumentation*. 5th ed. Baltimore, MD: Lippincott Williams & Wilkins; 2004 (burnished calculus, dental implant radiograph, dentist-retrievable prosthesis, effective calculus removal, explorers, sickle scalers).

From Nield-Gehrig JS. *Fundamentals of Periodontal Instrumentation & Advanced Root Instrumentation*. 6th ed. Baltimore, MD: Lippincott Williams & Wilkins; 2008 (abutment, concavity on mesial surface of maxillary premolar tooth, curette, dental handpiece and prophylaxis angle, dentinal tubules: drawing, detection of supragingival calculus deposits, diastema, facial and lingual aspects, Gracey curette series, implant superstructure, indirect vision, line angle, mesial furcation of maxillary first molar, modified pen grasp, mouth mirror, odontoblastic processes, parts of the periodontal instrument, periodontal attachment system, periodontal files, periodontal probes, probing depth, recession, retraction, rubber cup and polishing agent, unpaired and paired working-ends).

From Nield-Gehrig JS. *Patient Assessment Tutorials: A Step-by-Step Guide for the Dental Hygienist*. 1st ed. Baltimore, MD: Lippincott Williams & Wilkins; 2007 (location of lymph nodes, overjet).

From Oatis, CA. *Kinesiology: The Mechanics and Pathomechanics of Human Movement*. Baltimore, MD: Lippincott Williams & Wilkins; 2004 (arcs: maxillary and mandibular).

Courtesy of Dr. Joe Petrey. Langlais RP, Miller CS, Nield-Gehrig JS. *Color Atlas of Common Oral Diseases*. 4th ed. Baltimore, MD: Lippincott Williams & Wilkins; 2009 (Angle classification of malocclusion: class II division 2, center).

Courtesy of Potter B, DDS. School of Dentistry, Medical College of Georgia, Augusta, GA (amalgam restorations and fixed bridge, endosteal implants, panoramic radiograph: adult and mixed dentition, radiolucent area, recurrent decay, root canal filling, unerupted 3rd molar).

From Reece RM, Ludwig S. *Child Abuse: Medical Diagnosis and Management*. 2nd ed. Philadelphia, PA: Lippincott Williams & Wilkins; 2001 (oral trauma).

From Robinson HBG, Miller AS. *Colby, Kerr, and Robinson's Color Atlas of Oral Pathology*. Philadelphia, PA: JB Lippincott; 1990 (candidiasis, Hutchinson incisors).

Courtesy of Dr. Elias Romero. From Langlais RP, Miller CS, Nield-Gehrig JS. *Color Atlas of Common Oral Diseases*. 4th ed. Baltimore, MD: Lippincott Williams & Wilkins; 2009 (complex odontoma).

From Rubin E, Gorstein F, Schwarting R, Strayer DS. *Rubin's Pathology: Clinicopathologic Foundations of Medicine*. 4th ed. Philadelphia, PA: Lippincott Williams & Wilkins; 2004 (intracranial cavity infection routes, teeth and odontogenic tumor development).

From Sadler T PhD. *Langman's Medical Embryology Image Bank*. 9th ed. Baltimore, MD: Lippincott Williams & Wilkins; 2003 (development of permanent teeth, secondary palate development, tooth: antenatal and after eruption, tooth formation).

From Scheid RC. *Woelfel's Dental Anatomy: Its Relevance to Dentistry*. 7th ed. Baltimore, MD: Lippincott Williams & Wilkins; 2007 (class II caries: mesial surface of mandibular second premolar, maxilla, measurements for clinical attachment loss, oropharynx and tonsillar pillars, radiograph of completed endodontic treatment).

Courtesy of Dr. Paul Schnitman and Nobel Biocare. From Gladwin M, Bagby M. *Clinical Aspects of Dental Materials: Theory, Practice, and Cases*. 3rd ed. Baltimore, MD: Lippincott Williams & Wilkins; 2009 (implant-supported prosthesis).

Courtesy of Sheen G, DDS and Schuster GS, DDS, PhD. School of Dentistry, Medical College of Georgia, Augusta, GA (transillumination).

From *Stedman's Medical Dictionary*. 25th ed. Baltimore, MD: Williams & Wilkins; 1990 (impacted mandibular third molar).

From *Stedman's Medical Dictionary*. 28th ed. Baltimore, MD: Lippincott Williams & Wilkins; 2006 (nomenclature of viral hepatitis antigens and antibodies).

From Taylor C, Lillis C, LeMone P, Lynn P. *Fundamentals of Nursing: The Art and Science of Nursing Care*. 6th ed. Philadelphia, PA: Lippincott Williams & Wilkins; 2008 (Z-tract injection technique).

Courtesy of Dr. Geza Terezhalmy. From Langlais RP, Miller CS, Nield-Gehrig JS. *Color Atlas of Common Oral Diseases*. 4th ed. Baltimore, MD: Lippincott Williams & Wilkins; 2009 (infectious mononucleosis, melanoma).

Courtesy of Ultradent Products, Inc. Gladwin M, Bagby M. *Clinical Aspects of Dental Materials: Theory, Practice, and Cases*. 3rd ed. Baltimore, MD: Lippincott Williams & Wilkins; 2009 (veneers).

From Weber J RN EdD, Kelley J RN PhD. *Health Assessment in Nursing*. 2nd ed. Philadelphia, PA: Lippincott Williams & Wilkins; 2003 (lower gingiva, permanent secondary dentition).

From Wilkins EM. *Clinical Practice of the Dental Hygienist*. 9th ed. Baltimore, MD: Lippincott Williams & Wilkins; 2005 (abfraction, anesthesia: dental injections, debanding and debonding armamentarium, dentin tubules and pulpal nerve endings, fiber groups of the periodontium, fixed appliance system, gemination, gingiva, Hawley retainer, systemic fluoride).

From Wilkins EM. *Clinical Practice of the Dental Hygienist*. 10th ed. Baltimore, MD: Lippincott Williams & Wilkins; 2009 (direct digital imaging system, magnetostrictive ultrasonic device, parts of endosseous implant with crown, subgingival scaling and root planing, types of sutures).

From Yokum TR, Rowe LJ. *Essentials of Skeletal Radiology*. 2nd ed. Baltimore, MD: Williams & Wilkins; 1996 (dental film techniques: panoramic, cephalometric).

# Artwork Credits

Artwork in this edition of *Stedman's Dental Dictionary* was created or adapted by the following companies and artists (see Illustration Sources for sources of adaptions):

**Anatomical Chart Company**: facial muscles, mastication muscles, mandible, mesioangular impaction, nerves: temporomandibular region, oral cavity: anterior view, oral cavity: lateral view, periodontal disease, permanent teeth with approximate eruption ages, primary teeth with approximate eruption ages, teeth types, tooth anatomy. All rights reserved.

**Susan R. Caldwell**, Riva, MD: nomenclature of viral hepatitis antigens and antibodies.

**Neil O. Hardy**, Westport, CT: caries, dentition, Le Fort fractures, paranasal sinuses.

# A

**A** Abbreviation for alanine; ampere.

**Å** Abbreviation for Ångström.

**Ā** Abbreviation for anion.

**aa** Abbreviation for amino acid.

**AAP** Abbreviation for American Academy of Periodontics.

**Aar·on sign** (ar′ŏn sīn) In acute appendicitis, a referred pain or feeling of distress in the epigastrium or precordial region.

**AB** Abbreviation for abortion.

**Ab** Abbreviation for antibody.

♻ **ab-, abs-** *Do not confuse words formed with this prefix with words formed with the prefix ad-.* Prefixes meaning from, away from, off. [L. *ab*, from, usually *abs-* before c, q, and t; often *a-* before m, p, or v]

**a·bac·te·ri·al** (ā′bak-tēr′ē-ăl) Not caused by or characterized by the presence of bacteria.

**a·bap·i·cal** (ă-bap′i-kăl) Opposite the apex.

**a·bar·og·no·sis** (ā-bar′ŏg-nō′sis) *In the diphthong gn, the g is silent only at the beginning of a word.* Loss of ability to appreciate weight of handheld objects, or differentiate among objects of different weights. [G. *a-* priv. + *baros*, weight, + *gnōsis*, knowledge]

**a·bate·ment** (ă-bāt′ment) 1. A diminution or easing. 2. Reduction, ultimately elimination, of public-health nuisances such as smoke or loud noise. [abate, fr. M.E. *abaten*, fr. O.Fr. *abattre*, to beat down, fr. L. L. *batto*, to beat, + *-ment*]

**abax·i·al, ab·ax·ile** (ab-ak′sē-ăl, -ak′sīl) 1. Lying outside the axis of any body or body part. 2. Situated at the opposite extremity of the axis of a part.

**Abbe-Est·land·er op·e·ra·tion** (ab′ē-āst′lahn-der op′ĕr-ā′shŭn) Operation involving graft of flap of tissue from one lip of the oral cavity to the other lip to correct a defect.

**Ab·be flap** (ab′ē flap) Triangular wedge of lower lip (usually midline) transferred into upper lip and vascularized by labial artery.

**ab·do·men** (ab′dŏ-mĕn) [TA] The part of the trunk that lies between thorax and pelvis; does not include the vertebral region posteriorly but is considered by some anatomists to include the pelvis (abdominopelvic cavity). It includes the greater part of the abdominal cavity (cavitas abdominis [TA]) and is divided by arbitrary planes into nine regions. [L. *abdomen*, etym. uncertain]

**ab·dom·i·nal an·gi·na, an·gi·na ab·do·m·i·nis** (ab-dom′i-năl an′ji-nă, an′ji-nă ab-dō′mi-nis) Intermittent abdominal pain, frequently occurring at a fixed time after eating, caused by inadequate mesenteric circulation. SYN intestinal angina.

**ab·dom·i·nal ap·o·plexy** (ab-dom′i-năl ap′ŏ-plek′sē) Mesenteric hemorrhage, thrombosis, or embolus involving the mesenteric or abdominal blood vessels.

**ab·dom·i·nal au·ra** (ab-dom′i-năl awr′ă) Epileptic aura characterized by abdominal discomfort, including nausea, malaise, pain, and hunger.

**ab·dom·i·nal guard·ing** (ab-dom′i-năl gahrd′ing) Spasm of abdominal wall muscles, detected on palpation, to protect inflamed abdominal viscera from pressure.

**ab·dom·i·nal mi·graine** (ab-dom′i-năl mī′grān) 1. Migraine in children accompanied by paroxysmal abdominal pain. This must be distinguished from similar symptoms requiring surgical attention. 2. Disorder that causes intermittent abdominal pain and is believed to be related to migraines.

**ab·dom·i·nal pres·sure** (ab-dom′i-năl presh′ŭr) Pressure surrounding the bladder.

**ab·dom·i·nal pulse** (ab-dom′i-năl pŭls) Soft, compressible aortic pulse occurring in some abdominal disorders.

**ab·dom·i·nal re·flexes** (ab-dom′i-năl rē′fleks-ĕz) Contraction of abdominal wall muscles on stimulation of skin or tapping on neighboring bony structures.

**ab·dom·i·nal thrust** (ab-dom′i-năl thrŭst) SYN Heimlich manuever.

**ab·dom·i·no·car·di·ac re·flex** (ab-dom′i-nō-kahr′dē-ak rē′fleks) Mechanical stimulation (usually distention) of abdominal viscera causing changes (usually a slowing) in the heart rate or the occurrence of extrasystoles.

**ab·du·cens** (ab-dū′senz) SYN abducent. [L.]

**ab·du·cent** (ab-dū′sĕnt) Abducting; drawing away, especially away from the median plane. SYN abducens. [L. *abducens*]

**ab·du·cent nerve [CN VI]** (ab-dū′sĕnt nĕrv) [TA] Small motor nerve supplying lateral rectus muscle of the eye. SYN nervus abducens [CN VI], sixth cranial nerve [CN VI].

**ab·duct** (ab-dŭkt′) *Do not confuse this word with adduct.* To move away from the median plane.

**ab·duc·tion** (ab-dŭk′shŭn) *Do not confuse this word with adduction.* 1. Movement of a body part away from the median plane. 2. Monocular rotation (duction) of the eye toward the temple. 3. A position resulting from such movement. [L. *abductio*]

**ab·er·rant** (ab-er′ănt) 1. Differing from the

usual or norm; in botany or zoology, used for certain atypical individuals in a species; abnormal. **2.** Wandering off; used to describe certain ducts, vessels, or nerves that deviate from the usual or normal course or pattern. [L. *aberrans*]

**ab·er·ra·tion** (ab′ĕr-ā′shŭn) **1.** Deviation from the usual or normal course or pattern. **2.** Deviant development or growth. SEE ALSO chromosome. [L. *aberratio*]

**abetalipoproteinaemia** [Br.] SYN abetalipoproteinemia.

**a·be·ta·lip·o·pro·tein·e·mi·a** (ā-bā′tă-lip′ō-prō′tē-nē′mē-ă) A disorder characterized by an absence of low-density β-lipoprotein, presence of acanthocytes in blood, retinal pigmentary degeneration, malabsorption, engorgement of upper intestinal absorptive cells with dietary triglycerides, and neuromuscular abnormalities. SYN abetalipoproteinaemia. [G. *a-*, priv., + *β*, + lipoprotein + *-emia*, blood]

**a·bey·ance** (ă-bā′ăns) A state of temporary cessation of function. [fr. O. Fr.]

**ab·frac·tion** (ab-frak′shŭn) Loss of tooth structure considered due to combined stress on tooth, resulting from flexure and chemical factors; usually evident as a notch on the buccal surface just occlusal to the adjacent gingiva. See this page. [*ab-* + L. *fractio*, a breaking, Fr. *frango*, *fractum*, to break]

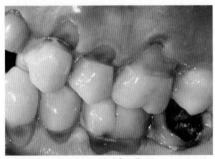

**toothbrush abrasion and abfraction**

**ab·frac·tion le·sion** (ab-frak′shŭn lē′zhŭn) Loss of tooth structure, usually in a wedge-shaped pattern in the cervical area of the tooth, attributed to flexure and fatigue in an area away from the point of loading (usually cervical).

**a·bil·i·ty** (ă-bil′i-tē) The physical or legal competence to function. [L. *habilitas*, aptitude]

**a·bi·ot·ic** (ā-bī-ot′ik) **1.** Incompatible with life. **2.** Without life.

**a·blas·te·mic** (ā′blas-tē′mik) Not germinal or blastemic. [G. *a-* priv. + *blastēma*, sprout]

**ab·late** (ab-lāt′) *Avoid the mispronunciation ab′late.* To remove or destroy function of something. [L. *au-fero*, pp. *ab- latus*, to take away]

**ab·la·tion** (ab-lā′shŭn) Removal of a body part or the destruction of its function, procedure

or morbid process, or the presence or application of a noxious substance.

**ab·lu·ent** (ab′lū-ĕnt) *Avoid the mispronunciation ablu′ent.* **1.** Cleansing. **2.** Anything with cleansing properties. [L. *abluens*, fr. *ab-luo*, to wash off]

**ab·lu·tion** (ă-blū′shŭn) An act of washing or bathing. [L. *ablutio*, washing off, cleansing]

**ab·nor·mal** (ab-nōr′măl) Not normal; differing in any way from the usual.

**ab·nor·mal·i·ty** (ab′nōr-mal′i-tē) **1.** State or quality of being abnormal. **2.** An anomaly, deformity, malformation, or dysfunction.

**ab·nor·mal oc·clu·sal re·la·tion·ship** (ab-nōr′măl ŏ-klū′zăl rĕ-lā′shŭn-ship) SYN abnormal occlusion.

**ab·nor·mal oc·clu·sion** (ab-nōr′măl ŏ-klū′zhŭn) Arrangement of teeth not considered to be within normal range of variation. SYN abnormal occlusal relationship.

**ab·o·rad, ab·o·ral** (ab-ōr′ad, -ăl) In a direction away from the mouth; opposite of orad. [L. *ab*, from, + *os* (*or-*), mouth]

**a·bort** (ă-bōrt′) **1.** To arrest a disease in its earliest stages. **2.** To arrest anything before completion. [L. *aborior*, to fail at onset]

**a·bor·tion (AB)** (ă-bōr′shŭn) The arrest of any action or process before its completion.

**a·bor·tive** (ă-bōr′tiv) Not reaching completion. [L. *abortivus*]

**ABR** Abbreviation for auditory brainstem response.

**a·brade** (ă-brād′) **1.** To wear away by mechanical action. **2.** To scrape away part or all of the surface layer from a part. [L. *ab-rado*, pp. *-rasus*, to scrape off]

**a·bra·sion** (ă-brā′zhŭn) **1.** In dentistry, the pathologic grinding or wearing away of tooth substance by incorrect tooth-brushing methods, the presence of foreign objects, bruxism, or similar causes. SYN grinding. **2.** An excoriation or circumscribed removal of the superficial layers of skin or mucous membrane. See this page and page A4.

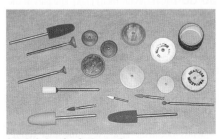

**bonded abrasion instruments**

**a·bra·sion re·sis·tance** (ă-brā′zhŭn rĕ-zis′tăns) Ability of a tooth or a material to avoid being worn away by abrasive forces.

**a·bra·sive** (ă-brā′siv) 1. Causing abrasion. 2. Any material used to produce abrasions. 3. A substance used in dentistry for abrading, grinding, or polishing.

**a·bra·sive discs** (ă-brā′siv disks) Paper, metal, or plastic flat, circular pads covered with particles to grind or abrade.

**a·bra·sive·ness** (ă-brā′siv-nes) 1. Those properties of a substance that cause surface wear by friction. 2. The quality of being able to scratch or wear away another material.

**a·bra·sive pol·ish·ing a·gent** (ă-brā′siv pol′ish-ing ā′jĕnt) SYN abrasive system.

**a·bra·sive ro·ta·ry point** (ă-brā′siv rō′tăr-ē poynt) A pointed device used to grind or polish a tooth or restoration.

**a·bra·sive strip** (ă-brā′siv strip) Ribbonlike piece of linen with bonded abrasive particles on one side; used in dentistry to contour and polish proximal surfaces of restorations.

**a·bra·sive sys·tem** (ă-brā′siv sis′tĕm) Substances with cleaning and polishing properties used to formulate a dentifrice; must be compatible with other ingredients and must not alter tooth structure unfavorably.

**ab·rup·tion** (ab-rŭp′shŭn) Separation or detachment. [L. abruptio, Fr. abrumpo, to break off]

**ab·scess** (ab′ses) 1. Circumscribed collection of purulent exudate. 2. Cavity formed by liquefactive necrosis within solid tissue. See this page and page A2. [L. abscessus, a going away]

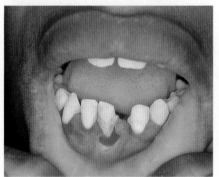

**gingivitis:** adolescent patient presented with oral pain, mild jaundice, and generalized gingivitis and gingival hemorrhage; results of complete blood count were consistent with hemolytic anemia and thrombocytopenia; final diagnosis was Evans syndrome

**ab·scis·sa** (ab-sis′ă) In a plane cartesian coordinate system, the horizontal axis (x). [L. ab-scindo, pp. -scissus, to cut away from]

**ab·scis·sion** (ab-sĭ′zhŭn) Cutting away. [L. ab-scindo, pp. -scissus, to cut away from]

**ab·scon·si·o** (ab-skon′sē-ō) A recess, cavity, or depression. [Mod. L. fr. abs-condo, pp. -con-ditus or -consus, to hide]

**ab·sco·pal** (ab-skō′păl) Denoting the effect that irradiation of a tissue has on remote nonirradiated tissue. [ab- + G. skopos, target, + -al]

**ab·sence** (ab′sahnz′) Paroxysmal attacks of impaired consciousness, occasionally accompanied by spasm or twitching of cephalic muscles, which usually can be brought on by hyperventilation. [L. absentia]

**ab·sence sei·zure** (ab′sĕns sē′zhŭr) A seizure characterized by impaired awareness of interaction with, or memory of, ongoing events external or internal to the person; may comprise the following elements: mental confusion, diminished awareness of environment, inability to respond to internal or external stimuli, and amnesia.

**ab·so·lute** (ab′sō-lūt) Although the traditional pronunciation is as shown, the word is often stressed on the last syllable in the U.S. Unconditional; unlimited; uncombined; undiluted (as in reference to alcohol); certain. [L. absolutus, complete, pp. of ab- solvo, to loosen from]

**ab·so·lute al·co·hol** (ab-sō-lūt′ al′kō-hol) A 100% alcohol, water having been removed. SYN anhydrous alcohol.

**ab·so·lute thresh·old** (ab-sō-lūt′ thresh′ōld) Lowest limit of any perception.

**ab·sorb** (ăb-sōrb′) Do not confuse this word with adsorb. 1. To take in by absorption. 2. To reduce the intensity of transmitted light. [L. ab-sorbeo, pp. -sorptus, to suck in]

**ab·sorb·a·ble gel·a·tin sponge** (ăb-sōr′bă-bĕl jel′ă-tin spŭnj) A sterile, absorbable, water-insoluble, gelatin-based sponge, used to control capillary bleeding in surgical operations; it is left in situ and absorbed within 4–6 weeks.

**ab·sorb·a·ble sur·gi·cal su·ture** (ab-sōr′bĕnt sŭr′ji-kăl sū′chŭr) One made of material prepared from a substance that can be dissolved by body tissues and is therefore not permanent; it is available in various diameters and tensile strengths; rate of diminution of strength depends on the characteristics of the suture material.

**ab·sorb·a·ble su·ture** (ăb-sōr′bă-bĕl sū′chŭr) Suture material dissolved by the body's enzymes during the healing process; used when deep tissue requires inner layers of suture to close a wound.

**ab·sorbed dose** (ab-sōrbd′ dōs) Amount of energy absorbed per unit mass of irradiated material at the target site; in radiation therapy, the former unit for absorbed dose is the rad (100 ergs/g); the current (SI) unit is the gray (1 J/kg or 100 rad).

**ab·sor·be·fa·cient** (ăb-sōr′bĕ-fā′shĕnt) **1.** Causing absorption. **2.** Any substance possessing such quality. [L. *ab-sorbeo*, to suck in, + *facio*, to make]

**ab·sor·bent** (ab-sōr′bĕnt) *Avoid the misspelling absorbant.* **1.** Having the power to absorb, soak up, or incorporate a gas, liquid, light rays, or heat. SYN absorptive. **2.** Any substance possessing such power.

**ab·sor·bent cot·ton** (ab-sōr′bĕnt kot′ŏn) Cotton from which all fatty matter has been extracted, so that it readily takes up fluids.

**ab·sor·bent points** (ăb-sōr′bĕnt poynts) Cones of paper or paper products used to dry or maintain medicaments during root canal therapy. SYN paper point.

**ab·sorb·er head** (ab-sōr′ber hed) Portion of a rebreathing anesthesia circuit that contains carbon dioxide absorbent; often referred to as a canister.

**ab·sorp·tion** (ab-sōrp′shŭn) *Do not confuse this word with adsorption.* **1.** The taking in, incorporation, or reception of gases, liquids, light, or heat. Cf. adsorption. **2.** In radiology, the uptake of energy from radiation by the tissue or medium through which it passes. **3.** Removal of a particular antibody from a mixture on addition of the complementary antigen. [L. *absorptio*, fr. *absorbeo*, to swallow]

**ab·sorp·tion co·ef·fi·cient** (ab-sōrp′shŭn kō-ĕ-fish′ĕnt) **1.** The milliliters of a gas at standard temperature and pressure that will saturate 100 mL of liquid. **2.** The amount of light absorbed in passing through 1 cm of a 1 molar solution of a given substance, expressed as a constant in Beer-Lambert law. **3.** RADIOLOGY a measure of the rate of decrease of intensity of a beam in its passage through matter, resulting from a combination of scattering and conversion to other forms of energy. SEE ALSO attenuation.

**ab·sorp·tive** (ăb-sōrp′tiv) SYN absorbent (1).

**ab·sti·nence** (ab′sti-nĕns) Refraining from the use of certain foods, alcoholic beverages, or illegal drugs, or from sexual or other activity. [L. *abstineo*, to hold back, fr. *teneo*, to hold]

**ab·sti·nence syn·drome** (ab′sti-nĕns sin′drōm) Constellation of physiologic changes undergone by people or animals who have become physically dependent on a drug or chemical who are abruptly deprived of that substance.

**ab·stract** (ab′strakt) **1.** Preparation made by evaporating a fluid extract to a powder and triturating with milk sugar. **2.** Condensation or summary of a scientific or literary article or address. [L. *ab-traho*, pp. *-tractus*, to draw away]

**ab·strac·tion** (ăb-strak′shŭn) Malocclusion in which the teeth or associated structures are lower than their normal occlusal plane. [L. *abstraho*, pp. *-tractus*, to draw away]

**ab·ter·mi·nal** (ab-ter′mi-năl) In a direction away from the end and toward the center; denoting the course of an electrical current in a muscle. [L. *ab*, from, + *terminus*, end]

**a·bu·li·a** (ă-bū′lē-ă) **1.** Loss or impairment of the ability to perform voluntary actions or to make decisions. **2.** Reduction in speech, movement, thought, and emotional reaction. [G. *a*-priv. + *boulē*, will]

**a·bu·lic** (ă-bū′lĭk) Relating to, or suffering from, abulia.

**a·buse** (ă-byūs′) **1.** Misuse or wrongful use of anything. **2.** Injurious, harmful, or offensive treatment.

**a·bused stim·u·lant** (ă-byūzd′ stim′yū-lănt) SYN drug abuse.

**a·but·ment** (ă-bŭt′mĕnt) In dentistry, a natural tooth or implanted tooth substitute, used to support or anchor a fixed or removable prosthesis. See this page.

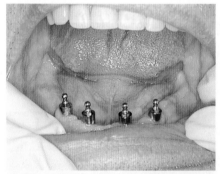

**abutment:** patient has 4 implants with abutment posts that support removable prosthesis on the mandibular arch

**a·but·ment im·plant sub·struc·ture** (ă-bŭt′mĕnt im′plant sŭb′strŭkshŭr) SYN implant substructure.

**a·but·ment screw** (ă-bŭt′mĕnt skrū) A screw that fits into a dental implant.

**a·but·ment splint** (ă-bŭt′mĕnt splint) A support formed by uniting multiple tooth restorations rigidly at their proximal contacts to form a single abutment.

**a·but·ment tooth** (ă-bŭt′mĕnt tūth, ă-bŭt′ mĕnt tūth) SYN abutment.

**AC** Abbreviation for acetate.

**aC** Symbol for arabinosylcytosine.

**AC, a.c.** Abbreviation for alternating current; ante cibum.

**A·cad·e·my of Gen·e·ral Den·tis·try (AGD)** (ă-kad´ĕ-mē jen´ĕr-ăl den´tis-trē) Organization meant to serve professional needs, provide continuing education, and represent interests of general dentists.

**acanthaesthesia** [Br.] SYN acanthesthesia.

**a·can·thes·the·si·a** (ă-kan´thes-thē´zē-ă) Paresthesia of a pinprick. [G. *akantha,* thorn, + *aisthēsis,* sensation]

**a·can·thi·on** (ă-kan´thē-on) Tip of anterior nasal spine. [G. *akantha,* thorn]

♻ **acantho-** Combining form denoting a spinous process; spiny, thorny. [G. *akantha,* a thorn, the backbone, the spine, fr. *akē,* a point, + *anthos,* a flower]

**a·can·thoid** (ă-kan´thoyd) Spine-shaped.

**ac·an·thol·y·sis** (ak´an-thol´i-sis) Separation of individual epidermal keratinocytes from their neighbors. [*acantho-* + G. *lysis,* loosening]

**ac·an·tho·ma·tous am·e·lo·blas·to·ma** (ak´an-thō´mă-tŭs am´ĕ-lō-blas-tō´mă) An ameloblastoma similar to a simple ameloblastoma except usually seen in the third to fourth decade.

**ac·an·tho·sis** (ak-an-thō´sis) Increased thickness of epidermal stratum spinosum. [G. fr. *acantho-,* thorn + G. *-osis,* condition]

**ac·an·tho·sis ni·gri·cans** (ak-an-thō´sis nī´gri-kanz) Eruption of velvety, warty benign growths and hyperpigmentation on the skin of the axillae, neck, anogenital area, and groin. [L. fr. *niger,* black]

**ac·an·thot·ic** (ak-an-thot´ik) Pertaining to or characteristic of acanthosis.

**a·cap·ni·a** (ă-kap´nē-ă) Absence of carbon dioxide in the blood. [G. *a-* priv. + *kapnos,* smoke]

**a·cat·a·la·se·mi·a** (ā-kat´ă-lă-sē´mē-ă) SYN acatalasia.

**a·cat·a·la·si·a** (ā-kat´ă-lā´zē-ă) Absence or deficiency of catalase from blood and tissues, often manifested by recurrent infection or ulceration of the gingivae (gums) and related oral structures. SYN acatalasemia.

**ac·cel·er·at·ed e·rup·tion** (ak-sel´ĕr-ā-tĕd ē-rŭp´shŭn) Dental eruption pattern that is chronologically advanced in comparison with the average pattern of dental eruption.

**ac·cel·er·at·ed re·ac·tion** (ak-sel´ĕr-ā-tĕd rē-ak´shŭn) Response occurring in a shorter time than expected; the cutaneous manifestations occurring during the period between the second and tenth days following smallpox vaccination; because it is intermediate between a primary reaction and an immediate reaction, regarded as evidence of a degree of resistance.

**ac·cel·er·a·tion** (ak-sel-er-ā´shŭn) *Avoid the mispronunciation uh-sel-er-ā´shŭn.* **1.** The act of accelerating. **2.** The rate of increase in velocity per unit of time; commonly expressed in *g* units; also expressed in centimeters or feet per second squared. **3.** The rate of increasing deviation from a rectilinear course.

**ac·cel·er·a·tor** (ak-sel´ĕr-ā-tŏr) *Avoid the mispronunciation uh-sel´er-ā-ter.* **1.** Anything that increases rapidity of action or function. **2.** That which activates developing agents in x-ray film processing chemicals or increases alkalinity, or softens the emulsion in film. [L. *accelerans,* pres. p. of *ac-celero,* to hasten, fr. *celer,* swift]

**ac·cel·er·in** (ak-sel´er-in) Obsolete term for what was once considered an intermediary product of coagulation but is no longer thought to exist.

**ac·cess** (ak´ses) *Do not confuse this word with assess or axis.* **1.** In dentistry, space required for visualization and manipulation of instruments to remove decay and prepare a tooth for restoration. **2.** SYN access cavity. **3.** A way or means of approach or admittance. SYN access opening. [L. *accessus*]

**ac·cess cav·i·ty** (ak´ses kav´i-tē) Removal of the pulp roof to gain direct access to the pulp chamber and all root canals SYN access (2).

**ac·cess flap** (ak´ses flap) An incision through soft tissue made in an effort to approximate bony structures during surgical procedures.

**ac·ces·si·bil·i·ty stan·dards** (ak´ses-ĭ-bil´ĭ-tē stan´dărdz) The U.S. Americans with Disabilities Act prohibits discrimination on the basis of a disability and requires places of public accommodation and commercial facilities to meet federally mandated requirements of accessibility.

**ac·cess open·ing** (ak´ses ō´pĕn-ing) SYN access.

**ac·ces·so·ry** (ak-ses´ŏr-ē) ANATOMY denoting structures (muscles, arteries, nerves, glands, and others) that are auxiliary (normally present) or supernumerary (anomalous) to another more typical or larger structure of the same type. SYN accessorius. [L. *accessorius,* fr. *ac-cedo,* pp. *-cessus,* to move toward]

**ac·ces·so·ry branch of mid·dle me·nin·ge·al ar·te·ry** (ak-ses´ŏr-ē branch mid´ĕl mĕ-nin´jē-ăl ahr´tĕr-ē) [TA] Branch of either the middle meningeal or maxillary artery in the infratemporal fossa that passes superiorly through the foramen ovale to supply the trigeminal ganglion, dura mater, and inner table of bone.

**ac·ces·so·ry ca·nal** (ak-ses´ŏr-ē kă-nal´) In the tooth, channel leading from the root pulp laterally through dentin to the periodontal tissue; may be found anywhere in the tooth root but is more common in apical third of the root. SYN lateral canal.

**ac·ces·so·ry cusp** (ak-ses´ŏr-ē kŭsp) Tubercle or extra tooth cusp. Cf. Carabelli cusp, talon cusp. See this page.

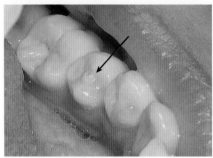

**accessory cusp:** dens evaginatus (Leong tubercle)

**ac·ces·so·ry gland** (ak-ses´ŏr-ē gland) Small mass of glandular structure, detached from but lying near another and larger gland, to which it is similar in structure and probably in function.

**ac·ces·so·ry lac·ri·mal glands** (ak-ses´ŏr-ē lak´ri-măl glandz) [TA] Small, compound, branched, tubular glands located sometimes in the middle part of the lid or along the superior and inferior fornices of the conjunctival sac. These accessory glands are ectopic portions of the lacrimal gland tissue; all produce the same kind of tears, secreting onto the conjunctival surface.

**ac·ces·so·ry lymph node** (ak-ses´ŏr-ē limf nōd) Lymphoid tissue or node located near the larger lymph node with same function.

**ac·ces·so·ry na·sal car·ti·la·ges** (ak-ses´ŏr-ē nā´zăl kahr´ti-lăj-ĕz) [TA] Variable small plates of cartilage located in the interval between the greater alar and lateral nasal cartilages.

**ac·ces·so·ry nerve [CN XI]** (ak-ses´ŏr-ē nĕrv) [TA] One that arises by two sets of roots: the presumed cranial, emerging from the side of the medulla, and the presumed spinal, emerging from the ventrolateral part of the first five cervical segments of the spinal cord; these roots unite to form the accessory nerve trunk. SYN eleventh cranial nerve [CN XI], nervus accessorius [CN XI].

**ac·ces·so·ry nerve trunk** (ak-ses´ŏr-ē nĕrv trŭngk) [TA] Part of the accessory nerve formed within the cranial cavity by the union of the traditional cranial and spinal roots, which then divides within the jugular foramen into internal and external branches, the former uniting with the vagus, the latter exiting the foramen as an independent branch commonly considered to be the accessory nerve. Validity of the concept of a cranial root of the accessory nerve has been questioned as well as the common existence of its trunk. Recent studies claim the "cranial root" is always part of the vagus nerve.

**ac·ces·so·ry or·gans of the eye** (ak-ses´ŏr-ē ōr´gănz ī) SYN accessory visual structures.

**ac·ces·so·ry pa·rot·id gland** (ak-ses´ ŏr-ē pă-rot´id gland) [TA] Occasional islet of parotid tissue separate from the mass of the gland, lying anteriorly just above the commencement of the parotid duct.

**ac·ces·so·ry phren·ic nerves** (ak-ses´ ŏr-ē fren´ik nĕrvz) [TA] Accessory nerve strands that arise from the fifth cervical nerve, often as branches of the nerve to the subclavius, passing downward to join the phrenic nerve.

**ac·ces·so·ry pro·cess of lum·bar ver·te·bra** (ak-ses´ŏr-ē pro´ses lŭm´bahr vĕr´tĕ-bră) [TA] A small apophysis at the posterior part of the base of the transverse process of each lumbar vertebra. SYN accessory tubercle (1).

**ac·ces·so·ry quad·rate car·ti·lage** (ak-ses´ŏr-ē kwahd´rāt kahr´ti-lăj) SYN minor alar cartilage of nose.

**ac·ces·so·ry root of tooth** (ak-ses´ŏr-ē rūt tūth) [TA] An anomalous additional tooth root.

**ac·ces·so·ry sign** (ak-ses´ŏr-ē sīn) Finding frequently but not consistently present in a disease.

**ac·ces·so·ry symp·tom** (ak-ses´ŏr-ē simp´ tŏm) Symptom that usually but not always accompanies a specific disease, as distinguished from a pathognomonic symptom. SYN concomitant symptom.

**ac·ces·so·ry thym·ic tis·sue** (ak-ses´ ŏr-ē thī´mik tish´ū) Isolated mass of tissue that arises from the developing thymus and enters the neck.

**ac·ces·so·ry thy·roid gland** (ak-ses´ŏr-ē thī´royd gland) [TA] Isolated mass of thyroid tissue, sometimes present in the side of the neck, or ranging in position from just superior to the hyoid bone (suprahyoid accessory thyroid gland) to the arch of the aorta inferiorly.

**ac·ces·so·ry thy·roid tis·sue** (ak-ses´ ŏr-ē thī´royd tish´ū) Isolated mass of tissue that arises from the developing thyroid gland and appears in the tongue or the thymus gland.

**ac·ces·so·ry tooth** (ak-ses´ŏr-ē tūth) Any malformed supernumerary tooth.

**ac·ces·so·ry tu·ber·cle** (ak-ses´ŏr-ē tū´bĕr-kĕl) **1.** SYN accessory process of lumbar vertebra. **2.** SYN dens evaginatus.

**ac·ces·so·ry vis·u·al struc·tures** (ak-ses´ŏr-ē vizh´ū-ăl strŭk´shŭrz) [TA] Eyelids, with lashes and eyebrows, lacrimal apparatus, conjunctival sac, and extrinsic muscles of the eyeball. SYN accessory organs of the eye.

**ac·cess prep·a·ra·tion** (ak´ses prep´ăr-ā´shŭn) SYN access cavity.

**ac·ci·dent** (ak´si-dĕnt) An unplanned or unintended but sometimes predictable event leading to injury, or such an event developing in the course of a disease. [L. ac-cido, to happen]

**ac·ci·den·tal hy·po·ther·mi·a** (ak-si-den´tăl hī´pō-thĕr´mē-ă) Unintentional decrease in body temperature, especially in neonates, infants, and the elderly, particularly during surgery.

**ac·ci·den·tal my·i·a·sis** (ak-si-den´tăl mī-ī´ă-sis) Gastrointestinal infection due to ingestion of contaminated food.

**ac·ci·den·tal symp·tom** (ak´si-den´tăl simp´tŏm) Any morbid phenomenon coincidentally occurring in the course of a disease, but having no relation with it.

**ac·ci·dent-prone** (ak´si-dĕnt-prōn) **1.** Experiencing a greater number of accidents than would be expected of the average person in similar circumstances. **2.** Having personality characteristics predisposing one to accidents.

**ac·cli·mat·ing fe·ver** (ak´li-māt-ing fē´vĕr) Elevated body temperature with malaise that affects people working in a very hot environment.

**ac·com·mo·da·tion** (ă-kom´ŏ-dā´shŭn) **1.** Act or state of adjustment or adaptation. **2.** In sensorimotor theory, the alteration of schemata or cognitive expectations to conform with experience. [L. ac-commodo, pp. -atus, to adapt, fr. modus, a measure]

**ac·com·mo·da·tion of nerve** (ă-kom´ŏ-dā´shŭn nĕrv) Property of a nerve by which it adjusts to a slowly increasing level of stimulus, so that its threshold of excitation is greater than it would be were the stimulus level to have risen more drastically.

**ac·com·mo·da·tive** (ă-kom´ŏ-dā-tiv) Relating to accommodation.

**ac·cred·i·ta·tion** (ă-kred´i-tā´shŭn) Approval, certification, or formal recognition of a program or institution by an authority. [F. ac-créditation, fr. L. ad-, to, + credo, creditum, to believe, trust]

**ac·cre·men·ti·tion** (ak´rĕ-men-ti´shŭn) Re-

production by budding or germination. [L. ac-cresco, pp. -cretus, to increase]

**ac·cre·tion** (ă-krē´shŭn) In dentistry, foreign material (usually plaque or calculus) collecting on the surface of a tooth or in a cavity. [L. ac-cretio, fr. ad, to, + crescere, to grow]

**ac·cre·tion·ar·y growth** (ă-krē´shŭn-ar-ē grōth) Growth by an increase of intercellular material.

**ac·cre·tion lines** (ak´rē-shŭn līnz) Striations seen in microscopic sections of dental enamel.

**ACE in·hi·bi·tor** (ās in-hib´i-tŏr) Class of drugs (angiotensin–converting enzyme inhibitors) that blocks conversion of angiotensin I to angiotensin II; used to treat hypertension and other disorders.

**a·cel·lu·lar** (ā-sel´yū-lăr) Devoid of cells. [G. a- priv. + L. cellula, a small chamber]

**a·cel·lu·lar ce·men·tum** (ā-sel´yū-lăr sĕ-men´tŭm) Cementum that is devoid of cells; it cannot regenerate itself.

**a·cen·tric oc·clu·sion** (ā-sen´trik ŏ-klū´zhŭn) SYN eccentric occlusion.

**a·cen·tric re·la·tion** (ā-sen´trik rĕ-lā´shŭn) SYN eccentric relationship.

**ace·sul·fame po·tas·si·um** (ā´sĕ-sŭl´fām pŏ-tas´ē-ŭm) A potassium salt that is sweeter than table sugar.

**ac·e·tab·u·lum,** pl. **ac·e·tab·u·la** (as-ĕ-tab´yū-lŭm, -lă) [TA] A cup-shaped depression on the external surface of the hip bone, with which the head of the femur articulates. SYN cotyloid cavity. [L. a shallow vinegar vessel]

**ac·et·a·min·o·phen (APAP)** (as-et-ă-min´ō-fen) An antipyretic and analgesic, with potency similar to that of aspirin.

**ac·e·tate (AC)** (as´ĕ-tāt) A salt or ester of acetic acid.

**a·cet·a·zol·a·mide** (as´ĕ-tă-zol´ă-mīd) Agent that inhibits action of carbonic anhydrase in the kidney.

**a·ce·tic** (a-sē´tik, -set´ik) **1.** Denoting the presence of the two-carbon fragment of acetic acid. **2.** Relating to vinegar; sour. [L. acetum, vinegar]

**a·ce·tic ac·id** (a-sē´tik as´id) Product of oxidation of ethanol and of the destructive distillation of wood; used locally as a counterirritant and occasionally internally, and also as a reagent; contained in vinegars. SYN ethanoic acid.

**a·ce·ti·fy** (ă-set´i-fī) To cause acetic fermentation; to make vinegar or become vinegar. [L. acetum, vinegar, + facio, to make; or fieri, to be made, to become]

**acetonaemia** [Br.] SYN acetonemia.

**ac·e·tone** (as′ĕ-tōn) A colorless, volatile, flammable liquid; extremely small amounts are found in normal urine, but larger quantities occur in the urine and blood of people with diabetes, sometimes imparting an ethereal odor to the urine and breath.

**ac·e·tone breath** (as′ĕ-tōn breth) Odor of acetone on the breath; suggestive of diabetes.

**ac·e·to·ne·mi·a** (as′ĕ-tŏ-nē′mē-ă) Presence of acetone or acetone bodies in relatively large amounts in the blood, manifested at first by excitability, and later by a progressive depression. SYN acetonaemia. [*acetone* + G. *haima,* blood]

**ac·e·to·ne·mic** (as′ĕ-tō-nē′mik) Relating to or caused by acetonemia.

**ac·e·tone test** (as′ĕ-tōn test) A laboratory evaluation of blood or urine to determine the organic synthesis of ketone bodies.

**ac·e·to·nu·ri·a** (as′e-tō-nyūr′ē-ă) Excretion in urine of large amounts of acetone; commonly occurs in diabetic acidosis. [*acetone* + G. *ouron,* urine]

**a·ce·tum,** pl. **a·ce·ta** (a-sē′tŭm, -tă) SYN vinegar. [L. *vinum acetum,* soured wine, vinegar]

**a·ce·tyl·cho·line (ACH)** (as′ĕ-til-kō′lēn) Acetic ester of choline, the neurotransmitter substance at cholinergic synapses.

**a·ce·tyl·cho·lin·es·ter·ase** (as′ĕ-til-kō′lin-es′tĕr-ās) Cholinesterase that hydrolyzes acetylcholine to acetate and choline within the central nervous system and at peripheral neuroeffector junctions (e.g., motor endplates and autonomic ganglia).

**a·ce·tyl·cys·te·ine, N-a·ce·tyl·cys·te·ine** (as′ĕ-til-sis′tē-in) A mucolytic agent that reduces the viscosity of mucous secretions.

**a·ce·tyl group** (as′ĕ-til grūp) An acetic acid molecule from which the hydroxyl group has been removed.

**a·ce·tyl·sal·i·cyl·ic ac·id (ASA)** (as′ĕ-til-sal-i-sil′ik as′id) SYN aspirin.

**ACH** Abbreviation for acetylcholine.

**a·cha·la·sia** (ak-ă-lā′zē-ă) Failure to relax; referring especially to visceral openings. [G. *a-* priv. + *chalasis,* a slackening]

**ache** (āk) A dull, poorly localized pain, usually of less than severe intensity.

**a·chei·li·a** (ă-kī′lē-ă) Congenital absence of the lips. [G. *a-* priv. + *cheilos,* lip]

**a·chei·lous, a·chi·lous** (ă-kī′lŭs) Characterized by or relating to acheilia.

**a·chei·ri·a** (ă-kī′rē-ă) Anesthesia in one or both hands with loss of the sense of possession of the hand or hands. [G. *a-* priv. + *cheir,* hand]

**a·chlor·hy·dri·a** (ā-klōr-hī′drē-ă) Absence of hydrochloric acid from the gastric juice. [G. *a-* priv. + chlorhydric (acid)]

**a·chlor·hy·dric a·ne·mi·a** (ā-klōr-hī′drik ă-nē′mē-ă) Chronic hypochromic microcytic anemia associated with achlorhydria or achylia gastrica.

**a·cho·lu·ric jaun·dice** (ā-kō-lyūr′ik jawn′dis) Jaundice with excessive amounts of unconjugated bilirubin in plasma but no bile pigments in the urine.

**a·chon·dro·pla·si·a** (ā-kon-drō-plā′zē-ă) Hereditary chondrodystrophy characterized by an abnormality in conversion of cartilage into bone. [G. *a-* priv. + *chondros,* cartilage, + *plasis,* a molding]

**a·chon·dro·plas·tic dwarf·ism** (a-kon-drō-plas′tik dwōrf′izm) SYN achondroplasia.

**achrestic anaemia** [Br.] SYN achrestic anemia.

**a·chres·tic a·ne·mi·a** (ă-kres′tik ă-nē′mē-ă) A form of chronic progressive macrocytic anemia, potentially fatal, in which the changes in bone marrow and circulating blood closely resemble those of pernicious anemia, but in which there is, at best, only transient response to therapy with vitamin B12. SYN achrestic anaemia. [G. *a-* priv. + *chrēsis,* use]

**ach·ro·ma·si·a** (ak′rō-mā′zē-ă) Pallor associated with hippocratic facies, emaciation, and weakness, often heralding a moribund state. SYN cachectic pallor. [G. *achrōmos,* colorless]

**ach·ro·ma·top·si·a, ach·ro·ma·top·sy** (ă-krō-mă-top′sē-ă, ă-krō′mă-top-sē) A severe congenital deficiency in color perception, often associated with nystagmus and reduced visual acuity. SYN monochromatism (2). [G. *a-* priv. + *chrōma,* color, + *opsis,* vision]

**ach·y·li·a** (ă-kī′lē-ă) Absence of gastric juice or chyle. [G. *a-* priv. + *chylos,* juice]

**ac·id** (as′id) **1.** A compound yielding a hydrogen ion in a polar solvent; acids form salts by replacing all or part of the ionizable hydrogen with an electropositive element or radical. **2.** Colloquially, any chemical compound that has a sour taste. **3.** Sour; sharp to the taste. **4.** Relating to acid; giving an acid reaction. **5.** A substance with a pH between 0 and 7. [L. *acidus,* sour]

**acidaemia** [Br.] SYN acidemia.

**ac·id al·co·hol** (as′id al′kŏ-hol) Ethyl alcohol (70%) containing 1% hydrochloric acid.

**ac·id-ash di·et** (as′id-ash dī′ĕt) SYN alkaline-ash diet.

**ac·id-base bal·ance** (as′id-bās bal′ăns) Normal balance between acid and base in the blood plasma, expressed in the hydrogen ion concentration or pH, resulting from the relative amounts of acidic and basic materials ingested and produced by body metabolism, compared with the relative amounts of acidic and basic materials excreted from the body and consumed by body metabolism.

**ac·id-base buf·fer sys·tem** (as′id-bās bŭf′ĕr sis′tĕm) Regulation of balance of fluids through chemical buffers.

**ac·id con·di·tion·ing** (as′id kŏn-dish′ŭn-ing) SYN acid etching.

**ac·id dys·pep·sia** (as′id dis-pep′sē-ă) Upset stomach due to excess gastric acidity.

**ac·i·de·mi·a** (as-i-dē′mē-ă) An increase in the H⁺ ion concentration of the blood or a fall below normal in pH. SYN acidaemia. [*acid* + G. *haima*, blood]

**ac·id etch** (as′id ech) Application of phosphoric acid to enamel or dentin surface of a tooth to improve mechanical retention for sealant or resin restoration.

**acid etch·ant** (as′id ech′ănt) Material used to acid etch a tooth. SEE acid etch.

**ac·id etch ce·ment·ed splint** (as′id ech sĕ-men′tĕd splint) Piece of heavy wire cemented to the labial surfaces of teeth with any of the acid etch cement techniques.

**ac·id-etch·ed res·to·ra·tion** (as′id echt res′tŏr-ā′shŭn) Restoration of tooth structure with a resin after surface of tooth has been etched with an acid solution to increase retention of the restoration.

**🖐ac·id etch·ing** (as′id ech′ing) Treatment of tooth surfaces with phosphoric acid solution to roughen tooth structure microscopically to create retention, usually for resin-type restorations. See this page.

**ac·id-fast** (as′id-fast) Denoting bacteria that are not decolorized by acid-alcohol after having been stained with dyes such as basic fuchsin.

**ac·id·ic** (ă-sid′ik) **1.** Sour; sharp to the taste **2.** Relating to an acid.

**ac·id in·di·ges·tion** (as′id in′di-jes′chŭn) Dyspepsia due to hyperchlorhydria; used colloquially as a synonym for pyrosis.

**ac·id in·tox·i·ca·tion** (as′id in-tok′si-kā′shŭn) Poisoning by acid products formed as a result of faulty metabolism (e.g., uncontrolled diabetes mellitus) or by nonphysiologic acids; marked by epigastric pain, headache,

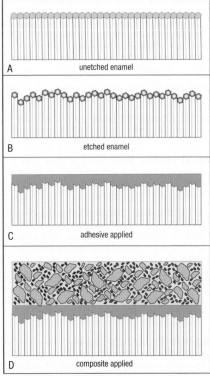

A　　unetched enamel

B　　etched enamel

C　　adhesive applied

D　　composite applied

**acid etching process for enamel:** (A) vertical bars represent clean surface composed of enamel rods; (B) etching dissolves some of the enamel rods, creating interrod spaces at surface; (C) adhesive flows between rods, sets, and then covers surface with resin; (D) composite restorative material is applied and then bonds to underlying resin

other symptoms, and an odor of acetone on the breath.

**ac·id·i·ty** (ă-sid′i-tē) **1.** The state of being acid. **2.** The acid content of a fluid.

**ac·i·do·gen·ic** (as′i-dō-jen′ik) Acid producing.

**ac·id·o·gen·ic bac·te·ria** (as′id-ō-jen′ik bak-tēr′ē-ă) Producers of acid from fermentable carbohydrates, found in dental biofilm (q.v.); may be related to caries development.

**ac·i·do·phil, ac·i·do·phile** (ă-sid′ŏ-fil, ă-sid′ŏ-fīl) A structure, cell, or other histologic element staining readily with acidic dyes. [*acid* + G. *philos*, fond]

**ac·i·do·phil ad·e·no·ma** (ă-sid′ŏ-fil ad′ĕ-nŏ′mă) A lesion with cells that have have an affinity for and stain with an acidic dye (e.g., eosin). SYN eosinophil adenoma.

**ac·i·do·phil·ic** (as′i-dŏ-fil′ik) Having an affinity for acid dyes; denoting a cell or tissue element that stains with an acid dye.

**ac·i·do·sis** (as-i-dō′sis) A pathologic state characterized by an increase in the concentration of hydrogen ions in the arterial blood above the normal level, 40 nmol/L, or pH less than 7.4; may be caused by increased carbon dioxide or by decreased alkaline compounds. [*acid* + G. *-ōsis,* condition]

**ac·i·dot·ic** (as′i-dot′ik) Pertaining to or indicating acidosis.

**ac·id phos·pha·tase** (as′id fos′fă-tās) A phosphatase with an optimal pH of less than 7.0, notably present in the prostate gland.

**ac·id re·flux test** (as′id rē′flŭks test) Assessment of gastroesophageal reflux by monitoring esophageal pH either basally or after acid is instilled into the stomach.

**ac·i·dul·a·ted phos·phate flu·o·ride (APF)** (ă-sid′yū-lā-tĕd fos′fāt flōr′ĭd) Sodium fluoride solution with phosphoric acid added to lower its pH; intended to increase dental fluoroapatite.

**ac·i·du·ria** (as′i-dyūr′ē-ă) Excretion of an abnormal amount of any specified acid. Individual types of aciduria are prefixed by the specific acid; e.g., aminoaciduria, ketoaciduria. [*acid* + G. *ouron,* urine]

***Ac·i·ne·to·bac·ter*** (as-i-nē′tō-bak′tĕr) A genus of nonmotile, non-spore-forming aerobic bacteria containing gram-negative or -variable coccoid or short rods, or cocci, often occurring in pairs; a frequent cause of nosocomial infections; often resistant to many antibiotics, can also cause severe primary infections in immunocompromised people.

**a·cin·ic cell ad·e·no·car·ci·no·ma** (ă-sin′ik sel ad′ĕ-nō-kahr-si-nō′mă) Lesion arising from secreting cells of a racemose gland.

**ac·i·nous, ac·i·nose** (as′i-nŭs, -nōs) Resembling an acinus or grape-shaped structure.

**ac·i·nus,** pl. **ac·i·ni** (as′i-nŭs, -nī) [TA] One of the minute grape-shaped secretory portions of an acinous gland. [L. berry, grape]

**ac·me** (ak′mē) Period of greatest intensity of any symptom, sign, or process.

**ac·ne** (ak′nē) An inflammatory follicular, papular, and pustular eruption involving the pilosebaceous apparatus.

**ac·ne ro·sa·ce·a** (ak′nē rō-sā′shē-ă) SYN rosacea.

**ac·ne vul·ga·ris** (ak′nē vŭl-gā′ris) Eruption, predominantly of the face, upper back, and chest, composed of comedones, cysts, papules, and pustules on an inflammatory base; the condition occurs in most people during puberty and adolescence, due to androgenic stimulation of sebum secretion, with plugging of follicles by keratinization, associated with proliferation of *Propionibacterium acnes.*

**a·cou·stic me·a·tus** (ă-kūs′tik mē-ā′tŭs) **1.** SYN external acoustic meatus. **2.** SYN external auditory canal.

**a·cous·tic pa·pil·la** (ă-kūs′tik pă-pil′ă) SYN spiral organ.

**a·cous·tic teeth** (ă-kūs′tik tēth) [TA] Tooth-shaped formations or ridges occurring on the vestibular lip of the limbus laminae spiralis of the cochlear duct. SYN dentes acustici [TA], auditory teeth, Huschke auditory teeth.

**a·cous·tic tur·bu·lence** (ă-kū′stik tŭr′byū-lens) Swirling effect produced within the confined space of a periodontal pocket by continuous stream of fluid flowing over an electronically powered instrument tip, which disrupts plaque biofilm.

**ac·quired** (ă-kwīrd′) Denoting a disease, predisposition or abnormality that is not inherited. See this page. [L. *ac-quiro (adq-),* to obtain, fr. *quaero,* to seek]

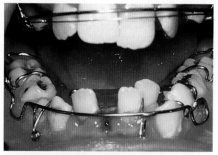

acquired hypodontia: creation of space for orthodontic requirements by selectively extracting primary teeth

**ac·quired cen·tric** (ă-kwīrd sen′trik) SYN centric occlusion.

**ac·quired cen·tric re·la·tion** (ă-kwīrd′ sen′trik rĕ-lā′shŭn) Relationship of the maxilla and the mandible that is not centric, although teeth are in contact.

**ac·quired char·ac·ter** (ă-kwīrd′ kar′ăk-tĕr) Character developed due to environmental influences.

**ac·quired char·ac·ter·is·tics** (ă-kwīrd′ kar′ăk-tĕr-is′tiks) SYN acquired character.

**ac·quired cu·ti·cle, ac·quired e·nam·el cu·ti·cle** (ă-kwīrd′ kyū′ti-kĕl, ĕ-nam′ĕl) SYN brown pellicle.

**ac·quired ec·cen·tric jaw re·la·tion** (ă-kwīrd′ ek-sen′trik rĕ-lā′shŭn) SYN acquired eccentric relation.

**ac·quired ec·cen·tric re·la·tion** (ă-kwīrd′ ek-sen′trik rĕ-lā′shŭn) An eccentric relation that is assumed by habit to bring the teeth into occlusion.

**ac·quired he·mo·lyt·ic a·ne·mi·a** (ă-kwīrd´ hē´mō-lit´ik ă-nē´mē-ă) Nonhereditary acute or chronic anemia associated with or caused by extracorpuscular factors, e.g., certain infectious agents, chemicals, burns, or toxic materials from higher plant and animal forms.

**ac·quired he·mo·lyt·ic ic·te·rus** (ă-kwīrd´ hē´mō-lit´ik ik´tĕr-ŭs) Icterus and anemia with moderate splenomegaly, increased fragility of red blood cells, and increased urinary urobilin.

**ac·quired im·mu·ni·ty** (ă-kwīrd´ i-myū´ni-tē) Resistance due to previous exposure of the individual in question to an infectious agent or antigen; may be active, due to naturally acquired infection or vaccination; or passive, acquired from transfer of antibodies from another person or animal, either from mother to fetus or by inoculation.

**ac·quired meg·a·co·lon** (ă-kwīrd´ meg´ă-kō-lŏn) Megacolon associated with disease; occurs in inflammatory bowel disease and Chagas disease.

**ac·quired me·the·mo·glo·bi·ne·mi·a** (ă-kwīrd´ met-hē´mō-glō´bi-nē´mē-ă) Form caused by various chemical agents.

**ac·quired pel·li·cle** (ă-kwīrd´ pel´i-kĕl) SYN brown pellicle.

**ac·quired sen·si·tiv·i·ty** (ă-kwīrd´ sen´si-tiv´i-tē) SYN allergy (1).

**ac·ral** (ak´răl) Relating to peripheral body parts. [G. akron, extremity]

**ac·rid** (ak´rid) Sharp, pungent, biting, or irritating. [L. acer (acr-), pungent]

**ac·rid poi·son** (ak´rid poy´zŏn) Poison that causes local irritation and systemic destruction.

**ac·ri·mo·ny** (ak´rĭ-mō-nē) Being intensely irritant, biting, or pungent.

♻ **acro-** Combining form meaning: Extremity, tip, end, peak, topmost, extreme.

**acroaesthesia** [Br.] SYN acroesthesia.

**ac·ro·ag·no·sis** (ak´rō-ag-nō´sis) 1. Loss or impairment of the sensory recognition of a limb. 2. Absence of acrognosis.

**acroanaesthaesia** [Br.] SYN acroanaesthesia.

**ac·ro·an·es·the·si·a** (ak´rō-an-es-thē´zē-ă) Anesthesia of the limbs. SYN acroanaesthaesia. [acro- + G. an- priv. + aisthēsis sensation]

**ac·ro·as·phyx·i·a** (ak´rō-as-fik´sē-ă) Impaired digital circulation, marked by a discoloration of the fingers, with subnormal local temperature and paresthesia.

**ac·ro·a·tax·i·a** (ak´rō-ă-tak´sē-ă) Ataxia affecting the distal portion of limbs.

**ac·ro·ce·pha·li·a** (ak´rō-se-fā´lē-ă) SYN oxycephaly.

**ac·ro·ceph·a·ly** (ak´rō-sef´ă-lē) SYN oxycephaly. [acro- + G. kephalē, head]

**ac·ro·ci·ne·si·a, ac·ro·ci·ne·sis, ac·ro·ki·ne·si·a** (ak´rō-si-nē´zē-ă, -si-nē´sis, -ki-nē´sē-ă) Excessive movement.

**ac·ro·cy·a·no·sis** (ak´rō-sī-ă-nō´sis) Circulatory disorder in which the hands, and less commonly the feet, are persistently cold and blue. [acro- + G. kyanos, blue, + -osis, condition]

**ac·ro·cy·a·not·ic** (ak´rō-sī-ă-not´ik) Characterized by acrocyanosis.

**ac·ro·der·ma·ti·tis** (ak´rō-dĕr-mă-tī´tis) Inflammation of the skin of limbs. [acro- + G. derma, skin, + -itis, inflammation]

**ac·ro·der·ma·ti·tis en·ter·o·path·i·ca** (ak´rō-dĕr´mă-tī´tis en´tĕr-ō-path´i-kă) Progressive hereditary defect of zinc metabolism in young children; often manifests first as a blistering, oozing, and crusting eruption on a limb or around an orifice; relieved by lifelong oral zinc supplementation.

**ac·ro·dont** (ak´rō-dont) Tooth attachment in some lower vertebrates in which the teeth rest on the edge of the jaw bone. [acro- + G. odous, tooth]

**ac·ro·dyn·i·a** (ak´rō-din´ē-ă) Pain in peripheral or acral body parts. SYN Feer disease. [acro- + G. odynē, pain]

**ac·ro·es·the·si·a** (ak´rō-es-thē´zē-ă) 1. Extreme hyperesthesia. 2. Hyperesthesia of the limbs. [acro- + G. aisthēsis, sensation]

**ac·ro·fa·cial dys·os·to·sis** (ak´rō-fā´shăl dis´os-tō´sis) Mandibulofacial dysostosis associated with malformations of extremities and radioulnar synostosis. SYN acrofacial syndrome.

**ac·ro·fa·cial syn·drome** (ak´rō-fā´shăl sin´drōm) SYN acrofacial dysostosis.

**ac·ro·meg·a·lo·gi·gan·tism** (ak´rō-meg´ă-lō-jī´gan-tizm) Gigantism with enlarged facial features and limbs and other signs of acromegaly. [acro- + G. megas, great, + gigas, giant]

**ac·ro·meg·a·ly** (ak´rō-meg´ă-lē) Disorder marked by progressive enlargement of peripheral body parts due to excessive secretion of somatotropin; organomegaly and metabolic disorders occur; diabetes mellitus may develop. SYN hyperpituitarism. [acro- + G. megas, large]

**ac·ro·mi·al a·nas·to·mo·sis of the thor·a·co·a·cro·mi·al ar·te·ry** (ă-krō´mē-ăl ă-nas´tō-mō´sis thōr´ă-kō-ă-krō´mē-ăl ahr´

tĕr-ē) [TA] Vascular network between the acromion and skin shoulder formed by anastomoses of the acromial branch of the suprascapular artery with the acromial branch of the thoracoacromial artery.

**ac·ro·mi·al an·gle** (ă-krō′mē-ăl ang′gĕl) [TA] Prominent angle at the junction of the posterior and lateral borders of the acromion.

**ac·ro·mic·ria** (ak′rō-mik′rē-ă, ak′rō-mī′krē-ă) Antithesis of acromegaly; condition in which bones of the face and limbs are small and delicate. [*acro-* + G. *mikros,* small]

**ac·ro·mi·o·hu·mer·al** (ă-krō′mē-ō-hyū′ mĕr-ăl) Relating to acromion and humerus.

**ac·rop·e·tal** (ă-krop′ĕ-tăl) In a direction toward the summit. [*acro-* + L. *peto,* to seek]

**ac·ro·scle·ro·sis, ac·ro·scle·ro·der·ma** (ak′rō-skler-ō′sis, -ō-dĕr′mă) Stiffness and tightness of the skin of the fingers, with atrophy of the soft tissue and osteoporosis of the distal phalanges of the hands and feet. SYN sclerodactyly.

**ac·ro·ter·ic** (ak′rō-ter′ik) Relating to the extreme peripheral or apical parts, such as the tips of the fingers and the toes or the end of the nose. [G. *akrōtērion,* the topmost point]

**a·crot·ic** (ă-krot′ik) Marked by great weakness or absence of the pulse; pulseless. [G. *a-* priv. + *krotos,* a striking]

**ac·ro·tism** (ak′rō-tizm) Absent or imperceptible pulse. [G. *a-* priv. + *krotos,* a striking]

**a·cryl·ic** (ă-kril′ik) Denoting certain synthetic plastic resins derived from acrylic acid.

**a·cryl·ic res·in** (ă-kril′ik rez′in) Resinous material of various esters of acrylic acid; used as a denture base material, dental restorations, and trays.

**a·cryl·ic res·in base** (ă-kril′ik rez′in bās) Form made of acrylic resin molded to conform to alveolar process tissues to support prosthetic teeth.

**a·cryl·ic res·in bite-guard splint** (ă-kril′ik rez′in bīt′gahrd splint) A dental appliance that is fabricated using acrylic resin material that protects teeth from excessive occlusal forces and bruxism.

**a·cryl·ic res·in den·ture** (ă-kril′ik rez′in den′chŭr) A dental appliance that replaces natural teeth that is fabricated using acrylic resin material.

**a·cryl·ic res·in tooth** (ă-kril′ik rez′in tūth)

Tooth made of acrylic resinous material. See this page.

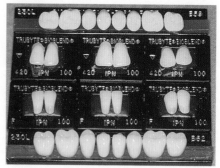

**acrylic teeth for maxillary and mandibular dentures:** (top to bottom) maxillary posterior, maxillary anterior, mandibular anterior, and mandibular posterior teeth

**a·cryl·ic res·in tray** (ă-kril′ik rez′in trā) Plastic impression tray used in dentistry; usually fashioned for the individual patient from an autopolymerizing acrylic resin.

**ACS** Abbreviation for acute coronary syndrome.

**ACTH** Abbreviation for adrenocorticotropic hormone.

**ACTH stim·u·la·tion test** (stim′yū-lā′ shŭn test) Measurement of adrenal cortical function.

**ac·tin·ic chei·li·tis** (ak-tin′ik kī-lī′tis) SYN solar cheilitis.

**ac·tin·ic chei·lo·sis** (ak-tin′ik kī-lō′sis) SEE chelitis, fissured labial mucosa. See page A8. SYN solar cheilitis.

**ac·tin·ic ker·a·to·sis** (ak-tin′ik ker′ă-tō′ sis) A premalignant warty lesion occurring on the sun-exposed skin of the face or hands in aged light-skinned people.

**ac·tin·ic ra·di·a·tion** (ak-tin′ik rā′dē-ā′ shŭn) Light radiation toward and beyond the violet end of the spectrum.

**actino-** Combining form meaning a ray, as of light; applied to any form of radiation or to any structure with radiating parts. [G. *aktis, aktinos,* a ray of light, a beam.]

**Ac·ti·no·ba·cil·lus** (ak′tin-ō-bă-sil′ŭs) A genus of nonmotile, non-spore-forming, aerobic, facultatively anaerobic bacteria containing gram-negative rods interspersed with coccal elements. They are pathogenic to animals. The type species is *A. lignieresii.* [*actino-* + L. *bacillus,* a little rod]

**Ac·ti·no·ba·cil·lus ac·ti·no·my·ce·tem·com·i·tans** (ak′ti-nō-bă-sil′ŭs ak′ti-nō-mī-sĕ-tem-kom´i-tanz) Species of doubtful taxonomic position; frequently associated with some forms of human periodontal disease as well as subacute and chronic endocarditis.

**Ac·ti·no·my·ces** (ak´ti-nō-mī´sēz) A genus of slow-growing, nonmotile, non-spore-forming, anaerobic to facultatively anaerobic bacteria containing gram-positive, irregularly staining filaments; diphtheroid cells may be predominant. Most species produce a filamentous microcolony. May have characteristic sulfur granules in purulent drainage. Pathogenic for humans and other animals and can cause chronic suppurative infection in humans. [*actino-* + G. *mykēs,* fungus]

**Ac·ti·no·my·ces naes·lun·di·i** (ak´ti-nō-mī´sēz nēs-lŭn´dē-ī) Bacterial pathogen found in human oral cavity that may lead to periodontitis.

**Ac·ti·no·my·ces o·don·to·ly·ti·cus** (ak´ti-nō-mī´sēz ō-don´tō-lit´i-kŭs) Species in the human oral cavity; isolated from deep dental caries.

**Ac·ti·no·my·ces vis·co·sus** (ak´ti-nō-mī´sēz vis-kō´sŭs) Species isolated from oral cavity of humans and some species of other animals; produces periodontal disease in animals and has been isolated from human dental calculus and root surface caries.

**ac·ti·no·my·cins** (ak´tin-ō-mī´sinz) A group of peptide antibiotic agents, isolated from several species of *Streptomyces* (originally *Actinomyces*), which are active against gram-positive bacteria, fungi, and neoplasms.

**⬛ac·ti·no·my·co·sis** (ak´ti-nō-mī-kō´sis) Disease primarily of cattle and humans caused by the bacterium *Actinomyces bovis* in cattle and by *A. israelii* and *Arachnia propionica* in humans. Part of the normal bacterial flora of the mouth and pharynx, but when introduced into tissue they may produce chronic destructive abscesses or granulomas that eventually discharge a viscid pus containing minute yellowish granules (sulfur granules). In humans, commonly affects cervicofacial area, abdomen, or thorax. See page A11. [*actino-* + G. *mykēs,* fungus, + *-osis,* condition]

**ac·ti·no·my·cot·ic** (ak´ti-nō-mī-kot´ik) Relating to actinomycosis.

**ac·ti·no·phy·to·sis** (ak´ti-nō-fī-tō´sis) SYN botryomycosis.

**ac·tion** (ak´shŭn) 1. The performance of any of the vital functions; manner or result of such performance. 2. The exertion of any force or power: physical, chemical, or mental. [L. *actio,* from *ago,* pp. *actus,* to do]

**ac·tion po·ten·ti·al** (ak´shŭn pŏ-ten´shăl) The change in membrane potential occurring in nerve, muscle, or other tissue excitation.

**ac·tion trem·or** (ak´shŭn trem´ŏr) SYN intention tremor.

**ac·ti·vate** (ak´ti-vāt) 1. To render active. 2. To make radioactive.

**ac·ti·vat·ed char·coal** (ak´ti-vā-tĕd chahr´kōl) Residue from destructive distillation of various organic materials, treated to increase its adsorptive power; used to treat diarrhea, as an antidote to various poisons, and in purification processes in industry and research.

**ac·ti·vat·ed resin** (ak´ti-vā-tĕd rez´in) SYN autopolymer resin.

**ac·ti·va·tion** (ak´ti-vā´shŭn) 1. Act of rendering active. 2. Act of making something radioactive.

**ac·ti·va·tor** (ak´ti-vā-tŏr) 1. A substance that renders another substance active, or accelerates a process or reaction. 2. A removable type of myofunctional orthodontic appliance that acts as a passive transmitter of force, produced by the function of the activated muscles, to the teeth and alveolar process that are in contact with it. SEE ALSO accelerator.

**ac·tive ca·ries** (ak´tiv kar´ēz) Microbially induced lesions of growing teeth.

**ac·tive con·ges·tion** (ak´tiv kŏn-jes´chŭn) Congestion due to an increased flow of arterial blood to a part.

**ac·tive e·lec·trode** (ak´tiv ē-lek´trōd) Small electrode with an exciting effect used to stimulate or record localized potentials.

**active hyperaemia** [Br.] SYN active hyperemia.

**ac·tive hy·per·e·mi·a** (ak´tiv hī´pĕr-ē´mē-ă) Hyperemia due to an increased afflux of arterial blood into dilated capillaries. SYN fluxionary hyperemia, active hyperaemia.

**ac·tive pla·ce·bo** (ak´tiv plă-sē´bō) SYN placebo.

**ac·tive prin·ci·ple** (ak´tiv prin´si-pĕl) Constituent of a drug, usually an alkaloid or glycoside; largely responsible for conferring its characteristic therapeutic properties.

**ac·tive tip ar·e·a** (ak´tiv tip ar´ē-ă) Portion of an electronically powered instrument tip capable of doing work; ranges from approximately 2–4 mm of the length of the instrument tip.

**ac·tive trans·port** (ak´tiv trans´pōrt) Passage of ions or molecules across a cell membrane by an energy-consuming process at the expense of catabolic processes proceeding within the cell.

**ac·tive treat·ment** (ak´tiv trēt´mĕnt) Therapeutic substance or course intended to ameliorate the basic disease problem, as opposed to supportive or palliative treatment.

**ac·tiv·i·ty** (ak-tiv′i-tē) **1.** ELECTROENCEPHAL-OGRAPHY the presence of neurogenic electrical energy. **2.** PHYSICAL CHEMISTRY an ideal concentration for which the law of mass action will apply perfectly; the ratio of the activity to the true concentration is the activity coefficient (γ), which becomes 1.00 at infinite dilution. **3.** For enzymes, the amount of substrate consumed (or product formed) in a given time under given conditions; turnover number. **4.** The number of nuclear transformations (disintegrations) in a given quantity of a material per unit time. Units: curie (Ci), millicurie (mCi), becquerel (Bq), megabecquerel (MBq).

**ac·tu·al cau·te·ry** (ak′chū-ăl kaw′tĕr-ē) Cautery using heat not chemicals.

**a·cu·i·ty** (ă-kyū′i-tē) **1.** Sharpness, clearness, distinctness. **2.** Severity. [thr. Fr., fr. L. *acuo*, pp. *acutus*, sharpen]

**a·cu·le·ate** (ă-kyū′lē-āt) Pointed; covered with sharp spines. [L. *aculeatus*, pointed, fr. *acus*, needle]

**a·cu·mi·nate** (ă-kyū′mi-nāt) Pointed; tapering to a point. [L. *acumino*, pp. -*atus*, to sharpen]

**ac·u·ol·o·gy** (ak′yū-ol′ŏ-jē) Study of the use of needles for therapeutic purposes, as in acupuncture. [L. *acus*, needle, + G. *logos*, study]

**ac·u·pres·sure** (ak′yū-presh-ŭr) Application of pressure in sites used for acupuncture with therapeutic intent.

**ac·u·punc·ture** (ak′yū-pŭngk′shŭr) Ancient Asian system of therapy in which long, fine needles are inserted into discrete areas of the body that are considered linked to symptoms or disease. [L. *acus*, needle, + *puncture*]

**ac·u·punc·ture an·es·the·si·a** (ak′yū-pŭngk′shŭr an′es-thē′zē-ă) Percutaneous insertion of, and stimulation by, needles placed in critical areas of the body to produce loss of sensation in another area.

**a·cute** (ă-kyūt′) **1.** Referring to a health effect, usually of rapid onset, brief, not prolonged; sometimes loosely used to mean severe. **2.** Referring to exposure, brief, intense, short-term; sometimes specifically referring to brief exposure of high intensity. [L. *acutus*, sharp]

**a·cute ab·do·men** (ă-kyūt′ ab′dŏ-mĕn) Any serious acute intraabdominal condition with pain, tenderness, and muscular rigidity and for which emergency surgery must be considered.

**a·cute ab·scess** (ă-kyūt′ ab′ses) Newly formed abscess with little or no fibrosis in the wall of the cavity.

**a·cute a·dre·no·cor·ti·cal in·suf·fi·cien·cy** (ă-kyūt′ ă-drē′nō-kōr′ti-kăl in′sŭ-fish′ĕn-sē) Disorder due to intercurrent illness that increases demand for adrenocortical hormones in a patient with adrenal insufficiency; can be fatal if untreated. SYN addisonian crisis, adrenal crisis.

**a·cute al·co·hol·ism** (ă-kyūt′ al′kŏ-hol-izm) Temporary deterioration in mental function, with muscular incoordination due to rapid ingestion of alcoholic beverages.

**a·cute an·gle** (ă-kyūt′ ang′gĕl) Angle measuring less than 90 degrees.

**a·cute ap·pen·di·ci·tis** (ă-kyūt′ ă-pen′di-sī′tis) Inflammation of the appendix, usually resulting from bacterial infection, which may be precipitated by obstruction of the lumen by a fecalith; symptoms include periumbilical colicky pain, vomiting, among others.

**a·cute bul·bar po·li·o·my·e·li·tis** (ă-kyūt′ bŭl′bahr pō′lē-ō-mī-ĕ-lī′tis) Viral infection affecting nerve cells in the medulla oblongata and paralyzing the lower motor cranial nerves.

**a·cute cor·o·nar·y syn·drome (ACS)** (ă-kyūt′ kōr′ŏ-nar-ē sin′drōm) A general term for clinical syndromes due to reduction of blood flow in coronary arteries. SYN preinfarction angina, unstable angina.

**a·cute de·li·ri·um** (ă-kyūt′ dĕ-lir′ē-ŭm) Delirium of recent, rapid onset.

**a·cute glo·mer·u·lo·ne·phri·tis** (ă-kyūt′ glō-mer′yū-lō-nef-rī′tis) Glomerulonephritis that frequently occurs as a late complication of pharyngitis or skin infection, characterized by abrupt onset of hematuria, edema of the face, oliguria, and variable azotemia and hypertension.

**a·cute her·pet·ic gin·gi·vo·sto·ma·ti·tis** (ă-kyūt′ hĕr-pet′ik jin′ji-vō-stō′mă-tī′tis) SYN primary herpetic gingivostomatitis.

**a·cute her·pet·ic sto·ma·ti·tis** (ă-kyūt hĕr-pet′ik stō-mă-tī′tĭs) Inflammation and ulceration of the oral cavity caused by herpes simplex virus infection.

**a·cute in·flam·ma·tion** (ă-kyūt′ in′flă-mā′shŭn) Any rapid-onset inflammation that quickly worsens but resolves in a few days to weeks; characterized histologically by edema, hyperemia, and inflitrates of polymorphonuclear leukocytes.

**a·cute ma·la·ri·a** (ă-kyūt′ mă-lar′ē-ă) Intermittent or remittent form of malaria, consisting of a chill accompanied and followed by fever with its attendant general symptoms and terminating in sweating.

**a·cute my·o·car·di·al in·farc·tion** SYN acute coronary syndrome.

**a·cute nec·ro·tiz·ing ul·cer·a·tive gin·gi·vi·tis (ANUG)** (ă-kyūt′ nek′rō-tīz-ing ŭl′sĕr-ă-tiv jin′ji-vī′tis) An acute or recurrent gingivitis of young and middle-aged adults characterized clinically by gingival erythema and pain, fetid odor, necrosis, and sloughing of interdental papillae and marginal gingiva that gives rise to a gray pseudomembrane; fever, regional lymphadenopathy, and other systemic manifestations also may be present. A fusiform bacillus and *Treponema vincentii* can be isolated from the gingival tissues in large numbers and are thought to play a significant but poorly defined role in the pathogenesis.

**a·cute per·i·o·don·ti·tis** (ă-kyūt´ per´ē-ō-don-tī´tis) Rapid inflammatory process of the periodontium involving moderate to severe pain that may be caused by infectious, chemical, or physical factors.

**a·cute pri·mar·y her·pe·tic gin·gi·vo·sto·ma·ti·tis** (ă-kyūt prī´mar-ē hĕr-pet´ik jin´ji-vō-stō-mă-tī´tis) First infection of oral tissues with herpes simplex virus; characterized by gingival inflammation, vesicles, and ulcers. SYN primary herpetic gingivostomatitis.

**acute promyelocytic leukaemia** [Br.] SYN acute promyelocytic leukemia.

**a·cute pro·my·e·lo·cyt·ic leu·ke·mi·a** (ă-kyūt´ prō´mī-ĕ-lō-sit´ik lū-kē´mē-ă) Leukemia as a severe bleeding disorder, with infiltration of the bone marrow by abnormal promyelocytes and myelocytes, a low plasma fibrinogen level, and defective coagulation. SYN acute promyelocytic leukaemia.

**a·cute ra·di·a·tion syn·drome** (ă-kyūt´ rā´dē-ā´shŭn sin´drōm) Syndrome caused by exposure of the body to large amounts of radiation; divided into three major forms that are, in ascending order of severity, the hematologic, gastrointestinal, and central nervous system–cardiovascular forms.

**a·cute rheu·mat·ic ar·thri·tis** (ă-kyūt´ rū-mat´ik ahr-thrī´tis) Arthritis due to rheumatic fever.

**a·cute rhi·ni·tis** (ă-kyūt´ rī-nī´tis) Acute inflammation of the mucous membranes, marked by sneezing, lacrimation, and profuse secretion of watery mucus; usually associated with infection by one of the common cold viruses of acute allergic rhinitis. SYN coryza.

**a·cute stress re·ac·tion** (ă-kyūt´ stres rē-ak´shŭn) SYN anxiety reaction.

**a·cy·a·not·ic** (ā-sī´ă-not´ik) Characterized by absence of cyanosis.

**acyclovir** (ā-sī´klō-vir) A synthetic nucleoside medication used to treat chicken pox, shingles, and the genital form of herpes simplex symptoms.

♻ **-ad** In anatomic nomenclature, a suffix synonymous with -ward; toward or in the direction of the part indicated by the main portion of the word. [L. *ad,* to]

**AD** Abbreviation for Alzheimer disease.

**Ad** Abbreviation for adduction.

♻ **ad-** *Do not confuse words formed with this prefix and words formed with the prefix ab-.* Prefix

denoting increase, adherence, to, toward; near; very. [L. *ad,* to, toward;]

**ADA** Abbreviation for American Dental Association.

**ADA** Abbreviation for Americans with Disabilities Act.

**ad·a·man·tine** (ad´ă-man´tēn) Exceedingly hard; formerly used denoting tooth enamel. [G. *adamantinos,* very hard]

**ad·a·man·tine mem·brane** (ad´ă-man´tēn mem´brān) SYN enamel cuticle.

**Ad·am's ap·ple** (ad´ămz ap´ĕl) SYN laryngeal prominence.

**Ad·ams clasp** (ad´ămz klasp) Wire gripping device of modified arrowhead design using undercuts on mesial and distal proximal and buccal surfaces of a tooth for retention.

**Ad·ams-Stokes syn·drome** (ad´ămz-stōks sin´drōm) A disorder characterized by slow or absent pulse, vertigo, syncope, convulsions, and sometimes Cheyne-Stokes respiration; usually as a result of advanced atrioventricular block or sick sinus syndrome. SYN Morgagni disease, Spens syndrome, Stokes-Adams syndrome.

**ad·ap·ta·tion** (ad´ap-tā´shŭn) *Avoid the incorrect form adaption.* **1.** The fitting, condensing, or contouring of a restorative material, foil, or shell to a tooth or cast to ensure close contact. **2.** Alignment of an instrument against a tooth before activation of an exploratory or working stroke. **3.** An advantageous change in function or constitution of an organ or tissue to meet new conditions. **4.** A homeostatic response. [L. *adapto,* pp. *-atus,* to adjust]

**ad·ap·ta·tion dis·eas·es** (ad´ap-tā´shŭn di-zēz´ĕz) Diseases falling theoretically into the Selye concept of the general-adaptation syndrome. The courses of these diseases lay within the organism's excessive and prolonged or deficient (i.e., maladaptive) responses to stressors. SEE ALSO general adaptation syndrome.

**ad·ap·ta·tion syn·drome of Sel·ye** (ad´ap-tā´shŭn sin´drōm sel´yĕ) SYN general adaptation syndrome.

**a·dapt·er, a·dap·tor** (ă-dap´tĕr, -tŏr) **1.** A connecting part, joining two pieces of apparatus. **2.** A converter of electric current to a desired form. **3.** A single- or double-stranded digodeoxynucleotide used to join two incompatible ends of restriction fragments.

**ADA Seal of Ac·cept·ance** (sēl ak-sep´tăns) An award by a voluntary self-regulatory program administered by the American Dental Association (ADA) to ensure safety and effectiveness of dental products.

**ad·ax·i·al** (ad-ak´sē-ăl) Toward an axis, or on one or other side of an axis.

**ADC** Abbreviation for AIDS dementia complex.

**ADD** Abbreviation for attention deficit disorder.

**ad·dict** (ad′ikt) A person who is habituated to a substance or practice.

**ad·dic·tion** (ă-dik′shŭn) Habitual psychological or physiologic dependence on a substance or practice that is beyond voluntary control. [L. *ad-dico*, pp. *-dictus*, consent, fr. *ad- + dico*, to say]

**ad·dic·tive drug** (ă-dik′tiv drŭg) Any drug that creates a certain degree of euphoria and has a strong potential for addiction.

**Addison anaemia** [Br.] SYN Addison anemia.

**Ad·di·son a·ne·mi·a** (ad′i-sŏn ă-nē′mē-ă) SYN pernicious anemia, Addison anaemia.

**Ad·di·son-Bier·mer dis·ease** (ad′i-sŏn bēr′měr di-zēz′) SYN pernicious anemia.

🔲**Ad·di·son dis·ease** (ad′i-sŏn di-zēz′) See page A14. SYN chronic adrenocortical insufficiency.

**ad·di·so·ni·an a·ne·mi·a** (ad′i-sō′nē-ăn ă-nē′mē-ă) SYN pernicious anemia.

**ad·di·tion pol·y·me·ri·za·tion** (ă-dish′ŭn pol′i-měr-ī-zā′shŭn) A chemical reaction in which a higher molecular weight product is produced by addition of simpler compounds.

**ad·di·tive** (ad′i-tiv) A substance not naturally part of a material (e.g., food) but deliberately added to fulfill some specific purpose (e.g., preservation).

**ad·di·tive ef·fect** (ad′i-tiv e-fekt′) Any effect wherein two or more substances or actions used in combination produce a total effect.

**ad·di·tive mod·el** (ad′i-tiv mod′ĕl) One in which the combined effect of several factors is the sum of the effects that would be produced by each of the factors in the absence of the others.

**ad·di·tiv·i·ty** (ad′i-tiv′i-tē) The quality or state of being additive.

**ad·du·cent** (ă-dū′sĕnt) Bringing toward. [L. *adducens*, pres. p. of *ad-duco*, to bring]

**ad·duct** (ă-dŭkt′) 1. To draw toward the median plane. 2. An addition product, or complex, or one part of the same. [L. *ad-duco*, pp. *-ductus*, to bring toward]

**ad·duc·tion (Ad)** (ă-dŭk′shŭn) Movement of a body part toward the median plane (of the body, in the case of limbs; of the hand or foot, in the case of digits).

**ad·duc·tor mus·cle** (ă-dŭk′tŏr mŭs′ĕl) [TA] Muscle that causes movement toward the median plane of the body, the axis of the third finger or second toe, or the plane of the palm.

**ad·duc·tor re·flex** (ă-dŭk′tŏr rē′fleks) Contraction of the adductors of the thigh caused by tapping the tendon of the adductor magnus muscle while the thigh is abducted.

**ADE** Abbreviation for adverse drug effect.

**ad·e·nine** (ad′ĕ-nēn) A purine found in both RNA and DNA, and also in various free nucleotides of importance to the body.

**ad·e·ni·tis** (ad′ĕ-nī′tis) Inflammation of a lymph node or of a gland. [*aden-* + G. *-itis*, inflammation]

🌀**adeno-, aden-** *Do not confuse these with ad-reno-.* Combining forms denoting gland, glandular; corresponds to L. glandul-, glandi-. [G. *adēn, adenos,* a gland]

**ad·e·no·am·e·lo·blas·to·ma** (ad′ĕ-nō-am′el-ō-blas-tō′mă) SYN adenomatoid odontogenic tumor.

**ad·e·no·car·ci·no·ma** (ad′ĕ-nō-kahr′si-nō′mă) A malignant neoplasm of epithelial cells with a glandular or glandlike pattern.

**ad·e·no·hy·po·phy·si·al** (ad′ĕ-nō-hī-pō-fiz′ē-ăl) Relating to the adenohypophysis.

**ad·e·no·hy·poph·y·sis** (ad′ĕ-nō-hī-pof′i-sis) [TA] The anterior pituitary gland; it consists of the distal, intermediate, and infundibular parts. SEE ALSO pituitary gland.

**ad·e·noid** (ad′ĕ-noyd) *Avoid the misspelling/mispronunciation adnoid.* 1. Glandlike; of glandular appearance. 2. Epithelial and lymphatic unencapsulated structure located on the posterior wall of the nasopharynx; enlargement is associated with otitis media, nasal obstruction, sinusitis, and obstructive sleep apnea. SYN tonsilla pharyngealis. [G. *adeno-*, gland + G. *eidos*, appearance]

🔲**ad·e·noid cys·tic car·ci·no·ma** (ad′ĕ-noyd sis′tik kahr′si-nō′mă) Histologic type of carcinoma characterized by large epithelial masses containing round, glandlike spaces or cysts that frequently contain mucus or collagen; most common in salivary glands and skin. See this page.

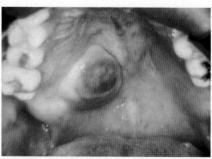

**adenoid cystic carcinoma:** surface ulceration

**ad·e·noid·ec·to·my** (ad′ĕ-noyd-ek′tŏ-mē) An operation for the removal of adenoid growths in the nasopharynx. [*adenoid* + G. *ektomē,* excision]

**ad·e·noid fa·ci·es** (ad′ĕ-noyd fā′shē-ēz) The open-mouthed and often dull appearance seen in children with adenoid hypertrophy, associated with a pinched nose.

**ad·e·noids** (ad′ĕ-noydz) **1.** A normal collection of unencapsulated lymphoid tissue in the nasopharynx. Also called pharyngeal tonsils. **2.** Common terminology for the large pharyngeal tonsils of children. [G. *adēn,* gland, + *-eidos,* resemblance]

**ad·e·noid tis·sue** (ad′ĕ-noyd tish′ū) Lymphatic tissue intimately associated with epithelium. SEE epithelium.

**▣ad·e·no·ma,** pl. **ad·e·no·mas,** pl. **ad·e·no·ma·ta** (ad′ĕ-nō′mă, -măz, -mă-tă) A benign epithelial neoplasm in which the tumor cells form glands or glandlike structures; usually well circumscribed, tending to compress rather than infiltrate or invade adjacent tissue. See this page. [*adeno-* + G. *-oma,* tumor]

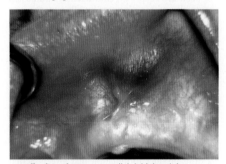

canalicular adenoma: purplish labial nodule

**▣ad·e·no·ma·toid o·don·to·gen·ic tu·mor** (ad′ĕ-nō′mă-toyd ō-don′tŏ-jen′ik tū′mŏr) Benign epithelial type lesion appearing radiographically as a well-circumscribed, radiolucent-radiopaque lesion usually surrounding crown of an impacted tooth in an adolescent or young adult. See page A16. SYN adenoameloblastoma, ameloblastic adenomatoid tumor.

**ad·e·no·ma·to·sis** (ad′ĕ-nō′mă-tō′sis) A condition characterized by multiple glandular overgrowths.

**ad·e·no·ma·to·sis o·ris** (ad′ĕ-nō-mă-tō′sis ōr′is) Nonpathologic hypertrophy of the mucous glands of the lips.

**ad·e·no·meg·a·ly** (ad′ĕ-nō-meg′ă-lē) Enlargement of a gland. [*adeno-* + G. *megas,* large]

**ad·e·nop·a·thy** (ad′ĕ-nop′ă-thē) Swelling or morbid enlargement of the lymph nodes. [*adeno-* + G. *pathos,* suffering]

**ad·e·no·phleg·mon** (ad′ĕ-nō-fleg′mon) Acute inflammation of a gland and the adjacent connective tissue. [*adeno-* + G. *phlegmonē,* inflammation]

**ad·e·nose** (ad′ĕ-nōs) Relating to a gland or like a gland.

**a·den·o·sine** (ă-den′ō-sēn) Condensation product of adenine and D-ribose.

**a·den·o·sine tri·phos·pha·tase** (ă-den′ō-sēn trī-fos′fă-tās) Enzyme that catalyzes release of the terminal phosphate group of adenosine 5′-triphosphate.

**a·den·o·sine tri·phos·phate** (ă-den′ō-sen trī-fos′făt) SYN adenosine 5′-triphosphate (ATP).

**a·den·o·sine 5′-tri·phos·phate (ATP)** (ă-den′ō-sēn trī-fos′făt) Adenosine with triphosphoric acid esterified at its 5′ position; immediate precursor of adenine nucleotides in RNA; the promary energeny of a cell.

**ad·e·no·sis** (ad′ĕ-nō′sis) Glandular tissue in sites in which it is not usually found.

**ad·e·no·vi·rus** (ad′ĕ-nō-vī′rŭs) Adenoidal-pharyngeal-conjunctival or A-P-C virus; many types infect humans, causing upper respiratory symptoms, acute respiratory disease (ARD), conjunctivitis, and other diseases. [G. *adēn,* gland, + virus]

**ad·e·nyl cy·clase** (ad′e-nil sī′klās) An enzyme that converts adenosine monophosphate to 3′,5′-cyclic adenosine monophosphate, an intracellular second messenger of neural and hormonal activation.

**ad·e·nyl·ic ac·id** (ad′ĕ-nil′ik as′id) A condensation product of adenosine and phosphoric acid; a nucleotide found among the hydrolysis products of all nucleic acids. SEE ALSO AMP. SYN adenine nucleotide.

**a·deps,** pl. **a·di·pes** (ad′eps, -i-pēz) **1.** Denoting fat or adipose tissue. **2.** The rendered fat of swine, lard, used in the preparation of ointments. [L. lard, fat]

**ad·e·quate stim·u·lus** (ad′ĕ-kwăt stim′yū-lŭs) Stimulus to which a particular receptor responds effectively and gives rise to a characteristic sensation.

**ADHA** Abbreviation for American Dental Hygienists Association.

**ADHD** Abbreviation for attention deficit hyperactivity disorder.

**ad·her·ence** (ad-hēr′ĕns) **1.** Act or quality of sticking to something. **2.** Extent to which a patient continues an agreed-on mode of treatment without close supervision. Cf. compliance, maintenance. [L. *adhaereo,* to stick to]

**ad·he·si·o,** pl. **ad·he·si·o·nes** (ad-hē′ zē-ō, -ō′nēz) SYN adhesion. [L.]

**ad·he·sion** (ad-hē′zhŭn) Process of binding to a surface or binding two surfaces using chemical bonds or micromechanical interlocks. SYN adhesio. [L. *adhaesio,,* fr. *adhaereo,* to stick to]

**ad·he·sive** (ad-hē′siv) 1. Relating to, or having the characteristics of, an adhesion. 2. Any material that adheres to a surface or causes adherence between surfaces.

**ad·he·sive a·tel·ec·ta·sis** (ad-hē′siv at′ ĕ-lek′tă-sis) Alveolar collapse in the presence of patent airways, especially when surfactant is inactivated or absent, particularly in respiratory distress syndrome of the newborn, acute radiation pneumonitis, or viral pneumonia.

**ad·hesive foil** (ăd-hē′siv foyl) SYN cohesive foil.

**ad·he·sive tape** (ad-hē′siv tāp) Fabric or film evenly coated on one side with a pressure-sensitive adhesive mixture.

**a·di·a·pho·ret·ic** (ā-dī′ă-fō-ret′ik) SYN anhidrotic.

**A·die syn·drome, A·die pu·pil** (a′dē sin′drōm, pyū′pil) An idiopathic postganglionic denervation of the parasympathetically innervated intraocular muscles.

**ad·i·poid** (ad′i-poyd) SYN lipoid. [adipo- + G. *eidos,* resemblance]

**ad·i·pose** (ad′i-pōs) Denoting fat.

**ad·i·pose tis·sue** (ad′i-pōs tish′ū) Form of connective tissue consisting chiefly of fat cells. SYN fat (1).

**ad·i·pos·i·ty** (ad′i-pos′i-tē) 1. SYN obesity. 2. Excessive accumulation of lipids in a site or organ.

**ad·i·po·so·gen·i·tal dys·tro·phy** (ad′i-pō-sō-jen′i-tăl dis′trŏ-fē) SYN dystrophia adiposogenitalis.

**a·dip·si·a, a·dip·sy** (ă-dip′sē-ă, -dip′sē) *Avoid the misspelling adypsia.* Absence of thirst or the lack of desire to drink. [G. *a-* priv. + *dipsa,* thirst]

**ad·i·tus,** pl. **ad·i·tus** (ad′i-tŭs) [TA] SYN aperture. [L. access, fr. *ad-eo,* pp. *-itus,* go to]

**ad·i·tus glot·ti·dis in·fe·ri·or** (ad′i-tŭs glot′i-dis in-fēr′ē-ŏr) SYN infraglottic cavity.

**ad·i·tus glot·ti·dis su·per·i·or** (ad′i-tŭs glot′i-dis sŭ-pēr′ē-ŏr) SYN intermediate laryngeal cavity.

**ad·i·tus la·ryn·gis** (ad′i-tŭs lă-rin′jŭs) [TA] SYN laryngeal inlet.

**ad·i·tus to mas·toid an·trum** (ad′i-tŭs mas′toyd an′trŭm) [TA] Orifice leading from epitympanic recess to mastoid antrum.

**ad·ja·cent an·gle** (ă-jā′sĕnt ang′gĕl) Angle with a line in common with another angle.

**ad·just** (ă-jŭst′) To reshape a dental prosthesis, restoration, or oral appliance to improve effectiveness, function, or appearance.

**ad·just·a·ble an·te·ri·or guide** (ă-jŭs′ tă-bĕl an-tēr′ē-ŏr gīd) SYN incisal guide.

**ad·just·a·ble ar·tic·u·la·tor** (ă-jŭs′tă-bĕl ahr-tik′yū-lā-tŏr) 1. Articulator that may be adjusted to permit movement of the casts into recorded eccentric relationships; 2. Articulator capable of adjustment to more than one eccentric position.

**ad·just·a·ble ax·is face-bow** (ă-jŭs′tă-bĕl ak′sis fās′bō) Face-bow with caliper ends that can be adjusted to permit location of the axis of rotation of the mandible. SYN kinematic face-bow.

**ad·just·a·ble oc·clu·sal pi·vot** (ă-jŭs′tă-bĕl ŏ-klū′zăl piv′ŏt) One that may be adjusted vertically with a screw or by other means.

**ad·just·ment** (ă-jŭst′mĕnt) Modification made to a restoration, denture, or oral appliance.

**ad·just·ment dis·or·ders** (ă-jŭst′mĕnt dis-ōr′dĕrz) A group of mental and behavioral disorders in which the development of symptoms is related to the presence of some environmental stressor or life event and is expected to remit when the stress ceases.

**ad·ju·vant** (ad′jū-vănt) 1. Substance added to a drug product formulation that affects action of the active ingredient in a predictable way. 2. Additional therapy given to enhance or extend primary therapy's effect, as in chemotherapy's addition to a surgical regimen. [L. *adjuvo,* pres. p. *-juvans,* to give aid to]

**ad·me·di·al, ad·me·di·an** (ad-mē′dē-ăl, -dē-ăn) Toward or near the median plane.

**ad·mi·nic·u·lum,** pl. **ad·mi·nic·u·la** (ad-mi-nik′yū-lŭm, -yū-lă) That which gives support to a part. [L. a hand-rest, prop, fr. *ad + manus,* hand]

**ad·min·i·stra·tion** (ad-min′ĭ-strā′shŭn) 1. The management of the affairs and activities of a group or entity. 2. Persons charged with executive functions. 3. The giving of a medicine or other treatment. [L. *administro,* to manage]

**ad·min·i·stra·tor** (ad-min′i-strā-tŏr) A person or entity managing executive duties.

**ad·neu·ral, ad·ner·val** (ad-nūr′ăl, -nĕr′ văl) 1. Lying near a nerve. 2. In the direction of a nerve; said of an electric current passing through muscular tissue toward the point of entrance of the nerve.

**ad·nex·al** (ad-nek′săl) Relating to the adnexa.

**ad·o·les·cence** (ad′ŏ-les′ĕns) The period of life beginning with puberty and ending with completed growth and physical maturity. [L. *adolescentia*]

**ad·o·les·cent** (ad′ŏ-les′ĕnt) **1.** Pertaining to adolescence. **2.** A person in that stage of development.

**ad·o·les·cent growth spurt** (ad′ŏ-les′ĕnt grōth spŭrt) Growth characterized by rapid gains in height and weight, as much as 3 inches in a single year; occurs 2 years earlier in girls.

**ad·o·les·cent med·i·cine** (ad′ŏ-les′ĕnt med′i-sin) Branch of medicine concerned with treatment of youth ages 13–21 years.

**ADR** Abbreviation for adverse drug reaction.

**a·dre·nal bod·y** (ă-drē′năl bod′ē) SYN suprarenal gland.

**ad·re·nal cor·tex** (ă-drē′năl kōrteks) SYN cortex of suprarenal gland.

**ad·re·nal cor·ti·coid** (ă-drē′năl kōr′ti-koid) SYN corticosteroid.

**ad·re·nal cor·ti·cos·te·roid** (ă-drē′năl kōr′ti-kō-ster′oyd) SYN corticosteroid. adrenal [*ad-*, at, near, + L. *ren*, kidney, + *-al*, adj. suffix] corticosteroid [L. *cortex*, gen. *corticis*, bark, + *ster-* fr. cholesterol, + *-oid*, noun suffix]

**ad·re·nal·ec·to·my** (ă-drē′năl-ek′tŏ-mē) Removal of one or both suprarenal glands, may be total or partial. Preoperative steroid replacement therapy may be required. [*adrenal* + G. *ektomē,* excision]

**ad·re·nal gland** (ă-drē′năl gland) SYN suprarenal gland.

**ad·ren·a·line** (ă-dren′ă-lin) SYN epinephrine.

**ad·re·nal·ism** (ă-drē′năl-izm) SYN hypercorticoidism.

**a·dre·nal leu·ko·dys·tro·phy** (ă-drē′năl lū′kō-dis′trŏ-fē) A metabolic disorder of young males, characterized by widespread myelin degeneration and associated adrenal insufficiency. Symptoms include bronzing of the skin, dysarthria, and cortical blindness.

**ad·re·na·lop·a·thy** (ă-drē′nă-lop′ă-thē) Any pathologic condition of the suprarenal glands. [*adrenal* + G. *pathos,* suffering]

**ad·re·nal ste·roids** (ă-drē′năl ster′oydz) SYN corticosteroid.

**ad·ren·ar·che** (ad-ren-ahr′kē) *Avoid the mispronunciation ad′renarche.* **1.** Growth of axillary and pubic hair induced by hyperactivity of the suprarenal cortex in early puberty. **2.** Physiologic change at puberty caused by adrenocortical secretion of androgenic hormones or their precursors. [*adren-* + G. *archē,* beginning]

**ad·re·ner·gic** (ad′rĕ-nĕr′jik) **1.** Relating to nerve cells or fibers of the autonomic nervous system that use norepinephrine as their neurotransmitter. **2.** Relating to drugs that mimic actions of the sympathetic nervous system. [*adren-* + G. *ergon,* work]

**ad·re·ner·gic a·gent** (ad′rĕ-nĕr′jik ā′jĕnt) A drug that mimics the action of the sympathetic nervous system.

**ad·re·ner·gic ag·o·nist** (ad′rĕ-nĕr′jik ag′ŏ-nist) An agent capable of combining with receptors to initiate actions of or like epinephrine. SEE agonist. SEE ALSO epinephrine.

**ad·re·ner·gic a·mine** (ad′rĕ-nĕr′jik ă-mēn′) SYN sympathomimetic amine.

**ad·re·ner·gic block·ade** (ad′rĕ-nĕr′jik blok-ād′) Selective inhibition by a drug of the responses of effector cells to adrenergic sympathetic nerve impulses (sympatholytic) and to epinephrine and related amines (adrenolytic).

**ad·re·ner·gic block·ing a·gent** (ad′rĕ-nĕr′jik blok′ing ā′jĕnt) Compound that selectively blocks or inhibits responses to sympathetic adrenergic nerve activity (sympatholytic agent) and to epinephrine, norepinephrine, and other adrenergic amines (adrenolytic agent); two distinct classes exist, α- and β-adrenergic receptor blocking agents.

**ad·re·ner·gic fi·bers** (ad′rĕ-nĕr′jik fī′bĕrz) Nerve fibers that transmit nervous impulses to other nerve cells (or smooth muscle or gland cells) by medium of the adrenalinelike transmitter substance norepinephrine (noradrenaline). SYN adrenergic fibres.

**adrenergic fibres** [Br.] SYN adrenergic fibers.

**ad·re·ner·gic neu·ro·nal block·ing a·gent** (ad′rĕ-nĕr′jik nūr-ō′năl blok′ing ā′jĕnt) Drug that prevents release of norepinephrine from sympathetic nerve terminals; does not inhibit responses of adrenergic receptors to circulating epinephrine, norepinephrine, and other adrenergic amines.

**ad·re·ner·gic neu·ro·trans·mit·ter** (ad′rĕ-nĕr′jik nūr′ō-trans′mit-ĕr) Neurotransmitter formed in sympathetic postganglionic synapses (e.g., norepinephrine).

**α-ad·re·ner·gic re·cep·tors** (ad′rĕ-nĕr′jik rĕ-sep′tŏrz) Those in effector tissues capable of selective activation and blockade by drugs; conceptually derived from the ability of certain agents, such as phenoxybenzamine, to block only some adrenergic receptors and of other agents, such as methoxamine, to activate only the same adrenergic receptors. Such receptors are designated as α-receptors. Their activation results in physiologic responses such as increased peripheral vascular resistance, mydriasis, and contraction of pilomotor muscles.

**β-ad·re·ner·gic re·cep·tors** (ad′rĕ-nĕr′jik rĕ-sep′tŏrz) Those in effector tissues capable of selective activation and blockade by drugs.

**ad·re·ner·gic re·cep·tors** (ad′rĕ-nĕr′jik rĕ-sep′tŏrz) Reactive components of effector tissues, most of which are innervated by adrenergic postganglionic fibers of the sympathetic nervous system. Such receptors can be activated by norepinephrine and/or epinephrine and by various adrenergic drugs. SYN adrenoceptor.

**a·dren·ic** (ă-drē′nik) Relating to the suprarenal gland.

**a·dre·no·cep·tive** (ă-drē′nō-sep′tiv) Referring to chemical sites in effectors with which the adrenergic mediator unites.

**a·dre·no·cep·tor** (ă-drē′nō-sep′tŏr) SYN adrenergic receptors.

**a·dre·no·cor·ti·cal hor·mones** (ă-drē′nō-kōr′ti-kăl hōr′mōnz) Hormones secreted by the human cortex of the suprarenal gland, e.g., cortisol, aldosterone, corticosterone.

**ad·re·no·cor·ti·cal in·suf·fi·cien·cy** (ă-drē′nō-kōr′ti-kăl in′sŭ-fish′ĕn-sē) Loss, to varying degrees, of adrenocortical function.

**ad·re·no·cor·ti·co·tro·pic, ad·re·no·cor·ti·co·tro·phic** (ă-drē′nō-kōr′ti-kō-trō′pik, -trō′fik) Stimulating growth of the suprarenal cortex or secretion of its hormones. SYN adrenotropic, adrenotrophic. [*adrenal cortex* + G. *trophē*, nurture; *tropē*, a turning]

**ad·re·no·cor·ti·co·tro·pic hor·mone (ACTH)** (ă-drē′nō-kōr′ti-kō-trō′pik hōr′mōn) Hormone of anterior lobe of hypophysis that governs nutrition and growth of the adrenal cortex, stimulates it to functional activity. SYN corticotropic hormone.

**a·dre·no·cor·ti·co·tro·pic pep·tide** (ă-drē′nō-kōr′ti-kō-trō′pik pep′tīd) Peptide with adrenocorticotropic hormone activity, isolated from pituitary extracts.

**a·dre·no·cor·ti·co·tro·pin re·leas·ing factor** (ă-drē′nō-kōr′ti-kō-trō′pin rĕ-lēs′ing fak′tŏr) Hormone produced by the hypothalamus that causes the pituitary to secrete adrenocorticotropic hormone.

**a·dre·no·gen·ic, a·dre·nog·e·nous** (ă-drē′nō-jen′ik, ad′rĕ-noj′ĕ-nŭs) Of suprarenal origin. [*adreno-* + G. *-gen*, producing]

**ad·re·no·gen·i·tal syn·drome** (ă-drē′nō-jen′i-tal sin′drōm) Group of disorders caused by congenital adrenocortical hyperplasia characterized by masculinization of women, feminization of men, and sexual ambiguity or precocious sexual development of children.

**ad·re·no·lyt·ic** (ă-drē′nō-lit′ik) Denoting antagonism to or inhibition or blockade of the action of epinephrine, norepinephrine, and related sympathomimetics. SEE ALSO adrenergic blocking agent. [*adreno-* + G. *lysis,* loosening, dissolution]

**ad·re·no·med·ul·lar·y hor·mones** (ă-drē′nō-med′ŭ-lar-ē hōr′mōnz) Hormones produced by the adrenal medulla, particularly epinephrine and norepinephrine.

**ad·re·no·mi·met·ic** (ă-drē′nō-mi-met′ik) Having an action similar to that of the compounds epinephrine and norepinephrine. Cf. adrenergic. [*adreno-* + G. *mimētikos,* imitative]

**a·dre·no·mi·met·ic a·mine** (ă-drē′nō-mi-met′ik ă-mēn′) SYN sympathomimetic amine.

**a·dre·no·re·ac·tive** (ă-drē′nō-rē-ak′tiv) Responding to the catecholamines.

**a·dre·no·re·cep·tor** (ă-drē′nō-rē-sep′tŏr) SEE adrenergic receptors.

**ad·re·no·tox·in** (ă-drē-nō-tok′sin) Any substance toxic to the suprarenal glands.

**ad·re·no·tro·pic, a·dre·no·tro·phic** (ă-drē-nō-trō′pik, -trō′fik) SYN adrenocorticotropic.

**ad·sorb** (ad-sōrb′) *Do not confuse this word with absorb.* To take up by adsorption. [L. *ad,* to, + *sorbeo,* to suck in]

**ad·sorb·ate** (ad-sōr′bāt) Any adsorbed substance.

**ad·sorb·ent** (ad-sōr′bĕnt) **1.** Substance that adsorbs, i.e., a solid substance endowed with the property of attaching other substances to its surface without any covalent bonding, e.g., activated charcoal. **2.** An antigen or antibody used in immune adsorption.

**ad·sorp·tion** (ad-sōrp′shŭn) *Do not confuse this word with absorption.* The property of a solid substance of attracting and holding to its surface a gas, liquid, or a substance in solution or in suspension. [L. *ad,* to, + *sorbeo,* to suck in]

**ad·sorp·tion the·o·ry of nar·co·sis** (ad-sōrp′shŭn thē′ŏr-ē nahr-kō′sis) That a drug becomes concentrated at the surface of the cell as a result of adsorption, and thus alters permeability and metabolism.

**ad·ter·mi·nal** (ad-tĕr′mi-năl) In a direction toward the nerve endings, muscular insertions, or the extremity of any structure. SEE anterograde.

**a·dult** (ă-dŭlt′) **1.** Fully grown and physically mature. **2.** A fully grown and mature individual. [L. *adultus,* grown up fr. *adolesco,* to grow up]

**a·dul·ter·ant** (ă-dŭl′tĕr-ănt) An impurity; an

additive that is considered to have an undesirable effect or to dilute the active material so as to reduce its therapeutic value.

**ad·ul·ter·a·tion** (ă-dŭl'tĕr-ā'shŭn) The alteration of any substance by the deliberate addition of a component not ordinarily part of that substance; usually used to imply that the substance is debased as a result.

**a·dult-on·set di·a·be·tes** (ă-dŭlt' on'set dī'ă-bē'tēz) Former designation for Type 2 diabetes (q.v.).

**a·dult res·pi·ra·to·ry dis·tress syn·drome (ARDS)** (ă-dŭlt' res'pir-ă-tōr-ē distres' sin'drōm) Acute lung injury from a variety of causes, characterized by interstitial or alveolar edema and hemorrhage as well as perivascular pulmonary edema associated with hyaline membrane formation, proliferation of collagen fibers, and swollen epithelium with increased pinocytosis.

**a·dult ric·kets** (ă-dŭlt' rik'ĕts) SYN osteomalacia.

**a·dult T-cell lym·pho·ma (ATL)** (ă-dŭlt' sel lim-fō'mă) Acute or subacute disease associated with a human T-cell virus, with lymphadenopathy, hepatosplenomegaly, skin lesions, peripheral blood involvement, and hypercalcemia.

**ad·vance** (ad-vans') To move forward. [Fr. ♻ *avancer,* to set forward]

**ad·vanced ful·crum** (ad-vanst' ful'krŭm) Variation of an intraoral or extraoral finger rest used to gain access to root surfaces within deep periodontal pockets (e.g., modified intraoral, cross arch, opposite arch, finger-on-finger, and finger assist fulcrums).

**ad·vance di·rec·tive** (ăd-vans' dĭr-ek'tiv) Legal document giving instructions as to the type and degree of medical care to be administered in the event that the person signing the document becomes mentally incompetent during the course of a terminal illness, or becomes permanently comatose.

**ad·ven·ti·ti·a** (ad'vĕn-tish'ă) [TA] Outermost connective tissue covering of any organ, vessel, or other structure not covered by a serous coat. [L. *adventicius,* coming from abroad, foreign, fr. *ad,* to + *venio,* to come]

**ad·ven·ti·tial** (ad'vĕn-tish'ăl) Relating to outer coat or adventitia of a blood vessel or other structure. SYN adventitious (3).

**ad·ven·ti·tious** (ad'vĕn-tish'ŭs) 1. Arising from an external source or occurring in an unusual place or manner. 2. Occurring accidentally or spontaneously, as opposed to naturally or through heredity. 3. SYN adventitial.

**ad·ven·ti·tious breath sounds** (ad' vĕn-tish'ŭs breth sowndz) Noise heard on auscultation of abnormal lungs.

**ad·verse drug re·ac·tion (ADR)** (ad-vĕrs' drŭg rē-ak'shŭn) Any noxious, unintended, and undesired effect of a drug after its administration for prophylaxis, diagnosis, or therapy. Also called adverse drug effect.

**ad·verse ef·fect** (ad'vers e-fekt') 1. Result of drug or other therapy in addition to or in extension of the desired therapeutic effect; usually but not necessarily, connoting an undesirable effect. 2. Although technically the therapeutic effect carried beyond the desired limit (e.g., a hemorrhage from an anticoagulant) is a side effect, the term more often refers to pharmacologic results of therapy unrelated to the usual objective (e.g., a development of signs of Cushing syndrome with steroid therapy). SYN side effect.

**a·dy·nam·i·a** (ā-dī-nam'ē-ă, ad-i-nā'mē-ă) 1. SYN asthenia. 2. Lack of motor activity or strength. [G. *a-* priv. + *dynamis,* power]

**a·dy·nam·ic** (ā-dī-nam'ik) Relating to adynamia.

**Ae·by plane** (ā'bē plān) In craniometry, a plane perpendicular to the median plane of the cranium, cutting the nasion and the basion.

**AED** Abbreviation for automatic external defibrillator.

♻ **aer-, aero-** Combining forms denoting the air, a gas; aerial, gassy. [G. *aēr* (L. *aer*), air]

**aer·ate** (ār'āt) 1. To supply (blood) with oxygen. 2. To expose to the circulation of air for purification. 3. To supply or charge (liquid) with a gas, especially carbon dioxide.

**aer·a·tion** (ār-ā'shŭn) Charging a liquid with air or gas.

**aer·obe** (ār'ōb) 1. An organism that can live and grow in the presence of oxygen. 2. An organism that uses oxygen as a final electron acceptor in a respiratory chain. [*aero-* + G. *bios,* life]

**aer·o·bic** (ār-ō'bik) 1. Living in air. 2. Relating to an aerobe.

**aer·o·bic bac·te·ria** (ār-ō'bik bak-tēr'ē-ă) Bacteria that can live and grow in the presence of oxygen. SEE aerobe, aerobic.

**aer·o·bi·o·sis** (ār'ō-bī-ō'sis) Existence in an atmosphere containing oxygen. [*aero-* + G. *biōsis,* mode of living]

**aer·o·don·tal·gi·a** (ār'ō-don-tal'jē-ă) Dental pain caused by either increased or reduced atmospheric pressure. SYN aeroodontodynia. [*aero-* + G. *odous,* tooth, + *algos,* pain]

**aer·o·don·ti·a** (ār-ō-don'shē-ă) The science of the effect of either increased or reduced atmospheric pressure on the teeth. [*aero-* + G. *odous,* tooth]

**aer·o·dy·nam·ic size** (ār'ō-dī-nam'ik sīz) In aerosols, the particle size with unit density that best represents the aerodynamic behavior of a particle.

**aer·o·gas·tri·a** (ār-ō-gas'trē-ă) Distention of the stomach by gas.

**Aer·o·mo·nas** (ār-ō-mō'năs) Genus of water-borne bacteria also found in sewage.

**aer·o·o·don·tal·gi·a** (ār'ō-ō-don-tal'jē-ă) SYN aerodontalgia.

**aer·o·o·don·to·dyn·i·a** (ār'ō-ō-don-tō-din' ē-ă) SYN aerodontalgia.

**aer·o·phil, aer·o·phile** (ār'ō-fil, -fīl) An organelle, cell, organ, or organism that needs air. [*aero-* + G. *philos,* fond]

**aer·o·pi·e·so·ther·a·py** (ār'ō-pī-ē'sō-thār' ă-pē) Treatment of disease with compressed (or rarified) air. [*aero-* + G. *piesis,* pressure, + *therapeia,* medical treatment]

**aer·o·si·al·oph·a·gy** (ār'ō-sī-ă-lof'ă-jē) SYN sialoaerophagy.

**aer·o·si·nus·i·tis** (ār'ō-sī'nŭ-sī'tis) Inflammation of the paranasal sinuses caused by pressure differences within the sinus relative to ambient pressure, secondary to obstruction of the sinus orifice, sometimes due to high altitude flying or by descent from high altitude.

**aer·o·sis** (ār-ō'sis) Generation of gas in the tissues. [*aero-* + G. *-osis,* condition]

**aer·o·sol** (ār'ō-sol) **1.** Invisible airborne particles dispersed into the surrounding environment by dental equipment (e.g., handpieces, electronic instruments). Microorganisms in aerosols have been shown to survive up to 24 hours. **2.** Liquid or particulate matter dispersed in air, gas, or vapor in the form of a fine mist for therapeutic, insecticidal, or other purposes. **3.** A product that is packaged under pressure and contains therapeutically or chemically active ingredients intended for topical application, inhalation, or introduction into body orifices. [*aero-* + *solution*]

**aer·o·sol gen·er·a·tor** (ār'ō-sol jen'ĕr-ā-tŏr) Device for producing airborne suspensions of small particles for inhalation therapy or experimental work.

**aesthesia** [Br.] SYN esthesia.

**aesthesiophysiology** [Br.] SYN esthesiophysiology.

**aesthetic** [Br.] SYN esthetic.

**aesthetics** [Br.] SYN esthetics.

**a·fe·brile** (ā-feb'ril) Without fever, denoting apyrexia; having a normal body temperature. SYN apyretic, apyrexial.

**af·fect** (a'fekt) *Do not confuse this word with*

*effect.* The emotional feeling, tone, and mood attached to a thought, including its external manifestations. [L. *affectus,* state of mind, fr. *afficio,* to have influence on]

**af·fec·tive** (a-fek'tiv) Pertaining to mood, emotion, feeling, sensibility, or a mental state.

**af·fec·to·mo·tor** (a-fek'tō-mō'tŏr) Pertaining to muscular manifestations associated with affective tone.

**af·fer·ent** (af'ĕr-ĕnt) Inflowing; conducting toward a center. Opposite of efferent. SYN centripetal (1). [L. *afferens,* fr. *af-fero,* to bring to]

**af·fer·ent nerve** (af'ĕr-ĕnt nĕrv) Nerve conveying impulses from the periphery to the central nervous system.

**af·fer·ent ves·sel** (af'ĕr-ĕnt ves'ĕl) Artery conveying blood or fluid to a body part.

**af·flux** (af'lŭks) Flowing to or toward a body part. [L. *af-fluo, af-fluxus,* to flow toward]

**af·fric·a·tive** (a-frik'ă-tiv) Speech sound composed of plosion, occlusion, and frication (an audible rush of air) as in the 'ts' sound of mats or the 'ch' sound of church. [L. *af-frico,* pp. *af-fricatus,* fr. *ad-* toward, against, + *frico,* to rub, + *-ive,* adj. suffix]

**af·fu·sion** (ă-fyū'zhŭn) Pouring water on body parts for therapeutic purposes. [L. *af-fundo,* to pour into]

**AFH** Abbreviation for anterior facial height.

**a·fi·bril·lar ce·ment** (ā-fī'bri-lăr sĕ-ment') Cementum that, using an electron microscope, appears as laminated, electron-dense reticular material.

**af·la·tox·i·co·sis** (af'lă-toks-ē-cō'sis) Disease caused by ingestion of aflatoxin, a toxin due to *Aspergillus.*

**af·ter·care, af·ter-care** (af'tĕr-kār) Treatment of a patient after an operation procedure, delivery, or convalescence from an illness.

**af·ter·cur·rent, af·ter-cur·rent** (af'tĕr-kŭr'ĕnt) An electrical current induced in a muscle on termination of a constant current that has been passed through it.

**af·ter·dis·charge, af·ter-dis·charge** (af'tĕr-dis'chahrj) Persistance of response of muscle or neural elements after cessation of stimulation. Myotonia is a clinical manifestation of prolonged muscle afterdischarge.

**af·ter·ef·fect, af·ter-ef·fect** (af'tĕr-ĕ-fekt') A physical, physiologic, psychological, or emotional effect that continues after removal of a stimulus.

**af·ter·per·cep·tion, af·ter-per·cep·tion,** (af'tĕr-pĕr-sep'shŭn) Subjective persistence of a stimulus after its cessation. Cf. pali-nopsia.

**af·ter·po·ten·tial, af·ter·po·ten·tial** (af'tĕr-pŏ-ten'shăl) The small change in electrical potential in a stimulated nerve that follows the main, or spike, potential.

**af·ter·sen·sa·tion, af·ter·sen·sa·tion,** (af'tĕr-sen-sā'shŭn) Subjective persistence of sensation after a stimulus stops.

**af·ter·sound, af·ter·sound** (af'tĕr-sownd) Subjective persistence of an auditory sensation after cessation of the acoustic stimulus.

**af·ter·taste, af·ter·taste** (af'tĕr-tāst) Subjective persistence of a gustatory sensation after contact with the taste stimulus has ceased.

**af·ter·touch, af·ter·touch,** (af'ter-tŭch) Subjective persistence of tactile sensation after cessation of stimulus; a form of aftersensation.

**a·func·tion·al oc·clu·sion** (ā-fŭngk'shŭn-ăl ŏ-klū'zhŭn) Malocclusion that does not permit normal function of the dentition.

**a·gar** (ā'gahr) A complex polysaccharide (a sulfated galactan) derived from seaweed (various red algae); used as a solidifying agent in culture media. [Bengalese]

**a·gas·tro·neu·ri·a** (ă-gas'trō-nyū'rē-ă) Lessened nervous control of the stomach. [G. *a*-priv. + *gastēr*, belly, + *neuron*, nerve]

**AGD** Abbreviation for Academy of General Dentistry.

**age** (āj) **1.** In dentistry materials–related science, treatment of a material to stabilize or strengthen it by forming a coherent precipitate that is particle formation caused by clustering of atoms of one type as part of a lattice consisting of more than one atom type. **2.** One of the periods into which human life is divided. [F. *âge*, L. *aetas*]

**age har·den·ing** (āj hahr'dĕn-ing) Heat treatment that increases the strength and hardness of some dental alloys.

**a·gen·e·sis** (ā-jen'ĕ-sis) Absence or failure to form of any part. [G. *a*- priv. + *genesis*, production]

**a·gent** (ā'jĕnt) **1.** An active force or substance capable of producing an effect. **2.** In disease, a factor such as a microorganism, chemical substance, or a form of radiation, the presence or absence of which (as in deficiency diseases) results in disease or in more advanced form of disease. [L. *ago*, pres. p. *agens* (*agent*-), to perform]

**a·geu·si·a** (ă-gū'sē-ă) Loss or absence of the sense of taste. Also called ageustia. [G. *a*- priv. + *geusis*, taste]

**ag·ger,** pl. **ag·ger·es** (ah'gĕr, -ēz) [TA] An

eminence, projection, or shallow ridge. [L. mound]

**ag·ger na·si** (ah'gĕr nā'sī) [TA] Elevation on the lateral wall of the nasal cavity lying between the atrium of the middle meatus and the olfactory sulcus.

**ag·ger per·pen·di·cu·la·ris** (ah'gĕr pĕr' pĕn-dik'yū-lā'ris) SYN eminence of triangular fossa of auricle.

**ag·glom·er·ate, ag·glom·er·at·ed** (ă-glom'ĕr-ăt, -ā'tĕd) SYN aggregated. [L. *ag-glom-ero,* to wind into a ball; from *ad,* to, + *glomus,* a ball]

**ag·glu·ti·nant** (ă-glū'ti-nănt) A substance that holds parts together or causes agglutination. [L. *ad,* to + *gluten,* glue]

**ag·glu·ti·na·tion** (ă-glū'ti-nā'shŭn) **1.** The process by which suspended bacteria, cells, or other particles are caused to adhere and form into clumps. **2.** Adhesion of the surfaces of a wound. **3.** The process of adhering. [L. *ad,* to, + *gluten,* glue]

**ag·glu·ti·nin** (ă-glū'ti-nin) Antibody that causes clumping or agglutination of the bacteria or other cells that either stimulated the formation of the agglutinin or contain immunologically similar, reactive antigen.

**ag·gre·gat·ed** (ag'rĕ-gā-tĕd) Collected together, thereby forming a cluster, clump, or mass of individual units. SYN agglomerate.

**ag·gres·sive per·i·o·don·tal dis·ease** (ă-gres'iv per'ē-ō-don'tăl dĭz-ēz') Rapid periodontal attachment loss and bone destruction in people who are otherwise clinically healthy; familial tendency. It can be either a localized form, in which molars and incisors are affected, or generalized. Associated bacteria are *Actinobacillus actinomycetemcomitans* and *Porphyromonas gingivalis.*

**ag·ing** (āj'ing) The process of growing old, especially by failure of replacement of cells in sufficient number to maintain full functional capacity; particularly affects cells (e.g., neurons) incapable of mitotic division.

**a·glos·si·a** (ā-glos'ē-ă) Congenital absence of the tongue. [G. *a*- priv. + *glōssa,* tongue]

**a·glos·si·a-a·dac·tyl·i·a syn·drome** (ā-glos'ē-ă ā-dak-til'ē-ă sin'drōm) Congenital absence or hypoplasia of the tongue, associated with absence of the digits.

**a·glos·so·sto·mi·a** (ā'glos-ō-stō'mē-ă) Congenital absence of the tongue, with a malformed (usually closed) mouth. [G. *a*- priv. + *glōssa,* tongue, + *stoma,* mouth]

**ag·na·thi·a** (āg-nāth'ē-ă) Congenital absence of the mandible, usually accompanied by approximation of the ears. [G. *a*- priv. + *gnathos,* jaw]

✿**-agogue, -agog** *Avoid the misspellings -ogog and -ogogue.* Suffixes denoting leading, promoting, stimulating; a promoter or stimulant of something. [G. *agōgos,* leading forth, fr. *agō,* to lead]

**a·gom·phi·ous** (ă-gom′-fē-us) SYN edentulous.

**ag·o·nist** (ag′ŏn-ist) **1.** Denoting a muscle in a state of contraction, with reference to its opposing muscle, or antagonist. **2.** A drug capable of combining with receptors to initiate drug actions; it possesses affinity and intrinsic activity. [G. *agōn,* a contest]

**ag·o·ny** (ag′ŏ-nē) Intense pain or anguish of body or mind. [G. *agōn,* a struggle, trial]

**ag·or·a·pho·bi·a** (ag′ŏr-ă-fō′bē-ă) Mental disorder characterized by irrational fear of leaving the familiar setting of home or venturing into the open. [G. *agora,* marketplace, + *phobos,* fear]

✿**-agra** Suffix denoting sudden onslaught of acute pain. [G. *agra,* a hunting, a catching, a trap]

**a·gran·u·lo·cy·to·sis** (ā′gran′yŭ-lō-sī-tō′sis) An acute potentially lethal condition characterized by pronounced leukopenia with great reduction in the number of polymorphonuclear leukocytes; infected ulcers are likely to develop in the throat, intestinal tract, and other mucous membranes, as well as in the skin; increases patients' risk of infection.

**a·gree·ment** (ă-grē′měnt) The act or result of concurring in a belief, opinion, or plan of action. [O.Fr. *agreer,* fr. L.L. *aggrato,* to make onself pleasing]

**a·gue** (ā′gyū) *Avoid the mispronunciation āg.* **1.** Malarial fever. **2.** A chill. [Fr. *aigu,* acute]

**Ai·car·di syn·drome** (ī-kahr′dē sin′drōm) X-linked dominant disorder lethal in hemizygous males; characterized by agenesis of corpus callosum, chorioretinal abnormality with "holes," cleft lip with or without cleft palate, seizures, and characteristic electroencephalographic changes.

**aid** (ād) **1.** Help; assistance. **2.** A device that helps in the performance of an action. [M.E. *aiden,* fr. O.Fr. *aider,* fr. L. *adjutare,* to help]

**AIDS** (ādz) Acronym for acquired immune deficiency (or immunodeficiency) syndrome; disorder of the immune system characterized by opportunistic diseases, including candidiasis, *Pneumocystis jiroveci* and others. Caused by the human immunodeficiency virus, which is transmitted in body fluids (notably breast milk, blood, and semen) through sexual contact, sharing of contaminated needles (by injecting drug abusers), accidental needle sticks, and contact with contaminated blood.

**AIDS de·men·ti·a com·plex (ADC)** (ādz dĕ-men′shē-ă kom′pleks) Subacute or chronic HIV-1 encephalitis, the most common neurologic complication in the later stages of HIV infection.

**AIDS-re·lat·ed com·plex (ARC)** (ādz-rē-lāt′ĕd kom′pleks) Manifestations of AIDS in patients who have not yet developed major deficient immune function, characterized by fever with generalized lymphadenopathy, diarrhea, weight loss, minor opportunistic infections, and cytopenias.

**air** (ār) **1.** A mixture of odorless gases found in the atmosphere in the following approximate percentages by volume after water vapor has been removed: oxygen, 20.95; nitrogen, 78.08; argon 0.93; carbon dioxide, 0.03; other gases, 0.01. Formerly used to mean any respiratory gas, regardless of its composition. **2.** SYN ventilate. [G. *aēr;* L. *aer*]

**air a·bra·sion** (ār ă-brā′zhŭn) Use of abrasive particles such as aluminum oxide under high pressure to abrade and sometimes remove dentin and enamel. SYN air pointing.

**air a·bra·sive** (ār ă-brā′siv) SYN air-powder polisher.

**air-bone gap** (ār-bōn gap) An abnormal condition in which the auditory threshold for an air-conducted test tone is higher than that for a bone-conducted test tone of the same frequency. SEE ALSO conductive hearing loss.

**air·borne** (ār′bōrn, ār′bōrn) Carried by air. [air, fr. M.E., fr. O.Fr., fr. L., fr. G. *aēr* + borne, pp. fr. bear, fr. O.E. *beren,* fr. O.E. *beran*]

**air·borne con·tam·i·nant** (ār′bōrn kŏntam′i-nănt) An extraneous material (e.g., a chemical or bacterium) carried by air. SEE ALSO contaminant.

**air·borne in·fec·tion** (ār′bōrn in-fek′shŭn) A mechanism of transmission of an infectious agent by particles, dust, or droplet nuclei suspended in the air.

**air·bra·sive** (ār′brā′siv) SYN air-powder polisher.

**air-con·di·tion·er lung** (ār′kŏn-dish′ŭn-ĕr lŭng) Extrinsic allergic alveolitis caused by forced air contaminated by thermophilic actinomycetes and other organisms.

**air con·duc·tion** (ār kŏn-dŭk′shŭn) In relation to hearing, the transmission of sound to the inner ear through the external auditory canal and the structures of the middle ear.

**air em·bo·lism** (ār em′bŏ-lizm) Obstruction that occurs when air enters a blood vessel, usually a vein, as a result of trauma, surgery, or deliberate injection; a large air embolism can cause lethal derangement of cardiac function.

**air hun·ger** (ār hŭng′ĕr) Extremely deep ventilation such as occurs in patients with acidosis attempting to increase ventilation of alveoli and exhale more carbon dioxide. SEE ALSO Kussmaul respiration.

**air point·ing** (ār poynt′ing) SYN air abrasion.

**air pol·ish·ing** (ār pol′ish-ing) SYN air-powder polisher.

**air pow·der pol·ish** (ār pow′dĕr pol′ish) Method of skin removal involving water, powdered sodium bicarbonate, and air. Powder acts abrasively; action varies with grit's coarseness.

**air-pow·der pol·ish·er** (ār-pow′dĕr pol′ish-ĕr) Air-powered device combining air and water pressure to deliver a controlled stream of abrasive through the handpiece nozzle to roughen or polish a tooth surface, depending on coarseness of agent. SYN air abrasive, air polishing, air-powered abrasive, airbrasive.

**air-pow·der pol·ish·ing** (ār pow′dĕr pol′ish-ing) Technique for extrinsic stain removal that uses a mixture of warm water, sodium bicarbonate powder (as an abrasive to remove stains), and air. Action of sodium bicarbonate varies with grit used.

**air-pow·er·ed a·bra·sive** (ār-pow′ĕrd ă-brā′siv) SYN air-powder polisher.

**air·sick·ness** (ār′sik-nĕs) Condition resembling seasickness due to erratic stimulation of the inner ear.

**air·space** (ār′spās) Pertaining to the lung portion distal to the conducting airways or bronchi.

**air sy·ringe** (ār sĭr-inj′) Dental device that supplies a focused stream of compressed air.

**air tip** (ār tip) The tip of an air or air-water syringe used to wash or remove debris from a tooth during dental treatment.

**air-trap·ping** (ār′trap-ing) Slow or incomplete emptying of gas from all or part of a lung on expiration; implies obstruction of regional airways or emphysema.

**air tube** (ār tūb) The trachea, a bronchus, or any of its branches conveying air to the lungs.

**air-turbine hand·piece** (ār-tŭr′bĭn hand′pēs) A dental handpiece that uses air pressure to rotate cutting, grinding, or polishing dental instruments. SEE ALSO handpiece.

**air-wa·ter sy·ringe** (ār-waw′tĕr sĭr-inj′) A dental device that supplies a focused stream of compressed air, water, or a combination of both. Frequently used to clean a tooth or surface during dental treatment. SEE ALSO air syringe.

**air·way** (ār′wā) **1.** Any part of the respiratory tract through which air passes during breathing. **2.** In anesthesia or resuscitation, device to correct obstruction to breathing, especially an oro-pharyngeal and nasopharyngeal airway, endotracheal airway, or tracheotomy tube.

**air·way ob·struc·tion** (ār′wā ŏb-strŭk′shŭn) Respiratory dysfunction that reduces airflow, usually on expiration; can be localized or generalized.

**air·way pat·tern** (ār′wā pat′ĕrn) Chest radiographic appearance of thickened bronchial walls, bronchiectasis, bronchiolitis, or acinar consolidation.

**air·way re·sis·tance** (ār′wā rĕ-zis′tăns) PHYSIOLOGY Impendance to flow of gases during ventilation due to obstruction or turbulent flow in the upper and lower airways; to be differentiated during inhalation from resistance to inflation due to decreases in pulmonary or thoracic compliance.

**akinaesthesia** [Br.] SYN akinesthesia.

**a·ki·ne·si·a, a·ki·ne·sis** (ā′ki-nē′sē-ă, -nē′sis) Absence or loss of the power of voluntary movement, due to an extrapyramidal disorder. [G. *a-* priv. + *kinēsis,* movement]

**a·kin·es·the·si·a** (ā-kin′es-thē′zē-ă) Inability to perceive movement or position. [G. *a-* priv. + *kinēsis,* motion, + *aisthēsis,* sensation]

**a·ki·net·ic mut·ism** (ā′ki-net′ik myū′tizm) Persistent state of intermittently alert altered consciousness, caused by lesions of various cerebral structures.

**Ala** Abbreviation for alanine.

**a·la,** pl. **a·lae** (ā′lă, ā′lē) SYN wing. [L. wing]

**a·la·li·a** (ă-lā′lē-ă) Mutism; inability to speak. SEE aphonia. [G. *a-* priv. + *lalia,* talking]

**a·lal·ic** (ă-lal′ik) Relating to alalia.

**a·la ma·jor os·sis sphe·noi·da·lis** (ā′lă mā′jŏr os′is sfē′noy-dā′lis) [TA] SYN greater wing of sphenoid (bone).

**a·la mi·nor os·sis sphe·noi·da·lis** (ā′lă mī′nŏr os′is sfē-noyd-dā′lis) [TA] SYN lesser wing of sphenoid (bone).

**a·la na·si** (ā′lă nā′sī) [TA] *The plural of this word is alae nasi, not alae nasae.* SYN ala of nose.

**al·a·nine (A, Ala)** (al′ă-nēn) 2-Aminopropionic acid; α-aminopropionic acid; one of the amino acids widely occurring in proteins.

**a·la of cris·ta gal·li** (ā′lă kris′tă gal ī) [TA] Small lateral expansion of the ethmoid bone from anterior aspect of crista galli on each side that articulates with the frontal bone and forms the foramen cecum. SYN alar process.

**a·la of nose** (ā′lă nōz) [TA]The lateral, mobile, more or less flaring, wall of each naris. SYN ala nasi [TA].

**a·la of vo·mer** (ā´lă vō´mĕr) [TA] Everted lips on either side of upper border of the vomer, between which fits the sphenoidal rostrum.

**a·lar** (ā´lăr) Relating to the wings (ala) of such structures as the nose, sphenoid, and sacrum.

**ALARA** (ă-lahr´ă, ă-lar´ă) Acronym for a philosophy of radiation use based on keeping dosages as low as reasonably achievable to attain the desired diagnostic, therapeutic, or other type of goal.

**a·lar ar·te·ry of nose** (ā´lăr ahr´tĕr-ē nōz) Branch of the angular artery that supplies the ala of the nose.

**a·lar part of na·sa·lis mus·cle** (ā´lăr pahrt nā-sā´lis mŭs´ĕl) [TA] SEE nasalis (muscle).

**a·lar pro·cess** (ā´lăr pros´es) SYN ala of crista galli.

**a·lar spine** (ā´lăr spīn) SYN spine of sphenoid bone.

**Al·bers-Schön·berg dis·ease** (ahl´berz-shern´bĕrg di-zēz´) SYN osteopetrosis.

**Al·brecht bone** (ahl´brekt bōn) Small bone between the basioccipital and basisphenoid.

**Al·bright dis·ease** (awl´brīt di-zēz´) SYN McCune-Albright syndrome.

**Al·bright he·red·i·tar·y os·te·o·dys·tro·phy** (awl´brīt hĕr-ed´i-tar-ē os´tē-ō-dis´trŏ-fē) Inherited form of hyperparathyroidism associated with ectopic calcification, ossification, and skeletal defects.

**al·bu·min** (al-bū´min) *Avoid the mispronunciation al′byū-men.* A type of simple protein, varieties of which are widely distributed throughout the tissues and fluids of plants and animals. [L. *albumen* (*-min-*), the white of egg]

**al·bu·mi·nop·ty·sis** (al-bū´mi-nop´ti-sis) Albuminous expectoration. [*albumin* + G. *ptysis,* a spitting]

**al·bu·mi·nu·ria** (al-bū´mi-nyūr´ē-ă) *Avoid substituting this word for the more precise proteinuria.* Presence of protein in urine, chiefly albumin but also globulin; usually indicates disease, but may be due to transient dysfunction. [*albumin* + G. *ouron,* urine]

**al·bu·ter·ol** (al-bū´ter-ol) Sympathomimetic inhalable bronchodilator with relatively selective effects on $\beta_2$ receptors.

**Al·ca·lig·e·nes** (al-kā-lij´en-ēz) A genus of gram-negative, rod-shaped, nonfermenting bacteria that are either motile and peritrichous or nonmotile. Found mostly in the intestinal canal, decaying materials, dairy products, water, and soil; they can be isolated from human respiratory and gastrointestinal tracts and wounds in hospitalized patients with compromised immune systems; occasionally the cause of opportunistic infections, including nosocomial septicemia. Type species is *A. faecalis.* [*alkali* + G. *-gen,* producing]

**al·co·hol** (al´kŏ-hol) Agent made from sugar, starch, and other carbohydrates by fermentation with yeast, and synthetically from ethylene or acetylene; used in beverages and as a solvent, vehicle, and preservative; medicinally, used externally and internally. Known chemically as ethanol. [Ar. *al,* the, + *kohl,* fine antimonial powder, the term being applied first to a fine powder, then to anything impalpable (spirit)]

**al·co·hol am·nes·tic syn·drome** (al´kŏ-hol am-nes´tik sin´drōm) Syndrome of memory loss resulting from alcoholism.

**al·co·hol·ate** (al-kŏ-hol´āt) A tincture or other preparation containing alcohol.

**al·co·hol·ic** (al´kŏ-hol´ik) 1. Relating to, containing, or produced by alcohol. 2. One who abuses alcohol or depends on alcohol ingestion.

**al·co·hol·ic car·di·o·my·op·a·thy** (al-kō-hol´ik kahr´dē-ō-mī-op´ă-thē) Myocardial disease in some patients with long-term alcoholism; may result from alcohol toxicity, or thiamin deficiency, or unknown pathogenesis.

**al·co·hol·ic cir·rho·sis** (al´kŏ-hol´ik sir-ō´sis) Disorder that frequently develops in chronic alcoholism, characterized in an early stage by enlargement of the liver due to fatty change with mild fibrosis, and later by Laënnec cirrhosis with contraction of the liver.

**al·co·hol·ism** (al´kŏ-hol-ism) Chronic alcohol abuse, dependence, or addiction; chronic excessive drinking of alcoholic beverages resulting in impairment of health or of social or occupational functioning, and increasing tolerance requiring increasing doses to achieve and sustain the desired effect. Symptoms of withdrawal may occur on sudden cessation of alcohol intake.

**al·co·hol with·draw·al de·lir·i·um** (al´kŏ-hol with-draw´ăl dĕ-lir´ē-ŭm) Mental state experienced by a person habituated to alcohol consumption that is caused by the abrupt cessation of alcohol intake. Cf. delirium tremens.

**al·de·hyde** (al´dĕ-hīd) A compound containing the radical —CH=O, reducible to an alcohol (—CH₂OH), oxidizable to a carboxylic acid (—COOH); e.g., acetaldehyde.

**al·dos·ter·one** (al-dos´tĕr-ōn) *Avoid the mispronunciation aldoster′one.* Mineralocorticoid hormone produced by the zona glomerulosa of the cortex of the suprarenal gland that facilitates potassium exchange for sodium in the distal renal tubule, causing sodium reabsorption and potassium and hydrogen loss.

**al·dos·ter·one an·tag·o·nist** (al-dos' tĕr-ōn an-tag'ŏ-nist) Agent that opposes action of the adrenal hormone aldosterone on renal tubular mineralocorticoid retention.

**al·dos·ter·on·ism** (al-dos'tĕr-ŏn-izm) A disorder caused by excessive secretion of aldosterone.

**al·do·ste·ron·o·gen·e·sis** (al-dos-tĕr-on' ō-jen'ĕ-sis) Formation of aldosterone. [*aldosterone* + G. *genesis*, production]

**alendronate** (ă-len'drŏ-nāt) A bisphosphonate drug used to treat osteoporosis. [coined term based on parts of the chemical name]

**a·lex·i·a** (ă-lek'sē-ă) Inability to comprehend the meaning of written or printed words and sentences, caused by a cerebral lesion. [G. *a-* priv. + *lexis*, a word or phrase]

**algaesthesia** SYN algesthesia.

♻ **alge-, algesi-, algio-, algo-** Combining forms denoting pain; corresponds to L. dolor-. [G. *algos*, a pain]

**al·ge·sic** (al-jē'zik) **1.** Painful; related to or causing pain. **2.** Relating to hypersensitivity to pain. SYN algetic.

**al·ge·si·chro·nom·e·ter** (al-jē'zē-krō-nom' ĕ-ter) An instrument for recording the time required to perceive a painful stimulus. [G. *algēsis*, sense of pain, + *chronos*, time, + *metron*, measure]

**al·ge·si·me·try, al·ge·siometry** (al'jē-sim'ĕ-trē) Use of an algesiometer to measure the degree of sensitivity to a painful stimulus. [G. *algēsis*, pain, + *metron*, measure]

**al·ge·si·o·gen·ic** (al'jē'zē-ō-jen'ik) Pain-producing. SYN algogenic. [G. *algēsis*, sense of pain, + *-gen*, production]

**al·ge·si·om·e·ter** (al'jē-zē-om'ĕ-tĕr) An instrument for measuring the degree of sensitivity to a painful stimulus. [G. *algēsis*, sense of pain, + *metron*, measure]

**al·ges·the·sia** (al'jes-thē'zē-ă) **1.** The appreciation of pain. **2.** Hypersensitivity to pain. SYN algesia, algesthesis, algaesthesia. [G. *algos*, pain, + *aisthēsis*, sensation]

**al·get·ic** (al-jet'ik) SYN algesic.

♻ **-algia** Suffix denoting pain, painful condition. [G. *algos*, a pain]

**al·gid** (al'jid) Chilly, cold. [L. *algidus*, cold]

**al·gin** (al'jin) A carbohydrate product of a seaweed, *Macrocystis pyrifera;* used as a gel in pharmaceutical preparations.

▣ **al·gi·nate** (al'ji-nāt) Elastic dental impression material composed of potassium alginate from kelp, calcium sulfate, and other ingredients; usually a powder to mix with water. Setting re-

action cross-links alginic acid to form a semi-solid. See this page.

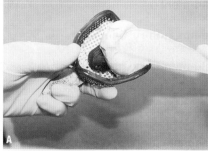

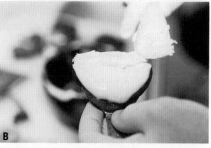

**loading maxillary tray with alginate impression material:** (A) posterior aspect; (B) anterior aspect

**al·go·gen·e·sis, al·go·ge·ne·si·a** (al-gō-jen'ĕ-sis, -jĕ-nē'zē-ă) The production or origin of pain. [*algo-* + G. *genesis*, origin]

**al·go·gen·ic** (al-gō-jen'ik) SYN algesiogenic.

**al·gol·o·gy** (al-gō'lŏ-jē) **1.** The study of pain. **2.** The scientific study of algae. [G. *algos*, pain, + *-logy*]

**al·gom·e·try** (al-gom'ĕ-trē) The process of measuring pain.

**al·go·pho·bi·a** (al'gō-fō'bē-ă) Abnormal fear of pain. [*algo-* + G. *phobos*, fear]

**al·go·rithm** (al'gŏr-idhm) A systematic process consisting of an ordered sequence of steps, each step depending on the outcome of the previous one. [Mediev. L. *algorismus*, after Muhammad ibn-Musa *al-Khwarizmi*, Persian mathematician, + G. *arithmos*, number]

**al·go·spasm** (al'gō-spazm) Spasm produced by pain. [G. *algos*, pain, + *spasmos*, convulsion]

**al·i·form** (al'i-fōrm) Wing-shaped. [L. *ala*, + *forma*, shape]

**a·lign·ment** (ă-līn'mĕnt) In dentistry, the arrangement of the teeth in relation to the supporting structures and the adjacent and opposing dentitions. [Fr. *aligner*, to line up, fr. L. *linea*, line]

**a·lign·ment curve** (ă-līn'mĕnt kŭrv) Line

passing through the center of the teeth laterally in the direction of the curve of the dental arch.

**al·i·ment** (al'i-mĕnt) SYN nourishment. [L. *alo*, to nourish]

**al·i·men·ta·ry ca·nal** (al'i-men'tăr-ē kă-nal') SYN digestive tract.

**al·i·men·ta·ry gly·co·su·ria** (al'i-men' tăr-ē glī-kō-syūr'ē-ă) Glycosuria developing after ingestion of a moderate amount of sugar or starch because the rate of intestinal absorption exceeds the capacity of the liver and the other tissues to remove the glucose.

**al·i·men·ta·ry hy·per·in·su·lin·ism** (al'i-men'tăr-ē hī'pĕr-in'sŭ-lin-izm) Elevated levels of insulin in the plasma after ingestion of meals by people with abnormally rapid gastric emptying.

**al·i·men·ta·ry li·pe·mi·a** (al'i-men'tăr-ē li-pē'mē-ă) Transient lipemia occurring after ingestion of foods with a high fat content.

**al·i·men·ta·ry os·te·op·a·thy** (al'i-men' tăr-ē os'tē-op'ă-thē) Bone disease resulting from dietary deficiency.

**al·i·men·ta·ry pen·to·su·ria** (al'i-men' tăr-ē pen-tō-syūr'ē-ă) Urinary excretion of L-arabinose and L-xylose, as result of excessive ingestion of fruits containing these pentoses.

**al·i·men·ta·ry sys·tem** (al-i-men'tăr-ē sis' tĕm) [TA] Digestive tract from the mouth to the anus with all its associated glands and organs.

**al·i·men·ta·ry tract** (al'i-men'tăr-ē trakt) SYN digestive tract.

**al·i·men·ta·ry tract smear** (al'i-men'tăr-ē trakt smēr) Cytologic specimens containing material from the mouth (oral smear), esophagus and stomach (gastric smear), duodenum (paraduodenal smear), and colon, obtained by specialized lavage techniques.

**al·i·na·sal** (al'i-nā'zăl) Relating to the wings of the nose (alae nasi), or flaring portions of the nostrils. [L. *ala*, + *nasus*, nose]

**a·lip·o·tro·pic** (ā'lip-ō-trōp'ik) Having no effect on fat metabolism or movement of fat to the liver. [G. *a-* priv. + *lipos*, fat, + *tropos*, a turning]

**al·i·sphe·noid** (al'i-sfē'noyd) Relating to the greater wing of the sphenoid bone. [L. *ala*, + *sphēn*, wedge]

**al·ka·li**, pl. **al·ka·lies**, pl. **al·ka·lis** (al'kă-lī, -līz) **1.** A strongly basic substance yielding hydroxide ions (OH⁻) in solution; e.g., sodium hydroxide, potassium hydroxide. **2.** SYN base (3). **3.** SYN alkali metal. [Ar., *al*, the, + *qalīy*, soda ash]

**al·ka·li met·al** (al'kă-lī met'ăl) An alkali of the families Li, Na, K, Rb, Cs, and Fr, all of which have highly ionized hydroxides. SYN alkali (3).

**al·ka·line** (al'kă-lin) Relating to or having the reaction of an alkali.

**al·ka·line-ash di·et** (al'kă-lin-ash dī'ĕt) Diet consisting mainly of fruits, vegetables, and milk (with minimal amounts of meat, fish, eggs, cheese, and cereals), which, when catabolized, produces alkaline residue excreted in urine. SYN acid-ash diet.

**al·ka·line phos·pha·tase** (al'kă-lin fos' fă-tās) A phosphatase with an optimal pH of above 7.0 present in many tissues; low levels of this enzyme are seen in cases of hypophosphatasia.

**al·ka·line re·flux gas·tri·tis** (al'kă-lin rē'fluks gas-trī'tis) Inflammation of gastric mucosa believed to be caused by irritating factors that reflux from the intestine into the stomach.

**al·ka·line wa·ter** (al'kă-lin waw'tĕr) Water that contains appreciable amounts of the bicarbonates of calcium, lithium, potassium, or sodium.

**al·ka·li re·serve** (al'kă-lī rē-zĕrv') The sum total of the basic ions (mainly bicarbonates) of the blood and other body fluids that, acting as buffers, maintain the normal pH of the blood.

**al·ka·li·ther·a·py** (al'kă-lī-thār'ă-pē) Therapeutic use of a basic substance for local or systemic effect.

**al·ka·liz·er** (al'kă-līz-ĕr) Agent that neutralizes acids or renders a solution alkaline.

**al·ka·loid** (al'kă-loyd) Heterocyclic nitrogenous and often complex structures possessing pharmacologic activity; synthesized by plants and are found in the leaf, bark, seed, or other parts, usually constituting the active principle of the crude drug; they comprise a loosely defined group.

**al·ka·lo·sis** (al-kă-lō'sis) *Do not confuse this word with ankylosis.* A state characterized by a decrease in the hydrogen ion concentration of arterial blood below the normal level, 40 nmol/L, or pH over 7.4.

**al·lele** (ă-lēl') Any one of a series of two or more different genes that may occupy the same locus on a specific chromosome. [G. *allēlōn*, reciprocally]

**al·ler·gen** (al'ĕr-jĕn) Antigen that induces an allergic or hypersensitive response. [*allergy* + G. *-gen*, producing]

**al·ler·gen im·mu·no·ther·a·py** (al'ĕr-jen im'yū-nō-thār'ă-pē) Process of administering allergenic extracts to patients who suffer from allergic rhinoconjunctivitis and allergic asthma to decrease the degree of hypersensitivity and symptoms by reducing immunologic responses to environmental allergens like pollen, dust, animal dander, and molds.

**al·ler·gic** (ă-lĕr′jik) Relating to any response stimulated by an allergen.

**al·ler·gic bron·cho·pul·mo·na·ry as·per·gil·lo·sis** (ă-lĕr′jik brong′kō-pul′mŏ-nar-ē as′pĕr-ji-lō′sis) Disease in which the fungus grows in mucus.

**al·ler·gic con·junc·ti·vi·tis** (ă-lĕr′jik kŏn-jŭngk′ti-vī′tis) Immunologic conjunctival reaction mediated by immunoglobulin E; associated with itching, redness, and tearing.

**al·ler·gic con·tact der·ma·ti·tis** (ă-lĕr′jik kon′takt dĕr′mă-tī′tis) Delayed type IV allergic reaction of the skin with varying degrees of erythema, edema, and vesiculation resulting from cutaneous contact with a specific allergen.

**al·ler·gic pur·pu·ra** (ă-lĕr′jik pŭr′pyŭr-ă) Nonthrombocytopenic purpura due to hypersensitivity to foods, drugs, and insect bites. SYN anaphylactoid purpura (1).

**al·ler·gic re·ac·tion** (ă-lĕr′jik rē-ak′shŭn) Local or general reaction of an organism after contact with a specific allergen to which it has been previously exposed and sensitized. SYN hypersensitivity reaction.

**al·ler·gic rhi·ni·tis** (ă-lĕr′jik rī-nī′tis) Rhinitis associated with hay fever; manifest by sneezing, rhinorrhea, nasal congestion, pruritus of the nose, ears, palate; may also occur concurrently with allergic conjunctivitis.

**al·ler·gic sto·ma·ti·tis** (ă-lĕr′jik stō′mă-tī′tis) A type I hypersensitivity reaction to a systemically administered drug or to a food. Oral manifestations vary and may resemble erythema multiforme, lichen planus, or lupus erythematosus, with a dry shiny red patch and sometimes white patches as well. Painful condition often involves buccal and labial mucosa and gingiva, but may affect the complete oral cavity.

**al·ler·gized** (al′er-jīzd) State of being specifically altered in reactivity; rendered capable of exhibiting one or another aspect of allergy.

**al·ler·gy** (al′ĕr-jē) 1. Hypersensitivity caused by exposure to a particular antigen (allergen) resulting in a marked increase in reactivity to that antigen on subsequent exposure, sometimes resulting in harmful immunologic consequences. 2. An acquired hypersensitivity to certain drugs and biologic materials. SEE ALSO allergic reaction, anaphylaxis. SYN acquired sensitivity. [G. allos, other, + ergon, work]

**al·lied health pro·fes·sion·al** (al′īd helth prŏ-fesh′ŭn-ăl) Someone trained to perform services in the care of patients other than a physician or registered nurse; includes therapy technicians (e.g., pulmonary), dental technicians, and physical therapists.

**al·lo·chi·ri·a, al·lo·chei·ri·a** (al′ō-kī′rē-ă) A form of allachesthesia in which the sensation of a stimulus in one limb is referred to the contralateral limb. [allo- + G. cheir, hand]

**al·lo·dyn·ia** (al′ō-din′ē-ă) Pain due to stimulus that does not normally elicit any (e.g., response to percussion of tooth with pulpitis). [allo- + G. odynē, pain]

**al·lo·gen·ic, al·lo·ge·ne·ic** (al-ō-jen′ik, -jĕ-nē′ik) As used in transplantation biology, it pertains to different gene constitutions within the same species; antigenically distinct.

**al·lo·graft** (al′ō-graft, al′ō-graft) A graft transplanted between genetically nonidentical individuals of the same species. SYN homograft, homologous graft, homoplastic graft. [G. allos, other, + graft, fr. M.E., fr. O.Fr. graffe, stylus, scion, fr. L. graphium, fr. G. graphō, to write]

**al·lo·im·mune** (al′ō-im-yūn′) Immune to an allogenic antigen. [allo- + immune]

**al·lo·la·lia** (al′ō-lā′lē-ă) Any speech defect, especially one caused by a cerebral disorder. [allo- + G. lalia, talking]

**al·loph·a·sis** (al-of′ă-sis) Speech that is incoherent, disordered. [allo- + G. phasis, speech]

**al·lo·plast** (al′ō-plast) 1. A graft of an inert metal or plastic material. 2. A relatively inert foreign body used for implantation into tissues. [allo- + G. plastos, formed]

**al·lo·plas·ty** (al′ō-plas-tē) Repair of defects by allotransplantation.

**al·lo·pu·ri·nol** (al′ō-pū′ri-nol) Inhibitor of xanthine oxidase to inhibit uric acid formation; used treat gout and retard rapid metabolic degradation of 6-mercaptopurine.

**al·lot·ri·o·don·ti·a** (al-ot′rē-ō-don′shē-ă) 1. Growth of a tooth in some abnormal location. 2. Transplantation of teeth. [G. allotrios, foreign, + odous (odont-), tooth]

**al·lot·ri·os·mi·a** (al-ot-rē-oz′mē-ă) Incorrect or inaccurate recognition of odors. [G. allotrios, foreign, + osmē, smell]

**al·lo·tro·phic** (al′o-trō′fik) Having an altered nutritive value. [allo- + G. trophē, nourishment]

**al·lox·an (AX)** (ă-loks′an) An oxidation product of uric acid.

**al·loy** (al′oy) A combination of metals formed when they are miscible in the liquid state.

**al·lyl al·co·hol** (al′il al′kŏ-hol) A colorless liquid of pungent odor used in making resins and plasticizers; highly irritating to mucous membranes and readily absorbed.

**al·ma gauge** (ăl′mă gāj) Mechanical device

used to provide accurate measurement in the reconstruction of existing dentures by determining the position of teeth within the arch and the precise width of the arch itself.

**al·oe** (al′ō) The dried juice from the leaves of plants of the genus *Aloe* (family Liliaceae), from which are derived aloin, resin, emodin, and volatile oils.

**al·o·pe·ci·a** (al-ō-pē′shē-ă) Absence or loss of hair. [G. *alōpekia,* a disease resembling fox mange, fr. *alōpēx,* a fox]

**al·pha am·y·lase** (al′fă am′i-lās) A starch-splitting enzyme obtained from a nonpathogenic bacterium of the *Bacillus subtilis* class; used to treat inflammatory conditions and edema of soft tissues associated with traumatic injury.

**al·pha-hem·i·hy·drate** (al′fă-hem′ē-hī′drāt) The porous and irregular crystal form of $CaSO_4$ · ½ $H_2O$, commonly known as dental plaster or type II gypsum product. [*hemi-,* half, + hydrate]

**al·pha par·ti·cle** (al′fă pahr′ti-kĕl) A particle consisting of two neutrons and two protons, with a positive charge; emitted energetically from the nuclei of unstable isotopes of mass number 82 and up. SYN alpha ray.

**al·pha ray** (al′fă rā) SYN alpha particle.

**al·pra·zo·lam** (al-prā′zō-lam) A benzodiazepine used to manage anxiety disorders and panic attack; tolerance, habituation, or dependency may result from increased dosage.

**al·pros·ta·dil** (al-pros′tă-dil) A vasodilator used for palliative therapy to maintain patency of the ductus arteriosus in neonates with congenital heart defects temporarily. SYN prostaglandin $E_1$.

**ALS** Abbreviation for amyotrophic lateral sclerosis.

**ALT:AST ra·ti·o** (rā′shē-ō) Ratio of serum alanine aminotransferase to serum aspartate aminotransferase; elevated serum levels of both enzymes characterize hepatic disease.

**al·ter·ed cast** (awl′tĕrd kast) Model of dental structures that are modified before fabrication of the final prosthesis. SYN corrected cast.

**al·ter·nate hem·i·an·es·the·sia** (awl′tĕr-năt hem′ē-an′es-thē′zē-ă) Hemianesthesia affecting the head on one side and the body and extremities on the other side.

**al·ter·nat·ing cur·rent (AC, a.c.)** (awl′tĕr-nāt-ing kŭr′rĕnt) Electric current that reverses direction (positive-negative polarity) many times each second (with each rotation of the armature of the dynamo generating the current).

**al·ter·nat·ing hem·i·ple·gi·a** (awl′tĕr-năt-ing hem′ē-plē′jē-ă) Unilateral cranial nerve paresis caused by lesion of brainstem with contralateral cranial nerve palsies.

**al·um** (al′ŭm) Agent used locally as a styptic. [L. *alumen*]

**a·lu·mi·na** (ă-lū′mi-nă) One of the strongest white ceramic materials used in dental practice; an abrasive employed to strengthen porcelain or as a substructure for all ceramic crowns and bridges. [L. *alumen,* alum]

**a·lu·mi·nat·ed** (ă-lū′mi-nā-tĕd) Containing alum.

**a·lu·mi·num** (ă-lū′min-ŭm) Light, white, silvery metal widely used in dentistry and other branches of health care. [L. *alumen,* alum]

**a·lu·mi·num as·pi·rin** (ă-lū′mi-nŭm as′pĭr-in) Analgesic and antipyretic. SYN aluminum acetylsalicylate.

**a·lu·mi·num hy·drox·ide** (ă-lū′mi-nŭm hī-drok′sīd) Astringent dusting powder; also used internally as a mild astringent antacid.

**a·lu·mi·num hy·drox·ide gel** (ă-lū′mi-nŭm hī-drok′sīd jel) Suspension containing aluminum hydroxide, used as an antacid.

**a·lu·mi·num pen·i·cil·lin** (ă-lū′mi-nŭm pen′i-sil′in) Trivalent aluminum salt of an antibiotic substance or substances produced by the growth of the molds *Penicillium notatum* or *P. chrysogenum;* used in oral or sublingual administration.

**a·lu·mi·num phe·nol·sul·fo·nate** (ă-lū′mi-nŭm fē-nol-sŭl′fŏ-nāt) Antiseptic and astringent for local application, usually for cutaneous ulcers.

**a·lu·mi·num phos·phate** (ă-lū′mi-nŭm fos′fāt) Infusible powder used for dental cements with calcium sulfate and sodium silicate.

**a·lu·mi·num sub·ac·e·tate** (ă-lū′mi-nŭm sŭb-as′ē-tāt) Compound of aluminum used in solution as an astringent and as an ingredient in mouthwashes.

**al·ve·o·al·gi·a** (al-vē′ō-al′jē-ă) A postoperative complication of tooth extraction in which the blood clot in the socket disintegrates, resulting in focal osteomyelitis and severe pain. SYN alveolalgia, alveolar osteitis, dry socket. [*alveolus* + G. *algos,* pain]

**al·ve·o·lal·gia** (al-vē′ō-lal′jē-ă) SYN alveoalgia.

**al·ve·o·lar** (al-vē′ŏ-lăr) Relating to an alveolus.

▪**al·ve·o·lar ab·scess** (al-vē'ŏ-lăr ab'ses) Abscess situated within the alveolar process of the jaws, most often caused by extension of infection from an adjacent nonvital tooth. See this page. SYN dental abscess, dentoalveolar abscess, root abscess.

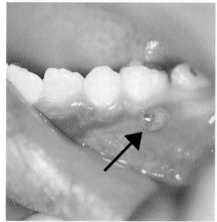

**alveolar abscess:** this 8-year-old girl had fever, dental pain, and a "bump" for 2 days; bump is localized gingival swelling caused by an alveolar abscess

**al·ve·o·lar an·gle** (al-vē'ŏ-lăr ang'gĕl) Angle between the horizontal plane and a line connecting the base of the nasal spine and the middle point of the projection of the alveolus of the maxilla.

**al·ve·o·lar arch of man·di·ble** (al-vē'ŏ-lăr ahrch man'di-bĕl) [TA] Free margin of alveolar process of mandible from which mandibular teeth emerge.

**al·ve·o·lar arch of max·il·la** [TA] Free border of alveolar process of maxilla from which maxillary teeth emerge.

**al·ve·o·lar at·ro·phy** (al-vē'ŏ-lăr at'rŏ-fē) Loss or diminution of supportive alveolar bone due to loss of teeth or to function, trauma, reduced blood supply, or unknown cause.

**al·ve·o·lar body** (al-vē'ŏ-lăr bod'ē) SYN alveolar process of maxilla.

**al·ve·o·lar bone** (al-vē'ŏ-lăr bōn) **1.** In dentistry, specialized bony structure that supports teeth; consists of cortical bone that comprises the tooth socket into which roots of tooth fit; supported by trabecular bone. SYN alveolar supporting bone. **2.** SYN alveolar process of maxilla.

**al·ve·o·lar bone loss** (al-vē'ŏ-lăr bōn laws) Resorption of bone that surrounds and supports teeth.

**al·ve·o·lar bor·der** (al-vē'ŏ-lăr bōr'dĕr)

**1.** Most occlusal edge of alveolar bone. **2.** SYN alveolar process of maxilla.

**al·ve·o·lar ca·nals of max·il·la** (al-vē'ŏ-lăr kă-nalz' mak-sil'ă) [TA] Canals in body of maxilla that transmit nerves and vessels from the alveolar foramina to maxillary teeth. SYN alveolodental canals, dental canals.

**al·ve·o·lar crest** (al-vē'ŏ-lăr krest) **1.** Portion of alveolar bone (i.e., coronal portion) extending beyond periphery of socket, lying interproximally. **2.** Top of residual alveolar bone.

**al·ve·o·lar for·a·mi·na of max·il·la** (al-vē'ŏ-lăr fōr-am'i-nă mak-sil'ă) [TA] Openings of posterior dental canals on infratemporal surface of maxilla.

**al·ve·o·lar gin·gi·va** (al-vē'ŏ-lăr jin'ji-vă) Gingival tissue applied to the alveolar bone.

**al·ve·o·lar in·dex** (al-vē'ŏ-lăr in'deks) **1.** SYN gnathic index. **2.** SYN basilar index.

**al·ve·o·lar mac·ro·phage** (al-vē'ŏ-lăr mak'rō-fāj) A vigorously phagocytic macrophage on the epithelial surface of lung alveoli where it ingests inhaled particulate matter. SYN coniophage, dust cell.

**al·ve·o·lar mu·co·sa** (al-vē'ŏ-lăr myū-kō'să) Mucous membrane apical to attached gingiva.

**al·ve·o·lar os·te·i·tis** (al-vē'ŏ-lăr os'tē-ī'tis) SYN alveolalgia.

**al·ve·o·lar part of man·di·ble** (al-vē'ŏ-lăr pahrt man'di-bĕl) [TA] Portion of body of mandible that surrounds and supports lower teeth.

**al·ve·o·lar per·i·os·te·um** (al-vē'ŏ-lăr per'ē-os'tē-ŭm) SYN periodontium.

**al·ve·o·lar point** (al-vē'ŏ-lăr poynt) SYN prosthion.

**al·ve·o·lar pro·cess** (al-vē'ŏ-lăr pros'es) That portion of bone in either maxilla or mandible that surrounds and supports teeth.

**al·ve·o·lar pro·cess of max·il·la** (al-vē'ŏ-lăr pro'ses mak-sil'ă) [TA] Projecting ridge on inferior surface of body of maxilla that contains the tooth sockets; also denotes superior aspect of body of mandible, containing tooth sockets of the lower jaw. SYN alveolar body, alveolar bone (2), alveolar border (2), alveolar ridge, basal ridge (1), dental process.

**al·ve·o·lar ridge** (al-vē'ŏ-lăr rij) SYN alveolar process of maxilla.

**al·ve·o·lar sep·tum** (al-vē'ŏ-lăr sep'tŭm) SYN interalveolar septum.

**al·ve·o·lar sup·port·ing bone** (al-vē'ŏ-lăr sŭ-pōrt'ing bōn) SYN alveolar bone (1).

**al·ve·o·lar yokes** (al-vē'ŏ-lăr yōks) [TA]

One of the eminences on the outer surface of the alveolar process of maxilla or mandible, formed by roots of incisor teeth.

**al·ve·o·late** (al-vē′ō-lāt) Pitted like a honeycomb.

**al·ve·o·lec·to·my** (al′vē-ō-lek′tŏ-mē) Surgical excision of a portion of dentoalveolar process, for recontouring of alveolar ridge during tooth removal. [*alveolus* + G. *ektomē*, excision]

**al·ve·o·lin·gual** (al′vē-ō-ling′gwăl) SYN alveololingual.

**al·ve·o·li·tis** (al′vē-ō-lī′tis) Inflammation of a tooth socket.

♻ **alveolo-** Combining form denoting an alveolus, the alveolar process; alveolar. [L. *alveolus*, a concave vessel, a bowl, a basin, fr. *alveus*, a trough, + *-olus*, small, little; akin to *alvus*, the belly, the womb]

**al·ve·o·lo·buc·cal groove** (al-vē′ŏ-lō-bŭk′ăl grūv) Upper and lower portions of buccal vestibule on each side; portions between cheek and superior and inferior bursal gingivae, excluding portion of vestibule between cheek and teeth. SYN alveolobuccal sulcus, gingivobuccal groove, gingivobuccal sulcus.

**al·ve·o·lo·buc·cal sul·cus** (al-vē′ŏ-lō-bŭk′ĕl sŭl′kŭs) SYN alveolobuccal groove.

**al·ve·o·lo·den·tal** (al-vē′ŏ-lō-den′tăl) Relating to the alveoli and the teeth.

**al·ve·o·lo·den·tal ca·nals** (al-vē′ŏ-lō-den′tăl kă-nalz′) SYN alveolar canals of maxilla.

**al·ve·o·lo·den·tal lig·a·ment** (al-vē′ŏ-lō-den′tăl lig′ă-mĕnt) SYN periodontal ligament.

**al·ve·o·lo·den·tal mem·brane** (al-vē′ŏ-lō-den′tăl mem′brān) SYN periodontium.

**al·ve·o·lo·gin·gi·val fi·ber group** (al-vē′ŏ-lō-jin′ji-văl fī′bĕr grūp) Type I collagen fibers collected into fiber bundles within the subepithelial connective tissue of the gingiva; they extend from the crest of the alveolus to insert into the connective tissue of the free and attached gingiva.

**al·ve·o·lo·la·bi·al** (al-vē′ŏ-lō-lā′bē-ăl) Relating to the labial or vestibular surface of the alveolar processes of the upper or lower jaw.

**al·ve·o·lo·la·bi·al groove** (al-vē′ŏ-lō-lā′bē-ăl grūv) Indentation between maxillary and mandibular halves of labial vestibule. SYN alveololabial sulcus, gingivolabial groove, gingivolabial sulcus.

**al·ve·o·lo·la·bi·a·lis** (al-vē′ŏ-lō-lā′bē-ā′lis) Relating to the alveololabial groove or region.

**al·ve·o·lo·la·bi·al sul·cus** (al-vē′ŏ-lō-lā′bē-ăl sŭl′kŭs) SYN alveololabial groove.

**al·ve·o·lo·lin·gual** (al-vē′ŏ-lō-ling′gwăl) Re-

lating to the lingual (inner) surface of the alveolar process of the lower jaw. SYN alveolingual.

**al·ve·o·lo·lin·gual groove** (al-vē′ŏ-lō-ling′gwăl grūv) Part of the oral cavity proper, on each side of the frenulum of the tongue, between the tongue and the mandibular alveolar process or ridge. SYN alveololingual sulcus, gingivolingual groove, gingivolingual sulcus.

**al·ve·o·lo·lin·gual sul·cus** (al-vē′ŏ-lō-ling′gwăl sŭl′kŭs) SYN alveololingual groove.

**al·ve·o·lo·na·sal line** (al-vē′ŏ-lō-nā′zăl līn) Line connecting alveolar point and nasion.

**al·ve·o·lo·pal·a·tal** (al-vē′ŏ-lō-pal′ă-tăl) Relating to the palatal surface of the alveolar process of the upper jaw.

**al·ve·o·lo·plas·ty** (al-vē′ŏ-lō-plas-tē) Surgical preparation of the alveolar ridges for the reception of dentures; shaping and smoothing of socket margins after extraction of teeth with subsequent suturing to ensure optimal healing. SYN alveoplasty. [*alveolo-* + G. *plassō*, to form]

**al·ve·o·los·chi·sis** (al′vē-ō-los′ki-sis) A cleft of the alveolar process. [*alveolo-* + G. *schisis*, cleaving]

**al·ve·o·lot·o·my** (al′vē-ō-lot′ŏ-mē) Surgical opening into a dental alveolus to allow drainage of pus from a periapical or other intraosseous abscess. [*alveolo-* + G. *tomē*, incision]

**al·ve·o·lus** (al-vē′ō-lŭs, -lī) [TA] **1.** SYN tooth socket. **2.** A small cell, cavity, or socket. [L. dim. of *alveus*, trough, hollow sac, cavity]

**al·ve·o·lus den·ta·lis,** pl. **al·ve·o·li den·ta·les** (al-vē′ō-lŭs den-tā′lis, al-vē′ō-lī den-tā′lēz) [TA] SYN tooth socket.

**al·ve·o·plas·ty** (al-vē′ŏ-plas′tē) SYN alveoloplasty.

**al·ve·us,** pl. **al·ve·i** (al′vē-ŭs, -ī) A channel or trough. [L. tray, trough, cavity, fr. *alvus*, belly]

**a·lym·phi·a** (ă-lim′fē-ă) Absence or deficiency of lymph. [G. *a-* priv + lymph +-ia]

**Alz·hei·mer dis·ease, Alz·heim·er de·men·tia (AD)** (awlts′hī-mĕr di-zēz′, dĕmen′shē-ă) Progressive degenerative disease of the brain that causes impairment of memory and dementia manifested by confusion, visual-spatial disorientation, and other conditions.

**am** Abbreviation for ammeter.

**a·mal·gam** (ă-mal′găm) An alloy of an element or a metal with mercury. In dentistry, primarily of two types: silver-tin alloy, containing small amounts of copper, zinc, and perhaps other metal, and a second type containing more copper (12–30% by weight); amalgams are used in restoring teeth and making dies. See this page. SYN amalgam alloy, dental amalgam alloy. [G. *malagma,* a soft mass]

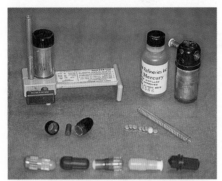

**forms of amalgam alloy:** (top row, left to right) alloy pellet and mercury dispenser, bulk mercury, mercury dispenser; (center row) reusable capsule and amalgam alloy pellets; (bottom row) preencapsulated amalgam products

**a·mal·gam al·loy** (ă-mal´găm al´oy) SYN amalgam.

**a·mal·ga·mate** (ă-mal´gă-māt) To make an amalgam.

**a·mal·ga·ma·tion** (ă-mal´gă-mā´shŭn) Process of combining mercury with a metal or alloy to form a new alloy.

**a·mal·ga·ma·tor** (ă-mal´gă-mā-tŏr) A device for combining mercury with a metal or an alloy to form a new alloy.

**a·mal·gam car·ri·er** (ă-mal´găm kar´ē-ĕr) Tool used to transport triturated amalgam to a cavity preparation and to deposit it therein.

**a·mal·gam con·den·ser** (ă-mal´găm kŏn-den´sĕr) Instrument used to impress unset amalgam into a cavity preparation of a tooth. SYN amalgam plugger.

**a·mal·gam core** (ă-mal´găm kōr) Restoration intended to replace lost tooth structure under a crown and to provide support and retention for the crown.

**a·mal·gam ma·trix** (ă-mal´găm mā´triks) Tool used during placement of amalgam mass within a compound cavity preparation, facilitating proper condensation and contour of the mass by providing a confining wall.

**a·mal·gam pig·men·ta·tion** (ă-mal´găm pig´mĕn-tā´shŭn) SYN amalgam tattoo.

**a·mal·gam plug·ger** (ă-mal´găm plŭg´ĕr) SYN amalgam condenser.

**a·mal·gam res·to·ra·tion** (ă-mal´găm res´tŏr-ā´shŭn) A dental restoration made of an alloy of an element or metal with mercury. SEE amalgam, restoration. SYN silver filling.

**a·mal·gam strip** (ă-mal´găm strip) Linen strip without abrasive used to smooth proximal contours of newly placed amalgam restorations.

▣**a·mal·gam tat·too** (ă-mal´găm ta-tū´) Dark macular lesion of oral mucous membrane caused by accidental implantation of silver amalgam into the tissue during tooth restoration or extraction. See this page. SYN focal argyrosis.

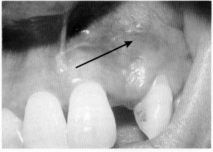

**amalgam tattoo caused by retrograde amalgam**

**a·man·ta·dine hy·dro·chlor·ide** (ă-man´tă-dēn hī´drŏ-klōr´īd) An antiviral agent used to treat influenza; also used to treat parkinsonism.

**am·ba·geu·si·a** (am´bă-gū´sē-ă) Loss of taste on both sides of the tongue. [L. *ambo,* both, + G. *a-* priv. + *geusis,* taste]

**Am·berg lat·er·al si·nus line** (am´bĕrg lat´ĕr-ăl sī´nŭs līn) Line dividing the angle formed by the anterior edge of the mastoid process and the temporal line.

♦**ambi-** *Do not confuse this prefix with the combining form ambly-.* Prefix meaning around; on all (both) sides; both, double; corresponds to G. *amphi-.* SEE ALSO ambo-. [L., around, about, akin to *ambo,* both]

**am·bi·lat·er·al** (am´bi-lat´ĕr-ăl) Relating to both sides. [*ambi-* + L. *latus,* side]

♦**ambly-** *Do not confuse this combining form with the prefix ambi-.* Combining form denoting dullness, dimness; blunt, dull, dim, dimmed. [G. *amblys,* blunt, dulled; faint, dim]

**am·bly·ge·us·ti·a** (am´blē-gū´stē-ă) Diminution in sense of taste. [*ambly-* + G. *geusis,* taste]

♦**ambo-** Prefix meaning around; on all (both) sides; corresponds to G. ampho-. SEE ALSO ambi-. [L. *ambo,* both]

**am·bu·la·to·ry care** (am´byū-lă-tōr-ē kār) Treatment provided during an episode of care that does not require an overnight stay in a medical facility and from which the patient goes home.

**am·bu·la·to·ry sur·gery** (am'byū-lă-tōr-ē sŭr'jĕr-ē) Operative procedures performed on patients admitted to and discharged from a hospital the same day.

**a·me·ba,** pl. **a·me·bae,** pl. **a·me·bas** (ă-mē'bă, -bē, -băz) Common name for *Amoeba* and similar naked, lobose, sarcodine protozoa. SYN amoeba.

**a·me·bi·cide** (ă-mē'bi-sīd) Any agent that causes the destruction of amebae. [*ameba* + L. *caedo*, to kill]

**a·me·li·a** (ă-mē'lē-ă) Congenital absence of a limb or limbs. [G. *a-* priv. + *melos*, a limb]

**am·e·lo·blast** (am'ĕl'ō-blast) One of the columnar epithelial cells of the inner layer of the enamel organ of a developing tooth, involved with the formation of enamel matrix. SYN enamel cell, enameloblast. [Early E. *amel*, enamel, + G. *blastos*, germ]

**am·e·lo·blas·tic ad·e·no·ma·toid tu·mor** (am'el'ō-blas'tik ad'ĕ-nō'mă-toyd tū'mŏr) SYN adenomatoid odontogenic tumor.

🔲**am·e·lo·blas·tic fi·bro·ma** (am´ĕ-lō-blas´tik fī-brō´mă) Benign mixed odontogenic tumor characterized by neoplastic proliferation of both epithelial and mesenchymal components of the tooth bud without the production of dental hard tissue; presents clinically as a slow-growing painless radiolucency occurring most commonly in the mandibles of children and adolescents. See page A16.

**am·e·lo·blas·tic fi·bro·sar·co·ma** (am´ĕ-lō-blas´tik fī´brō-sahr-kō´mă) Fast-growing, painful, destructive, radiolucent odontogenic tumor that usually arises through malignant change in the mesenchymal component of a preexisting ameloblastic fibroma. SYN ameloblastic sarcoma.

**am·e·lo·blas·tic lay·er** (am´ĕ-lō-blas´tik lā´ĕr) Innermost layer of the enamel organ. SYN enamel layer.

**am·e·lo·blas·tic o·don·to·ma** (am'ĕl'ō-blas'tik ō'don-tō'mă) Benign mixed odontogenic tumor composed of an undifferentiated component histologically identical to an ameloblastoma and a well-differentiated component identical to an odontoma; appears as a mixed radiolucent-radiopaque lesion and presents clinically as an ameloblastoma. SYN odontoameloblastoma.

**am·e·lo·blas·tic sar·co·ma** (am´ĕ-lō-blas´tik sahr-kō´mă) SYN ameloblastic fibrosarcoma.

🔲**am·e·lo·blas·to·ma** (am'el'ō-blas-tō'mă) Benign odontogenic epithelial neoplasm that histologically mimics the embryonal enamel organ but does not differentiate from it to the point of forming dental hard tissues; behaves as a slowly growing expansile radiolucent tumor; occurs most commonly in the posterior regions of the mandible and tends to recur if inadequately excised. See this page and page A16. [*ameloblast* + G. *-oma*, tumor]

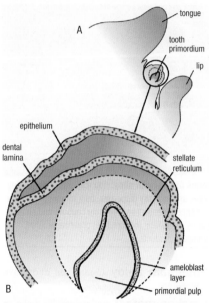

development of teeth and odontogenic tumors: schematic representation of normal tooth development and development of a dentigerous cyst and ameloblastoma; (A) sagittal section of lower jaw of embryo at 14 weeks, viewed through primordium of lower central incisor; (B) stronger magnification of circled area in panel A

**am·e·lo·den·tin·al** (am'ĕ-lō-den'ti-năl) SYN dentinoenamel.

**am·e·lo·gen·e·sis** (am'ĕ-lō-jen'ĕ-sis) The deposition and maturation of enamel. SYN amelogenesis.

🔲**am·e·lo·gen·e·sis im·per·fec·ta** (am´ĕ-lō-jen´ĕ-sis im-pĕr-fek´tă) Group of hereditary ectodermal disorders in which tooth enamel is defective in structure or deficient in quantity. Three major groups are recognized. See page 35 and page A3. SYN enamel dysplasia.

**am·e·lo·gen·ins** (am'ĕ-lō-jen'inz) Class of proteins that form much of the organic matrix during early development of tooth enamel. [*amelogenesis* + *-in*]

**a·men·or·rhe·a** (ā-men'ō-rē´ă) Absence or abnormal cessation of the menses. SYN amenorrhea. [G. *a-* priv. + *mēn*, month, + *rhoia*, flow]

**amenorrhoea** [Br.] SYN amenorrhea.

**A·mer·i·can A·cad·e·my of Per·i·o·don·tics** (ă-mer´i-kăn ă-kad´ĕ-mē per´ē-ŏ-don´tiks) A professional organization of dentists who specialize in periodontics.

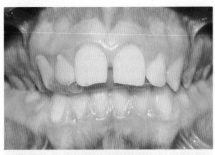

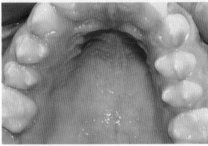

**amelogenesis imperfecta**

**A·mer·i·can Den·tal As·so·ci·a·tion (ADA)** (ă-mer´i-kăn den´tăl ă-sō´si-ā´shŭn) Professional organization of dentists in the United States with a mission to promote the public's oral health and to advance the science of dentistry.

**A·mer·i·can Den·tal Hy·gien·ists As·so·ci·a·tion (ADHA)** (ă-mer´i-kăn den´tăl hī-jē´nists ă-sō´sē-ā´shŭn) Professional organization in the United States; its mission is to promote the public's oral health and to advance the practice and techniques of dental hygiene.

**Amer·i·can Man·u·al Al·pha·bet** (ă-mer´i-kăn man´yū-ăl al´fă-bet) Specific hand and finger positions used to represent each letter of the alphabet, used in conjunction with American Sign Language and other sign languages.

**A·mer·i·can Na·tion·al Stand·ards In·sti·tute (ANSI)** (ă-mer´i-kăn den´tăl hī-jē´nists ă-sō´sē-ā´shŭn) Organization that sets standards for physical measures in the United States.

**Amer·i·cans with Dis·a·bil·i·ties Act (ADA)** (ă-mer´i-kănz dis´ă-bil´i-tēz akt) Federal legislation that prohibits discrimination of services or employment opportunities against people with disabilities.

**am·ide** (am´īd) A substance formally derived from ammonia through the substitution of one or more of the hydrogen atoms by acyl groups, $R—CO—NH_2$, or from a carboxylic acid by replacement of a carboxylic OH by $NH_2$.

**a·mine** (ă-mēn´) *Although this word is correctly stressed on the first syllable, U.S. usage often stresses it on the last syllable as shown here.* A substance formally derived from ammonia by the replacement of one or more of the hydrogen atoms by hydrocarbon or other radicals.

**ami·no ac·id (aa)** (ă-mē´nō as´id) An organic acid in which one of the hydrogen atoms on a carbon atom has been replaced by $NH_2$. Usually refers to an aminocarboxylic acid. However, taurine is also an amino acid. SEE ALSO alpha (α)-amino acid.

**a·mi·no·gly·co·side** (ă-mē´nō-glī´kō-sīd) Any bacteriocidal antibiotic derived from species of *Streptomyces* or *Micromonosporum*; effective against aerobic gram-negative bacilli and *Mycobacterium tuberculosis*.

**a·mi·no·pen·i·cil·lins** (ă-mē´nō-pen-i-sil´ inz) A class of penicillinlike antibiotics that includes ampicillin and amoxicillin; used to treat upper respiratory infections, meningitis, and *Salmonella* infections.

**a·mi·no·pher·ase** (ă-mi-nō´phĕr-āz) SYN aminotransferase.

**am·i·trip·ty·line hy·dro·chlor·ide** (am´ i-trip´ti-lēn hī´drŏ-klōr´ īd) A tricyclic antidepressant that can be used to treat some sleep disorders and neurogenic pain syndromes.

**am·me·ter (am)** (am´ē-tĕr) An instrument for measuring strength of electric current in amperes.

**am·mo·nia** (ă-mō´nē-ă) A colorless volatile gas, $NH_3$, highly soluble in water, capable of forming a weak base, which combines with acids to form ammonium compounds. [fr. L. *sal ammoniacus*, salt of Amen (G. *Ammōn*), obtained near a temple of Amen in Libya]

**am·mo·ni·um car·bon·ate** (ă-mō´nē-ŭm kahr´bŏ-nāt) Cardiac and respiratory stimulant and carminative expectorant.

**am·mo·ni·um chlo·ride** (ă-mō´nē-ŭm klōr´ īd) Stimulant expectorant and cholagogue; used to relieve alkalosis and promote lead excretion and acidify urine.

**am·ne·si·a** (am-nē´zē-ă) A disturbance in the memory of stored information of very variable durations, minutes to months. [G. *amnēsia*, forgetfulness]

**am·ne·si·ac** (am-nē´sē-ak) One suffering from amnesia.

**am·ne·sic** (am-nē´sik) Relating to or characterized by amnesia. SYN amnestic (1).

**am·nes·tic** (am-nes´tik) **1.** SYN amnesic. **2.** An agent causing amnesia.

**amnio-** Combining form denoting the amnion. [G. *amnion*]

**am·ni·on·ic** (am´nē-on´ik) Relating to the amnion. SYN amniotic.

**am·ni·ot·ic** (am'nē-ot'ik) SYN amnionic.

**am·o·bar·bi·tal** (am'ō-bahr'bi-tahl) A central nervous system depressant with an intermediate duration of action.

**A·moe·ba** (ă-mē'bă) A genus of naked, lobose, pseudopod-forming protozoa of the class Sarcodina (or Rhizopoda), which are abundant soil-dwellers, especially in rich organic debris, and are also commonly found as parasites. The typical amebic parasites in humans are placed in the genera *Entamoeba, Endolimax,* and *Iodamoeba*. [Mod. L. fr. G. *amoibē* change]

**amoeba** [Br.] SYN ameba.

**a·mor·phous** (ā-mōr'fŭs) **1.** Without definite shape or visible differentiation in structure. **2.** Not crystallized.

**a·mox·i·cil·lin** (ă-mok'si-sil'in) A semisynthetic penicillin antibiotic with an antimicrobial spectrum similar to that of ampicillin.

**AMP** Abbreviation for adenosine monophosphate.

**am·pere (A)** (am'pēr) **1.** The practical unit of electrical current. **2.** Scientific (SI) definition: the current that, if maintained in two straight parallel conductors of infinite length and of negligible circular cross-sections and placed 1 m apart in a vacuum, produces between them a force of $2 \times 10^{-7}$ N/m of length. [André-Marie *Ampère*]

⚕**amph-** SEE amphi-.

**am·phet·a·mine** (am-fet'ă-mēn) Structurally a sympathomimetic amine, considered a psychostimulant, and approved by the U.S. Food and Drug Administration to treat narcolepsy and attention deficit hyperactivity disorder.

⚕**amphi-** Combining form denoting on both sides, surrounding, double; corresponds to L. *ambi-*. [G. *amphi-*, on both sides, about, around]

**am·pho·my·cin** (am'fō-mī'sin) Antibiotic substance produced by *Streptomyces canus;* used topically for skin infections.

**am·phor·ic res·o·nance** (am-fōr'ik rez' ŏ-năns) A percussion sound, like that produced by striking a large empty bottle, obtained by percussing over a pulmonary cavity.

**am·pho·ter·i·cin, am·pho·ter·i·cin B** (am'fō-ter'i-sin) An amphoteric antibiotic and nephrotoxic antifungal agent used extensively to treat systemic mycoses.

**am·pi·cil·lin** (am'pi-si'lin) An acid-stable semisynthetic penicillin that inhibits the growth of gram-positive and gram-negative bacteria and is not resistant to penicillinase.

**am·pli·tude** (am'pli-tūd) Largeness, extent, breadth, or range. [L. *amplitudo,* fr. *amplus,* large]

**ampoule** [Br.] SYN ampule.

**am·pule** (am'pyūl) A hermetically sealed container, usually made of glass, containing a sterile medicinal solution, or powder to be made up in solution, to be used for subcutaneous, intramuscular, or intravenous injection. SYN ampoule. [L. *ampulla*]

**am·pul·la,** pl. **am·pul·lae** (am-pul'ă, -ē) [TA] A saccular dilation of a canal or duct. [L. a two-handled bottle]

**am·pul·la mem·bra·na·ce·a** (am-pul'ă mem-bră-nā'shē-ă) [TA] SYN membranous ampullae of the semicircular ducts.

**am·pul·la of lac·ri·mal can·a·lic·u·lus** [TA] Slight dilation at angle of lacrimal canaliculus just beyond lacrimal punctum.

**am·pul·la·ry crest (of sem·i·cir·cu·lar ducts)** (am'pŭ-lar-ē krest sem'ē-sĭr'kyū-lăr dŭkts) [TA] Crescentic ridge invaginating lumen of ampullae of semicircular ducts bearing sensory epithelium on a base of nerve fibers and connective tissue.

**am·pul·la·ry cru·ra of sem·i·cir·cu·lar ducts** (am'pŭ-lar-ē krūr'ă sem'ē-sĭr'kyū-lăr dŭkts) SYN ampullary membranous limbs of semicircular ducts.

**am·pul·la·ry mem·bra·nous limbs of sem·i·cir·cu·lar ducts** (am'pŭ-lar-ē mem' bră-nŭs limz sem'ē-sĭr'kyū-lăr dŭkts) [TA] The dilated ends of the three semicircular ducts, each of which contains a specialized thickening of the epithelium known as the ampullary crest. SYN ampullary crura of semicircular ducts.

**am·pul·li·tis** (am'pul-ī'tis) Inflammation of any ampulla, especially of the dilated extremity of the ductus deferens or of the ampulla of Vater. [*ampulla* + G. *itis*, inflammation]

**am·pu·ta·tion** (amp'yū-tā'shŭn) **1.** In dentistry, removal of the root of a tooth, or of the pulp, or of a nerve root or ganglion; a modifying adjective is therefore used (pulp amputation; root amputation). **2.** The severing of a limb or part of a limb, the breast, or other projecting part. [L. *amputatio,* fr. *am-puto*, pp. *-atus*, to cut around, prune]

**am·pu·ta·tion neu·ro·ma** (amp'yū-tā' shŭn nūr-ō'mă) SYN traumatic neuroma.

**a·my·e·li·na·tion** (ā-mī'ĕ-li-nā'shŭn) Failure of formation of myelin sheath of a nerve.

**a·myg·da·line** (ă-mig'dă-līn) [TA] **1.** [TA] Relating to an almond. **2.** [TA] Relating to a tonsil, or to the brain structure called amygdala or amygdaloid complex. **3.** SYN tonsillar.

**a·myg·da·loid** (ă-mig'dă-loyd) Resembling an almond or a tonsil. [*amygdala* + G. *eidos*, appearance]

**a·myg·da·loid fos·sa** (ă-mig′dă-loyd fos′ ă) SYN tonsillar fossa.

**α-am·y·lase** (am′il-ās) A glucanohydrolase that has been used clinically as a digestive aid.

**am·yl·ene** (am′i-lēn) Flammable liquid hydrocarbon formed by the decomposition of amyl alcohol; has anesthetic properties but undesirable side effects.

**am·y·loid** (am′i-loyd) Any of a group of chemically diverse proteins that appears microscopically homogeneous but is composed of linear nonbranching aggregated fibrils arranged in sheets when seen under the electron microscope; occurs characteristically as pathologic extracellular deposits (amyloidosis), especially in association with reticuloendothelial tissue; the chemical nature of the proteinaceous fibrils, depends on the underlying disease process. [*amylo-* + G. *eidos*, resemblance]

**am·y·loi·do·sis** (am′i-loy-dō′sis) **1.** Disease characterized by extracellular accumulation of amyloid in various organs and tissues of the body; may be local or generalized, primary or secondary. **2.** The process of deposition of amyloid protein. [*amyloid* + G. *-osis,* condition]

**am·y·loid tongue** (am′i-loyd tŭng) Macroglossia associated with amyloidosis.

**am·y·lor·rhe·a** (am′i-lō-rē′ă) Passage of undigested starch in the stools. SYN amylorrhoea. [*amylo-* + G. *rhoia,* flow]

**amylorrhoea** [Br.] SYN amylorrhea.

**am·y·lo·su·ri·a, am·y·lu·ri·a** (am′i-lō-syūr′ē-ă, -i-lyūr′ē-ă) Excretion of starch in the urine.

**am·y·lum** (am′i-lŭm) SYN starch.

**am·y·o·es·the·si·a, a·my·o·es·the·sis** (ă-mī′ō-es-thē′zē-ă, -thē′sis) Absence of muscle sensation. SYN amyaesthesia. [G. *a-* priv. + *mys,* muscle, + *aisthēsis,* perception]

**a·my·o·to·ni·a** (ă-mī′ō-tō′nē-ă) Generalized absence of muscle tone, usually associated with flabby musculature and increased range of passive movement at joints. [G. *a-* priv. + *mys,* muscle, + *tonos,* tone]

**amy·o·tro·phic lat·er·al scle·ro·sis (ALS)** (ă-mī′ō-trō′fik lat′ĕr-ăl skler-ō′sis) Fatal degenerative disease involving the corticobulbar, corticospinal, and spinal motor neurons, generally manifested by progressive weakness and wasting of muscles innervated by the affected neurons. Sometimes called Lou Gehrig disease. SYN motor neuron disease (1).

**amy·ot·ro·phy, amy·o·tro·phi·a** (ā′mī-ot′rō-fē, ă-mī′ō-trō′fē-ă) Muscular wasting or atrophy. [G. *a-* priv. + *mys,* muscle, + *trophē,* nourishment]

**a·myx·or·rhe·a** (ă-mik′sōr-ē′ă) Absence of the normal secretion of mucus. [G. *a-* priv. + *myxa,* mucus, + *rhoia,* flow]

**ANA** Abbreviation for antinuclear antibody.

**✿ana-** *Do not confuse words formed with this prefix and similar words formed with the prefix an-. CAUTION: an- before a vowel usually stands for a- — meaning not; sometimes ana- becomes am- before p, b, or ph.* Combining form denoting up, again, back; sometimes *an-* before a vowel; corresponds to L. sursum-. [G. *ana,* up]

**an·a·bi·ot·ic** (an′ă-bī-ot′ik) *Do not confuse this word with antibiotic.* **1.** Resuscitating or restorative. **2.** A revivifying remedy; a powerful stimulant. [*ana-* + G. *bios,* life]

**an·a·bol·ic** (an′ă-bol′ik) Relating to or promoting anabolism.

**an·a·bol·ic ster·oid** (an′ă-bol′ik ster′oyd) Compound with androgenic properties that increases muscle mass and stimulated protein production; used to treat emaciation; sometimes used by athletes in an effort to increase size, strength, and endurance of muscle. Examples include methyltestosterone, nandrolone, methandrostenolone, and stanozolol.

**a·nab·o·lism** (ă-nab′ŏ-lizm) The building up in the body of complex chemical compounds from smaller simpler compounds (e.g., proteins from amino acids), usually with the use of energy. Cf. catabolism, metabolism. [G. *anabolē,* a raising up]

**a·nab·o·lite** (ă-nab′ŏ-līt) Any substance formed as a result of anabolic processes.

**an·ac·id·i·ty** (an′ă-sid′i-tē) Absence of acidity; used especially to denote absence of hydrochloric acid in the gastric juice.

**anaemia** [Br.] SYN anemia.

**anaemic** [Br.] SYN anemic.

**an·aer·obe** (an-ār′ōb) A microorganism that can live and grow in the absence of oxygen. [G. *an-* priv. + *aēr,* air, + *bios,* life]

**an·aer·ob·ic bac·te·ri·a** (an′ār-ō′bik baktēr′ē-ă) Bacteria that can live and grow in the absence of oxygen. Some anaerobic bacteria are inhibited or killed by oxygen.

**an·aer·o·bic cel·lu·li·tis** (an′ă-rō′bik sel′ yū-lī′tis) Infection of subcutaneous soft tissues by anaerobic bacteria, usually a mixed culture including *Bacteroides* species, anaerobic cocci, and clostridia.

**an·aer·o·bic pneu·mo·ni·a** (an′ă-rō′bik nū-mō′nē-ă) Pneumonia caused by bacteria usually originating in the mouth, especially in the presence of periodontal disease; cavitation common.

**anaesthekinesia** [Br.] SYN anesthekinesia.

**anaesthesia** [Br.] SYN anesthesia.

**anaesthesia dolorosa** [Br.] SYN anesthesia dolorosa.

**anaesthesia record** [Br.] SYN anesthesia record.

**anaesthesiologist** [Br.] SYN anesthesiologist.

**anaesthesiology** [Br.] SYN anesthesiology.

**anaesthetic** [Br.] SYN anesthetic.

**anaesthetist** [Br.] SYN anesthetist.

**an·a·lep·tic** (an'ă-lep'tik) A central nervous system stimulant, particularly used to denote agents that reverse depressed central nervous system function. [G. *analēptikos*, restorative]

**an·al·ge·si·a** (an'ăl-jē'zē-ă) *Do not confuse this word with anesthesia.* A neurologic or pharmacologic state in which painful stimuli are moderated such that, although still perceived, they are no longer painful. [G. insensibility, fr. *an-* priv. + *algēsis*, sensation of pain]

**an·al·ge·sic** (an'ăl-jē'zik) **1.** A compound capable of producing analgesia, i.e., one that relieves pain by altering the perception of nociceptive stimuli without producing anesthesia or loss of consciousness. **2.** Characterized by reduced response to painful stimuli.

**an·al·ge·sim·e·ter** (an'ăl-jē-zim'i-ter) A device for eliciting painful stimuli to measure pain under experimental conditions. [*analgesia* + G. *metron*, measure]

**an·al·get·ic** (an'ăl-jet'ik) Associated with decreased pain perception.

**an·al·gi·a** (an-al´jē-ă) Absence of pain. [G. *an-* negative prefix, + *algos*, pain, + *-ia*, noun suffix]

**a·nal·o·gous** (ă-nal'ŏ-gŭs) Possessing a functional resemblance, but having a different origin or structure.

**analphalipoproteinaemia** [Br.] SYN analphalipoproteinemia.

**an·al·pha·lip·o·pro·tein·e·mi·a** (an'al'fă-lip'ŏ-prō'tēn-ē'mē-ă) High-density lipoprotein deficiency. SYN analphalipoproteinaemia. [G. *an-*, priv., + *alpha*,α, + lipoprotein + *-emia*, blood]

**a·nal·y·sis,** pl. **a·nal·y·ses** (ă-nal'i-sis, -sēz) The breaking up of a chemical compound or mixture into simpler elements; a process by which the composition of a substance is determined. [G. a breaking up, fr. *ana*, up, + *lysis*, a loosening]

**an·a·lyz·ing rod** (an'ă-līz-ing rod) Tool used with a surveyor to determine the relative positions of parallel surfaces and undercuts when removable partial dentures are designed.

**an·am·ne·sis** (an'am-nē'sis) **1.** The act of remembering. **2.** The medical or developmental history of a patient. [G. *anamnēsis*, recollection]

**an·a·phy·lac·tic** (an'ă-fi-lak'tik) Relating to anaphylaxis; manifesting extremely great sensitivity to foreign protein or other material.

**an·a·phy·lac·tic shock** (an'ă-fi-lak'tik shok) Severe, often fatal form of shock characterized by respiratory compromise from laryngeal edema or bronchospasm, hypotension or shock, from cardiac arrhythmias, or peripheral vasodilation and vascular permeability. SEE ALSO anaphylaxis, serum sickness.

**an·a·phy·lac·toid** (an'ă-fi-lak'toyd) Resembling anaphylaxis. [*anaphylaxis* + G. *eidos*, resemblance]

**an·a·phy·lac·toid pur·pu·ra** (an'ă-fi-lak'toyd pŭr'pyŭr-ă) **1.** SYN allergic purpura. **2.** SYN Henoch-Schönlein purpura.

**an·a·phy·lac·toid shock** (an'ă-fi-lak'toyd shok) Reaction that is similar to anaphylactic shock, but does not require the incubation period characteristic of induced sensitivity (anaphylaxis); it is a non-IgE mediated reaction.

**an·a·phy·lax·is** (an'ă-fi-lak'sis) An induced systemic or generalized sensitivity; at times the term anaphylaxis is used for anaphylactic shock. The physiologic manifestations reflect the biologic effects of these mediators. Cutaneous symptoms include pruritus, erythema, urticaria, and angioedema. Respiratory compromise can come from laryngeal obstruction or bronchospasm. Cardiac effects include arrhythmia, hypotension, and shock. The reaction may be fatal if asphyxiation or cardiovascular collapse occurs. [G. *ana*, away from, back from, + *phylaxis*, protection]

**an·a·pla·si·a** (an'ă-plā'zē-ă) Loss of structural differentiation, especially as seen in most, but not all, malignant neoplasms. SYN dedifferentiation (2). [G. *ana*, again, + *plasis*, a molding]

**an·a·sar·ca** (an'ah-sahr'kă) A generalized infiltration of edematous fluid into subcutaneous connective tissue. [G. *ana*, through, + *sarx* (*sark-*), flesh]

**a·nas·to·mo·sis,** pl. **a·nas·to·mo·ses** (ă-nas'tŏ-mō'sis, -mō'sēz) **1.** A natural communication, direct or indirect, between two blood vessels or other nonneural tubular structures. **2.** An opening created by surgery, trauma, or disease between two or more normally separate spaces or organs. [G. *anastomōsis*, from *anastomoō*, to furnish with a mouth]

**a·nas·to·mot·ic branch** (ă-nas'tŏ-mot'ik branch) [TA] A blood vessel that interconnects two neighboring vessels.

**an·a·tom·ic, an·a·tom·i·cal** (an-ă-tom´ik, -i-kăl) **1.** Relating to anatomy. **2.** SYN structural. **3.** Denoting a strictly morphologic feature distinct from its physiologic or surgical considerations, e.g., anatomic neck of humerus, anatomic dead space, anatomic lobulation of the liver.

**an·a·tom·i·c crown** (an'ă-tom'ik krown) Portion of a tooth covered with enamel. SYN crown of tooth.

**an·a·tom·i·c dead space** (an'ă-tom'ik ded spās) The volume of the conducting airways from the external environment (at the nose and mouth) down to the level at which inspired gas exchanges oxygen and carbon dioxide with pulmonary capillary blood.

**an·a·tom·ic height of con·tour** (an'ă-tom'ik hīt kon'tūr) SYN height of contour.

**an·a·tom·ic im·pres·sion** (an'ă-tom'ik im-presh'ŭn) An impression of dental structures in a passive state.

**an·a·tom·ic land·mark** (an'ă-tom'ik land'mahrk) A morphologic feature of the anatomy that is readily recognizable and may be used as a reference point for other body features.

**an·a·tom·i·co·med·i·cal** (an'ă-tom'i-kō-med'i-kăl) Referring to both medicine and anatomy.

**an·a·tom·i·co·path·o·log·ic** (an'ă-tom'i-kō-path'ŏ-loj'ik) Relating to anatomic pathology.

**an·a·tom·i·co·sur·gi·cal** (an'ă-tom'i-kō-sŭr'ji-kăl) Relating to surgical anatomy.

**an·a·tom·ic po·si·tion** (an'ă-tom'ik pŏ-zish'ŏn) Standing erect, arms at the sides, with palms facing forward.

**an·a·tom·ic root** (an'ă-tom'ik rūt) Portion of a tooth extending from the cervical line to its apical extremity.

**an·a·tom·ic teeth** (an'ă-tom'ik tēth) Artificial teeth in a dental appliance that retain the functional anatomy of natural teeth.

**a·nat·o·my** (ă-nat'ŏ-mē) [TA] Morphologic structure of an organism. See this page. [G. *anatomē,* dissection, from *ana,* apart, + *tomē,* a cutting]

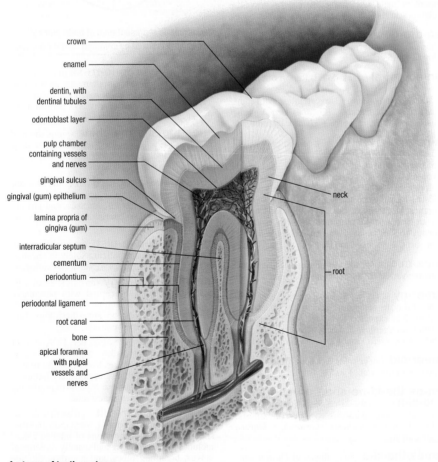

crown

enamel

dentin, with dentinal tubules

odontoblast layer

pulp chamber containing vessels and nerves

gingival sulcus

gingival (gum) epithelium

lamina propria of gingiva (gum)

interradicular septum

cementum

periodontium

periodontal ligament

root canal

bone

apical foramina with pulpal vessels and nerves

neck

root

**features of tooth anatomy**

**ANB an·gle** (ang′gĕl) Cephalometric area, formed by A point, nasion, and B point, which describes (i.e., informs) the anteroposterior relationship of the mandible to the maxilla.

**an·chor·age** (ang′kŏr-ăj) **1.** In dentistry, a tooth or an implanted tooth substitute with which a fixed or removable partial denture, crown, or restoration is retained. **2.** The nature and degree of resistance to displacement offered by an anatomic unit when used for the purpose of effecting tooth movement. [L. *ancora,* fr. G. *ankyra,* anchor]

**an·chor splint** (ang′kŏr splint) Splint used to set a fractured jaw, with wires around the teeth and a rod to hold it in place.

**an·cip·i·tal, an·cip·i·tate, an·cip·i·tous** (an-sip′i-tăl, -i-tāt, -i-tŭs) Two-headed; two-edged. [L. *anceps,* two-headed]

**an·dro·gen** (an′drŏ-jen) Generic term for an agent, usually a hormone (e.g., androsterone, testosterone), which stimulates activity of the accessory male sex organs, encourages development of male sex characteristics, or prevents changes in the latter due to castration.

**an·dro·gen·ic hor·mone** (an′drō-jen′ik hōr′mōn) Any hormone that produces a masculinizing effect.

**an·ec·dot·al** (an′ek-dō′tăl) Report of clinical experiences based on individual experience, rather than an organized investigation with standard research features. [G. *anekdota,* unpublished items, fr. *an-* priv + *ekdido,* to publish]

**a·ne·mi·a** (ă-nē′mē-ă) Any condition in which the number of red blood cells/mm$^3$, the amount of hemoglobin in 100 mL of blood, and/or the volume of packed red blood cells/100 mL of blood are less than normal; frequently manifested by pallor of the skin and mucous membranes, shortness of breath, palpitations of the heart, soft systolic murmurs, lethargy, and tendency to fatigue. SYN anaemia. [G. *anaimia,* fr. *an-* priv. + *haima,* blood]

**a·ne·mic** (ă-nē′mik) Pertaining to or manifesting the various features of anemia. SYN anaemic.

**an·er·gy** (an′ĕr-jē) **1.** In a person, absence of the ability to generate a sensitivity reaction to substances expected to be antigenic (immunogenic, allergenic). **2.** Lack of energy. [G. *an-* priv. + *energeia,* energy, from *ergon,* work]

**an·er·oid** (an′ĕr-oyd) Without fluid. [G. *a-* priv. + *nēros,* wet, + *eidos,* form]

**an·es·the·ki·ne·si·a, an·es·the·ci·ne·si·a** (an-es′thē-ki-nē′zē-ă) Combined sensory and motor paralysis. SYN anaesthekinesia. [G. *an-* priv. + *aisthēsis,* sensation, + *kinēsis,* movement]

▉**an·es·the·si·a** (an′es-thē′zē-ă) *Do not confuse this word with analgesia or hypesthesia.*

**1.** Loss of sensation due to pharmacologic depression of nerve function or from neurogenic dysfunction. **2.** Broad term for anesthesiology as a clinical specialty. See this page. [G. *anaisthēsia,* fr. *an-* priv. + *aisthēsis,* sensation]

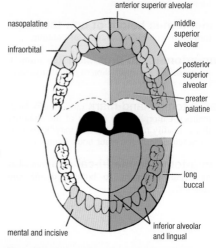

diagram labels: anterior superior alveolar, nasopalatine, middle superior alveolar, infraorbital, posterior superior alveolar, greater palatine, long buccal, mental and incisive, inferior alveolar and lingual

**diagrammatic representation of teeth and soft tissues anesthetized by common dental injections**

**an·es·the·si·a do·lo·ro·sa** (an′es-thē′zē-ă dō-lō-rō′să) Severe spontaneous pain occurring in an anesthetic area; paradoxic result may occur in cases of neuropathy. SYN painful anesthesia, anaesthesia dolorosa.

**an·es·the·si·a ma·chine** (an′es-thē′zē-ă mă-shēn′) Equipment used for inhalation anesthesia, including flowmeters, vaporizers, and sources of compressed gases.

**an·es·the·si·a rec·ord** (an′es-thē′zē-ă rek′ŏrd) Written or electronic account of drugs administered, procedures undertaken, and physiologic responses noted during anesthesia. SYN anaesthesia record.

**an·es·the·si·ol·o·gist** (an′es-thē′zē-ol′ŏ-jist) A physician specializing solely in anesthesiology and related areas. SYN anaesthesiologist.

**an·es·the·si·ol·o·gy** (an′es-thē′zē-ol′ŏ-jē) Medical specialty concerned with pharmacologic, physiologic, and clinical bases of anesthesia and related fields. SYN anaesthesiology. [*anesthesia* + G. *logos,* treatise]

**an·es·thet·ic** (an′es-thet′ik) **1.** Agent or compound that reversibly depresses neuronal function, which produces loss of ability to perceive pain and/or other sensations. **2.** Characterized by loss of sensation or capable of producing loss of sensation. SYN anaesthetic.

**an·es·thet·ic cir·cuit** (an′es-thet′ik sĭr′kŭt) Equipment used during inhalation anesthesia to regulate concentrations of inhaled gases; includes a reservoir bag and usually directional valves, breathing tubes, and a carbon dioxide absorber.

**an·es·thet·ic depth** (an'es-thet'ik depth) Degree of central nervous system depression produced by a general anesthetic agent; function of potency of anesthetic and the concentration in which it is administered.

**an·es·thet·ic eth·er** (an'es-thet'ik ē'thĕr) General designation for many ethers.

**an·es·thet·ic in·dex** (an'es-thet'ik in'deks) Ratio of the number of units of anesthetic required for anesthesia to the number of units of anesthetic required to produce respiratory or cardiovascular failure.

**an·es·thet·ic va·por** (an'es-thet'ik vā'pŏr) Gaseous phase of a liquid anesthetic with sufficient partial pressure at room temperature to produce general anesthesia when inhaled.

**a·nes·the·tist** (ă-nes'thĕ-tist) One who administers an anesthetic, whether an anesthesiologist, a physician who is not an anesthesiologist, a nurse anesthetist, or an anesthesia assistant. SYN anaesthetist.

**a·nes·the·tize** (ă-nes'thĕ-tīz) To produce loss of sensation. SYN anaesthetize.

**an·eu·rysm** (an'yūr-izm) *Avoid the misspelling aneurism.* Circumscribed dilation of an artery or a cardiac chamber, in direct communication with the lumen, usually resulting from an acquired or congenital weakness of the wall of the artery or chamber. [G. *aneurysma* (*-mat-*), a dilation, fr. *eurys,* wide]

**an·eu·rys·mal bone cyst** (an'yūr-iz'măl bōn sist) A solitary benign osteolytic lesion expanding a long bone or within a vertebra, consisting of blood-filled spaces, and separated by fibrous tissue containing multinucleated giant cells; such cysts cause swelling, pain, and tenderness.

**ANF** Abbreviation for antinuclear antibody.

**An·gel·man syn·drome** (an'jĕl-măn sin' drōm) Microdeletion of 15q-13, of maternal origin, resulting in mental retardation, ataxia, paroxysms of laughter, seizures, characteristic facies, and minimal speech.

**an·gi·i·tis, an·gi·tis** (an'jē-ī'tis, an-jī'tis) Inflammation of a blood vessel (arteritis, phlebitis) or lymphatic vessel (lymphangitis). [*angio-* + G. *-itis,* inflammation]

**an·gi·na** (an'ji-nă) *Although the correct classical pronunciation stresses the first syllable (an'gina), the stress is often placed on the second syllable (angi'na) in the U.S.* Severe, often constricting pain or sensation of pressure, usually referring to angina pectoris. [L. quinsy]

**an·gi·nal** (an'ji-năl) Relating to angina in any sense.

**an·gi·na pec·to·ris** (an'ji-nă pek-tō'ris) Severe constricting chest pain or pressure, often radiating from precordium to shoulder (usually left) and down the arm, resulting from ischemia of the heart muscle.

**an·gi·o·e·de·ma** (an'jē-ō-ĕ-dē'mă) Recurrent large circumscribed areas of subcutaneous or mucosal edema of sudden onset, usually disappearing within 24 hours; often due to an allergic reaction to foods or drugs. See this page. SYN angioneurotic edema.

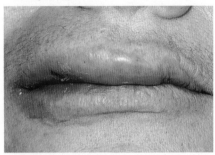

**angioedema:** unilateral swelling of upper lip

**an·gi·o·gen·e·sis fac·tor** (an'jē-ō-jen'ĕ-sis fak'tŏr) Substance secreted by several types of cells that stimulates neovascularization in healing wounds or stroma of tumors.

**an·gi·og·ra·phy** (an'jē-og'ră-fē) Radiography of vessels after injecting radiopaque contrast material; usually requires percutaneous insertion of a radiopaque catheter and positioning under fluoroscopic control. SEE ALSO arteriography, venography. [*angio-* + G. *graphō,* to write]

**an·gi·o·ker·a·to·ma** (an'jē-ō-ker-ă-tō'mă) Superficial, intradermal, capillary-acquired telangiectasis, with hyperkeratosis and acanthosis. [*angio-* + G. *keras,* horn, + *-ōma,* tumor]

**an·gi·o·ma** (an'jē-ō'mă) Swelling or tumor due to proliferation, with or without dilation, of blood vessels (hemangioma) or lymphatics (lymphangioma). [*angio-* + G. *-ōma,* tumor]

**an·gi·o·ma·to·sis** (an'jē-ō-mă-tō'sis) A condition characterized by multiple angiomas.

**an·gi·o·my·op·a·thy** (an'jē-ō-mī-op'ă-thē) Any disease of blood vessels involving the muscular layer. [*angio-* + G. *mys,* muscle, + *pathos,* suffering]

**an·gi·o·neu·rop·a·thy** (an'jē-ō-nūr-op'ă-thē) Vascular disorder attributed to abnormality of autonomic nervous system fibers supplying blood vessels.

**an·gi·o·neu·rot·ic e·de·ma** (an'jē-ō-nūr-ot'ik ĕ-dē'mă) SYN angioedema.

**an·gi·op·a·thy** (an'jē-op'ă-thē) Any disease of the blood vessels or lymphatics. [*angio-* + G. *pathos,* suffering]

**an·gi·o·plas·ty** (an'jē-ō-plas-tē) Reconstitution or recanalization of a blood vessel; may involve balloon dilation, mechanical stripping of intima, forceful injection of fibrinolytics, or placement of a stent. SEE percutaneous coronary intervention. [*angio-* + G. *plastos,* formed, shaped]

**an·gi·o·some** (an'je-ō-sōm) Composite anatomic vascular territories of skin and underlying muscles, tendons, nerves, and bones, based on segmental or distributing arteries.

**an·gle** (ang'gĕl) [TA] Meeting point of two lines or planes; figure formed by the junction of two lines or planes; space bounded on two sides by converging lines or planes. [L. *angulus*]

🄰**An·gle clas·si·fi·ca·tion of mal·oc·clu·sion** (ang'gĕl klas'i-fi-kā'shŭn mal'ŏ-klū'zhŭn) *Because Angle is a proper name, it is spelled with a capital A.* System for classifying different types of malocclusion, based on mesiodistal relationship of permanent molars in their eruption and locking, and consisting of three classes; *Class I:* normal relationship of the jaws, wherein the mesiobuccal cusp of the maxillary first molar occludes in the buccal groove of the mandibular first permanent molar; *Class II:* distal relationship of the mandible, wherein the distobuccal cusp of the maxillary first permanent molar occludes in buccal groove of the mandibular first molar, and further classified as Division 1, labioversion of maxillary incisor teeth, and Division 2, linguoversion of maxillary central incisors, both of which may be unilateral conditions; *Class III:* mesial relationship of the mandible, wherein the mesiobuccal cusp of the maxillary first molar occludes in the embrasure between the mandibular first and second permanent molars, further classified as a unilateral condition. See this page.

**an·gle of man·di·ble** (ang'gĕl man'di-bĕl) [TA] The angle formed by the inferior border of the mandible and the posterior edge of the ramus of the lower jaw. SYN mandibular angle.

**an·gle of mouth** (ang'gĕl mowth) [TA] The lateral limit of the oral fissure. SEE ALSO labial commissure (of mouth). SYN angulus oris.

**an·gle of re·tro·ver·sion** (ang'gĕl ret'rō-vĕr'zhŭn) Angle formed by a line drawn through center of longitudinal axis of neck and head of the humerus meeting a line drawn along the transverse axis of the condyles, when the base is viewed from above, looking straight down from above the head of the humerus.

**Ångström (Å)** (ang'strŏm) A unit of wavelength, 10-10 m, equivalent to 0.1 nm. [Anders J. *Ångström*, Swedish physicist]

**an·gu·lar ar·te·ry** (ang'gyŭ-lăr ahr'tĕr-ē) [TA] The terminal branch of the facial artery; *distribution*, muscles and skin of side of nose; *anastomoses*, lateral nasal, and dorsal artery of nose and palpebrals from the ophthalmic artery, thereby providing an external-internal carotid arterial anastomosis.

🄰**an·gu·lar chei·li·tis** (ang'gyŭ-lăr kī-lī'tis) Inflammation and fissuring radiating from commissures of mouth secondary to predisposing factors such as lost vertical dimension in denture wearers, nutritional deficiencies, atopic dermatitis, or *Candida albicans* infection. See page A8. SYN commissural cheilitis, perlèche.

**an·gu·lar chei·lo·sis** (ang'gyŭ-lăr kī-lō'sis) Reddish inflammation of the lips and pro-

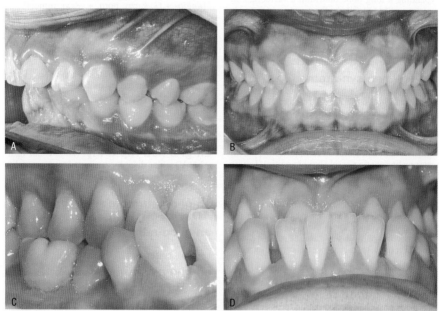

**Angle classification of malocclusion:** (A) class II division 1, left; (B) class II division 2, center; (C) class III, right; (D) class III, center

duction of fissures that radiate from the angles of the mouth.

**an·gu·lar vein** (ang′gyŭ-lăr vān) [TA] Short vein at medial angle of the eye, formed by supraorbital and supratrochlear veins and continuing as facial vein.

**⊞an·gu·la·tion** (ang′gyū-lā′shŭn) **1.** In dentistry, description of alignment of entire tooth, tooth roots, or anatomic crown of tooth to a vertical axis in both anteroposterior and lateral planes of jaws. **2.** Variable spatial (i.e., angular) relationship that exists between tooth surface and face of instrument used to remove calculus. See this page.

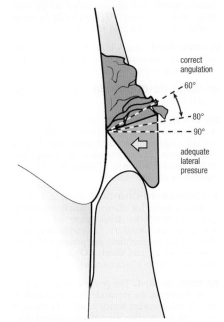

correct angulation

60°

80°

90°

adequate lateral pressure

**effective calculus removal:** combination of correct angulation and adequate lateral pressure is required to fracture deposited dental calculus from tooth surface

**an·gu·lus mas·toi·de·us os·sis pa·ri·e·tal·is** (ang′gyū-lŭs mas-toy′dē-ŭs os′is pă-rī′ĕ-tā′lis) [TA] SYN mastoid angle of parietal bone.

**an·gu·lus oc·ci·pi·ta·lis os·sis pa·ri·e·tal·is** (ang′gyū-lŭs ok-sip′i-tā′lis os′is pă-rī′ĕ-tā′lis) [TA] SYN occipital angle of parietal bone.

**an·gu·lus o·ris** (ang′gyū-lŭs ōr′is) [TA] SYN angle of mouth.

**an·gu·lus sphe·noi·da·lis os·sis pa·ri·e·tal·is** (ang′gyū-lŭs sfĕ′noy-dā′lis os′is pă-rī′ĕ-tā′lis) [TA] SYN sphenoidal angle of parietal bone.

**an·hi·dro·sis, an·i·dro·sis** (an′hī-drō′sis, -i-drō′sis) Absence of sweat glands or absence of sweating. [G. *an-* priv. + *hidrōs,* sweat]

**an·hi·drot·ic** (an′hī-drot′ik) Relating to, or characterized by, anhidrosis. SYN adiaphoretic.

**an·hi·drot·ic ec·to·der·mal dys·pla·si·a** (an′hī-drot′ik ek′tō-dĕr′măl dis-plā′zē-ă) Disorder characterized by absent or defective sweat glands, saddle-shaped nose, hyperpigmentation around the eyes, malformed or missing teeth, sparse hair, dysplastic nails, smooth finely wrinkled skin, syndactyly, absent mammary gland tissue, and occasionally mental retardation.

**an·hy·drous** (an-hī′drŭs) Containing no water, especially water of crystallization.

**an·hy·drous al·co·hol** (an-hī′drŭs al′kŏ-hol) SYN absolute alcohol (1).

**an·ic·ter·ic vi·ral hep·a·ti·tis** (an′ik-ter′ik vī′răl hep′ă-tī′tis) A relatively mild hepatitis, without jaundice, caused by a virus.

**an·i·mal** (an′i-măl) **1.** A living, sentient organism that has membranous cell walls, requires oxygen and organic foods, and is capable of voluntary movement, as distinguished from a plant or mineral. **2.** One of the lower animal organisms as distinguished from humans. [L.]

**an·i·mal starch** (an′i-măl stahrch) SYN glycogen.

**an·i·on (Ā)** (an′ī-on) An ion that carries a negative charge, going therefore to the positively charged anode; in salts, acid radicals are anions.

**an·i·on·ic de·ter·gent** (an′ī-on′ik dĕ-tĕr′jĕnt) Cleansing agent that carries a net negative charge on a lipidlike molecule and exerts a limited antibacterial effect (e.g., a soap).

**an·ise** (an′is) Fruit of *Pimpinellla anisum;* an aromatic and carminative resembling fennel. [L. *anisum,* fr. G. *anēson,*]

**♦ aniso-** Combining form denoting unequal, dissimilar, unlike. [G. *anisos,* unequal, fr. *an-,* not, + *isos,* equal]

**an·i·so·cy·to·sis** (an-ī′sō-sī-tō′sis) Variation in the size of cells that are normally uniform, especially red blood cells. [*aniso-* + G. *kytos,* cell, + *-osis,* condition]

**an·i·sog·na·thous** (an′i-sog′nă-thŭs) *In the diphthong gn, the g is silent only at the beginning of a word.* Having jaws of unequal size, the upper being wider than the lower. [*aniso-* + G. *gnathos,* jaw]

**an·i·sos·then·ic** (an-ī′sos-then′ik) Of unequal strength; denoting two muscles or groups of muscles that are either paired or antagonistic. [*aniso-* + G. *sthenos,* strength]

**an·i·so·tro·pic** (an-ī′sō-trō′pic) Not having properties that are the same in all directions. [*aniso-* + G. *tropos,* a turning]

**an·ky·lo·glos·si·a** (ang′ki-lō-glos′ē-ă) Partial or complete fusion of the tongue to the floor of the mouth; abnormal shortness of the frenulum linguae. See this page. See [*ankylo-* + G. *glōssa*, tongue]

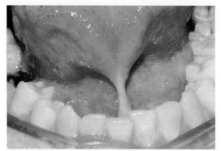

**ankyloglossia:** speech of this patient was not impaired

**an·ky·lo·glos·si·a su·pe·ri·or syn·drome** (ang′ki-lō-glos′ē-ă sŭ-pēr′ē-ŏr sin′drōm) Congenital condition in which tongue adheres to hard palate; no evidence of genetic factors.

**an·ky·losed tooth** (ang′ki-lōst tŭth) SEE dental ankylosis.

**an·ky·lo·sis** (ang′ki-lō′sis) Bony union of the radicular surface of a tooth to the surrounding alveolar bone in an area of previous partial root resorption. See this page. [G. *ankylōsis*, stiffening of a joint]

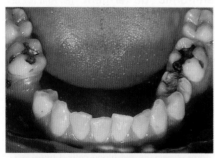

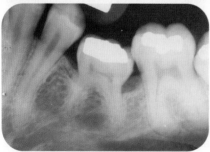

**ankylosis:** second primary molar

**an·ky·los·to·ma** (ang′ki-los′tŏ-mă) SYN trismus. [*ankylo-* + G. *stoma*, mouth]

**an·la·ge**, pl. **an·la·gen** (ahn′lah-ge, -gen) SYN primordium. [Ger. plan, outline]

**an·neal** (ă-nēl′) In dentistry, to heat gold leaf preparatory to its insertion into a cavity to remove adsorbed gases and other contaminants. [A.S. *anaelan*, to burn]

**an·neal·ing lamp** (ă-nēl′ing lamp) Alcohol lamp with a soot-free flame used in dentistry to drive off protective $NH_3$ gas coating from the surface of cohesive gold foil.

**an·neal·ing tray** (ă-nēl′ing trā) Electrically heated, thermostatically controlled device used to drive off protective $NH_3$ gas coating from the surface of cohesive gold foil.

**an·nec·tent** (ă-nek′tĕnt) Connected with; joined. [L. *an-necto*, pres. p. *-nectere*, pp. *-nexus*, to join to]

**an·nu·al de·duc·ti·ble** (an′yū-ăl dĕ-dŭk′ti-bel) SYN deductible.

**an·o·chro·ma·si·a** (an′ō-krō-mā′zē-ă) **1.** Failure of cells or other elements of tissue to acquire color in the usual manner when treated with a stain. **2.** Accumulation of hemoglobin in the peripheral zone of erythrocytes. [G. *anō*, upward, + *chrōma*, color]

**a·no·ci·as·so·ci·a·tion** (ă-nō′sē-ă-sō′sē-ā′shŭn) Theory that afferent stimuli, especially pain, contribute to development of surgical shock, and, as a corollary, that conduction anesthesia at the surgical field and presurgical sedation protect against shock. [G. *a-* priv. + L. *noceo*, to injure, + *association*]

**an·ode** (an′ōd) **1.** The positive pole of a galvanic battery or the electrode connected with it; an electrode toward which negatively charged ions (anions) migrate; a positively charged electrode. **2.** The portion of an x-ray tube from which x-rays are released by bombardment by cathode rays. [G. *anodos*, a way up, fr. *ana*, up, + *hodos*, a way]

**an·o·don·ti·a** (an′ō-don′shē-ă) Congenital absence of the teeth; developmental, not due to extraction or impaction. [G. *an-* priv. + *odous*, tooth + *ia* n. suffix]

**an·o·dont·ism** (an′ō-dont′izm) Congenital absence of tooth bud development.

**an·o·dyne** (an′ō-dīn) A compound less potent than an anesthetic that is capable of relieving pain. [G. *an-* priv. + *odynē*, pain]

**a·nom·a·lous tu·ber·cle of tooth** (ă-nom′ă-lŭs tū′bĕr-kĕl tŭth) [TA] An atypical tubercle on a tooth.

**a·nom·a·ly** (ă-nom′ă-lē) Birth defect caused by structural abnormality or marked deviation from the average or norm; anything structurally unusual or irregular or contrary to a general rule e.g., a congenital defect. [G. *anōmalia,* irregularity]

**an·oph·thal·mi·a, an·oph·thal·mos** (an'of-thal'mē-ă, -mŏs) Congenital absence of all tissues of the eyes. [G. *an-* priv. + *ophthalmos,* eye]

**an·o·rec·tic, an·o·ret·ic, an·o·rex·ic** (an'ŏ-rek'tic, -ret'ik, -rek'sik) **1.** Relating to, characteristic of, or suffering from anorexia, especially anorexia nervosa. **2.** An agent that causes anorexia.

**an·o·rex·i·a** (an'ŏ-rek'sē-ă) *Avoid substituting the simple word anorexia for anorexia nervosa.* Diminished appetite; aversion to food. [G. fr. *an-* priv. + *orexis,* appetite]

**an·o·rex·ia ner·vo·sa** (an'ŏ-rek'sē-ă nĕr-vō'să) Mental disorder manifested by extreme fear of becoming obese and an aversion to food, usually occurring in young women and often resulting in life-threatening weight loss, accompanied by a disturbance in body image, hyperactivity, and amenorrhea. Cf. bulimia nervosa.

**an·os·mi·a** (an-oz'mē-ă) Loss or absence of the sense of smell. [G. *an-* priv. + *osmē,* sense of smell]

**a·no·so·di·a·pho·ri·a** (ă-nō'sō-dī-ă-fōr'ē-ă) Indifference to disease, specifically paralysis. [G. *a-* priv. + *nosos,* disease, + *diaphora,* difference]

**anoxaemia** [Br.] SYN anoxemia.

**an·ox·e·mi·a** (an'ok-sē'mē-ă) Absence of oxygen in arterial blood; formerly often used to include moderate decrease in oxygen now properly distinguished as hypoxemia. SYN anoxaemia. [G. *an-* priv. + oxygen + G. *haima,* blood]

**an·ox·i·a** (an-ok'sē-ă) *Avoid the careless substitution of this word for hypoxia or hypoxemia.* Absence or almost complete absence of oxygen from inspired gases, arterial blood, or tissues. [G. *an-* priv. + *oxygen*]

**an·ox·ic an·ox·i·a** (an-ok'sik an-ok'sē-ă) Severe cases of hypoxic hypoxia in which oxygen is almost completely lacking.

**ANS** Abbreviation for autonomic nervous system.

**ANSI** Abbreviation for American National Standards Institute.

**an·si·form** (an'si-fōrm) In the shape of a loop or arc. [L. *ansa,* handle, + *forma,* shape]

**ant·ac·id** (ant-as'id) Any agent that reduces or neutralizes acidity, as of the gastric juice or any other secretion (e.g., calcium carbonate, magnesium hydroxide).

**an·tag·o·nist** (an-tag'ŏ-nist) Something opposing or resisting the action of another; certain

structures, agents, diseases, or physiologic processes that tend to neutralize or impede the action or effect of others. Cf. synergist.

**ant·a·tro·phic** (ant'ă-trō'pik) Preventing or curing atrophy.

**an·te·ced·ent** (an'tĕ-sē'dĕnt) A precursor. [L. *antecedo,* to go before]

**an·te ci·bum (AC, a.c.)** (an'tē sī'bŭm) Before a meal. [L.]

**an·te·go·ni·al notch** (an'tĕ-gō'nē-ăl noch) Concavity in the lower border of the mandible immediately anterior to its angle.

**an·te·grade** (an'tĕ-grād) In the direction of normal movement. [*ante-* + L. *gradior,* to walk]

**an·te·po·si·tion** (an'tē-pō-zi'shŭn) Forward or anterior position.

**an·te·py·ret·ic** (an'tē-pī-ret'ik) Before the occurrence of fever; before the period of reaction after shock. [*ante-* + G. *pyretos,* fever]

**an·te·ri·or** (an-tēr'ē-ŏr) [TA] In human anatomy, denoting the front surface of the body; often used to indicate the position of one structure relative to another, i.e., situated nearer the front part of the body. SYN ventral (2) [TA]. [L.]

**an·te·ri·or am·pul·lary nerve** (an-tēr'ē-ŏr am'pŭ-lar-ē nĕrv) [TA] A branch of the utriculoampullar nerve that supplies the crista ampullaris of the anterior semicircular duct.

**an·te·ri·or ar·tic·u·lar sur·face of dens** (an-tēr'ē-ŏr ahr-tik'yū-lăr sŭr'făs denz) [TA] The curved articular facet on the anterior aspect of the dens of the axis that articulates with the facet for the dens of the axis on the anterior arch of the atlas. SYN facies articularis anterior dentis.

**an·te·ri·or au·ric·u·lar branch·es of su·per·fi·cial tem·po·ral ar·te·ry** (an-tēr'ē-ŏr aw-rik'yū-lăr branch'ĕz sū'pĕr-fish'ăl tem'pŏr-ăl ahr'tĕr-ē) [TA] *Distribution,* auricle, earlobe, and external acoustic meatus.

**an·te·ri·or au·ric·u·lar mus·cle** (an-tēr'ē-ŏr awr-ik'yū-lăr mŭs'ĕl) SYN auricularis anterior (muscle).

**an·te·ri·or au·ric·u·lar nerves** (an-tēr'ē-ŏr awr-ik'yū-lăr nĕrvz) [TA] Branches of the auriculotemporal nerve that supply tragus and upper part of auricle.

**an·te·ri·or au·ric·u·lar vein** (an-tēr'ē-ŏr aw-rik'yū-lăr vān) [TA] One of several veins draining the auricle and acoustic meatus and emptying into the retromandibular vein.

**an·te·ri·or bor·der** (an-tēr'ē-ŏr bōr'dĕr) [TA] Ventral or most forward margin of a structure.

**an·te·ri·or branch** (an-tēr′ē-ŏr branch) [TA] Anatomic branch passing ventral or toward the front.

**an·te·ri·or can·al·ic·u·lus of chor·da tym·pa·ni** (an-tēr′ē-ŏr kan′ă-lik′yū-lŭs kōr′dă tim-pan′ī) Canal in the petrotympanic fissure, near its posterior edge, through which the chorda tympani nerve issues from the skull.

**an·te·ri·or ce·re·bral ar·te·ry** (an-tēr′ē-ŏr ser′ĕ-brăl ahr′tĕr-ē) [TA] One of two terminal branches (with middle cerebral artery) of internal carotid; passes anteriorly, loops around the genu of the corpus callosum, and then passes posteriorly in the longitudinal fissure along with its fellow of the opposite side, the two being joined by the anterior communicating artery [TA].

**an·te·ri·or ce·re·bral veins** (an-tēr′ē-ŏr ser′ĕ-brăl vānz) [TA] Small veins that parallel the anterior cerebral artery and drain into the basal vein.

**an·te·ri·or cer·vic·al re·gion** (an-tēr′ē-ŏr sĕr′vi-kăl rē′jŏn) [TA] Area of the neck bounded by the mandible, anterior border of the sternocleidomastoid muscle, and the anterior midline of the neck. SYN anterior triangle of the neck, regio cervicalis anterior, trigonum cervicale anterius, trigonium colli anterius, amterior region of the neck.

**an·te·ri·or cham·ber of eye·ball** (an-tēr′ē-ŏr chăm′bĕr ī′bawl) [TA] Space between cornea anteriorly and the iris/pupil posteriorly, filled with a watery fluid (aqueous humor).

**an·te·ri·or cham·ber tra·bec·u·la** (an-tēr′ē-ŏr chăm′bĕr tră-bek′yū-lă) Tissue at the angle of the anterior chamber through which aqueous humor exits from the eye.

**an·te·ri·or cli·noid pro·cess** (an-tēr′ē-ŏr klin′oyd pros′es) [TA] Posteriorly directed projection that is the medial end of the sphenoidal ridge (lesser wing of sphenoid); it provides attachment for the free edge of the tentorium cerebelli.

**an·te·ri·or com·po·nent of force** (an-tēr′ē-ŏr kŏm-pō′nĕnt fōrs) Force operating to move teeth anteriorly.

**an·te·ri·or con·dy·loid fo·ra·men** (an-tēr′ē-ŏr kon′di-loyd fōr-ā′mĕn) SYN hypoglossal canal.

**an·te·ri·or cra·ni·al fos·sa** (an-tēr′ē-ŏr krā′nē-ăl fos′ă) [TA] Portion of internal base of skull, anterior to the sphenoidal ridges and limbus, in which cerebral frontal lobes rest.

**an·te·ri·or cross-bite** (an-tēr′ē-ŏr kraws′bīt) An abnormal relationship wherein the maxillary and mandibular anterior teeth occlude with the opposing teeth in an opposite relationship with the opposing (i.e., antagonistic) teeth.

**an·te·ri·or eth·moi·dal ar·te·ry** (an-tēr′ē-ŏr eth-moyd′ăl ahr′tĕr-ē) [TA] *Origin*, ophthalmic; *distribution*, central dura mater of anterior cranial fossa, anterior ethmoidal cells, frontal sinus, anterior upper part of nasal mucous membrane, skin of dorsum of nose.

**an·te·ri·or eth·moid·al cells** (an-tēr′ē-ŏr eth-moy′dăl selz) [TA] Group of air cells of the ethmoidal sinuses; each communicates with the middle meatus of the nasal cavity.

**an·te·ri·or eth·moid·al nerve** (an-tēr′ē-ŏr eth-moyd′ăl nĕrv) [TA] Branch of the nasociliary nerve; passes through the anterior ethmoidal foramen on the superomedial wall of orbit into the cranial cavity, giving rise to anterior meningeal nerves, then passes through the cribriform plates into the nasal cavity, supplying the anterosuperior nasal mucosa.

**an·te·ri·or fa·cial height (AFH)** (an-tēr′ē-ŏr fā′shăl hīt) In cephalometrics, linear measurement from nasion to menton.

**an·te·ri·or fa·cial vein** (an-tēr′ē-ŏr fā′shăl vān) SYN facial vein.

**an·te·ri·or fas·ci·cle of pa·la·to·pha·ryn·ge·us (mus·cle)** (an-tēr′ē-ŏr fas′i-kĕl pal′ă-tō-fă-rin′jē-ŭs mŭs′ĕl) [TA] Thicker portion of the muscle of the palatopharyngeal arch that passes forward between the levator and tensor veli palatini muscles to attach to posterior border of hard palate and palatine aponeurosis.

**an·te·ri·or glan·du·lar branch of su·pe·ri·or thy·roid ar·te·ry** (an-tēr′ē-ŏr gland′yū-lăr branch sŭ-pēr′ē-ŏr thī′royd ahr′tĕr-ē) One of three branches of the superior thyroid artery to the thyroid gland; anterior glandular branch supplies anterosuperior portion.

**an·te·ri·or guide** (an-tēr′ē-ŏr gīd) SYN incisal guide.

**an·te·ri·or horn** (an-tēr′ē-ŏr hōrn) [TA] **1.** [TA] Frontal or anterior division of the lateral ventricle of the brain, extending forward from the interventricular (Monro) foramen. **2.** Anterior horn or anterior (ventral) gray column of the spinal cord as appearing in cross-section.

**an·te·ri·or in·fe·ri·or cer·e·bel·lar ar·te·ry** (an-tēr′ē-ŏr in-fēr′ē-ŏr ser′ĕ-bel′ăr ahr′tĕr-ē) [TA] *Origin*, basilar artery; *distribution*, inferior surface of lateral lobes of cerebellum, choroid plexus in cerebellopontine angle; *anastomoses*, posterior inferior cerebellar; usual source of labyrinthine artery.

**an·te·ri·or lac·ri·mal crest** (an-tēr′ē-ŏr lak′ri-măl krest) [TA] Vertical ridge on lateral surface of frontal process of maxilla that forms part of medial rim of orbit.

**an·te·ri·or la·ter·al na·sal branch·es of an·te·ri·or eth·moid·al ar·te·ry** (an-tēr′ē-ŏr lat′ĕr-ăl nā′zăl branch′ĕz an-tēr′ē-ŏr eth-moy′dăl ahr′tĕr-ē) [TA] Branches of the intracranial part of the anterior ethmoidal artery that pass through the cribriform plates of the ethmoid bone, descending into the nasal cavity with the anterior ethmoidal nerves, to run in a groove on the deep surface of the nasal bone and supply the anterosuperior aspect of the lateral wall of the cavity.

**an·te·ri·or lig·a·ment of mal·le·us** (an-tēr´ē-ŏr lig´ă-mĕnt mal´ē-ŭs) [TA] Ligament consisting of two portions: Meckel band, passing from the base of the anterior process to the spine of the sphenoid through the petrotympanic fissure and anterior ligament of Helmholtz, extending from the anterior aspect of the neck of the malleus to the anterior boundary of the tympanic notch.

**an·te·ri·or lin·gual gland** (an-tēr´ē-ŏr ling´gwăl gland) Small mixed gland deeply placed near the apex of the tongue on each side of the frenulum. SYN apical gland, Bauhin gland, Blandin gland.

**an·te·ri·or me·nin·ge·al branch (of an·te·ri·or eth·moid·al ar·te·ry)** (an-tēr´ē-ŏr mĕ-nin´jē-ăl branch an-tēr´ē-ŏr ethmoy´dăl ahr´tĕr-ē) [TA] *Origin*, anterior ethmoidal; *distribution*, meninges in anterior cranial fossa; *anastomoses*, branches of middle meningeal and meningeal branches of internal carotid and lacrimal.

**an·te·ri·or na·ris** (an-tēr´ē-ŏr nar´is) SYN naris.

**an·te·ri·or na·sal spine of max·il·la** (an-tēr´ē-ŏr nā´zăl spīn mak-sil´ă) [TA] Pointed projection at anterior extremity of the intermaxillary suture.

**an·te·ri·or notch of aur·i·cle** (an-tēr´ē-ŏr noch awr´i-kĕl) [TA] Notch between the supratragic tubercle and the crus of the helix. SYN anterior auricular groove.

**an·te·ri·or oc·clu·sion** (an-tēr´ē-ŏr ŏ-klū´zhŭn) **1.** Occlusion of anterior teeth. **2.** SYN mesial occlusion.

**an·te·ri·or pal·a·tal bar** (an-tēr´ē-ŏr pal´ă-tăl bahr) Part of a partial denture framework that rests against the anterior palate. [L., before, fr. *ante-*, before, + *-ior*, comparative suffix]

**an·te·ri·or pal·a·tal ma·jor con·nec·tor** (an-tēr´ē-ŏr pal´ă-tăl mā´jŏr kŏ-nek´tŏr) Thin plate in the region of the anterior palate connecting opposite sides of a maxillary removable partial denture.

**an·te·ri·or pal·a·tine arch** (an-tēr´ē-ŏr pal´ă-tīn ahrch) SYN palatoglossal arch.

**an·te·ri·or pal·a·tine for·a·men** (an-tēr´ē-ŏr pal´ă-tīn fōr-ā´mĕn) SYN greater palatine foramen.

**an·te·ri·or pa·ri·e·tal ar·te·ry** (an-tēr´ē-ŏr pă-rī´ē-tăl ahr´tĕr-ē) [TA] One of terminal branches of insular part of middle cerebral artery, distributed to anterior part of parietal lobe.

**an·te·ri·or part** (an-tēr´ē-ŏr pahrt) [TA] Portion of a structure that lies most forward, or closest to the front surface, relative to other parts; in human anatomy, the ventral portion of a structure.

**an·te·ri·or part of tongue** (an-tēr´ē-ŏr pahrt tŭng) [TA] Portion (about two thirds) of tongue anterior to the sulcus terminalis, distinct from the posterior part in embryologic origin and innervation.

**an·te·ri·or pil·lar of fau·ces** (an-tēr´ē-ŏr pil´ăr faw´sēz) SYN palatoglossal arch.

**an·te·ri·or pi·tu·i·tar·y go·nad·o·tro·pin** (an-tēr´ē-ŏr pi-tū´i-tār-ē gō-nad´ō-trō´pin) Gonadotropin of hypophysial origin.

**an·te·ri·or ra·mus of la·ter·al cer·e·bral sul·cus** (an-tēr´ē-ŏr rā´mŭs lat´ĕr-ăl ser´ē-brăl sŭl´kŭs) Those portions of the lateral sulcus extending into, and dividing, the inferior frontal gyrus into its parts.

**an·te·ri·or seg·ment** (an-tēr´ē-ŏr seg´mĕnt) [TA] Delimited part or section of an organ or other structure that lies in front of or ventral to similar parts or sections.

**an·te·ri·or sem·i·cir·cu·lar ca·nal** (an-tēr´ē-ŏr sem´ē-sĭr´kyū-lăr kă-nal´) SEE semicircular canals (of bony labyrinth).

**an·te·ri·or sep·tal branch·es of an·te·ri·or eth·moid·al ar·te·ry** (an-tēr´ē-ŏr sep´tăl branch´ĕz an-tēr´ē-ŏr eth-moy´dăl ahr´tĕr-ē) [TA] Branches of intracranial part of the anterior ethmoidal artery that pass through the cribriform plate of the ethmoid bone, descending into the nasal cavity with the anterior ethmoidal nerves and supply anterosuperior aspect of the nasal septum.

**an·te·ri·or su·pe·ri·or al·ve·o·lar ar·te·ries** (an-tēr´ē-ŏr sŭ-pēr´ē-ŏr al-vē´ō-lăr ahr´tĕr-ēz) [TA] *Origin*, infraorbital artery within intraorbital canal; *distribution*, through anterior alveolar canals to upper incisors and canine teeth, mucous membrane of maxillary sinus. SYN anterior superior dental arteries, arteriae alveolares superiores anteriore.

**an·te·ri·or su·pe·ri·or al·ve·o·lar branch·es of in·fra·or·bit·al nerve** (an-tēr´ē-ŏr sŭ-pēr´ē-ŏr al-vē´ō-lăr branch´ĕz in´fră-ŏr´bi-tăl nĕrv) SYN anterior superior alveolar branches of superior alveolar nerve.

**an·te·ri·or su·pe·ri·or al·ve·o·lar branch·es of su·pe·ri·or al·ve·o·lar nerve** (an-tēr´ē-ŏr sŭ-pēr´ē-ŏr al-vē´ō-lăr branch´ĕz sŭ-pēr´ē-ŏr al-vē´ō-lăr nĕrv) [TA] Branches of superior alveolar nerve that supply the incisors, canines, premolars, and first molars by their contributions to the superior dental plexus. SYN anterior superior alveolar branches of infraorbital nerve.

**an·te·ri·or su·pe·ri·or den·tal ar·te·ries** (an-tēr′ē-ŏr sŭ-pēr′ē-ŏr den′tăl ahr′tĕr-ēz) SYN anterior superior alveolar arteries.

**an·te·ri·or su·pe·ri·or il·i·ac spine** (an-tēr′ē-ŏr sŭ-pēr′ē-ŏr il′ē-ak spīn) [TA] Anterior extremity of iliac crest, which provides attachment for the inguinal ligament and the sartorius muscle.

**an·te·ri·or sur·face of max·il·la** (an-tēr′ē-ŏr sŭr′făs mak-sil′ă) [TA] Surface of maxilla below the orbit and lateral to the nasal aperture.

**an·te·ri·or sur·face of pet·rous part of tem·po·ral bone** (an-tēr′ē-ŏr sŭr′făs pet′rŭs pahrt tem′pŏr-ăl bōn) [TA] Surface of the petrous part of the temporal bone contributing to floor of middle cranial fossa.

**an·te·ri·or tem·po·ral di·plo·ic vein** (an-tēr′ē-ŏr tem′pŏr-ăl dip-lō′ik vān) [TA] Vein with tributaries in spongy bone of posterior part of frontal and anterior part of parietal bones that penetrates inner table of bone of greater wing of sphenoid to enter sphenoparietal dural venous sinus or anterior deep temporal vein.

**an·te·ri·or tooth** (an-tēr′ē-ŏr tūth) Central incisor, lateral incisor, or cuspid tooth. Such teeth are the organs for incision and are located in the front portion of the jaws. SYN oral teeth.

**an·te·ri·or tym·pan·ic ar·te·ry** (an-tēr′ē-ŏr tim-pan′ik ahr′tĕr-ē) [TA] *Origin*, first (retromandibular) part of the maxillary; *distribution*, middle ear; *anastomoses*, tympanic branches of internal carotid and ascending pharyngeal and stylomastoid.

**an·te·ri·or vein** (an-tēr′ē-ŏr vān) [TA] Tributary of right or left superior pulmonary vein draining oxygenated blood from the anterior part of the superior lobe of the right or left lung.

**an·te·ri·or ves·ti·bu·lar ar·te·ry** (an-tēr′ē-ŏr ves-tib′yŭ-lăr ahr′tĕr-ē) [TA] *Origin:* as a terminal branch, with common cochlear artery, of labyrinthine artery; *branch:* vestibulocochlear artery; *distribution:* to vestibular ganglion, utricle and (especially the ampullae of the) lateral and posterior semicircular ducts.

**an·te·ri·or wall of mid·dle ear** (an-tēr′ē-ŏr wawl mid′ĕl ēr) SYN carotid wall of tympanic cavity.

♻ **antero-** Combining form denoting anterior. [L. *anterior*, more before, earlier, fr. *ante*, before, + -r- *-ior*, more]

**an·ter·o·ex·ter·nal** (an′tĕr-ō-eks-tĕr′năl) In front and to the outer side.

**an·ter·o·fa·cial dys·pla·si·a** (an′tĕr-ō-fā′shăl dis-plā′zē-ă) Abnormal growth of the face or cranium in an anteroposterior direction

as seen and measured with a cephalogram. SYN anteroposterior facial dysplasia, anteroposterior dysplasia.

**an·ter·o·grade** (an′tĕr-ō-grād) Moving forward. Cf. antegrade. [L. *gradior*, pp. *gressus*, to step, go]

**an·ter·o·in·fe·ri·or, an·ter·i·or-in·fer·i·or** (an′tĕr-ō-in-fēr′ē-ŏr, an-tēr′ē-ŏr-in-fēr′ē-ŏr) In front of and below.

**an·ter·o·in·ter·nal** (an′tĕr-ō-in-tĕr′năl) In front of and to the inner side.

**an·ter·o·lat·er·al** (an′tĕr-ō-lat′ĕr-ăl) In front of and away from the middle line.

**an·ter·o·me·di·al** (an′tĕr-ō-mē′dē-ăl) In front of and toward the middle line.

**an·ter·o·me·di·al fron·tal branch of cal·lo·so·mar·gi·nal ar·te·ry** (an′tĕr-ō-mē′dē-ăl frŭn′tăl branch kă-lō′sō-mahr′ji-năl ahr′tĕr-ē) [TA] Branch of initial portion of callosomarginal artery to anteroinferior portion of medial aspect of frontal lobe of cerebrum.

**an·ter·o·me·di·al in·ter·mus·cu·lar sep·tum** [TA] Dense fascial triangle extending from the inferior medial border of the adductor magnus muscle to the vastus medialis muscle.

**an·ter·o·me·di·an** (an′tĕr-ō-mē′dē-ăn) In front of and in the central line.

**an·ter·o·pos·te·ri·or, an·te·ri·or-pos·te·ri·or (AP)** (an′tĕr-ō-pos-tēr′ē-ŏr, an-tē′rē-ŏr-pos-tē′rē-ŏr) 1. Relating to both front and rear. 2. In x-ray imaging, describing the direction of the beam through the patient (projection) from anterior to posterior.

**an·ter·o·pos·te·ri·or dis·crep·an·cy** (an′tĕr-ō-pos-tēr′ē-ŏr dis-krep′ăn-sē) Misalignment of maxilla and mandible or their teeth in an anteroposterior direction.

**an·ter·o·pos·te·ri·or dys·pla·si·a** (an′tĕr-ō-pos-tēr′ē-ŏr dis-plā′zē-ă) SYN anterofacial dysplasia.

**an·ter·o·pos·te·ri·or fa·cial dys·pla·si·a** (an′tĕr-ō-pos-tēr′ē-ŏr fā′shăl dis-plā′zē-ă) SYN anterofacial dysplasia.

**an·ter·o·su·pe·ri·or** (an′tĕr-ō-sŭ-pēr′ē-ŏr) In front of and above.

**an·te·ver·sion** (an′tĕ-vĕr′zhŭn) Forward displacement or turning forward of a body segment. [*ante*- + Mediev. L. *versio*, a turning]

**an·thrax** (an′thraks) A disease in humans caused by infection with *Bacillus anthracis;* marked by hemorrhage and serous effusions and symptoms of extreme prostration. [G. *anthrax* (*anthrak*-), charcoal, coal, a carbuncle]

**anthropo-** *Distinguish this combining form from andro-.* Combining form denoting involving human beings. [G. *anthrōpos,* a human being (of either sex)]

**an·thro·pol·o·gy** (an'thrŏ-pol'ŏ-jē) Branch of science concerned with origin and development of humans in all their physical, social, and cultural relationships. [*anthropo-* + G. *logos,* treatise]

**an·thro·pom·e·try** (an'thrŏ-pom'ĕ-trē) The branch of anthropology concerned with comparative measurements of the human body. [*anthropo-* + G. *metron,* measure]

**anti-** *Do not confuse this prefix with ante-.* **1.** Combining form meaning against, opposing, or, in relation to symptoms and diseases, curative. **2.** Combining form denoting an antibody (immunoglobulin) specific for the thing indicated; e.g., antitoxin (antibody specific for a toxin). [G. *anti,* against, opposite, instead of]

**an·ti·bi·ot·ic** (an'tē-bī-ot'ik) *Avoid the jargonistic use of the plural antibiotics when the reference is to a single drug.* Soluble substance derived from a mold or bacterium that kills or inhibits growth of other microorganisms.

**an·ti·bi·ot·ic en·ter·o·col·i·tis** (an'tē-bī-ot'ik en'tĕr-ō-kŏ-lī'tis) Disorder caused by oral administration of broad-spectrum antibiotics.

**an·ti·bi·ot·ic pre·med·i·ca·tion** (an'tē-bī-ot'ik prē-med'i-kā'shŭn) Antibiotic therapy given before clinical procedures that can induce transient bacteremia, which, in turn, can cause infective endocarditis or other serious infection.

**an·ti·bi·ot·ic proph·y·lax·is** (an'tē-bī-ot'ik prō'fi-lak'sis) SYN prophylactic antibiotic.

**an·ti·bi·ot·ic sen·si·tiv·i·ty** (an'tē-bī-ot'ik sen'si-tiv'tē) Microbial susceptibility to antibiotics.

**an·ti·bi·ot·ic spec·trum** (an'tē-bī-ot'ik spek'trŭm) The range of microorganisms that an antibiotic agent inhibits or kills. SEE antibiotic, antimicrobial agent, dental plaque, biofilm.

**an·ti·bi·ot·ic tongue** (an'tē-bī-ot'ik tŭng) Glossitis caused by antibiotics; may result from hypersensitivity or disturbance of oral microflora.

**an·ti·blen·nor·rhag·ic** (an'tē-blen-ō-raj'ik) Agent to prevent or resolve mucous discharge (blennorrhagia).

**an·ti·bod·y (Ab)** (an'ti-bod-ē) *Avoid the jargonistic use of the plural antibodies when the reference is to a single antibody species.* An immunoglobulin molecule produced by B-lymphoid cells that combine specifically with an immunogen or antigen. Antibodies may be present naturally; their specificity is determined through gene rearrangement or somatic replacement or may be synthesized in response to stimulus provided by the introduction of an antigen.

**an·ti·cal·cu·lous** (an'tē-kal'kyū-lŭs) SYN antilithic.

**an·ti·car·i·o·gen·ic** (an'tē-kar'ē-ō-jen'ik) Denotes those foods or medications that inhibit caries development and may encourage mineralization.

**an·ti·car·i·ous** (an'tē-kār'ē-ŭs) Preventing or inhibiting caries.

**an·ti·cho·lin·er·gic** (an'tē-kō'li-nĕr'jik) Antagonistic to the action of parasympathetic or other cholinergic nerve fibers (e.g., atropine).

**an·ti·cho·lin·er·gic a·gent** (an'tē-kō-li-nĕr'jik ā'jĕnt) Drug that inhibits action of acetylcholine or cholinergic drugs at cholinergic receptors. SYN cholinergic blocking agent.

**an·ti·cho·lin·es·ter·ase** (an'tē-kō-lin-es'tĕr-ās) A drug that inhibits or inactivates acetylcholinesterase, either reversibly (e.g., physostigmine) or irreversibly (e.g., tetraethyl pyrophosphate).

**an·ti·cli·nal** (an'tē-klī'năl) Inclined in opposite directions, as two sides of a pyramid. [*anti-* + G. *klinō,* to incline]

**an·ti·co·ag·u·lant** (an'tē-kō-ag'yŭ-lănt) An agent that prevents coagulation (e.g., warfarin).

**an·ti·co·ag·u·lant ther·a·py** (an'tē-kō-ag'yŭ-lănt thār'ă-pē) Use of anticoagulant drugs to reduce or prevent intravascular or intracardiac clotting.

**an·ti·con·vul·sant** (an'tē-kŏn-vŭl'sănt) **1.** Preventing or arresting seizures. **2.** An agent having such action. SYN anticonvulsive.

**an·ti·con·vul·sive** (an'tē-kŏn-vŭl'siv) SYN anticonvulsant.

**an·ti·de·pres·sant** (an'tē-dĕ-pres'ănt) **1.** Counteracting depression. **2.** A pharmacologic agent used in treating depression.

**an·ti·di·a·bet·ic** (an'tē-dī-ă-bet'ik) Counteracting diabetes; denoting an agent that reduces blood sugar (e.g., tolbutamide, insulin).

**an·ti·di·ar·rhe·al, an·ti·di·ar·rhet·ic** (an'tē-dī-ă-rē'ăl, an'tē-dī'ă-ret'ik) **1.** Having the property of opposing or correcting diarrhea. **2.** An agent having such action (e.g., loperamide). SYN antidiarrhoeal.

**antidiarrhoeal** [Br.] SYN antidiarrheal.

**an·ti·di·u·ret·ic hor·mone** (an'tē-dī-yŭr-et'ik hōr'mōn, an'tē-dī-yŭr-et'ik hōr'mōn) SEE ALSO vasopressor. SYN vasopressin.

**an·ti·dot·al** (an'ti-dō'tăl) Relating to or acting as an antidote.

**an·ti·dote** (an'ti-dōt) An agent that neutralizes a poison or counteracts its clinical or physiologic effects. [G. *antidotos,* fr. *anti,* against, + *dotos,* what is given, fr. *didōmi,* to give]

**an·ti·e·met·ic** (an'tē-ĕ-met'ik) **1.** Preventing or arresting vomiting. **2.** A remedy that tends to control nausea and vomiting. [*anti-* + G. *emetikos,* emetic]

**an·ti·feb·rile** (an'tē-feb'ril) SYN antipyretic (1). [*anti-* + L. *febris,* fever]

**an·ti·flux** (an'tē-flŭks) In dentistry, a material that prevents flow of solder.

**an·ti·fun·gal** (an'tē-fŭng'ăl) SYN antimycotic.

**an·ti·gen** (an'ti-jen) Any substance that, as a result of coming in contact with appropriate cells, induces a state of sensitivity or immune responsiveness and reacts in a demonstrable way with antibodies or immune cells of the sensitized subject in vivo or in vitro. [*anti*(body) + G. *-gen,* producing]

**an·ti·gen·ic drift** (an'ti-jen'ik drift) The process of "evolutionary" changes in molecular structure of DNA/RNA in microorganisms during their passage from one host to another; affecting the immunologic responses of people and populations to exposure to the microorganism concerned.

**an·ti-HB$_s$** (an'tē) Antibody to the hepatitis B surface antigen (HB$_s$Ag).

**an·ti·he·li·cal fos·sa** (an'tē-hel'ĭ-kăl fos'ă) [TA] SYN fossa antihelica.

**an·ti·he·lix, ant·he·lix** (an'tē-hē'liks, anthē'liks) [TA] An elevated ridge of cartilage anterior and roughly parallel to the posterior portion of the helix of the external ear.

**an·ti·his·ta·mines** (an'tē-his'tă-mēnz) Drugs having an action antagonistic to that of histamine on either H$_1$ or H$_2$ receptors.

**an·ti·his·ta·min·ic** (an'tē-his-tă-min'ik) **1.** An agent that antagonizes actions of histamine. **2.** An agent that relieves symptoms of allergy (H$_1$ antagonist) or gastric hyperacidity (H$_2$ antagonist).

**an·ti·hy·per·ten·sive** (an'tē-hī-pĕr-ten'siv) Indicating a drug or treatment that reduces the blood pressure of hypertensive patients.

**an·ti·hyp·not·ic, ant·hyp·not·ic** (an'tē-hip-not'ik, ant'hip-) **1.** Preventing or tending to prevent sleep. **2.** An arousing agent, or one antagonistic to sleep.

**an·ti·hy·po·ten·sive** (an'tē-hī'pō-ten'siv) Any measure or medication that tends to raise reduced blood pressure.

**an·ti·in·flam·ma·to·ry** (an'tē-in-flam'ă-tōr-ē) Reducing inflammation by acting on body responses, without directly antagonizing the causative agent; denoting agents such as glucocorticoids and aspirin.

**an·ti·leu·ko·tri·ene** (an'tē-lū-ko-trī'ēn) A drug that prevents or alleviates bronchoconstriction in asthma by blocking the production or action of naturally occurring leukotrienes; may also be useful in psoriasis.

**an·ti·lith·ic** (an'tē-lith'ik) **1.** Preventing the formation of calculi or promoting their dissolution. **2.** An agent so acting. SYN anticalculous. [*anti-* + G. *lithos,* stone]

**an·ti·mi·cro·bi·al** (an'tē-mī-krō'bē-ăl) Tending to destroy microbes, to prevent their multiplication or growth, or to prevent their pathogenic action.

**an·ti·mi·cro·bi·al a·gent** (an'tē-mī-krō'bē-ăl ā'jĕnt) Therapeutic that kills or suppresses the growth of microorganisms.

**an·ti·mi·cro·bi·al soap** (an'tē-mī-krō'bē-ăl sōp) Cleansing agent containing an ingredient inhibitory to microorganisms.

**an·ti·mi·cro·bi·al ther·a·py** (an'tē-mī-krō'bē-ăl thār'ă-pē) Use of specific chemical or pharmaceutical agents to control or destroy microorganisms, either systemically or at specific sites.

**an·ti-Mon·son curve** (an'tē-mon'sŏn kŭrv) SYN reverse curve.

**an·ti·mo·ny** (an'ti-mō-nē) *Do not confuse this word with antinomy.* A metallic element used in alloys; toxic and irritating to the skin and mucous membranes. [G. *anti + monos,* not found alone]

**an·ti·mo·ny po·tas·si·um tar·trate** (an'ti-mō-nē pŏ-tas'ē-ŭm tahr'trāt) A potentially toxic compound used as an expectorant and to treat schistosomiasis japonicum.

**an·ti·my·cot·ic** (an'tē-mī-kot'ik) Antagonistic to fungi. SYN antifungal. [*anti-* + G. *mykēs,* fungus]

**an·ti·nau·se·ant** (an'tē-naw'zē-ănt) Having properties or action to prevent nausea.

**an·ti·ne·o·plas·tic** (an'tē-nē'ō-plas'tik) Preventing the development, maturation, or spread of neoplastic cells.

**an·tin·i·on** (an-tin'ē-on) Space between eyebrows; point on cranium opposite inion. [*anti-* + G. *inion,* nape of the neck]

**an·tin·o·my** (an-tin'ŏ-mē) *Do not confuse this word with antimony.* A contradiction between two principles, each of which is considered true. [*anti-* + G. *nomos,* law]

**an·ti·nu·cle·ar an·ti·bod·y, an·ti·nu·cle·ar fac·tor (ANA, ANF)** (an'tē-nū'klē-ăr an'ti-bod-ē, fak'tŏr) An antibody showing an affinity for cell nuclei, demonstrated by exposing a cell substrate to the serum to be tested, followed by exposure to an antihuman-globulin serum; found in the serum of a high proportion of patients with systemic lupus erythematosus, rheumatoid arthritis, and some collagen diseases.

**an·ti·o·don·tal·gic** (an'tē-ō'don-tăl'jik) **1.** Relieving toothache. **2.** A toothache remedy. [*anti-* + G. *odous,* tooth, + *algos,* pain]

**an·ti·ox·i·dant** (an'tē-ok'si-dănt) An agent that inhibits oxidation; one of many chemical substances including some natural body products that can neutralize the oxidant effect of free radicals and other substances.

**an·ti·par·a·sit·ic** (an'tē-par-ă-sit'ik) Destructive to parasites.

**an·ti·pe·ri·od·ic** (an'tē-pēr'ē-od'ik) Preventing the regular recurrence of a disease (e.g., malaria) or symptom.

**an·ti·phlo·gis·tic** (an'tē-flō-jis'tik) **1.** Older term denoting the capacity to prevent or relieve inflammation. **2.** Agent that reduces inflammation and fever. [*anti-* + G. *phogistos,* burnt up]

**an·ti·plaque** (an'tē-plak') A drug or compound that inhibits or prevents buildup of dental plaque. SEE dental plaque, biofilm. [G. *anti-* against, + plaque, fr. Middle D. *plakke*]

**an·ti·pru·rit·ic** (an'tē-prūr-it'ik) **1.** Preventing or relieving itching. **2.** An agent that relieves itching.

**an·ti·psy·chot·ic** (an'tē-sī-kot'ik) **1.** SYN antipsychotic agent. **2.** Denoting the actions of such an agent (e.g., chlorpromazine).

**an·ti·psy·chot·ic a·gent** (an'tē-sī-kot'ik ā'jĕnt) Category of neuroleptic drugs that are helpful in the treatment of psychosis and have a capacity to ameliorate thought disorders. SYN antipsychotic (1).

**an·ti·py·o·gen·ic** (an'tē-pī'ō-jen'ik) Preventing suppuration. [*anti-* + G. *pyon,* pus, + *-gen,* production]

**an·ti·py·ret·ic** (an'tē-pī-ret'ik) **1.** Reducing fever. SYN antifebrile, febrifugal. **2.** An agent that reduces fever (e.g., acetaminophen, aspirin). [*anti-* + G. *pyretos,* fever]

**an·ti·py·rine** (an'tē-pī'rin) An analgesic and antipyretic, used topically as an analgesic in acute otitis media and to loosen cerumen from the external auditory canal.

**an·ti·py·rine sal·i·cyl·ac·e·tate** (an'tē-pī'rin să-lis'il-as'ĕ-tāt) An analgesic, antirheumatic, and antipyretic.

**an·ti·scor·bu·tic** (an'tē-skōr-byū'tik) **1.** Preventing or curing scurvy (scorbutus). **2.** A treatment for scurvy (e.g., vitamin C).

**an·ti·se·cre·to·ry** (an'tē-sĕ-krē'tŏr-ē) Inhibitory to secretion.

**an·ti·sep·sis** (an'ti-sep'sis) Prevention of infection by inhibiting the growth of infectious agents. SEE ALSO disinfection. [*anti-* + G. *sēpsis,* putrefaction]

**an·ti·sep·tic** (an'ti-sep'tik) *Do not confuse this word with aseptic.* **1.** Relating to antisepsis. **2.** An agent or substance capable of effecting antisepsis.

**an·ti·sep·tic dress·ing** (an'ti-sep'tik dres' ing) Sterile gauze bandage impregnated with an antiseptic.

**an·ti·si·al·a·gogue** (an'tē-sī-al'ă-gog) *Avoid the misspelling antisialogogue.* An agent that diminishes or arrests the flow of saliva (e.g., atropine). [*anti-* + G. *sialon,* saliva, + *agōgos,* drawing forth]

**an·ti·spas·mod·ic** (an'tē-spaz-mod'ik) **1.** Preventing or alleviating muscle spasms (cramps). **2.** An agent that quiets spasm.

**an·ti·te·tan·ic** (an'tē-te-tan'ik) *Avoid the mispronunciation antitet'anic.* Preventing or alleviating muscular contraction.

**an·ti·ton·ic** (an'tē-ton'ik) Diminishing muscular or vascular tonus.

**an·ti·tox·ic** (an'tē-tok'sik) Neutralizing the action of a poison; specifically, relating to an antitoxin. SEE ALSO antidotal.

**an·ti·tox·in** (an'tē-tok'sin) Antibody formed in response to antigenic poisonous substances of biologic origin; in general usage, antitoxin refers to whole, or globulin fraction of, serum from people immunized by injections of the specific toxoid. [*anti-* + G. *toxikon,* poison]

**an·ti·trag·i·cus (mus·cle)** (an'tē-traj'ĭ-kŭs mŭs'ĕl) [TA] Band of transverse muscular fibers on outer surface of antitragus, arising from border of intertragic notch and inserted into antihelix and tail of helix.

**an·ti·tra·go·hel·i·cine fis·sure** (an'tē-trā'gō-hel'ĭ-sēn fish'ŭr) SYN fissura antitrago-helicina.

**an·ti·tra·gus** (an'tē-trā'gŭs) [TA] Projection of cartilage of auricle, in front of tail of helix, just above lobule, and posterior to tragus from which it is separated by intertragic notch. [G. *anti-tragos,* the eminence of the external ear, fr. *anti,* opposite, + *tragos,* a goat, the tragus]

**an·ti·tris·mus** (an'tē-triz'mŭs) A condition of tonic muscular spasm that prevents closing of the mouth.

**an·ti·tus·sive** (an'tē-tŭs'iv) **1.** Relieving cough. **2.** A cough remedy (e.g., codeine). [*anti-* + L. *tussis,* cough]

**an·ti·vi·ral** (an'tē-vī'răl) Opposing a virus; interfering with its replication; weakening or halting its action (e.g., zidovudine, acyclovir).

**an·tral** (an'trăl) Relating to an antrum.

**an·tro·na·sal** (an'trō-nā'zăl) Relating to a maxillary sinus and the corresponding nasal cavity.

**an·tro·scope** (an'trō-skōp) An instrument used to visualize a cavity, particularly the maxillary sinus. [G. *antron*, cave + G. *skopeō*, to view]

**an·tros·co·py** (an-tros'kŏ-pē) Examination of any cavity, particularly the maxillary sinus, by means of an antroscope.

**an·tros·to·my** (an-tros'tŏ-mē) Formation of a permanent opening into any antrum. [G. *antron*, cave + G. *stoma*, mouth]

**an·tro·tym·pan·ic** (an'trō-tim-pan'ik) Relating to the mastoid antrum and the tympanic cavity.

**an·trum,** pl. **an·tra** (an'trŭm, -tră) [TA] *Do not confuse this word with atrium.* Any nearly or relatively closed cavity. [L. fr. G. *antron*, a cave]

**an·trum au·ris** (an'trŭm aw'ris) SYN external acoustic meatus.

**an·trum mas·toi·de·um** (an'trŭm mastoy'dē-ŭm) [TA] SYN mastoid antrum.

**an·trum of High·more** (an'trŭm hī'mōr) SYN maxillary sinus.

**ANUG** Abbreviation for acute necrotizing ulcerative gingivitis.

**an·u·lar, an·nu·lar** (an'yū-lăr) Ring-shaped.

**an·u·ric** (ă-nyūr'ik) Relating to anuria.

**an·vil** (an'vil) SYN incus.

**anx·i·e·ty** (ang-zī'ĕ-tē) Experience of fear or apprehension in response to anticipated internal or external danger accompanied by a range of findings. It may be transient and adaptive or pathologic in intensity and duration. [L. *anxietas*, anxiety, fr. *anxius*, distressed, fr. *ango*, to press tight, to torment]

**anx·i·e·ty at·tack** (ang-zī'ĕ-tē ă-tak') Acute episode of anxiety.

**anx·i·e·ty dis·or·ders** (ang-zī'ĕ-tē dis-ōr'dĕrz) Disorders involving various manifestations of panic or nervosity.

**anx·i·e·ty neu·ro·sis** (ang-zī'ĕ-tē nūr-ō'sis) Chronic abnormal distress and worry to the point of panic followed by a tendency to avoid or run from the feared situation, associated with overaction of the sympathetic nervous system.

**anx·i·e·ty re·ac·tion** (ang-zī'ĕ-tē rē-ak'shŭn) Psychological reaction or experience involving the apprehension of danger accompanied by a feeling of dread and such physical symptoms. SYN acute stress reaction.

**anx·i·o·lyt·ic** (ang'zē-ō-lit'ik) **1.** SYN antianxiety agent. **2.** Denoting the actions of such an agent (e.g., diazepam). [*anxiety* + G. *lysis,* a dissolution or loosening]

**a·or·ta,** pl. **a·or·tae** (ā-ōr'tă, -tē) [TA] Large elastic artery that is the main trunk of the systemic arterial system, arising from base of left ventricle and ending at left side of body of fourth lumbar vertebra by dividing to form right and left common iliac arteries. [Mod. L. fr. G. *aortē*, from *aeirō*, to lift up]

**a·or·tic an·eur·ysm** (ā-ōr'tik an'yūr-izm) Diffuse or circumscribed dilation of a portion of the aorta (e.g., abdominal aortic aneurysm, aortic arch aneurysm).

**a·or·tic mur·mur** (ā-ōr'tik mŭr'mŭr) A murmur produced at the aortic orifice, either obstructive or regurgitant.

**a·or·tic valve** (ā-ōr'tik valv) [TA] The valve between the left ventricle and the ascending aorta, consisting of three fibrous semilunar cusps (valvules).

**a·or·ti·tis** (ā'ōr-tī'tis) Inflammation of the aorta.

**AP** Abbreviation for anteroposterior.

**apallaesthesia** [Br.] SYN apallesthesia.

**a·pall·es·the·si·a** (ă-pal'es-thē'zē-ă) SYN pallanesthesia, apallaesthesia. [G. *a-* priv. + *pallo,* to tremble, quiver, + *aisthēsis,* feeling]

**APAP** Abbreviation for acetaminophen.

**ap·a·thism** (ap'ă-thizm) A sluggishness of reaction.

**ap·a·thy** (ap'ă-thē) Indifference; absence of interest in the environment. Often one of the earliest signs of cerebral disease. [G. *apatheia,* fr. *a-* priv. + *pathos,* suffering]

**ap·a·tite** (ap'ă-tīt) Generic name for a class of minerals with compositions that are variants of the formula $D_5T_3M$, where D is a divalent cation, T is a trivalent tetrahedral compound ion, and M is a monovalent anion; calcium phosphate apatites are important mineral constituents of bones and teeth.

**a·per·i·od·ic** (ā'pēr-ē-od'ik) Not occurring periodically.

**a·per·i·tive** (ă-per'i-tiv) Stimulating the appetite. [Fr. *apéritif,* from L. *aperio,* to open]

**a·per·tog·nath·i·a** (a-per'tog-nā'thē-ă) *In the diphthong gn, the g is silent only at the beginning of a word.* An open-bite deformity, a type of malocclusion characterized by premature posterior occlusion and the absence of anterior occlusion. SYN open bite (2). [L. *apertus,* open, + G. *gnathos,* jaw]

**A·pert syn·drome** (ah-pār' sin´drōm) Disorder characterized by craniosynostosis and syndactyly of all the fingers and usually the toes as well; the thumbs are free; mental retardation is a variable feature. Autosomal dominant mutation with most cases sporadic, caused by mutation in the fibroblast growth factor receptor 2 gene (*FGFR2*) on 10q.

**ap·er·tu·ra,** pl. **ap·er·tu·rae** (ap-ĕr-tū´ră, -rē) [TA] SYN aperture (1). [L. fr. *aperio,* pp. *apertus,* to open]

**ap·er·tu·ra in·ter·na ca·nal·ic·u·li coch·le·ae** (ap´ĕr-tyūr´ă in-ter´nă kan´ă-lik´yū-lī kok´lē-ē) [TA] SYN internal opening of cochlear canaliculus.

**ap·er·tu·ra in·ter·na ca·nal·ic·u·li ves·tib·u·li** (ap´ĕr-tyūr´ă in-ter´nă kan´ă-lik´yū-lī ves-tib´yū-lī) [TA] SYN internal opening of vestibular canaliculus.

**ap·er·tu·ra in·ter·na ca·nal·is ca·rot·i·ci** (ap´ĕr-tyūr´ă in-ter´nă kā-nā´lis kah-rot´i-sī) [TA] SYN internal opening of carotid canal.

**ap·er·tu·ra na·sa·lis pos·te·ri·or** (ap´ĕr-tyūr´ă nā-sā´lis pos-tēr´ē-ŏr) SYN choana.

**ap·er·ture** (ap´ĕr-chŭr) [TA] **1.** [TA] Opening. An inlet or entrance to a cavity or channel. In anatomy, a gap or hole. SYN apertura. **2.** The diameter of the objective of a microscope. SEE ALSO fossa, ostium, orifice. SYN aditus [TA]. [L. *apertura,* an opening]

**a·pex,** pl. **ap·i·ces** (ā´peks, -i-sēz) [TA] The extremity of a conic or pyramidal structure. [L. summit or tip]

**a·pex au·ric·u·lae** (ā´peks aw-rik´yū-lē) [TA] SYN apex of auricle.

**a·pex cus·pi·dis den·tis** (ā´peks kŭs´pi-dis den´tis) [TA] SYN apex of cusp of tooth.

**a·pex den·tis** (ā´peks den´tis) [TA] SYN apex of dens.

**a·pex·i·fi·ca·tion** (ā-pek´si-fi-kā´shŭn) Treatment to induce formation of an incomplete apex with a necrotic pulp.

**a·pex·i·graph** (ā-pek´si-graf) Device for determining size and position of the apex of a tooth root. [*apex* + G. *graphō,* to write]

**a·pex lo·ca·tor** (ā´peks lō´kā-tŏr) Electronic device used to identify the vertex of the root canal.

**a·pex na·si** (ā´peks nā´sī) [TA] SYN apex of nose.

**a·pex of ar·y·te·noid car·ti·lage** (ā´peks ar´i-tē´noyd kahr´ti-lăj) [TA] Pointed upper end of cartilage that supports the corniculate cartilage and aryepiglottic fold.

**a·pex of au·ri·cle** (ā´peks aw´ri-kĕl) [TA] Point projecting upward and posteriorly from the free outcurved margin of the helix slightly posterior to its upper end. SEE ALSO auricular tubercle. SYN apex auriculae, apex satyri.

**a·pex of cusp of tooth** (ā´peks kŭsp tūth) [TA] Tip of the peaklike projections from the crown of a tooth. SYN apex cuspidis dentis.

**a·pex of dens** (ā´peks denz) [TA] Tip of dens of axis to which is attached the apical ligament of the dens. SYN apex dentis.

**a·pex of nose** (ā´peks nōz) [TA] Anteriormost pointed end of the external nose. SYN apex nasi.

**a·pex of or·bit** (ā´peks ōr´bit) Posterior part of orbit into which optic canal opens; forms tip of pyramidal space.

**a·pex of pet·rous part of tem·po·ral bone** (ā´peks pet´rŭs pahrt tem´pŏr-ăl bōn) [TA] The irregular anteromedial extremity of the petrous part on which the anterior end of the carotid canal opens. SYN apex partis petrosae ossis temporalis.

**a·pex of tongue** (ā´peks tŭng) [TA] Anterior extreme of tongue that can be made pointed for sensing or probing; rests against the lingual aspect of the incisor teeth.

**a·pex·o·gen·e·sis** (ā-pek´sō-jen´ĕ-sis) Normal development of apex of tooth root. [*apex-* + G. *genesis,* origin, birth]

**a·pex par·tis pe·tro·sae os·sis tem·po·ra·lis** (ā´peks pahr´tis pe-trō´sē os´is tem´pō-rā´lis) [TA] SYN apex of petrous part of temporal bone.

**a·pex ra·di·cis den·tis** (ā´peks rad´i-sis den´tis) [TA] SYN root apex.

**a·pex sat·y·ri** (ā´peks sā-tir´ī) SYN apex of auricle.

**APF** Abbreviation for acidulated phosphate fluoride.

**a·pha·gi·a** (ă-fā´jē-ă) Difficulty with or incapacity for eating. [G. *a-* priv. + *phagō,* to eat]

**a·pha·si·a** (ă-fā´zē-ă) Impaired or absent comprehension or production of, or communication by, speech, reading, writing, or signs. [G. speechlessness, fr. *a-* priv. + *phasis,* speech]

**a·pher·e·sis, pher·e·sis** (ă´fĕr-ē´sis, fĕr-ē´sis) Infusion of a patient's own blood from which elements (e.g., plasma, leukocytes, or platelets) have been removed. [G. *aphairesis,* withdrawal]

**a·phra·si·a** (ă-frā´zē-ă) Inability to speak, from any cause. [G. *a-* priv. + *phrasis,* speaking]

**aph·tha,** pl. **aph·thae** (af′thă, -thē) *Avoid the misspelling/mispronunciation aptha.* **1.** In the singular, a small ulcer on a mucous membrane. **2.** In the plural, stomatitis characterized by intermittent episodes of painful oral ulcers of unknown etiology that are covered by gray exudate, are surrounded by an erythematous halo, and range from several millimeters to 2 cm in diameter; they are limited to oral mucous membranes that are not bound to periosteum, occur as solitary or multiple lesions, and heal spontaneously in 1–2 weeks. See this page. SYN aphthae minor, aphthous stomatitis, canker sores, recurrent aphthous stomatitis, recurrent aphthous ulcers, recurrent ulcerative stomatitis, ulcerative stomatitis. [G. ulceration]

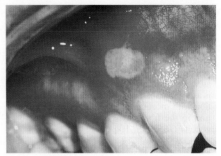
**aphthous ulcer:** alveolar mucosa

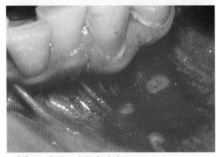
**aphthae:** clustered, typical shapes

**aph·thae ma·jor** (af′thē mā′jŏr) SYN periadenitis mucosa necrotica recurrens.

**aph·thae mi·nor** (af′thē mī′nŏr) SYN aphtha (2).

**aph·thoid** (af′thoyd) Resembling aphthae.

**aph·tho·sis** (af-thō′sis) Any condition characterized by the presence of aphthae.

**aph·thous** (af′thŭs) *Avoid the misspelling/ mispronunciation apthous.* Characterized by or relating to aphthae or aphthosis.

**aph·thous sto·ma·ti·tis** (af′thŭs stō′mă-tī′tis) See page A7. SYN aphtha (2).

**aph·thous ul·cer** (af′thŭs ŭl′sĕr) Stomatitis with intermittent episodes of painful oral ulcers of unknown etiology. See this page and page A6.

**ap·i·cal** (ap′i-kăl) [TA] Relating to the apex or tip of a root or tooth. SYN apicalis [TA].

**ap·i·cal ab·scess** (ap′i-kăl ab′ses) SYN periapical abscess.

**ap·i·cal a·re·a** (ap′i-kăl ar′ē-ă) Area surrounding root end of a tooth.

**ap·i·cal den·tal fo·ra·men** (ap′i-kăl den′tăl fōr-ā′mĕn) SYN apical foramen of tooth.

**ap·i·cal fo·ra·men of tooth** (ap′i-kăl fōr-ā′mĕn tūth) [TA] Opening at apex of tooth root that gives passage to the nerve and blood ves-

sels. See page 55. SYN apical dental foramen, root foramen.

**ap·i·cal gland** (ap′i-kăl gland) SYN anterior lingual gland.

**ap·i·cal gran·u·lo·ma** (ap′i-kăl gran′yū-lō′mă) SYN periapical granuloma.

**ap·i·cal in·fec·tion** (ap′i-kăl in-fek′shŭn) Implantation of microorganisms at tooth apex, usually due to migration of microorganisms from pulp canal through apical foramen.

**ap·i·ca·lis** (ap-i-kā′lis) [TA] SYN apical. [L.]

**ap·i·cal lig·a·ment of dens** (ap′i-kăl lig′ă-mĕnt denz) [TA] Ligament that extends from apex of dens of the axis to anterior margin of the foramen magnum; includes vestiges of notochord.

**ap·i·cal per·i·o·don·tal ab·scess** (ap′i-kăl per′ē-ō-don′tăl ab′ses) SYN periapical abscess.

**ap·i·cal per·i·o·don·tal cyst** (ap′i-kăl per′ē-ō-don′tăl sist) Inflammatory odontogenic cyst derived histogenetically from Malassez epithelial rests surrounding root apex of a nonvital tooth. SYN periapical cyst, radicular cyst, root end cyst.

**ap·i·cal per·i·o·don·ti·tis** (ap′i-kăl per′ē-ō-don-tī′tis) Inflammation of periodontal ligament surrounding root apex of a tooth; usually due to pulpal inflammation or necrosis. See page 55.

**ap·i·cal space** (ap′i-kăl spās) Space between alveolar wall and apex of tooth root where an alveolar abscess usually has its origin.

**ap·i·cec·to·my** (ap′i-sek′tŏ-mē) **1.** In dental surgery, an obsolete synonym for apicoectomy. **2.** Opening and exenteration of air cells in the apex of the petrous part of the temporal bone. [L. *apex*, summit or tip, + G. *ektomē*, excision]

**apico-** Combining form meaning an apex; apical. [L. *apex, apicis*, a summit or a tip + -*o*-]

**ap·i·co·ec·to·my** (ap′i-kō-ek′tŏ-mē) Surgical removal of a tooth root apex. SYN root resection. [*apico-* + G. *ektomē*, tooth excision]

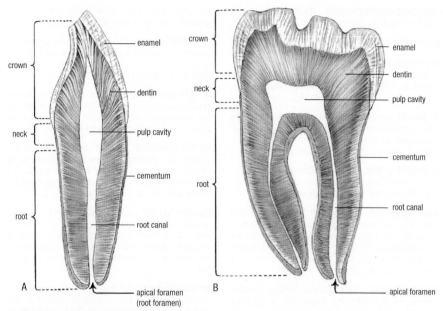

**longitudinal sections of teeth:** (A) incisor; (B) molar. Pulp cavity (tooth cavity) is a hollow space within the crown and neck of tooth that contains pulpal soft tissue, connective tissue, blood vessels, and nerves. It narrows down to root canal in single-rooted tooth or to one canal for each root of a multirooted tooth. Blood vessels and nerves enter or leave through the apical (root) foramen

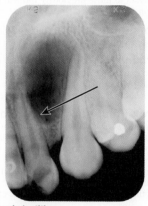

**apical periodontitis**

**ap·i·co·lo·ca·tor** (ap′i-kō-lō′kā-tŏr) A device for locating the root apex of a tooth.

**ap·i·co·stome** (ap′i-kō-stōm) Type of trocar and cannula used in apicostomy.

**ap·i·cos·to·my** (ap′i-kos′tō-mē) An operation in which the labial or buccal alveolar plate is perforated with a trocar and cannula; performed to reach the root apex and to take bacterial cultures from this area. [*apico-* + G. *stoma*, mouth]

**ap·i·cot·o·my, ap·i·ce·ot·o·my** (ap-i-

kot′ŏ-mē, ă-pis′ē-ot′ŏ-mē) Incision into an apical structure. [*apico-* + G. *tomē*, a cutting]

**ap·i·cu·ret·tage** (ap′i-kur-ě-tahzh′) Apical curettage after removal of an infected tooth.

**a·pla·si·a** (ă-plā′zē-ă) Defective development or congenital absence of an organ or tissue. [G. *a-* priv. + *plasis*, a molding]

**a·plas·tic** (ā-plas′tik) Pertaining to aplasia, or conditions characterized by defective regeneration, as in aplastic anemia.

**a·plas·tic a·ne·mi·a** (ā-plas′tik ă-nē′mē-ă) Disorder characterized by a greatly decreased formation of erythrocytes and hemoglobin.

**ap·ne·a** (ap′nē-ă) Absence of breathing. [G. *apnoia*, want of breath]

**ap·ne·a-hy·pop·ne·a in·dex** (ap′nē-ă-hī-pop′nē-ă in′deks) SYN respiratory disturbance index, apnoea-hypopnoea index.

**ap·ne·ic** (ap′nē-ik) Related to or suffering from apnea. SYN apnoeic.

**ap·ne·ic ox·y·gen·a·tion** (ap′nē-ik ok′sĭ-jě-nā′shŭn) Diffusion of oxygen to alveoli in absence of ventilation.

**ap·neus·tic breath·ing** (ap-nū′stik brēdh′ing) Pauses in respiratory cycle at full inspiration, caused by damage to respiratory control centers in the more caudal pons.

**apnoea-hypopnoea index** [Br.] SYN apnea-hypopnea index.

**apnoeic** [Br.] SYN apneic.

**a·po·gee** (ap′ō-jē) The peak of severity of the clinical manifestations of an illness. [Fr., fr. Mod. L. *apogaeum,* fr. G. *apogaios,* far from the earth, fr. *apo,* + *gaia,* earth]

**A point** (poynt) The most posterior delimit on the cephalometric profile between the nasal spine and the maxillary incisors. [Fr., fr. L. *punctum,* fr. *pungo,* pp. *punctum,* to pierce]

**a·poph·y·sis,** pl. **a·poph·y·ses** (ă-pof′i-sis, -sēz) Outgrowth or projection, especially one from bone. [G. an offshoot]

**ap·o·pto·sis** (ap′ŏ-tō′sis) Programmed cell death; deletion of individual cells by fragmentation into membrane-bound particles, which are phagocytized by other cells. SYN programmed cell death. [G. a falling or dropping off, fr. *apo,* off, + *ptosis,* a falling]

**ap·o·stax·is** (ap′ō-staks′is) Slight hemorrhage, or bleeding by drops. [G. a trickling down]

**a·poth·e·car·ies' weights** (ă-poth′ĕ-kar-ēz wāts) System of weight measurement based on the weight of a grain of wheat. This system has been largely superseded by the metric system (based on grams). One grain is the equivalent of 64.8 milligrams. One scruple contains 20 grains; one dram contains 60 grains; one apothecary ounce contains 8 drams (480 grains); one apothecary pound contains 12 ounces (5760 grains).

**ap·ox·e·sis** (ap′ok-sē′sis) SYN subgingival curettage. [G. *apo,* away, + *xeein,* to scrape]

**ap·pa·ra·tus** (ap′ă-rat′ŭs) *The plural of this word is apparatus, not apparati.* **1.** [TA] A collection of instruments adapted for a special purpose. **2.** An instrument made up of several parts. **3.** [TA] A group or system of glands, ducts, blood vessels, muscles, or other anatomic structures involved in the performance of some function. SEE ALSO system. [L. equipment. fr. *apparo,* pp. *-atus,* to prepare]

**ap·par·ent** (ă-par′ĕnt) **1.** Manifest; obvious; evident (e.g., a clinically apparent infection). **2.** Frequently used (confusingly) to mean ''seeming to be,'' ostensible, pseudo-. [L. *apparens,* visible, fr. *appareo,* to come in sight]

**ap·pend·age** (ă-pen′dăj) Any part, subordinate in function or size, attached to a main structure. [L. *appendix*]

**ap·pen·di·ci·tis** (ă-pen′di-sī′tis) Inflammation of the vermiform appendix. [*appendix* + G. *-itis,* inflammation]

**ap·pen·dix,** pl. **ap·pen·dix·es, ap·pen·di·ces** (ă-pen′diks, -dik-sĕz, -di-sēz) [TA] An appendage or appendixlike structure. [L. appendage, fr. *ap-pendo,* to hang something on]

**ap·pe·tite** (ap′ĕ-tīt) A desire derived from a biologic or psychological need for food, water, sex, or affection. [L. *ad-peto,* pp. *-petitus,* to seek after, desire]

**ap·pli·ance** (ă-plī′ăns) Device used by dental professionals to improve function of a part or for therapeutic purposes. [fr. O. Fr. *aplier,* to apply, fr. L. *applico,* to fold together]

**ap·pli·ca·tion** (ap′li-kā′shŭn) **1.** Act of applying, as in bringing a medicine, dressing, or device into contact with the body surface. **2.** Act of putting to specific use, or such capacity. [L. *applicatio,* fr. *ap-plico,* to affix]

**ap·pli·ca·tor** (ap′li-kā-tŏr) Slender rod of wood, flexible metal, or synthetic material, at one end of which is attached a pledget of cotton or other substance for making local applications to any accessible surface. [L. *ap-plico,* to attach to]

**ap·po·si·tion** (ap′ŏ-zish′ŭn) **1.** SYN appositional growth. **2.** The placing in contact of two substances or structures. **3.** The condition of being placed or fitted together. [L. *ap-pono,* pp. *-positus,* to place at or to]

**ap·po·si·tion·al growth** (ap′ŏ-zish′ŭn-ăl grōth) Growth accomplished by the addition of new layers to those previously formed. SYN apposition (1).

**ap·po·si·tion su·ture** (ap′ŏ-zish′ŭn sū′-chŭr) SYN suture apposition.

**ap·proach** (ă-prōch′) The path or method used to expose the operative field during an operation. [M.E., fr. O. Fr., fr L.L. *appropio,* to come nearer, fr. *ad,* to + *propius,* nearer]

**ap·prox·i·mal sur·face of tooth** (ă-prok′si-măl sŭr′făs tūth) [TA] Surface of a tooth that faces an adjacent tooth in the dental arch; the contact surface closest to anterior midline of the dental arch is the mesial surface of a tooth; that farthest is the distal surface. SYN contact surface of tooth, facies approximalis dentis, facies contactus dentis, interproximal surface of tooth.

**ap·prox·i·mate** (ă-prok′si-măt) **1.** Proximate, denoting the contact surfaces, either mesial or distal, of two adjacent teeth. **2.** Close together; denoting the teeth in the human jaw, as distinguished from the separated teeth in certain lower animals. [L. *ad,* to, + *proximus,* nearest]

**ap·prox·i·ma·tion su·ture** (ă-prok′si-mā′shŭn sū′chŭr) Suture that pulls together the deep tissues.

**a·py·ret·ic** (ā′pī-ret′ik) SYN afebrile.

**a·py·rex·i·a** (ā′pī-rek′sē-ă) Absence of fever. [G. *a-* priv. + *pyrexis,* fever]

**a·py·rex·i·al** (ā′pī-rek′sē-ăl) SYN afebrile.

**aq·ua,** pl. **aq·uae** (ah′kwă, -kwē) Water (H₂O). Pharmaceutical waters, aquae, are aqueous solutions of volatile substances. SEE water (3), solution (3). [L.]

**a·que·ous** (ā′kwē-ŭs) Watery; of, like, or containing water.

**a·que·ous so·lu·tion** (ā′kwē-ŭs sŏ-lū′shŭn) Solution containing water as the solvent.

**a·quip·ar·ous** (ă-kwip′er-ŭs) Secreting or excreting a watery fluid. [L. *aqua,* water, + *pario,* to bring forth]

**ar·a·chi·don·ic ac·id** (ar′ă-ki-don′ik as′id) An unsaturated fatty acid, usually essential in nutrition; the biologic precursor of the prostaglandins, the thromboxanes, and the leukotrienes (collectively known as eicosanoids).

**ar·bo·ri·za·tion** (ahr′bŏr-ī-zā′shŭn) The terminal branching of nerve fibers or blood vessels in a treelike pattern.

**ARC** Abbreviation for AIDS-related complex.

**arc** (ahrk) **1.** A curved line or segment of a circle. SEE arch, arcus, arcade. **2.** Continuous luminous passage of an electric current in a gas or vacuum between two or more separated electrodes. See this page. [L. *arcus,* a bow]

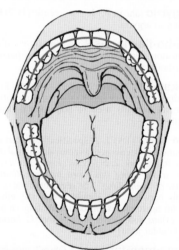

**arcs formed by maxillary and mandibular teeth:** mandibular arc is smaller than maxillary, so that maximum contact requires lateral mandibular deviation

---

***Ar·can·o·bac·te·ri·um hae·mo·ly·ti·cum*** (ahr-kan′ō-bak-tēr′ē-ŭm hē′mō-lit′i-kŭm) Species that causes pharyngitis and chronic skin ulcers in humans and farm animals.

**ar·cate** (ahr′kāt) SYN arcuate.

**arch** (ahrch) [TA] Any structure resembling a bent bow or an arc. In anatomy, any vaulted or archlike structure. Cf. dental arch. SYN arcus [TA]. [thru O. Fr. fr. L. *arcus,* bow]

**arch bar** (ahrch bahr) One of several types of wires, bars, or splints conforming to the arch of the teeth, extending from one side of the arch to the other and located labially, or lingually; used to treat jaw fractures and stabilize injured teeth.

**arch form** (ahrch fōrm) Shape and contour of a dental arch (e.g., ovoid, tapering, trapezoidal, U-shaped, square) or of an orthodontic wire formed to the shape of that arch.

**arch length** (ahrch length) Amount of space required for permanent teeth as measured from mesial aspect of first molar on one side to mesial aspect of first molar on opposite side, as measured through contact points along an imaginary dental arch line, as they curve around the arch.

**arch length de·fi·ci·en·cy** (ahrch length dĕ-fish′ĕn-sē) Difference between the available circumference of the dental arch and that required to accommodate the succedaneous teeth in proper alignment.

**arch of the pal·ate** (ahrch pal′ăt) Vaulted roof of the mouth.

**arch width** (ahrch width) Distance in a straight line between canine teeth.

**arch wire** (ahrch wīr) A device with a wire conforming to the alveolar or dental arch, used as an anchorage in correcting irregularities in the position of the teeth, so as to move teeth orthodontically into a more satisfactory position.

**ar·ci·form** (ahr′si-fōrm) SYN arcuate.

**arc of clo·sure** (ahrk klō′zhŭr) Area defined by closure of mandible when viewed using reference point on mandible; viewed most often in midsagittal plane.

**ar·con ar·tic·u·la·tor** (ahr′kon ahr-tik′yū-lā-tŏr) **1.** Articulator with the equivalent condylar guides fixed to the upper member and the hinge axis to the lower member. **2.** Instrument that maintains a constant relationship between the occlusal plane and the arcon guides at any position of the upper member, thereby making possible more accurate reproductions of mandibular movements.

**ar·cu·al** (ar′kyū-ăl) Relating to an arch.

**ar·cu·ate** (ahrk′yū-ăt) Denoting a form that is arched or has the shape of a bow. SYN arcate, arciform. [L. *arcuatus,* bowed]

**ar·cu·ate crest of ar·y·te·noid car·ti·lage** (ahr′kyū-ăt krest ar′i-tē′noyd kahr′ti-lăj) [TA] The ridge on the anterior surface of the arytenoid cartilage that separates the triangular from the oblong fovea.

**ar·cu·ate em·i·nence** (ahr´kyū-ăt em´ĭ-nĕns) [TA] Prominence on anterior surface of the petrous portion of the temporal bone indicating position of the superior semicircular canal.

**ar·cu·ate line** (ahr´kyū-ăt līn) [TA] An arching or bow-shaped line.

**ar·cu·ate zone** (ahrk´yū-ăt zōn) Inner third of the basilar membrane of the cochlear duct extending from tympanic lip of osseous spiral lamina to outer pillar cell of the spiral organ (of Corti).

**ar·cu·a·tion** (ahr´kyū-ā´shŭn) A bending or curvature.

**ar·cus** (ahr´kŭs) [TA] *The plural of this word is arcus, not arci.* SYN arch. [L. a bow]

**ar·cus cor·ne·a·lis** (ahr´kŭs kōr-nē-ā´lis) SYN arcus senilis.

**ar·cus den·ta·lis in·fe·ri·or** (ahr´kŭs den-tā´lis in-fēr´ē-ŏr) SYN mandibular dental arcade.

**ar·cus den·ta·lis su·pe·ri·or** (ahr´kŭs den-tā´lis sŭ-pēr´ē-ŏr) SYN maxillary dental arcade.

**ar·cus se·ni·lis** (ahr´kŭs sĕ-nil´is) An opaque, grayish ring at the periphery of the cornea just within the sclerocorneal junction; frequent occurrence in old people. SYN anterior embryotoxon, gerontoxon.

**ar·cus zy·go·mat·i·cus** (ahr´kŭs zī´gō-mat´i-kŭs) [TA] SYN zygomatic arch.

**ARDS** Abbreviation for adult respiratory distress syndrome.

**ar·e·a** (ār´ē-ă) **1.** [TA] Any circumscribed surface or space. **2.** All of the part supplied by a given artery or nerve. **3.** A part of an organ having a special function, as the motor area of the brain. SEE ALSO region, space, zone. [L. a courtyard]

**ar·e·a of Lai·mer** (ār´ē-ă lī´mĕr) A triangular (or V-shaped) area on the posterior aspect of the proximal esophagus.

**ar·e·a-spe·ci·fic cu·rettes** (ār´ē-ă spĕ-sif´ik kyūr-ets´) Periodontal instruments used to remove calculus deposits from crowns and roots of teeth. Each is designed for use only on certain teeth and certain surfaces and thus have long functional shanks created at specific angles; one working cutting edge is used for calculus removal.

**ar·e·a-spe·cif·ic in·stru·ment** (ār´ē-ă-spĕ-sif´ik in´strŭ-mĕnt) Tool or device designed for use on specific dental surfaces.

**a·re·flex·i·a** (ā-rĕ-flek´sē-ă) Absence of reflexes.

**A·re·na·vi·ri·dae** (ă-rē´nă-vir´i-dē) A family of RNA viruses, many of which are parasites of rodents, which includes Lassa virus. [L. *arena* (*harena*), sand]

**a·re·o·la,** pl. **a·re·o·lae** (ă-rē´ō-lă, -lē) *Avoid the mispronunciation areo'la.* **1.** Any small area. **2.** Pigmented, depigmented, or erythematous zone surrounding a papule, pustule, wheal, or cutaneous neoplasm. [L. dim. of *area*]

**ar·gen·tic** (ahr-jen´tik) **1.** Relating to silver. SYN argyric (1). **2.** Denoting a chemical compound containing silver.

**ar·gi·nine** (ahr´ji-nēn) An amino acid occurring among the hydrolysis products of proteins, particularly abundant in the basic proteins.

**Ar·gyll Ro·bert·son pu·pil** (ahr´gīl rob´ĕrt-sŏn pyū´pil) *Do not hyphenate Argyll Robertson.* A form of reflex iridoplegia characterized by miosis, irregular shape, and a loss of the direct and consensual pupillary reflex to light.

**ar·gyr·ia, ar·gy·rism, ar·gy·ro·sis** (ahr-jir´ē-a, ahr´jir-izm, -jir-ō´sis) A slate-gray or bluish discoloration of the skin and deep tissues caused by deposits of insoluble albuminate of silver; occurs after a long period of medicinal administration of a soluble silver salt. SYN silver poisoning. [G. *argyros,* silver]

**ar·gyr·ic** (ahr-jir´ik) **1.** SYN argentic (1). **2.** Relating to argyria.

**a·ri·bo·fla·vin·o·sis** (ă-rī´bō-flā-vi-nō´sis) Nutritional condition produced by a deficiency of riboflavin in the diet.

**Ar·kan·sas stone** (ahr´kăn-saw stōn) Fine-grained sharpening block quarried from natural mineral deposits used to hone dental instruments.

**arm** (ahrm) [TA] **1.** A specifically shaped and positioned extension of a removable partial denture framework. **2.** *In technical speech and writing, avoid using this word in the colloquial sense of 'upper limb.'* The segment of the upper limb between the shoulder and the elbow. **3.** An anatomic extension resembling an arm. [L. *armus,* forequarter of an animal; G. *harmos,* a shoulder joint]

**ar·ma·men·tar·i·um** (ahrm´ă-men-tar´ē-ŭm) All therapeutic means available to the health care practitioner for professional practice. [L. an arsenal, fr. *armamenta,* implements, tackle, fr. *arma,* armor, arms]

**ar·o·mat·ic** (ar´ō-mat´ik) **1.** Having an agreeable, somewhat pungent, spicy odor. **2.** One of a group of vegetable-based drugs having a fragrant odor and slightly stimulant properties. [G. *arōmatikos,* fr. *arōma,* spice, sweet herb]

**ar·rest·ed den·tal car·ies** (ă-res´tĕd den´tăl kar´ēz) Carious lesions that have become inactive and stopped progressing; may change color and consistency.

**ar·rhin·i·a, ar·hin·i·a** (ă-rī′nē-ă) Congenital absence of the nose. [G. *a*- priv. + *rhis* (*rhin*-), nose]

**ar·rhyth·mi·a** (ā-ridh′mē-ă) *Avoid the misspelling arhythmia.* Loss or abnormality of rhythm; denoting especially an irregularity of the heartbeat. Cf. dysrhythmia. [G. *a*- priv. + *rhythmos*, rhythm]

**ar·row clasp** (ar′ō klasp) SYN arrowhead clasp.

**ar·row·head clasp** (ar′ō-hed klasp) Device made by forming a single piece of wire into arrowhead shape to engage mesial and distal proximal undercuts on buccal areas of adjacent teeth to stabilize a removable appliance. SYN arrow clasp.

**ar·row point trac·ing** (ar′ō poynt trās′ing) SYN intraoral tracing.

**ar·sen·i·cal sto·ma·ti·tis** (ahr-sen′i-kăl stō′mă-tī′tis) Inflammation of the oral mucosa due to exposure to a drug or agent that contains arsenic. SEE arsenical, stomatitis.

**ar·sen·ic tri·ox·ide** (ahr′sĕ-nik trī-ok′sīd) $H_3AsO_3$; used in the treatment of skin diseases and historically for malaria and as a tonic; also used externally as a caustic.

**ar·te·ri·a**, pl. **ar·te·ri·ae** (ahr-tēr′ē-ă, -ē) [TA] SYN artery. [L. from G. *artēria*, the windpipe, later an artery as distinct from a vein]

**ar·te·ri·ae al·ve·o·la·res su·pe·ri·o·resan·te·ri·o·res**(ahr-tēr′ē-ēal′vē-ō-lā′ rēz sū-pēr′ē-ō′rēz an-tēr′ē-ō′rēz) SYN anterior superior alveolar arteries.

**ar·te·ri·al** (ahr-tēr′ē-ăl) Relating to one or more arteries or to the entire system of arteries.

**ar·te·ri·al blood** (ahr-tēr′ē-ăl blŭd) Blood that is oxygenated in the lungs, found in the left chambers of the heart and in the arteries; colored a relatively bright red.

**ar·te·ri·al scler·o·sis** (ahr-tēr′ē-ăl skler-ō′sis) SYN arteriosclerosis.

**ar·te·ri·al ten·sion** (ahr-tēr′ē-ăl ten′shŭn) Blood pressure within an artery.

**ar·te·ri·a men·ta·lis** (ahr-tēr′ē-ă men-tā′lis) [TA] SYN mental artery.

**ar·te·ries of brain** (ahr′tĕr-ēz brān) [TA] Arteries and arterial branches supplying brain; derived from cerebral arterial circle and anterior choroidal artery.

♻ **arterio-, arteri-** Combining form denoting artery. [L. *arteria*, fr. G. *artēria*, a windpipe, an artery]

**ar·te·ri·o·cap·il·lar·y** (ahr-tēr′ē-ō-kap′i-lar-ē) Relating to both arteries and capillaries.

**ar·te·ri·og·ra·phy** (ahr-ter′ē-og′ră-fē) Demonstration of an artery or arteries by x-ray im-

aging after injection of a radiopaque contrast medium. [L. *arteria*, + G. *graphō*, to write]

**ar·te·ri·ole** (ahr-tēr′ē-ōl) [TA] A minute artery with a tunica media comprising only one or two layers of smooth muscle cells; a terminal artery continuous with the capillary network.

♻ **arteriolo-** Combining form denoting the arterioles. [Modern L. *arteriola*, arteriole]

**ar·te·ri·ol·o·gy** (ahr-tēr′ē-ol′ŏ-jē) Anatomy of arteries. [L. *arteria*, artery, + G. *logos*, study]

**ar·te·ri·o·lo·ve·nous** (ahr-tēr′ē-ō-lō-vē′nŭs) Involving both arterioles and the veins. SYN arteriolovenular.

**ar·te·ri·o·lo·ven·u·lar** (ahr-tēr′ē-ō-lō-ven′yū-lăr) SYN arteriolovenous.

**ar·te·ri·om·e·ter** (ahr-tēr′ē-om′ē-tĕr) Instrument for measuring the diameter of an artery or its change in size during pulsation. [L. *arteria*, + G. *metron*, measure]

**ar·te·ri·o·scle·ro·sis** (ahr-tēr′ē-ō-skler-ō′sis) Hardening of the arteries; types generally recognized are: atherosclerosis, Mönckeberg arteriosclerosis, and arteriolosclerosis. SYN arterial sclerosis. [L. *arteria*, + G. *sklērōsis*, hardness]

**ar·te·ri·o·scle·rot·ic an·eur·ysm** (ahr-tēr′ē-ō-skler-ot′ik an′yūr-izm) SYN atherosclerotic aneurysm.

**ar·te·ri·o·ve·nous (AV)** (ahr-tēr′ē-ō-vē′nŭs) Relating to both an artery and a vein or both arteries and veins in general.

**ar·te·ri·o·ve·nous an·eur·ysm** (ahr-tēr′ē-ō-vē′nŭs an′yūr-izm) **1.** A dilated arteriovenous shunt. **2.** Communication between an artery and a vein, sometimes congenital.

**ar·te·ri·o·ve·nous fis·tu·la** (ahr-tēr′ē-ō-vē′nŭs fis′tyū-lă) An abnormal communication between an artery and a vein, usually resulting in the formation of an arteriovenous aneurysm.

**ar·te·ri·o·ve·nous shunt** (ahr-tēr′ē-ō-vē′nŭs shŭnt) The passage of blood directly from arteries to veins, without going through the capillary network.

**ar·te·ri·tis** (ahr′tĕr-ī′tis) Inflammation or infection involving an artery or arteries. [L. *arteria*, artery, + G. *-itis*, inflammation]

**ar·te·ry** (ahr′tĕr-ē) [TA] A relatively thick-walled, muscular, pulsating blood vessel conveying blood away from the heart. SYN arteria [TA]. [L. *arteria*, fr. G. *artēria*]

**ar·te·ry of lab·y·rinth** (ahr′tĕr-ē lab′i-rinth) SYN labyrinthine artery.

**ar·te·ry of post·cen·tral sul·cus** (ahr′tĕr-ē pōst-sen′trăl sŭl′kŭs) [TA] Branch of terminal part of middle cerebral artery distributing to cortex on either side of postcentral sulcus.

**ar·te·ry of pre·cen·tral sul·cus** (ahr´těr-ē pre-sen´trăl sŭl´kŭs) [TA] Branch of terminal part of middle cerebral artery distributed to cortex on either side of precentral sulcus.

**ar·te·ry of pter·y·goid ca·nal** (ahr´těr-ē ter´i-goyd kă-nal´) [TA] Arises from the third part of maxillary artery, supplying contents and wall of the canal, mucous membrane of the upper pharynx, auditory tube, and tympanic cavity.

**ar·thral** (ahrth´răl) SYN articular.

**ar·thral·gi·a** (ahr-thral´jē-ă) Pain in a joint. [G. *arthron*, joint, + *algos*, pain]

**ar·thrit·ic** (ahr-thrit´ik) Relating to arthritis.

**ar·thri·tis**, pl. **ar·thrit·i·des** (ahr-thrī´tis, ahr-thrit´i-dēz) Inflammation of a joint; state characterized by inflamed joints. [G. fr. *arthron*, joint, + *-itis*, inflammation]

**ar·thri·tis de·for·mans** (ahr-thrī´tis dē-fōr´manz) SYN rheumatoid arthritis.

**ar·thri·tis mu·ti·lans** (ahr-thrī´tis myŭ´ti-lanz) Chronic rheumatoid arthritis in which osteolysis occurs with extensive destruction of joint cartilages and bony surfaces with pronounced deformities, chiefly of hands and feet.

🔄 **arthro-, arthr-** Combining forms denoting a joint, an articulation; corresponds to L. articul-. [G. *arthron*, a joint, fr. *arariskō*, to join, to fit together]

***Arth·ro·bac·ter*** (ahrth´rō-bak´těr) Genus of strictly aerobic, gram-positive bacteria the cells of which change from a coccoid form to a rod shape after transfer to fresh complex growth medium. *Arthrobacter* species have been found in the advancing front of lesions of dental caries. [G. *arthron*, joint, + *baktron*, staff or rod]

**ar·thro·cen·te·sis** (ahr´thrō-sen-tē´sis) 1. Aspiration of fluid from a joint by needle puncture. 2. Sometimes used for a procedure in which an affected joint is flushed with a corticosteroid. [G. *arthron*, joint + G. *kentēsis*, puncture]

**ar·thro·cla·si·a** (ahr´thrō-klā´zē-ă) The forcible breaking up of the adhesions in ankylosis. [G. *arthron*, joint + G. *klasis*, a breaking]

**ar·throg·e·nous** (ar-throj´ĕ-nŭs) Of articular origin; starting from a joint.

**ar·throl·o·gy** (ahr-throl´ŏ-jē) Branch of anatomy concerned with joints. [G. *arthron*, joint + G. *logos*, study]

**ar·throl·y·sis** (ahr-throl´i-sis) Restoration of mobility in stiff and ankylosed joints through the process of disrupting intraarticular and ex-

traarticular adhesions. [*arthro-* + G. *lysis*, a loosening]

**ar·thro·pa·thol·o·gy** (ahrth´rō-pă-thol´ŏ-jē) Study of diseases of the joints.

**ar·throp·a·thy** (ahr-throp´ă-thē) Any disease affecting a joint. [*arthro-* + G. *pathos*, suffering]

**ar·thro·plas·ty** (ahr´thrō-plas-tē, ahr´thrō-plas-tē) 1. Creating an artificial joint to correct ankylosis. 2. An operation to restore the integrity and functional power of a joint. [G. *arthron*, joint, + *-plasty*, reparative procedure, fr. *plassō*, to shape]

**ar·thro·scope** (ahr´thrŏ-skōp) An endoscope for examining the internal anatomy of a joint.

**ar·thros·co·py** (ahr-thros´kŏ-pē) Endoscopic examination of the interior of a joint. [*arthro-* + G. *skopeō*, to view]

**ar·thro·sis**, pl. **ar·thro·ses** (ahrth-rō´sis, -sēz) 1. Degenerative joint changes. 2. SYN osteoarthritis. [G. *arthrōsis*, a jointing]

**ar·thros·to·my** (ahr-thros´tŏ-mē) Establishment of a temporary opening into a joint cavity. [G. *arthron*, joint + G. *stoma*, mouth]

**ar·ti·caine** (ahr´ti-kān) Local anesthetic, usually in a 4% solution, commonly used in dentistry. [coined term incl. *-caine*, local anesthetic, fr. *cocaine*, fr. *coca* + *-ine*, chem. suffix]

**ar·tic·u·lar** (ahr-tik´yū-lăr) Relating to a joint. SYN arthral.

**ar·tic·u·lar branch·es** (ahr-tik´yū-lăr branch´ēz) [TA] Branches distributed to joints; most vessels related to a joint will supply articular rami.

**ar·tic·u·lar car·ti·lage** (ahr-tik´yū-lăr kahr´ti-lăj) The cartilage covering the articular surfaces of the bones participating in a synovial joint.

**ar·tic·u·lar disc** (ahr-tik´yū-lăr disk) [TA] A plate or ring of fibrocartilage attached to the joint capsule and separating the articular surfaces of the bones for a varying distance, sometimes completely; it serves to adapt two articular surfaces that are not entirely congruent.

**ar·tic·u·lar disc of tem·po·ro·man·dib·u·lar joint** (ahr-tik´yū-lăr disk tem´pŏr-ō-man-dib´yū-lăr joynt) [TA] Fibrocartilaginous plate that separates the temporomandibular joint into upper and lower cavities. SYN mandibular disc.

**ar·tic·u·la·re** (ahr-tik´yū-lā´rē) In cephalometrics, the point of intersection of the external dorsal contour of the mandibular condyle and the temporal bone; the midpoint is used when a profile radiograph shows double projections of the rami.

**ar·tic·u·lar fac·et** (ahr-tik′yū-lăr fas′ĕt) Relatively small articular surface of a bone, especially a vertebra.

**ar·tic·u·lar fos·sa of the tem·po·ral bone** (ahr-tik′yū-lăr fos′ă tem′pŏr-ăl bōn) SYN mandibular fossa.

**ar·tic·u·lar frac·ture** (ahr-tik′yū-lăr frak′ shŭr) Fracture involving joint surface of a bone.

**ar·tic·u·lar gout** (ahr-tik′yū-lăr gowt) Usual form of gout attacking one or more joints.

**ar·tic·u·lar la·mel·la** (ahr-tik′yū-lăr lă-mel′ă) Layer of compact bone comprising articular surface of a bone; firmly attaches to the overlying articular cartilage.

**ar·tic·u·lar lip** (ahr-tik′yū-lăr lip) SYN labrum (3).

**ar·tic·u·lar mus·cle** (ahr-tik′yū-lăr mŭs′ĕl) Muscle that inserts directly onto joint capsule, acting to retract the capsule in certain movements.

**ar·tic·u·lar nerve** (ahr-tik′yū-lăr nĕrv) Branch of a nerve supplying a joint.

**ar·tic·u·lar sur·face** (ahr-tik′yū-lăr sŭr′ făs) [TA] Any surface of a skeletal formation (bone, cartilage) that makes normal direct contact with another skeletal structure as part of a synovial joint.

**ar·tic·u·lar sur·face of man·dib·u·lar fos·sa of tem·po·ral bone** (ahr-tik′yū-lăr sŭr′făs man-dib′yū-lăr fos′ă tem′pŏr-ăl bōn) [TA] Smooth portion of mandibular articular fossa and eminence of the temporal bone that articulates with the disc of the temporomandibular joint. SYN facies articularis fossae mandibularis ossis temporalis.

**ar·tic·u·lar sys·tem** (ahr-tik′yū-lăr sis′ tĕm) [TA] All the arthroses of the body, collectively.

**ar·tic·u·lar tu·ber·cle of tem·po·ral bone** (ahr-tik′yū-lăr tū′bĕr-kĕl tem′pŏr-ăl bōn) [TA] Articular eminence of the temporal bone that bounds the mandibular fossa anteriorly; forms anterior root of the zygomatic process.

**ar·tic·u·lar veins** (ahr-tik′yū-lăr vānz) [TA] Tributaries of the pterygoid plexus draining blood from the temporomandibular joint.

**ar·tic·u·late** (ahr-tik′yū-lăt) **1.** Capable of distinct and connected meaningful speech. **2.** To join or connect together loosely to allow motion between the parts. **3.** To speak distinctly and precisely. [L. *articulo,* pp. *-atus,* to articulate]

**ar·tic·u·lat·ing pa·per** (ahr-tik′yū-lăt-ing pā′pĕr) SYN occluding paper.

**ar·tic·u·la·ti·o,** pl. **ar·tic·u·la·ti·o·nes** (ahr-tik-ū-lā′shē-ō) [TA] SYN synovial joint. [L. a forming of vines]

**ar·tic·u·la·tion** (ahr-tik′yū-lā′shŭn) **1.** In dentistry, the contact relationship of the occlusal surfaces of the teeth during jaw movement. **2.** SYN joint. **3.** A joining or connecting together loosely to allow motion between parts. [L. a forming of vines]

**ar·tic·u·la·tion dis·or·ders** (ahr-tik′yū-lā′shŭn dis-ōr′dĕrz) Pronunciation errors including phoneme omissions and distortions.

**ar·tic·u·la·tor** (ahr-tik′yū-lā-tŏr) Mechanical device that represents temporomandibular joints and jaw members to which maxillary and mandibular casts may be attached. See this page. SYN occluding frame.

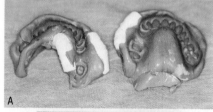

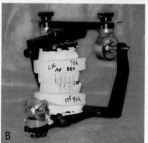

articulator: (A) maxillary and mandibular permanent impressions; (B) casts mounted on articulator

**ar·tic·u·lo·stat** (ahr-tik′yū-lō-stat) A research instrument that positions the dentition of a patient and the head of an x-ray machine such that films made at separate times may be accurately superimposed. [*articulo-* + G. *stasis,* a standing still]

**ar·ti·fact, ar·te·fact** (ahr′ti-fakt) Anything, especially in a histologic specimen or a graphic record or x-ray, caused by the technique used that does not reflect the original specimen or experiment. [L. *ars,* art, + *facio,* pp. *factus,* to make]

**ar·ti·fac·tu·al, ar·ti·fac·ti·tious** (ahr′ti-fak′chū-ăl, -fak-tish′ŭs) Produced or caused by an artifact.

**ar·ti·fi·cial crown** (ahr-ti-fish′ăl krown) Fixed restoration of the major part of the entire coronal part of a natural tooth; usually of gold, porcelain, or acrylic resin.

**ar·ti·fi·cial den·ti·tion** (ahr´ti-fish´ăl den-tish´ŭn) SYN denture (1).

**ar·ti·fi·cial heart** (ahr´ti-fish´ăl hahrt) A mechanical pump used to replace the function of a damaged heart, either temporarily or as a permanent prosthesis.

**ar·ti·fi·cial stone** (ahr-ti-fish´ăl stōn, ahr´ti-fish´ăl stōn) A specially calcined gypsum derivative similar to plaster of Paris but stronger because its grains are nonporous.

**ar·ti·fi·ci·al tooth** (ahr´ti-fish´ăl tūth) A tooth made of plastic, porcelain, or metal used in a prosthetic device (e.g., a fixed or removable partial denture).

**ar·ti·fi·cial ven·ti·la·tion** (ahr´ti-fish´ăl ven´ti-lā´shŭn) Any means of producing gas exchange mechanically or manually between the lungs and the surrounding air, but not performed entirely by the person's own respiratory system.

**ar·y·cor·ni·cul·ate syn·chon·dro·sis** (ar´i-kōr-nik´yū-lăt sin´kon-drō´sis) Junction of corniculate cartilage with arytenoid.

**ar·y·ep·i·glot·tic** (ar´ē-ep-i-glot´ik) Relating to arytenoid cartilage and epiglottis; denoting a fold of mucous membrane (aryepiglottic fold) and a muscle contained in it (aryepiglottic muscle). SYN arytenoepiglottidean.

**ar·y·ep·i·glot·tic fold** (ar´ē-ep-i-glot´ik fōld) [TA] Prominent fold of mucous membrane stretching between lateral margin of the epiglottis and arytenoid cartilage on either side; encloses the aryepiglottic muscle. SYN arytenoepiglottidean fold.

**ar·y·ep·i·glot·tic mus·cle** (ar´ē-ep-i-glot´ik mŭs´ĕl) SYN aryepiglottic part of oblique arytenoid (muscle).

**ar·y·ep·i·glot·tic part of o·blique ar·y·ten·oid (mus·cle)** (ar´ē-ep´i-glot´ik pahrt ō-blēk´ ar´i-tē´noyd mŭs´ĕl) [TA] Fibers of oblique arytenoid muscle that continue past summit of arytenoid cartilage to side of epiglottis; *action,* constricts the laryngeal aperture in a "purse-string" manner. SYN aryepiglottic muscle.

**ar·y·te·no·ep·i·glot·tid·e·an** (ă-rit´ē-nō-ep´i-glo-tid´ē-ăn) SYN aryepiglottic.

**ar·y·te·no·ep·i·glot·tid·e·an fold** (ă-rit´ē-nō-ep´i-glo-tid´ē-ăn fōld) SYN aryepiglottic fold.

**ar·y·te·noid** (ar´i-tē´noyd) [TA] *Avoid the mispronunciations a´rytenoid and aryt´enoid.* Denoting a cartilage (arytenoid cartilage) and muscles (oblique and transverse arytenoid muscles) of the larynx.

**ar·y·te·noi·d ar·tic·u·lar sur·face of lam·i·na of cri·coid car·ti·lage** (ar´i-tē´noyd ahr-tik´yū-lăr sŭr´făs lam´i-nă krī´koyd kahr´ti-lăj) [TA] One of two oval facets on the superolateral margin of the cricoid lamina for articulation with the arytenoid cartilages.

**ar·y·te·noid car·ti·lage** (ar´i-tē´noyd kahr´ti-lăj) [TA] One of a pair of small triangular pyramidal laryngeal cartilages that articulate with lamina of cricoid cartilage.

**ar·y·te·noid glands** (ar´i-tē´noyd glandz) Mucosal glands in the region of laryngeal arytenoid cartilages.

**ASA** Abbreviation for acetylsalicylic acid. SEE aspirin.

**ASA class·i·fi·ca·tion** (klas´i-fi-kā´shŭn) American Society of Anesthesiologists' identification system for a patient's medical status.

**as·bes·tos** (as-bes´tŏs) The commercial product, after mining and processing, obtained from a family of fibrous hydrated silicates. Inhalation of such particles can cause asbestosis, pleural plaques, and other disorders. [G. unquenchable; so-called in the erroneous belief that when heated, its warmth could not be quenched]

**as·bes·to·sis** (as-bes-tō´sis) Pneumoconiosis resulting from inhalation of asbestos fibers suspended in ambient air.

**as·bes·tos lin·er** (as-bes´tŏs lī´nĕr) Material used to line a dental casting ring so that during heating and expansion of the investment the compression of the liner will free the investment from restraint of ring.

**as·car·i·cide** (as-kar´i-sīd) 1. Causing the death of ascarid nematodes. 2. An agent having such properties. [G. *askaris,* an intestinal worm + L. *caedo,* to kill]

**As·ca·ris** (as´kă-ris) A genus of large, heavy-bodied roundworms parasitic in the small intestine. [G. *askaris,* an intestinal worm]

**as·cen·dens** (ă-sen´denz) Ascending. Going upward, ascending, toward a higher position. [L.]

**Asch·er syn·drome** (ahsh´ĕr sin´drōm) A condition in which a congenital double lip is associated with blepharochalasis and nontoxic thyroid gland enlargement.

**as·ci·tes** (ă-sī´tēz) Accumulation of serous fluid in the peritoneal cavity. [L. fr. G. *askos,* a bag, + *-ites*]

**a·scit·ic** (ă-sit´ik) *Do not confuse this word with acetic or acidic.* Of or relating to ascites.

**a·scor·bic ac·id** (ă-skōr´bik as´id) Vitamin used to prevent scurvy, as a strong reducing agent, and as an antioxidant. SYN vitamin C. [G. *a-* priv. + Mod.L. *scorbutus,* scurvy, fr. Germanic]

**ASD** Abbreviation for atrial septal defect.

**a·se·cre·to·ry** (ă-sē′krĕ-tōr-ē) Without secretions.

**a·sep·sis** (ā-sep′sis) A condition in which living pathogenic organisms are absent; a state of sterility. [G. *a-* priv. + *sēpsis,* putrefaction]

**a·sep·tic** (ā-sep′tik) *Do not confuse this word with antiseptic.* Marked by or relating to asepsis.

**a·sep·tic fe·ver** (ă-sep′tik fē′vĕr) Pyrexia with malaise caused by absorption of dead but noninfected tissue after trauma.

**a·sep·tic ne·cro·sis** (ā-sep′tik nĕ-krō′sis) Necrosis occurring in the absence of infection.

**a·sep·tic tech·nique** (ā-sep′tik tek-nēk′) Medical treatment, usually involving surgery, which avoids contact with pathogenic microorganisms rather than actively destroying them.

**a·sex·u·al** (ā-sek′shū-ăl) **1.** Referring to reproduction without nuclear fusion in an organism. **2.** Having no sexual desire or interest. [G. *a-* priv. + sexual]

**a·si·al·ism** (ā-sī′ă-lizm, ā-sī′ă-lizm) Absence of saliva. [G. *a-* negative prefix, + *sialon,* saliva, + *-ism,* noun suffix]

**a·sit·i·a** (ă-sish′ē-ă) Disgust at the sight or thought of food. [G. *a-* priv. + *sitos,* food]

**as·par·a·gine** (as-par′ă-jin) The β-amide of aspartic acid, the L-isomer is a nutritionally nonessential amino acid occurring in proteins; a diuretic.

**as·par·a·gus** (ă-spar′ă-gŭs) *Asparagus officinalis* is an edible vegetable, the rhizome and roots of which, together with the young edible shoots, have been used as a diuretic. [L. fr. G. *asparagos*]

**as·par·tame** (as′pĕr-tām) Methyl-aspartyl-phenylalanine, a synthetic dipeptide with a high sweetness index but very low caloric content used as an artificial sweetner for some foods and beverages.

**as·par·tate** (as-pahr′tāt) A salt or ester of aspartic acid.

**as·par·tyl·gly·cos·a·mi·nu·ri·a** (as-par′ til-glī-kō′să-min-yū′rē-ă) A lysosomal disorder caused by deficiency of aspartoglucosaminidase; involves recurrent infections and diarrhea; mental retardation, seizures, coarse facial features, and skeletal abnormalities that become evident by adolescence.

**as·pect** (as′pekt) **1.** Manner of appearance; looks. **2.** Side of an object that is directed in any designated direction. [L. *aspectus,* fr. *a-spicio,* pp. *-spectus,* to look at]

**as·per·gil·lo·sis** (as′pĕr-ji-lō′sis) The presence of the fungus *Aspergillus* in the tissues (invasive aspergillosis) or air-containing body cavities. SEE ALSO aspergilloma.

**As·per·gil·lus** (as′pĕr-jil′ŭs ) A genus of fungi (class Ascomycetes) that contains about 300 species, some with black, brown, or green spores. A few species are pathogenic for humans, birds, and other animals. [Med. L. a sprinkler, fr. L. *aspergo,* to sprinkle]

**as·phyx·i·a** (as-fik′sē-ă) Impaired or absent exchange of oxygen and carbon dioxide on a ventilatory basis; combined hypercapnia and hypoxia or anoxia. [G. *a-* priv. + *sphyzō,* to throb]

**as·pi·rate** (as′pir-āt) **1.** To remove by aspiration. **2.** To inhale into the airways foreign particulate material, such as vomitus. **3.** Foreign body, food, gastric contents, or fluid, including saliva, which is inhaled. [L. *a-spiro,* pp. *-atus,* to breathe on, make the H sound]

**as·pi·rat·ing sy·ringe** (as′pir-āt-ing sĭr-inj′) A syringe, commonly used to inject local anesthetic in dentistry, which allows blood into the anesthetic capsule if the needle is in a blood vessel. SEE syringe.

**as·pi·ra·tion** (as′pir-ā′shŭn) **1.** Removal, by suction, of a gas, fluid, or tissue from a body cavity or organ from unusual accumulations, or from a container. **2.** The inspiratory sucking into the airways of fluid or any foreign material, especially gastric contents or food. [L. *aspiratio,* fr. *aspiro,* to breathe on]

**as·pi·ra·tion bi·op·sy** (as′pir-ā′shŭn bī′ op-sē) SYN needle biopsy.

**as·pi·ra·tor** (as′pir-ā-tŏr) An apparatus for removing fluid, air, or tissue by aspiration from body cavities.

**as·pi·rin** (as′pir-in) A widely used analgesic, antipyretic, and antiinflammatory agent; also used as an antiplatelet agent. SYN acetylsalicylic acid.

**as·pi·rin burn** (as′pir-in bŭrn) Oral tissue damage, resulting from aspirin being placed against the mucosa and allowed to dissolve there.

**as·say** (as′ā) **1.** The quantitative or qualitative evaluation of a substance for impurities, toxicity, or other characteristics; the results of such an evaluation. **2.** To examine; to subject to analysis. **3.** Test of purity; trial. [M.E., fr. O.Fr. *essaier,* fr. L.L. *exagium,* a weighing]

**as·sess·ment** (ă-ses′mĕnt) Evaluation of the patient using selected skills of history-taking; physical examination, laboratory, imaging, and social evaluation, to achieve a specific goal. [M.E. *assessen,* to evaluate, fr. Med.L. *assideo,* pp. *assessus,* to sit in judgment, as to estimate a charge or apportion a tax]

**as·sess·ment stroke** (ă-ses′mĕnt strōk) Instrumentation motion that is used to evaluate teeth or determine health of periodontal tissues.

**As·sé·zat tri·ang·le** (ah-sā-zah′ trī′ang-gĕl) Area formed by lines connecting the nasion with the alveolar and nasal points; used to indicate prognathism in comparative craniology.

**as·sign·ment** (ă-sīn′mĕnt) A dentist "accepts assignment" when the insurance fee is considered as payment in full. [*assign*, fr. O.Fr. *assigner*, fr. L. *adsigno*, to mark, label, + -*ment*]

**as·sign·ment of ben·e·fits** (ă-sīn′mĕnt ben′ĕ-fits) Authorization from an insured to allow any payment to go directly to the physician.

**as·sis·tant** (ă-sis′tănt) Provider of subordinate support services to patients under the guidance of a dental health care professional.

**as·sist-con·trol ven·ti·la·tion** (ă-sist′ kŏn-trōl′ ven′ti-lā′shŭn) Artificial positive-pressure ventilation by machine in which a full breath is produced automatically, following a patient's natural inspiratory effort.

**as·sist·ed cir·cu·la·tion** (ă-sis′tĕd sĭr′kyū-lā′shŭn) Application of external devices to improve pressure, flow, or both in the heart or arteries.

**as·sist·ed ven·ti·la·tion** (ă-sis′tĕd ven′ti-lā′shŭn) Use of mechanically or manually generated positive pressure to gas(es) in or about the airway during inhalation to augment movement of gases into lungs. Also called assisted respiration.

**as·so·ci·ate** (ă-sō′sē-ăt, -āt) **1.** Any item or person grouped with others by some common factor. **2.** To form an association.

**as·so·ci·at·ed move·ments** (ă-sō′sē-ā-tĕd mūv′mĕnts) Normal involuntary limb movements that accompany voluntary movement, e.g., arm swing with walking.

**as·so·ci·a·tion** (ă-sō′sē-ā′shŭn) A connection of people, things, or ideas by some common factor. [L. *as-socio*, pp. -*sociatus*, to join to; *ad* + *socius*, companion]

**as·so·ci·a·tion fi·bers** (ă-sō′sē-ā′shŭn fī′bĕrz) Nerve fibers interconnecting subdivisions of the cerebral cortex of the same hemisphere or different segments of the spinal cord on the same side.

**as·so·ci·a·tive re·ac·tion** (ă-sō′sē-ă-tiv rē-ak′shŭn) A secondary or side reaction.

**as·te·ri·on** (as-tē′rē-on) [TA] Craniometric point in region of posterolateral (mastoid) fontanelle, at junction of lambdoid, occipitomastoid, and parietomastoid sutures. [G. *asterios*, starry]

**as·the·ni·a** (as-thē′nē-ă) Weakness or debility. SYN adynamia (1). [G. *astheneia*, weakness, fr. *a-* priv. + *sthenos*, strength]

**as·then·ic** (as-then′ik) **1.** Relating to asthenia. **2.** Denoting a thin, delicate body habitus.

**asth·ma** (az′mă) Inflammatory lung disease characterized by (in most cases) reversible airway obstruction; now used to denote bronchial asthma. [G.]

**asth·mat·ic** (az-mat′ik) Relating to or suffering from asthma.

**asth·ma·toid wheeze** (az′mă-toyd wēz) Puffing or musical sound heard on exhalation in front of patient's open mouth in cases in which a foreign body is present in the trachea or a bronchus.

**a·stig·ma·tism** (ă-stig′mă-tizm) A condition of unequal curvatures along the different meridians in one or more of the refractive ocular surfaces. [G. *a-* priv. + *stigma* (*stigmat-*), a point]

**as·trin·gent** (ă-strin′jĕnt) **1.** Causing contraction or shrinkage of the tissues, arrest of secretion, or control of bleeding. **2.** An agent having these effects. [L. *astringens*]

**as·tro·cyte** (as′trō-sīt, as′trŏ-sīt) One of the large neuroglial cells of neural tissue. SEE neuroglia. [G. *astēr*, star, + *kytos*, chamber, cell]

**as·tro·cy·to·ma** (as′trō-sī-tō′mă) A glioma derived from astrocytes; in people younger than 20 years of age, usually arise in a cerebellar hemisphere; in adults, usually occur in the cerebrum, sometimes growing rapidly and invading extensively. [G. *astron*, star, + *kytos*, cell, + -*oma*, tumor]

**a·sym·met·ric, a·sym·met·ric·al** (ā′si-met′rik, -ri-kăl) Not symmetric; denoting a lack of symmetry between two or more like parts.

**a·sym·me·try** (ā-sim′ĕ-trē) Lack of symmetry; disproportion between two parts normally alike.

**a·symp·to·mat·ic** (ā′simp-tŏ-mat′ik) Without symptoms, or producing no symptoms.

**a·symp·to·mat·ic car·ri·er** (ā′simp-tŏ-mat′ik kar′ē-ĕr) One who harbors pathogenic organisms without clinically recognizable symptoms; may infect others.

**a·syn·cli·tism** (ă-sin′kli-tizm) Absence of parallelism in dental arches or cranial planes. [G. *a-* priv. + *syn-klinō*, to incline together]

**asyn·cli·tism of the skull** (ă-sin′kli-tizm skŭl) SYN plagiocephaly.

**a·syn·er·gic** (ā′sin-ĕr′jik) Characterized by asynergy.

**a·syn·er·gy, a·syn·er·gi·a** (ā-sin′ĕr-jē, ā′si-nĕr′jē-ă) Lack of coordination among various muscle groups during the performance of complex movements, resulting in loss of skill and speed.

**a·sys·to·le, a·sys·to·li·a** (ā-sis′tō-lē, -sis-tō′lē-ă) Absence of contractions of the heart. [G. *a-* priv, + *systolē,* a contracting]

**AT₁₀** Abbreviation for dihydrotachysterol.

**a·tac·til·i·a** (ā′tak-til′ē-ă) Loss of the sense of touch. [G. *a-* priv. + L. *tactilis,* relating to touch, fr. *tango,* pp. *tactus,* to touch]

**at·a·rac·tic** (at′ăr-ak′tik) 1. Having a calming or tranquilizing effect. 2. A tranquilizer. [G. *ataraktos,* calm]

**at·a·rax·i·a, at·a·rax·y** (at′ă-rak′sē-ă, -rak′sē) Calmness and peace of mind; tranquility. [G. *a-* priv. + *taraktos,* disturbed, + *-ia*]

**a·tax·i·a** (ă-tak′sē-ă) Inability to coordinate muscle activity during voluntary movement; results from disorders of the cerebellum or posterior columns of spinal cord; may involve limbs, head, or trunk. Also called ataxy. [G. *a-*prov. + *taxis,* order]

**at·el·ec·ta·sis** (at′ĕ-lek′tă-sis) Decrease or loss of air in all or part of the lung, with resulting loss of lung volume itself. [G. *atelēs,* incomplete, + *ektasis,* extension]

**at·el·ec·ta·sis of the mid·dle ear** (at′ĕ-lek′tă-sis mid′ĕl ēr) Reduction in the volume of the middle ear because of pharyngotympanic (auditory) tube obstruction followed by absorption of the oxygen in the middle ear and subsequent retraction of the tympanic membrane medially.

**ath·er·o·ma** (ath′ĕr-ō′mă) The lipid deposits in the intima of arteries, producing a yellow swelling on the endothelial surface; a characteristic of atherosclerosis. [G. *athērē,* gruel, + *-ōma,* tumor]

**ath·er·o·scle·ro·sis** (ath′ĕr-ō-skler-ō′sis) Arteriosclerosis characterized by irregularly distributed lipid deposits in the intima of large and medium-sized arteries, causing narrowing of arterial lumens and proceeding eventually to fibrosis and calcification. [G. *athērē,* gruel, + *sclerosis*]

**ath·er·o·scle·rot·ic an·eu·rysm** (ath′ĕr-ō-sklĕ-rot′ik an′yŭr-izm) Most common type of aneurysm, occurring in the abdominal aorta and other large arteries, primarily in old people. SYN arteriosclerotic aneurysm.

**ath·e·to·sis** (ath′ĕ-tō′sis) A condition involving a constant succession of slow, writhing, involuntary movements of flexion, extension, pronation, and supination of the fingers and hands, and sometimes of the toes and feet. [G. *athetos,* without position or place]

**a·throm·bi·a** (ă-throm′bē-ă) A hereditary bleeding disorder characterized by prolonged bleeding time, decreased platelet adhesion and aggregation, but normal plasma clotting and clot retraction, normal platelet count with platelet factor 3 availability; probably autosomal recessive inheritance. [G. *a-* priv. + *thrombin*]

**ATL** Abbreviation for adult T-cell leukemia; adult T-cell lymphoma.

▣**at·lan·to·ax·i·al joint** (at-lan′tō-ak′sē-ăl joynt) [TA] Complex joint between first and second cervical vertebrae, consisting of the median and lateral atlantoaxial joints. See this page.

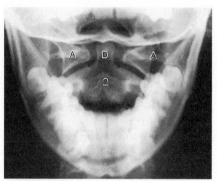

**atlantoaxial joint:** radiographic image viewed through open mouth; 2 = body of axis; D = dens; A = atlas

**at·lan·to·oc·cip·i·tal joint** (at-lan′tō-ok-sip′i-tăl joynt, at-lan′tō-ok-sip′i-tăl joynt) [TA] Articulation between the superior facets of the atlas and the condyles of the occipital joint. SYN articulatio atlantooccipitalis, atlanto-occipital articulation.

**at·las** (at′lăs) [TA] First cervical vertebra, articulating with the occipital bone and rotating around the dens of the axis. [G. *Atlas,* in Greek mythology, a Titan who supported the heavens on his shoulders]

**at·om** (at′ŏm) Formerly considered the ultimate particle of an element, discovery of radioactivity demonstrated the existence of subatomic particles, notably protons, neutrons, and electrons, the first two making up most of the mass of the atomic nucleus. Subatomic particles are now further classified into hadrons, leptons, and quarks. [G. *atomos,* indivisible, uncut]

**a·tom·ic** (ă-tom′ik) Relating to an atom.

**a·tom·ic mass num·ber** (ă-tom′ik mas nŭm′bĕr) The mass of the atom of a particular isotope relative to hydrogen 1 (or to one twelfth the mass of carbon 12), generally very close to the whole number represented by the sum of the protons and neutrons in the atomic nucleus of the isotope; it is not to be confused with the atomic weight of an element, which may include a number of isotopes in natural proportion.

**a·tom·ic weight (AW, at. wt.)** (ă-tom′ik wāt) The mass in grams of 1 mol (6.02 × 10²³, atoms) of an atomic species. SEE ALSO molecular weight.

**at·om·iz·er** (at′ŏm-ī-zĕr) Device used to reduce liquid medication to fine aerosol particles; used to deliver medication to lungs, nose, and throat. SEE ALSO nebulizer, vaporizer. [G. *atomos,* indivisible particle]

**a·ton·ic** (ā-ton′ik) Relaxed; without normal tone or tension.

**at·o·ny** (at′ŏ-nē) Relaxation, flaccidity, or lack of tone or tension. [G. *atonia,* languor]

**a·top·ic** (ā-top′ik) 1. Relating to or marked by atopy. 2. Allergic. [G. *atopos,* out of place; strange]

**a·top·ic der·ma·ti·tis** (ā-top′ik dĕr′mă-tī′tis) Dermatitis characterized by the distinctive phenomena of atopy, including infantile and flexural eczema.

**a·top·og·no·si·a, a·top·og·no·sis** (ā′top-og-nō′zē-ă, -nō′sis) Sensory inattention; inability to locate a sensation properly. [G. *a-* priv. + *topos,* place, + *gnōsis,* knowledge]

**at·o·py** (at′ŏ-pē) A genetically determined state of hypersensitivity to environmental allergens. [G. *atopia,* strangeness, fr. *a-* priv. + *topos,* a place]

**ATP** Abbreviation for adenosine 5′-triphosphate.

**a·tre·si·a** (ă-trē′zē-ă) Congenital absence of a normal opening or normally patent lumen. [G. *a-* priv. + *trēsis,* a hole]

**a·tri·al fi·bril·la·tion, au·ric·u·lar fi·bril·la·tion** (ā′trē-ăl fib′ri-lā′shŭn, aw-rik′yū-lăr) Fibrillation in which normal rhythmic contractions of the cardiac atria are replaced by rapid irregular twitchings of the muscular wall.

**a·tri·o·ven·tric·u·lar, au·ri·cu·lo·ven·tric·u·lar (AV)** (ā′trē-ō-ven-trik′yū-lăr, aw-rik′yū-lō-) Relating to both the atria and the ventricles of the heart, especially to the ordinary, orthograde transmission of conduction or blood flow.

**a·tri·um,** pl. **a·tri·a** (ā′trē-ŭm, -ă) [TA] *Do not confuse this word with antrum.* Chamber or cavity to which are connected several chambers or passageways. [L. entrance hall]

**a·tri·um me·a·tus me·di·i** (ā′trē-ŭm mē-ā′tŭs mē′dē-ī) [TA] SYN atrium of middle nasal meatus.

**a·tri·um of mid·dle na·sal me·a·tus** (ā′trē-ŭm mid′ĕl nā′zăl mē-ā′tŭs) [TA] The anterior expanded portion of the middle meatus of the nose, just above the vestibule. SYN atrium meatus medii, nasal atrium.

**a·troph·ic glos·si·tis** (ă-trō′fik glos-ī′tis) Erythematous, edematous, and painful tongue condition that appears smooth because of loss of the filiform and sometimes the fungiform papillae due to nutritional deficiencies. SYN smooth tongue.

**a·troph·ic rhi·ni·tis** (ā-trō′fik rī-nī′tis) Chronic rhinitis with thinning of the mucous membrane.

**at·ro·phy** (at′rŏ-fē) A wasting of tissues, organs, or the entire body, as from death and reabsorption of cells, diminished cellular proliferation, decreased cellular volume, pressure, ischemia, malnutrition, lessened function, or hormonal changes. [G. *atrophia,* fr. *a-* priv. + *trophē,* nourishment]

**at·ro·pine** (at′rŏ-pēn) Mixture of D- and L-hyoscyamine, alkaloids obtained from the leaves and roots of *Atropa belladonna;* an anticholinergic, with diverse effects attributable to reversible competitive blockade of acetylcholine at muscarinic type cholinergic receptors.

**at·tached gin·gi·va** (ă-tacht′ jin′ji-vă) That part of the oral mucosa firmly bound to the tooth and alveolar process. See this page.

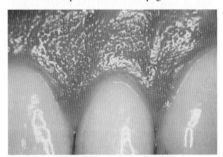

**attached gingiva:** stippled surface texture

**at·tach·ment** (ă-tach′mĕnt) 1. In dentistry, a mechanical device for the fixation and stabilization of a dental prosthesis. 2. A connection of one part with another.

**at·tach·ment ap·pa·ra·tus** (ă-tach′mĕnt ap′ă-rat′ŭs) Tissues that attach the tooth to the alveolar process: cementum, periodontal ligament, and alveolar bone.

**at·tach·ment loss** (ă-tach′mĕnt laws) A periodontal condition with loss of the tissues that attach the tooth to the alveolar process.

**at·ten·tion def·i·cit dis·or·der (ADD)** (ă-ten′shŭn def′i-sit dis-ōr′dĕr) Disorder of attention, organization, and impulse control appearing in childhood and often persisting to adulthood. Hyperactivity may be a feature but is not necessary for the diagnosis.

**at·ten·tion def·i·cit hy·per·ac·tiv·i·ty dis·or·der (ADHD)** (ă-ten′shŭn def′i-sit hī′pĕr-ak-tiv′i-tē dis-ōr′dĕr) A behavioral disorder manifested by developmentally inappropriate degrees of inattentiveness (short attention span, distractability, inability to complete tasks, difficulty in following directions), impulsiveness (acting without due reflection), and hyperactivity (restlessness, fidgeting, squirming, excessive loquacity).

**at·ti·tude** (at′i-tūd) **1.** Position of the body and limbs. **2.** Manner of behavior. [Mediev. L. *aptitudo,* fr. L. *aptus,* fit]

**at·ti·tu·di·nal** (at′i-tū′di-năl) Relating to body posture; e.g., attitudinal (statotonic) reflex.

**at·tri·tion** (ă-trish′ŭn) **1.** In dentistry, physiologic loss of tooth structure caused by normal wear inherent in the aging process, as well as by the abrasive character of food or by bruxism. **2.** Wearing away by friction or rubbing. See this page and page A4. [L. *at-tero,* pp. *-tritus,* to rub against, rub away]

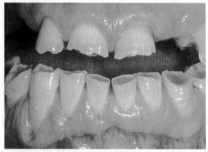

**attrition along incisal surfaces**

**at·tri·tion·al oc·clu·sion** (ă-trish′ŭn-ăl ŏ-klū′zhŭn) Occlusion that results in abnormal wearing away of tooth structure. attritional [L. *attritio,* gen. *attritionis,* fr. *attero,* pp. *attritus,* to rub, grind, + *-al,* adj. suffix] occlusion [L. *oc-cludo,* pp. *oc-clusus,* to shut up, fr. *ob-,* in the way of, + *claudo,* to close, + *-ion,* noun suffix]

**at. wt.** Abbreviation for atomic weight.

**a·typ·i·cal** (ā-tip′i-kăl) Denotes the unexpected or unanticipated; not corresponding to the normal form or type. [G. *a-* priv. + *typikos,* conformed to a type]

**a·typ·i·cal fa·cial neuralgia** (ā-tip′i-kăl fā′shăl nūr-al′jē-ă) SYN atypical trigeminal neuralgia.

**a·typ·i·cal gin·gi·vi·tis** (ā-tip′i-kăl jin′ji-vī′tis) SYN plasma cell gingivitis.

**a·typ·i·cal li·po·ma** (ā-tip′i-kăl li-pō′mă) Lesion, occurring primarily in older men on the posterior neck, shoulders, and back, which is benign but microscopically atypical, containing giant cells with multiple overlapping nuclei forming a circle. SYN pleomorphic lipoma.

**a·typ·i·cal my·co·bac·te·ri·a** (ā-tip′i-kăl mī′kō-bak-tēr′ē-ă) Species of *Mycobacte-*

*rium* other than *M. tuberculosis* that cause infections in both healthy and immunosuppressed people.

**a·typ·i·cal tri·gem·i·nal neu·ral·gi·a** (ā-tip′i-kăl trī-jem′i-năl nūr-al′jē-ă) Periodic pain in any region of the face, teeth, tongue, and occasionally in the occipital or shoulder area, which lasts several minutes to several days but has no trigger point and lacks the paroxysmal character of tic douloureux.

**Au** Symbol for gold.

**audio-** Combining form denoting the sense of hearing. [L. *audio,* to hear]

**au·di·o·an·al·ge·si·a** (aw′dē-ō-an-ăl-jē′zē-ă) Use of music or other sounds delivered through earphones to mask pain during dental or surgical procedures.

**au·di·o·gen·ic sei·zure** (aw′dē-ō-jen′ik sē′zhŭr) Reflex seizure precipitated by loud noises, rare in humans.

**au·di·o·gram** (aw′dē-ō-gram) The graphic record drawn from the results of hearing tests with the audiometer. [L. *audio,* to hear + G. *gramma,* a drawing]

**au·di·ol·o·gist** (aw′dē-ol′ŏ-jist) A specialist in evaluation and rehabilitation of patients whose communication disorders stem in whole or in part from hearing impairment.

**au·di·ol·o·gy** (aw′dē-ol′ŏ-jē) **1.** Study of hearing disorders through identification and measurement of hearing impairment. **2.** Rehabilitation of patients with hearing impairments.

**au·di·om·e·ter** (aw′dē-om′ĕ-tĕr) Electronic device used to measure hearing thresholds for pure tones, modulated tones, speech, and other acoustic stimuli. [L. *audio,* to hear + G. *metron,* measure]

**au·di·om·e·trist** (aw′dē-om′ĕ-trist) A person trained in the use of an audiometer in hearing testing.

**au·dit** (aw′dit) An examination or review to establish extent to which a condition or process conforms to predetermined standards or criteria. [L. *auditus,* a hearing, fr. *audio,* to hear]

**au·di·to·ry** (aw′di-tōr-ē) **1.** Pertaining to the sense of hearing or to the system that serves hearing. **2.** Used to describe a person who preferentially uses verbal mental imagery. [L. *audio,* pp. *auditus,* to hear]

**au·di·to·ry brain·stem re·sponse (ABR)** (aw′di-tōr-ē brān′stem rĕ-spons′) Electrophysiologic measure of auditory function using computer-averaged responses produced by the auditory nerve and the central auditory pathways principally in the brainstem to repetitive acoustic stimuli. SYN brainstem evoked response.

**au·di·to·ry gan·gli·on** (aw´di-tōr-ē gang´ glē-ŏn) SYN cochlear ganglion.

**au·di·to·ry os·si·cles** (aw´di-tōr-ē os´i-kĕlz) [TA] Small bones of middle ear articulated to form a chain for the transmission of sound from the tympanic membrane to the oval window. SYN ear bones.

**au·di·to·ry path·way** (aw´di-tōr-ē path´ wā) Neural paths and connections within the central nervous system, beginning at the hair cells of the spiral organ, continuing along the eighth cranial nerve, and ending at the auditory cortex.

**au·di·to·ry pro·cess** (aw´di-tōr-ē pro´ses) Roughened edge of tympanic plate giving attachment to cartilaginous portion of the external acoustic meatus.

**au·di·to·ry teeth** (aw´di-tōr-ē tēth) SYN acoustic teeth.

**au·di·to·ry tube** (aw´di-tōr-ē tūb) SYN pharyngotympanic (auditory) tube.

**aug·men·ta·tion** (awg´men-tā´shŭn) Process of increasing in size, amount, degree, or severity. [L. *augmentum,* growth, increase]

**au·ra,** pl. **au·rae** (awr´ă) **1.** Epileptic ictal phenomenon perceived only by the patient. **2.** Subjective symptom at onset of migraine headache. [L. breeze, odor, gleam of light]

**au·ral, au·ric·u·lar** (awr´ăl, aw-rik´yū-lăr) **1.** Relating to the ear (auris). **2.** Relating to an aura.

**au·ral my·i·a·sis** (awr´ăl mī-ī´ă-sis) Invasion of the external, middle, or inner ear by larvae of dipterous insects.

✿ **auri-** *Do not confuse words containing this combining form with words based on aurum 'gold' or os, oris 'mouth.'* Combining form denoting the ear. [L. *auris,* an ear.]

**au·ric** (awr´ik) Relating to gold (aurum).

**au·ri·cle** (awr´i-kĕl) [TA] *Avoid the outmoded use of this word in the sense of atrium.* The projecting shell-like structure on the side of the head, constituting, with the external acoustic meatus, the external ear.

**au·ric·u·lar** (awr-ik´yū-lăr) Relating to the ear, or to an auricle in any sense.

**au·ric·u·lar arc, bin·au·ric·u·lar arc** (aw-rik´yū-lăr ahrk, bin´) Line carried over the cranium from center of one external auditory meatus to that of the other.

**au·ric·u·lar branch of va·gus nerve** (aw-rik´yū-lăr branch vā´gŭs nĕrv) [TA] Branch of superior ganglion of vagus, merging with fibers from inferior ganglion of glossopharyngeal nerve supplying cranial surface of the auricle, external acoustic meatus, and lower part of external surface of tympanic membrane. Also called Arnold nerve.

**au·ric·u·lar car·ti·lage** (awr-ik´yū-lăr kahr´ti-lăj) [TA] Cartilage of the auricle (pinna) of external ear.

**au·ric·u·la·re,** pl. **au·ric·u·lar·i·a** (aw-rik´yū-lā´rē, -rē-ă) Craniometric point at center of opening of the external auditory meatus or, in certain cases, middle of upper edge of this opening. [L. *auricularis,* pertaining to the ear]

**au·ric·u·lar fis·sure** (aw-rik´yū-lăr fish´ŭr) SYN tympanomastoid fissure.

**au·ric·u·lar gan·gli·on** (aw-rik´yū-lăr gang´ glē-ŏn) SYN otic ganglion.

**au·ric·u·lar in·dex** (aw-rik´yū-lăr in´deks) Relation of the width to the height of the auricle or pinna: (width of pinna × 100)/length of pinna.

**au·ric·u·la·ris an·te·ri·or (mus·cle)** (aw-rik´yū-lā´ris an-tēr´ē-ŏr mŭs´ĕl) [TA] Facial muscle of external ear; considered by some to be the anterior part of the temporoparietalis muscle. SYN anterior auricular muscle.

**au·ric·u·la·ris pos·te·ri·or (mus·cle)** (aw-rik´yū-lā´ris pos-tēr´ē-ŏr mŭs´ĕl) [TA] Facial muscle of external ear.

**au·ric·u·la·ris su·pe·ri·or (mus·cle)** (aw-rik´yū-lā´ris sŭ-pēr´ē-ŏr mŭs´ĕl) [TA] Facial muscle associated with the external ear; considered by some to be posterior part of temporoparietal muscle.

**au·ric·u·lar lig·a·ments** (aw-rik´yū-lăr lig´ă-mĕnts) SYN ligaments of auricle.

**au·ric·u·lar mus·cles** (aw-rik´yū-lăr mŭs´ĕlz) [TA] Small muscles associated with the auricle, having little function in humans.

**au·ric·u·lar notch** (aw-rik´yū-lăr noch) SYN terminal notch of auricle.

**au·ric·u·lar tri·an·gle** (aw-rik´yū-lăr trī´ ang-gĕl) Area formed by base of auricle and by lines drawn from true tip of the auricle to extremities of the base.

**au·ric·u·lar tu·ber·cle** (aw-rik´yū-lăr tū´ bĕr-kĕl) [TA] Small inconstant projection from the upper end of the posterior portion of the incurved free margin of the helix of the auricle.

**au·ric·u·lo·cra·ni·al** (aw-rik´yū-lō-krā´nē-ăl) Relating to auricle or pinna of the ear and cranium.

**au·ric·u·lo·tem·po·ral** (awr-ik´yū-lō-tem´ pŏr-ăl) Relating to the auricle or pinna of the ear and the temporal region.

**au·ric·u·lo·tem·po·ral nerve** (awr-ik´ yū-lō-tem´pŏr-ăl nĕrv) [TA] A branch of the mandibular nerve, usually arising by two roots embracing the middle meningeal artery. SYN nervus auriculotemporalis [TA].

**au·ric·u·lo·tem·po·ral nerve syn·drome** (aw-rik′yū-lō-tem′pŏr-ăl nĕrv sin′drōm) Facial flushing and sweating resulting from eating spicy or acidic foods, due to damage of the parasympathetic fibers in the auriculotemporal nerve. SYN Frey syndrome, gustatory sweating.

**au·ris,** pl. **au·res** (awr′is, awr′ēz) [TA] SEE ear. [L.]

**au·ris ex·ter·na** (awr′is eks-tĕr′nă) [TA] SEE ear.

**au·ris in·ter·na** (awr′is in-tĕr′nă) [TA] SEE ear.

**au·ris me·di·a** (awr′is mē′dē-ă) [TA] SYN middle ear.

**au·ro·ther·a·py** (aw′rō-thār′ă-pē) SYN chrysotherapy. [L. *aurum,* gold]

**aus·cul·tate, aus·cult** (aws′kŭl-tāt, aws-kŭlt′) To perform auscultation.

**aus·cul·ta·tion** (aws′kŭl-tā′shŭn) Listening to the sounds made by various body structures as a diagnostic method. [L. *auscultatio,* fr. *ausculto,* pp. *auscultatus,* to listen, + *-io,* noun suffix]

**aus·cul·ta·to·ry per·cus·sion** (aws-kŭl′tă-tōr-ē pĕr-kŭsh′ŭn) Auscultation of chest or other body part at the same time that percussion is made, to facilitate hearing of sound made by percussion.

**aus·cul·ta·to·ry sound** (aw-skŭl′tă-tōr-ē sownd) Rale, murmur, bruit, fremitus, or other sound heard on auscultation of the chest or abdomen.

**au·thor·i·za·tion** (aw′thŏr-ī-zā′shŭn) 1. In dental accounting, guaranteed acceptance of a procedure or therapy and payment thereof by a third-party payer. 2. An agreement or acknowledgement, generally written, from a patient or caregiver that records and documents may be shared among other oral care providers.

**au·tism** (aw′tizm) Mental disorder characterized by severely abnormal development of social interaction and of verbal and nonverbal communication skills. Affected people may adhere to inflexible, nonfunctional rituals or routines. They may become upset with even trivial changes in their environment. [G. *autos,* self]

⟡ **auto-, aut-** Prefixes meaning self, same. [G. *autos,* self]

**au·to·a·nal·y·sis** (aw′tō-ă-nal′i-sis) Attempted analysis, or psychoanalysis, of oneself. SYN self-analysis.

**au·to·an·ti·body** (aw′tō-an′ti-bod-ē) Antibody occurring in response to antigenic constit-

uents of the host's tissue, and which reacts with the inciting tissue component.

**au·toc·la·sis, au·to·cla·si·a** (aw-tok′lă-sis, aw′tō-klā′zē-ă) 1. A breaking up or rupturing from intrinsic or internal causes. 2. Progressive immunologically induced tissue destruction. [*auto-* + G. *klasis,* breaking]

**au·to·clave** (aw′tō-klāv) 1. An apparatus for sterilization involving steam under pressure consisting of a strong closed boiler in which are placed a small quantity of water and a wire basket holding the articles to be sterilized. 2. To sterilize in an autoclave. [*auto-* + L. *clavis,* a key, in the sense of self-locking]

**au·to·drain·age** (aw′tō-drān-ăj) Drainage into contiguous tissues.

**au·to·e·ryth·ro·cyte sen·si·ti·za·tion syn·drome** (aw′tō-ē-rith′rō-sīt sen′si-ti-zā′shŭn sin′drōm) A condition that usually occurs primarily in women, in which the person bruises easily (purpura simplex). SYN Gardner-Diamond syndrome.

**au·tog·e·nous** (aw-toj′ĕ-nŭs) 1. SYN autologous. 2. Originating within the body, applied to vaccines prepared from bacteria or other materials obtained from the affected person. [G. *autogenēs,* self-produced]

**au·tog·e·nous u·ni·on** (aw-toj′ĕ-nŭs yūn′yŏn) In dentistry, union of two pieces of metal without solder.

**au·to·graft** (aw′tō-graft) Tissue or organ transferred into a new position in the body of the same patient. [*auto-* + A.S. *graef*]

**autohaemolysis** [Br.] SYN autohemolysis.

**au·to·he·mol·y·sis** (aw′tō-hē-mol′i-sis) Hemolysis occurring in certain diseases as a result of an autohemolysin. SYN autohaemolysis.

**au·to·im·mune** (aw′tō-i-myūn′) Arising from and directed against the person's own tissues, as in autoimmune disease.

**au·to·im·mune dis·ease** (aw′tō-i-myūn′ di-zēz′) Disorder in which loss of function or destruction of normal tissue arises from humoral or cellular immune responses to the body's own tissue constituents.

**au·to·im·mu·ni·ty** (aw′tō-i-myū′ni-tē) In immunology, the condition in which one's own tissues are subject to deleterious effects of actions of the immune system.

**au·to·in·fec·tion** (aw′tō-in-fek′shŭn) Reinfection by microbes or parasitic organisms that have already passed through an infective cycle.

**au·to·in·oc·u·la·tion** (aw′tō-in-ok-yū-lā′shŭn) Seeding or establishing an infection by transferring an organism from one area of the body to another. Patients who are asymptomatic nasal carriers of *Staphylococcus* may autoinoculate areas of breached skin, on other parts of the body, causing clinical infection and cellulites.

**au·to·in·tox·i·cant** (aw′tō-in-toks′i-kănt) An endogenous toxic agent that causes autointoxication.

**au·tol·o·gous** (aw-tol′ŏ-gŭs) Occurring naturally and normally in a certain type of tissue or in a specific structure of the body. SYN autogenous (1). [*auto-* + G. *logos,* relation]

**au·to·mated probe** (aw′tō-mā′tĕd prōb) An electronic device used to determine the depth of the periodontal sulcus or a periodontal probe.

**au·to·mat·i·cal·ly tuned** (aw′tō-mat′ik-lē tūnd) Denotes an ultrasonic device that does not allow the clinician to adjust the vibration frequency of the instrument tip. SEE ALSO tuning, manually tuned.

**au·to·mat·ic con·den·ser** (aw′tō-mat′ik kŏn-den′sĕr) SYN automatic plugger.

**au·to·mat·ic ex·ter·nal de·fib·ril·la·tor (AED)** (aw′tō-mat′ik eks-tĕr′năl dē-fib′ri-lā-tŏr) Device used to administer electric shock to arrest fibrillation of the atria or ventricles and restore normal heart rhythm; can be used by technicians without medical training.

**au·to·mat·ic plug·ger** (aw′tō-mat′ik plŭg′ĕr) Mechanically or electrically activated device used to provide condensing pressure in the placement of amalgam or gold foil in a cavity preparation. SYN automatic condenser.

**au·to·mat·ic tooth·brush** (aw′tō-mat′ik tūth′brŭsh) An electric device to facilitate cleaning of the teeth at home. SYN electric toothbrush.

**au·tom·a·tism** (aw-tom′ă-tizm) 1. State of being independent of the will or of central innervation; applicable, for example, to the heart's action. 2. A condition in which a person is consciously or unconsciously, but involuntarily, compelled to perform certain motor or verbal acts, often purposeless and sometimes foolish or harmful. [G. *automatos,* self-moving, + *-in*]

**au·to·nom·ic** (aw′tō-nom′ik) Relating to the autonomic nervous system.

**au·to·no·mic dys·re·flex·ia** (aw′tō-nom′ik dis-rē-flek′sē-ă) A syndrome occurring in some people with spinal cord lesions resulting from functional impairment of the autonomic nervous system.

**au·to·nom·ic ner·vous sys·tem (ANS)** (aw′tō-nom′ik nĕr′vŭs sis′tĕm) SYN autonomic (visceral motor) division of nervous system.

**au·to·no·mic sei·zure** (aw′tō-nom′ik sē′zhŭr) Seizure characterized by objectively documented dysfunction of the autonomic nervous system, usually involving cardiovascular, gastrointestinal, or sudomotor functions.

**au·to·no·mic (vis·cer·al mo·tor) di·vi·sion of ner·vous sys·tem** (aw′ tō-nom′ik vis′ĕr-ăl mō′tŏr di-vizh′ŭn nĕr′vŭs sis′tĕm) [TA] Part of the nervous system that represents motor innervation of smooth muscle, cardiac muscle, and gland cells. It consists of two physiologically and anatomically distinct, mutually antagonistic components: sympathetic and parasympathetic parts.

**au·to·nom·o·tro·pic** (aw′tō-nom-ō-trō′pik) Acting on the autonomic nervous system. [*autonomic* + G. *trepo,* to turn]

**au·ton·o·mous** (aw-ton′ŏ-mŭs) Having independence or freedom from control by external forces or, in a narrow sense, by the cerebrospinal nerve centers. Cf. heteronomous.

**au·ton·o·my** (aw-ton′ŏ-mē) Condition or state of being autonomous, able to make decisions unaided by others. [*auto-* + G. *nomos,* law]

**au·toph·o·ny** (aw-tof′ŏ-nē) Increased hearing of one's own voice, breath sounds, arterial murmurs, and other noises of the upper body; noted especially in disease of the middle ear or of the nasal fossae. [*auto-* + G. *phōnē,* sound]

**au·to·pol·ym·er·i·za·tion** (aw′tō-pol′i-mĕr-ī-zā′shŭn) Polymerization reaction initiated chemically rather than by application of heat or light. SYN cold-cure polymerization.

**au·to·pol·y·mer res·in, au·to·po·ly·mer·iz·ing res·in** (aw′tō-pol′i-mĕr rez′in, aw′tō-pol′i-mĕr-īz-ing) Any resin that can be polymerized by chemical catalysis rather than by application of heat or light; used in dentistry for dental restoration, denture repair, and impression trays. SYN activated resin, cold cure resin, self-curing resin.

**au·top·sy** (aw′top-sē) *Avoid the mispronunciation autop′sy.* Examination of the organs of a cadaver to determine the cause of death or to study the pathologic changes present. [G. *autopsia,* seeing with one's own eyes]

**au·to·ra·di·og·ra·phy** (aw′tō-rā-dē-og′ră-fē) The process of producing an autoradiograph. SYN radioautography.

**au·to·re·cep·tor** (aw′tō-rē-sep′tŏr) A site on a neuron that binds the neurotransmitter released by that neuron, which then regulates the neuron's activity. [*auto-* + *receptor*]

**au·to·sep·ti·ce·mi·a** (aw′tō-sep′ti-sē′mē-ă) Septicemia apparently originating from microorganisms existing within the individual and not introduced from without. [*auto-* + G. *sēpsis,* decay, + *haima,* blood]

**au·to·trans·plan·ta·tion** (aw′tō-trans-plan-tā′shŭn) The transfer of an organ or other tissue (skin, bone, muscle, tendon, nerve, arterial or venous segments) as grafts or vascularized (by pedicle or microanastomosis) structures from one location to another in the same person (e.g., a kidney moved from its original position to the pelvis, where the iliac vessels provide vascular supply).

**aux·il·ia·ry** (awg-zil′yă-rē) *Avoid the mispronunciation og-zil′ă-rē.* **1.** Functioning in an augmenting capacity; supplementary. **2.** Functioning as a subordinate; secondary.

**aux·il·ia·ry a·but·ment** (awg-zil′yă-rē ă-bŭt′mĕnt) Any tooth other than the one supporting the direct retainer, assisting in the overall support of a removable partial denture.

**aux·il·i·a·ry spring** (awg-zil′yă-rē spring) A short piece of wire attached to an orthodontic appliance used to apply force to the teeth.

**AV** Abbreviation for arteriovenous; atrioventricular; auriculoventricular.

**a·vail·a·ble arch length** (ă-vā′lă-bĕl ahrch length) Amount of space available for permanent teeth around dental arch from first permanent molar to first permanent molar.

**a·vas·cu·lar·i·za·tion** (ā-vas′kyū-lar-ī-zā′shŭn) **1.** Expulsion of blood from a part, as by means of a tourniquet or other method of arterial compression. **2.** Loss of vascularity, as by scarring.

**A·vel·lis syn·drome** (ah-vel′is sin′drōm) Unilateral paralysis of the larynx, pharynx, and velum palati with crossed hemianesthesia for pain and temperature, due to a lesion (most often infarct or neoplasm) involving either the vagal nuclei and the spinothalamic tract in the medullary tegmentum, or the vagus nerve and spinothalamic tract nerve near the jugular foramen.

**av·er·age life** (av′ĕr-ăj līf) SYN mean life.

**a·vi·a·tion med·i·cine** (ā′vē-ā′shŭn med′i-sin) Study and practice of medicine as it applies to physiologic problems peculiar to aviation.

**av·i·din** (av′i-din) Glycoprotein obtained from egg whites that possesses a high affinity for biotin; ingestion can cause biotin deficiency. [L. *avidus,* eager fr. *aveo,* to crave + *-in*]

**a·vi·ta·min·o·sis** (ā-vī′tă-min-ō′sis) SEE hypovitaminosis.

**a·void·ance** (ă-voy′dăns) In psychiatry, a term describing a decrease in strength of relationships or fear and withdrawal when conflict emerges. SEE attachment.

**a·vulsed tooth** (ă-vŭlst′ tūth) Tooth that has, as a result of trauma, been separated and completely dislodged from the alveolus.

**⬛a·vul·sion** (ă-vŭl′shŭn) Tearing away, forcible separation, or complete displacement of a

tooth from the alveolar bone. Cf. evulsion. See this page. [L. *a-vello,* pp. *-vulsus,* to tear away]

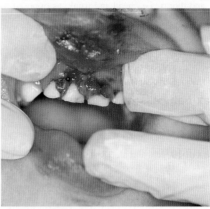

**gingival avulsion**

**a·vul·sion frac·ture** (ă-vŭl′shŭn frak′shŭr) Breakage that occurs when a joint capsule, ligament, or muscle insertion or origin is pulled from the bone as a result of a sprain, dislocation, or strong contracture of the muscle against resistance; as the soft tissue is pulled away from the bone, a fragment (or fragments) remains attached to the soft tissue of the bone.

**AW** Abbreviation for atomic weight.

**AX** Abbreviation for alloxan.

**ax·i·al** (ak′sē-ăl) [TA] **1.** In dentistry, relating to or parallel with the long axis of a tooth. **2.** In radiology, an axial image is one obtained by rotating around the axis of the body, producing a transverse planar image, i.e., a section transverse to the axis. **3.** Relating to an axis. **4.** Relating to or situated in the central part of the body, in the head and trunk as distinguished from the limbs, e.g., axial skeleton. [L. *axis,* axle, + *-al,* adj. suffix]

**ax·i·al an·gle** (ak′sē-ăl ang′gĕl) Angle formed by two surfaces of a body, the line of union of which is parallel with its axis; those of a tooth are the distobuccal, distolabial, distolingual, mesiobuccal, mesiolabial, and mesiolingual.

**ax·i·al in·clin·a·tion** (ak′sē-ăl in′kli-nā′shŭn) Angle formed by long axis of tooth with plane of the bone from which it arises.

**ax·i·al mus·cle** (ak′sē-ăl mŭs′ĕl) Skeletal muscle of the trunk or head.

**ax·i·al plane** (aks′ē-ăl plān) **1.** Plane parallel to long axis of tooth (or other elongated anatomic structure) that can be aligned mesiodistally or bucolingually. **2.** Plane perpendicular to body's sagittal and frontal reference planes.

**ax·i·al sec·tion** (ak′sē-ăl sek′shŭn) SYN transverse section.

**ax·i·al skel·e·ton** (ak′sē-ăl skel′ĕ-tŏn) [TA] Articulated bones of head, vertebral column, and thorax, i.e., head and trunk, as opposed to the appendicular skeleton, articulated bones of the upper and lower limbs.

**ax·i·al sur·fac·es** (ak′sē-ăl sŭr′făs-ĕz) Surfaces of a tooth parallel to its long axis; include vestibular (labial or buccal), lingual, and contact (mesial or distal).

**ax·i·al walls of the pulp cham·bers** (ak′sē-ăl wawlz pŭlp chăm′bĕrz) Walls parallel with the long axis of a tooth: the mesial, distal, buccal, and lingual walls.

**ax·il·la**, gen. and pl. **ax·il·lae** (ak-sil′ă, -sil′ē) [TA] The space below the shoulder joint, bounded by the pectoralis major anteriorly, the latissimus dorsi posteriorly, the serratus anterior medially, and the humerus laterally; it has a superior opening between the clavicle, scapula, and first rib (cervicoaxillary canal), and an inferior opening covered by the axillary fascia; it contains the axillary artery and vein, the infraclavicular part of the brachial plexus, axillary lymph nodes and vessels, and areolar tissue. SYN axillary cavity. [L.]

**ax·il·lar·y cavity** (ak′sil-ār-ē kav′i-tē) SYN axilla.

⚙ **axio-** Combining form denoting an axis. SEE ALSO axo-. [L. *axis*]

**ax·i·o·buc·cal** (ak′sē-ō-bŭk′ăl) Referring to the junction of the axial and buccal planes of a tooth, usually a line.

**ax·i·o·buc·co·gin·gi·val** (ak′sē-ō-bŭk′ō-jin′ji-văl) Referring to the junction of the axial, buccal, and gingival planes of teeth; usually a point.

**ax·i·o·buc·co·lin·gual plane** (ak′sē-ō-bŭk′ō-ling′gwăl plān) Plane parallel to the long axis of the tooth and aligned buccolingually.

**ax·i·o·in·ci·sal** (ak′sē-ō-in-sī′săl) Referring to the line angle formed by the junction of the incisal edge and axial walls of a tooth.

**ax·i·o·la·bi·al** (ak′sē-ō-lā′bē-ăl) Referring to the line angle of a cavity formed by the junction of the axial and the labial walls of a tooth.

**ax·i·o·la·bi·o·lin·gual** (ak′sē-ō-lā′bē-ō-ling′gwăl) Referring to a section from labial to lingual along the longitudinal axis of a tooth.

**ax·i·o·la·bi·o·lin·gual plane** (ak′sē-ō-lā′bē-ō-ling′gwăl plān) Plane parallel to the long axis of a tooth and extending in a labiolingual direction.

**ax·i·o·lin·gual** (ak′sē-ō-ling′gwăl) Referring to the line angle of a cavity formed by the junction of an axial and a lingual wall of a tooth.

**ax·i·o·lin·guo·cer·vi·cal** (ak′sē-ō-ling′gwō-sĕr′vi-kăl) Referring to the point angle formed by the junction of an axial, lingual, and cervical (gingival) wall of a tooth cavity.

**ax·i·o·lin·guo·clu·sal** (ak′sē-ō-ling′gwō-klū′zăl) Referring to the point angle formed by the junction of an axial, lingual, and occlusal wall of a tooth cavity.

**ax·i·o·lin·guo·gin·gi·val** (ak′sē-ō-ling′gwō-jin′ji-văl) Referring to the point angle formed by the junction of an axial, lingual, and gingival (cervical) wall of a tooth cavity.

**ax·i·o·me·si·al** (ak′sē-ō-mē′zē-ăl) Referring to the line angle of a tooth cavity formed by the junction of an axial and a mesial wall.

**ax·i·o·me·si·o·cer·vi·cal** (ak′sē-ō-mē′zē-ō-sĕr′vi-kăl) Referring to the point angle formed by the junction of an axial, mesial, and cervical (gingival) wall of a tooth cavity.

**ax·i·o·me·si·o·dis·tal** (ak′sē-ō-mē′zē-ō-dis′tăl) SEE axiomesiodistal plane.

**ax·i·o·me·si·o·dis·tal plane** (ak′sē-ō-mē′zē-ō-dis′tăl plān) Plane parallel to long axes of the teeth that extend mesiodistally.

**ax·i·o·me·si·o·gin·gi·val** (ak′sē-ō-mē′zē-ī′ō-jin′ji-văl) Referring to the point angle formed by an axial, mesial, and gingival (cervical) wall of a tooth cavity.

**ax·i·o·me·si·o·in·ci·sal** (ak′sē-ō-mē′zē-ō-in-sī′zăl) Referring to the point angle formed by the junction of an axial, a mesial, and an incisal wall of a tooth cavity.

**ax·i·o·oc·clu·sal** (ak′sē-ō-ŏ-klū′zăl) Pertaining to the line angle formed by the junction of the axial and occlusal walls of a tooth.

**ax·i·o·pul·pal** (ak′sē-ō-pŭl′păl) Referring to the line angle formed by the junction of an axial and pulpal wall of a tooth cavity.

**ax·i·o·ver·sion** (ak′sē-ō-vĕr′zhŭn) Abnormal inclination of the long axis of a tooth.

**ax·is**, pl. **ax·es** (ak′sis, ak′sēz) **1.** [TA] Straight line joining two opposing poles of a spheric body, about which the body may revolve. **2.** Central line of the body or any of its parts. **3.** [TA] Second cervical vertebra. **4.** Vertebral column. **5.** Central nervous system. **6.** Artery that divides, immediately on its origin, into a number of branches, e.g., celiac axis.

**ax·is de·vi·a·tion** (ak′sis dē-vē-ā′shŭn) Deflection of the electrical axis of the heart to the right or left of the normal. SEE ALSO axis. SYN axis shift.

**ax·is shift** (aks′is shift) SYN axis deviation.

⚙ **axo-** Combining form denoting axis; axion. [G. *axōn*, axis]

**ax·on** (ak′son) **1.** The single process of a nerve cell that under normal conditions conducts nervous impulses away from the cell body and its remaining processes (dendrites). [G. *axōn,* axis]

**ax·o·nal** (ak'sō-năl) Pertaining to an axon; most often used to describe the type of underlying nerve pathology responsible for generalized polyneuropathies. In this context, usually used incorrectly, i.e., "axonal polyneuropathy", rather than "axon loss polyneuropathy" (to distinguish the disorder from a "demyelinating polyneuropathy").

**ax·on ter·mi·nals** (ak'son těr'mi-nălz) The somewhat enlarged, often club-shaped endings by which axons make synaptic contacts with other nerve cells or with effector cells (muscle or gland cells). SYN end-feet, neuropodia, terminal boutons, boutons terminaux.

**a·za·thi·o·prine** (ā'ză-thī'ō-prēn) Deriva-tive of 6-mercaptopurine, used as cytotoxic and immunosuppressive agent.

**az·i·do·thy·mi·dine (AZT)** (az'i-dō-thī' mi-dēn) SEE zidovudine.

**a·zith·ro·my·cin** (ă-zith'rō-mī'sin) An antibiotic in the macrolide group. [azithromycin [coined from parts of the chemical name]]

**a·zo dyes** (ā'zō dīz) Dyes in which the azo group is the chromophore and joins benzene or naphthalene rings; they include a large number of biologic stains (e.g., Congo red and oil red O); also used clinically to promote epithelial growth in the treatment of ulcers, burns, and other wounds; many have anticoagulant action.

**AZT** Abbreviation for azidothymidine. SEE zidovudine.

# B

**Bab·bitt met·al** (bab´it met´ăl) Alloy of antimony, copper, and tin; used occasionally in dentistry.

***Ba·be·si·a mi·cro·ti*** (bă-bē´zē-ă mī´krō-tī) A malarialike protozoan naturally parasitizing certain rodents; several human cases have been reported from the islands of Nantucket and Martha's Vineyard and nearby coastal New England.

**ba·be·si·o·sis** (bă-bē´zē-ō´sis) An infectious disease caused by a species of *Babesia*, transmitted by ticks. Subclinical human infection may be common but symptomatic disease occurs only sporadically and in limited geographic distribution. Immunodeficient and asplenic people are at higher risk of infection.

**ba·by bot·tle syn·drome** (bā´bē bot´ĕl sin´drōm) SYN baby bottle tooth decay.

▪**ba·by bot·tle tooth de·cay** (bā´bē bot´ĕl tūth dĕ-kā´) Abnormally high level of dental caries affecting the teeth of children usually younger than 4 years of age, related to prolonged use of a baby bottle containing cariogenic liquids. See this page. SYN baby bottle syndrome, nursing bottle caries.

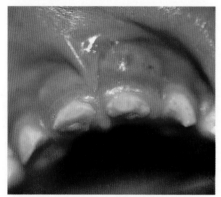

**baby bottle tooth decay (nursing bottle caries):** this 3-year-old boy was brought to emergency department due to mouth pain; eroded incisors resulted from bottle caries; gingival swelling above incisor is caused by a dentoalveolar abscess

**ba·by tooth** (bā´bē tūth) SYN deciduous tooth.

**bac·il·la·ry dys·en·ter·y** (bas´i-lar-ē dis´ ĕn-ter´ē) Infection with *Shigella dysenteriae, S. flexneri,* or other organisms.

**bac·il·lo·sis** (bas-i-lō´sis) General infection involving bacilli.

**bac·il·lu·ri·a** (bas-il-yūr´ē-ă) The presence of bacilli in the urine. [*bacillus* + G. *ouron,* urine]

***Ba·cil·lus*** (bă-sil´ŭs) A genus of aerobic or facultatively anaerobic, spore-forming, ordinar-ily motile bacteria; these organisms are chemoheterotrophic and are found primarily in soil. A few species are animal pathogens; some species evoke antibody production. [L. dim. of *baculus,* rod, staff]

**ba·cil·lus, ba·cil·li** (bă-sil´ŭs, -´ī) **1.** A vernacular term used to refer to any member of the bacterial genus *Bacillus.* **2.** Term used to refer to any rod-shaped bacterium. [L. dim. of *baculus,* a rod, staff]

***Ba·cil·lus an·thra·cis*** (bă-sil´ŭs an-thrā´sis) Bacterial species that causes anthrax in humans, cattle, swine, and other animals.

***Ba·cil·lus ste·a·ro·ther·moph·i·lus*** (ba-sil-´ŭs stē´ăr-ō-thĕr-mof´i-lŭs) A species in the genus Bacillus used as an indicator organism when testing the effectiveness of sterilization.

**bac·i·tra·cin** (bas´i-trā´sin) Antibacterial antibiotic polypeptide isolated from cultures of an aerobic, gram-positive, spore-bearing bacillus; active against hemolytic streptococci, staphylococci, and several types of gram-positive, aerobic, rod-shaped organisms; usually applied locally.

**back** (bak) [TA] **1.** Area on a débridement instrument where lateral surfaces meet or are continuous to its formation. **2.** Portion of instrument working-end opposite its face. Sickle scalers have a pointed back, curettes a rounded one. **3.** Posterior aspect of trunk, below neck and above buttocks. **4.** Vertebral column with associated muscles (erector spinae and transversospinalis) and overlying integument. SEE dorsum.

**back-ac·tion clasp** (bak-ak´shŭn klasp) Device that is placed on one tooth surface and then passes over suprabulge area to another surface where it is supported by remainder of occlusal surface. It then continues to encircle tooth on a third surface; terminates in infrabulge area beyond angle of originating surface.

**back-ac·tion con·den·ser** (bak-ak´shŭn kŏn-den´sĕr) Dental instrument with the end of the shank bent into a U-shape so that condensing force is achieved by pulling rather than pushing. SYN reverse condenser, reverse plugger.

**back-ac·tion plug·ger** (bak-ak´shŭn plŭg´ ĕr) Instrument for condensing gold foil or amalgam in areas that cannot be reached directly.

**back·ground ra·di·a·tion** (bak´grownd rā´ dē-ā´shŭn) Irradiation from environmental sources, including the earth's crust, the atmosphere, cosmic rays, and ingested radionuclides.

**back·ing** (bak´ing) In dentistry, metal support that serves to attach a facing to a prosthesis.

**back-pres·sure por·os·i·ty** (bak´presh-ŭr pōr-os´i-tē) Voids in a casting due to the inability of the air inside the mold to be adequately displaced by the incoming molten metal.

**back·scat·ter ra·di·a·tion** (bak´skat˝ĕr rā´ dē-ā´shŭn) Secondary radiation deflected more than 90 degrees from the primary beam.

**back tooth** (bak tūth) Any tooth posterior to the canines.

**back·wash il·e·i·tis** (bak´wawsh il˝ē-ī´tis) Involvement of terminal ileum by inflammatory and ulcerative changes seen in chronic ulcerative colitis; distinguished from involvement of ileum and proximal colon by regional (granulomatous) enteritis (e.g., Crohn disease of terminal ileum and proximal colon).

**bacteraemia** [Br.] SYN bacteremia.

**bac·te·re·mi·a** (bak´tĕr-ē´mē-ă) Presence of viable bacteria in circulating blood; may be transient following trauma such as dental or other iatrogenic manipulation or may be persistent or recurrent as a result of infection. SYN bacteraemia. [*bacteria* + G. *haima*, blood]

**bac·te·ri·a** (bak-tēr´ē-ă) *Do not use this word as a singular noun.* Plural of bacterium.

**bacteriaemia** [Br.] SYN bacteriemia.

**bac·te·ri·al al·ler·gy** (bak-tēr˝ē-ăl al˝ĕr-jē) **1.** Type I hypersensitivity allergic reaction caused by bacterial allergens. **2.** Delayed type of skin test (type IV hypersensitivity reaction), so called because of its early association with bacterial antigens (e.g., the tuberculin test).

**bac·te·ri·al an·tag·o·nism** (bak-tēr˝ē-ăl an-tag´ŏ-nizm) Inhibition of one bacterium by another.

**bac·te·ri·al en·ceph·a·li·tis** (bak-tēr´ē-ăl en-sef˝ă-lī´tis) Encephalitis caused by bacterial activity.

**bac·te·ri·al end·ar·ter·i·tis** (bak-tēr˝ē-ăl end´ahr-tĕr-ī´tis) Implantation and growth of bacteria with formation of vegetation on the arterial wall.

**bac·te·ri·al en·do·car·di·tis** (bak-tēr´ē-ăl en´dō-kahr-dī´tis) Condition caused by the direct invasion of bacteria and leading to deformity and destruction of the valve leaflets.

**bac·te·ri·al food poi·son·ing** (bak-tēr´ē-ăl fūd poy´zŏn-ing) Term commonly used to refer to conditions limited to enteritis or gastroenteritis (excluding the enteric fevers and the dysenteries) caused by bacterial multiplication itself or by a soluble bacterial exotoxin.

**bac·te·ri·al in·ter·fer·ence** (bak-tēr˝ē-ăl in˝tĕr-fēr´ĕns) Condition in which colonization by one bacterial strain prevents colonization by another strain.

**bac·te·ri·al plaque** (bak-tēr˝ē-ăl plak) In dentistry, mass of filamentous microorganisms and a large variety of smaller forms attached to the tooth surface that, depending on bacterial activity and environmental factors, may give rise to caries, calculus, or inflammatory changes in adjacent tissue. SYN dental plaque (2).

**bac·te·ri·al spore** (bak-tēr˝ē-ăl spōr) A quiescent form of some bacteria that is resistant to environmental stress and difficult to destroy.

**bac·te·ri·al tox·in** (bak-tēr˝ē-ăl tok´sin) Any intracellular or extracellular toxin formed in or elaborated by bacterial cells.

**bac·te·ri·cid·al** (bak-tēr´i-sī´dăl) Causing the death of bacteria. Cf. bacteriostatic.

**bac·te·ri·cide** (bak-tēr´i-sīd) An agent that destroys bacteria. [*bacteria* + L. *caedo*, to kill]

**bac·ter·id** (bak´tĕr-id) **1.** A recurrent or persistent eruption of discrete sterile pustules of the palms and soles, thought to be an allergic response to bacterial infection at a remote site. **2.** A dissemination of a previously localized bacterial skin infection. [*bacteria* + -*id* (1)]

**bac·te·ri·o·cid·in** (bak-tēr˝ē-ō-sī´din) Antibody having bactericidal activity.

**bac·te·ri·ol·o·gy** (bak-tēr˝ē-ol´ŏ-jē) The branch of science concerned with the study of bacteria. [*bacterio-* + G. *logos*, study]

**bac·te·ri·o·lyt·ic** (bak-tēr˝ē-ō-lit´ik) Destruction of bacteria by disruption of its cell structure.

**bac·te·ri·o·phage** (bak-tēr˝ē-ō-fāj) A virus with specific affinity for bacteria; found in essentially all groups of bacteria; like other viruses, they contain either RNA or DNA (but never both) and vary in structure from simple to complex; their relationships to host bacteria are specific and may be genetically intimate. SYN phage. [*bacterio-* + G. *phagō*, to eat]

**bac·te·ri·o·stat·ic** (bak-tēr˝ē-ō-stat´ik) Inhibiting or retarding the multiplication of bacteria.

**Bac·te·roi·des** (bak-ter-oy´dēz) A genus that includes many species of obligate anaerobic, non-spore-forming bacteria containing gram-negative rods. Both motile and nonmotile species occur; motile cells are peritrichous. They are part of the normal flora of the intestinal tract and to a lesser degree, the respiratory and urogenital cavities of humans and animals; many species formerly classified as *Bacteroides* have been reclassified as belonging to the genus *Prevotella*. Many species can be pathogenic. [G. *bacterion* + *eidos*, form]

**bad breath** (bad breth) SYN halitosis.

**badge** (baj) SEE film badge.

**BAER** Abbreviation for brainstem auditory evoked response.

**baked tongue** (bākt tŭng) Dry blackish tongue noted when patients with typhoid fever or other disorders are allowed to become dehydrated.

**bak·ing so·da** (bāk′ing sō′dă) SYN sodium bicarbonate.

**bal·ance** (bal′ăns) **1.** An apparatus for weighing (e.g., scales). **2.** The normal state of action and reaction between two or more parts or organs of the body. **3.** Quantities, concentrations, and proportionate amounts of bodily constituents. **4.** The difference between intake and use, storage, or excretion of a substance by the body. **5.** The act of maintaining an upright posture in standing or locomotion. **6.** The system that depends on vestibular function, vision, and proprioception to maintain posture, navigate in one's surroundings, coordinate motion of body parts, modulate fine motor control, and initiate vestibulo reflexes. [L. *bi-*, twice, + *lanx*, dish, scale]

**bal·ance bil·ling** (bal′ăns bil′ing) Sending a financial statement to the patient for the remainder of the amount charged and remaining unpaid after the third-party payer has submitted their financial contribution.

**bal·anced ar·tic·u·la·tion** (bal′ănst ahr-tik′yū-lā′shŭn) Dental occlusion in which the anterior and posterior teeth of both arches are in contact on both sides in both centric and eccentric positions

**bal·anced bite** (bal′ănst bīt) SYN balanced occlusion.

**bal·anced di·et** (bal′ănst dī′ĕt) Diet containing essential nutrients with a reasonable ration of all major food groups.

**bal·anced in·stru·ment** (bal′ănst in′strŭ-mĕnt) Periodontal device that has working-ends that are aligned with the long axis of the handle.

**bal·anced oc·clu·sion** (bal′ănst ŏ-klū′zhŭn) Simultaneous contacting of the upper and lower teeth on the right and left and in the anterior and posterior occlusal areas in centric and eccentric positions within the functional range; used primarily in reference to the mouth, but also arranged and observed on articulators, developed to prevent a tipping or rotating of the denture bases in relation to the supporting structures. Cf. balanced articulation. SYN balanced bite.

**bal·anc·ing con·tact** (bal′ăns-ing kon′takt) **1.** Contacts between upper and lower dentures on the balancing or mediotrusive side to stabilize dentures. **2.** Contacts between upper and lower dentures at the opposite side from the working or laterotrusive side (anteroposteriorly or laterally) to stabilize the dentures. SYN balancing occlusal surface.

**bal·anc·ing oc·clu·sal sur·face** (bal′ăn-sing ŏ-klū′zăl sŭr′făs) SYN balancing contact.

**bal·anc·ing side** (bal′ăns-ing sīd) In dentistry, nonfunctioning side from which the mandible moves during the working bite.

**bal·anc·ing side con·dyle** (bal′ăns-ing sīd kon′dīl) In dentistry, the mandibular condyle

on the side away from which the mandible moves in a lateral excursion.

**bald tongue** (bawld tŭng) SYN smooth tongue.

**ball-and-sock·et a·but·ment** (bawl-and-sok′ĕt ă-bŭt′ mĕnt) Abutment connected to a fixed partial denture by a ball and socket-shaped nonrigid connector.

**ball bur·nish·er** (bawl bŭr′ni-shĕr) A manual dental instrument with a round tip used for smoothing or polishing a restoration.

**bal·loon** (bă-lūn′) **1.** An inflatable spheric or ovoid device used to retain tubes or catheters in, or provide support to, various body structures. **2.** A distensible device used to stretch or occlude a viscus or blood vessel. **3.** To distend a body cavity with a gas or fluid to facilitate its examination, dilate a structure, occlude a lumen, or create a space for a retroperitoneal, laparoscopic procedure. [Fr. *ballon*, fr. It. *ballone*, fr. *balla*, ball, fr. Germanic]

**bal·loon-tip cath·e·ter** (bă-lūn′tip kath′ĕ-tĕr) **1.** A single- or double-lumen tube with a balloon at its tip that can be inflated or deflated without removal after installation; the balloon may be inflated to facilitate the passage of the tube through a blood vessel (propelled by the bloodstream) or to occlude the vessel in which the tube alone would allow free flow; such catheters are used to enter the pulmonary artery to facilitate hemodynamic measurements. SEE ALSO Swan-Ganz catheter. **2.** A tube with an inflatable balloon at its tip used to enter arteries and then removed while inflated to withdraw clots (embolectomy catheter) **3.** SYN Fogarty catheter.

**balm** (bawlm) **1.** SYN balsam. **2.** An ointment, especially a fragrant one. **3.** A soothing application. [L. *balsamum*, fr. G. *balsamon*, the balsam tree]

**bal·sam** (bawl′săm) A fragrant, resinous or thick, oily exudate from various trees and plants. SYN balm (1). [G. *balsamon*; L. *balsamum*]

**BANA as·say** (as′ā) Test for an enzyme that hydrolyzes a substrate, benzoyl-DL-arginine naphthylamide (BANA); reveals presence and general levels of bacteria that are risk factors for periodontal disease.

**band** (band) **1.** Any appliance or part of an apparatus that encircles or binds a part of the body or body structure. SEE ALSO zone. **2.** Any ribbon-shaped or cordlike anatomic structure that encircles or binds another structure or connects two or more parts.

**band a·dapt·er** (band ă-dap′tĕr) A dental instrument used to seat a matrix band more apically or more precisely on a tooth. SYN band pusher.

**ban·dage** (ban′dăj) *Avoid using this word in the incorrect sense of dressing.* **1.** Piece of cloth or other material, of varying shape and size, applied to a body part to provide compression, protect from external contamination, prevent drying, absorb drainage, prevent motion, and retain surgical dressings. **2.** To cover a body part by application of a bandage.

**band·box res·o·nance** (band´boks rez´ŏ-năns) SYN vesiculotympanitic resonance.

**band push·er** (band push´ĕr) SYN band adapter.

**band re·mov·er** (band rĕ-mūv´ĕr) Plierslike instrument used to detach an orthodontic band from a tooth. One beak rests on the occlusal surface while the other engages inferior edge of band. Squeezing the handles lifts the band in an occlusal direction.

**bar** (bahr) **1.** A metal segment of greater length than width that serves to connect two or more parts of a removable partial denture. SEE ALSO major connector. **2.** A segment of tissue or bone that unites two or more similar structures.

**bar·ag·no·sis** (bar-ag-nō´sis) *In the diphthong gn, the g is silent only at the beginning of a word. Do not confuse this word with barognosis.* Loss of ability to appreciate the weight of objects held in the hand, or to differentiate objects of different weights. [G. *baros,* weight + *a-* priv., + *gnōsis,* a knowing]

**barb·ed broach** (bahrbd brōch) Root canal instrument set with barbs; used for removing dental pulp, pulp tissue remnants, or dentinal debris.

**bar·bi·tal** (bar´bi-tawl) Hypnotic and sedative agent.

**bar·bi·tu·rate** (bahr-bich´ŭr-ăt) *Avoid the misspelling/mispronunciation barbituate.* Central nervous system depressant used for its tranquilizing, hypnotic, and antiseizure effects; most forms have potential for abuse.

**bar·bi·tu·ric ac·id** (bar´bi-chūr´ik as´id) A nonsedating crystalline dibasic acid from which barbital and other barbiturates are derived.

**bar·bi·tu·rism** (bahr-bich´ŭr-izm) Chronic poisoning by any of the derivatives of barbituric acid.

**bar clasp** (bahr klasp) **1.** Clasp with arms that are bar-type extensions from major connectors or from within denture base; arms pass adjacent to soft tissues and approach point of contact on the tooth in a gingivoocclusal direction. **2.** Clasp consisting of two or more separate arms located opposite each other on the tooth; bar arms arise from the framework or from a connector and may traverse the soft tissue; one arm (bar), the retentive arm, usually terminates in the infrabulge (gingival convergence) area of the tooth; the other, the reciprocal arm, usually terminates on the suprabulge (occlusal convergence) area. SYN Roach clasp.

**bar clasp arm** (bahr klasp ahrm) Appliance that has its origin in the denture base or major connector; consists of the arm that traverses but does not contact the gingival structures, and a terminal end that approaches its contact with the tooth in a gingivoocclusal direction.

**bar clip at·tach·ments** (bahr klip ă-tach´ mĕnts) SYN bar-sleeve attachments.

**bar con·nec·tor** (bahr kŏ-nek´tŏr) Portion of a removable partial denture framework that serves to join or connect parts of the framework.

**bar·i·um** (bar´ē-ŭm) A metallic, alkaline, divalent earth element. Its insoluble salts are often used in radiology. [G. *barys,* heavy]

**bar joint den·ture** (bahr joynt den´chŭr) SYN overlay denture.

**Bar·low dis·ease** (bahr´lō di-zēz´) SYN infantile scurvy.

**bar·o·cep·tor** (bahr´ō-sep´tŏr) SYN baroreceptor.

**bar·o·don·tal·gi·a** (bar´ō-don-tal´jē-ă) Pain in the soft tissue resulting from a disequilibrium in the air-filled spaces around a tooth caused by ascent or descent into places with differentiatial barometric pressure. SYN tooth squeeze.

**bar·o·re·cep·tor** (bar´ō-rĕ-sep´tŏr) In general, any sensor of atmospheric pressure changes. SYN pressoreceptor. [G. *baros,* weight, + *receptor*]

**Bar·rett syn·drome, Bar·rett e·soph·a·gus, Bar·rett met·a·pla·si·a** (bar´ĕt sin´ drōm, ĕ-sof´ă-gŭs, met´ă-plā´zē-ă) Chronic peptic ulceration of the lower esophagus, which is lined by columnar epithelium, resembling the mucosa of the gastric cardia, acquired as a result of long-standing chronic esophagitis.

**bar·ri·er** (bar´ē-ĕr) An obstacle or impediment. [M.E., fr. O. Fr. *barriere,* fr. L.L. *barraria*]

**bar·ri·er pro·tec·tion** (bar´ē-ĕr prŏ-tek´ shŭn) Placing a physical barrier between the patient's body fluids (e.g., blood, saliva) and dental care personnel to prevent disease transmission.

**bar·ri·ers for health care pro·vid·ers** (bar´ē-ĕrz helth kār prŏ-vī´dĕrz) Protective measures for dental providers during treatment of patients (e.g., gloves, mask, protective eyewear, protective clothing).

**bar·ri·ers for pa·tients** (bar´ē-ĕrz pā´shĕnts) Protective measures for patients during treatment (e.g., protective eyewear, head-covers during surgery, rubber dams during dental restorative and sealant procedures).

**bar-sleeve at·tach·ments** (bahr´slēv ă-tach´mĕnts) Fixed bar joints or rigid bar units used for splinting abutments with removable sleeves or clips within the partial denture for supporting and/or retaining the prosthesis. SYN bar clip attachments.

**Bar·tho·lin duct** (bahr′tō-lin dŭkt) Ducts of one of the major salivary glands, the sublingual gland.

🔲**Bar·ton ban·dage** (bahr′tŏn ban′dăj) A figure-of-8 bandage supporting the mandible inferiorly and anteriorly; used in mandibular fracture. See this page.

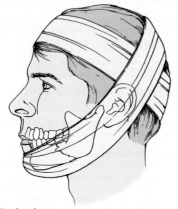

**Barton bandage**

*Bar·to·nel·la* (bahr-tō-nel′ă) A genus of bacteria found in humans and in arthropod vectors; grows slowly in artificial media and may be recovered from blood cultures from infected patients; a minute, gram-negative, coccobacillary organism; can cause an indolent, poorly defined, progressive disease in immunocompromised patients, including those with HIV infections. [A. L. *Barton*]

*Bar·to·nel·la* a·ne·mi·a (bahr-tō-nel′ă ă-nē′mē-ă) Anemia occurring in infection with *B. bacilliformis* and characterized by an acute febrile anemia of rapid onset and high mortality.

**ba·sal** (bā′săl) [TA] **1.** [TA] In dentistry, denoting the floor of a cavity in the grinding surface of a tooth. **2.** Situated nearer the base of a pyramidal organ in relation to a specific reference point. SYN basalis [TA]. **3.** Denoting a standard or reference state of a function, as a basis for comparison.

**ba·sal an·es·the·si·a** (bā′săl an′es-thē′zē-ă) Parenteral administration of one or more sedatives to produce a state of depressed consciousness short of general anesthesia.

**ba·sal bone** (bā′săl bōn) The osseus tissue of the mandible and maxillae except the alveolar processes.

**ba·sal cell** (bā′săl sel) Cell of the deepest layer of stratified epithelium.

**ba·sal cell car·ci·no·ma, ba·sal cell ep·i·the·li·o·ma** (bā′săl sel kahr′si-nō′mă, ep′i-thē-lē-ō′mă) A slow-growing, invasive, but usually nonmetastasizing neoplasm recapitulating normal basal cells of the epidermis or hair follicles; most commonly found in sun-damaged skin of old people and fair-skinned people of any age group.

**ba·sal cell lay·er** (bā′săl sel lā′ĕr) SYN stratum basale epidermidis.

**ba·sal cell ne·vus** (bā′săl sel nē′vŭs) A hereditary disease noted in infancy or adolescence, characterized by lesions of the eyelids, nose, cheeks, neck, and axillae, appearing as uneroded flesh-colored papules, some becoming pedunculated, and histologically indistinguishable from basal cell epithelioma.

**ba·sal cell pap·il·lo·ma** (bā′săl sel pap′i-lō′mă) SYN seborrheic keratosis.

**ba·sal crest of co·chle·ar duct** (bā′săl krest kok′lē-ăr dŭkt) [TA] Sharp extension of central portion of the spiral ligament that continues as the basilar membrane.

**ba·sal di·et** (bā′săl dī′ĕt) Diet with a caloric value equal to the basal heat production and sufficient quantities of essential nutrients to meet basic needs.

**ba·sa·lis** (bā-sā′lis) [TA] SYN basal (2). [L.]

**ba·sal lam·i·na** (bā′săl lam′i-nă) **1.** An amorphous extracellular layer applied to the basal surface of epithelium and also investing muscle cells, fat cells, and Schwann cells. Its principal component is a layer (consisting mostly of type IV collagen) called the lamina densa. On either side of the lamina densa are two less dense layers, called the laminae rarae. **2.** SYN lamina densa.

**ba·sal lam·i·na of co·chle·ar duct** (bā′săl lam′i-nă kok′lē-ăr dŭkt) [TA] The membrane extending from the bony spiral membrane to the basilar crest of the cochlea; it forms the greater part of the floor of the cochlear duct separating the latter from the scala tympani, and it supports the organ of Corti.

**ba·sal lay·er** (bā′săl lā′ĕr) SYN stratum basale (1).

**ba·sal mem·brane of sem·i·cir·cu·lar duct** (bā′săl mem′brān sem′ē-sĭr′kyū-lăr dŭkt) That underlying the epithelium of the semicircular duct.

**ba·sal met·a·bol·ic rate (BMR)** (bā′săl met′ă-bol′ik rāt) The minimal amount of energy required to sustain life in the waking state.

**ba·sa·loid mixed tu·mor** (bā′să-loyd mikst tū′mŏr) SYN cylindroma.

**ba·sal part** (bā′săl pahrt) [TA] Portion of a structure that forms its base—the bottom part or part opposite the apex of the structure—or a branch serving that portion of the structure; e.g., the basal part of the lungs (formed by the four basal bronchopulmonary segments of each side) served by basal parts of the right and left pulmonary arteries.

**ba·sal ra·tion** (bā′săl rā′shŭn) Minimal diet containing only essential components.

**ba·sal ridge** (bā′săl rij) **1.** SYN alveolar process of maxilla. **2.** SYN cingulum of tooth.

**ba·sal seat** (bā′săl sēt) SYN denture foundation area.

**ba·sal seat ar·e·a** (bā′săl sēt ar′ē-ă) SEE denture foundation. SYN denture foundation area.

**ba·sal sur·face** (bā′săl sŭr′făs) Surface of the denture of which the detail is determined by the impression and which rests on the basal seat.

**ba·sal vein** (bā′săl vān) [TA] Large vein originating from the confluence of veins from the orbital cortex and passing caudally and dorsally along the medial surface of the temporal lobe, eventually emptying into the great cerebral vein.

**base** (bās) [TA] **1.** The lower part or bottom; the part of a pyramidal or conic structure opposite the apex (e.g., heart); the foundation. SYN basement (1). **2.** PHARMACY the chief ingredient of a mixture. **3.** A substance with a pH over 7.0, in contrast to an acid. [L. and G. *basis*]

**Ba·se·dow dis·ease** (bahz′e-dō di-zēz′) SYN Graves disease.

**base·line** (bās′līn) **1.** A line approximating the base of the skull, passing from the infraorbital ridge to the midline of the occiput, intersecting the superior margin of the external auditory meatus. **2.** Level of performance or aggregate findings before therapy. SYN orbitomeatal line.

**base ma·te·ri·al** (bās mă-tēr′ē-ăl) Substance from which a denture base may be made (e.g., shellac, acrylic resin, vulcanite, polystyrene, metal).

**base·ment** (bās′mĕnt) **1.** SYN base (1). **2.** A cavity or space partly or completely separated from a larger space above it.

**base·ment mem·brane** (bās′mĕnt mem′brān) An amorphous extracellular layer closely applied to the basal surface of epithelium and also investing muscle cells, fat cells, and Schwann cells; composed of three successive layers (lamina lucida, lamina densa, and lamina fibroreticularis), a matrix of collagen.

**base met·al, ba·sic met·al** (bās met′ăl, bā′sik) A metal that is readily oxidized (e.g., iron, copper).

**base of ar·y·te·noid car·ti·lage** (bās ar′i-tē′noyd kahr′ti-lăj) [TA] Part of the arytenoid cartilage that articulates with the cricoid cartilage and from which the muscular process extends laterally and the vocal process projects anteriorly.

**base of co·chle·a** (bās kok′lē-ă) [TA] Enlarged part of cochlea directed posteriorly and medially; lies close to the internal acoustic meatus; planar surface underlies basal turn of cochlea.

**base of cra·ni·um** (bās krā′nē-ŭm) SYN cranial base.

**base of man·di·ble** (bās man′di-bĕl) [TA] Rounded inferior border of the body of the mandible.

**base of mo·di·o·lus of co·chle·a** (bās mō-dē-ō′lŭs kok′lē-ă) [TA] Part of the modiolus surrounded by the basal turn of the cochlea; faces lateral end of the internal acoustic meatus.

**base of tongue** (bās tŭng) SYN root of tongue.

**base·plate** (bās′plāt) Temporary form representing the base of a denture; used to record maxillomandibular (jaw) relationships and arrangement of teeth. SYN record base, temporary base, trial base.

**base·plate wax** (bās′plāt waks) Durable (usually pink) substance used to fabricate occlusion rims for dental construction into which denture teeth are arranged before laboratory processing of the denture.

**ba·si·al·ve·o·lar** (bā′sē-al-vē′ŏ-lăr) Relating to both basion and alveolar points; denoting especially basialveolar length, or the shortest distance between these two points.

**ba·si·breg·mat·ic ax·is** (bā′si-breg-mat′ik ak′sis) Line extending from basion to bregma.

**ba·sic** (bā′sik) Relating to a base.

**ba·sic ex·tra·or·al ful·crum** (bās′ik eks′tră-ōr′al ful′krŭm) An extraoral operative position in which the clinician's dominant hand rests against the patient's chin or cheek.

**ba·sic life sup·port** (bā′sik līf sŭ-pōrt′) Emergency cardiopulmonary resuscitation; control of bleeding; treatment of shock, acidosis, and poisoning; stabilization of injuries and wounds; and basic first aid.

**ba·si·cra·ni·al** (bā′si-krā′nē-ăl) Relating to the base of the skull.

**ba·si·cra·ni·al ax·is** (bā′si-krā′nē-ăl ak′sis) Line drawn from basion to midpoint of the sphenoethmoidal suture.

**ba·si·cra·ni·um** (bā′si-krā′nē-ŭm) SYN cranial base.

**ba·si·fa·cial** (bā′si-fā′shăl) Relating to lower portion of the face.

**ba·si·fa·cial ax·is** (bā′si-fā′shăl ak′sis) Line

drawn from subnasal point to midpoint of the sphenoethmoidal suture.

**bas·i·lar** (bas'i-lăr) [TA] Relating to base of a pyramidal or broad structure.

**bas·i·lar an·gle** (bas'i-lăr ang'gĕl) Area formed by intersection at basion of lines coming from nasal spine and nasal point.

**bas·i·lar bone** (bas'i-lăr bōn) Developmental basilar process of the occipital bone that unites with the condylar portions around the fourth or fifth year, becoming the basilar part of occipital bone. SYN basioccipital bone.

**bas·i·lar im·pres·sion** (bas'i-lăr impresh'ŭn) Invagination of the base of the skull into the posterior fossa with compression of brainstem and cerebellar structures into the foramen magnum.

**bas·i·lar in·dex** (bas'i-lăr in'deks) Ratio between the basialveolar line and the maximum length of the cranium, according to the formula: (basialveolar line × 100)/length of cranium. SYN alveolar index (2).

**bas·i·lar mi·graine** (bas'i-lăr mī'grān) Migraine accompanied by transient brainstem signs (e.g., vertigo, tinnitus, perioral numbness, diplopia) thought due to vasospastic narrowing of basilar artery.

**bas·i·lar part of oc·cip·i·tal bone** (bas'i-lăr pahrt ok-sip'i-tăl bōn) [TA] Wedgelike portion of occipital bone that lies anterior to foramen magnum and joins with body of sphenoid bone. SYN basilar process of occipital bone [TA].

**bas·i·lar pro·cess of oc·cip·i·tal bone** (bas'i-lăr pro'ses ok-sip'i-tăl bōn) [TA] SYN basilar part of occipital bone.

**bas·i·lar prog·na·thism** (bas'i-lăr prog'nă-thizm) Concave facial profile, or forward position of chin, resembling mandibular prognathism, created by the prominence of mandible at chin or menton.

**bas·i·lar si·nus** (bas'i-lăr sī'nŭs) SYN basilar venous plexus.

**bas·i·lar ve·nous plex·us** (bas'i-lăr vē'nŭs pleks'ŭs) [TA] Located on the clivus, connected with the cavernous and petrosal sinuses and the internal vertebral (epidural) venous plexus. SYN basilar sinus.

**ba·si·lat·er·al** (bas'i-lat'ĕr-ăl) Relating to base and one or more sides of any part.

**ba·sil·i·cus** (ba-sil'i-kŭs) Denoting a prominent or important part or structure. [L. fr. G. basilikos, royal]

**ba·si·na·sal** (bā'si-nā'zăl) Relating to the basion and the nasion; denoting especially the basinasal length, or the shortest distance between the two points.

**ba·si·na·sal line** (bā'si-nā'zăl līn) Line connecting basion and nasion.

**ba·si·oc·cip·i·tal** (bā'sē-ok-sip'i-tăl) Relating to basilar process of occipital bone.

**ba·si·oc·cip·i·tal bone** (bā'sē-ok-sip'i-tăl bōn) SYN basilar bone.

**ba·si·on** (bā'sē-on) Midpoint on anterior margin of foramen magnum, opposite opisthion. [G. basis, a base]

**ba·sip·e·tal** (bā'sip-ĕ-tăl) In a direction toward the base. [basi- + L. peto, to seek]

**ba·si·tem·po·ral** (bas'i-tem'pŏ-răl) Relating to lower part of temporal region.

**bas·ket** (bas'kĕt) 1. A basketlike arborization of the axon of cells in the cerebellar cortex, surrounding the cell body of Purkinje cells. 2. Any basketlike structure. [M.E., from Celtic]

**ba·so·phil, ba·so·phile** (bā'sō-fil, -fīl) A phagocytic leukocyte of the blood characterized by numerous basophilic granules containing heparin, histamine, and leukotrines. [baso- + G. phileō, to love]

**ba·so·phil·i·a** (bā'sō-fil'ē-ă) A condition in which there are more than the usual number of basophilic leukocytes in the circulating blood (basophilic leukocytosis) or an increase in the proportion of parenchymatous basophilic cells in an organ (in the bone marrow, basophilic hyperplasia).

**ba·so·squa·mous car·ci·no·ma, ba·si·squa·mous car·ci·no·ma** (bā'sō-skwā'mŭs kahr'si-nō'mă, bā'si) A carcinoma of the skin, considered transitional between basal cell and squamous cell carcinoma.

**bat·ter·y** (bat'ĕr-ē) Series of tests administered for analytic or diagnostic purposes. [M.E. batri, beaten metal, fr. O.Fr. batre, to beat]

**Bat·tle sign** (bat'ĕl sīn) Postauricular ecchymosis in cases of fracture of cranial base.

**Bau·hin gland** (bō'an[h] gland) SYN anterior lingual gland.

**bay** (bā) In anatomy, a recess containing fluid, but especially, the lacrimal bay.

**bay·o·net** (bā-ŏ-net') An instrument having a blade or nib that is offset and parallel to the shaft. [Fr. bayonette, fr. Bayonne, France, where first made]

**bay·o·net con·den·ser** (bā-ŏ-net' kŏnden'sĕr) Implement commonly used to compress gold foil in which the tip is offset from the shank by a series of bends near the end of the shank, although the force is approximated within the same long axis.

**BBB** Abbreviation for blood-brain barrier.

**BBP** Abbreviation for blood-borne pathogens.

**bead·ing** (bēd′ing) **1.** Rounded elevation along the border of the tissue surface of the major connectors of a maxillary dental prosthesis. **2.** Protection of the formed borders of final impressions for a dental prosthesis done by placement of wax sticks or a plaster-pumice combination adjacent to the borders prior to forming the master cast.

**beak** (bēk) **1.** Nose of pliers used in dentistry to contour and adjust wrought or cast metal dental appliances. **2.** Sometimes used to describe any beak-shaped anatomic structure. [L. *beccus*]

**beam** (bēm) **1.** Any bar the curvature of which changes under load; in dentistry, frequently used instead of "bar." **2.** A collimated emission of light or other radiation. [O.H.G. *Boum*]

**beam-in·di·cat·ing de·vice** (bēm in′di-kāt′ing dĕ-vīs′) SYN position-indicating device.

**beat** (bēt) **1.** To strike; to throb or pulsate. **2.** A stroke, impulse, or pulsation, as of the heart or pulse. **3.** Activity of a cardiac chamber produced by catching a stimulus generated elsewhere in the heart. **4.** The perception of a third tone when two tones of slightly different frequencies are presented. [A.S. *beatan*]

**Beck·with-Wie·de·mann syn·drome** (bek′with vē′de-mahn sin′drōm) An overgrowth syndrome characterized by exomphalos, macroglossia, and gigantism, often with neonatal hypoglycemia.

**bed** (bed) In anatomy, a base or structure(s) that support(s) another structure.

**Bed·nar aph·thae** (bed′nahr af′thē) Traumatic ulcers located bilaterally on either side of midpalatal raphe in infants.

**bed·sore, bed sore** (bed′sōr, bed sōr) SYN decubitus ulcer.

**beef·y tongue** (bē′fē tŭng) Erythematous or atrophic glossitis, often associated with ulcerations of the dorsal lingual surface.

**bees·wax** (bēz′waks) SYN wax (1).

**beet-tongue** (bēt′tŭng) Appearance of tongue in pellagra, in which intense erythema appears, first at the tip, then along the edges, and finally over the dorsum.

**be·hav·ior** (bē-hāv′yŏr) **1.** Any response emitted by or elicited from an organism. **2.** Any mental or motor act or activity. **3.** Specifically, parts of a total response pattern. SYN behaviour. [M.E., fr. O. Fr. *avoir*, to have]

**be·hav·ior·al med·i·cine** (bē-hāv′yŏr-ăl med′i-sin) Interdisciplinary field concerned with development and integration of behavioral and biomedical science knowledge and techniques relevant to health and illness, and to its application to prevention, diagnosis, treatment, and rehabilitation.

**be·hav·ior·al path·o·gen** (bē-hāv′yŏr-ăl path′ŏ-jĕn) Personal habits and lifestyle behaviors associated with an increased risk of physical illness and dysfunction. SEE ALSO risk factor.

**be·hav·ior·al sci·enc·es** (bē-hāv′yŏr-ăl sī′ĕns-ĕz) Collective term for disciplines or branches of science, such as psychology, sociology, and anthropology, which derive their theories, concepts, and approaches from observation and study of behavior of living organisms.

**be·hav·ior mod·i·fi·ca·tion** (bē-hāv′yŏr mod′i-fi-kā′shŭn) **1.** A systematic treatment technique that attempts to change a person's habitual maladaptive response by creating rewards for a new desired response or unrewarding outcomes for the habitual response; intended to teach certain skills or to extinguish undesirable behaviors, attitudes, or phobias. **2.** A psychological theory based on observation of behavior and operant principles of behavior change.

**be·hav·ior ther·a·py** (bē-hāv′yŏr thār′ă-pē) An offshoot of psychotherapy involving the use of procedures and techniques associated with conditioning and learning for the treatment of a variety of psychological conditions.

**behaviour** [Br.] SYN behavior.

**Beh·çet syn·drome** (be-shet′ sin′drōm) Syndrome characterized by simultaneously or successively occurring recurrent attacks of genital and oral ulcerations (aphthae) and uveitis or iridocyclitis with hypopyon, often with arthritis.

**be·hind-the-ear hear·ing aid** (bĕ-hīnd′ ēr hēr′ing ād) Hearing aid that rests on the medial aspect of the pinna.

**belch·ing** (belch′ing) SYN eructation. [A.S. *baelcian*]

**bel·la·don·na** (bel′ă-don′ă) *Atropa belladonna* (family Solanaceae); a perennial herb with dark or yellow purple flowers and shining purplish-black berries and tincture to treat diarrhea, asthma, colic, and hyperacidity. [It. *bella*, beautiful, + *donna*, lady]

**bell-crown·ed** (bel′krownd) Denoting a tooth with a crown that has a cross-sectional diameter much greater than that of the neck.

**Bell pal·sy** (bel pawl′zē) Paresis or paralysis, usually unilateral, of the facial muscles, caused by dysfunction of the facial nerve. See page 82.

**Bell pal·sy tests** (bel pawl′zē tests) Sensory and motor clinical assessments that involve movements of facial muscles and gauging of sweet, salt, sour, and bitter taste perception.

**Bell phe·nom·e·non** (bel fĕ-nom′ĕ-non) Reflex upper deviation of the eye on attempted eye closure; seen in facial mononeuropathies, Guillain-Barré syndrome, and myasthenia gravis.

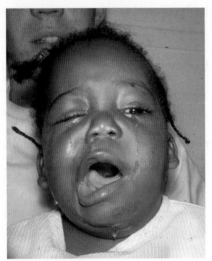

**patient with Bell palsy**

**bell-shaped crown** (bel´shăpt krown) Tooth crown that has an exaggerated occlusogingival contour; human deciduous molars exemplify the form.

**Bell spasm** (bel spazm) SYN facial tic.

**bell stage** (bel stāj) Third stage of tooth development, wherein cells form the inner enamel epithelium, the stratum intermedium, the stellate reticulum, and the outer enamel epithelium; the enamel organ assumes a bell shape.

**Ben·e·dict test** (ben´ĕ-dikt test) A copper-reduction test for glucose in urine.

**be·ne·fi·ci·ar·y** (ben´ĕ-fish´ē-ar-ē) A person with health care insurance coverage, usually through the Medicare program. SYN insured, recipient. [Med.L. *beneficiarius,* fr. *beneficium,* benefit]

**be·nign** (bĕ-nīn´) Denoting mild character of an illness or the nonmalignant character of a neoplasm. [through O.Fr., fr. L. *benignus,* kind]

**be·nign mi·gra·to·ry glos·si·tis** (bĕ-nīn´ mī´gră-tōr-ē glos-ī´tis) SYN geographic tongue.

**be·nign mu·cous mem·brane pem·phi·goid** (bĕ-nin´ myū´kŭs mem´brān pem´fi-goyd) Blistering disease chiefly involving the subepidermal mucous membranes of mouth and eye (ocular pemphigus); usually chronic, benign, and typically bilateral. Scarring can occur and may lead to progressive shrinkage and tightening of the affected mucous membranes and connective tissues. SYN cicatricial pemphigoid, ocular cicatricial pemphigoid.

**Ben·nett an·gle** (ben´ĕt ang´gĕl) Difference in direction of movement of nonworking condyle between protrusive and balancing movements, as viewed clinically in the horizontal plane.

**Ben·nett move·ment** (ben´ĕt mūv´mĕnt) Bodily lateral motion or lateral shift of the mandible during laterotrusive movement (i.e., toward working side).

**ben·zo·caine** (ben´zō-kān) Topical anesthetic agent.

**ben·zo·di·az·e·pine** (ben´zō-dī-az´ĕ-pēn) Class of compounds with antianxiety, hypnotic, anticonvulsant, and skeletal muscle relaxant properties.

**ben·zo·ic ac·id** (ben-zō´ik as´id) Natural agent in gum benzoin, used as a food preservative a fungistatic, and oral as an antiseptic.

**ben·zo·in** (ben´zō-in) Balsamic resin used as a stimulant expectorant, but more usually by inhalation in laryngitis and bronchitis. [It. *benzoino,* fr. Ar. *lubān jāwīy,* Javan incense]

**ben·zo·na·tate** (ben-zō´nă-tāt) Antitussive related chemically to tetracaine.

**ben·zoyl** (ben´zō-il) The benzoic acid radical that forms benzoyl compounds.

**ben·zoyl per·ox·ide** (ben´zō-il pĕr-ok´sīd) Compound applied to ulcers, burns, and scalds; promotes polymerization of dental resins and used as a keratolytic in the treatment of acne.

**ben·zyl·pen·i·cil·lin, ben·zyl pen·i·cil·lin** (ben´zil-pen´i-sil´in) SYN penicillin G.

**ber·i·ber·i** (ber´ē-ber´ē) A specific nutritional deficiency syndrome occurring in endemic form in eastern and southern Asia, sporadically in other parts of the world without reference to climate, and sometimes in alcoholic patients, resulting mainly from a dietary deficiency of thiamin. [Singhalese, extreme weakness]

**Ber·lin blue** (bĕr-lin´ blū) [CI 77510] A ferric ferrocyanide dye used to color injection masses for blood vessels and lymphatics. SYN Prussian blue.

**ber·yl·li·um** (bĕr-il´ē-ŭm) A white metal element belonging to the alkaline earths; a component of some alloys used in dentistry.

**Bes·nier-Boeck-Schau·mann dis·ease** (bā-nyā´ bĕrk show´mahn di-zēz´) SYN sarcoidosis.

**be·ta an·gle** (bā´tă ang´gĕl) Angle formed by a line connecting the bregma and hormion meeting the radius fixus.

**be·ta-lac·tam** (bā´tă lak´tam) Class of broad-spectrum antibiotics structurally and pharmacologically related to penicillins and cephalosporins.

**be·ta-lac·ta·mase** (bā´tă lak´tā-mās) An enzyme produced by many species of bacteria that disrupts the four-membered β-lactam ring of penicillin and cephalosporin groups of antibiotics, destroying their antimicrobial activity. SYN penicillinase.

**be·ta-lac·tam·ase in·hib·i·tors** (bā´tă lak´ti-mās in-hib´i-tŏrz) Drugs used to inhibit bacterial β-lactamases; often used with a penicillin or cephalosporin to overcome drug resistance.

**be·ta (β) par·ti·cle** (bā´tă-pahr´ti-kĕl) An electron, either positively (positron, β⁺) or negatively (negatron, β⁻) charged, emitted during beta decay of a radionuclide. SYN beta ray.

**beta-thalassaemia** [Br.] SYN beta-thalassemia.

**be·ta-thal·as·se·mi·a** (bā´tă thal´ă-sē´mē-ă) Thalassemia due to one of two or more genes that depress (partially or completely) synthesis of beta-globin chains by the chromosome bearing the abnormal gene.

**be·ta-tron** (bā´tă-tron) A circular electron accelerator that is a source of either high energy electrons or x-rays.

**be·tel** (bē´tĕl) Dried leaves of *Piper betle* used as a stimulant and narcotic. [Pg. *betel, betle,* fr. Malayalam or Tamil *vetila*]

**be·tel nut** (bē´tĕl nŭt) Nut of the areca palm, *Areca catechu,* of the East Indies, chewed by some local residents; contains arecoline; stains teeth and gums red.

**bev·el** (bev´ĕl) **1.** A surface having a sloped or slanting edge. **2.** The incline that one surface or line makes with another when not at right angles. **3.** The edge of a cutting instrument. **4.** To create a slanting edge on a body structure. [O.Fr.]

**be·zoar** (bē´zōr) A concretion formed in the alimentary canal of animals, and occasionally humans; formerly considered to be a useful medicine with magical properties and apparently still used for this purpose in some countries; according to the substance forming the ball, may be termed trichobezoar (hairball), trichophytobezoar (hair and vegetable fiber mixed), or phytobezoar (food ball). [Pers. *padzahr,* antidote]

**BHN** Abbreviation for Brinell hardness number.

**Bi** Symbol for bismuth.

**bi·as** (bī´ăs) **1.** Systematic discrepancy between a measurement and the true value; may be constant or proportionate and may adversely affect test results. **2.** Any trend in the collection, analysis, interpretation, publication, or review, which can lead to conclusions that differ systematically from the truth; deviation of results or inferences from the truth, or processes leading to deviation. [Fr. *biais,* obliquity, perh. fr. L. *bifax,* two-faced]

**bi·au·ric·u·lar** (bī´awr-ik´yū-lăr) Relating to both auricles, in any sense.

**bi·ax·i·al joint** (bī-ak´sē-ăl joynt) Joint with two principal axes of movement situated at right angles to each other; e.g., saddle joints.

**bib·u·lous** (bib´yū-lŭs) Absorbent; in medical terms, refers to materials used to soak up unwanted fluids, such as saliva during dental procedures. [L. *bibulus,* drinking freely, absorbent]

**bi·cam·er·al** (bī-kam´ĕr-ăl) Having two chambers; denoting especially an abscess divided by a more or less complete septum. [*bi*- + L. *camera,* chamber]

**bi·car·bon·ate** (bī-kahr´bŏn-āt) Ion remaining after first dissociation of carbonic acid; central buffering agent in blood.

**bi·cor·nous, bi·cor·nu·ate, bi·cor·nate** (bī-kōr´nŭs, -nū-āt, -nāt) Two-horned; having two processes or projections. [*bi*- + L. *cornu,* horn]

**bi·cus·pid** (bī-kŭs´pid) Having two points, prongs, or cusps, especially teeth with two cusps. Humans have eight bicuspid or premolar teeth: two in front of each group of molars. SEE premolar tooth. [*bi*- + L. *cuspis,* point]

**bid** Abbreviation for bis in die.

**Bier·mer a·ne·mi·a** (bēr´mĕr ă-nē´mē-ă) SYN pernicious anemia.

**bi·fid** (bī´fid) Split or cleft; separated into two parts. [L. *bifidus,* cleft in two parts]

***Bi·fi·do·bac·te·ri·um*** (bī´fī-dō-bak-tēr´ē-ŭm) A genus of anaerobic bacteria containing gram-positive rods of highly variable appearance. Rare infection in humans, although the bacterium has been found in the feces and alimentary tract of infants, some older people, and animals. [L. *bifidus,* cleft in two parts, + *bacterium*]

***Bi·fi·do·bac·te·ri·um den·ti·um*** (bī´fī-dō-bak-tēr´ē-ŭm den´shē-ŭm) Opportunistic bacterial species recovered in association with dental caries and periodontal disease, and with mixed infections associated with abscess formation.

**bi·fid tongue** (bī´fid tŭng) A congenital lingual structural defect in which its anterior part is divided longitudinally for a greater or lesser distance. SYN cleft tongue.

**bi·fid u·vu·la** (bī´fid yū´vyū-lă) Bifurcation of the uvula, constituting a partially cleft soft palate. See page 84.

**bi·fo·rate** (bī-fōr´āt) Having two openings. [*bi*- + L. *foro,* pp. -*atus,* to bore, pierce]

**bi·fur·cate, bi·fur·cat·ed** (bī´fŭr-kāt, -kā-tĕd) Forked; two-pronged; having two branches. [*bi*- + L. *furca,* fork]

**bi·fur·ca·tion** (bī´fŭr-kā´shŭn) [TA] A forking; a division into two branches.

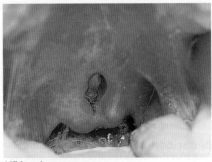

**bifid uvula:** severe case

**bi·fur·ca·tion in·volve·ment** (bī´fŭr-kā´shŭn in-volv´mĕnt) Colloq. for dental caries or periodontal disease extending into the area where the roots of a two-rooted tooth separate or divide; most common on mandibular molars.

**bi·lat·er·al** (bī-lat´ĕr-ăl) Relating to, or having, two sides. [*bi-* + L. *latus,* side]

**bi·lat·er·al·ism** (bī-lat´ĕr-ăl-izm) A condition in which the two sides are symmetric.

**bile** (bīl) *Avoid the jargonistic substitution of this word for bile pigment(s) in expressions such as bile in the urine and bile staining of tissues.* Yellowish-brown or green fluid secreted by the liver and discharged into the duodenum, where it aids in the emulsification of fats. SYN gall (1). [L. *bilis*]

**bil·har·zi·a·sis, bil·har·zi·o·sis** (bil´hahr-zī´ă-sis, zē-ō´sis) SYN schistosomiasis.

**bil·i·ar·y a·tre·si·a** (bil´ē-ar-ē ă-trē´zē-ă) Atresia of the major bile ducts, causing cholestasis and jaundice, which does not become apparent until several days after birth; periportal fibrosis develops and leads to cirrhosis, with proliferation of small bile ducts and giant cell transformation of hepatic cells.

**bilirubinaemia** [Br.] SYN bilirubinemia.

**bil·i·ru·bi·ne·mi·a** (bil´i-rū-bin-ē´mē-ă) The presence of increased amounts of bilirubin in the blood, where it is normally present in only relatively small amounts; usually used to describe various pathologic conditions in which there is excessive destruction of erythrocytes or interference with the mechanism of excretion in the bile. SYN bilirubinaemia. [*bilirubin* + G. *haima,* blood]

**bil·i·ru·bin en·ceph·a·lop·a·thy** (bil´i-rū´bin en-sef´a-lop´ă-thē) SYN kernicterus.

**bil·i·ru·bi·nu·ri·a** (bil´i-rū-bi-nyūr´ē-ă) The presence of bilirubin in the urine. [*bilirubin* + G. *ouron,* urine]

**bi·lob·u·lar** (bī-lob´yū-lăr) Having two lobules.

**bi·loc·u·lar, bi·loc·u·late** (bī-lok´yū-lăr,

-lăt) Having two compartments or spaces. [*bi-* + L. *loculus,* dim. of *locus,* a place]

**bi·man·u·al** (bī-man´yū-ăl) Relating to, or performed by, both hands. [*bi-* + L. *manus,* hand]

**bi·man·u·al pal·pa·tion** (bī-man´yū-ăl pal-pā´shŭn) Use of both hands to feel or examine dental structures.

**bi·mas·toid** (bī-mas´toyd) Relating to both mastoid processes.

**bi·max·il·lar·y** (bī-mak´si-lar-ē) Relating to both the right and left maxillae; sometimes used to describe something affecting both halves of the upper jaw.

**bi·max·il·lar·y den·to·al·ve·o·lar pro·tru·sion** (bī-mak´si-lar-ē den´tō-al-vē´ŏ-lăr prō-trū´zhŭn) Positioning of the entire dentition forward with respect to the facial profile.

**bi·max·il·lar·y pro·tru·sion** (bī-mak´si-lar-ē prō-trū´zhŭn) Excessive forward projection of both maxilla and mandible in relation to cranial base. SYN double protrusion.

**bi·max·il·lar·y pro·tru·sive oc·clu·sion** (bī-mak´si-lar-ē prō-trū´siv ŏ-klū´zhŭn) Occlusion in which both maxilla and mandible protrude, causing the long axes of the maxillary anterior teeth to be at an extremely acute angle to the mandibular teeth; may be secondary to a skeletal or dental deformity, or both.

**bin·an·gle** (bin-ang´gĕl) Dental instrument in which the second angle given the shank of an angled instrument to bring its working end close to the axis of the handle to prevent it from turning about the axis. [L. *bini,* pair, + *angulus,* angle]

**bin·an·gle chis·el** (bin-ang´gĕl chiz´ĕl) Chisel with an angled shank to which a second angle is added to bring the cutting edge nearly in line with the axis of the handle so as to restore balance and to prevent it from turning about the axis; used when a chisel must be angled for access.

**bin·au·ral** (bī-naw´răl) Relating to both ears. [L. *bini,* a pair, + *auris,* ear]

**bind·er** (bīnd´ĕr) **1.** A broad bandage, especially one encircling the abdomen. **2.** Anything that binds.

**bind·ing** (bīnd´ing) The perceptual connection between aspects of a visual experience, such that the color of a moving object appears to be unified with the object (e.g., whereas movement and color are processed in different brain regions).

**binge eat·ing and purg·ing** (binj ēt´ing pŭrj´ing) SYN bulimia nervosa.

**bin·oc·u·lar loupe** (bin-ok´yū-lăr lūp) A magnifying device, attached to spectacles or a headband, worn as a visual aid when doing procedures on small dental structures.

**bi·o·ac·tive glass** (bī'ō-ak'tiv glas) A fused silica-containing aluminum oxide that has a surface-reactive glass film compatible with tissues; used as a surface coating in some types of dental and medical implants. SYN bioglass.

**bi·o·a·vail·a·bil·i·ty** (bī'ō-ă-vāl'ă-bil'i-tē) Physiologic availability of a given amount of a drug, as distinct from its chemical potency.

**bi·o·bur·den** (bī'ō-bŭr'dĕn) Degree of microbial contamination or microbial load; the number of microorganisms contaminating an object.

**bi·o·chem·is·try** (bī'ō-kem'is-trē) The chemistry of living organisms and of the chemical, molecular, and physical changes occurring therein. SYN physiologic chemistry.

**bi·o·cid·al** (bī'ō-sī'dăl) Destructive of life; particularly pertaining to microorganisms. [bio- + L. caedo, to kill]

**bio·com·pat·i·bil·i·ty** (bī'ō-kŏm-pat'i-bil' i-tē) The relative ability of a inorganic material to interact favorably with a biologic system. The degree of biocompatibility depends on a material's stability over time, tendency to cause inflammation, cause disease, or be carcinogenic.

**bi·o·com·pat·i·ble ma·te·ri·al** (bī'ō-kŏm-pat'i-bĕl mă-tēr'ē-ăl) Substance that elicits no unfavorable reaction from tissues.

**bi·o·de·grad·a·ble** (bī'ō-dĕ-grād'ă-bĕl) Denoting a substance that can be chemically degraded or decomposed by natural effectors (e.g., weather, soil bacteria, plants, animals).

**bi·o·eth·ics** (bī'ō-eth'iks) Branch of ethics dealing with the use of the human body or body tissue in medical procedures (i.e., organ and fetal tissue transplant).

**bi·o·feed·back** (bī'ō-fēd'bak) A training technique that enables a patient to gain some element of voluntary control over autonomic body functions or involuntary unwanted behaviors or reactions; based on the principle that a desired response is learned when received information such as a recorded increase in skin temperature indicates that a specific thought complex or action has produced the desired physiologic response.

**bi·o·film** (bī'ō-film) A thin coating containing biologically active agents, which coats the surface of structures such as teeth or the inner surfaces of catheter, tube, or other implanted or indwelling device. It contains viable and nonviable microorganisms that adhere to the surface and are trapped within a matrix of organic matter (e.g., proteins, glycoproteins, and carbohydrates).

**bi·o·fix·ture** (bī'ō-fiks-chŭr) An item, bio-

logic or inert, affixed to or within a patient for permanent or long-term service (e.g., dental implant, prosthetic heart valve).

**bi·o·fla·vo·noids** (bī'ō-flāv'ŏn-oydz) Naturally occurring flavone or coumarin derivatives commonly found in citrus fruits.

**bi·o·gen·e·sis** (bī'ō-jen'ĕ-sis) **1.** The principle that life originates from only preexisting life and never from nonliving material. **2.** SYN biosynthesis. [bio- + G. genesis, origin]

**bi·o·glass** (bī'ō-glas) A fused silica-containing aluminum oxide that has a surface-reactive glass film compatible with tissues; used as a surface coating in some types of dental implants.

**bi·o·haz·ard** (bī'ō-haz'ărd) Any material, substance, or item usually contaminated with transmissible pathogenic microorganisms (e.g., bacteria, viruses) that poses a risk to health.

**bi·o·in·te·gra·tion** (bī'ō-in'tĕ-grā'shŭn) SYN integration.

**bi·o·log·ic, bi·o·log·i·cal** (bī'ŏ-loj'ik, -i-kăl) Relating to biology.

**bi·o·log·ic age** (bī'ŏ-loj'ik āj) Anatomic or physiologic age of a person as determined by organismic structure and function; takes into account features such as posture, skin texture, strength, speed, and sensory acuity.

**bi·o·log·ic half-life** (bī'ŏ-loj'ik haf'līf) The time required for one half of an amount of a substance to be lost through biologic processes.

**bi·o·log·ic in·di·ca·tor** (bī'ŏ-loj'ik in'di-kā-tŏr) A preparation of nonpathogenic microorganisms, usually bacterial spores, carried by an ampule or specially impregnated paper enclosed within a package during sterilization and subsequently incubated to verify that the spores were killed by the sterilization process.

**bi·o·log·ic vec·tor** (bī'ŏ-loj'ik vek'tŏr) A vector, such as the Anopheles mosquito for malarial agents or the tsetse fly for agents of African sleeping sickness, in which the agent multiplies before transmission to another host.

**bi·o·log·ic width of per·i·o·don·tal lig·a·ment** (bī'ŏ-loj'ik width per'ē-ō-don'tăl lig'ă-mĕnt) The width of the periodontal ligament under normal conditions. It is related to the functional forces to which it is subjected.

**bi·ol·o·gy** (bī-ol'ŏ-jē) Science concerned with phenomena of life and living organisms. [bio- + G. logos, study]

**bi·o·mark·er** (bī'ō-mahr-kĕr) A detectable cellular or molecular indicator of exposure, health effects, or susceptibility, which can be used to measure the absorbed, metabolized, or biologically effective dose of a substance, the response to the substance including susceptibility and resistance, idiosyncratic reactions, and other factors or conditions.

**bi·o·mass** (bī′ō-mas) The total weight of all living things in a given area, biotic community, species population, or habitat; a measure of total biotic productivity.

**bi·o·ma·te·ri·al** (bī′ō-mă-tēr′ē-ăl) A synthetic or semisynthetic material used in a biologic system to construct an implantable prosthesis and chosen for its biocompatibility.

**bi·o·me·chan·i·cal clean·ing** (bī′ō-mĕ-kan′i-kăl klēn′ing) Use of irrigating solutions, often antimicrobial, during process of enlarging and shaping a canal during root canal surgery.

**bi·o·me·chan·i·cal prep·a·ra·tion** (bī′ō-mĕ-kan′i-kăl prep′ăr-ā′shŭn) Colloq. for biomechanical cleaning (q.v.).

**bi·o·me·chan·ics** (bī′ō-mĕ-kan′iks) Science concerned with action of forces, internal or external, on the living body.

**bi·o·med·i·cal** (bī′ō-med′i-kăl) Pertaining to those aspects of the natural sciences, especially the biologic and physiologic sciences, which relate to or underlie medicine.

**bi·o·med·i·cal en·gi·neer·ing** (bī′ō-med′i-kăl en′ji-nēr′ing) Application of engineering principles to obtain solutions to biomedical problems.

**bi·o·med·i·cal mod·el** (bī′ō-med′i-kăl mod′ĕl) Concept of illness that excludes psychological and social factors and includes only biologic factors in an attempt to understand a person's medical illness or disorder.

**bi·on** (bī′on) A living thing.

**bi·o·na·tor** (bī′ō-nā-tŏr) Removable orthodontic appliance used to retrain the muscles of mastication.

**bi·on·o·my** (bī-on′ŏ-mē) Science concerned with the laws regulating the vital functions. [bio- + G. nomos, law]

**bi·o·phar·ma·ceu·tics** (bī′ō-fahr′mă-sū′tiks) Study of the physical and chemical properties of a drug, and its dosage form, as related to the onset, duration, and intensity of drug action.

**bi·o·phys·ics** (bī′ō-fiz′iks) **1.** The study of biologic processes and materials by means of the theories and tools of physics. **2.** The study of physical processes (e.g., electricity, luminescence) occurring in organisms.

**bi·o·pol·y·mer** (bī′ō-pol′i-mĕr) A naturally occurring compound that is a polymer containing identical or similar subunits.

**bi·op·sy** (bī′op-sē) **1.** Process of removing tissue from patients for diagnostic examination. **2.** A specimen obtained by biopsy. [bio- + G. opsis, vision]

**bi·or·bit·al** (bī-ōr′bi-tăl) Relating to both orbits. [bi- + G. orbita, orbit]

**bi·or·bit·al an·gle** (bī-ōr′bi-tăl ang′gĕl) Angle formed by meeting of the axes of the orbits.

**bi·o·reg·u·la·tor** (bī′ō-reg′yŭ-lā-tŏr) Any endogenous substance that modifies the rate or intensity of a biologic process so as to maintain homeostasis or meet changing needs of the organism. SYN melanocyte-stimulating hormone.

**bi·o·sis** (bī-ō′sis) Life in general.

**bi·o·syn·the·sis** (bī′ō-sin′thĕ-sis) Formation of a chemical compound by enzymes, either in the organism (in vivo) or by fragments or extracts of cells (in vitro). SYN biogenesis (2).

**bi·o·tech·nol·o·gy** (bī′ō-tek-nol′ō-jē) Field devoted to applying techniques of biochemistry, cellular biology, biophysics, and molecular biology to addressing practical issues related to human beings, agriculture, and the environment.

**bi·o·te·lem·e·try** (bī′ō-tĕ-lem′ĕ-trē) The technique of monitoring vital processes and transmitting data without wires to a point remote from the subject.

**bi·ot·ics** (bī-ot′iks) The science concerned with the functions of life, or vital activity and force. [G. biōtikos, relating to life]

**bi·o·tin** (bī′ō-tin) The D-isomer component of the vitamin B2 complex occurring in or required by most organisms and inactivated by avidin. SEE ALSO avidin.

**bi·o·trans·for·ma·tion** (bī′ō-trans′fŏr-mā′shŭn) The conversion of molecules from one form to another within an organism, often associated with change in pharmacologic activity.

**bi·pa·ri·e·tal** (bī′păr-ī′ĕ-tăl) Relating to both parietal bones of the cranium. [bi- + L. paries, wall]

**bi·par·tite** (bī-pahr′tīt) Consisting of two parts or divisions.

**bi·phase ex·ter·nal pin fix·a·tion** (bī′fāz eks-tĕr′năl pin fik-sā′shŭn) In oral surgery, stabilization of fractures of the mandible, maxilla, or zygoma by pins or screws drilled into the bony part through overlying skin and connected by a metal bar.

**bi·po·lar** (bī-pō′lăr) With two poles or ends.

**bi·po·lar cau·ter·y** (bī-pō′lăr kaw′tĕr-ē) Electrocautery by high frequency electrical current passed through tissue from an active to a passive electrode; used for hemostasis.

**bi·po·lar dis·or·der** (bī-pō′lăr dis-ōr′dĕr) Affective disorder characterized by occurrence of alternating manic, hypomanic, or mixed episodes and with major depresive episodes.

**bi·ra·mous** (bī-rā′mŭs) Having two branches. [*bi-* + L. *ramus,* branch]

**bird face** (bĭrd fās) SYN brachygnathia.

**Bird sign** (bĭrd sīn) The presence of a zone of dullness on percussion with absence of respiratory signs in hydatid cyst of the lung.

**birth con·trol** (bĭrth kŏn-trōl′) **1.** Limiting offspring by means of contraceptive measures. **2.** Projects, programs, or methods to control reproduction, by either controlling fertility.

**birth de·fect** (bĭrth dē′fekt) Defect present at birth; sometimes referred to as congenital defect or anomaly.

**birth weight** (bĭrth wāt) In humans, the first weight of an infant obtained within less than the first 60 completed minutes after birth; a full-size infant is one weighing 2500 g or more; a low birth weight is less than 2500 g.; very low birth weight is less than 1500 g.; and extremely low birth weight is less than 1000 g.

♻ **bis-** **1.** Prefix signifying two or twice. **2.** CHEMISTRY used to denote the presence of two identical but separated complex groups in one molecule. Cf. bi-, di-. [L.]

**bis·cuit** (bis′kit) A term associated with the firing of porcelain, and applied to the fired article before glazing. May be any stage after the fluxes have flowed enough to provide rigidity to the structure up to the stage where shrinkage is complete. Referred to as low, medium or high biscuit, depending on the completeness of vitrification, also as hard or soft biscuit.

**bis·cuit-bake** (bis′kit bāk) The initial bake(s) given fusing porcelain at lower than glazing temperature to control shrinkage during the process of building up the dental restoration. SYN biscuit-firing.

**bis·cuit bite** (bis′kit bīt) SYN maxillomandibular record.

**bis·cuit-fir·ing** (bis′kit fīr′ing) SYN biscuit-bake.

**bi·sect** (bī-sekt′) In anatomy, to divide a body part into equal halves — right and left halves in the case of the head, neck, or trunk; medial and lateral halves in the case of the limb.

**bi·sect·ing an·gle tech·nique** (bī-sekt′ing ang′gĕl tek-nēk′) Intraoral radiographic procedure wherein film is placed along lingual surface of the resting on palate or floor of mouth; central ray of the x-ray beam is perpendicular to imaginary plane that bisects angle formed by film and long axis of tooth at their contact point. SYN bisecting method, bisecting technique, digital method.

**bi·sect·ing meth·od** (bī-sekt′ing meth′ŏd) SYN bisecting angle technique.

**bi·sect·ing tech·nique** (bī-sekt′ing tek-nēk′) SYN bisecting angle technique.

**bis in di·e (bid)** (bis in dē′ā) Twice a day.

**bis·muth (Bi)** (biz′mŭth) A trivalent metallic element; its salts are used in medicine.

**bis·muth a·lu·mi·nate** (biz′mŭth ă-lū′mi-nāt) A gastric antacid.

**bis·muth gin·gi·vi·tis** (biz′mŭth jin′ji-vī′tis) Bismuth deposits in the gingival margin.

**bis·muth line** (biz′mŭth līn) Black zone on free marginal gingiva, often first sign of poisoning from prolonged parenteral administration of bismuth.

**bis·mu·tho·sis** (biz′mŭ-thō′sis) Chronic bismuth poisoning.

**bis·muth sto·ma·ti·tis** (biz′mŭth stō′mă-tī′tis) Inflammation of the oral cavity, especially the gingiva, due to deposition of bismuth in gingival tissues.The gingival margins discolor darkly.

**bis·phos·pho·nate** (bī-fos′fō-nāt) Member of a class of drugs used for treatment of osteoporosis; works by inhibiting osteoclast-mediate resorption of bone. bisphosphonate

**bis·phos·pho·nate-as·so·ci·a·ted os·te·o·ne·cro·sis** (bis-fos′fō-nāt ă-sō′sē-ā-tĕd os′tē-ō-nĕ-krō′sis) Osteonecronecrosis, frequently found in the jaws, associated with prolonged use of bisphosphonates.

**bi·ste·phan·ic** (bī′stĕ-fan′ik) Relating to both stephanions; denoting particularly the bistephanic width of the cranium, or bistephanic diameter, the shortest distance from one stephanion to the other.

**bite** (bīt) **1.** To incise or seize with the teeth. **2.** The act of incision or seizure with the teeth. **3.** A morsel of food held between the teeth. **4.** Term used to denote the amount of pressure developed in closing the jaws. **5.** Undesirable jargon for terms such as interocclusal record, maxillomandibular registration, denture space, and interarch distance. **6.** A wound or puncture of the skin made by animal or insect. [A.S. *bītan*]

**bite a·nal·y·sis** (bīt ă-nal′i-sis) SYN occlusal analysis.

**bite force** (bīt fōrs) SYN biting pressure.

**bite fork** (bīt fōrk) SYN face-bow fork.

**bite gauge** (bīt gāj) SYN gnathodynamometer.

**bite guard** (bīt gahrd) Occlusal appliance used for diagnosis or therapy of the maxillary-mandibular relationship. SYN bite guard splint.

**bite guard splint** (bīt gahrd splint) SYN bite guard.

**bite plane** (bīt plān) SYN occlusal plane.

**bite·plate** (bīt′plāt) Removable appliance that incorporates a plane of acrylic designed to occlude with opposing teeth.

**bite re·cord** (bīt rek′ŏrd) SYN maxillo-mandibular record.

**bite rim** (bīt rim) SYN occlusion rim.

**bites** (bīts) Multiple penetrations of the skin (puncture or laceration) causing reactions that result from 1) mechanical injury; 2) injection of toxic material such as snake or scorpion venom; 3) injection of antigenic substances, especially by insect or arthropod bites, capable of inducing and eliciting allergic sensitization; 4) introduction of otherwise indigenous mouth flora in the instance of human bites; 5) invasion of the tissue as in myiasis; 6) transmission of diseases.

**bite·wing** (bīt′wing) SEE bitewing radiograph.

**bite·wing ra·di·o·graph** (bīt′wing rā′dē-ō-graf) Intraoral dental film adapted to show coronal portion and cervical third of root of teeth in near occlusion; useful in detecting interproximal caries and determining alveolar septal height.

**bit·ing pres·sure** (bīt′ing presh′ŭr) Force applied between the maxillary and mandibular teeth resulting from contraction of the masticatory elevator muscles.

**bit·ing strength** (bīt′ing strength) SYN force of mastication.

**Black clas·si·fi·ca·tion** (blak klas′i-fi-kā′shŭn) Classification of dental cavities based on the tooth surface(s) involved.

**black·out** (blak′owt) **1.** Temporary loss of consciousness due to decreased blood flow to the brain. **2.** A transient episode that occurs during a state of intense intoxication.

**black stain** (blak stān) Black or gray discoloration of teeth near the gingival margins; may be caused by chromogenic bacteria or by orally inhaling silver or manganese dust.

**black tongue** (blak tŭng) Discoloration of the dorsum of the tongue due to staining by exogenous material such as the components of tobacco; usually superimposed on hairy tongue. SYN lingua nigra.

**blade** (blād) Working end of an instrument with special design for a particular clinical dental treatment.

**blade en·dos·te·al im·plant** (blād en-dos′tē-ăl im′plant) SYN blade implant.

🛈**blade im·plant** (blād im′plant) Flat form of implant, usually made of titanium covered with film to prevent corrosion; placed anteroposteriorly in jaw; osseointegration usually results. Prongs projecting through oral mucosa hold appliance (e.g., denture) in place. See this page.

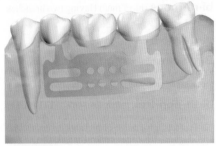

**blade implant**

**blade·vent** (blād′vent) A thin, wedged metal endosteal implant inserted into a surgically prepared groove in maxilla or mandible.

**Blan·din gland** (blahn-dan[h]′ gland) SYN anterior lingual gland.

**blan·ket stich** (blangk′ĕt stĭch) SYN blanket suture.

**blan·ket su·ture** (blangk′ĕt sū′chŭr) A continuous lock-stitch used to approximate the skin of a wound.

**blast** (blast) General term for immature or precursor cell. [G. *blastos,* germ]

***Blas·to·my·ces der·ma·tit·i·dis*** (blas′tō-mī′sēz dĕr′mă-tit′i-dis) A soil fungus that causes blastomycosis. [*blasto-* + G. *mykēs,* fungus]

**blas·to·my·cin** (blas′tō-mī′sin) An antigen for intradermal testing prepared from sterile filtrates of cultures of the filamentous form of *Blastomyces dermatitidis.*

**blas·to·my·co·sis** (blas′tō-mī-kō′sis) Chronic granulomatous and suppurative disease caused by *Blastomyces dermatitidis;* originates as a respiratory infection and disseminates, usually with pulmonary, osseous, or cutaneous involvement predominating.

**bleach, bleach·ing** (blēch, blēch′ing) Removal of color from an object using chemicals or light.

**bleed·er** (blē′dĕr) A blood vessel cut during a surgical procedure.

**bleed·ing** (blēd′ing) Losing blood as a result of the rupture or severance of blood vessels.

**bleed·ing time** (blēd′ing tīm) A screening procedure to detect congenital and acquired platelet disorders. Test is performed at bedside and usually lasts 1–3 minutes but may be prolonged in some cases.

**bleph·a·ri·tis** (blef′ă-rī′tis) Inflammation of the eyelids. [G. *blepharon,* eyelid + G. *-itis,* inflammation]

**bleph·a·ro·phi·mo·sis** (blef'ă-rō-fi-mō' sis) Decreased size of the palpebral aperture without fusion of lid margins. [G. *blepharon*, eyelid + G. *phimōsis*, an obstruction]

**bleph·a·rop·to·sis** (blef'ăr-op-tō'sis) Drooping of the upper eyelid. SYN ptosis (2). [G. *blepharon*, eyelid + G. *ptōsis*, a falling]

**bleph·a·ro·spasm, bleph·a·ro·spas·mus** (blef'ă-rō-spazm, -spaz'mŭs) Involuntary spasmodic contraction of the orbicularis oculi muscle; may occur in isolation or be associated with other dystonic contractions of facial, jaw, or neck muscles.

**blind na·so·tra·che·al in·tu·ba·tion** (blīnd nā'zō-trā'kē-ăl in'tū-bā'shŭn) Passage of a tube through nose into trachea without using a laryngoscope.

**blis·ter** (blis'tĕr) A fluid-filled, thin-walled structure under the epidermis or within the epidermis (subepidermal or intradermal).

**Bloch-Sulz·ber·ger syn·drome** (bloksults'ber-ger sin'drōm) Finding of patterned hyperpigmented lesions after development of bullous verrucous skin lesions.

**block** (blok) **1.** To obstruct; to arrest passage through. **2.** A condition in which the passage of an electric impulse is arrested, wholly or in part, temporarily or permanently. [Fr. *bloquer*]

**block an·es·the·si·a** (blok an'es-thē'zē-ă) SYN conduction anesthesia.

**block·ing** (blok'ing) Obstructing; arresting passage, conduction, or transmission.

**block·ing a·gent** (blok'ing ā'jĕnt) A class of drugs that inhibit (block) a biologic activity or process; frequently called "blockers."

**block-out** (blok'owt) Elimination of undercuts by filling such areas with a medium such as wax or wet pumice.

**blood** (blŭd) The "circulating tissue" of the body; the fluid and its suspended formed elements that are circulated through the heart, arteries, capillaries, and veins; blood is the means by which: 1) oxygen and nutritive materials are transported to the tissues, and 2) carbon dioxide and various metabolic products are removed for excretion. Blood consists of a pale yellow or gray-yellow fluid, plasma, in which are suspended red blood cells (erythrocytes), white blood cells (leukocytes), and platelets. SEE ALSO arterial blood, venous blood. [A.S. *blōd*]

**blood-borne path·o·gens (BBP)** (blŭd' bōrn path'ŏ-jĕnz) Disease-producing microorganisms transmitted by means of blood, tissue, and body fluids containing blood.

**blood-brain bar·ri·er (BBB)** (blŭd-brān bar'ē-ĕr) A selective mechanism opposing the passage of most ions and large-molecular weight compounds from the blood to brain tissue.

**blood cir·cu·la·tion** (blŭd sĭr-kyū-lā'shŭn) Course of the blood from the heart through the arteries, capillaries, and veins back again to the heart.

**blood clot** (blŭd klot) SYN thrombus.

**blood count** (blŭd kownt) Calculation of the number of red (RBC) or white (WBC) blood cells in a cubic millimeter of blood, by means of counting the cells in an accurate volume of diluted blood.

**blood cul·ture** (blŭd kŭl'chŭr) Microbiologic culture of a blood specimen.

**blood cyst** (blŭd sist) SYN hemorrhagic cyst.

**blood disc** (blŭd disk) SYN platelet.

**blood dys·cra·si·a** (blŭd dis-krā'zē-ă) Diseased state of the blood; usually refers to abnormal cellular elements of a permanent character.

**blood gas a·nal·y·sis** (blŭd gas ă-nal'i-sis) The direct electrode measurement of the partial pressure of oxygen and carbon dioxide in the blood.

**blood group** (blŭd grŭp) **1.** A system of antigens under the control of closely linked allelic loci on the surface of the erythrocyte. Often used as synonymous with blood type. **2.** The classification of blood samples by means of laboratory tests of their agglutination reactions with respect to one or more blood groups.

**blood poi·son·ing** (blŭd poy'zŏn-ing) SEE septicemia, pyemia.

**blood pres·sure (BP)** (blŭd presh'ŭr) Pressure or tension of the blood within the systemic arteries, maintained by the contraction of the left ventricle, the resistance of the arterioles and capillaries, the elasticity of the arterial walls, as well as the viscosity and volume of the blood; expressed as relative to the ambient atmospheric pressure.

**blood·stream** (blŭd'strēm) Flowing blood as it is encountered in the circulatory system, as distinguished from blood that has been removed from the circulatory system or sequestered in a part; thus, something added to the bloodstream may be expected to become distributed to all parts of the body through which blood is flowing.

**blood sug·ar** (blŭd shug'ăr) SEE glucose.

**blood u·re·a ni·tro·gen (BUN)** (blŭd yūr-ē'ă nī'trŏ-jĕn) Nitrogen, in the form of urea, in the blood.

**blood ves·sel** (blŭd ves'ĕl) [TA] Any vessel conveying blood: arteries, arterioles, capillaries, venules, veins.

**blow-out frac·ture** (blŏ′owt frak′shŭr) Breakage in floor or medial wall of the orbit, without a fracture of the rim, produced by a blow on the globe.

**blue line** (blū līn) Bluish line along free border of gingiva, occurring in chronic heavy metal poisoning.

**⊞blue ne·vus** (blū nē′vŭs) A dark blue or blue-black nevus covered by smooth skin and formed by heavily pigmented spindle-shaped or dendritic melanocytes in the reticular dermis. See this page.

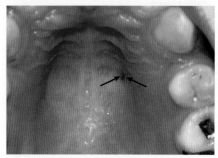

blue nevus: uniform slate-blue color, hard palate

**blun·der·buss a·pex** (blŭn′dĕr-bŭs ā′peks) A tooth root apex that widens at its end.

**B lym·pho·cyte** (lim′fō-sīt) Immunologically important lymphocyte that is not thymus dependent, is short lived, and resembles the bursa-derived lymphocyte of birds in that it is responsible for the production of immunoglobulins.

**BMR** Abbreviation for basal metabolic rate.

**board cer·ti·fi·ca·tion** (bōrd sĕr′ti-fi-kā′shŭn) A specialty designation typically obtained by the successful completion of an examination signifying the possession of expert knowledge in a field; eligibility requires completion of prerequisites.

**board cer·ti·fied** (bōrd sĕr′ti-fīd) Referring to someone certified in a specialty area.

**board dip·lo·mate** (bōrd dip′lŏ-māt) A specialist in an area who has completed the academic and clinical requirements to practice as a specialist and has successfully completed the examination(s) required by the specialty.

**board el·i·gi·ble** (bōrd el′i-ji-bĕl) Referring to someone who is not yet certified in a specialty but who has met the requirements to sit for the examination.

**board qua·li·fied** (bōrd kwah′li-fīd) A specialist who is qualified by completion of appropriate academic and clinical work to take a specialty board examination but who has not as yet successfully completed that examination.

**Boch·da·lek gan·gli·on** (bok′dă-lek gang′glē-ŏn) Ganglion of plexus of dental nerve lying in the maxilla just above root of canine tooth.

**Boch·da·lek valve** (bok′dă-lek valv) Fold of mucous membrane in the lacrimal canaliculus at the lacrimal punctum.

**Bö·deck·er in·dex** (bod′ĕ-kĕr in′deks) Modification of the DMF caries index (q.v.).

**bod·y** (bod′ē) 1. The human body, consisting of head (caput), neck (collum), trunk (truncus), and limbs (membra). SYN corpus (1) [TA]. 2. The material part of a human, as distinguished from the mind and spirit. SEE ALSO soma. [A.S. *bodig*]

**bod·y bur·den** (bod′ē bŭr′dĕn) The amount of a harmful substance that is permanently present in a person's body.

**bod·y dys·mor·phic dis·or·der** (bod′ē dis-mōr′fik dis-ōr′dĕr) Psychosomatic disorder characterized by preoccupation with some imagined defect in appearance.

**bod·y im·age** (bod′ē im′ăj) 1. Cerebral representation of all body sensation organized in the parietal cortex. 2. Personal conception of one's own body as distinct from one's actual anatomic body.

**bod·y mass in·dex** (bod′ē mas in′deks) Anthropometric measure of body mass, defined as weight in kilograms divided by height in meters squared.

**bod·y me·chan·ics** (bod′ē mĕ-kan′iks) The application of physical principles to achieve maximum efficiency and to limit risk of physical stress or injury to the practitioner of physical therapy and other specialties.

**bod·y of man·di·ble** (bod′ē man′di-bĕl) [TA] Heavy, U-shaped, horizontal portion of the mandible extending posteriorly to the angle where it is continuous with the ramus; supports lower teeth.

**bod·y of max·il·la** (bod′ē mak-sil′ă) [TA] Central portion of maxilla hollowed out by maxillary sinus; presents orbital, nasal, anterior, and infratemporal surfaces and supports four processes: frontal, zygomatic, palatine, and alveolar.

**bod·y of tongue** (bod′ē tŭng) [TA] Oral part of the tongue anterior to the terminal sulcus.

**bod·y sur·face ar·e·a (BSA)** (bod′ē sŭr′făs ār′ē-ă) Area of external surface of the body, expressed in square meters ($m^2$).

**Boeck dis·ease** (bĕrk di-zēz′) SYN sarcoidosis.

**Bohn nod·ules** (bon nod′yūlz) Tiny multiple cysts in newborns found at junction of the hard and soft palates and along buccal and lingual parts of the dental ridges.

**boil** (boyl) SYN furuncle. [A.S. *byl,* a swelling]

**Bo·ley gauge** (bō′lē gāj) Caliper-type gauge (in mm.) used to measure thickness of various dental materials.

**Bol·ton point** (bōl′tŏn poynt) Apex of the retrocondylar fossa, interposed between it and the basal surface of the occipital bone.

**Bol·ton tri·an·gle** (bōl′tŏn trī′ang-gĕl) Area formed by the nasion, the sella turcica, and the Bolton point.

**bo·lus** (bō′lŭs) **1.** A single, relatively large quantity of a substance, usually one intended for therapeutic use (e.g., dose of an intravenous drug). **2.** A masticated morsel of food or another substance ready to be swallowed. [L. fr. G. *bōlos,* lump, clod]

**bond** (bond) CHEMISTRY the force holding two neighboring atoms in place and resisting their separation.

**bond·ing** (bond′ing) **1.** Process by which orthodontic brackets are affixed to tooth surfaces; fluoride-releasing light-activated resin is commonly used. **2.** Physical adherence of sealant to enamel surface is done using an acid-etching technique that leaves microspaces between enamel rods.

**bond strength** (bond strength) Expression of degree of adherence between tooth surface and another material.

**bone** (bōn) [TA] Hard connective tissue consisting of cells embedded in a matrix of mineralized ground substance and collagen fibers. Fibers are impregnated with inorganic components, including crystals of calcium phosphate, such that using X-ray defraction, they are seen to be organized in a hydroxyapatite pattern (calcium phosphate is 85% by weight) as well as calcium carbonate (10%), and magnesium; by weight, bone is composed of 65–75% inorganic and 25–35% organic material; humans have approximately 200 distinct bones in the skeleton, not including the auditory ossicles of the tympanic cavity or the sesamoid bones other than the two patellae. [A.S. *bān*]

**bone ache** (bōn āk) Dull pain in one or more bones, often severe; extreme variety occurs in dengue.

**bone aug·men·ta·tion** (bōn awg-men-tā′shŭn) Increase in osseus dimensions by addition of material or tissue.

**bone chips** (bōn chips) Small pieces of cancellous bone generally used to fill bony defects and to promote reossification.

**bone con·duc·tion** (bōn kŏn-dŭk′shŭn) AUDIOLOGY the transmission of sound to the

inner ear through vibrations applied to the bones of the skull.

**bone cyst** (bōn sist) SEE solitary bone cyst. See this page.

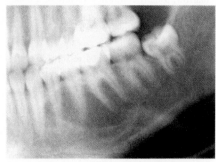

**traumatic bone cyst:** interradicular extension

**bone den·si·ty** (bōn den′si-tē) Quantitative measurement of the mineral content of bone, used as an indicator of the structural strength of the bone and as a screen for osteoporosis.

**bone for·ceps** (bōn fōr′seps) A strong forceps used for seizing or removing fragments of bone.

**bone graft** (bōn graft) Bone transplanted from a donor site to a recipient site, without anastomosis of nutrient vessels; bone can be transplanted within the same person (i.e., autograft) or between different people (i.e., allograft).

**bone im·plant** (bōn im′plant) Use of natural or artificial materials for osseous reconstruction.

**bone loss** (bōn laws) In dentistry, resorption of alveolar bone due to disease, trauma, or irritants. SEE ALSO bone resorption. See this page.

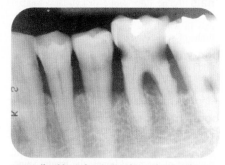

**generalized bone loss:** extrusion and root caries

**bone mar·row** (bōn mar′ō) [TA] The tissue filling the cavities of bones, having a stroma of reticular fibers and cells.

**bone mar·row dose** (bōn mar′ō dōs) Cumulative dose to the blood-forming organ from therapeutic or nuclear fallout irradiation; the presumed leukemogenic dose.

**bone mar·row em·bo·lism** (bōn mar´ō em´bŏ-lizm) Obstruction of a vessel by bone marrow, usually following fracture of a bone.

**bone plate** (bōn plāt) Metal bar with perforations for the insertion of screws; used to immobilize fractured segments.

**bone re·sorp·tion** (bōn rē-sōrp´shŭn) Removal of osseous tissue by osteoclasts; can be part of the normal balance of bone resorption and deposition or part of a pathologic process.

**bones of cra·ni·um, bones of skull** (bōnz krā´nē-ŭm, skŭl) Paired inferior nasal concha, lacrimal, maxilla, nasal, palatine, parietal, temporal, and zygomatic; and the unpaired ethmoid, frontal, occipital, sphenoid, and vomer.

**Bon·will tri·an·gle** (bon´wil trī´ang-gĕl) Equilateral triangle formed by lines from contact points of the lower central incisors or the medial line of residual ridge of mandible, to condyle on either side and from one condyle to the other.

**bon·y am·pul·lae of sem·i·cir·cu·lar ca·nals** (bō´nē am-pul´ē sem´ē-sĭr´kyū-lăr kă-nalz´) Circumscribed dilation of one extremity of each of the three bony semicircular canals, anterior, posterior, and lateral; each contains a membranous ampulla of the semicircular ducts.

**bon·y an·ky·lo·sis** (bō´nē ang´ki-lō´sis) SYN synostosis.

**bon·y lab·y·rinth** (bō´nē lab´i-rinth) Series of cavities (e.g., cochlea, vestibule, and semicircular canals) contained within otic capsule of petrous portion of the temporal bone; filled with perilymph, in which the delicate, endolymph-filled membranous labyrinth is suspended.

**bon·y limbs of sem·i·cir·cu·lar ca·nals** (bō´nē limz sem´ē-sĭr´kyū-lăr kă-nalz´) [TA] Extremities of the bony semicircular canals in which the corresponding membranous limbs of semicircular ducts are located.

**bon·y na·sal cav·i·ty** (bō´nē nā´zăl kav´i-tē) [TA] Skeletal nasal depression with walls of bone and cartilage (vs. the nasal cavity of a person or cadaver), lined with nasal mucosa or respiratory epithelium.

**bon·y na·sal sep·tum** (bō´nē nā´zăl sep´tŭm) [TA] Bones supporting the bony part of the nasal septum; they are the perpendicular plate of the ethmoid, the vomer, the sphenoidal rostrum, the crest of the nasal bones, the frontal spine, and the median crest formed by the apposition of the maxillary and palatine bones.

**bon·y pal·ate** (bō´nē pal´ăt) Concave elliptic plate that contributes to roof of oral cavity.

**bon·y part of ex·ter·nal a·cous·tic me·a·tus** (bō´nē pahrt eks-tĕr´năl ă-kū´stik mē-ā´tŭs) Medial two thirds of external acoustic

meatus, which is formed as the tympanic plate of the temporal bone develops.

**bon·y part of na·sal sep·tum** (bō´nē pahrt nā´zăl sep´tŭm) [TA] Major portion of the nasal septum including (supported by) the vomer and the perpendicular plate of the ethmoid.

**bon·y part of pha·ryn·go·tym·pan·ic (au·di·to·ry) tube** (bō´nē pahrt fă-ring´gō-tim-pan´ik aw´di-tōr-ē tūb) [TA] Portion of the pharyngotympanic (auditory) tube formed by petrous part of temporal bone passing anteromedially from the tympanic cavity, gradually narrowing to terminate at the junction of the petrous and squamous parts.

**bon·y part of skel·e·tal sys·tem** (bō´nē pahrt skel´ē-tăl sis´tĕm) [TA] Portion of the skeleton composed of cortical, compact, or spongy bone.

**Böök syn·drome** (buk sin´drōm) Premolar aplasia, hyperhidrosis, and premature canities.

**boost·er dose** (bū´stĕr dōs) Dose given at some time after an initial dose to enhance the effect.

**bo·rax** (bō´raks) SYN sodium borate. [Pers. *būraq*]

**bor·der** (bōr´dĕr) The part of a surface that forms its outer boundary. SEE ALSO edge, margin.

**bor·der·line case** (bōr´dĕr-līn kās) Patient, whose clinical findings are suggestive, but not fully convincing, of a specific diagnosis.

**bor·der·line hy·per·ten·sion** (bōr´dĕr-līn hī´pĕr-ten´shŭn) By consensus, that blood pressure zone between highest acceptable ''normal'' and hypertensive blood pressure.

**bor·der mold·ing** (bōr´dĕr mōld´ing) Impression technique to record the oral muscles in an active state to determine the delimits of a removable denture. SYN tissue molding, tissue-trimming.

**bor·der move·ment** (bōr´dĕr mūv´mĕnt) The limit of movement of the lower jaw as recorded in the sagittal and horizontal planes; often referred to as the envelope of motion.

**bor·der seal** (bōr´dĕr sēl) Contact of denture border with underlying or adjacent tissues to prevent passage of air or other substances.

**bor·der tis·sue move·ments** (bōr´dĕr tish´ū mūv´mĕnts) Action of muscles and other tissues adjacent to borders of a denture.

***Bor·de·tel·la per·tus·sis*** (bōr-dĕ-tel´ă pĕr-tŭs´is) A bacterial species that causes whooping cough.

**bo·ric ac·id** (bōr´ik as´id) A weak acid, used as an antiseptic dusting powder, in saturated solution as a collyrium, and with glycerin in cases of aphthae and stomatitis.

⊞**bo·try·oid o·don·to·gen·ic cyst** (bot´rē-oyd ō-don´tō-jen´ik sist) Lateral periodontal cyst that shows a multilocular growth pattern. See page A6.

**bo·try·o·my·co·sis** (bot´rē-ō-mī-kō´sis) A chronic granulomatous condition of horses, cattle, swine, and humans, usually involving the skin but occasionally also the viscera. SYN actinophytosis (2). [fr. *Botryomyces*]

**Böt·tcher cells** (bĕrt´shĕr selz) Cells of the basilar membrane of the cochlea.

**Bött·cher gan·gli·on** (bĕrt´shĕr gang´glē-ŏn) Ganglion on cochlear nerve in internal acoustic meatus.

**bot·u·li·nus tox·in** (bot-yū-lī´nŭs toks´in) Potent exotoxin that is highly neurotoxic derived from *Clostridium botulinum*.

**bouche de ta·pir** (būsh dĕ tah-pir´) SYN tapir mouth. [Fr.]

**bound** (bownd) **1.** Limited; circumscribed; enclosed. **2.** Denoting a substance which is not in readily diffusible form but exists in combination with a high molecular weight substance, especially protein.

**bou·ton** (bū-tōn[h]´) A button, pustule, or knoblike swelling. [Fr. button]

**Bow·en dis·ease** (bō´ĕn di-zēz´) A form of intraepidermal carcinoma characterized by the development of slowly enlarging pinkish or brownish papules or eroded plaques covered with a thickened horny layer.

**Bow·man cap·sule** (bō´măn kap´sŭl) SYN glomerulus.

**box·ing** (boks´ing) In dentistry, building up vertical walls, usually with wax, around a dental impression after beading, to produce desired size and form of the dental cast and preserve certain landmarks of the impression.

**box·ing strip** (boks´ing strip) SYN boxing wax.

⊞**box·ing wax** (boks´ing waks) Wax used to create an enclosure for pouring a mold or cast, such as boxing impressions. SEE ALSO boxing. See this page. SYN boxing strip.

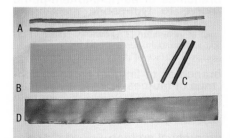

**dental waxes:** (A) beading or periphery wax; (B) baseplate wax; (C) inlay wax; (D) boxing wax

**BP** Abbreviation for blood pressure.

**B point** (poynt) The most posterior point on the cephalometric profile between the chin and mandibular incisors.

**Br** Symbol for bromine.

**brace** (brās) An orthosis or orthopedic appliance that supports or holds in correct position any movable part of the body and that allows motion of the part. [M.E., fr. O.Fr., fr. L. *brachium*, arm, fr. G. *brachion*]

**brac·es** (brās´ĕz) Colloquialism for orthodontic appliances.

**bra·chi·al pulse** (brā´kē-ăl pŭls) A palpable rhythmic expansion of the brachial artery in the antecubital space.

**bra·chi·o·ce·phal·ic ar·ter·i·tis** (brak´ē-ō-se-fal´ik ahr´tĕr-ī´tis) Giant-cell arteritis seen in older adults; characterized by inflammatory lesions in medium-sized arteries, most commonly in the head, neck, and/or pectoral girdle.

**bra·chi·o·ra·di·al re·flex** (brak´ē-ō-rā´dē-ăl rē´fleks) With the arm supinated to 45°, a tap near the lower end of the radius causes contracts of the brachioradial muscle. SYN styloradial reflex.

♲**brachy-** *Do not confuse this combining form with brachi-.* Combining form meaning short. [G. *brachys*, short]

**brach·y·ceph·a·ly** (brak´ē-sef´ă-lē) Disproportionate shortness of head, the cranium having a cephalic index over 80; among the brachycephalic races are Native Americans, Malays, and Burmese. [*brachy-* + G. *kephalē*, head]

**brach·y·chei·li·a, brach·y·chi·li·a** (brak´ē-kī´lē-ă) Abnormal shortness of the lips. [*brachy-* + G. *cheilos*, lip]

**brach·y·dac·ty·ly** (brak´ē-dak´ti-lē) Abnormal shortness of the fingers. [*brachy-* + G. *daktylos*, finger]

**brach·y·glos·sal** (brak´ē-glos´ăl) Denoting an abnormally short tongue. [*brachy-* + G. *glōssa*, tongue]

**brach·yg·na·thi·a** (brak´ig-nā´thē-ă) *In the diphthong gn, the g is silent only at the beginning of a word.* Abnormal shortness or recession of the mandible. SEE ALSO micrognathia. SYN bird face. [*brachy-* + G. *gnathos*, jaw]

**brach·y·o·dont** (brak´ē-ō-dont) Having abnormally short teeth. [*brachy-* + G. *odous*, tooth]

**brach·y·rhyn·chus** (brak´ē-ring´kŭs) Abnormal shortness of the nose and maxilla, often associated with cyclopia. [*brachy-* + G. *rhynchos*, snout]

**brach·y·staph·y·line** (brak´ē-staf´i-lin) Having a short palate. [*brachy-* + G. *staphylē*, uvula]

**brac·ing** (brās'ing) In dentistry, resistance to horizontal components of masticatory force.

**■brack·et** (brak'ĕt) In dentistry, a small metal attachment soldered or welded to an orthodontic band or alternatively bonded directly to teeth, serving to fasten arch wire to band or tooth. See this page.

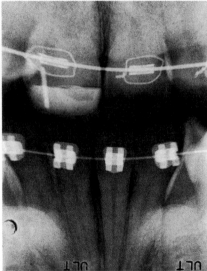

anterior vertical bitewing radiograph showing brackets, wires, and stainless-steel ligatures: threaded pin and composite have restored fractured incisal edge; bilateral mandibular tori are present and appear radiopaque

**♻brady-** Combining form meaning slow. [G. *bradys*, slow]

**bradyaesthesia** [Br.] SYN bradyesthesia.

**bra·dy·car·di·a** (brad'ē-kahr'dē-ă) Slowness of the heartbeat, usually under 50 beats/minute. [*brady-* + G. *kardia*, heart]

**bra·dy·di·as·to·le** (brad'ē-dī-as'tŏ-lē) Prolongation of the diastole of the heart.

**bra·dy·es·the·si·a** (brad'ē-es-thē'zē-ă) Slow sensory perception. SYN bradyaesthesia. [*brady-* + G. *aisthēsis*, sensation]

**bra·dy·glos·si·a** (brad'ē-glaws'ē-ă) Slow or difficult tongue movement. [*brady-* + G. *glōssa*, tongue]

**bra·dy·ki·ne·si·a** (brad'ē-kin-ē'sē-ă) A decrease in spontaneity and movement. [*brady-* + G. *kinēsis*, movement]

**bra·dy·ki·net·ic** (brad'ē-ki-net'ik) Characterized by or pertaining to slow movement.

**bra·dy·ki·nin** (brad'ē-kī'nin) One of several plasma kinins, a potent vasodilator; physiologic mediator of anaphylaxis released from cytotropic antibody-coated mast cells following reaction with antigen (allergen) specific for the antibody. [*brady-* + G. *kineō*, to move]

**bra·dyp·ne·a** (brad'ip-nē'ă) *In the diphthong pn*, the *p* is silent only at the beginning of a word. Although *bradypne'a* is correct pronunciation, alternative pronunciation *bradyp'nea* is widespread in the U.S. Abnormal slowness of respiration, specifically a low respiratory frequency. [*brady-* + G. *pnoē*, breathing]

**brain** (brān) [TA] That part of the central nervous system contained within the cranium. [A.S. *braegen*]

**brain con·cus·sion** (brān kŏn-kŭsh'ŭn) Clinical syndrome usually due to head trauma, characterized by immediate but transient impairment of cerebral function, principally alteration of consciousness, but also disturbance of vision and equilibrium, without any detectable structural brain damage.

**brain death** (brān deth) SYN cerebral death.

**brain e·de·ma** (brān ĕ-dē´mă) SYN cerebral edema.

**brain·stem, brain stem** (brān'stem) [TA] Originally, the entire unpaired subdivision of the brain, composed of the rhombencephalon, mesencephalon, and diencephalon as distinguished from the brain's only paired subdivision, the telencephalon. More recently, the connotation of the term has undergone several arbitrary modifications: some use it to denote no more than rhombencephalon plus mesencephalon, distinguishing that complex from the prosencephalon (diencephalon plus telencephalon); others restrict it even further to refer exclusively to the rhombencephalon. From both developmental and architectural viewpoints, the original interpretation seems preferable.

**brak·ing ra·di·a·tion** (brāk'ing rā'dē-ā' shŭn) SYN Bremsstrahlung radiation.

**branch** (branch) [TA] An offshoot; in anatomy, one of the primary divisions of a nerve or blood vessel. SEE ramus, artery, nerve, vein. [Fr. *branche*, related to L. *brachium*, arm]

**branch·es of au·ric·u·lo·tem·po·ral nerve to tym·pan·ic mem·brane** (branch'ĕz ahr-tik´yū-lō-tem'pŏr-ăl nĕrv tim-pan'ik mem'brān) [TA] Sensory branch of the auriculotemporal nerve (from CN V₃) supplying external surface of the tympanic membrane.

**branch·es of lin·gual nerve to isth·mus of fau·ces** (branch'ĕz ling'gwăl nĕrv is'mŭs faw'sēz) [TA] Branches of lingual nerve of CN V, conveying general sensation from oral mucosa between oral cavity and oropharynx.

**bran·chi·al arch·es** (brang'kē-ăl ahr'chĕz) Typically, six arches in vertebrates; in lower vertebrates, they bear gills; they are pharyngeal arches (q.v.) in human embryos.

**bran·chi·o·mer·ic mus·cles** (brang´kē-ō-mer´ik mŭs´ĕlz) Muscles associated with the pharyngeal arches; provide large portion of the musculature for face and neck.

**branch to an·gu·lar gy·rus** (branch ang´ gyū-lăr jī´rŭs) [TA] The last branch of the terminal part of the middle cerebral artery distributed to parts of the temporal parietal and occipital lobes.

**braz·ing** (brāz´ing) In dentistry, to solder.

**break-e·ven point** (brāk-ē´vĕn poynt) The point in sales volume at which total revenue equals total costs; indicating a balance. Sales volume below the break-even point will cause a negative cash flow (loss); sales volume above the break-even point will result in a profit.

**breast bone** (brest bōn) SYN sternum.

**breath** (breth) 1. The respired air. 2. An inspiration. [A.S. *braeth*]

**breath·ing** (brēdh´ing) Inhalation and exhalation of air or gaseous mixtures.

**breath·ing bag** (brēdh´ing bag) A collapsible reservoir from which gases are inhaled and into which gases may be exhaled during general anesthesia or artificial ventilation. SYN reservoir bag.

**breath test** (breth test) Any diagnostic test in which endogenous or exogenous materials are measured in samples of breath as a means of identifying pathologic processes.

**breg·ma** (breg´mă) Point on the cranium corresponding to the junction of coronal and sagittal sutures. [G. the forepart of the head]

**breg·mat·o·lamb·doid arc** (breg-mat´ō-lam´doyd ahrk) Line running along the sagittal suture from the bregma to the apex of the lambdoid suture.

**breg·mo·car·di·ac re·flex** (breg´mō-kahr´ dē-ak rē´fleks) In infants, pressure on the anterior fontanelle causing cardiac slowing.

**brems·strah·lung ra·di·a·tion** (bremz´ shtrah-lung rā´dē-ā´shūn) When a high-speed electron from the cathode stream is slowed down and pulled off course by the positive pull of the target, this represents a loss of energy which is given up as heat and an x-ray photon. Most x-rays in medicine and dentistry are of bremsstrahlung origin. SYN braking radiation. [Ger. *Brems*, brake, + *Strahlung*, radiation]

**brev·i·col·lis** (brev´i-kol´is) Abnormal shortness of the neck.

▪**bridge** (brij) 1. The upper part of the ridge of the nose formed by the nasal bones. 2. One of the threads of protoplasm that appear to pass from one cell to another. See this page. 3. SYN fixed partial denture.

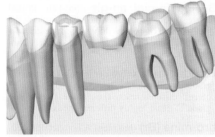

**bridge:** three-unit bridge attached to teeth

**bridge·work** (brij´wŏrk) SYN partial denture.

**Bri·nell hard·ness num·ber (BHN)** (bri-nel´ hahrd´nĕs nŭm´bĕr) Number related to the size of the permanent impression made by a ball indenter of specified size (usually 10 mm in diameter) pressed into the surface of the material under a specified load: where $P$ = applied load in kg, $D$ = diameter of the ball in mm, and $d$ = diameter of the impression in mm.

**Bri·nell hard·ness test** (bri-nel´ hahrd´ nĕs test) Common dental measurement to determine hardness of ductile materials (e.g., metals). A hardened steel ball of specific diameter is pressed into the polished surface of the material under a specified load. The result, determined from the area of the surface of the indentation, is an index of hardness (e.g., Brinell hardness number).

**Bris·saud-Ma·rie syn·drome** (brē-sō´ mah-rē´ sin´drōm) Functional spasms of the lips and glossolabial paralysis (related to conversion disorder).

**Bris·saud-Si·card syn·drome** (brē-sō´ sē-kahr´ sin´drōm) Hemiparesis and contralateral hemifacial spasm resulting from a pontine lesion.

**bris·tle** (bris´ĕl) Traditionally, individual short, stiff, natural hair of an animal taken from domestic swine or wild boars, but today most toothbrush bristles are made of nylon and thus are more properly called filaments.

**brit·tle di·a·be·tes** (brit´ĕl dī´ă-bē´tēz) Diabetes with refractory fluctuations in glucose.

**broach** (brōch) A dental instrument for removing the pulp of a tooth or exploring the canal.

**broad spec·trum** (brawd spek´trŭm) Term indicating a wide range of activity of an antibiotic against a variety of microorganisms.

**Bro·ca an·gles** (brō-kah´ ang´gĕlz) 1. SYN Broca basilar angle. 2. SYN Broca facial angle. 3. SYN occipital angle of parietal bone (1).

**Bro·ca bas·i·lar an·gle** (brō-kah´ bas´i-lăr ang´gĕl) Area formed at the basion of lines drawn from the nasion and the alveolar point. SYN Broca angles (1).

**Bro·ca fa·cial an·gle** (brō-kah´ fā´shăl ang´gĕl) Area formed by the intersection at the biauricular axis of lines drawn from the supraorbital point and the alveolar point. SYN Broca angles (2).

**Bro·der in·dex** (brō´dĕr in´deks) System for grading epidermoid carcinomas. I–IV on basis of cell differentiation (i.e., grade I most and grade IV least highly differentiated).

**bro·mine (Br)** (brō´mēn) A nonmetallic, reddish, volatile, liquid element; unites with hydrogen to form hydrobromic acid, and this reacts with many metals to form bromides, some of which are used in medicine. [Fr. *brome,* bromine, fr. G. *bromos,* stench]

**bro·mism, bro·min·ism** (brō´mizm, -minizm) Chronic bromide intoxication, characterized by headache, drowsiness, confusion and occasionally violent delirium, muscular weakness, cardiac depression, an acneform eruption, foul breath, anorexia, and gastric distress.

**bron·chi·a** (brong´kē-ă) The smaller divisions of the bronchi. SEE ALSO bronchus, bronchiole. [G. pl. of *bronchion,* dim. of *bronchos,* trachea]

**bron·chi·al asth·ma** (brong´kē-ăl az´mă) An acute or chronic disorder characterized by widespread and largely reversible reduction in the caliber of bronchi and bronchioles, due in varying degrees to smooth muscle spasm, mucosal edema, and excessive mucus in the lumens of airways. Cardinal symptoms are dyspnea, wheezing, and cough.

**bron·chi·ec·ta·sis** (brong´kē-ek´tă-sis) Chronic dilation of bronchi or bronchioles as a sequel of inflammatory disease or obstruction.

**bron·chi·ole** (brong´kē-ōl) One of approximately six generations of increasingly finer subdivisions of the bronchi, all smaller than 1 mm in diameter.

**bron·chi·tis** (brong-kī´tis) Inflammation of the mucous membrane of the bronchi.

**bron·chi·um,** pl. **bron·chi·a** (brong´kē-ŭm, -ă) A term sometimes used for a subdivision of a bronchus that is larger than a bronchiole. SEE ALSO bronchus, bronchiole. [Mod. L. fr. G. *bronchion*]

♻**broncho-** Combining form meaning bronchus, and, in ancient usage, the trachea. [G. *bronchos,* windpipe]

**bron·cho·con·stric·tion** (brong´kō-kŏnstrik´shŭn) Constriction of the bronchi.

**bron·cho·di·la·tion** (brong´kō-dī-lā´shŭn) Increase in caliber of bronchi and bronchioles in response to pharmacologically active substances or autonomic nervous activity.

**bron·cho·di·la·tor** (brong´kō-dī´lā-tŏr) Agent that increases caliber of a bronchus or bronchial tube.

**bron·cho·my·co·sis** (brong´kō-mī-kō´sis) Any fungal disease of the bronchial tubes or bronchi. [*broncho-* + G. *mykēs,* fungus]

**bron·cho·pneu·mo·ni·a** (brong´kō-nū-mō´nē-ă) Acute inflammation of the walls of the smaller bronchial tubes, with varying amounts of pulmonary consolidation due to spread of the inflammation into peribronchiolar alveoli and the alveolar ducts; may become confluent or may be hemorrhagic.

**bron·cho·scope** (brong´kō-skōp) An endoscope for inspecting the interior of the tracheobronchial tree. [*broncho-* + G. *skopeō,* to view]

**bron·chos·co·py** (brong-kos´kŏ-pē) Inspection of the interior of the tracheobronchial tree through a bronchoscope.

**bron·cho·spasm** (brong´kō-spazm) Contraction of smooth muscle in the walls of the bronchi and bronchioles, causing narrowing of the lumen.

**bron·cho·spas·mo·lyt·ic** (brong´kō-spaz´mō-lit-ik) Relieving a bronchospasm.

**bron·cho·spi·rog·ra·phy** (brong´kō-spī-rog´ră-fē) Use of a single-lumen endobronchial tube for measurement of ventilatory function of one lung. [*broncho-* + L. *spiro,* to breathe, + G. *graphō,* to write]

**bron·cho·ste·no·sis** (brong´kō-stĕ-nō´sis) Chronic narrowing of a bronchus.

**bron·cho·ve·sic·u·lar** (brong´kō-vĕ-sik´yū-lăr) Relating to the bronchi and alveoli in the lungs, especially as regards lung sounds heard by auscultation.

**bron·cho·ve·sic·u·lar res·pi·ra·tion** (brong´kō-vĕ-sik´yū-lăr res´pir-ā´shŭn) Combined bronchial and vesicular respiration.

**bron·chus,** pl. **bron·chi** (brong´kŭs, -kī) One of two subdivisions of the trachea serving to convey air to and from the lungs. [Mod. L., fr. G. *bronchos,* windpipe]

**bronze di·a·be·tes, bronzed dis·ease** (bronz dī-ă-bē´tēz, bronzd di-zēz´) Diabetes mellitus associated with hemochromatosis, with iron deposits in the skin, liver, pancreas, and other viscera, often with severe liver damage and glycosuria. SEE ALSO hemochromatosis.

**bronzed skin** (bronzd skin) Dark skin produced by Addison disease.

**brown pel·li·cle** (brown pel´i-kĕl) A thin discolored film (about 1 mcm), derived mainly from salivary glycoproteins, which forms over the surface of a cleansed tooth crown when it is exposed to the saliva; may result from poor oral hygiene. SYN acquired cuticle, acquired pellicle.

**brown stri·ae** (brown strī´ē) SYN Retzius striae.

**bru·isse·ment** (brū-ēs-mon[h]′) A purring auscultatory sound. [Fr.]

**bru·it** (brū-ē′) A harsh or musical intermittent auscultatory sound, especially an abnormal one. [Fr.]

**brush** (brŭsh) An instrument made of some flexible material, such as bristles or filaments, attached to a handle or to the tip of a catheter.

**brush bi·op·sy** (brŭsh bī′op-sē) Use of a stiff brush to abrade surface cells of a lesion for automated microscopic analysis; generally used in screening for oral cancer.

**brush·ite** (brŭsh′īt) A naturally occurring acid calcium phosphate occasionally found in dental calculus and renal calculi.

**brux·ism** (brŭk′sizm) A clenching of the teeth, associated with forceful lateral or protrusive jaw movements, resulting in rubbing, gritting, or grinding together of the teeth, usually during sleep. [G. *bruchō*, to grind the teeth]

**BSA** Abbreviation for body surface area.

**bu·bo** (bū′bō) Inflammatory swelling of lymph nodes, usually in the groin; confluent mass of nodes suppurates and drains pus.

**bu·bon·ic** (bū-bon′ik) Relating in any way to a bubo.

**buc·ca,** pl. **buc·cae** (bŭk′ă, -ē) SYN cheek. [L.]

**buc·cal** (bŭk′ăl) *Avoid the mispronunciation byū′kăl.* Pertaining to, adjacent to, or in the direction of the cheek. See this page.

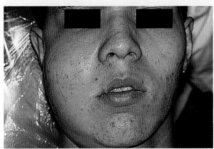

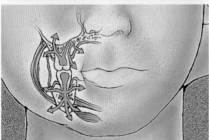

**buccal space infection:** infected mandibular molar

**buc·cal bi·fur·ca·tion cyst** (bŭk′ăl bī′fŭr-kā′shŭn sist) Dentoalveolar lesion located on facial side of tooth at bifurcation of a two-rooted tooth. See this page.

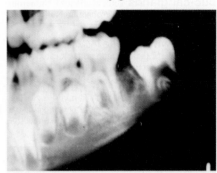

**buccal bifurcation cyst**

**buc·cal branch·es of fa·cial nerve** (bŭk′ăl branch′ĕz fā′shăl nĕrv) Motor branches of the parotid plexus of the facial nerve distributed to buccinator muscle and other muscles of facial expression below orbit and above chin.

**buc·cal car·ies** (bŭk′ăl kar′ēz) Caries beginning with decay on the buccal surface of a tooth.

**buc·cal cav·i·ty** (bŭk′ăl kav′i-tē) SYN oral vestibule.

**buc·cal con·tour** (bŭk′ăl kon′tūr) Shape of the facial (buccal) surface of a tooth.

**buc·cal cross·bite** (bŭk′ăl kraws′bīt) Buccal displacement of the affected posterior tooth or teeth as related to the opposing (i.e., antagonistic) tooth or teeth.

**buc·cal curve** (bŭk′ăl kŭrv) The line of the dental arch from the canine, or cuspid tooth to the third molar.

**buc·cal cusp** (bŭk′ăl kŭsp) Elevation of the crown of a tooth located toward the cheek. May be single, as on a premolar or multiple, as on a molar. If multiple, designated as to mesial or distal (e.g., mesiobuccal or distobuccal).

**buc·cal di·ges·tion** (bŭk′ăl di-jes′chŭn) Part of digestion carried on in the mouth, e.g., the action of salivary amylases.

**buc·cal em·bra·sure** (bŭk′ăl em-brā′shŭr) Space on facial aspect of interproximal contact area between adjacent posterior teeth.

**buc·cal fat-pad** (bŭk′ăl fat pad) Encapsuled fat mass in the cheek on outer side of buccinator muscle, especially marked in the infant; supposed to strengthen and support the cheek during the act of sucking.

**buc·cal flange** (bŭk′ăl flanj) Portion of denture flange that occupies buccal vestibule of the mouth.

**buc·cal gin·gi·va** (bŭk´ăl jin´ji-vă) Portion of gingiva that covers the buccal surfaces of teeth and alveolar process.

**buc·cal glands** (bŭk´ăl glandz) Numerous racemose, mucous, or serous glands in the submucous tissue of the cheeks.

**buc·cal lymph node** (bŭk´ăl limf nōd) One of the chain of facial lymph nodes located superficial to the buccinator muscle. SYN buccinator node.

**buc·cal mu·co·sa** (bŭk´ăl myū-kō´ză) Tissue lining that covers inside of cheeks; consists mainly of epithelium and subjacent connective tissue. See this page.

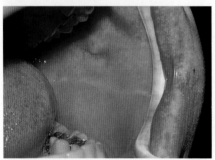

linea alba buccalis: buccal mucosa

**buc·cal nerve** (bŭk´ăl nĕrv) Sensory branch of mandibular division of the trigeminal nerve. SYN buccinator nerve, long buccal nerve.

**buc·cal notch** (bŭk´ăl noch) Indentation in an impression or denture flange formed by a buccal frenum.

**buc·cal oc·clu·sion** (bŭk´ăl ŏ-klū´zhŭn) **1.** Malposition of a tooth toward the cheek. **2.** The occlusion as seen from the buccal side of the teeth.

**buc·cal pit** (bŭk´ăl pit) Structural depression found on the buccal enamel of molars.

**buc·cal re·gion** (bŭk´ăl rē´jŭn) [TA] Area of the cheek, corresponding approximately to the outlines of the underlying buccinator muscle.

**buc·cal root of tooth** (bŭk´ăl rūt tūth) [TA] Root of a multirooted tooth located toward the buccal side of the alveolar ridge.

**buc·cal shelf** (bŭk´ăl shelf) Broad flat surface of the posterior mandible buccal to the teeth or alveolar ridge that provides denture support.

**buc·cal smear** (bŭk´ăl smēr) Cytologic smear containing material obtained by scraping the lateral buccal mucosa above the dentate line, smearing, and fixing immediately; used principally for determining somatic sex as indicated by the presence of the sex chromocenter (Barr body).

**buc·cal sur·face** (bŭk´ăl sŭr´făs) **1.** Mucosa of cheek. **2.** In prosthodontics, side of a denture adjacent to the cheek.

**buc·cal sur·face of tooth** (bŭk´ăl sŭr´făs tūth) Cheek portion of vestibular surface of tooth. SYN facies buccalis dentis.

**buc·cal tab·let** (bŭk´ăl tab´lĕt) Small, flat tablet intended to be inserted in the buccal pouch, where the active ingredient is absorbed directly through oral mucosa; dissolves or erodes slowly.

**buc·cal tube** (bŭk´ăl tūbe) A metal tube affixed to the facial (buccal) surface of an orthodontic molar band or directly to the surface of the tooth that allows the archwire to pass through while exerting either a torquing force or allowing the wire to slide as tooth movement occurs. See this page.

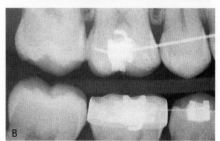

A

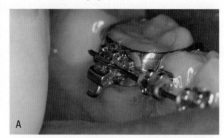

B

buccal tube: device as part of orthodontic fixed appliance; (A) note hook for attachment of elastics; (B) posterior bitewing of same area; note mandibular tube uses a band, whereas maxillary tube is bonded to molar directly

**buc·cal ves·ti·bule** (bŭk´ăl ves´ti-byūl) Part of the oral vestibule related to the cheek.

**buc·ci·na·tor** (buk´si-nā´tŏr) SEE buccinator muscle.

**buc·ci·na·tor crest** (bŭk´si-nā´tŏr krest) Ridge passing from base of the coronoid process of mandible to the region of last molar tooth; attaches to the mandibular part of the buccinator muscle.

**buc·ci·na·tor mus·cle** (bŭk´si-nā´tŏr mŭs´ĕl) *Origin*, posterior portion of alveolar portion of maxilla and mandible and pterygomandibular raphe; *insertion*, orbicularis oris at angle of mouth; *action*, flattens cheek, retracts angle of mouth; *nerve supply*, facial. Plays an important role in mastication, working with tongue to keep food between teeth; when it is paralyzed, food accumulates in the oral vestibule. SYN musculus buccinator [TA].

**buc·ci·na·tor nerve** (bŭk´si-nā´tŏr nĕrv) SYN buccal nerve.

**buc·ci·na·tor node, buc·cal node** (bŭk´si-nā´tŏr nōd, bŭk´ăl) SYN buccal lymph node.

♻ **bucco-** Combining form meaning cheek. [L. *bucca*]

**buc·co·ax·i·al** (bŭk´ō-ak´sē-ăl) Referring to the line angle formed by the buccal and axial walls of a cavity.

**buc·co·ax·i·o·cer·vi·cal** (bŭk´ō-ak´sē-ō-sĕr´vi-kăl) Referring to the point angle formed by the junction of the buccal, axial, and cervical (gingival) walls of a cavity.

**buc·co·ax·i·o·gin·gi·val** (bŭk´ō-ak´sē-ō-jin´ji-văl) Referring to the point angle formed by the junction of buccal, axial, and gingival (cervical) walls.

**buc·co·cer·vi·cal** (bŭk´ō-sĕr´vi-kăl) 1. Relating to the cheek and the neck. 2. In dental anatomy, referring to that portion of the buccal surface of a bicuspid or molar tooth adjacent to its cementoenamel junction.

**buc·co·cer·vi·cal ridge** (bŭk´ō-sĕr´vi-kăl rij) Convexity within cervical third of buccal surface of molars.

**buc·co·clu·sal** (bŭk´ō-klū´zăl) Incorrect term referring to the line angle formed by the junction of a buccal and pulpal wall. SEE buccopulpal.

**buc·co·dis·tal** (buk´ō-dis´tăl) Referring to the line angle formed by the junction of a buccal and distal wall of a cavity.

**buc·co·gin·gi·val** (bŭk´ō-jin´ji-văl) Relating to the cheek and the gum.

**buc·co·gin·gi·val ridge** (bŭk´ō-jin´ji-văl rij) Distinct ridge on buccal surface of a deciduous molar tooth, approximately 1.5 mm from the crown-root junction.

**buc·co·la·bi·al** (bŭk´ō-lā´bē-ăl) 1. In dentistry, referring to that aspect of the dental arch or those surfaces of the teeth in contact with the mucosa of lip and cheek. 2. Relating to both cheek and lip.

**buc·co·lin·gual** (bŭk´ō-ling´gwăl) 1. In dentistry, referring to that aspect of the dental arch or those surfaces of the teeth in contact with the mucosa of the lip or cheek and the tongue. 2. Pertaining to the cheek and the tongue.

**buc·co·lin·gual di·am·e·ter** (bŭk´ō-ling´gwăl dī-am´ĕ-tĕr) Diameter of tooth crown measured from buccal to lingual surfaces.

**buc·co·lin·gual di·men·sion** (bŭk´ō-ling´gwăl di-men´shŭn) Diameter of a premolar or molar tooth from buccal to lingual surface.

**buc·co·lin·gual re·la·tion** (bŭk´ō-ling´gwăl rĕ-lā´shŭn) Position of a space or tooth in relation to tongue and cheek.

**buc·co·me·si·al** (bŭk´ō-mē´zē-ăl) Referring to the line angle formed by the junction of a buccal and mesial wall of a cavity.

**buc·co·na·sal mem·brane** (bŭk´ō-nā´zăl mem´brān) Thin, transient epithelial sheet separating the primordial nasal cavity from the stomodeum in the 7-week-old human embryo. SYN oronasal membrane.

**buc·co·oc·clu·sal an·gle** (bŭk´ō-ŏ-klū´zăl ang´gĕl) Line of junction of buccal and occlusal surfaces of a tooth.

**buc·co·pha·ryn·ge·al** (bŭk´ō-făr-in´jē-ăl) Relating to both cheek or mouth and pharynx.

**buc·co·pha·ryn·ge·al fas·ci·a** (bŭk´ō-făr-in´jē-ăl fash´ē-ă) [TA] Fascia that covers muscular layer of pharynx and is continued forward onto the buccinator muscle.

**buc·co·pha·ryn·ge·al mem·brane** (bŭk´ō-făr-in´jē-ăl mem´brān) A bilaminar (ectoderm and endoderm) membrane derived from the prechordal plate; after the embryonic head fold has evolved, it lies at the caudal limit of the stomodeum. SYN oral membrane, oropharyngeal membrane.

**buc·co·pul·pal** (bŭk´ō-pŭl´păl) Referring to the line angle formed by the junction of a buccal and pulpal wall of a cavity.

**buc·co·ver·sion** (bŭk´ō-vĕr-zhŭn) Malposition of a posterior tooth from normal line of occlusion toward the cheek.

**buc·cu·la** (bŭk´yū-lă) A fatty puffing under the chin. SYN double chin. [L. dim. of *bucca*, cheek]

**Buck knife** (bŭk nīf) A narrow, pointed surgical implement used to excise interproximal tissue during periodontal surgery procedures.

**buck tooth** (bŭk tūth) Anterior tooth in labioversion.

**Buck·y di·a·phragm** (bŭk´ē dī´ă-fram) In radiography, a diaphragm with a moving grid that avoids grid shadows. SYN Potter-Bucky diaphragm.

**bud stage** (bŭd stāj) Initiation of tooth development; development of the primordia of the enamel organs, the tooth buds.

**buff·ered crys·tal·line pen·i·cil·lin G** (bŭf´ĕrd kris´tă-lin pen´i-sil´in) Penicillin buffered with not less than 4% and not more than 5% sodium citrate.

**bug** (bŭg) **1.** Any insect of the order Hemiptera. **2.** More colloquially, any insect or arachnid. **3.** (slang) An acute febrile illness such as influenza or the common cold. [of uncertain origin]

**bulb** (bŭlb) Any globular or fusiform structure. [L. *bulbus,* a bulbous root]

**bul·bus ol·fac·to·ri·us** (bŭl′bŭs ōl-fak-tō′rē-ŭs) [TA] SYN olfactory bulb.

**bu·lim·i·a** (bŭ-lē′mē-ă) SYN bulimia nervosa. [G. *bous,* ox, + *limos,* hunger]

**bu·lim·i·a ner·vo·sa** (bŭ-lē′mē-ă nĕr-vō′să) Chronic morbid disorder involving repeated and secretive episodic bouts of eating characterized by uncontrolled rapid ingestion of large quantities of food over a short period of time, followed by self-induced vomiting and other means. See this page. SYN bulimia, hyperotexia.

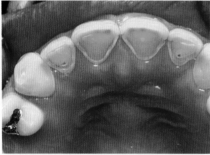

**erosion:** due to chronic induced vomiting associated with bulimia nervosa

**bu·lim·ic** (bŭ-lē′mik) Relating to, or suffering from, bulimia nervosa.

**bul·la,** pl. **bul·lae** (bul′ă, -ē) A fluid-filled dermatologic blister greater than 1 cm in diameter. See this page. [L. bubble]

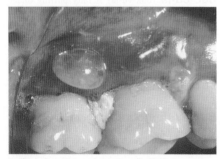

**bulla:** bullous lichen planus (rare finding)

**BUN** Abbreviation for blood urea nitrogen.

**bun·dle** (bŭn′dĕl) [TA] A structure composed of a group of fibers; a fasciculus.

**bu·no·dont** (bū′nō-dont) Having molar teeth with rounded or low conic cusps, in contrast to lophodont. [G. *bounos,* mound, + *odous* (*odont-*), tooth]

**bu·no·loph·o·dont** (bū′nō-lof′ō-dont) Having molar teeth with transverse ridges and rounded cusps on the occlusal surface. [G. *bounos,* mound, + *lophos,* ridge, + *odous,* tooth]

**bu·no·se·le·no·dont** (bū′nō-sĕ-len′ō-dont) Having molar teeth with crescentic ridges and rounded cusps on the occlusal surface. [*bounos,* mound + *selēnē,* moon, + *odous,* tooth]

**Bun·ya·vir·i·dae** (bŭn′yă-vir′i-dē) A family of arboviruses involved in several diseases in the tropics.

**bur** (bŭr) A rotary cutting instrument, used in dentistry, consisting of a small metal shaft and a head designed in various shapes; used at various rotational velocities to excavate decay, shape cavity forms, and reduce tooth structure.

**bur·ied su·ture** (ber′ēd sū′chŭr) Suture placed entirely below the surface of the skin.

**Bur·kitt lym·pho·ma** (bŭr′kit lim-fō′mă) A form of malignant lymphoma reported in African children, frequently involving the jaw and abdominal lymph nodes. Occasional cases of lymphoma with similar features have been reported in the United States.

**Bur·lew disc** (bŭr′lū disk) SYN Burlew wheel.

**Bur·lew wheel** (bŭr′lū wēl) Abrasive-impregnated, knife-edged rubber polishing wheel used in dentistry. SYN Burlew disc.

**burn** (bŭrn) **1.** A sensation of pain caused by excessive heat, or similar pain from any cause. **2.** A lesion caused by heat or any cauterizing agent, including friction, caustic agents, electricity, or electromagnetic energy; types of burns resulting from different agents are relatively specific and diagnostic. The division of burns into three levels (superficial, partial thickness, full-thickness, [q.v.]) reflects the severity of skin damage (erythema, blisters, charring, respectively). [A.S. *baernan*]

**burn·ing mouth syn·drome** (bŭrn′ing mowth sin′drōm) Clinical condition in which the patient complains of a burning sensation in the oral cavity although the appearance of the oral mucosa is normal; cause not determined.

**burn·ing tongue** (bŭrn′ing tŭng) SYN glossodynia.

**burn·ing tongue syn·drome** (bŭrn′ing tŭng sin′drōm) Idiopathic lingual pain without apparent lesions, often associated with ageusia; more common in elderly women.

**bur·nish** (bŭrn′ish) To smooth and polish (e.g., when a dental instrument is rubbed over a rough surface).

**bur·nished cal·cu·lus** (bŭrn′isht kal′kyū-lŭs) Deposit that has had the outermost layer removed so the surface is smooth; difficult to remove because the cutting edge tends to slip over the smooth surface of the deposit. See this page.

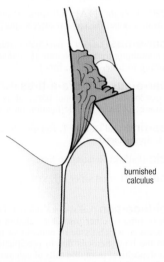

burnished
calculus

**burnished calculus:** inadequate lateral pressure alone or combined with incorrect angulation may result in incomplete removal of dental calculus; in this case, only outermost layer of deposit is removed, balance remains unfractured, and will be more difficult to detect and remove

**bur·nish·er** (bŭr′nish-ĕr) Instrument for smoothing and polishing surface or edge of a dental restoration. [O.F. *burnir*, to polish]

**bur·nish·ing** (bŭr′nish-ing) Smoothing the surface of a dental amalgam after initial carving, or adapting margins of gold restorations by rubbing with a broad-surfaced metal instrument; refers to rubbing a medication into dentinal tubules. [O.Fr. *burnir*, to polish]

**burn·out** (bŭrn′owt) In dentistry, the elimination, by heat, of an invested pattern from a set investment to prepare the mold to receive casting metal.

**Bur·ton line** (bŭr′tŏn līn) Bluish striation on gingival border, seen in lead poisoning.

**butt** (bŭt) **1.** In dentistry, to place a restoration directly against the tissues covering the alveolar ridge. **2.** To bring any two square-ended surfaces in contact so as to form a joint.

**but·ton** (bŭt′ŏn) A structure, lesion, or device of knob shape. [M.E., fr. O.Fr. *bouton*, fr. *bouter*, to thrust, fr. Germanic]

**but·ton su·ture** (bŭt′ŏn sū′chŭr) A suture in which the threads are passed through the holes of a button and then tied; used to reduce the danger of the threads cutting through the flesh.

**By·zan·tine arch pal·ate** (biz′in-tēn ahrch pal′ăt) Incomplete fusion of palatal process with nasal spine.

# C

$\chi^2$ Abbreviation for chi-square.

**C** Abbreviation for cathode; carbon; curie; cysteine.

**CA** Abbreviation for chronologic age; cancer; carcinoma; cardiac arrest; calcium.

**ca·chec·tic di·ar·rhe·a** (kă-kek′tik dī′ă-rē′ă) Diarrhea in patients with severe wasting.

**ca·chec·tic e·de·ma** (kă-kek′tik ĕ-dē′mă) Swelling occurring in diseases characterized by wasting and hypoproteinemia.

**ca·chec·tic pal·lor** (kă-kek′tik pal′ŏr) SYN achromasia.

**ca·chet** (kă-shā′) A seal-shaped capsule or wafer made of flour for enclosing powders of disagreeable taste. The sealed dosage form is wetted and swallowed. [Fr. a seal]

**ca·chex·i·a** (kă-kek′sē-ă) General weight loss and wasting in the course of a chronic disease or emotional disturbance. [G. *kakos*, bad, + *hexis*, condition of body]

**CAD** Abbreviation for coronary artery disease.

**ca·dav·er** (kă-dav′ĕr) Dead body. [*Usage note:* In common use, this term has come to specify a dead body used for a particular purpose, such as dissection.] [L. fr. *cado*, to fall]

**ca·dav·er·ine** (kă-dav′ĕr-in) A foul-smelling diamine formed by bacterial decarboxylation of lysine; poisonous and irritating to the skin.

**CAD/CAM** Abbreviation for computer-aided design/computer-aided manufacturing.

**cad·mi·um** (kad′mē-ŭm) Metallic element; its salts are poisonous and little used in medicine but are frequently employed in the basic sciences. [L. *cadmia*, fr. G. *kadmeia* or *kadmia*, an ore of zinc, calamine]

**caecum** [Br.] SYN cecum.

**caesium** [Br.] SYN cesium.

**ca·fé-au-lait spots** (ka-fā′ō-lā′ spots) Pigmented cutaneous lesions, ranging from light to dark brown; due to excess of melanosomes in the malpighian cells, rather than to an excess of melanocytes; major cutaneous manifestation of neurofibromatosis (von Recklinghausen disease).

**caf·feine** (kaf′ēn) An alkaloid obtained from the dried leaves of *Thea sinensis*, tea, or the dried seeds of *Coffea arabica*, coffee; used as a central nervous system stimulant, diuretic, and circulatory and respiratory stimulant.

**caf·feine and so·di·um sa·lic·y·late** (kaf′ēn sō′dē-ŭm să-lis′i-lāt) Mixture of sodium salicylate and caffeine formerly used for the relief of headache and neuralgia.

**caf·fein·ism** (kaf′ēn-izm) Caffeine intoxication characterized by tremulousness, nervousness, and other disorders; due to ingestion of excess of substances containing caffeine.

**cal·car** (kal′kahr) [TA] Dull spine or projection from a bone. [L. spur, rooster's spur]

**cal·car·e·ous** (kal-kar′ē-ŭs) Chalky; relating to or containing lime or calcium. [L. *calcarius*, pertaining to lime, fr. *calx*, lime]

**cal·car·e·ous pan·cre·a·ti·tis** (kal-kar′ē-ŭs pan′krē-ă-tī′tis) Chronic pancreatitis with appearance of areas of calcification on x-ray.

**cal·ca·rine** (kal′kă-rēn) 1. Relating to a calcar. 2. Spur-shaped.

**cal·cic** (kal′sik) Relating to lime.

**cal·cif·er·ol** (kal-sif′ĕr-ol) SYN ergocalciferol.

**cal·ci·fi·ca·tion** (kal′si-fi-kā′shŭn) 1. Deposition of lime or other insoluble calcium salts. 2. Process in which tissue or noncellular material in the body hardens due to precipitates or larger deposits of insoluble salts of calcium, especially calcium carbonate and phosphate normally occurring only in the formation of bone and teeth. [L. *calx*, lime, + *facio*, to make]

**cal·ci·fi·ca·tion lines of Ret·zi·us** (kal′si-fi-kā′shŭn līnz ret′zē-ŭs) Incremental lines of rhythmic deposition of successive layers of normally calcified and hypocalcified enamel during tooth development.

**cal·ci·fy·ing ep·i·the·li·al o·don·to·gen·ic tu·mor** (kal′si-fī′ing ep′i-thē′lē-ăl ō-don′tō-jen′ik tū′mŏr) Benign epithelial odontogenic neoplasm derived from the stratum intermedium of the enamel organ.

**cal·ci·fy·ing o·don·to·gen·ic cyst, cal·ci·fy·ing and ker·a·tin·iz·ing o·don·to·gen·ic cyst** (kal′si-fī-ing ō-don′tō-jen′ik sist, ker′ă-ti-nī′zing) Mixed radiolucent-radiopaque jaw lesion with features of both a cyst and a solid neoplasm. SYN Gorlin cyst.

**cal·ci·no·sis** (kal′si-nō′sis) Condition characterized by deposition of calcium salts in nodular foci in various tissues other than the parenchymatous viscera. [*calcium* + *-osis*, condition]

**cal·ci·pe·ni·a** (kal′si-pē′nē-ă) Disorder with insufficient calcium in body tissues and fluids. [*calcium* + G. *penia*, poverty]

**cal·ci·priv·ia** (kal′si-priv′ē-ă) Absence or deprivation of calcium in diet.

**cal·cite** (kal′sīt) Naturally occurring mineral used as a dental abrasive.

**cal·ci·to·nin** (kal-si-tō′nin) A peptide hormone formed in parathyroid, thyroid, and thymus glands; increases deposition of calcium and phosphate in bone and lowers blood levels of calcium. [*calci-* + G. *tonos,* stretching, + -in]

**cal·ci·um (Ca)** (kal′sē-ŭm) A metallic bivalent element; salts useful in metabolism and in medicine; responsible for radiopacity of bone, calcified cartilage, and arteriosclerotic arterial plaques in arteries. [Mod. L. fr. L. *calx,* lime]

**cal·ci·um car·bon·ate** (kal′sē-ŭm kahr′bŏ-nāt) Astringent, antacid, and dietary supplement. SEE ALSO calcite. SYN chalk.

**cal·ci·um chan·nel block·er** (kal′sē-ŭm chan′ĕl blok′ĕr) Drug that stops calcium ions from passing through biologic membranes; used to treat hypertension, angina pectoris, and cardiac arrhythmias.

**cal·ci·um chlo·ride** (kal′sē-ŭm klōr′īd) Agent that reduces calcium deficiencies; used to treat hypocalcemia, hyperkalemia, cardiac failure, and drug overdose.

**cal·ci·um glyc·er·o·phos·phate** (kal′sē-ŭm glis′ĕr-ō-fos′fāt) Calcium and phosphorus dietary supplement.

**cal·ci·um hy·drox·ide** (kal′sē-ŭm hī-drok′sīd) Cavity liner material made of calcium hyroxide and salicylate to stimulate formation of secondary dentin.

**cal·cu·lo·gen·e·sis** (kal′kyū-lō-jen′ĕ-sis) Formation of calculus. [L. *calculus,* small stone, + G. *genesis,* formation]

**cal·cu·lo·gen·ic** (kalk′yū-lō-jen′ik) Denotes that which encourages formation of calculus (e.g., dental biofilm conducive to formation of calculus).

**cal·cu·lus,** pl. **cal·cu·li** (kal′kyū-lŭs, -lī) **1.** SYN dental calculus. **2.** Concretion formed in any part of the body, most commonly in passages of biliary and urinary tracts; usually composed of salts of inorganic or organic acids, or of other material such as cholesterol. See this page. SYN stone (1). [L. a pebble]

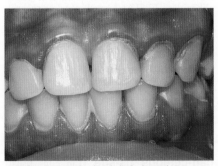
**calculus:** interproximal and gingival margins

**cal·cu·lus bridge** (kal-kyū′lŭs brij) Colloq. term for dental calculus that has accreted such that it forms an outer layer that completely covers the teeth and interdental spaces. See this page.

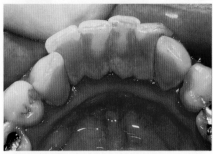
**calculus bridge:** lingual face of incisors

**cal·cu·lus re·mov·al work stroke** (kal′kyū-lŭs rĕ-mū′văl wŏrk strōk) Instrumentation maneuver used to remove calculus deposits.

**Cal·cu·lus Sur·face In·dex (CSI)** (kalk′yū-lŭs sŭr′făs in′deks) Measurements of dental calculus, used for evaluating new calculus formation within a large group of test subjects.

**Cald·well-Luc op·er·a·tion** (kawld′wel lūk op-ĕr-ā′shŭn) Intraoral procedure for opening into the maxillary antrum through the supradental (canine) fossa above the maxillary premolar teeth.

**cal·i·ber** (kal′i-bĕr) Diameter of a hollow tubular structure. [Fr. *calibre,* of uncert. etym.]

**cal·i·brate** (kal′i-brāt) **1.** To graduate or standardize any measuring instrument. **2.** To measure the diameter of a tubular structure.

**cal·i·brat·ed per·i·o·don·tal probe** (kal′i-brā-tĕd per′ē-ō-don′tăl prōb) Type of periodontal tool marked in millimeter increments used to evaluate the depth of the periodontal sulcus.

**cal·i·bra·tion** (kal′i-brā′shŭn) Standardizing an instrument or laboratory procedure.

**Cal·i·ci·vi·ri·dae** (kal′i-sē-vir′i-dē) A family of RNA viruses associated with epidemic viral gastroenteritis and some forms of hepatitis.

**ca·lic·u·lus,** pl. **ca·lic·u·li** (kă-lik′yū-lŭs, -lī) A bud-shaped or cup-shaped structure. [L. dim. from G. *kalyx,* the cup of a flower]

**ca·lic·u·lus an·gu·lar·is** (kă-lik′yū-lŭs ang-gyū-lā′ris) Small keratinized projections of oral mucosa at labial termination of a torus buccalis. See this page.

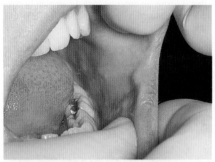

**buccal mucosa and caliculus angularis**

**cal·lo·so·mar·gin·al ar·te·ry** (ka′lō-sō-mahr′ji-năl ahr′těr-ē) [TA] Second branch of the pericallosal artery running in the cingulate sulcus and sending branches to supply medial and superolateral surfaces of cerebral hemisphere.

**cal·lus** (kal′ŭs) **1.** SYN callosity. **2.** A composite mass of tissue that forms at a fracture site to establish continuity between the bone ends.

**cal·mod·u·lin** (kal-mod′yū-lin) Protein that binds calcium ions. [*cal*cium + *modul*ate]

**ca·lor** (kā′lōr) Heat, as one of the four signs of inflammation (the others are rubor, tumor, dolor) enunciated by Celsius. [L.]

**ca·lor·ic val·ue** (kă-lōr′ik val′yū) Heat produced by food when burnt or metabolized.

**cal·o·rie** (kal′ŏr-ē) *As used in nutrition and dietetics, this word ordinarily means kilogram calorie* (*kilocalorie*). Unit of heat content or energy; amount of heat necessary to raise 1 g of water from 14.5–15.5°C (small calorie). [L. *calor,* heat]

**cal·o·rim·e·try** (kal′ŏr-im′ě-trē) Measurement of the amount of heat given off by a reaction or group of reactions (as by an organism).

**cal·var·i·a,** pl. **cal·var·i·ae** (kal-var′ē-ă, -ē) [TA] *Avoid the incorrect form calvarium.* Skull's upper domelike portion. [L. a skull]

**calx,** pl. **cal·ces** (kalks, kal′sēz) **1.** SYN lime (1). **2.** The posterior rounded extremity of the foot. SYN heel (2). [L. limestone]

**CAM** Abbreviation for complementary and alternative medicine.

**Camp·er line** (kahm′pěr līn) Line running from inferior border of nasal ala to superior border auricular tragus.

**Camp·er plane** (kahm′pěr plān) Plane running from tip of the anterior nasal spine (acanthion) to center of bony external auditory meatus on the right and left sides.

**cam·phor** (kam′fŏr) A ketone distilled from the bark and wood of *Cinnamonum camphora;* used as a topical antiinfective and antipruritic.

**cam·phor·at·ed men·thol** (kam′fŏr-ā-těd men′thol) Liquid obtained by triturating equal parts of camphor and menthol; used as a counterirritant.

**cam·phor·a·ted par·a·chlor·o·phe·nol** (kam′fŏr-āt-ěd par′ă-klōr-ō-fē′nol) Combination of parachlorophenol and camphor used in endodontics as an intracanal medication.

**cam·phor·at·ed phe·nol** (kam′fŏr-ā-těd fē′nol) Camphorated carbolic acid, (phenol, camphor, and liquid petrolatum); used as a local anesthetic.

**Cam·py·lo·bac·ter** (kam′pi-lō-bak′těr) A genus of bacteria containing gram-negative, nonspore-forming, spiral or S-curved rods. [G. *campylos,* curved, + *baktron,* staff or rod]

**Ca·na·di·an Den·tal As·so·ci·a·tion (CDA)** (kă-nā′dē-ăn den′tăl ă-sō′sē-ā′shŭn) Professional organization of dentists in Canada whose mission is to promote the public's oral health and the science of dentistry.

**Ca·na·di·an Den·tal Hy·gien·ists As·so·ci·a·tion (CDHA)** (kă-nā′dē-ăn den′tăl hī-gēn′ists ă-sō′sē-ā′shŭn) Professional organization of dental hygienists in Canada; its mission is to promote the public's oral health and to advance the practice and techniques of dental hygiene.

**Ca·na·di·an Jour·nal of Den·tal Hy·giene (CJDH)** (kă-nā′dē-ăn jŭr′năl den′tăl hī′jēn) Prominent Canadian and subscription-based peer-reviewed journal, which strives to relate studied information about dental hygiene.

**ca·nal** (kă-nal′) [TA] Duct or channel; tubular structure. SEE ALSO channel, duct. [L. *canalis*]

**ca·nal for phar·yn·go·tym·pan·ic (aud·i·tor·y) tube** (kă-nal′ fă-ring′gō-tim-pan′ik aw′di-tōr-ē tūb) [TA] Inferior division of musculotubal canal that forms the bony part of the pharyngotympanic (auditory) tube.

**can·a·lic·u·lus,** pl. **can·a·lic·u·li** (kan-ă-lik′yū-lŭs, -lī) [TA] A small canal or channel. [L. dim. fr. *canalis,* canal]

**ca·na·lis nu·tri·ci·us** (kă-nā′lis nū′tri-sī′ ŭs) [TA] SYN nutrient canal.

**ca·nals of Scar·pa** (kă-nalz′ skahr′pă) Nasopalatine nerves and vessels.

**can·cel·lous** (kan′sě-lŭs) Denoting bone that has a latticelike or spongy structure.

**can·cel·lous bone** (kan′sě-lŭs bōn) SYN substantia spongiosa.

**can·cel·lous tis·sue** (kan′sě-lŭs tish′ū) Latticelike or spongy osseous tissue.

**can·cer (CA)** (kan'sĕr) General term frequently used to indicate any of various types of malignant neoplasms, most of which invade surrounding tissues, may metastasize to several sites, and are likely to recur after attempted removal and kill the patient unless adequately treated. [L. a crab, a cancer]

**can·crum,** pl. **can·cra** (kang'krŭm, -krǎ) A gangrenous, ulcerative, inflammatory lesion. [Mod. L., fr. L. *cancer,* crab]

**can·crum o·ris** (kang'krŭm ō'ris) SYN noma.

**Can·di·da** (kan'di-dǎ) Common genus of yeastlike fungi; species are isolated from the skin, feces, and vaginal and pharyngeal tissue, but gastrointestinal tract is the source of the most important species. [L. *candidus,* dazzling white]

**Can·di·da al·bi·cans** (kan'di-dǎ al'bi-kanz) Fungal species ordinarily a part of humans' normal gastrointestinal flora, which only becomes pathogenic with a disturbance in balance of flora or impairment of the host defenses from other causes.

◼**can·di·di·a·sis** (kan'di-dī'ǎ-sis) Infection with, or disease caused by, *Candida,* especially *C. albicans.* Commonly affected areas include skin, oral mucous membranes, respiratory tract, and vagina. SYN moniliasis. See this page and page A11.

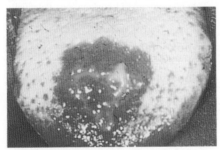

**candidiasis:** thick white coat on tongue is due to Candida infection, raw red surface is where coat was scraped off

**ca·nine** (kā'nīn) **1.** Relating to the canine teeth. **2.** SYN canine tooth. **3.** Referring to the cuspid tooth. [L. *caninus*]

**ca·nine em·i·nence** (kā'nīn em'i-nĕns) Elevation on maxilla corresponding to root and socket of canine tooth. SYN canine prominence.

**ca·nine fos·sa** (kā'nīn fos'ǎ) [TA] Depression on anterior surface of the maxilla below infraorbital foramen and on lateral side of canine eminence.

**ca·nine groove** (kā'nīn grūv) Longitudinal sulcus on mesial aspect of the first premolar.

**ca·nine guid·ance** (kā'nīn gī'dǎns) Occlu-

sion in which occlusal contacts of the cuspids cause contacts of posterior teeth to separate in excursive mandibular movements.

**ca·nine prom·i·nence** (kā'nīn prom'i-nĕns) SYN canine eminence.

**ca·nine tooth** (kā'nīn tūth) [TA] Tooth with a thick conic crown and a long, slightly flattened conic root; there are two canine teeth in each jaw, one on either side adjacent to the distal surface of the lateral incisors, in both the deciduous and the permanent dentition. SYN dens caninus [TA], canine (2), cuspid tooth, cuspid (2), dens angularis, dens cuspidatus, eye tooth.

**ca·ni·ni·form** (kā-nī'ni-fōrm) Resembling a canine tooth.

**can·ker** (kang'kĕr) SEE aphtha. [L. *cancer,* crab, malignant growth]

**can·ker sores** (kang'kĕr sōrz) SYN aphtha (2).

**can·na·bis** (kan'ǎ-bis) The dried flowering tops of the pistillate plants of *Cannabis sativa;* in restricted use in management of iatrogenic anorexia, especially that associated with cancer therapy. [L., fr. G. *kannabis,* hemp]

**can·nu·la** (kan'yū-lǎ) Tube that can be inserted into a cavity, usually by means of a trocar filling its lumen. [L. dim. of *canna,* reed]

**can·tho·me·a·tal plane** (kan'thō-mē-ā'tǎl plān) Plane passing through two lateral angles of the eye and center of external acoustic meatus.

**can·ti·le·ver beam** (kan'ti-lē-vĕr bēm) In dentistry, beam supported by only one fixed support at only one of its ends.

**can·ti·le·ver bridge** (kan'ti-lē-vĕr brij) Fixed partial denture in which pontic is retained on only one side by an abutment tooth. SYN extension bridge.

**cap** (kap) **1.** A protective covering for an incomplete tooth. **2.** Colloquialism for restoration of the coronal part of a natural tooth with an artificial crown.

**ca·pac·i·ty** (kǎ-pas'i-tē) **1.** The potential cubic contents of a cavity or receptacle. SEE ALSO volume. **2.** Power to do. [L. *capax,* able to contain; fr. *capio,* to take]

**cap·il·lar·i·ty** (kap'i-lar'i-tē) The rise of liquids in narrow tubes or through the pores of a loose material, as a result of capillary action.

**cap·il·la·rop·a·thy** (kap'i-lǎ-rop'ǎ-thē) Any disease of the capillaries. SYN microangiopathy. [*capillary* + G. *pathos,* disease]

**cap·il·lar·y** (kap'i-lar-ē) [TA] **1.** Resembling a hair; fine; minute. **2.** A capillary vessel; e.g., blood capillary, lymph capillary. [L. *capillaris,* relating to hair]

**cap·il·lar·y at·trac·tion** (kap'i-lar-ē ă-trak'shŭn) The force that causes fluids to rise up very fine tubes or pass through the pores of a loose material.

**cap·il·lar·y fra·gil·i·ty test** (kap'i-lar-ē fră-jil'i-tē test) Test used to determine vitamin C deficiency. SYN Rumpel-Leede test, vitamin C test.

**cap·i·ta·tion** (kap'i-tā'shŭn) A system of dental reimbursement wherein the health care provider is paid an annual fee per covered patient by an insurer or other financial source, which aggregate fees are intended to reimburse all provided services. [L.L. *capitatio*, fr. *caput*, head]

**ca·pit·u·lum,** pl. **ca·pit·u·la** (kă-pit'yū-lŭm, -lă) [TA] Small osseous articular extremity of a bone. [L. dim. of *caput*, head]

*Cap·no·cy·to·pha·ga* (kap'nō-sī-tof'ă-gă) Genus of gram-negative, fusiform bacteria associated with human periodontal disease.

**cap·ping** (kap'ing) Covering. SEE direct pulp capping, indirect pulp capping.

**cap·sa·i·cin** (kap-sā'i-sin) Alkaloid used for analgesia. [Irreg. fr. *capsicum*, + *-in*]

**cap splint** (kap splint) Plastic or metallic fracture appliance designed to cover crowns of the teeth and usually cemented to them.

**cap stage** (kap stāj) Second level of dental development involving inner and outer enamel epithelium.

**cap·sule** (kap'sŭl) **1.** [TA] A membranous anatomic structure, usually dense, irregular, collagenous connective tissue, which envelops a body part. **2.** A fibrous tissue layer enveloping an organ or a tumor, especially if benign. **3.** A solid dosage form in which a drug is enclosed in a hard or soft soluble container or ''shell'' of a suitable form of gelatin. [L. *capsula*, dim. of *capsa*, box]

**ca·put,** pl. **ca·pi·ta** (kah'put, -pi-tă) [TA] SYN head. [L.]

**Ca·ra·bel·li cusp** (kah-rĕ-bel'lē kŭsp) Cusp on lingual surface of mesiolingual cusp of upper first molars.

**Ca·ra·bel·li tu·ber·cle** (kahr-ră-bel'lē tū'bĕr-kĕl) Small tubercle, found on lingual surface of the mesiolingual cusp of a permanent maxillary first molar.

**car·ba·pen·ems** (kahr'bă-pen'emz) Broad-spectrum bactericidal β-lactam antibiotics that bind to penicillin-binding protein and thereby interfere with cell wall structure.

**car·ben·i·cil·lin** (kahr-ben'i-sil'in) Semi-synthetic extended-spectrum penicillin active against many bacteria.

**car·bo·hy·drates (CHO)** (kahr-bō-hī'drāts) Compound that includes simple sugars and macromolecular (polymeric) substances (e.g., starch, glycogen).

**car·bo·lat·ed** (kahr'bŏ-lā-tĕd) SYN phenolated.

**car·bon (C)** (kahr'bŏn) Nonmetallic tetravalent element found in all living tissues; the study of its vast number of compounds constitutes most of organic chemistry. [L. *carbo*, coal]

**car·bon·ate** (kahr'bŏn-āt) A salt of carbonic acid.

**car·bon di·ox·ide (CO$_2$)** (kahr'bŏn dī-oks'īd) Product of the combustion of carbon with an excess of oxygen.

**car·bon di·sul·fide (CS$_2$) poi·son·ing** (kahr'bŏn dī-sŭl'fīd poy'zŏn-ing) Acute or chronic intoxication by $CS_2$; an industrial disease encountered among rubber workers and makers of artificial silk (rayon).

**car·bon mon·ox·ide (CO)** (kahr'bŏn mŏ-noks'īd) Colorless, practically odorless, and poisonous gas formed by the incomplete combustion of carbon.

**car·bon mon·ox·ide poi·son·ing** (kahr'bŏn mŏ-noks'īd poy'zŏn-ing) Potentially fatal acute or chronic intoxication caused by inhalation of carbon monoxide gas.

**car·box·y·late** (kahr-bok'si-lāt) A salt or ester of the carboxylic acid group.

**car·box·yl·a·tion** (kahr-bok'si-lā'shŭn) Addition of $CO_2$ to an organic acceptor to yield a —COOH group; catalyzed by carboxylases.

**car·box·y·meth·yl·cel·lu·lose** (kahr-bok'sē-meth'il-sel'yū-lōs) Cellulose derivative that forms a colloidal dispersion in water; used as a bulk laxative and suspending agent.

**car·bun·cle** (kahr'bŭng-kĕl) Deep-seated pyogenic infection of the skin and subcutaneous tissues. [L. *carbunculus*, dim. of *carbo*, a live coal, a carbuncle]

**car·cin·o·gen** (kahr-sin'ŏ-jen) Any cancer-producing substance or organism. [*carcino-* + G, *-gen*, producing]

**car·ci·no·ma (CA),** pl. **car·ci·no·mas,** pl. **car·ci·no·ma·ta** (kahr'si-nō'mă, -măz, -mă-tă) Various types of malignant neoplasm derived from epithelial cells, chiefly glandular or squamous; most common type of cancer. [G. *karkinōma*, fr. *karkinos*, cancer, + *-oma*, tumor]

**car·ci·no·ma in si·tu (CIS)** (kahr'si-nō'mă in sit'ū) A lesion characterized by cytologic changes of the type associated with invasive carcinoma, but with pathology limited to the lining epithelium and without histologic evidence of extension to adjacent structures.

**car·ci·no·ma·to·sis** (kahr´si-nō´mă-tō´sis) A condition resulting from widespread dissemination of carcinomas in multiple sites in various organs or tissues of the body.

**car·ci·no·stat·ic** (kahr´si-nō-stat´ik) Agent with an arresting or inhibitory effect on the development or progression of a carcinoma.

**car·di·a** (kahr´dē-ă) [TA] Opening of the esophagus into the stomach. [G. *kardia,* heart]

**car·di·ac** (kahr´dē-ak) 1. Pertaining to heart. 2. Pertaining to esophageal opening of stomach. [L. *cardiacus*]

**car·di·ac ar·rest (CA)** (kahr´dē-ak ă-rest´) Complete cessation of cardiac activity.

**car·di·ac asth·ma** (kahr´dē-ak az´mă) Asthmatic attack, with bronchoconstriction secondary to pulmonary congestion and edema.

**car·di·ac com·pe·tence** (kahr´dē-ak kom´pĕ-tĕns) Ability of ventricles to pump the blood returning to the atria.

**car·di·ac dys·rhyth·mi·a** (kahr´dē-ak dis-ridh´mē-ă) Any abnormality in the rate, regularity, or sequence of cardiac activation.

**car·di·ac in·dex** (kahr´dē-ak in´deks) Amount of blood ejected by heart in a unit of time divided by the body surface area.

**car·di·ac in·suf·fi·cien·cy** (kahr´dē-ak in´sŭ-fish´ĕn-sē) SYN heart failure (1).

**car·di·ac mas·sage** (kahr´dē-ak mă-sahzh´) SYN heart massage.

**car·di·ac mur·mur** (kahr´dē-ak mŭr´mŭr) A sound generated by blood flow through the heart, at one of its valvular orifices or across ventricular septal defects.

**car·di·ac out·put** (kahr´dē-ak owt´put) Amount of blood ejected by the heart in a unit of time in liters per minute (L/min).

**car·di·ac re·serve** (kahr´dē-ak rē-zĕrv´) The work the heart is able to perform beyond that required under the ordinary circumstances of daily life.

**card·ing** (kahrd´ing) Procedure of placing individual sets of anterior or posterior teeth in trays lined with a wax strip.

**car·di·o·dy·nam·ics** (kahr´dē-ō-dī-nam´iks) Mechanics of the heart's action, including its movement and the forces generated thereby.

**car·di·o·e·soph·a·ge·al re·lax·a·tion** (kahr´dē-ō-ē-sof´ă-jē´ăl rē-lak-sā´shŭn) Easing of the lower esophageal sphincter, which can allow reflux of acidic gastric contents into the lower esophagus, producing esophagitis.

**car·di·o·fa·cial syn·drome** (kahr´dē-ō-fā´shăl sin´drōm) 1. Transient or persistent unilateral partial lower facial paresis accompanying congenital heart disease. 2. Syndromes characterized by congenital cardiovascular, bone, soft tissue, and facial abnormalities.

**car·di·o·in·hib·i·to·ry** (kahr´dē-ō-in-hib´i-tōr-ē) Arresting or slowing cardiac action.

**car·di·ol·o·gy** (kahr´dē-ol´ŏ-jē) The medical specialty concerned with heart disease. [*cardio-* + G. *logos,* study]

**car·di·o·meg·a·ly** (kahr´dē-ō-meg´ă-lē) Enlarged heart. [*cardio-* + G. *megas,* large]

**car·di·o·my·op·a·thy** (kahr´dē-ō-mī-op´ă-thē) Disease of the myocardium. [*cardio-* + G. *mys,* muscle, + *pathos,* disease]

**car·di·o·pul·mo·nar·y** (kahr´dē-ō-pul´mŏ-nar-ē) Relating to the heart and lungs. SYN pneumocardial.

**car·di·o·pul·mo·nar·y re·sus·ci·ta·tion** (kahr´dē-ō-pul´mŏ-nar-ē rē-sŭs´i-tā´shŭn) Therapeutic restoration of cardiac output and pulmonary ventilation after cardiac arrest and apnea.

**car·di·o·tox·ic** (kahr´dē-ō-tok´sik) Denotes with deleterious effect on action of heart, due to poisoning of the cardiac muscle or of its conducting system. [*cardio-* + G. *toxikon,* poison]

**car·di·o·vas·cu·lar (CV)** (kahr´dē-ō-vas´kyū-lăr) [TA] Relating to heart and blood vessels or circulation. [*cardio-* + L. *vasculum,* vessel]

**car·di·o·vas·cu·lar sys·tem (CVS)** (kahr´dē-ō-vas´kyū-lăr sis´tĕm) [TA] Heart and blood vessels considered as a whole.

**car·di·tis** (kahr-dī´tis) Inflammation of the heart.

**care** (kār) In medicine and public health, general term for application of knowledge to benefit a community or individual patient.

**care·giv·er** (kār´giv-ĕr) General term for a physician, nurse, other health care practitioner, or family member/friend who cares for patients.

**care plan** (kār plan) Outline of nursing care showing all of the patient's needs and the ways of meeting them. SYN plan of care.

▉**car·ies,** pl. **car·ies** (kar´ēz) Microbial destruction or necrosis of teeth. See page 108 and page A1. [L. dry rot]

**car·ies risk as·sess·ment** (kar´ēz risk ă-ses´mĕnt) Procedure to predict future dental caries development before the onset of disease.

**ca·ries sus·cep·ti·ble** (kar´ēz sŭ-sep´ti-bĕl) 1. Tooth surfaces that present a risk for

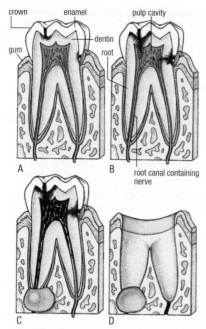

caries: (A) acid, enzymes, or both produced by oral bacteria break down enamel to form cavities; (B) bacteria penetrate dentin to invade pulp cavity; (C) infection destroys pulp and extends through left root canal to cause periapical disease; (D) tooth has been lost, leaving periapical cyst on the left

developing decay **2.** Said of an individual who is at risk for developing decay of the teeth

✿ **cario-** Prefix meaning caries. [L. *caries*]

**car·i·o·gen·e·sis** (kar′ē-ō-jen′ĕ-sis) Process of producing caries; mechanism of caries production.

**car·i·o·gen·ic** (kar′ē-ō-jen′ik) Producing caries; usually said of diets.

**car·i·o·gen·ic chal·lenge** (kar′ē-ō-jen′ik chal′ĕnj) Exposure of a tooth surface to an acid attack that may lead to caries.

**car·i·o·ge·nic·i·ty** (kar′ē-ō-jĕ-nis′i-tē) Potential for caries production.

**car·i·ol·o·gy** (kar′ē-ol′ŏ-jē) Study of dental caries and cariogenesis.

**car·i·o·stat·ic** (kar′ē-ō-stat′ik) Exerting inhibitory action on progress of dental caries. [L. *caries,* decay, + G. *statikos,* bringing to a stop]

**car·i·ous** (kar′ē-ŭs) Relating to or affected with caries.

**car·i·ous ex·po·sure** (kar′ē-ŭs eks-pō′zhŭr) Uncovering of the tooth pulp due to breakdown of the mineralized tooth structures by acidogenic bacteria.

**car·i·ous le·sion** (kar′ē-ŭs lē′zhŭn) Decayed area on the tooth crown or root.

**car·min·a·tive** (kahr-min′ă-tiv) Agent to prevent formation or cause expulsion of flatus. [L. *carmino,* pp. *-atus,* to card wool; special Mod. L. usage, to expel wind]

**Car·mo·dy-Bat·son op·er·a·tion** (kar′ mŏ-dē bat′sŏn op-ĕr-ā′shŭn) Reduction of fractures of the zygoma and zygomatic arch through intraoral incision above maxillary molar teeth.

**car·mus·tine** (kahr-mŭs′tēn) An antineoplastic agent.

**car·nas·si·al** (kahr-nas′ē-ăl) Adapted for shearing flesh; denoting teeth so designed. [Fr. *carnassier,* carnivorous, fr. L. *caro,* flesh]

**car·nas·si·al tooth** (kahr-nas′ē-ăl tūth) Last maxillary premolar or first mandibular molar tooth of some carnivores. SYN sectorial tooth.

**car·nau·ba wax** (kahr-naw′bă waks) Wax used in pharmaceuticals and in dentistry.

**car·ni·tine** (kahr′ni-tēn) Compound found in dairy and meat that stimulates fatty acid oxidation. [G. *karnin,* an alkali derived from meat]

**car·no·si·ne·mia** (kahr′nō-si-nē′mē-ă) Congenital disease, characterized by excess carnosine in the blood and urine and caused by a genetic deficiency of the enzyme carnosinase. [*carnosine* + G. *haima,* blood + *-ia*]

**carotenaemia** [Br.] SYN carotenemia.

**car·o·tene** (kar′ō-tēn) Yellow-red pigments widely distributed in plants and animals, notably in carrots; include precursors of vitamin A.

**car·o·ten·e·mi·a** (kar′ŏ-tĕ-nē′mē-ă) Surfeit of blood carotene, which sometimes causes a pale yellow-red dermal pigmentation. SYN carotinaemia.

**ca·rot·id** (kă-rot′id) Pertaining to any carotid structure.

**ca·rot·id bi·fur·ca·tion** (kă-rot′id bī′fŭr-kā′shŭn) [TA] Division of the common carotid artery into internal and external carotid arteries.

**ca·rot·id bod·y** (kă-rot′id bod′ē) [TA] Small epithelioid structure located just above the bifurcation of the common carotid artery on each side.

**ca·rot·id ca·nal** (kă-rot′id kă-nal′) [TA] A passage through the petrous part of the temporal bone from its inferior surface upward, medially, and anteriorly to the apex where it opens posterior and superior to the site of the foramen lacerum.

**ca·rot·id for·a·men** (kă-rot′id fōr-ā′měn) SYN openings of carotid canal.

**ca·rot·id pulse** (kă-rot′id pŭls) A palpable

**cd**

rhythmic expansion of the common carotid artery in the neck; palpated during adult cardiopulmonary resuscitation.

**ca·rot·id sheath** (kă-rot′id shēth) [TA] Dense fibrous investment of carotid artery, internal jugular vein, and vagus nerve on each side of the neck.

**ca·rot·id si·nus** (kă-rot′id sī′nŭs) [TA] Slight dilation of common carotid artery at its bifurcation into external and internal carotids.

**ca·rot·id si·nus branch** (kă-rot′id sī′nŭs branch) SYN carotid branch of glossopharyngeal nerve (CN IX).

**ca·rot·id si·nus nerve** (kă-rot′id sī′nŭs něrv) SYN carotid branch of glossopharyngeal nerve (CN IX).

**ca·rot·id si·nus re·flex** (kă-rot′id sī′nus rē′fleks) Bradycardia resulting from increased pressure within, or external manipulation of, the carotid sinus in the neck.

**ca·rot·id si·nus syn·co·pe** (kă-rot′id sī′nŭs sing′kŏ-pē) Syncope resulting from overactivity of the carotid sinus; attacks may be spontaneous or produced by pressure on a sensitive carotid sinus.

**ca·rot·id si·nus syn·drome** (kă-rot′id sī′nŭs sin′drōm) Confustion or syncope due to decreased cerebral perfusion caused by a hyperactive carotid sinus, producing marked bradycardia.

**ca·rot·id sul·cus** (kă-rot′id sŭl′kŭs) Groove on body of sphenoid bone in which internal carotid artery lies in its course through the cavernous sinus.

**ca·rot·id tri·an·gle** (kă-rot′id trī′ang-gĕl) [TA] A space bounded by the superior belly of the omohyoid muscle, anterior border of the sternocleidomastoid, and posterior belly of the digastric; it contains the bifurcation of the common carotid artery.

**ca·rot·id wall of tym·pan·ic cav·i·ty** (kă-rot′id wawl tim-pan′ik kav′i-tē) [TA] Entity of carotid canal and opening of pharyngotympanic tube. SYN anterior wall of middle ear.

**car·pal** (kahr′păl) Relating to the carpus.

**car·pal tun·nel syn·drome** (kahr′păl tŭn′ĕl sin′drōm) Most common nerve entrapment syndrome, characterized by sensory loss and wasting in the median nerve distribution in the hand; due to chronic entrapment of median nerve at wrist within carpal tunnel.

**carp mouth** (kahrp mowth) Orifice like that of this large fish, with downturning of the corners.

**car·ri·er** (kar′ē-ĕr) Being that harbors a specific infectious agent in the absence of discerni-

ble clinical disease and serves as a potential source of infection.

**car·ti·lage** (kahr′ti-lăj) [TA] Connective tissue characterized by its nonvascularity and firm consistency; consists chondrocytes of collagen, and proteoglycans. [L. *cartilago* (*cartilagin-*), gristle]

**car·ti·lage bone** (kahr′ti-lăj bōn) SYN endochondral bone.

**car·ti·lage of a·cous·tic me·a·tus** (kahr′ti-lăj ă-kū′stik mē-ā′tŭs) [TA] Cartilage that forms wall of lateral part of external acoustic meatus.

**car·ti·lage of pha·ryn·go·tym·pan·ic tube** (kahr′ti-lăj fă-ring′gō-tim-pan′ik tūb) [TA] Trough-shaped cartilage that forms medial wall, roof, and part of lateral wall of pharyngotympanic tube.

**car·ti·lag·i·nous part of ex·ter·nal a·cous·tic me·a·tus** (kahr′ti-laj′i-nŭs pahrt eks-těr′năl ă-kū′stik mē-ā′tŭs) Lateral third of external acoustic meatus; continuous with auricular cartilage and attached to circumference of the bony part.

**car·ti·lag·i·nous part of na·sal sep·tum** (kahr′ti-laj′i-nŭs pahrt nā′zăl sep′tŭm) [TA] Portion of nasal septum supported by cartilage (instead of bone).

**car·ti·lag·i·nous part of phar·yn·go·tym·pan·ic (au·di·to·ry) tube** (kahr′ti-laj′i-nŭs pahrt fă-ring′gō-tim-pan′ik aw′di-tōr-ē tūb) Portion of auditory tube supported by cartilage; continues anteromedially from osseous part to open into the nasopharynx.

**ca·run·cle** (kar′ŭng-kĕl) [TA] Small, fleshy protuberance.

**car·ver** (kahr′věr) Dental hand instrument, available in a wide variety of end shapes, used to form and contour wax, filling materials, and other material.

**carv·ing** (kahrv′ing) In dentistry, removal of excess filling material, using special instruments to produce accurate anatomic contours and restore form and function to the tooth.

**caryo-** Combining form meaning nucleus. [G. *karyon,* nut, kernel]

**car·y·o·phyl·lus, car·y·o·phyl·lum** (kar′ē-ō-fī′lŭs, -lŭm) Clove. [G. *karyophyllon,* clove tree, fr. *karyon,* nut, + *phyllon,* leaf]

**case** (kās) An instance of disease with its attendant circumstances. [L. *casus,* occurrence]

**case-con·trol study** (kās-kŏn-trōl′ stŭd′ē) Epidemiologic method that begins by identifying people with a disease or condition of interest and compares their past history of exposure to identified or suspected risk factors with the past history of similar exposures among those who resemble the cases but do not have the disease or condition of interest.

**case his·to·ry** (kās his'tŏr-ē) Detailed recension, generally written, of all particulars of a patient's familial, medical, and social involvements related to a condition or disease process.

**case man·age·ment** (kās man'ăj-mĕnt) A process in the U.S. whereby covered people with specific health care needs are identified and an efficient treatment plan is formulated and implemented to produce the most cost-effective outcomes.

**ca·se·ous ab·scess** (kā'sē-ŭs ab'ses) Abscess containing solid or semisolid material of cheeselike consistency.

**ca·se·ous ne·cro·sis, ca·se·a·tion ne·cro·sis** (kā'sē-ŭs nĕ-krō'sis, kā-sē-ā' shŭn) Necrosis characteristic of some inflammations; affected tissue manifests the crumbly consistency and dull opaque quality of cheese. Also called caseous degeneration.

**case pre·sen·ta·tion** (kās prez-ĕn-tā' shŭn) Consultation with a patient outlining diagnosis, proposed dental treatment, alternative treatments, risks, costs, and responsibilities.

**cas·sette** (kă-set') Plate, film, or tape holder for use in photography or radiography. A radiographic cassette contains two intensifying screens and a sheet of radiographic film. [Fr., dim. of *casse,* box]

**cast** (kast) **1.** In dentistry, a positive reproduction of the form of the tissues of the upper or lower jaw, which is made by the solidification of plaster, metal, or other materials, poured into an impression and over which denture bases or other dental restorations may be fabricated. **2.** An object formed by the solidification of a liquid poured into a mold. **3.** Rigid encasement of a part, as with plaster, plastic, or fiberglass, for purposes of immobilization. [M.E. *kasten,* fr. O.Norse *kasta*]

**cast bar splint** (kast bahr splint) A temporary-use support with cast clasps that follow the contours of the teeth at the height of contour. SYN Friedman splint.

**cast clasp** (kast klasp) Fitting on a removable partial denture molded into the form desired.

**cast core** (kast kōr) Restoration, usually a gold alloy, intended to replace lost tooth structure under a crown; provides support and retention for the crown.

▣**cast·ing** (kast'ing) A metal structure, such as an artificial tooth crown, produced by forcing molten metal into a mold. See this page.

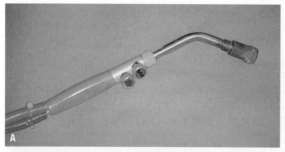
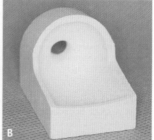
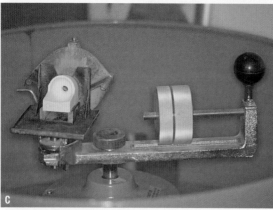
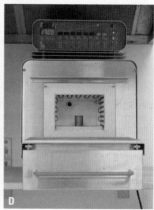

**dental casting equipment:** (A) torch; (B) crucible; (C) centrifugal casting machine; (D) burnout oven with casting ring inside it

**cast·ing shrink·age** (kast′ing shringk′ăj) Volumetric change of cast metal as it sets; counteracted by thermal and setting expansion of the investment material.

**cast·ing tem·per·a·ture** (kast′ing tem′pĕr-ă-chŭr) The degree of heating required to make a metal fluid so it can be introduced into a refractory cast.

**cast·ing wax** (kast′ing waks) Soft solid wax used in dentistry for patterns of many types; most are basically paraffin but are modified by addition of other ingredients, to meet various requirements. SYN inlay wax.

**cat·a·ba·si·al** (kat′ă-bā′sē-ăl) Denoting a skull in which the basion is lower than the opisthion.

**ca·tab·o·lism** (kă-tab′ō-lizm) Breaking down in the body of complex chemical compounds into simpler ones. [G. *katabolē*, a casting down]

**ca·tal·y·sis** (kă-tal′i-sis) The effect that a catalyst exerts on a chemical reaction. [G. *katalysis*, dissolution]

**cat·a·lyst** (kat′ă-list) A substance that accelerates a chemical reaction but is not consumed or changed permanently thereby.

**cat·a·me·ni·a** (kat′ă-mē′nē-ă) Menses; pertaining to menses. [G. the menses, ntr. pl. of *katamēnios*, monthly, fr. *mēn*, month]

**cat·a·ract** (kat′ăr-akt) Complete or partial opacity of the ocular lens.

**ca·tarrh** (kă-tahr′) SEE catarrhal inflammation. [G. *katarrheō*, to flow down]

**ca·tar·rhal in·flam·ma·tion** (kă-tahr′ăl in′flă-mā′shŭn) Term for inflammatory process that is most frequently seen in the respiratory tract, but may occur in any mucous membrane; characterized by hyperemia of the mucosal vessels, edema of the interstitial tissue, enlargement of the secretory epithelial cells (which proliferate and form conspicuous globules of mucus), and an irregular layer of viscous, mucinous material on the surface.

**cat·gut** (kat′gŭt) Absorbable surgical suture material made from the collagenous fibers of the submucosa of certain animals (e.g., sheep or cows); name is misnomer. [probably from *kit*, a small violin, through confusion with *kit*, a small cat]

**cath·e·ter** (kath′ĕ-tĕr) A tubular instrument to allow passage of fluid from or into a body cavity or blood vessel. [G. *kathetēr*, fr. *kathiēmi*, to send down]

**catheterisation** [Br.] SYN catheterization.

**cath·e·ter·i·za·tion** (kath′ĕ-tĕr-ī-zā′shŭn) Passage of a catheter to move fluid.

**cath·ode (C)** (kath′ōd) **1.** The negative pole of a galvanic battery or the electrode connected with it; the electrode to which positively charged ions (cations) migrate. Cf. anode. **2.** Negatively charged part of the x-ray tube head; it contains the tungsten filament. SYN negative electrode. [G. *kathodos,* a way down, fr. *kata,* down, + *hodos,* a way]

**cat·i·on** (kat′ī-on) An ion carrying a charge of positive electricity, therefore going to the negatively charged cathode. [G. *katiōn,* going down]

**cat·i·on·ic de·ter·gent** (kat′ī-on′ik dĕ-tĕr′jĕnt) Cleansing agent that has positively charged group(s) attached to the larger hydrophobic portion.

**cat·scratch dis·ease, cat·scratch fe·ver (CSD)** (kat′skrach di-zēz′, fē′vĕr) Benign, subacute illness caused by *Bartonella henselae;* characterized by regional lymphadenitis following the scratch (occasionally the bite) of a cat.

**cau·da,** pl. **cau·dae** (kaw′dă, -dē) [TA] SYN tail. [L. a tail]

**cau·dad** (kaw′dad) In a direction toward the tail.

**cau·dal** (kaw′dăl) [TA] Pertaining to the tail. [Mod. L. *caudalis* ]

**caul, cowl** (kawl, kowl) **1.** The amnion, either as a piece of membrane capping the baby's head at birth or the whole membrane when delivered unruptured with the baby. SYN galea (4), veil (2), velum (2). **2.** SYN greater omentum. [Gaelic, *call,* a veil]

**cau·sal·i·ty** (kaw-zal′i-tē) The relating of causes to the effects they produce; the pathogenesis of disease and epidemiology are largely concerned with causality.

**caus·al treat·ment** (kaw′zăl trēt′mĕnt) Therapy aimed at reversing the causal factor in a disease.

**caus·tic** (kaws′tik) **1.** Chemically exerting an effect resembling a burn. **2.** An agent producing this effect. [G. *kaustikos,* fr. *kaiō,* to burn]

**cauterise** [Br.] SYN cauterize.

**cau·ter·ize** (kaw′tĕr-īz) To apply a cautery; to burn with a cautery. SYN cauterise.

**cau·ter·y** (kaw′tĕr-ē) Agent or device for scarring, burning, or cutting the skin or other tissues with heat, cold, electric current, ultrasound, or caustic chemicals. [G. *kautērion,* a branding iron]

**cau·ter·y knife** (kaw′tĕr-ē nīf) Cutting tool that sears while cutting to diminish bleeding.

**cav·ern·ous an·gi·o·ma** (kav′ĕr-nŭs an′jē-ō′mă) Vascular malformation composed of sinusoidal vessels without a large feeding artery.

**ca·vern·ous branch·es of ca·ver·nous part of in·ter·nal ca·rot·id ar·te·ry** (kav′ĕr-nŭs branch′ĕz kav′ĕr-nŭs pahrt in-tĕr′năl kă-rot′id ahr′tĕr-ē) [TA] Small branches arising from the internal carotid artery as it traverses the cavernous sinus, distributed to the trigeminal ganglion, the walls of the cavernous and inferior petrosal sinuses, and the nerves contained within them.

**cav·ern·ous si·nus** (kav′ĕr-nŭs sī′nŭs) [TA] A paired dural venous sinus on either side of the sella turcica. It is sometimes described as a plexus because of its unique internal structure.

**cav·ern·ous si·nus syn·drome** (kav′ĕr-nŭs sī′nŭs sin′drōm) Partial or complete external ophthalmoplegia. Multiple causes, the most common today are neoplasms and trauma.

**cav·i·tar·y** (kav′i-tar-ē) 1. Relating to a cavity or having a cavity or cavities. 2. Denoting any animal parasite that has an enteric canal or body cavity and lives within the host's body.

**cav·i·tas**, pl. **cav·i·ta·tes** (kav′i-tahs, -tah′tēz) SYN cavity. [Mod. L.]

**cav·i·tas den·tis** (kav′i-tahs den′tis) [TA] SYN pulp cavity.

**cav·i·ta·tion** (kav-i-tā′shŭn) 1. Formation of tiny bubbles in water exiting tip of an electronic instrument; when collapsing, these bubbles produce bactericidal shock waves that act by tearing bacterial cell walls. 2. Formation of a cavity.

**cav·i·ty** (kav′i-tē) 1. A hollow space; hole. 2. Lay term for the loss of tooth structure resulting from dental caries. SYN cavitas. [L. *cavus, hollow*]

**cav·i·ty line an·gle** (kav′i-tē līn ang′gĕl) In dentistry, angle formed by two walls of a cavity, e.g., a tooth cavity, meeting along a line.

**cav·i·ty lin·er** (kav′i-tē lī′nĕr) SYN dental varnish.

**cav·i·ty mar·gin** (kav′i-tē mahr′jin) Periphery of a filling, line of junction between restoration and external surface of a tooth.

**cav·i·ty of con·cha** (kav′i-tē kong′kă) [TA] Space within lower, larger portion of the concha below crus helicis; forms vestibule leading into external acoustic meatus.

**cav·i·ty of lar·ynx** (kav′i-tē lar′ingks) SYN laryngeal cavity.

**cav·i·ty of mid·dle ear** (kav′i-tē mid′ĕl ēr) SYN tympanic cavity.

**cav·i·ty of phar·ynx** (kav′i-tē far′ingks) [TA] Area of a nasal part (nasopharynx) continuous anteriorly with nasal cavity and receiving openings of the auditory tubes, an oral part (oropharynx) opening through the fauces into the oral cavity, and a laryngeal part (laryngopha-

rynx) leading into the vestibule of the larynx and to the esophagus.

**cav·i·ty of tooth** (kav′i-tē tūth) SYN pulp cavity.

**cav·i·ty prep·a·ration** (kav′i-tē prep′ăr-ā′shŭn) 1. Removal of dental caries and surgical preparation of remaining tooth structure to receive, support, and retain a dental restoration. 2. Final form of an excavation in a tooth resulting from such preparation.

**cav·i·ty prep·a·ra·tion base** (kav′i-tē prep′ăr-ā′shŭn bās) SYN cement base.

**cav·i·ty prep·a·ra·tion form** (kav′i-tē prep′ăr-ā′shŭn fŏrm) Configuration or shape of a cavity preparation.

**cav·i·ty wall** (kav′i-tē wawl) A surface bounding a cavity.

**ca·vo·sur·face** (kā′vō-sŭr′făs) Relating to a cavity and the surface of a tooth.

**ca·vo·sur·face an·gle** (kā′vō-sŭr′făs ang′gĕl) Angle formed by junction of a cavity wall and tooth surface.

**ca·vo·sur·face bev·el** (kā′vō-sŭr′făs bev′ĕl) Incline of cavosurface angle of a prepared cavity wall in relation to the plane of the enamel wall.

**ca·vo·sur·face junc·tion** (kā′vō-sŭr′făs jŭngk′shŭn) Point of conjunction between any wall of a cavity preparation with the unprepared tooth structure.

**cav·um den·tis** (kā′vŭm den′tis) SYN pulp cavity.

**cav·um o·ris** (kā′vŭm ōr′is) SYN oral cavity.

**C.C.** Abbreviation for chief complaint.

**CD** Abbreviation for cluster of differentiation.

**CDA** Abbreviation for Canadian Dental Association.

**CDAC** Abbreviation for Commission of Dental Accreditation of Canada.

**CDC** Abbreviation for (U.S.) Centers for Disease Control and Prevention.

**CDHA** Abbreviation for Canadian Dental Hygienists Association.

**CDT** Abbreviation for *Current Dental Terminology*.

**Ce** Symbol for cerium.

**ce·as·mic ter·a·to·sis** (sē-az′mik ter′ă-tō′sis) Teratosis with failure of lateral halves of a part to unite, as in cleft palate.

**ce·cal for·a·men of tongue** (sē′kăl fŏr-ā′mĕn tŭng) SYN foramen cecum.

**ce·cum,** pl. **ce·ca** (sē′kŭm, -kă) [TA] **1.** The cul-de-sac, about 6 cm in depth, lying below the terminal ileum and forming first part of large intestine. **2.** Any similar structure ending in a cul-de-sac. SYN caecum. [L. ntr. of *caecus* blind]

**CEJ** Abbreviation for cementoenamel junction.

**ce·li·ac dis·ease** (sē′lē-ak di-zēz′) A disease occurring in children and adults characterized by sensitivity to gluten, with chronic inflammation and atrophy of the mucosa of the upper small intestine. SYN gluten enteropathy, coeliac disease.

**ce·li·ac rick·ets** (sē′lē-ak rik′ĕts) Arrested growth and osseous deformities associated with defective absorption of fat and calcium in celiac disease.

**cell** (sel) **1.** Smallest unit of living structure capable of independent existence, composed of a membrane-enclosed mass of protoplasm and containing a nucleus or nucleoid; highly variable and specialized in both structure and function, although all must at some stage replicate proteins and nucleic acids, use energy, and reproduce themselves. **2.** Small closed or partly closed cavity; compartment or hollow receptacle. [L. *cella,* a storeroom, a chamber]

**cel·la,** pl. **cel·lae** (sel′ă, -ē) A room or cell. [L. storeroom, or compartment]

**cell cul·ture** (sel kŭl′chŭr) The maintenance or growth of dispersed cells after removal from the body, commonly on a glass surface immersed in nutrient fluid.

**cell cy·cle** (sel sī′kĕl) The periodic biochemical and structural events occurring during proliferation of cells, such as in tissue culture.

**cell-me·di·at·ed im·mu·ni·ty, cel·lu·lar im·mu·ni·ty** (sel′mē′dē-āt-ĕd i-myū′ni-tē, sel′yū-lăr) SYN delayed hypersensitivity.

**cell mem·brane** (sel mem′brān) The protoplasmic boundary of all cells that controls permeability and may serve other functions through surface specializations. SYN plasma membrane, plasmalemma, Wachendorf membrane (2).

**cel·lu·lar im·mu·ni·ty de·fi·cien·cy syn·drome** (sel′yū-lăr i-myū′ni-tē dĕ-fish′ĕn-sē sin′drōm) Disorder with increased susceptibility to infection, especially to viral, fungal, parasitic, and opportunistic infections. Associated with defective functioning of the mechanism responsible for acquired cell-mediated immunity. SEE ALSO immunodeficiency.

**cel·lu·li·tis** (sel′yū-lī′tis) Inflammation of subcutaneous, loose connective tissue.

**cel·lu·loid strip** (sel′yū-loyd strip) Clear plastic ribbon used as a matrix when inserting a cement or resin in proximal cavity preparations of teeth.

**cel·lu·lose** (sel′yū-lōs) A linear B1→4 glu-

can; forms the basis of vegetable and wood fiber and is the most abundant organic compound. [L. *cellula,* cell, + -*ose*]

**cell wall** (sel wawl) **1.** Outer layer or membrane of some animal and plant cells. **2.** In bacteria, the rigid structure that provides osmotic protection and defines bacterial shape and staining properties.

■**ce·ment** (sĕ-ment′) [TA] **1.** In dentistry, nonmetallic material used for luting, filling, or permanent or temporary restorative purposes, made by mixing components into a plastic mass that sets, or as an adherent sealer in attaching various dental restorations in or on the tooth. SYN cementum [TA]. **2.** A layer of bonelike, mineralized tissue covering dentin of root and neck of a tooth that anchors fibers of the periodontal ligament. See this page. [L. *caementum,* rough quarry stone, fr. *caedo,* to cut]

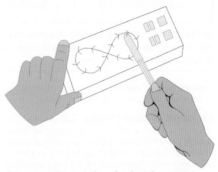

figure 8 mixing technique for dental cements

**ce·ment·al ca·ries** (sĕ-men′tăl kar′ēz) Caries of cementum of a tooth.

**ce·men·ta·tion** (sē′men-tā′shŭn) **1.** In dentistry, attaching a restoration to natural teeth by means of a cement. **2.** Process of attaching parts by means of a cement.

■**ce·ment base** (sĕ-ment′ bās) In dentistry, layer of dental cement, sometimes medicated, placed in deep portion of a cavity preparation to protect pulp, reduce bulk of a metallic restoration, or eliminate undercuts. See page 114. SYN cavity preparation base.

**ce·ment·ed pin** (sĕ-men′tĕd pin) Cylindric metal pin used for retention of a dental restoration and cemented into a hole of corresponding size placed in dentin.

**ce·ment·i·cle** (sĕ-men′ti-kel) Calcified spheric body, composed of cementum lying free within periodontal membrane, attached to cementum or imbedded within it.

**ce·ment line** (sĕ-ment′ līn) Thin visible layer of cement at the margin of a crown.

**ce·ment·o·blast** (sĕ-men′tō-blast) Cell of ectomesenchymal origin concerned with forma-

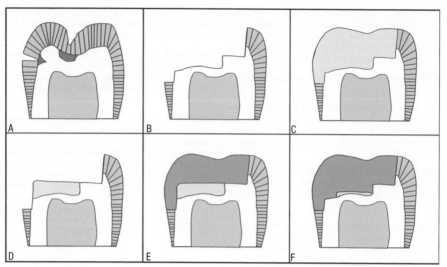

**dental cement in pulpal protection:** (A) carious lesions present; (B) prepared tooth; (C) temporary filling placed; (D) temporary filling cut back, leaving cement base; (E) base is covered with permanent restoration; (F) liner is much thinner than base

tion of layer of cementum on roots of teeth. [L. *cementum,* cement, + G. *blastos,* germ]

**ce·ment·o·blas·to·ma** (sĕ-men′tō-blas-tō′mă) A benign odontogenic tumor of functional cementoblasts; appears as a mixed radiolucent-radiopaque lesion attached to a tooth root and may cause expansion of the bone cortex or be associated with pain.

**ce·ment·o·cla·si·a** (sĕ-ment′ō-klā′zē-ă) Destruction of cement by cementoclasts. [L. *cementum,* cement, + G. *klasis,* fracture]

**ce·ment·o·clast** (sĕ-men′tō-klast) One of the multinucleated giant cells, similar or identical to osteoclasts, which are associated with the resorption of cementum. [L. *cementum,* cement, + G. *klastos,* broken]

**ce·ment·o·cyte** (sĕ-men′tō-sīt) An osteocytelike cell with numerous processes, trapped in a lacuna in the cement of the tooth. [L. *cementum,* cement, + G. *kytos,* cell]

**ce·ment·o·den·tin·al** (sē-men′tō-den′ti-năl) SYN dentinocemental.

**ce·men·to·e·nam·el junc·tion (CEJ)** (sĕ-men′tō-ĕ-nam′ĕl jŭngk′shŭn) Surface at which enamel of crown and cementum of tooth root are joined. SEE ALSO cervical line.

**ce·men·to·gen·e·sis** (sē-men′to-jen′ĕ-sis) Development of cementum over tooth root dentin. [*cementum* + G. *genesis,* production]

**ce·men·to·ma** (sē′mĕn-tō′mă) Nonspecific term referring to any benign cementum-producing tumor; four types are recognized: periapical cemental dysplasia, central ossifying fibroma, cementoblastoma, and sclerotic cemental mass. When the type is not specified, cementoma usually refers to periapical cemental dysplasia. [L. *cementum,* cement, + G. -*ōma,* tumor]

**ce·men·tum** (sĕ-men′tŭm) [TA] SYN cement (1), tooth cement. [L. *caementum,* rough quarry stone, fr. *caedo,* to cut]

**ce·men·tum hy·per·pla·si·a** (sĕ-men′ tŭm hī′pĕr-plā′zē-ă) SYN hypercementosis.

**cen·ter** (sen′tĕr) [TA] **1.** The middle point of a body; loosely, the interior of a body, especially an anatomic center. **2.** A group of nerve cells governing a specific function. [L. *centrum;* G. *kentron*]

**cen·ter of ridge** (sen′tĕr rij) Buccolingual midline of residual ridge.

**Cen·ters for Dis·ease Con·trol and Pre·ven·tion (CDC)** (sen′tĕrz di-zēz′ kŏntrōl′ prĕ-ven′shŭn) The U.S. federal facility for disease eradication, epidemiology, and education with headquarters in Atlanta, Georgia.

**cen·trad** (sen′trad) Toward the center.

**cen·tral ap·ne·a** (sen′trăl ap′nē-ă) Apnea due to medullary depression that inhibits respiratory movement.

**cen·tral bear·ing** (sen′trăl ber′ing) In dentistry, application of forces between the maxillae and mandible at a single point located as near as possible to center of supporting areas of upper and lower jaws; used to distribute closing forces evenly throughout areas of the supporting structures during recording of maxillomandibular (jaw) relations and correction of occlusal errors.

**cen·tral-bear·ing de·vice** (sen′trăl-ber′ ing dĕ-vīs′) In dentistry, device that provides a central point of bearing, or support, between upper and lower record bases; consists of a contacting point attached to one base and plate attached to the other that provides surface on which bearing point rests or moves.

**cen·tral-bear·ing point** (sen′trăl ber′ing poynt) Contact point of a central-bearing tracing device; must be positioned close to the center of the supporting areas of the mandible and maxilla to distribute closing forces evenly throughout the areas of the supporting structures during the registration and recording of interjaw relationhips.

**cen·tral-bear·ing trac·ing de·vice** (sen′trăl ber′ing trās′ing dĕ-vīs′) In dentistry, a device used for making a tracing and/or for support between upper and lower bases.

**cen·tral deaf·ness** (sen′trăl def′nĕs) Deafness due to disorder of the auditory system of brainstem or cerebral cortex.

**cen·tral in·ci·sor** (sen′trăl in-sī′zŏr) First tooth in maxilla and mandible on either side of the midsagittal cranial plane.

**cen·tral·i·za·tion phe·nom·e·non** (sen′ trăl-ī-zā′shŭn fĕ-nom′ĕ-non) Relatively rapid change in the perceived location of pain, from more peripheral, or distal, to a more proximal, or central, location.

**cen·tral ner·vous sys·tem (CNS)** (sen′ trăl nĕr′vŭs sis′tĕm) [TA] The brain and the spinal cord.

**cen·tral os·si·fy·ing fi·bro·ma** (sen′trăl os′i-fī-ing fī-brō′mă) Painless, slow-growing, expansile, sharply circumscribed benign fibroosseus tumor of the jaws that is derived from cells of periodontal ligament; presents initially on radiographs as a radiolucency that becomes progressively more opaque as it matures.

**cen·tral os·te·it·is** (sen′trăl os-tē-ī′tis) 1. SYN osteomyelitis. 2. SYN endosteitis.

**cen·tral vi·sion** (sen′trăl vizh′ŭn) Vision stimulated by an object imaged on the fovea centralis. SYN direct vision.

**centre** [Br.] SYN center.

✪ **centri-** Combining form denoting center.

**cen·tric** (sen′trik) Having a center (of a specific kind or number) or having a specific thing as its center. [G. *kentron*, center]

**cen·tric check·bite** (sen′trik chek′bīt) Colloq. for centric relation record (q.v.).

**cen·tric con·tact** (sen′trik kon′takt) SYN centric occlusion.

**cen·tric·i·put** (sen-tris′i-put) Central portion of upper surface of the cranium, between occiput and sinciput. [L. *centrum*, center, + *caput*, head]

**cen·tric jaw re·la·tion** (sen′trik jaw rĕ-lā′shŭn) Position of the mandible with respect to the maxilla where the condyles articulate with the thinnest portion of the disc and are positioned in the most anterosuperior part of the temporal fossa. This position is typically used as a reproducible jaw position by the clinician when such a position cannot be determined by the intercuspation of teeth. SEE ALSO eccentric relationship. SYN median retruded relation.

**cen·tric oc·clu·sion** (sen′trik ŏ-klū′zhŭn) 1. Relation of opposing occlusal surfaces that provides maximal planned contact and/or intercuspation. 2. Occlusion of the teeth when mandible is in centric relation to the maxillae. SYN acquired centric, centric contact, habitual centric.

**cen·tric path of clo·sure** (sen′trik path klō′zhŭr) Direction taken by mandible during closure of the mouth into centric relation.

**cen·tric po·si·tion** (sen′trik pŏ-zish′ŏn) Position of the mandible in its most retruded unstrained relation to maxillae. SEE ALSO centric jaw relation.

**cen·tric re·la·tion** (sen′trik rĕ-lā′shŭn) 1. The most retruded physiologic relation of the mandible to the maxillae to and from which the individual can make lateral movements; it is a condition that can exist at various degrees of jaw separation, and it occurs around the terminal hinge axis. 2. The most posterior relation of the mandible to the maxillae at the established vertical relation.

**cen·trif·u·gal** (sen-trif′yū-găl) Denoting direction of the force pulling an object outward (away) from an axis of rotation. [L. *centrum*, center, + *fugio*, to flee]

**cen·trif·u·gal cast·ing** (sen-trif′yū-găl kast′ing) Casting molten metal into a mold by spinning the metal from a crucible at the end of a revolving arm.

**cen·trip·e·tal** (sen-trip′ĕ-tăl) SYN afferent. [L. *centrum*, center, + *peto*, to seek]

✪ **centro-** Combining form denoting center. [G. *kentron*]

**ceph·a·lad** (sef′ă-lad) In a direction toward the head. SEE ALSO cranial.

**ce·phal·ic** (sĕ-fal′ik) SYN cranial.

**ce·phal·ic an·gle** (sĕ-fal′ik ang′gĕl) One of several angles formed by intersection of two lines passing through certain points of face or cranium.

**ce·phal·ic ar·te·ri·al ra·mi** (sĕ-fal′ik ahr-tēr′ē-ăl rā′mī) Parietal branches of sympathetic trunks conveying postsynaptic sympathetic fibers from superior cervical ganglion to carotid arteries for distribution within the head.

**ce·phal·ic in·dex** (sĕ-fal´ik in´deks) Ratio of maximal breadth to maximal length of the head.

**ce·phal·ic tri·an·gle** (sĕ-fal´ik trī´ang-gĕl) Triangle on cranium formed by lines connecting metopion, pogonion, and occipital point.

**ceph·a·lo·gy·ric** (sef´ă-lō-jī´rik) Relating to head rotation. [*cephalo-* + G. *gyros,* a circle]

**ceph·a·lo·meg·a·ly** (sef´ă-lō-meg´ă-lē) Enlargement of the head. [*cephalo-* + G. *megas,* great]

**ceph·a·lom·e·ter** (sef´ă-lom´ĕ-tĕr) An instrument used to position the head to produce oriented lateral and posteroanterior head films. [*cephalo-* + G. *metron,* measure]

**ceph·a·lo·met·ric a·nal·y·sis** (sef´ă-lō-met´rik ă-nal´ă-sis) Study of skeletal and dental relationships used in orthodontic case analysis.

**ceph·a·lo·me·tric land·mark** (sef´ă-lō-met´rik land´mahrk) A structure of the head viewed in cephalometric radiographs used to obtain measurements of the cranium and face to assess facial growth, trauma, and abnormalities in orthodontia and oral surgery.

**ceph·a·lo·met·ric ra·di·o·graph** (sef´ă-lō-met´rik rā´dē-ō-graf) X-ray view of jaws and cranium to allow their measurement.

**ceph·a·lo·met·rics** (sef´ă-lō-met´riks) ORAL SURGERY, ORTHODONTICS scientific measurement of bones of cranium and face, using a fixed, reproducible position for lateral radiographic exposure of skull and facial bones. [*cephalo-* + G. *metron,* measure]

**ceph·a·lo·met·ric trac·ing** (sef´ă-lō-met´rik trās´ing) Overlay drawing of the teeth, facial bones, and anthropometric landmarks made directly from a cephalometric radiograph and used as a basis for cephalometric analysis.

**ceph·a·lom·e·try** (sef´ă-lom´ĕ-trē) Scientific measurements, often taken by means of radiographic imaging, of the head in the living, or of the cadaveric, head with soft tissues in place, using specific reference points and sufficient standardization to allow reproducible results. [*cephalo-* + G. *metron,* measure]

**ceph·a·lo·mo·tor** (sef´ă-lō-mō´tŏr) Relating to movements of the head.

**ceph·a·lo·or·bit·al in·dex** (sef´ă-lō-ōr´bi-tăl in´deks) Ratio of cubic content of the two orbits to that of the cranial cavity multiplied by 100.

**ceph·a·lo·pal·pe·bral re·flex** (sef´ă-lō-pal-pē´brăl rē´fleks) Contraction of the orbicu-

laris muscle elicited by tapping the vertex of the skull.

**ceph·a·lor·rha·chid·i·an** (sef´ă-lō-ră-kid´ē-ăn) Relating to the head and the spine. [*cephalo-* + G. *rhachis,* spine]

**ceph·a·lo·spor·an·ic ac·id** (sef´ă-lō-spōr-an´ik as´id) The basic chemical nucleus on which cephalosporin antibiotic derivatives are based.

**ceph·a·lo·spo·rin** (sef´ă-lō-spōr´in) Antibiotic produced by a *Cephalosporium.*

**ceph·a·lo·spo·rin C** (sef´ă-lō-spōr´in) Antibiotic effective against gram-positive and gram-negative bacteria.

**ceph·a·my·cins** (sef´ă-mī´sinz) A family of β-lactam antibiotics (similar to penicillin and cephalosporins) produced by various *Streptomyces* species.

**ce·ra** (sē´ră) SYN wax (1). [L.]

**ce·ra·ceous** (se-rā´shŭs) Waxen. [L. *cera,* wax]

**cer·a·mic** (sĕr-am´ik) A product made primarily from nonmetallic mineral(s) by firing at a high temperature.

**cer·a·mo·met·al cast·ing** (ser´ă-mō-met´ăl kast´ing) Casting made of alloys containing or excluding precious metals, to which dental porcelain can be fused.

**cer·e·bel·lar ar·te·ries** (ser´ĕ-bel´ăr ahr´tĕr-ēz) Those related to and supplying the cerebellum.

**cer·e·bel·lar at·ro·phy** (ser´ĕ-bel´ăr at´rŏ-fē) Degeneration of cerebellum due to abiotrophy or alcoholism.

**cer·e·bel·lar gait** (ser´ĕ-bel´ăr gāt) Wide-based gait with lateral veering, unsteadiness, and irregularity of steps; often with a tendency to fall to one side, forward, or backward. SYN ataxic gait.

**cer·e·bel·lo·pon·tine an·gle** (ser´ĕ-bel´ō-pon´tēn ang´gĕl) Angle formed at junction of cerebellum, pons, and medulla.

**cer·e·bel·lum,** pl. **cer·e·bel·la,** pl. **cer·e·bel·lums** (ser´ĕ-bel´ŭm, -ă, -ŭmz) [TA] The large posterior brain mass lying dorsal to the pons and medulla and ventral to the posterior portion of the cerebrum; it consists of two lateral hemispheres united by a narrow middle portion, the vermis. [L. dim. of *cerebrum,* brain]

**ce·re·bral ar·te·ries** (ser´ĕ-brăl ahr´tĕr-ēz) Those related to and supplying cerebral cortex. SEE anterior cerebral artery.

**ce·re·bral cor·tex** (ser´ĕ-brăl kōr´teks) [TA] The gray cellular mantle (1–4 mm thick) covering the entire surface of the cerebral hemisphere of mammals characterized by a laminar organization of cellular and fibrous components. Based on local differences in the arrangement of nerve cells, there are multiple areas that, on the basis of function, can be categorized into three general groups: motor cortex, sensory cortex, and association cortex.

**ce·re·bral death** (ser'ĕ-brăl deth) Clinical syndrome characterized by permanent loss of cerebral and brainstem function, manifested by absence of responsiveness to external stimuli, absence of cephalic reflexes, and apnea. SYN brain death.

**ce·re·bral e·de·ma** (ser'ĕ-brăl ĕ-dē'mă) Brain swelling due to increased volume of extravascular compartment from uptake of water in neuropil and white matter. SYN brain edema.

**ce·re·bral falx** (ser'ĕ-brăl fawlks) SYN falx cerebri.

**ce·re·bral hem·is·phere** (ser'ĕ-brăl hem'is-fēr') [TA] Large mass of telencephalon, on either side of midline, consisting of the cerebral cortex and its associated fiber systems, together with the deeper-lying subcortical telencephalic ŏnuclei (i.e., basal nuclei [ganglia]).

**ce·re·bral hem·or·rhage** (ser'ĕ-brăl hem'ŏr-ăj) Hemorrhage into substance of cerebrum.

**ce·re·bral her·ni·a** (ser'ĕ-brăl hĕr'nē-ă) Protrusion of brain substance due to cranial defect.

**ce·re·bral in·dex** (ser'ĕ-brăl in'deks) Ratio of transverse to anteroposterior diameter of cranial cavity multiplied by 100.

**ce·re·bral pal·sy** (ser'ĕ-brăl pawl'zē) Generic term for nonprogressive motor dysfunction present at birth or beginning in early childhood. Causes are both hereditary and acquired.

**ce·re·bral sur·face** (ser'ĕ-brăl sŭr'făs) [TA] The internal surface of certain cranial bones; they are (the greater wing of) the sphenoid (facies cerebralis alae majoris ossis sphenoidale [TA]) and (the squamous part of) the temporal bone (facies cerebralis partis squamosae ossis temporale [TA]).

**ce·re·bral sur·face of tem·po·ral bone** (ser'ĕ-brăl sŭr'făs tem'pŏr-ăl bōn) Concave inner surface of the squamous portion of the temporal bone, which forms the lateral wall of the middle cranial fossa.

**ce·re·bral veins** (ser'ĕ-brăl vānz) [TA] SEE anterior cerebral veins.

**ce·re·bral vom·it·ing** (ser'ĕ-brăl vom'it-ing) Vomiting due to intracranial disease, especially elevated intracranial pressure.

**cer·e·bra·tion** (ser'ĕ-brā'shŭn) Activity of the mental processes; thinking. SEE ALSO mentation, cognition.

**cer·e·bri·form** (se-rē'bri-fōrm) Resembling brain's external fissures and convolutions.

**cer·e·bro·men·in·gi·tis** (ser'ĕ-brō-men-in-jī'tis) SYN meningoencephalitis.

**cer·e·bro·si·do·sis** (ser'ĕ-brō-sī-dō'sis) A lipidosis as found in Gaucher disease.

**cer·e·bro·spi·nal flu·id (CSF)** (ser'ĕ-brō-spī'năl flū'id) [TA] A fluid largely secreted by the choroid plexuses of the ventricles of the brain, filling the ventricles and the subarachnoid cavities of the brain and spinal cord.

**cer·e·bro·spi·nal flu·id o·tor·rhe·a** (ser'ĕ-brō-spī'năl flū'id ō'tō-rē'ă) Discharge of cerebrospinal fluid through external auditory canal or pharyngotympanic (auditory) tube into nasopharynx.

**cer·e·bro·spi·nal flu·id rhi·nor·rhe·a** (ser'ĕ-brō-spī'năl flū'id rī-nōr-ē'ă) Discharge of cerebrospinal fluid from the nose.

**cer·e·bro·spi·nal men·in·gi·tis** (ser'ĕ-brō-spī'năl men-in-jī'tis) SYN meningitis.

**cer·e·bro·spi·nal sys·tem** (ser'ĕ-brō-spī'năl sis'tĕm) Combined central nervous and peripheral nervous systems.

**cer·e·bro·ten·di·nous xan·tho·ma·to·sis** (ser'ĕ-brō-ten'di-nŭs zan'thō'mă-tō'sis) Metabolic disorder associated with bodily deposition of cholestanol and cholesterol.

**cer·e·bro·vas·cu·lar** (ser'ĕ-brō-vas'kyū-lăr) Relating to blood supply to brain, particularly with reference to pathologic changes.

**cer·e·bro·vas·cu·lar dis·ease** (ser'ĕ-brō-vas'kyū-lăr di-zēz') Brain dysfunction caused by an abnormality of cerebral blood supply.

**cer·e·brum,** pl. **cer·e·bra** (ser'ĕ-brŭm, -bră) [TA] Cerebral parts derived from the telencephalon; includes mainly the cerebral cortex and basal ganglia. [L., brain]

**cer·e·sin, cer·in, cer·o·sin** (ser'ĕ-sin, -in, -ō-sin) Mixture of hydrocarbons of high molecular weight; used in dentistry for impressions. SYN earth wax, mineral wax (1).

**ce·ri·um (Ce)** (sēr'ē-ŭm) A metallic element, atomic no. 58, atomic wt. 140.115. [fr. *Ceres,* the planetoid]

**ce·ro·plas·ty** (sē'rō-plas'tē) Manufacture of wax models of anatomic and pathologic specimens or of skin lesions. [G. *kēros,* wax, + *plassō,* to mold]

**cer·ti·fi·a·ble** (sĕr'ti-fī'ă-bĕl) Denoting a person showing disordered behavior of sufficient gravity to justify involuntary mental hospitalization.

**cer·ti·fi·ca·tion** (sĕr'ti-fi-kā'shŭn) Acknowledgment by a medical specialty board of successful completion of requirements for recognition as a specialist.

**cer·ti·fied milk** (sĕr'ti-fīd milk) Cow's milk that does not have more than the maximal permissible limit of 10,000 bacteria per mL at any time prior to delivery to the consumer.

**cer·ti·fied pas·teur·ized milk** (sĕr'ti-fīd pas'chŭr-īzd milk) Cow's milk in which the maximum permissible limit for bacteria should not be more than 10,000 bacteria per mL before pasteurization and not more than 500 bacteria per mL after pasteurization.

**cer·ti·fied reg·is·ter·ed nurse a·nes·the·tist (CRNA)** (sĕr'ti-fīd rej'ĭ-stĕrd nŭrs ă-nes'thĕ-tist) Clinician with additional education in administration of anesthetics.

**ce·ru·mi·nous glands** (sĕ-rū'mi-nŭs glandz) Tubuloalveolar apocrine glands in external auditory meatus; secrete cerumen ("earwax").

**cer·vi·cal** (sĕr'vi-kăl) Relating to a neck, or cervix, in any sense. [L. *cervix* (*cervic*-), neck]

**cer·vi·cal an·chor·age** (sĕr'vi-kăl ang' kŏr-ăj) Anchorage in which back of the neck is used for resistance by means of a cervical strap.

**cer·vi·cal branch of fa·cial nerve** (sĕr'vi-kăl branch fā'shăl nĕrv) [TA] Most inferior branch of parotid plexus of facial nerve; descends to innervate platysma muscle.

**cer·vi·cal clamp** (sĕr'vi-kăl klamp) Double-bowed grasping device used to help retract gingiva during restorative procedures near gingival margin. [L. *cervix*, neck, necklike structure + -*al*, adj. suffix]

**cer·vi·cal col·lar** (sĕr'vi-kăl kol'ăr) Splinting device used to stabilize the neck.

**cer·vi·cal con·ver·gence** (sĕr'vi-kăl kŏn-vĕr'jĕns) Angle formed between the axial inclination of a tooth surface and the stylus of the surveying instrument in contact with the height of contour of the tooth.

**cer·vi·cal den·ti·nal tri·an·gle** (sĕr'vi-kăl den'ti-năl trī'ang-gĕl) Three-sided overhanging projection of dentin from the wall of the pulp chamber of a tooth that impedes the dentist's access to the root canals.

**cer·vi·cal hy·per·es·the·si·a** (sĕr'vi-kăl hī'pĕr-es-thĕ'zē-ă) Hypersensitivity in cervical area of teeth due to exposure of dentin to oral environment.

**cer·vi·cal line** (sĕr'vi-kăl līn) Continuous anatomic irregular curved line marking cervical end of tooth crown and cementoenamel junction.

**cer·vi·cal mar·gin** (sĕr'vi-kăl mahr'jin) **1.** SYN gingival margin. **2.** Termination of a restoration in the gingival area.

**cer·vi·cal mar·gin of tooth** (sĕr'vi-kăl mahr'jin tūth) SYN neck of tooth.

**cer·vi·cal part of in·ter·nal ca·rot·id ar·te·ry** (sĕr'vi-kăl pahrt in-tĕr'năl kă-rot'id ahr'tĕr-ē) [TA] Unbranched portion located in the neck.

**cer·vi·cal ver·te·brae [C1–C7]** (sĕr'vi-kăl vĕr'tĕ-brē) [TA] The seven segments of the vertebral column located in the neck. See this page.

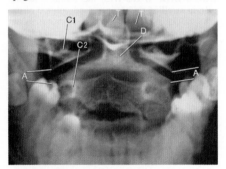

cervical vertebra: (A) normal anteroposterior (open-mouth, odontoid) view of C1 and C2. C1 = first cervical vertebra (lateral mass); C2 = second cervical vertebra; T = central incisors overlying dens, indicated by D. This panel shows normal relationship between lateral mass of C1 and vertebral body of C2

**cer·vi·cal zone of tooth** (sĕr'vi-kăl zōn tūth) SYN neck of tooth.

**cer·vi·co·buc·cal** (sĕr'vi-kō-bŭk'ăl) Relating to buccal region of neck of a premolar or molar tooth.

**cer·vi·co·dyn·ia** (sĕr'vi-kō-din'ē-ă) Neck pain. [*cervico*- + G. *odynē*, pain]

**cer·vi·co·fa·cial** (sĕr'vi-kō-fā'shăl) Relating to neck and face.

**cer·vi·co·la·bi·al** (sĕr'vi-kō-lā'bē-ăl) Relating to labial region of neck of an incisor or canine tooth.

**cer·vi·co·lin·gual** (sĕr'vi-kō-ling'gwăl) Relating to lingual region of the cervix of a tooth.

**cer·vi·co·lin·guo·ax·i·al** (sĕr'vi-kō-ling' gwō-ak'sē-ăl) Referring to point angle formed by junction of cervical (gingival), lingual, and axial walls of a cavity.

**cer·vi·co·oc·cip·i·tal** (sĕr'vi-kō-ok-sip'i-tăl) Relating to neck and occiput.

**cer·vi·co·tho·rac·ic** (sĕr'vi-kō-thōr-as'ik)

*Relating to:* **1.** Neck and thorax. **2.** Transition between the neck and thorax.

**cer·vix,** pl. **cer·vi·ces** (sĕr'viks, -vi-sēz) [TA] **1.** SYN neck. **2.** Any necklike structure. [L. neck]

**cer·vix den·tis** (sĕr'viks den'tis) [TA] SYN neck of tooth.

**cer·vix of tooth** (sĕr'viks tūth) SYN neck of tooth.

**ce·si·um (Cs)** (sē'zē-ŭm) A metallic element used in treatment of some malignancies. SYN caesium. [L. *caesius,* bluish gray]

**ce·tyl·pyr·i·din·i·um chlor·ide** (sē'til-pī'ri-din'ē-ŭm klōr'īd) The monohydrate of the quaternary salt of pyridine and cetyl chloride; a cationic detergent with antiseptic action against nonsporulating bacteria.

**Cha·gas dis·ease, Cha·gas-Cruz dis·ease** (shah'găs di-zēz', krūz) SYN South American trypanosomiasis.

**chain** (chān) BACTERIOLOGY a linear arrangement of living cells that have divided in one plane and remain attached to each other.

**chain of a·sep·sis** (chān ā-sep'sis) Procedure that avoids transfer of infection.

**chalk** (chawk) SYN calcium carbonate. [L. *calx*]

**chal·lenge di·et** (chal'ĕnj dī'ĕt) A diet in which one or more specific substances are included for the purpose of determining whether an abnormal reaction occurs.

**cham·e·ce·phal·ic, cham·e·ceph·a·lous** (kam'ĕ-se-fal'ik, -sef'ă-lŭs) Having a flat head.

**cham·e·pro·sop·ic, cham·ae·pro·sop·ic** (kam'ĕ-prō-sop'ik, kam'ĕ-) Having a broad face. [G. *chamai* (adv.), on the ground (low, spread out), + *prosōpikos,* facial]

**cham·fer** (sham'fĕr) Marginal finish on an extracoronal cavity preparation of a tooth that describes a curve from an axial wall to the cavosurface. [fr. O.Fr. *chanfrein(t),* beveled edge]

**chan·cre** (shang'kĕr) Primary lesion of syphilis. Finding *Treponema pallidum* on dark-field examination is diagnostic, except in oral ulcers, in which *T. microdentium* is normally present. [Fr. indirectly from L. *cancer*]

**chan·cre re·dux** (shang'kĕr rē'dŭks) Second chancre in a patient with syphilis.

**chan·croid** (shang'kroyd) An infectious, painful, ragged venereal ulcer at the site of infection by *Haemophilus ducreyi,* beginning after an incubation period of 3–7 days.

**chan·nel** (chan'ĕl) A furrow, gutter, or groovelike passageway. [L. *canalis*]

**char·ac·ter** (kar'ăk-tĕr) An attribute in individuals that is amenable to formal and logical analysis and may be used as the basis of generalizations about classes and other statements that transcend individuality. [G. *charakter,* stamp, mark, fr. *charassō,* to engrave]

**char·ac·ter·is·tic ra·di·a·tion** (kar'ăk-tĕr-is'tik rā'dē-ā'shŭn) When an incoming electron from the cathode stream that has enough energy to overcome the binding energy of electrons in the inner shells of the target material knocks the electron out of its shell, the outer electrons fall into the inner shell, giving up energy in the form of x-radiation.

**char·coal** (chahr'kōl) Carbon obtained by heating or burning wood with restricted access of air.

**Char·cot joint** (shahr-kō' joynt) SYN neuropathic joint.

**char·la·tan** (shahr'lă-tăn) A medical imposter claiming to cure disease by useless procedures, secret remedies, and worthless diagnostic and therapeutic machines. SYN quack. [Fr., fr. It. *ciarlare,* to prattle]

**Charles law** (shahrl law) All gases expand equally on heating, namely, 1/273.16 of their volume at 0°C for every degree Celsius. SYN Gay-Lussac law. [Jacques *Charles*]

**chart** (chahrt) Recording of clinical dental (or medical) data relating to a patient's case. [L. *charta,* sheet of papyrus]

**Char·ters meth·od** (chahr'tĕrz meth'ŏd) A method of toothbrushing using a restricted circular motion with the bristles inclined coronally at a 45-degree angle.

**chart·ing** (chahrt'ing) Making a written record of the progress of a patient's condition.

**Chayes at·tach·ment** (shayz ă-tach'mĕnt) *Avoid the incorrect forms Chaye and Chaye's.* Device that fastens a dental prosthesis to an abutment or supporting tooth by means of a mechanical device for fixation of the prosthesis; allows movement during functioning of abutment teeth.

**Chayes meth·od** (shayz meth'ŏd) Replacing lost teeth using a mechanical device for fixation and stabilization of the dental prosthesis that allows "movement in function" of abutment teeth.

**Chea·dle dis·ease** (chē'dĕl di-zēz') SYN infantile scurvy.

**check·bite** (chek'bīt) SYN interocclusal record.

**cheek** (chēk) Side of face forming lateral wall of the mouth. SYN bucca, mala (1). [A. S. *ceáce*]

**cheek bone** (chēk bōn) 1. SYN zygomatic bone. 2. SYN zygomatic arch.

**cheek mus·cle** (chēk mŭs´ĕl) SYN buccinator (muscle).

**cheek tooth** (chēk tūth) SYN molar tooth.

**chei·li·on** (kī´lē-on) Cephalometric point at angle (corner) of mouth. [G. *cheilos,* lips]

**▤chei·li·tis, chi·li·tis** (kī-lī´tis) Inflammation of the lips or of a lip. See page A8. [G. *cheilos,* lips + G. *-itis,* inflammation]

**chei·li·tis ex·fo·li·a·ti·va** (kī-lī´tis eks-fō-lē-ă-tī´vă) An exfoliative dermatitis; it may be related to atopic dermatitis or to contact sensitivity.

**▤chei·li·tis glan·du·la·ris** (kī-lī´tis gland´yū-lā´ris) An acquired disorder, of unknown etiology, of the lower lip characterized by swelling, ulceration, crusting, mucous gland hyperplasia, abscesses, and sinus tracts. See page A8. SYN Volkmann cheilitis.

**▤chei·li·tis gran·u·lo·ma·to·sa** (kī-lī´tis gran´yū-lō-mă-tō´să) Chronic, diffuse, soft swelling of the lips, of unknown etiology. See page A8. SEE ALSO Melkersson-Rosenthal syndrome.

**♻cheilo-, cheil-** Combining forms meaning lips. SEE ALSO chilo-, labio-. [G. *cheilos,* lip]

**chei·lo·gnath·o·glos·sos·chi·sis** (kī´lōg-nath´ō-glos-os´ki-sis) Associated condition of cleft lower lip and mandible and bifid tongue. [*cheilo-* + G. *gnathos,* jaw, + *glōssa,* tongue, + *schisis,* cleft]

**chei·lo·gnath·o·u·ra·nos·chi·sis** (kī-lōg-nath´ō-yū-ră-nos´ki-sis) Cleft lip, alveolar ridge, and palate. [*cheilo-* + G. *gnathos,* jaw, + *ouranos,* sky (roof of mouth), + *schisis,* cleft]

**chei·lo·pha·gi·a, chi·lo·pha·gi·a** (kī´lō-fā´jē-ă) Biting of the lips. [*cheilo-* + G. *phagō,* to eat]

**chei·lo·plas·ty, chi·lo·plas·ty** (kī´lō-plas-tē) Surgical repair of the lips. [*cheilo-* + G. *plastos,* formed]

**chei·lo·rhi·no·plas·ty** (kī´lō-rī´nō-plas-tē) Reconstructive surgery of nose and lips.

**chei·lor·rha·phy, chi·lor·rha·phy** (kī-lōr´ă-fē) Repair of the lip, most commonly used to refer to procedures for median, unilateral, or bilateral clefts. [*cheilo-* + G. *rhaphē,* suture]

**chei·lo·sis, chi·lo·sis** (kī-lō´sis) Condition characterized by dry scaling and fissuring of lips, attributed by some clinicians to riboflavin deficiencies and other nutritional requirements. SEE ALSO cheilitis. [*cheil-* + G. *-osis,* condition]

**chei·lot·o·my, chi·lot·o·my** (kī-lot´ō-mē) Incision into the lip. [*cheilo-* + G. *tomē,* incision]

**che·la·tion** (kē-lā´shŭn) Complex formation involving a metal ion and two or more polar groupings of a single molecule. [G. *chēlē,* claw]

**chem·i·cal cure** (kem´i-kăl kyūr) Mode of setting or polymerization in which the ingredients of the material unite in a chemical process that starts as soon as the blending is complete.

**chem·i·cal de·pen·dence** (kem´i-kăl dĕpen´dĕns) Psychological or physical reliance on drugs; withdrawal symptoms generally ensue if the agent is not available.

**chem·i·cal in·di·ca·tor** (kem´i-kăl in´di-kā-tŏr) A color change or appearance of a mark indicating that a chemical reaction has occurred.

**chem·i·cal ir·ri·tant** (kem´i-kăl ir´i-tănt) Any such agent capable of causing irritation or inflammation of tissues.

**chem·ic·al·ly cured re·sin** (kem´i-kăl-ē kyūrd rez´in) Resin that contains an initiator and an activator in separate pastes. When mixed, amine reacts with the benzoyl peroxide to form free radicals and polymerization occurs.

**chem·i·cal ster·il·i·za·tion** (kem´i-kăl ster´i-lī-zā´shŭn) Disinfection of instruments and devices by immersing them in liquid chemical germicides.

**chem·is·try** (kem´is-trē) Science concerned with atomic composition of substances, the elements, and their interreactions. [G. *chēmeia,* alchemy]

**che·mo·pro·phy·lax·is** (kē´mō-prō´fi-lak´sis) Prevention of disease using chemicals or drugs.

**che·mo·re·cep·tor, che·mo·ceptor** (kē´mō-rĕ-sep´tŏr, kē´mō-sep´tŏr) Any cell that responds to a change in its chemical milieu with a nerve impulse.

**che·mo·tax·is, pos·i·tive che·mo·tax·is, neg·a·tive che·mo·tax·is** (kē´mō-tak´sis, poz´i-tiv, neg´ă-tiv) Movement of cells in response to chemicals, whereby the cells are attracted or repelled by substances exhibiting chemical properties.

**che·mo·ther·a·peu·tic a·gent** (kē´mō-thār-ă-pyū´tik ā´jĕnt) Chemical that is used for therapeutic reasons.

**che·mo·ther·a·py** (kē´mō-thār´ă-pē) Treatment of disease by means of chemical substances or drugs; usually used in reference to neoplastic disease. SEE ALSO pharmacotherapy.

**che·no·de·ox·y·cho·lic ac·id** (kē´nō-dē-oks´ē-kō´lik as´id) A major bile acid in many vertebrates; facilitates cholesterol excretion and fat absorption; administered to dissolve cholesterol gallstones.

**che·rub·ic fa·ci·es** (chĕ-rū´bik fā´shē-ēz)

Characteristic childlike facies seen in cherubism; also seen in glycogenosis.

**che·rub·ism** (cher′ŭb-izm) Hereditary giant cell lesions of the jaws beginning in early childhood involving swelling. SYN fibrous dysplasia of jaws. [Hebr. *kerubh,* cherub]

**chew·ing** (chū′ing) Mandibular action during mastication of food to make it soft enough to swallow. [O.E. *cēowan*]

**chew·ing cy·cle** (chū′ing sī′kĕl) Complete course of movement of the mandible during a single masticatory stroke.

**chew·ing force** (chū′ing fōrs) SYN force of mastication.

**chew·ing to·bac·co** (chū′ing tŏ-bak′ō) SYN smokeless tobacco.

**chew-in tech·nique** (chū′in tek-nēk′) A method of generating and recording the occlusal paths of teeth in wax patterns of restorations wherein the patient moves her or his jaws to mark the pathways.

**Cheyne-Stokes res·pi·rat·ion** (chān stōks res′pir-ā′shŭn) Pattern of breathing with gradual increase in depth and sometimes in rate to a maximum, followed by a decrease resulting in apnea.

**CHF** Abbreviation for congestive heart failure.

**Chi·a·ri syn·drome** (kē-ah′rē sin′drōm) Thrombosis of the hepatic vein with great enlargement of the liver and extensive development of collateral vessels, intractable ascites, and severe portal hypertension.

**chi·asm, chi·as·ma** (kī′azm, kī-az′mă) In anatomy, decussation or crossing of two fibrous bundles, such as tendons, nerves, or tracts. [G. *chiasma*]

**chick·en·pox** (chik′ĕn-poks) SYN varicella.

**chi·cle** (chik′ĕl) Mixture of gutta with triterpene alcohols; used in manufacture of chewing gum. [Sp., from Nahuatl *chictli*]

**chief com·plaint (C.C.)** (chēf kŏm-plānt′) Primary symptom that a patient states as the reason for seeking dental care.

**child a·buse** (chīld ă-byūs′) Psychological, emotional, and sexual abuse of a child, typically by a parent, stepparent, or parent surrogate. SEE domestic violence.

**chill** (chil) A feeling of cold with shivering or shaking and pallor, accompanied by an elevation of temperature in the interior of the body; usually a symptom of an infectious disease. [A.S. *cele,* cold]

♻ **chilo-, chil-** Combining forms meaning lips. SEE ALSO cheilo-. [G. *cheilos,* lip]

**chin** (chin) [TA] Prominence formed by anterior projection of the mandible, or lower jaw. [A.S. *cin*]

**chin cap** (chin kap) Extraoral appliance designed to exert an upward and backward force on the mandible by applying pressure to the chin, thereby preventing forward growth.

**chin cup** (chin kŭp) Orthopedic device that fits over the chin and is attached to a head cap; directs force to the mandible in a vertical and/or posterior direction.

**chip sy·ringe** (chip sĭr-inj′) Tapered metal tube through which air is forced from a rubber bulb or pressure tank to blow debris from, or to dry, a cavity in preparing teeth for restoration. Also called chip blower.

**chi·rop·o·dy** (kī-rop′ŏ-dē) SYN podiatry.

**chi·ro·prac·tic** (kī′rō-prak′tik) A system that, in theory, uses the recuperative powers of the body and the relationship between the musculoskeletal structures and functions of the body, particularly of the spinal column and the nervous system, in the restoration and maintenance of health. [*chiro-* + G. *praktikos,* efficient]

**chis·el** (chiz′ĕl) Single beveled end-cutting blade with straight or angled shank used with a thrust along axis of handle for cutting or splitting dentin and enamel.

**chi-square ($\chi^2$)** (kī′skwār) A statistical technique whereby variables are categorized to determine whether a distribution of scores is due to chance or experimental factors.

***Chla·myd·i·a*** (klă-mid′ē-ă) Obligatory intracellular spheric or ovoid pathogenic bacteria with a complex intracellular life cycle; infective form is the elementary body, which penetrates the host cell, replicating as the rediculate body by binary fission.

**chla·myd·i·al** (klă-mid′ē-ăl) Relating to a bacterium of the genus *Chlamydia.*

***Chla·myd·i·a pneu·mo·ni·ae*** (klă-mi′ dē-a nū-mō′nē-ē) A species recognized as a common cause of pneumonia, bronchitis, rhinosinusitis, and pharyngitis. SYN TWAR.

**chlo·ral be·ta·ine** (klōr′ăl bā′tă-ēn) Combined chloral hydrate and betaine used as a hypnotic and sedative.

**chlo·ral hy·drate** (klōr′ăl hī′drāt) Hypnotic and sedative; also used externally as a rubefacient, anesthetic, and antiseptic.

**chlor·am·phen·i·col** (klōr′am-fen′i-kol) An antibiotic effective against several pathogenic microorganisms.

**chlor·hex·i·dine** (klōr-hek′si-dēn) A bis-biguanide useful as a topical antiseptic. The gluconate form is used as an oral rinse to inhibit oral bacteria in some conditions.

**chlor·hex·i·dine stain** (klōr-hek´si-dēn stān) Yellowish-brown stain on the tooth surfaces, restorations, and the surface of the tongue caused by the use of antimicrobial mouth rinses that contain chlorhexidine.

**chlo·ride** (klōr´īd) A compound containing chlorine, (e.g., salts of hydrochloric acid).

**chlo·ride shift** (klōr´īd shift) When $CO_2$ enters the blood from the tissues, it passes into the red blood cell and is converted by carbonate dehydratase to bicarbonate. SYN Hamburger phenomenon.

**chlo·rine** (klōr´ēn) A greenish, toxic, gaseous element used as a disinfectant and bleaching agent in the form of hypochlorite or of chlorine water. [G. *chloros*, greenish yellow]

**chlo·rine di·ox·ide** (klōr´ēn dī-ok´sīd) An oxidizing agent used to sterilize medical and dental instruments and in oral health care to decrease volatile sulfur compounds that could cause halitosis.

**chlor·o·form** (klōr´ō-fōrm) Formerly used inhalation agent to produce general anesthesia; also used as a solvent.

**chlor·o·per·cha** (klōr´ō-pĕr´chă) Solution of gutta-percha in chloroform, used in dentistry as an agent to lute gutta-percha filling material to the wall of a prepared root canal.

**chlor·o·per·cha meth·od** (klōr´ō-pĕr´chă meth´ŏd) Means of filling root canals of teeth by dissolving gutta-percha cones in a chloroform-resin solution within the root canal and forcing it to the apex as a plastic mass to provide a seal. SYN Johnson method.

**chlor·o·phyll** (klōr´ō-fil) Light-absorbing green plant pigments that, in living plants, convert light energy into oxidizing and reducing power, thus fixing $CO_2$ and evolving $O_2$.

**chlo·ro·pro·caine pen·i·cil·lin O** (klōr´ō-prō´kān pen´i-sil´in) An agent with antibacterial activity is similar to that of penicillin O and G.

**chlor·o·quine** (klōr´ō-kwīn) An antimalarial agent used for the treatment and suppression of *Plasmodium vivax, P. malariae,* and *P. falciparum;* also used for hepatic amebiasis and some skin diseases.

**chlor·o·thi·a·zide** (klōr´ō-thī´ă-zīd) An orally effective diuretic used to treat edema.

**CHO** Abbreviation for carbohydrates.

**cho·a·na,** pl. **cho·a·nae** (kō´ă-nă, -nē) The right or left opening from the nasal cavity into the nasopharynx. SYN apertura nasalis posterior. [Mod. L. fr. G. *choanē,* a funnel]

**cho·a·nal a·tre·si·a** (kō´ă-năl ă-trē´zē-ă) Atresia due to congenital failure of one or both choanae to open owing to the failure of the

bucconasal membrane to involute; results in nasal obstruction.

**cho·a·noid** (kō´ă-noyd) Funnel-shaped. [G. *choanē,* funnel, + *eidos,* resemblance]

**choice of path of place·ment** (choys path plās´mĕnt) Determination, at the design stage of prosthesis fabrication, of the direction of insertion (and removal); dictated by soft and hard tissue morphology, including undercuts, and can be modified with the placement of guide planes on teeth.

**choked disc** (chōkt disk) SYN papilledema.

**cho·la·gogue** (kō´lă-gog) Agent that promotes flow of bile into the intestine. [*chol-* + G. *agōgos,* drawing forth]

**cho·lem·e·sis** (kō-lem´ĕ-sis) Vomiting of bile. [*chole-* + G. *emesis,* vomiting]

**chol·er·a** (kol´ĕr-ă) An acute epidemic infectious disease caused by the bacterium *Vibrio cholerae* that causes profuse watery diarrhea, extreme loss of fluid and electrolytes, and dehydration and collapse. [L. a bilious disease, fr. G. *cholē,* bile]

**cho·le·ret·ic** (kō´lĕr-et´ik) An agent that stimulates liver to increase output of bile.

**cho·le·stat·ic** (kō´lĕ-stat´ik) Tending to diminish or stop the flow of bile.

**cho·les·te·a·to·ma** (kō´lĕ-stē´ă-tō´mă) A mass of keratinizing squamous epithelium and cholesterol in the middle ear, usually caused by chronic otitis media, with squamous metaplasia or extension of squamous epithelium inward to line an expanding cystic cavity that may involve the mastoid and erode surrounding bone. [*cholesterol* + G. *stear (steat-),* tallow, + *-ōma,* tumor]

**cho·les·ter·ol** (kŏ-les´tĕr-ol) The most abundant steroid in animal tissues; circulates in the plasma complexed to proteins of various densities; plays an important role in the pathogenesis of atheroma formation in arteries.

**cho·le·styr·a·mine res·in** (kō-les´tĕr-ă-mēn rez´in) Anion exchange resin used to bind dietary cholesterol and prevent its systemic absorption. Used to treat hypercholesteremia.

**cho·line** (kō´lēn) Agent found in most animal tissues either free or in combination as lecithin, acetate, or cytidine diphosphate; included in vitamin B complex.

**cho·lin·er·gic** (kō´li-nĕr´jik) **1.** Relating to nerve cells or fibers that use acetylcholine as their neurotransmitter. **2.** Drug or chemical with physiologic effects similar to those of acetylcholine. [*choline* + G. *ergon,* work]

**cho·lin·er·gic a·gent** (kō´li-nĕr´jik ā´jĕnt) Agent that mimics action of acetylcholine or parasympathetic nervous system.

**cho·lin·er·gic block·ing a·gent** (kō′li-nĕr′jik blok′ing ā′jĕnt) SYN anticholinergic agent.

**cho·line sal·i·cyl·ate** (kō′lēn să-lis′i-lāt) Choline salt of salicyclic acid, an analgesic and antipyretic (because of the salicylate moiety).

**cho·lin·es·ter·ase** (kō′lin-es′tĕr-ās) One of a family of enzymes capable of catalyzing the hydrolysis of acylcholines and a few other compounds. In mammals, found in white matter of brain, liver, heart, pancreas, and serum.

**cho·li·no·lyt·ic** (kō′lin-ō-lit′ik) Preventing the action of acetylcholine.

**chon·dri·tis** (kon-drī′tis) Inflammation of cartilage. [G. *chondros,* cartilage, + *-itis,* inflammation]

**chon·dro·dys·tro·phy with sen·sor·i·neu·ral deaf·ness** (kon′drō-dis′trŏ-fē sen′sŏr-ē-nūr′ăl def′nĕs) Skeletal dysplasia characterized by dwarfism, flat nasal bridge, cleft palate, sensorineural deafness, large epiphyses, and flattening of vertebral bodies.

**chon·dro·ec·to·der·mal dys·pla·si·a** (kon′drō-ek-tō-dĕr′măl dis-plā′zē-ă) Disorder involving chondrodysplasia, ectodermal dysplasia, and polydactyly with congenital heart defects, dwarfism, and abnormalities in teeth, hair, and nails. SYN Ellis-van Creveld syndrome.

**chon·dro·i·tin** (kon-drō′i-tin) Dietary supplement made from bovine cartilage; widely used for its purported efficacy against osteoarthritis; some clinical studies suggest its value, others make no such confirmation. Association with spontaneous internal bleeding. [*chondroit-* fr. *chondroitic acid,* + *-in*]

**chon·dro·ma** (kon-drō′mă) A benign neoplasm derived from mesodermal cells that form cartilage. [*chondro-* + G. *-ōma,* tumor]

**chon·dro·sar·co·ma** (kon′drō-sahr-kō′mă) A malignant neoplasm derived from cartilage cells.

**CHOP** (chop) Acronym for cyclophosphamide, doxorubicin, Oncovin (vincristine), and prednisone, a chemotherapeutic regimen.

**chor·da,** pl. **chor·dae** (kōr′dă, -dē) [TA] A tendinous or a cordlike structure. [L., cord]

**chor·da sa·li·va** (kōr′dă să-lī′vă) Secretion of submaxillary gland obtained by stimulation of the chorda tympani nerve.

**chor·da tym·pa·ni** (kōr′dă tim′pan-ī) [TA] Nerve given off from the facial nerve in the facial canal; conveys taste sensation from the anterior two thirds of the tongue and carries parasympathetic preganglionic fibers to the submandibular ganglion, for innervation of submandibular and sublingual salivary glands.

**cho·ri·on·ic go·nad·o·tro·pin** (kōr′ē-

on′ik gō-nad′ō-trō′pin) Glycoprotein with carbohydrate fraction composed of D-galactose and hexosamine, extracted from the urine of pregnant women.

**Chris·tian dis·ease, Chris·tian syn·drome** (kris′chĕn di-zēz′, sin′drōm) 1. SYN Hand-Schller-Christian disease. 2. SYN relapsing febrile nodular nonsuppurative panniculitis.

**Christ·mas dis·ease** (kris′măs di-zēz′) SYN hemophilia B.

**Christ·mas fac·tor** (kris′măs fak′tŏr) SYN factor IX.

**chro·ma·tin** (krō′mă-tin) The genetic material of the nucleus, consisting of deoxyribonucleoprotein. During mitotic division, the chromatin condenses into chromosomes. [G. *chrōma,* color]

**chro·ma·tog·ra·phy** (krō′mă-tog′ră-fē) The separation of chemical substances and particles by differential movement through a two-phase system of analysis.

**chrome-co·balt al·loys** (krōm-kō′bawlt al′oyz) Alloys of cobalt and chromium containing molybdenum alone or combined with tungsten plus trace elements; used in dentistry for denture bases and frameworks and other structures.

**chro·mic cat·gut, chro·mic gut** (krō′mik kat′gŭt) Catgut suture material impregnated with chromium salts to prolong its tensile strength and retard its absorption.

**chro·mi·um** (krō′mē-ŭm) A metallic element and essential dietary bioelement; used as diagnostic aid in many disorders (e.g., gastrointestinal protein loss). [G. *chroma,* color]

**chro·mi·um-co·balt-mol·yb·de·num** (krō′mē-ŭm-kō′bawlt-mŏ-lib′dĕ-nŭm) Stainless alloy used in dental prostheses.

**chro·mo·gen·ic** (krō′mō-jen′ik) 1. Denoting a chromogen. 2. Relating to chromogenesis.

**chro·mo·som·al** (krō′mŏ-sō′măl) Pertaining to chromosomes.

**chro·mo·some** (krō′mŏ-sōm) One of the bodies (normally 46 in somatic cells in humans) in the cell nucleus that is the bearer of genes, has the form of a delicate chromatin filament during interphase, contracts to form a compact cylinder segmented into two arms by the centromere during metaphase and anaphase stages of cell divison, and is capable of reproducing its physical and chemical structure through successive cell divisons.

**chro·mo·some ab·er·ra·tion** (krō′mŏ-sōm ab-ĕr-ā′shŭn) Any deviation from the normal number or morphology of chromosomes; also the phenotypic consequences thereof.

**chron·ic** (kron′ik) *Avoid the jargonistic use of*

*this word to refer to prolonged therapy, as in chronic estrogen replacement.* **1.** Referring to a health-related state, lasting a long time. **2.** Referring to exposure, prolonged or long-term, sometimes meaning also low intensity. Cf. acute. [G. *chronos,* time]

**chron·ic act·ive hep·a·ti·tis** (kron´ik ak´tiv hep-ă-tī´tis) Liver disease with portal inflammation that extends into the parenchyma, and usually progresses to a coarsely nodular postnecrotic cirrhosis.

**chron·ic al·co·hol·ism** (kron´ik al´kŏ-hol-izm) Pathologic condition, affecting chiefly the nervous and gastroenteric systems, associated with impairment in social and occupational functioning, caused by the habitual use of alcoholic beverages in toxic amounts.

**chron·ic bron·chi·tis** (kron´ik brong-kī´tis) Disorder of the bronchial tree characterized by cough, hypersecretion of mucus, and expectoration of sputum over a long period of time, associated with frequent bronchial infections; usually due to inhalation, over a prolonged period, of air contaminated by dust or by noxious gases of combustion.

**chron·ic des·qua·ma·tive gin·gi·vi·tis** (kron´ik des-kwahm´ă-tiv jin´ji-vī´tis) Clinical term for gingival condition of unknown etiology, usually encountered in middle-aged and older women, characterized by erythema, mucosal atrophy, and desquamation, and generally accompanied by a burning sensation and pain; diagnosis is usually made by biopsy and direct immunofluorescence. SYN gingivosis.

**chron·ic dif·fuse scle·ros·ing os·te·o·my·e·li·tis** (kron´ik di-fyūs´ skler-ōs´ing os´tē-ō-mī´ē-lī´tis) Proliferative reaction of bone to low-grade infection of the jaws; most often seen in middle-aged or older black women as extensive, often bilateral, radioopacities of the mandible and maxilla.

**chron·ic en·dem·ic fluor·o·sis** (kron´ik en-dem´ik flōr-ō´sis) Fluorosis caused by excessive fluorine in the natural water supply, as seen in parts of India.

**chron·ic fa·mil·i·al ic·te·rus** (kron´ik fă-mil´ē-ăl ik´tĕr-ŭs) SYN hereditary spherocytosis.

**chron·ic fa·mil·i·al jaun·dice** (kron´ik fă-mil´ē-ăl jawn´dis) SYN hereditary spherocytosis.

**chron·ic in·flam·ma·tion** (kron´ik in´flă-mă´shŭn) Inflammation that may begin with relatively rapid onset or in slow, insidious, and even unnoticed manner, and tends to persist for several weeks, months, or years and has a vague and indefinite termination; occurs when the injuring agent persists in the lesion, and the host's tissues respond in a manner insufficient to overcome its continuing effects.

**chron·ic ob·struc·tive pul·mo·nar·y dis·ease (COPD)** (kron´ik ŏb-strŭk´tiv pul´mŏ-nar-ē di-zēz´) General term for the diseases with permanent or temporary narrowing of small bronchi, in which forced expiratory flow is slowed, especially when no etiologic or other more specific term can be applied.

**chron·ic per·sist·ing hep·a·ti·tis** (kron´ik pĕr-sist´ing hep´ă-tī´tis) Form of disorder that does not progress to cirrhosis, usually benign and is usually asymptomatic without physical findings but with continuing abnormalities of tests of liver status.

**chron·ic pneu·mo·ni·a** (kron´ik nū-mō´nē-ă) Indefinite usage for long-term inflammation of pulmonary tissue of any etiology.

**chron·ic re·lap·sing pan·cre·a·ti·tis** (kron´ik rē-lap´sing pan´krē-ă-tī´tis) Repeated exacerbations of pancreatitis in patients with chronic inflammation of that organ.

**chro·no·log·ic age (CA)** (kron´ŏ-loj´ik āj) Age expressed in years and months from date of birth.

**chrys·o·ther·a·py** (kris´ō-thār´ă-pē) Treatment of disease by administration of gold salts. SYN aurotherapy. [G. *chrysos,* gold]

**Chvos·tek sign** (kvos´tek sīn) Facial irritability in tetany with unilateral spasm of the orbicularis oculi or oris muscle elicited by slight tap over facial nerve just anterior to external auditory meatus.

**chyme, chy·mus** (kīm, kī´mŭs) Semifluid mass of partly digested food passed from stomach into duodenum. [G. *chymos,* juice]

**chy·mo·poi·e·sis** (kī´mō-poy-ē´sis) Production of chyme; physical state of food (semifluid) brought about by digestion in stomach. [G. *chymos,* juice, chyme, + *poiesis,* a making]

**cic·a·tri·cial pem·phi·goid** (sik´ă-trish´ăl pem´fi-goyd) See page A11. SYN benign mucous membrane pemphigoid.

**cic·a·trix,** pl. **cic·a·tri·ces** (sik´ă-triks, -trish´ēz) A scar. [L.]

**cic·a·tri·za·tion** (sik´ă-trī-zā´shŭn) **1.** The process of scar formation. **2.** The healing of a wound otherwise than by first intention.

**cig·a·rette drain** (sig´ă-ret´ drān) A wick of gauze wrapped in rubber tissue, providing capillary drainage.

**cil·i·ar·y gan·gli·on** (sil´ē-ar-ē gang´glē-ŏn) [TA] A small parasympathetic ganglion lying in the orbit between the optic nerve and the lateral rectus muscle.

**cil·i·ar·y mus·cle** (sil´ē-ar-ē mŭs´ĕl) [TA] The smooth muscle of the ciliary body; *action,* in contracting, its diameter is reduced (like a sphincter), reducing tensile (stretching) forces on ocular lens, allowing it to thicken for near vision (accommodation). SYN musculus ciliaris [TA].

**ci·met·i·dine** (si-met'i-dēn) Histamine analogue and antagonist used to treat peptic ulcer and hypersecretory conditions.

**cin·e·ra·di·og·ra·phy, cin·e·roent·gen·og·ra·phy** (sin'ĕ-rā-dē-og'ră-fē, -rent' gen-og'ră-fē) Radiography of a moving organ.

**cin·e·seis·mog·ra·phy** (sin'ĕ-sīz-mog'ră-fē) Technique for measuring body movements by continuous photographic recording of shaking or vibration.

**cin·gu·late** (sing'gyū-lāt) Relating to a cingulum.

**cin·gu·lum,** pl. **cin·gu·la** (sing'gyū-lŭm, -lă) [TA] SYN girdle. [L. girdle, fr. *cingo,* to surround]

**cin·gu·lum mod·i·fi·ca·tion** (sing'gyū-lŭm mod'i-fi-kā'shŭn) Alteration of lingual cingulum of anterior tooth to form seat to support rest of metal framework of removable partial denture.

**cin·gu·lum of tooth** (sing'gyū-lŭm tūth) [TA] U- or W-shaped ridge at the base of the lingual surface of the crown of the maxillary incisors and cuspid teeth, the lateral limbs running for a short distance along the linguoproximal line angles, the central portion just above the gingiva. SYN basal ridge (2), lingual lobe.

**cin·gu·lum rest** (sing'gyū-lŭm rest) Rigid part of a removable partial denture supported by a prepared rest area on cingulum of an anterior tooth or crown.

**cin·na·mon** (sin'ă-mŏn) Dried aromatic bark of *Cinnamomum loureirii* used as a spice and, in medicine, as an adjuvant, carminative, and aromatic stomachic. [L. fr. G. *kinnamōmon,* cinnamon]

**cir·ca·di·an** (sĭr-kā'dē-ăn) Relating to biologic variations or rhythms with a cycle of about 24 hours. [L. *circa,* about, + *dies,* day]

**cir·cle** (sĭr'kĕl) ANATOMY ring-shaped or anular structure or group of structures, as formed by anastomosing arteries or veins, or by connected (communicating) nerves. [L. *circulus*]

**cir·cuit scal·ing** (sĭr'kŭt skāl'ing) SYN gross scaling.

**cir·cu·lar fi·bers** (sĭr'kyū-lăr fī'bĕrz) SYN circumferential fibers.

**cir·cu·lar si·nus** (sĭr'kyū-lăr sī'nŭs) Dural venous formation that surrounds the hypophysis, composed of right and left cavernous sinuses and the intercavernous sinuses;

**cir·cu·la·tion** (sĭr'kyū-lā'shŭn) Movements in a circle, or through a circular course, or

through a course that leads back to the same point. [L. *circulatio*]

**cir·cu·la·to·ry over·load** (sĭr'kyū-lă-tōr-ē ō'vĕr-lōd) SYN hypervolemia.

**cir·cum·al·ve·o·lar fix·a·tion** (sĭr'kŭm-al-vē'ŏ-lăr fik-sā'shŭn) Stabilization of a fracture segment or surgical splint by wire passed through and around the dental alveolar process.

**cir·cum·fer·en·tial clasp** (sĭr'kŭm-fĕr-en'shăl klasp) **1.** Appliance that encircles more than 180 degrees of a tooth, including opposite angles and usually contacts the tooth throughout the extent of the clasp, at least one terminal being in the infrabulge (gingival convergence) area; **2.** Clasp consisting of two circumferential clasp arms, both of which originate from the same minor connector and are located on opposite surfaces of the abutment tooth.

**cir·cum·fer·en·tial clasp arm** (sĭr'kŭm-fĕr-en'shăl klasp ahrm) One that has its origin in a minor connector and follows tooth contour approximately in a plane perpendicular to path of insertion of partial denture.

**cir·cum·fer·en·tial fi·bers** (sĭr'kŭm-fĕr-en'shăl fī'bĕrz) Fibers in free gingiva that encircle neck of the tooth. SYN circular fibers.

**cir·cum·fer·en·tial wir·ing** (sĭr'kŭm-fĕr-en'shăl wīr'ing) Fixation of mandibular fractures by passing wires around a section of bone and intraoral splint; i.e., circummandibular wiring.

**cir·cum·man·dib·u·lar** (sĭr'kŭm-man-dib'yū-lăr) Around or about the mandible.

**cir·cum·man·dib·u·lar fix·a·tion** (sĭr'kŭm-man-dib'yū-lăr fik-sā'shŭn) Stabilization of fracture segment or surgical splint by wire passed around mandible.

**cir·cum·oc·u·lar** (sĭr'kŭm-ok'yū-lăr) Around the eye. [*circum-* + L. *oculus,* eye]

**cir·cum·or·bit·al** (sĭr'kŭm-ōr'bi-tăl) Around the orbit.

**cir·cum·val·late** (sĭr'kŭm-val'āt) Denoting a structure surrounded by a wall (e.g., circumvallate [lingual] papillae).

**cir·cum·zy·go·mat·ic fix·a·tion** (sĭr'kŭm-zī'gō-mat'ik fik-sā'shŭn) Stabilization of fracture segment or surgical splint by wire passed around zygomatic arch.

**cir·rho·sis** (sĭr-ō'sis) A chronic liver disease of highly various etiology characterized by inflammation, degeneration, and regeneration in differing proportions. [G. *kirrhos,* yellow (liver), + *-osis,* condition]

**CIS** Abbreviation for carcinoma in situ.

**cis·tern** (sis'tĕrn) [TA] Any cavity or enclosed

space serving as a reservoir, especially for chyle, lymph, or cerebrospinal fluid.

**cit·rate** (sit′rāt) A salt or ester of citric acid; used as anticoagulant.

**cit·rat·ed cal·ci·um car·bi·mide** (sit′ rā-tĕd kal′sē-ŭm kahr′bă-mīd) Agent used in the treatment of alcoholism.

**cit·ric ac·id** (sit′rik as′id) The acid of citrus fruits, widely distributed in nature and a key intermediate in intermediary metabolism.

**cit·rin** (sit′rin) SYN vitamin P.

**CJD** Abbreviation for Creutzfeldt-Jakob disease.

**CJDH** Abbreviation for Canadian Journal of Dental Hygiene.

**CK** Abbreviation for creatine kinase.

**claim** (clām) A statement from a patient of a health care provider presented to an insurance company or HMO for payment.

**claim form** (klām fōrm) Document that gives necessary information about patient, treating provider, and coded treatment, including charges; filed for payment of benefits by carrier of dental insurance. [L. *forma*, shape, contour]

**clamp** (klamp) An instrument used to compress or hold in a place a bodily structure. Cf. forceps. [M.E., fr. Middle D. *klampe*]

**clamp for·ceps** (klamp fōr′seps) Forceps with pronged jaws designed to engage the jaws of a rubber dam clamp so that they may be separated to pass over the widest buccolingual contour of a tooth. SYN rubber dam clamp forceps.

**cla·po·tage, cla·pote·ment** (kla-pō-tahzh′, kla-pōt-mon[h]′) Splashing sound heard on succussion of a dilated stomach. [Fr.]

**Clap·ton line** (klap′tŏn līn) Greenish discoloration of the marginal gingiva in cases of chronic copper poisoning.

**clasp** (klasp) **1.** Part of a removable partial denture that acts as a direct retainer or stabilizer for denture by partially surrounding or contacting an abutment tooth. **2.** Direct retainer of a removable partial denture, usually consisting of two arms joined by a body that connects with an occlusal rest; at least one arm usually terminates in the infrabulge (gingival convergence) area of the tooth enclosed.

**clasp arm** (klasp ahrm) Portion of clasp of removable partial denture that projects from clasp body and helps retain the partial denture in position in the mouth. SEE clasp (2).

**clasp bar** (klasp bahr) SEE clasp.

**clasp flex·ure** (klasp flek′shŭr) Ability of retentive clasp arm to bend and then return to proper shape to permit its passage over surveyed

height of contour, thus allowing seating or removal of partial denture. [L. *flexura*, a bending, fr. *flecto, pp. flexum*, to bend]

**clasp guide·line** (klasp gīd′līn) SYN survey line.

**clasp-knife spas·ti·ci·ty, clasp-knife ri·gid·i·ty** (klasp′nīf′ spas-tis′i-tē, ri-jid′i-tē) Initial increased resistance to stretch of the extensor muscles of a joint that give way rather suddenly, allowing the joint then to be easily flexed; the rigidity is due to an exaggeration of the stretch reflex.

**clas·si·cal con·di·tion·ing** (klas′i-kăl kŏn-dish′ŭn-ing) A form of learning, as in pavlovian experiments, in which a previously neutral stimulus becomes a conditioned stimulus when presented together with an unconditioned stimulus.

**clas·sic hae·mo·phil·ia** [Br.] SYN classic hemophilia.

**clas·si·c he·mo·phil·ia** (klas′ik hē′mō-fil′ē-ă) SYN hemophilia A, classic haemophilia.

**clas·sic mi·graine** (klas′ik mī′grān) Hemicranial migraine preceded by a scintillating scotoma (teichopsia).

**clas·si·fi·ca·tion** (klas′i-fi-kā′shŭn) A systematic arrangement into classes or groups based on perceived common characteristics; a means of giving order to a group of disconnected facts.

**clas·si·fi·ca·tion of par·tial den·tures** (klas′i-fi-kā′shŭn pahr′shăl den′chŭrz) Diagnosis of a partially edentulous dental arch based on the area of edentulous space, remaining teeth, possible clasp design, and anatomic ability to support a partial denture.

**clas·si·fi·ca·tion of per·i·o·don·tal pock·ets** (klas′i-fi-kā′shŭn per′ē-ō-don′tăl pok′ĕts) Scheme to subcharacterize these openings into two classes: suprabony and infrabony

**claus·trum,** pl. **claus·tra** (klaws′trŭm, -tră) [TA] One of several anatomic structures bearing a resemblance to a barrier.

**clav·i·cle** (klav′i-kĕl) [TA] A doubly curved long bone that forms part of the shoulder girdle. SYN collar bone.

**clav·u·lan·ic ac·id** (klav′yū-lan′ik as′id) A β-lactam structurally related to the penicillins that inactivates β-lactamase enzymes in penicillin-resistant organisms.

**clean·ing** (klēn′ing) SYN dental prophylaxis.

**clear·ance** (klēr′ăns) Removal of something from an area.

**clear·ance time** (klēr′ăns tīm) Temporal duration from ingestion until food is cleared from the oral cavity; influenced by consistency and quantity of saliva; by action of tongue, lips, and cheeks; and by consistency of food.

**clear la·yer of ep·i·der·mis** (klēr lā′ĕr ep′i-dĕrm′is) SYN stratum lucidum.

**cleat** (klēt) A fixed anchorage, usually metal, embedded in the acrylic resin base of an orthodontic retainer or soldered to an arch wire. An elastic device is attached during tooth movement.

**cleft** (kleft) [TA] A fissure or, groove.

**cleft jaw** (kleft jaw) Congenital jaw anomaly resulting from failure of fusion of the mandibular prominences. SYN gnathoschisis.

**cleft lip** (kleft lip) Congenital abnormality of the lip (usually upper) resulting from failure of union of the medial and nasal prominences with maxillary prominence; may be unilateral, bilateral, or median. See this page. SYN harelip.

**cleft nose** (kleft nōz) Nose with furrow caused by failure of complete convergence of the paired embryonic primordia. Fissures of the soft tissues ordinarily signal coexistent underlying skeletal clefts.

**cleft pal·ate** (kleft pal′ăt) Congenital fissure in median line of the palate, often, but not necessarily associated with cleft lip. See this page.

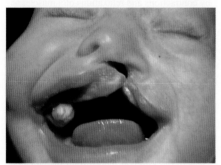
cleft lip and cleft palate

**cleft pal·ate pros·the·sis** (kleft pal′ăt pros-thē′sis) SYN speech aid prosthesis.

**cleft tongue** (kleft tŭng) SYN bifid tongue.

**clei·do·cra·ni·al dys·o·sto·sis, cli·do·cra·ni·al dys·o·sto·sis** (klī′dō-krā′nē-ăl dis-os-tō′sis) Developmental disorder characterized by absence or hypoplasia of clavicles, box-shaped cranium with open sutures, frontal bossing and missing teeth. See this page.

**clench·ing** (klench′ing) Nonfunctional tooth clamping in centric occlusion. See page A7.

**cle·oid** (klē′oyd) Dental instrument with pointed elliptic cutting end, used in excavating cavities or carving fillings and waxes. [A. S. cle, claw + G. eidos, resemblance]

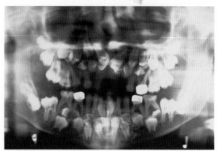
**cleidocranial dysostosis:** retention of primary teeth

**click·ing** (klik′ing) Snapping, crepitant noise noted on excursions of temporomandibular articulation due to asynchronous movement of disc and condyle.

**cli·mac·ter·ic, cli·mac·te·ri·um** (klī-mak′tĕr-ik, -mak-tē′rē-ŭm) The period of endocrinal, somatic, and transitory psychological changes occurring in the menopause. [G. klimaktēr, the rung of a ladder]

**cli·max** (klī′maks) **1.** The height or acme of a disease; its stage of greatest severity. **2.** Colloq. an orgasm. [G. klimax, staircase]

**clin·ic** (klin′ik) **1.** An institution, building, or part of a building where ambulatory patients receive health care. **2.** An institution, building, or part of a building in which medical instruction is given to students by means of demonstrations in the presence of the sick. **3.** A lecture or symposium on a subject relating to disease. [G. klinē, bed]

**clin·i·cal** (klin′i-kăl) Denoting symptoms and course of a disease, as distinguished from laboratory findings of anatomic changes. [G. klinē, bed, + -al]

**clin·i·cal a·ttach·ment lev·el** (klin′i-kăl ă-tach′mĕnt lev′ĕl) Estimated position of structures that support tooth as measured by periodontal probe; estimates tooth's stability and indicates loss of bone support.

**clin·i·cal at·tach·ment loss** (klin′i-kăl ă-tach′mĕnt laws) Extent of lost periodontal support about a tooth. See page 128.

**clin·i·cal chem·is·try** (klin′i-kăl kem′is-trē) **1.** The chemistry of human health and disease. **2.** Chemistry in connection with the management of patients, as in a hospital laboratory.

**clin·i·cal clerk·ship** (klin′i-kăl klĕrk′ship) Situation in which someone works for and under supervision of a more experienced dentist.

**clin·i·cal crown** (klin′i-kăl krown) Part of tooth crown visible in oral cavity.

**clin·i·cal di·ag·no·sis** (klin′i-kăl dī-ăg-nō′sis) Diagnosis made from a study of signs and symptoms of a disease or condition.

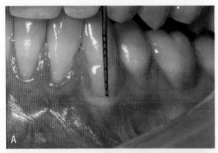
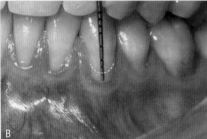

**measurements for clinical attachment loss:**
(A) first, sulcus is probed; (B) next, level of gingiva margin level from cementoenamel junction is measured. When the two numbers are added together, the amount of attachment loss is determined

**clin·i·cal end point** (klin′i-kăl end poynt) Traditional medical measures of a diagnostic or therapeutic impact that may or may not be perceived by the patient.

**clin·i·cal e·rup·tion** (klin′i-kăl ē-rŭp′shŭn) Development of tooth crown that can be observed clinically.

**clin·i·cal fit·ness** (klin′i-kăl fit′nĕs) Absence of frank disease or subclinical precursors.

**clin·i·cal le·thal** (klin′i-kăl lē′thăl) Denotes a disorder that culminates in premature death.

**clin·i·cal med·i·cine** (klin′i-kăl med′i-sin) Study and practice of medicine in relation to care of patients.

**clin·i·cal phar·ma·col·o·gy** (klin′i-kăl fahr′mă-kol′ŏ-jē) Branch of pharmacology concerned with the pharmacology of therapeutic agents.

**clin·i·cal phar·ma·cy** (klin′i-kăl fahr′mă-sē) Branch of pharmacy practice that emphasizes therapeutic use of drugs rather than their preparation and dispensing.

**clin·i·cal root of tooth** (klin′i-kăl rūt tūth) [TA] Portion of a tooth embedded in investing structures; portion not visible in oral cavity.

**clin·i·cal ther·mom·e·ter** (klin′i-kăl thĕr-mom′ĕ-tĕr) Device for measuring temperature of human body.

**cli·ni·cian** (klin-ish′ŭn) A health care professional engaged in the care of patients.

**clin·i·co·path·o·log·ic, clin·i·co·path·o·log·ic·al** (klin′i-kō-path-ŏ-loj′ik, -i-kăl) Pertaining to the signs and symptoms manifested by a patient, and also the results of laboratory studies.

**cli·nog·ra·phy** (klin-og′ră-fē) Graphic representation of the signs and symptoms exhibited by a patient. [G. *klinē*, bed, + *graphō*, to write]

**clo·nic** (klon′ik) Relating to or characterized by clonus.

**clo·nic con·vul·sion** (klon′ik kŏn-vŭl′shŭn) Convulsion with intermittent contractions; the muscles alternately contract and relax.

**clon·i·co·ton·ic** (klon′i-kō-ton′ik) Both clonic and tonic; said of certain forms of muscular spasm.

**clo·nic sei·zure** (klon′ik sē′zhŭr) Seizure characterized by repetitive rhythmic jerking of all or part of the body.

**clo·nic state** (klon′ik stāt) Movement marked by repetitive muscle contractions and relaxations in rapid succession.

**clo·nus** (klō′nŭs) A form of movement marked by contractions and relaxations of a muscle, occurring in rapid succession seen with, among other conditions, spasticity and some seizure disorders. [G. *klonos*, a tumult]

**close bite** (klōs bīt) SYN small interarch distance.

**closed an·es·the·si·a** (klōzd an′es-thē′zē-ă) Inhalation anesthesia with total rebreathing of all exhaled gases, except carbon dioxide.

**closed an·gle** (klōzd ang′gĕl) Angulation of the working-end of an instrument at an angle between 0 degrees and 40 degrees for insertion beneath the gingival margin into the sulcus or pocket.

**closed bite** (klōzd bīt) Form of reduced vertical bite in which the mandibular incisors are positioned near the lingual gingiva of the maxillary incisors. Cf. deep bite.

***Clos·trid·i·um*** (klos-trid′ē-ŭm) Genus of anaerobic, spore-forming, motile bacteria that may cause disease in intestinal tract.

**clo·sure** (klō′zhŭr) Bringing together the margins of a wound.

**clot** (klot) **1.** To coagulate (e.g., blood). **2.** A soft, nonrigid, insoluble mass formed when a liquid congeals. [O.E. *klott*, lump]

**clot·ting fac·tor** (klot′ing fak′tŏr) Any plasma components involved in clotting.

**clot·ting time** (klot′ing tīm) SYN coagulation time.

**clus·ter** (klŭs´tĕr) A group of similar or identical objects occurring naturally in close proximity (as grapes) or so assembled (as beads). [O.E. *clyster*]

**clus·ter head·ache** (klŭs´tĕr hed´āk) Headache possibly due to a hypersensitivity to histamine.

**clus·ter of dif·fer·en·ti·a·tion (CD)** (klŭs´tĕr dif´ĕr-en-shē-ā´shŭn) Cell membrane molecules that are used to classify leukocytes into subsets. CD molecules are classified by monoclonal antibodies.

**CNS** Abbreviation for central nervous system.

**c/o** Abbreviation for complains of.

**CO** Abbreviation for carbon monoxide.

**CO$_2$** Abbreviation for carbon dioxide.

**co·ag·u·lant** (kō-ag´yū-lĕnt) An agent that causes, stimulates, or accelerates coagulation, especially with reference to blood.

**co·a·gu·la·ting cur·rent** (kō-ag´yū-lāting kŭr´ĕnt) Electricity delivered to tissue to induce coagulation; often used in electrosurgery.

**co·ag·u·la·tion** (kō-ag´yū-lā´shŭn) **1.** Clotting; the process of changing from a liquid to a solid, said especially of blood (i.e., blood coagulation). **2.** A clot or coagulum.

**co·ag·u·la·tion time** (kō-ag´yū-lā´shŭn tīm) Temporal duration required for blood to coagulate. SYN clotting time.

**co·ap·ta·tion** (kō´ap-tā´shŭn) Joining or fitting together of two surfaces; e.g., the lips of a wound or the ends of a broken bone. [L. *co-apto,* pp. *-aptatus,* to fit together]

**coat** (kōt) **1.** The outer covering or envelope of an organ or part. **2.** One of the layers of membranous or other tissues forming the wall of a canal.

**coat·ed tongue** (kōt´ĕd tŭng) Tongue with a whitish layer on its upper surface, composed of epithelial debris, food particles, and bacteria; often an indication of indigestion or of fever. SYN furred tongue.

**co·bal·a·min** (kō-bal´ă-min) General term for compounds containing the dimethylbenzimidazolylcobamide nucleus of vitamin B12.

**co·balt** (kō´bawlt) A steel-gray metallic element; constituent of vitamin B12; some compounds are pigments. [Ger. *kobalt,* goblin or evil spirit]

**co·balt-chro·mi·um al·loy** (kō´bawlt-krō´mē-ŭm al´oy) Alloys of cobalt and chromium containing molybdenum alone or combined with tungsten plus trace elements; used in dentistry for denture bases and frameworks, and other structures.

**cob·ble·stone tongue** (kob´ĕl-stōn tŭng) Interstitial glossitis with hypertrophy of the papillae and a white surface coating.

**COBRA** (kō´bră) Acronym for U.S. federal Consolidated Omnibus Budget Reconciliation Act, which allowed fired workers to continue with group health insurance coverage for a period.

**co·caine** (kō-kān´) Benzoylmethylecgonine; a crystalline alkaloid obtained from the leaves of *Erythroxylon coca* and other species of *Erythroxylon,* or by synthesis from ecgonine or its derivatives; a potent central nervous system stimulant, vasoconstrictor, and topical anesthetic, widely abused as a euphoriant and associated with the risk of severe adverse physical and mental effects.

**co·caine hy·dro·chlo·ride** (kō-kān´ hī´drō-klōr´īd) Water-soluble salt used for local anesthesia of the eye or mucous membranes.

**coc·cid·i·oi·do·my·co·sis** (kok-sid´ē-oy´dō-mī-kō´sis) A variable, benign, severe, or sometimes fatal systemic mycosis due to inhalation of arthroconidia of *Coccidioides immitis.*

**coc·cus,** pl. **coc·ci** (kok´ŭs, -sī) A bacterium of round, spheroid, or ovoid form. [G. *kokkos,* berry]

**coch·lea,** pl. **coch·le·ae** (kok´lē-ă, -ē) [TA] Snail shell–shaped dense bone in the petrous portion of the temporal bone, forming anterior division of the labyrinth or internal ear. [L. snail shell]

**coch·le·ar a·que·duct** (kok´lē-ăr ah´kwă-dŭkt) [TA] Fine canal in temporal bone, opening superior to the tympanic canaliculus, connecting the perilymphatic space of the cochlea with the subarachnoid space in the region of the bulb of the internal jugular vein.

**co·chle·ar ar·ea** (kok´lē-ăr ar´ē-ă) [TA] Space inferior to transverse crest of the fundus of the internal acoustic meatus through which the filaments of the cochlear nerve pass to enter the cochlea. SEE base of modiolus of cochlea.

**coch·le·ar branch of ves·tib·u·lo·coch·le·ar ar·te·ry** (kok´lē-ăr branch vestib´yū-lō-kok´lē-ăr ahr´tĕr-ē) [TA] Terminal branch of vestibulocochlear artery.

**coch·le·ar can·al·ic·u·lus** (kok´lē-ăr kan´ă-lik´yŭ-lŭs) [TA] Minute canal in temporal bone that passes from the cochlea inferiorly to open in front of the medial side of the jugular fossa; contains perilymphatic duct.

**coch·le·ar cu·pu·la** (kok´lē-ăr kū´pū-lă) [TA] Domelike apex of cochlea.

**coch·le·ar duct** (kok´lē-ăr dŭkt) [TA] Spiral membranous tube suspended within the cochlea, lying between and separating the scala vestibuli and scala tympani. SYN ductus cochlearis.

**co·chle·ar gan·gli·on** (kok´lē-ăr gang´

cd

glē-ŏn) [TA] Elongated ganglion of bipolar sensory nerve cell bodies on the cochlear part of the vestibulocochlear nerve in the spiral canal of the modiolus. SYN auditory ganglion.

**coch·le·ar joint** (kok′lē-ăr joynt) Hinge joint in which elevation and depression, respectively, on the opposing articular surfaces form part of a spiral.

**coch·le·ar lab·y·rinth** (kok′lē-ăr lab′i-rinth) [TA] Part of membranous labyrinth concerned with hearing (vs. the vestibular labyrinth, which is concerned with equilibration) and innervated by the cochlear nerve.

**coch·le·ar nerve** (kok′lē-ăr něrv) [TA] Section of vestibulocochlear nerve [CN VIII] peripheral to the cochlear root.

**co·chle·ar re·cess** (kok′lē-ăr rē′ses) [TA] Small depression on inner wall of the vestibule of the labyrinth at the portion of the pyramid of vestibule, between the two limbs into which the vestibular crest divides posteriorly.

**coch·le·ate** (kok′lē-āt) 1. Resembling a snail shell. 2. Denoting the appearance of a form of plate culture. [L. cochlea, a snail shell]

**coch·le·o·ves·tib·u·lar** (kok′lē-ō-ves-tib′yū-lăr) Relating to cochlea and vestibule of ear.

**code** (kōd) 1. Any system devised to convey information or facilitate communication. 2. A numeric system for ordering and classifying information. [L. codex, book]

**co·deine** (kō′dēn) Alkaloid obtained from opium; analgesic and antitussive; drug dependence may develop, but codeine is more addictive than morphine.

**cod·ing** (kōd′ing) Assigning a number to a disease process, surgical procedure, or other type of health care service for the purpose of reimbursement, health care planning, and research.

**co·do·cyte** (kō′dō-sīt) SYN target cell.

**coeliac disease** [Br.] SYN celiac disease.

**co·en·zyme** (kō-en′zīm) A substance (excluding solo metal ions) that enhances or is necessary for the action of enzymes; coenzymes are of smaller molecular size than the enzymes themselves; several vitamins are coenzyme precursors.

**co·fac·tor** (kō′fak′tŏr) An atom or molecule essential for the action of a large molecule.

**cog·ni·tion** (kog-ni′shŭn) Generic term embracing mental activities associated with thinking, learning, and memory. [L. cognitio]

**cog·ni·tive** (kog′ni-tiv) Pertaining to cognition.

**cog·wheel res·pi·ra·tion** (kog′wēl res′

pir-ā′shŭn) Inspiratory sound interrupted by one or two silent intervals.

**co·he·sion** (kō-hē′zhŭn) The attraction between molecules that holds them together. [L. co-haereo, pp. -haesus, to stick together]

**co·he·sive foil** (kō-hē′siv foyl) An extremely thin pliable sheet of metal, the surface of which has been chemically treated so as to adhere to another like material.

**co·he·sive gold** (kō-hē′siv gōld) Nearly pure gold treated so as to be free of adsorbed surface gases and impurities so that it will weld under pressure at room temperature; in dentistry, used as a restorative material placed directly into a prepared cavity and welded by pressure.

**co·hort** (kō′hōrt) Designated group followed or traced over a period. [L. cohors, retinue, military unit]

**co·in·sur·ance** (kō-in-shŭr′ăns) The amount or percentage the insured is responsible for after the deductible has been met.

**co·i·tus** (kō′i-tŭs) Sexual union. SYN pareunia, sexual intercourse. [L.]

**col** (kol) Craterlike area of interproximal oral mucosa joining lingual and buccal interdental papillae.

**col·chi·cine** (kol′chi-sin) [USP] An alkaloid obtained from Colchicum autumnale; used to treat gout.

**cold** (kōld) 1. A low temperature; the sensation produced by a temperature noticeably below an accustomed norm or a comfortable level. 2. Popular term for viral infection involving upper respiratory tract.

**cold bend test** (kōld bend test) Measurement of ability of a wire to be shaped; performed by counting number of times a wire can be bent to a right angle and reversed at the same point before breaking; important for orthodontic wires.

**cold-cure pol·y·mer·i·za·tion** (kōld′ kyūr pol′i-měr-ī-zā′shŭn) SYN autopolymerization.

**cold cure res·in** (kōld kyūr rez′in) SYN autopolymer resin.

**cold pack** (kōld pak) Pouch of cloth or other material soaked in cold water or encasing ice.

**cold sore** (kōld sōr) Colloq. usage for labial lesion due to herpes simplex virus infection.

**co·li·bac·il·lo·sis** (kō′li-bas-i-lō′sis) Diarrheal disease caused by the bacterium Escherichia coli. Often called enteric colibacillosis.

**col·ic** (kol′ik) Spasmodic pains in the abdomen. [G. kōlikos, relating to the colon]

**co·li·tis** (kō-lī′tis) Inflammation of the colon. [G. *kōlon,* colon, + *-itis,* inflammation]

**col·la·gen** (kol′ă-jen) Major protein (comprising over half of that in mammals) of white fibers of connective tissue, cartilage, and bone. [G. *koila,* glue, + *-gen,* producing]

**col·lag·en·ase** (kŏ-laj′ĕ-nās) A proteolytic enzyme that acts on collagens.

**col·la·gen dis·ease, col·la·gen-vas·cu·lar dis·ease** (kol′ă-jen di-zēz′, kol′ă-jen-vas′kyū-lăr) Generalized disorder affecting connective tissue.

**col·la·gen fi·ber, col·lag·e·nous fi·ber** (kol′ă-jen fī′bĕr, kŏ-laj′ĕ-nŭs) Individual fiber that varies in diameter from less than 1 mcm to about 12 mcm and is composed of fibrils; constitutes the principal element of irregular connective tissue, tendons, aponeuroses, and most ligaments, and occurs in the matrix of cartilage, dentin, cementum, and osseous tissue. SYN collagen fibre.

**collagen fibre** [Br.] SYN collagen fiber.

**col·lapse** (kŏ-laps′) **1.** Condition of extreme prostration, similar or identical to hypovolemic shock and due to same causes. **2.** State of profound physical depression. **3.** Failure of a physiologic system. **4.** Falling away of an organ from its surrounding structure. [L. *col-labor,* pp. *-lapsus,* to fall together]

**col·lap·se of den·tal arch** (kŏ-laps′ den′tăl ahrch) Movement of teeth to fill a space normally filled by another, missing tooth, and so a malpositioning adjacent and opposing teeth.

**col·lar** (kol′ăr) *In most contexts, the phrase cervical collar is redundant.* A band, usually denoting one encircling the neck. [L. *collare,* fr. *collum,* neck]

**col·lar bone** (kol′ăr bōn) SYN clavicle.

**col·lic·u·lus,** pl. **col·lic·u·li** (kŏ-lik′yū-lŭs, -lī) [TA] Small elevation above surrounding parts. [L. mound, dim. of *collis,* hill]

**col·li·ma·tion** (kol′i-mā′shŭn) The method, in radiology, of restricting and confining the x-ray beam to a given area and, in nuclear medicine, of restricting the detection of emitted radiations from a given area of interest. [L. *collineo,* to direct in a straight line]

**col·li·ma·tor** (kol′i-mă-tŏr) A device of high absorption coefficient material used in collimation.

**col·loid** (kol′oyd) Aggregates of atoms or molecules in a finely divided state, dispersed in a gaseous, liquid, or solid medium, and resisting sedimentation, diffusion, and filtration, thus differing from precipitates. [G. *kolla,* glue, + *eidos,* appearance]

**co·lon** (kō′lŏn) [TA] Large intestine extending from the cecum to the rectum. [G. *kolon*]

**col·on·i·za·tion** (kol′ŏn-ī-zā′shŭn) Formation of compact population groups of same type of microorganism.

**col·or blind·ness** (kŏl′ŏr blīnd′nĕs) Misleading term for anomalous or deficient color vision; complete color blindness is the absence of one of the primary cone pigments of the retina. SYN colour blindness.

**col·or-co·ded re·fer·ence mark·ing** (kŏ′lŏr-kō′dĕd ref′ĕr-ĕns mahrk′ing) Colored band on the World Health Organization probe located 3.5–5.5 mm from the probe tip, used when examining using the Periodontal Screening and Recording System.

**col·or taste** (kŏl′ŏr tāst) Synesthesia in which color sense and taste are associated, with stimulation of either sense inducing a subjective sensation in the associated sense. SYN colour taste.

**colour blindness** [Br.] SYN color blindness.

**colour taste** [Br.] SYN color taste.

**col·u·mel·la coch·le·ae** (kol′yū-mel′ă kok′lē-ē) SYN modiolus of angle of mouth.

**col·u·mel·la na·si** (kol′ū-mel′ă nā′sī) Nasal skin investing medial crura of the lower lateral cartilages and separating the nostrils.

**co·ma** (kō′mă) Profound unconsciousness from which one cannot be roused; may be due to the action of an ingested toxic substance or of one formed in the body, to trauma, or to disease. [G. *kōma,* deep sleep, trance]

**co·ma·tose** (kō′mă-tōs) *Avoid the illegitimate form comatosed.* In a state of coma.

**com·bi·na·tion clasp** (kom′bi-nā′shŭn klasp) Fitting on a removable partial denture with both wrought-wire and cast stabilizing arms.

**com·bi·na·tion res·to·ra·tion** (kom′bi-nā′shŭn res′tŏr-ā′shŭn) Dental therapy with two or more materials applied in layers.

**com·mi·nut·ed frac·ture** (kom′i-nū′tĕd frak′shŭr) A fracture in which the bone is broken into pieces.

**Com·mis·sion of Den·tal Ac·cred·i·ta·tion of Can·a·da (CDAC)** (kŏ-mish′ŏn den′tăl ă-kred′i-tā′shŭn kan′ă-dă) Established by the Canadian Dental Association, this nongovernmental body is responsible for accrediting dental, dental hygiene, and dental assisting programs across Canada.

**com·mis·sur·al chei·li·tis** (kom′i-shŭr′ăl kī-lī′tis) SYN angular cheilitis.

**com·mis·sure** (kom′i-shŭr) [TA] **1.** Angle or corner of the eye, lips, or labia. **2.** A bundle of nerve fibers passing from one side in the brain or spinal cord to the other.

**com·mis·sure of lips (of mouth)** (kom´i-shŭr lips mowth) SYN labial commissure (of mouth).

**com·mon coch·le·ar ar·te·ry** (kom´ŏn kok´lē-ăr ahr´tĕr-ē) [TA] *Origin:* as a terminal branch, with the anterior vestibular artery, of the labyrinthine artery; *distribution:* runs in the cochlear axis of modiolus serving the spiral ganglia; sends the proper cochlear artery to the cochlear duct and supplies the apical two turns of the spiral modiolar artery.

**com·mon fa·cial vein** (kom´ŏn fā´shăl vān) Short vessel formed by union of facial vein and the retromandibular vein, emptying into jugular vein.

**com·mon mi·graine** (kom´ŏn mī´grān) Migraine headache without the visual prodrome, which is not limited to one side of head but nevertheless recognizable because of stereotyped course; relief is produced by sleep.

**com·mon salt** (kom´ŏn sawlt) SYN sodium chloride.

**com·mu·ni·ca·ble dis·ease** (kŏ-myūn´i-kă-bĕl di-zēz´) Disorder that is transmissible by infection or contagion directly or through the agency of a vector.

**com·mu·ni·ca·ble pe·ri·od (of a dis·ease)** (kŏ-myūn´i-kă-bĕl pēr´ē-ŏd di-zēz´) Temporal interval during which an infectious agent may be transferred directly or indirectly from an infected person to a susceptible host; may include, or may overlap, the incubation period of a disease.

**com·mu·ni·ca·ting branch of chor·da tym·pa·ni with lin·gual nerve** (kŏ-myūn´i-kāt-ing branch kōr´dă tim´pă-nī ling´gwăl nĕrv) [TA] Terminal branch of chorda tympani joining the lingual nerve in the infratemporal fossa.

**com·mu·ni·ca·tion** (kŏ-myūn´i-kā´shŭn) **1.** An opening or connecting passage between two structures. **2.** In anatomy, a joining or connecting, said of fibrous solid structures.

**com·mu·ni·ty den·tis·try** (kŏ-myū´ni-tē den´tis-trē) Public health dentistry, with an academic base, emphasizing the professional obligation to foster the delivery of prevention, education, and care to populations.

**com·mu·ni·ty nurse** (kŏ-myū´ni-tē nŭrs) SYN public health nurse.

**Com·mu·ni·ty Pe·ri·o·don·tal In·dex of Treat·ment Needs (CPITN)** (kŏ-myū´ni-tē per´ē-ō-don´tăl in´deks trēt´mĕnt nēdz) An assessment of periodontal requirements that divides mouth into sextants and uses a standard probe for examinations.

**com·pact bone** (kŏm-pakt´ bōn) [TA] Noncancellous portion of bone that consists largely of concentric lamellar osteons and interstitial lamellae. SYN substantia compacta [TA].

**com·pac·tion** (kŏm-pak´shŭn) Act of compression or squeezing together. [L. *compactio,* fr. *com-pingo,* pp. *com-pactus,* to press together]

**com·part·ment** (kŏm-pahrt´mĕnt) Partitioned-off portion of a larger bound space; a separate section or chamber.

**com·part·ment syn·drome** (kŏm-pahrt´mĕnt sin´drōm) Condition in which increased pressure in a confined anatomic space adversely affects circulation and threatens function and viability of structures therein.

**com·pat·i·ble** (kŏm-pat´i-bĕl) Capable of being mixed without undergoing destructive chemical change. [L. *con-,* with, + *patior,* to suffer]

**com·pen·sat·ed ac·i·do·sis** (kom´pĕn-sāt-ĕd as´i-dō´sis) An acidosis in which the pH of body fluids is normal; compensation is achieved by respiratory or renal mechanisms.

**com·pen·sat·ed al·ka·lo·sis** (kom´pĕn-sāt-ĕd al´kă-lō´sis) Disorder in which there is a change in bicarbonate but the pH of body fluids approaches normal.

**com·pen·sat·ed met·a·bol·ic al·ka·lo·sis** (kom´pĕn-sā-tĕd met´ă-bol´ik al´kă-lō´sis) Retention of acid, primarily carbon dioxide by lung and acid ions by the renal tubules, to reduce the effect on blood pH of excess alkali produced by ingestion or metabolism of alkali-producing substances.

**com·pen·sat·ed res·pi·ra·to·ry ac·i·do·sis** (kom´pĕn-sā-tĕd res´pir-ă-tōr-ē as´i-dō´sis) Retention of bicarbonate by renal tubules to minimize the effect on blood pH of carbon dioxide retention by the lungs.

**com·pen·sat·ed res·pi·ra·to·ry al·ka·lo·sis** (kom´pĕn-sā-tĕd res´pir-ă-tōr-ē al´kă-lō´sis) Increased excretion of acid ions by the kidney to minimize the effect on blood pH of excessive loss of carbon dioxide through the lungs.

**com·pen·sat·ing curve** (kom´pĕn-sāt´ing kŭrv) Anteroposterior and lateral curvature in alignment of occluding surfaces and incisal edges of artificial teeth; used to develop balanced occlusion.

**com·pen·sa·tion** (kom´pĕn-sā´shŭn) A process in which a tendency for a change in a given direction is counteracted by another change so that the original change is not evident.

**com·pe·tence** (kom´pĕ-tĕns) The quality of being competent or capable of performing an allotted function.

**com·pe·tent** (kom′pĕ-tĕnt) Capable or qualified; able to perform a task or function. [L. *competo,* to be suitable]

**com·plaint** (kŏm-plānt′) A disorder, disease, or symptom, or the description of it. [O.Fr. *complainte,* fr. L. *complango,* to lament]

**com·ple·ment** (kom′plĕ-mĕnt) Thermolabile substance, normally present in serum, which is destructive to bacteria and other cells sensitized by a specific complement-fixing antibody. [L. *complementum,* that which completes, fr. *com-pleo,* to fill up]

**com·ple·men·tal air** (kom′plĕ-ment′ăl ār) SYN inspiratory reserve volume.

**com·ple·men·ta·ry and al·ter·na·tive med·i·cine (CAM)** (kom′plĕ-men′ tăr-ē awl-tĕr′nă-tiv med′i-sin) Heterogeneous group of hygienic, diagnostic, and therapeutic philosophies and practices whose principles and techniques diverge from those of modern scientific medicine. SYN holistic medicine (2).

**com·ple·ment fix·a·tion** (kom′plĕ-mĕnt fik-sā′shŭn) A process in serum whereby an antigen-antibody combination is rendered unavailable to complete a reaction in a second antigen-antibody combination for which complement is necessary.

**com·plete blood count** (kŏm-plēt′ blŭd kownt) Laboratory-based combination of: red blood cell count, white blood cell count, erythrocyte indices, hematocrit, differential blood count, and often a platelet count.

**com·plete cross-bite** (kŏm-plēt′ kraws′ bīt) Abnormal displacement that is present when all the teeth in one arch are positioned either inside or outside of all the teeth of the opposing arch.

**com·plete crown** (kŏm-plēt′ krown) SYN full crown.

**com·plete den·ture** (kom′plēt den′chŭr) Dental prosthesis that is a substitute for the lost natural dentition and associated structures of the maxillae or mandible. SYN full denture.

**com·plete den·ture im·pres·sion** (kŏm-plēt′ den′chŭr im-presh′ŭn) 1. Impression of edentulous arch made to construct a complete denture. 2. Negative registration of entire denture-bearing, stabilizing area of either the maxillae or mandible. 3. Negative registration of entire denture foundation and border seal areas in an edentulous mouth.

▣**com·plete den·ture pros·the·sis** (kŏm-plēt′ den′chŭr pros-thē′sis) Removable prosthesis that replaces the entire dentition for function and aesthetics. See this page.

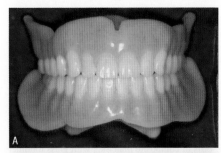
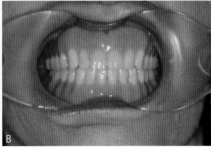

**complete denture prosthesis:** (A) as received from laboratory; (B) in place

**com·plete den·ture pros·tho·don·tics** (kŏm-plēt′ den′chŭr pros′thŏ-don′tiks) Knowledge and skills about restoration of the edentulous arch with a removable prosthesis.

**com·plex** (kom′pleks, kŏm-pleks′) 1. A structural anatomic entity made up of three or more interrelated parts. 2. An informal term used to denote a group of individual structures known or believed to be related anatomically, embryologically, or physiologically. [L. *complexus,* woven together]

**com·plex joint** (kŏm-pleks′ joynt) [TA] Joint composed of three or more skeletal elements, or in which two anatomically separate joints function as a unit.

▣**com·plex o·don·to·ma** (kŏm-pleks′ ō-′don-tō′mă) Odontoma in which various odontogenic tissues are organized in a haphazard arrangement with no resemblance to teeth. See page A16.

**com·plex par·tial sei·zure** (kŏm-pleks′ pahr′shăl sē′zhŭr) Seizure with impairment of consciousness, occurring in a patient with focal epilepsy.

**com·plex re·gion·al pain syn·drome (type I)** (kŏm-pleks′ rē′jŭn-ăl pān sin′drōm tīp) Diffuse persistent pain usually in a limb; frequently follows some local injury.

**com·plex shank** (kŏm-pleks′ shangk) Shank bent in two planes (front-to-back and side-to-side) to facilitate instrumentation of posterior teeth. SYN straight shank.

**com·pli·ance** (kŏm-plī′ăns) Consistency and accuracy with which a patient follows any regimen prescribed by dentist, physician, or other health care professional. [M.E. fr. O.Fr., fr. L. *compleo,* to fulfill]

**com·pli·ca·tion** (kom′pli-kā′shŭn) Morbid process or event that occurs during course of a disease but is not an essential part of it.

**com·po·mer** (kom′pŏ-mĕr) Material used for cementation of fixed crowns and bridges and also for some dental restorations; combines benefits of composite materials with glass ionomer cements. [*compo*site + poly*mer*]

**com·po·nent** (kŏm-pō′nĕnt) An element forming a part of the whole. [L. *com-pono,* pp. *-positus,* to place together]

**com·po·nent man·age·ment** (kŏm-pō′ nĕnt man′ăj-mĕnt) Approach to health care cost containment that involves trying to control individual components.

**com·po·nents of mas·ti·ca·tion** (kŏm-pō′nĕnts mas′ti-kā′shŭn) Various jaw movements made during act of chewing, as determined by the neuromuscular system, the temporomandibular articulations, the teeth, and the food being chewed; divided, for purposes of analysis or description, into opening, closing, left lateral, right lateral, and anteroposterior components.

**com·po·nents of oc·clu·sion** (kŏm-pō′ nĕnts ŏ-klū′zhŭn) Factors involved in occlusion (e.g., temporomandibular joint, associated neuromusculature, teeth, denture-supporting structures).

**com·pos·ite** (kŏm-poz′it) A colloquial term for resin materials used in restorative dentistry. [L. *compositus,* put together, fr. *compono,* to put together]

**com·pos·ite core** (kŏm-poz′it kōr) Restoration made of resin composite intended to replace lost tooth structure under a crown; provides support and retention for the crown.

**com·pos·ite den·tal ce·ment** (kŏm-poz′it den′tăl sĕ-ment′) Organic dental cement modified by inclusion of inorganic materials treated with a coupling agent to bond them to polymers. Colloq. term is composite cement.

**com·pos·ite graft** (kŏm-poz′it graft) A graft made up of several structures (e.g., skin and cartilage, full-thickness segment of the ear).

**com·pos·ite o·don·to·ma** (kŏm-poz′it ō′don-tō′mă) SYN compound odontoma.

**com·pos·ite res·in** (kŏm-poz′it rez′in) Synthetic resin usually acrylic based, to which a glass or natural silica filter has been added. Used mainly in dental restorative procedures. [L. *compositus,* put together, fr. *compono,* to put together]

**com·pos men·tis** (kom′pos men′tis) Of sound mind; usually used in its opposite form.

**com·pound** (kom′pownd) **1.** CHEMISTRY a substance formed by the covalent or electrostatic union of two or more atoms, generally differing entirely in physical characteristics from its components. **2.** PHARMACY denoting a preparation of several ingredients.

**com·pound ca·ries** (kom′pownd kar′ēz) **1.** Caries involving more than one surface of a tooth. **2.** Two or more carious lesions joined to form one cavity.

**com·pound frac·ture** (kom′pownd frak′ shŭr) SYN open fracture.

⊞**com·pound o·don·to·ma** (kom′pownd ō′don-tō′mă) Odontoma in which the odontogenic tissues are organized and resemble anomalous teeth. See page A16. SYN composite odontoma.

**com·pound res·tor·a·tion** (kom′pownd res′tŏr-ā′shŭn) Restoration of more than one surface of a tooth.

**com·pre·hen·sion** (kom′prē-hen′shŭn) Knowledge or understanding of something.

**com·pre·hen·sive den·tal care** (kom′ prē-hen′siv den′tăl kār) Concept that includes not only traditional treatment of dental disease but also prevention and early detection.

**com·pressed tab·let** (kŏm-prest′ tab′lĕt) Tablet prepared, usually as a large-scale production, by means of great pressure; most consist of the active ingredient and a diluent, binder, disintegrator, and lubricant.

**com·pres·sion** (kŏm-presh′ŭn) A squeezing together; the exertion of pressure on a body in such a way as to tend to increase its density.

**com·pres·sion mold·ing** (kŏm-presh′ŭn mōld′ing) **1.** Pressing or squeezing together to form a shape in a mold. **2.** Adaptation of a plastic material to the negative form of a split mold by pressure. SEE ALSO injection molding.

**com·pres·sion of tis·sue** (kŏm-presh′ŭn tish′ū) SYN tissue displaceability.

**com·pres·sive strength** (kŏm-pres′iv strength) Ability of a material to resist stress under compression.

**com·pres·sor** (kŏm-pres′ŏr) **1.** A muscle, the contraction of which causes compression of any structure. **2.** An instrument for placing pressure on a body part.

**com·pul·sion** (kŏm-pŭl′shŭn) Uncontrollable thoughts or impulses to perform an act, often repetitively, as an unconscious mechanism to avoid unacceptable ideas and desires that, by themselves, arouse anxiety. [L. *compello* pp. *-pulsus,* to drive together, compel]

**com·put·ed ra·di·og·ra·phy** (kŏm-pyū′

tĕd rā´dē-og´ră-fē) Converting transmitted x-rays into light, using a solid-state imaging device and recovering and processing the image using a digital computer; image may then be printed or displayed on a computer screen.

**com·put·ed to·mog·ra·phy (CT)** (kŏm-pyū´tĕd tŏ-mog´ră-fē) Imaging anatomic information from a cross-sectional plane of the body, each image generated by a computer synthesis of x-ray transmission data obtained in many different directions in a given plane.

**com·put·er** (kŏm-pyū´tĕr) A programmable electronic device that can be used to store and manipulate data to carry out designated functions.

**com·put·er-aid·ed de·sign/com·put·er-aid·ed man·u·fac·tur·ing (CAD/CAM)** (kŏm-pyū´tĕr-ā´dĕd dĕ-zīn´, man´yū-fak´chŭr-ing) Process by which an object is designed on a computer before information is transferred to a device that produces the item according to determined design specification; used in fabrication of crowns.

**con A** Abbreviation for concanavalin A.

**CO₂ nar·co·sis** (nahr-kō´sis) SYN hypoventilation coma.

**con·cam·er·a·tion** (kŏn-kam´ĕr-ā´shŭn) A system of interconnecting cavities. [L. *concameratio*, a vault; fr. *concamero*, pp. *-atus*, to vault over, fr. *camera*, a vault]

**con·ca·nav·a·lin A (con A)** (kon-kă-nav´ă-lin) A phytomitogen, extracted from the jack bean (*Canavalia ensiformis*), which agglutinates the blood of mammals and reacts with glucosans.

**⊞con·cav·i·ty** (kŏn-kav´i-tē) A hollow or depression, with more or less evenly curved sides, on any surface. See this page.

**con·ca·vo·con·vex** (kŏn-kā´vō-kon´veks) Concave on one surface and convex on the opposite surface.

**con·cen·tra·tion** (kon´sĕn-trā´shŭn) A preparation made by extracting a crude drug, precipitating it from the solution, and drying it. [L. *con-*, together, + *centrum*, center]

**con·cen·tric con·trac·tion** (kŏn-sen´trik kŏn-trak´shŭn) Muscular contraction producing movement as the result of shortening or decreasing the length of the muscle.

**con·cha,** pl. **con·chae** (kong´kă, -kē) [TA] In anatomy, a structure comparable with a shell in shape. [L. a shell]

**con·chal crest** (kong´kăl krest) [TA] Bony ridge that articulates with, or provides attachment for, the inferior nasal concha.

**con·chal crest of bod·y of max·il·la** (kong´kăl krest bod´ē mak-sil´ă) [TA] Ridge of

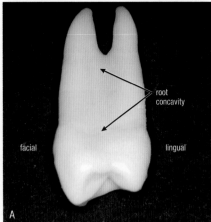

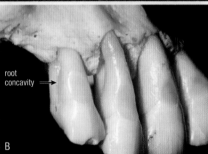

concavity on mesial surface of maxillary premolar tooth: (A) maxillary right first premolar showing linear mesial concavity commonly found on this tooth; (B) distal root concavity on maxillary first premolar exposed during a periodontal surgical procedure

the nasal surface of the body of the maxilla that articulates with the inferior nasal concha.

**con·chal crest of pal·a·tine bone** (kong´kăl krest pal´ă-tīn bōn) [TA] Ridge on nasal surface of the perpendicular part of palatine bone to which the inferior nasal concha attaches.

**con·cha of aur·i·cle** (kong´kă awr´i-kĕl) [TA] Large hollow, or floor of the auricle, between the anterior portion of the helix and the antihelix; it is divided by the crus of the helix into the cymba above and the cavum, below.

**con·choi·dal** (kŏn-koy´dăl) Shaped like a shell; having alternate convexities and concavities on the surface. [*concha* + G. *eidos*, appearance]

**con·com·i·tant symp·tom** (kŏn-kom´i-tănt simp´tŏm) SYN accessory symptom.

**con·cor·dance** (kŏn-kōr´dăns) A negotiated, shared agreement between dentist and patient concerning treatment regimen(s), outcomes, and behaviors; a more cooperative relationship than those based on issues of compliance and noncompliance. [L. *concordia,* agreeing, harmony]

**con·cres·cence** (kŏn-kres′ĕns) In dentistry, the union of the roots of two adjacent teeth by cementum. See this page.

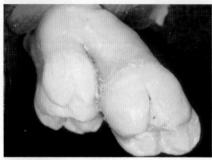

concrescence

**con·den·sa·tion** (kon′dĕn-sā′shŭn) In dentistry, the process of packing a filling material into a cavity, using such force and direction that no voids result. [L. *con-denso,* pp. *-atus,* to make thick, condense]

**con·dense** (kŏn-dens′) To pack; to increase density of something; applied particularly to insertion of gold foil or silver amalgam in a cavity prepared in a tooth. See this page.

**con·dens·er** (kŏn-den′sĕr) In dentistry, a manual or powered instrument used for packing a plastic or unset material into a cavity of a tooth; variation in sizes and shapes allows conformation of the mass to the cavity outline. SYN endodontic plugger, root canal plugger (2).

**con·di·tion·er** (kŏn-dish′ŭ-nĕr) A substance added to another to increase its suitability (e.g., in sealant placement, acid etchant is placed on the enamel to prepare it for bonding with the sealant).

**con·duct·ing air·way** (kŏn-dŭkt′ing ār′wā) Airway from nasal cavity to a terminal bronchiole.

**con·duc·tion** (kŏn-dŭk′shŭn) Transmitting or conveying energy, from one point to another, without evident movement in conducting body. [L. *con-duco,* pp. *ductus,* to lead, conduct]

**con·duc·tion an·es·the·si·a** (kŏn-dŭk′shŭn an′es-thē′zē-ă) Regional anesthesia in which local anesthetic solution is injected about nerves to inhibit nerve transmission. SYN block anesthesia.

**con·duc·tion block** (kŏn-dŭk′shŭn blok) Failure of impulse transmission at some point along a nerve fiber, although conduction along the segments proximal and distal to it are unaffected; clinically, most often the result of an area of focal demyelination or, less often, transient ischemia.

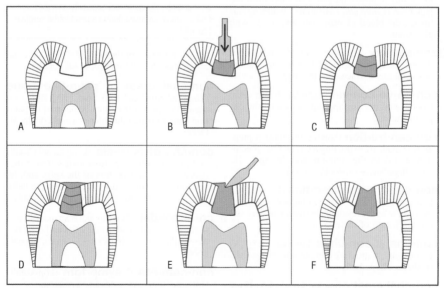

**condensing and carving procedures:** (A) cavity preparation; (B) first amalgam increment is placed in preparation and condensed to eliminate open spaces (voids); (C, D) second and sucessive increments are placed until preparation is overfilled; (E, F) while gel remains "soft", material is carved to reproduce correct anatomic contours

**con·duc·tive hear·ing loss** (kŏn-dŭk'tiv hēr'ing laws) Hearing loss caused by an obstruction in the outer ear, middle ear, or both.

**con·duc·tiv·i·ty** (kon'dŭk-tiv'i-tē) The power of transmission or conveyance of energy, without perceptible motion in the conducting body.

**con·duc·tor** (kŏn-dŭk'tŏr) **1.** A probe or sound with a groove along which a knife is passed in slitting open a sinus or fistula; a grooved director.

**con·dy·lar** (kon'di-lăr) Relating to a condyle.

**con·dy·lar ax·is** (kon'di-lăr ak'sis) A line through the two mandibular condyles around which the mandible may rotate during a part of the opening movement. SYN condyle cord, hinge-orbital axis, mandibular axis (2).

**con·dy·lar ca·nal** (kon'di-lăr kă-nal') [TA] Inconstant opening through the occipital bone posterior to the condyle on each side that transmits the occipital emissary vein.

**con·dy·lar guid·ance** (kon'di-lăr gī'dăns) The mechanical device on an articulator that is intended to produce guidance in articulator movement, similar to those produced by the paths of the condyles in the temporomandibular joints. SEE ALSO condylar guidance inclination.

**con·dy·lar guid·ance in·cli·na·tion** (kon'di-lăr gī'dăns in'kli-nā'shŭn) The angle of inclination of the condylar guidance to an accepted horizontal plane.

**con·dy·lar guide** (kon'di-lăr gīd) That portion of a mechanical articulation device intended to direct movement of those portions of the device that simulate the condylar processes of the mandible along pathways similar to those occurring when the mandibular condyles move about the temporomandibular joints.

**con·dy·lar guide in·cli·na·tion** (kon'di-lăr gīd in'kli-nā'shŭn) Angle of inclination in relation to the horizontal plane of the condylar guide apparatus of an articulation device.

**con·dy·lar hinge po·si·tion** (kon'di-lăr hinj pŏ-zish'ŭn) **1.** The position of the condyles in the temporomandibular joints from which a hinge movement is possible. **2.** The maxillomandibular relation from which a consciously stimulated true hinge movement can be executed.

**con·dy·lar pro·cess of man·di·ble** (kon'di-lăr pros'es man'di-bĕl) [TA] The articular process of the ramus of the mandible; it includes the head of the mandible, the neck of the mandible and pterygoid fovea.

**con·dy·lar pro·tru·sive path** (kon'di-lăr prō-trū'siv path) Direction of the condyle when the mandible is protruded from a centric position.

**con·dy·lar·thro·sis** (kon'dil-ahr-thrō'sis) A joint, like that of the knee, formed by condylar surfaces. [G. *kondylos,* condyle, + *arthrōsis,* a jointing]

**con·dyle** (kon'dīl) [TA] A rounded articular surface at the extremity of a bone.

**con·dyle cord** (kon'dīl kōrd) SYN condylar axis.

**con·dy·lec·to·my** (kon'di-lek'tŏ-mē) Excision of a condyle. [G. *kondylos,* condyle, + *ektomē,* excision]

**con·dyle path** (kon'dīl path) Trajectory of real or putative condylar point during movement. In research, image-defined condylar landmarks matched with jaw movement recordings will result in actual condylar paths. Clinically, a putative condylar point located by palpation for determining landmarks (e.g., terminal hinge axis) will be tracked during jaw movement to create a condyle path; also frequently used to describe movement of condylar sphere of an articulator.

**con·dyle rod** (kon'dīl rod) Adjustable fittings on a facebow that are placed over the patient's condyles or facial points marking the opening axis of the mandible.

**con·dyl·i·on** (kon-dil'ē-on) Point on lateral outer or medial inner surface of condyle of mandible. [G. *kondylion,* dim. of *kondylos,* condyle]

**con·dy·loid** (kon'di-loyd) Relating to or resembling a condyle. [G. *kondylōdēs,* like a knuckle, fr. *kondylos,* condyle, + *eidos,* resemblance]

🔲**con·dy·lo·ma a·cu·mi·na·tum** (kon-di-lō'mă ă-kū-mi-nā'tŭm) A warty growth on the external genitals or at the anus. See page A13. SYN genital wart, venereal wart.

**con·dy·lo·plas·ty** (kon'di-lō-plas-tē) A surgical procedure to alter the shape of a condyle.

**con·dy·lot·o·my** (kon'di-lot'ŏ-mē) Division, without removal, of a condyle. [G. *kondylos,* condyle, + *tomē,* incision]

✿**-cone** Suffix that denotes cusp of a tooth in upper jaw.

**cone** (kōn) **1.** A surface joining a circle to a point above the plane containing the circle. **2.** Metallic cylinder or truncated cone used to confine a beam of x-rays. [G. *kōnos,* cone]

🔲**cone-cut** (kōn'kŭt) Manifestation visible in a dental radiograph in which a portion of the image is missing due to the radiation beam's having been blocked by improper aim of the cone or position-indicating device (q.v.). See page 138.

**con·fi·den·ti·al·i·ty** (kon'fi-den-shē-al'i-tē) The legally protected right afforded to (and duty required of) specifically designated health care professionals not to disclose information dis-

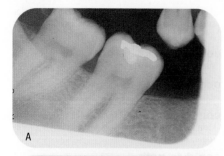

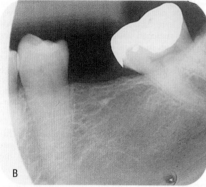

cone-cut: (A) rectangular position-indicating device (PID); (B) circular PID

tumor of the alveolar ridge, of unknown histogenesis. See this page.

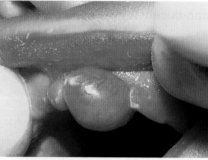

congenital epulis of newborn

cerned or communicated during consultation with a patient. [L. *con-fido,* to trust, be assured]

**con·flict of in·ter·est** (kon'flik in'tĕr-ĕst) Contradiction between the professional or personal interests and needs of a health care provider and his or her professional responsibilities toward a patient.

**con·flu·ence of si·nus·es** (kon-flū'ĕns sī'nŭs-ĕz) [TA] Meeting place, at the internal occipital protuberance, of the superior sagittal, straight, and occipital sinuses, drained by the two transverse sinuses of the dura mater.

**con·fu·sion** (kŏn-fyū'zhŭn) A mental state in which reactions to environmental stimuli are inappropriate. [L. *confusio,* a confounding]

**con·gen·i·tal** (kŏn-jen'i-tăl) *Do not confuse this word with hereditary, heredofamilial, familial, or genetic.* Existing at birth. [L. *congenitus,* born with]

**con·gen·i·tal ec·to·der·mal dys·pla·si·a** (kŏn-jen'i-tăl ek'tō-dĕr'măl dis-plā'zhē-ă) Incomplete development of epidermis and skin appendages; skin is smooth and hairless, the facies abnormal, and teeth and nails may be affected; sweating may be deficient.

**con·gen·i·tal ep·u·lis of new·born** (kŏn-jen'i-tăl ep-yū'lis nū'bōrn) Benign nodular

**con·gen·i·tal fa·cial di·ple·gi·a** (kŏn-jen'i-tăl fā'shăl dī-plē'jē-ă) SYN Moebius syndrome.

**con·gen·i·tal hy·po·phos·pha·ta·si·a** (kŏn-jen'i-tăl hī'pō-fos-fă-tā'zē-ă) Disorder associated with a low serum alkaline phosphatase, skeletal abnormalities, pathologic fractures, craniostenosis, premature loss of teeth, and often early death.

**con·gen·i·tal hy·po·thy·roid·ism** (kŏn-jen'i-tăl hī'pō-thī'royd-izm) Lack of thyroid secretion.

**con·gen·i·tal met·he·mo·glob·i·ne·mi·a** (kŏn-jen'i-tăl met-hē'mō-glō-bi-nē'mē-ă) 1. Methemoglobinemia due to formation of any one of a group of abnormal α chain or β chain hemoglobins collectively known as hemoglobin M. 2. Methemoglobinemia due to deficiency of cytochrome $b_5$ reductase or methemoglobin reductase.

**con·gen·i·tal syph·i·lis** (kŏn-jen'i-tăl sif'i-lis) Syphilis acquired by the fetus in utero, thus present at birth.

**con·ges·tion** (kŏn-jes'chŭn) Presence of an abnormal amount of fluid in the vessels or passages of a part or organ; especially, used of blood due to either increased influx or to an obstruction to outflow. [L. *congestio,* a bringing together, a heap, fr. *con-gero,* pp. *-gestus,* to bring together]

**con·ges·tive heart fail·ure (CHF)** (kŏn-jes'tiv hahrt fāl'yŭr) SYN heart failure (1).

**-conid** Suffix denoting cusp of tooth in lower jaw.

**con·ju·gate** (kon'jŭ-găt) [TA] Joined or paired, conjugated. [L. *conjugatus,* joined together]

**con·ju·ga·tion** (kon'jŭ-gā'shŭn) 1. An alternating sequence of multiple and single chemical bonds in a chemical compound. 2. Joining together of two compounds. [L. *con-jugo,* pp. *-jugatus,* to join together]

**con·junc·ti·va,** pl. **con·junc·ti·vae** (kŏn-jŭngk'tiv-ă, -ē) [TA] The mucous membrane investing the anterior surface of the eyeball and the posterior surface of the lids. [L. fem. of *conjunctivus,* from *conjungo,* pp. *-junctus,* to bind together]

**con·junc·ti·vi·tis** (kŏn-jŭngk'ti-vī'tis) Inflammation of conjunctiva.

**con·nec·tive tis·sue** (kŏ-nek'tiv tish'ū) Physical or functional supporting tissue of the animal body, a major constituent of which (in addition to various kinds of cells) is an extracellular matrix of ground substance, protein fibers, and structural glycoproteins; derived from the mesenchyme, which in turn is derived mainly from mesoderm.

**con·nec·tive-tis·sue dis·ease** (kŏ-nek' tiv-tish'ū di-zēz') One of a group of generalized diseases affecting connective tissue, especially those not inherited as mendelian characteristics.

**con·nec·tive tis·sue group** (kŏ-nek'tiv tish'ū grūp) Collective name for mucous tissue, dentin, bone, cartilage, and ordinary connective tissue, all derived from the mesenchyme.

**con·nec·tor** (kŏ-nek'tŏr) In dentistry, part of a partial denture that unites its components.

**con·nec·tor bar** (kŏn-nek'tŏr bahr) Piece of metal, longer than it is wide, which connects components of a removable partial denture. SEE major connector, minor connector.

**Conn syn·drome** (kon sin'drōm) SYN primary aldosteronism.

**con·san·guin·i·ty** (kon'sang-gwin'i-tē) Kinship because of common ancestry. [L. *consanguinitas,* blood relationship]

**con·scious** (kon'shŭs) **1.** Aware; having present knowledge or perception of oneself, one's acts, and surroundings. **2.** Denoting something occurring with the perceptive attention of the individual. [L. *conscius,* knowing]

**con·scious·ness** (kon'shŭs-nĕs) State of being aware, or perceiving physical facts or mental concepts; a state of general wakefulness and responsiveness to environment; a functioning sensorium. [L. *conscio,* to know, to be aware of]

**con·scious se·da·tion** (kon'shŭs sĕ-dā' shŭn) Sedation during which the subject is kept from losing consciousness and receives sufficient analgesia to allow the procedure for which sedation is essential to proceed.

**con·sen·su·al** (kŏn-sen'shū-ăl) With consent; by mutual agreement of all parties. [L. *consentio,* pp. *con-sensus,* to agree + *-al*]

**con·ser·va·tion** (kon'sĕr-vā'shŭn) **1.** Pres-

ervation from loss, injury, or decay. **2.** Retention of structure with a variation in environment or other conditions.

**con·ser·va·tive** (kŏn-sĕr'vă-tiv) Denoting treatment by gradual, limited, or well-established procedures, as opposed to radical.

**Con·sol·i·da·ted Om·ni·bus Bud·get Re·con·cil·i·a·tion Act (COBRA)** (kŏn-sol'i-dā-tĕd om'ni-bŭs bŭj'ĕt rek'ŏn-sil-ē-ā'shŭn akt) U.S. federal law that allows an employee to remain covered under employer's group health insurance plan for a given period of time after death of a spouse, divorce, termination, or having work hours reduced.

**con·so·nant** (kon'sŏ-nănt) A speech sound produced by partial or complete obstruction to the flow of air at any point in the vocal apparatus. [L. *consono,* to sound together]

**con·so·nat·ing rale** (kon'sŏ-nāt-ing rahl) Resonant rale produced in a bronchial tube and heard through consolidated lung tissue.

**con·sti·pa·tion** (kon'sti-pā'shŭn) A condition in which bowel movements are infrequent or incomplete. [L. *con-stipo,* pp. *-atus,* to press together]

**con·sti·tu·tion** (kon'sti-tū'shŭn) The physical makeup of a body, including the mode of performance of its functions, the activity of its metabolic processes, the manner and degree of its reactions to stimuli, and its power of resistance to the attack of pathogenic organisms or other disease processes. [L. *constitutio,* constitution, disposition, fr. *constituo,* pp. *-stitutus,* to establish, fr. *statuo,* to set up]

**con·sti·tu·tion·al symp·tom** (kon'sti-tū'shŭn-ăl simp'tŏm) Symptom indicating a systemic effect of a disease; e.g., weight loss.

**con·stric·tion** (kŏn-strik'shŭn) **1.** [TA] A normally or pathologically contracted or narrowed portion of a structure. **2.** The act or process of binding or contracting, becoming narrowed; the condition of being constricted or squeezed. [L. *con-stringo,* pp. *-strictus,* to draw together]

**con·struct** (kon'strŭkt) Combination of a bone graft, metal instrumentation, prosthetic devices, and/or bone cement applied to a specific level of the skeleton in the course of reconstructive, dental, or fracture surgery.

**con·sul·tant** (kŏn-sŭl'tănt) A physician or surgeon who does not take full responsibility for a patient, but acts in an advisory capacity. [L. *consulto,* pp. *-atus,* to deliberate, ask advice]

**con·sul·ta·tion** (kon'sŭl-tā'shŭn) Meeting of two or more dentists, physicians, or surgeons to evaluate the nature and progress of disease in a particular patient and to establish diagnosis, prognosis, and therapy.

**con·sump·tion** (kŏn-sŭmp'shŭn) The using up of something, especially the rate at which it is used. [L. *con-sumo*, pp. *-sumptus*, to take up wholly, use up, waste]

**con·sump·tion co·ag·u·lop·a·thy** (kŏn-sŭmp'shŭn kō-ag'yū-lop'ă-thē) A disorder in which marked reductions develop in blood concentrations of platelets with exhaustion of the coagulation factors in the peripheral blood due to disseminated intravascular coagulation.

**con·tact** (kon'takt) The touching or apposition of two bodies. [L. *con-tingo*, pp. *-tactus*, to touch, seize, fr. *tango*, to touch]

**con·tact al·ler·gy** (kon'takt al'ĕr-jē) SYN allergic contact dermatitis.

**con·tact ar·ea** (kon'takt ar'ē-ă) Part of proximal surface of a tooth that touches adjacent tooth mesially or distally. SYN point of proximal contact.

**con·tact chei·li·tis** (kon'takt kī-lī'tis) Inflammation of the lips resulting from contact with a primary irritant or specific allergen, including ingredients of lipsticks.

**con·tact der·ma·ti·tis** (kon'takt dĕr'mă-tī'tis) Inflammatory rash marked by itching and redness resulting from cutaneous contact with a specific allergen or irritant.

**con·tact point** (kon'takt poynt) Area of union or junction of surfaces that are not completely contiguous.

**con·tact sto·ma·ti·tis** (kon'takt stō'mă-tī'tis) Delayed hypersensitivity reaction with possible intraoral involvement; reaction to antiseptics, antibiotic lozenges, lipstick, lip balm, and sunscreens may cause the lips to swell, fissure, or roughen. Some dental appliances that contain heavy metals (e.g., cobalt, mercury, nickel, silver) may elicit mucosal reactions. Allergy to the free monomer found in dentures is rare.

**con·tact sur·face of tooth** (kon'takt sŭr'făs tūth) SYN approximal surface of tooth.

**con·ta·gion** (kŏn-tā'jŭn) Transmission of infection by direct contact, droplet spread, or contaminated fomites. [L. *contagio;* fr. *contingo*, to touch closely]

**con·ta·gious** (kŏn-tā'jŭs) Relating to contagion; communicable or transmissible by contact with the sick or their fresh secretions or excretions. SYN infectious (2).

**con·ta·gious dis·ease** (kŏn-tā'jŭs di-zēz') Infectious disease transmissible by direct or indirect contact; now used synonymously with communicable disease.

**con·tam·i·nant** (kŏn-tam'i-nănt) An impurity; any material of an extraneous nature associated with a pharmaceutical preparation, a principle, or infectious agent.

**con·tam·i·nate** (kŏn-tam'i-nāt) To cause or result in contamination. [L. *con-tamino*, to mingle, corrupt]

**con·tam·i·na·ted waste** (kŏn-tam'i-nā-tĕd wāst) Detritus that has been in contact with blood or other body secretions and must be discarded using specified procedures.

**con·tam·i·na·tion** (kŏn-tam'i-nā'shŭn) **1.** The presence of an infectious agent on or in something. **2.** In epidemiology, the situation that exists when a population being studied for one condition or factor also possesses other conditions or factors that modify results of the study. **3.** The presence of foreign material that adulterates or renders impure a material the composition of which is thereby degraded. [L. *contamino*, pp. *-atus*, to stain, defile]

**con·tent** (kon'tent) That which is contained within something else. [L. *contentus*, fr. *contineo*, pp. *-tentus*, to hold together, contain]

**con·ti·gu·i·ty** (kon'ti-gyū'i-tē) Contact without actual continuity. [L. *contiguus*, touching, fr. *contingo*, to touch]

**con·tin·u·ing ed·u·ca·tion** (kŏn-tin'yū-ing ed'yū-kā'shŭn) Systematic professional learning experiences designed to augment knowledge and skills of health care professionals.

**con·tin·u·ous bar con·nec·tor** (kon-tin'yū-ŭs bahr kŏ-nek'tŏr) In a mandibular removable partial denture, the bar that rests on the lingual surfaces of the anterior teeth and acts as an indirect retainer. SYN Kennedy bar.

**con·tin·u·ous bar re·tain·er** (kŏn-tin'yū-ŭs bahr rĕ-tān'ĕr) Metal bar, usually resting on lingual surfaces of teeth, to aid in their stabilization and act as indirect retainers.

**con·tin·u·ous beam** (kŏn-tin'yū-ŭs bēm) In dentistry, beam that continues over three or more supports, those supports not at the beam ends being equally free supports.

**con·tin·u·ous clasp** (kŏn-tin'yū-ŭs klasp) Circumferential clasp of a removable partial denture in which the body is attached to an occlusal rest and the clasp arms extend across the buccal or lingual surfaces of more than one tooth before engaging a proximal surface undercut. SYN continuous lingual clasp, secondary lingual bar.

**con·tin·u·ous clasp splint** (kŏn-tin'yū-ŭs klasp splint) A cast support to immobilize teeth temporarily.

**con·tin·u·ous e·rup·tion** (kŏn-tin'yū-ŭs ē-rŭp'shŭn) Eruption of tooth into mouth and its continuous movement in a vertical direction.

**con·tin·u·ous lin·gual clasp** (kŏn-tin'yū-ŭs ling'gwăl klasp) SYN continuous clasp.

**con·tin·u·ous loop wir·ing** (kŏn-tin'yū-ŭs lūp wīr´ing) Formation of wire loops on both maxillary and mandibular teeth, for placement of intermaxillary elastics; used in reduction and fixation of fractures.

**con·tin·u·ous su·ture** (kŏn-tin´yū-ŭs sū´ chŭr) An uninterrupted series of stitches using one suture; the stitching is fastened at each end by a knot. SYN uninterrupted suture.

🔲**con·tour** (kon´tūr) **1.** In dentistry, to restore normal outlines or form of a tooth or create external shape or form of a prosthesis. **2.** The outline of a part; the surface configuration. See this page. [L. *con-* (intens.), + *torno,* to turn (in a lathe), fr. *tornus,* a lathe]

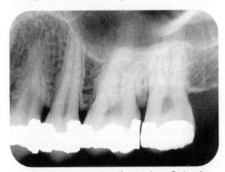

open contact, poor restoration contour: first molar

**con·tour·ing pli·ers** (kon´tūr-ing plī´ĕrz) Tool, usually fitted with curved beaks, to form contours or shape objects (e.g., metal temporary crowns, metal matrix bands).

**con·tra·an·gle** (kon´tră-ang-gĕl) **1.** One of the double or triple angles in the shank of a dental instrument by means of which the cutting edge or point is brought into the axis of the handle. **2.** Extension piece added to end of a dental handpiece, which, through a set of bevel gears, changes angle of axis of rotation of bur in relation to axis of handpiece.

**con·tra·an·gle chis·el** (kon´tră-ang-gĕl chiz´ĕl) Cutting tool with beveled end with blade that meets shank at an angle of ≥12 degrees.

**con·tra·bev·el** (kon´tră-bev´ĕl) Bevel located on the side opposite the customary side.

**con·tract** (kon´trakt, kŏn-trakt´) **1.** Explicit bilateral commitment by dentist and patient to a defined course of action to attain the goal of therapy. **2.** To acquire by contagion or infection. **3.** To shorten; to become reduced in size. [L. *con-traho,* pp. *-tractus,* to draw together]

**con·tract den·tist** (kon´trakt den´tist) One who provides care for a specific group of patients under preset guidelines.

**con·trac·tion** (kŏn-trak´shŭn) *Do not confuse this word with contracture.* **1.** Condition

wherein maxillary and mandibular structures are closer than normal to median plane. **2.** A shortening or increase in tension; denoting the normal function of muscle. **3.** Shrinkage or reduction in size. [L. *contractus,* drawn together]

**con·tract prac·tice** (kon´trakt prak´tis) A business wherein a third party contracts with the dental practice to provide care for a specific group of patients.

**con·trac·ture** (kŏn-trak´shŭr) *Do not confuse this word with contraction.* Static muscle shortening due to tonic spasm or fibrosis, to loss of muscular balance, to the antagonist being paralyzed, or to a loss of motion. [L. *contractura,* fr. *contraho,* to draw together]

**con·tra·fis·su·ra** (kon´tră-fi-sūr´ă) Fracture of a bone, as in the skull, at a point opposite that where the blow was received. [L. *contra,* against, counter, + *fissura,* fissure]

**con·tra·in·di·ca·tion** (kon´tră-in-di-kā´ shŭn) Any special symptom or circumstance that renders use of a remedy or carrying out of a procedure inadvisable, due to risk.

**con·tra·lat·er·al** (kon´tră-lat´ĕr-ăl) Relating to the opposite side, as when pain is perceived or paralysis occurs on the side opposite to that of the lesion. [L. *contra,* opposite, + *latus,* side]

**con·tra·lat·er·al part·ner** (kon´tră-lat´ĕr-ăl pahrt´nĕr) Corresponding structure on opposite side.

**con·trast** (kon´trast) **1.** A comparison in which differences are demonstrated or enhanced. **2.** In radiology, the difference between the image densities of two areas is the contrast between them. **3.** Contrast medium. **4.** Performed with a contrast medium. [L. *contra,* against, + *sto,* pp. *status,* to stand]

**con·trol** (kŏn-trōl´) To regulate, restrain, correct, or restore to normal.

**con·trol group** (kŏn-trōl´ grŭp) Subjects participating in the same experiment as another group, but not exposed to the variable under investigation.

**con·trolled re·lease** (kŏn-trōld´ rĕ-lēs´) Delivery of a chemotherapeutic agent to a site-specific area. The agent is released from the carrier device at a fixed rate (e.g., by a dermal patch or a polymeric fiber, such as that used to deliver a therapeutic agent to a periodontal pocket).

**con·trolled sub·stance** (kŏn-trōld´ sŭb´ stăns) Substance subject to U.S. Controlled Substances Act (1970), which regulates prescribing and dispensing, as well as manufacturing, storage, sale, or distribution of substances assigned to five schedules according to their 1) potential for or evidence of abuse, 2) potential for psychic or physiologic dependence, 3) contribution to a public health risk, 4) harmful pharmacologic effect, or 5) role as a precursor of other controlled substances.

**con·tu·sion** (kŏn-tū′zhŭn) Any mechanical injury (usually caused by a blow) resulting in hemorrhage beneath unbroken skin. [L. *contusio,* a bruising]

**con·ve·nience form** (kŏn-vēn′yĕns fōrm) Alterations in form or shape (outside the basic outline) of a cavity preparation to ease removal of decay and to enable proper instrumentation for the cavity preparation and insertion of a dental restoration.

**con·ver·gence** (kŏn-vĕr′jĕns) The tending of two or more objects toward a common point. [L. *con-vergere,* to incline together]

**con·ver·tin** (kon-vĕr′tin) Active form of factor VII designated VIIa.

**con·vex** (kon′veks) Denotes surface evenly curved outward, segment of a sphere. [L. *convexus,* vaulted, arched, convex, fr. *con-veho,* to bring together]

**con·vul·sion** (kŏn-vŭl′shŭn) **1.** A violent spasm or series of jerkings of the face, trunk, or extremities. **2.** SYN seizure (2). [L. *convulsio,* fr. *convello,* pp. *-vulsus,* to tear up]

**Coo·ley a·ne·mi·a** (kū′lē ă-nē′mē-ă) SYN thalassemia major.

**co·or·di·na·tion** (kō-ōr′di-nā′shŭn) Harmonious working together, especially of several muscles or muscle groups in the execution of complicated movements. [L. *co-,* together, + *ordino,* pp. *-atus,* to arrange, fr. *ordo* (*ordin-*), arrangement, order]

**co·or·di·na·tion of ben·e·fits** (kō-ōr′di-nā′shŭn ben′ĕ-fits) Process whereby two or more insurance companies or insuring entities apportion each's share of responsibility for payment of health care claims.

**co·pal res·in** (kō′păl rĕz′in) Brittle natural resin with a melting range that exceeds 149 degrees C. When deposited as a film from an organic solvent, it is used in dentistry as a liner for a cavity preparation before the restoration is placed.

**co·pay·ment, co·pay** (kō′pā-mĕnt, kō′pā) That portion of a dental care charge for which the patient herself, rather than a third party payor (i.e., insurer), is responsible.

**COPD** Abbreviation for chronic obstructive pulmonary disease.

**cope** (kōp) Upper half of flask in casting art; hence applicable to the upper or cavity side of a denture flask.

**cop·ing** (kōp′ing) Thin metal covering or cap.

**co·pol·y·mer** (kō′pol′i-mĕr) Polymer with two or more combined monomers or base units.

**co·pol·y·mer·i·za·tion** (kō′pol′i-mĕr-ī-zā′shŭn) Formation of a polymer from two or more monomers with different chemical structure so as to form the new structure with properties that vary from either discrete monomer.

**co·pol·y·mer res·in** (kō′pol′i-mĕr rez′in) Synthetic resin produced by joint polymerization of two or more different monomers or polymers.

**cop·per** (kop′ĕr) A metallic element; several of its salts are used in medicine. [L. *cuprum,* orig. *Cyprium,* fr. Cyprus, where it was mined]

**cop·per phos·phate ce·ment** (kop′ĕr fos′făt sĕ-ment′) Dental preparation, the combination of a solution of orthophosphoric acid with a cement powder (usually zinc oxide) modified with varying proportions of copper oxide.

**cop·ro·por·phyr·i·a** (kop′rō-pōr-fir′ē-ă) Presence of coproporphyrins in the urine.

**cop·ro·por·phy·rin** (kop′rō-pōr′fir-in) One of two porphyrin compounds found normally in feces as a decomposition product of bilirubin.

**cop·to·sis** (kop-tō′sis) A state of perpetual fatigue. [G. *kopto,* to tire, + *osis,* condition]

**cop·u·la** (kop′yū-lă) **1.** In anatomy, narrow part connecting two structures. **2.** Swelling formed during early development of the tongue by medial portions of second pharyngeal arches. [L. a bond, tie]

**cord** (kōrd) [TA] In anatomy, any long ropelike structure, composed of several to many longitudinally oriented fibers, vessels, ducts, or combinations thereof. [L. *chorda,* a string]

**cor·date** (kōr′dāt) *Do not confuse this word with chordate.* Heart-shaped.

**core** (kōr) **1.** Metal casting or resin form, usually with a post in the canal of a tooth root, designed to retain an artificial crown. **2.** Sectional record, usually of plaster of Paris or one of its derivatives, of the relationships of parts, such as teeth, metallic restorations, or copings. [L. *cor,* heart]

**core tem·per·a·ture** (kōr tem′pĕr-ă-chŭr) The temperature of the interior of the body.

**core-vent im·plant sys·tem** (kōr vent im′plant sis′tĕm) Endosseous appliance with a hollow apical portion that is submerged in bone.

**cor·ne·a** (kōr′nē-ă) [TA] Transparent tissue constituting the anterior sixth of the outer wall of the eye, with a 7.7-mm radius of curvature.[L. fem. of *corneus,* horny]

**cor·ne·al graft** (kōr′nē-ăl graft) SYN keratoplasty.

**cor·nic·u·late** (kōr-nik′yū-lăt) Resembling a horn. [L. *corniculatus,* horned]

**cor·nic·u·lum** (kōr-nik′yū-lŭm) A small cornu. [L. dim. of *cornu*, horn]

**cor·ni·fi·ca·tion** (kōr′ni-fi-kā′shŭn) SYN keratinization. [L. *cornu*, horn, + *facio*, to make]

**cor·nu,** pl. **cor·nu·a** (kōr′nū, -nū-ă) [TA] **1.** [TA] SYN horn. **2.** One of the coronal extensions of the dental pulp underlying a cusp or lobe. [L. horn]

**co·ro·na,** pl. **co·ro·nae** (kŏ-rō′nă, -nē) [TA] SYN crown (1). [L. garland, crown, fr. G. *korōnē*]

**cor·o·nad** (kōr′ŏ-nad) In a direction toward any corona.

**cor·o·nal** (kōr′ŏ-năl) [TA] *Do not confuse this word with coronary or coronoid.* **1.** Relating to a corona or the coronal plane. **2.** Relating to a crown of tooth.

**cor·o·nal plane** (kōr′ŏ-năl plān) A plane parallel to the long axis of the body in the anatomic (i.e., upright) position that divides the body into front and back parts; perpendicular to the sagittal and horizontal planes.

**cor·o·nal pol·ish·ing** (kōr′ŏ-năl pol′ishing) Burnishing of the anatomic crowns of the teeth to remove dental biofilm and extrinsic stains; process does not involve calculus removal, however. See this page.

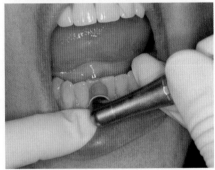

**rubber cup and polishing agent:** removal of extrinsic dental staining

**cor·o·nal pulp** (kōr′ŏ-năl pŭlp) SYN crown pulp.

**cor·o·nal su·ture** (kōr′ŏ-năl sū′chŭr) [TA] Line of junction of frontal with two parietal bones of skull.

**cor·o·nar·y ar·te·ry by·pass** (kōr′ŏ-nār-ē ahr′tĕr-ē bī′pas) Conduit, usually a vein graft or internal mammary artery, surgically interposed between the aorta and a coronary artery branch to coronary shunt blood beyond an obstruction.

**cor·o·nar·y ar·te·ry dis·ease (CAD)** (kōr′ŏ-nār-ē ahr′tĕr-ē di-zēz′) Narrowing of lumen of the coronary arteries; can cause congestive heart failure, angina pectoris, or myocardial infarction.

**cor·o·nar·y oc·clu·sion** (kōr′ŏ-nār-ē ŏ-klū′zhŭn) Blockage of a coronary vessel.

**cor·o·nar·y si·nus** (kōr′ŏ-nār-ē sī′nŭs) [TA] A short trunk receiving most of the cardiac veins.

**cor·o·nar·y throm·bo·sis** (kōr′ŏ-nār-ē throm-bō′sis) Coronary occlusion by thrombus formation, usually the result of atheromatous changes in the arterial wall and usually leading to myocardial infarction.

**Co·ro·na·vir·i·dae** (kō-rō′nă-vir′i-dē) A family of single-stranded RNA-containing viruses, some of which cause upper respiratory tract infections in humans. [L. *corona*, garland, crown]

**co·ro·ni·on** (kŏ-rō′nē-on) Tip of coronoid process of mandible; a craniometric point. SYN koronion. [G. *korōnē*, crow]

**cor·o·noid** (kōr′ŏ-noyd) *Do not confuse this word with coronal or coronary.* Shaped like a crow's beak. [G. *korōnē*, a crow, + *eidos*, resembling]

**cor·o·noi·dec·to·my** (kōr′ŏ-noyd-ek′tŏ-mē) Surgical removal of coronoid process of mandible. [*coronoid* + G. *ektomē*, excision]

**cor·o·noid pro·cess** (kōr′ŏ-noyd pros′es) A sharp triangular projection from a bone; coronoid process of the mandible, the triangular anterior process of the mandibular ramus, giving attachment to the temporal muscle.

**cor·o·noid pro·cess of man·di·ble** (kōr′ŏ-noyd pro′ses man′di-bĕl) [TA] Triangular anterior process of mandibular ramus, attaches to temporal muscle.

**cor·pus,** pl. **cor·po·ra** (kōr′pŭs, -pōr-ă) [TA] *The plural of this word is corpora, not corpi.* **1.** SYN body (1). **2.** Any body or mass. **3.** The main part of an organ or other anatomic structure, as distinguished from the head or tail.

**cor·pus cal·lo·sum** (kōr′pŭs ka-lō′sŭm) [TA] The great commissural plate of nerve fibers interconnecting the cortical hemispheres.

**cor·pus·cle** (kōr′pŭs-ĕl) **1.** A small mass or body. **2.** A blood cell. [L. *corpusculum*, dim. of *corpus*, body]

**cor·pus·cu·lar ra·di·a·tion** (kōr-pŭs′ kyū-lăr rā′dē-ā′shŭn) Radiation consisting of streams of subatomic particles such as protons, electrons, and neutrons.

**cor·rec·ted cast** (kŏ-rek′tĕd kast) SYN altered cast.

**cor·rec·tion** (kōr-ek′shŭn) The act of reducing a fault; the elimination of an unfavorable quality.

**cor·rec·tive** (kŏr-ek′tiv) 1. Counteracting, modifying, or changing what is injurious. 2. A drug that modifies or corrects an undesirable or injurious effect of another drug.

**cor·re·la·tion** (kōr′ĕ-lā′shŭn) 1. The mutual or reciprocal relation of two or more items or parts. 2. The act of bringing into such a relation. 3. The degree to which variables change together.

**cor·re·la·tion co·ef·fi·cient** (kōr′ĕ-lā′ shŭn kō′ĕ-fish′ĕnt) Measure of association that indicates degree to which two variables have a linear relationship.

**cor·re·spon·dence** (kōr′ĕ-spon′dĕns) OPTICS the points on each retina that have the same visual direction.

**cor·ro·sion** (kŏr-ō′zhŭn) 1. Gradual deterioration or consummation of a substance by another, especially by biochemical or chemical reaction. 2. That produced by corroding. [L. *corrodo* (*conr-*), pp. *-rosus*, to gnaw]

**cor·tex**, pl. **cor·ti·ces** (kōr′teks, -ti-sēz) [TA] The outer portion of an organ, as distinguished from the inner, or medullary, portion. [L. bark]

**cor·tex of su·pra·re·nal gland** (kōr′teks sū′pră-rē′năl gland) [TA] The outer part of the suprarenal gland. SYN adrenal cortex.

**cor·ti·cal** (kōr′ti-kăl) Relating to a cortex.

**cor·ti·cal bone** (kōr′ti-kăl bōn) [TA] Superficial thin layer of compact bone.

**cor·ti·cal hor·mones** (kōr′ti-kăl hōr′mōnz) Steroid hormones produced by the cortex of the suprarenal gland.

**cor·ti·cal os·te·ot·o·my** (kōr′ti-kăl os′ tē-ot′ŏ-mē) Osteotomy through cortex at base of the dentoalveolar segment, which serves to weaken osseous resistance to application of orthodontic forces.

**cor·ti·coid** (kōr′ti-koyd) 1. Having an action similar to that of a hormone of the cortex of the suprarenal gland. 2. SYN glucocorticoid (3).

**cor·ti·co·ste·roid** (kōr′ti-kō-ster′oyd) A steroid produced by the cortex of the suprarenal gland.

**cor·ti·cos·ter·one** (kōr′ti-kos′tĕr-ōn) A corticosteroid that induces some deposition of glycogen in the liver, sodium conservation, and potassium excretion.

**cor·ti·co·tro·pic hor·mone** (kōr′ti-kō-trō′pik hōr′mōn) SYN adrenocorticotropic hormone.

**β-cor·ti·co·tro·pin** (kōr′ti-kō-trō′pin) Acid-or pepsin-degraded β-corticotropin. SYN corticotropin (2).

**cor·ti·co·tro·pin** (kōr′ti-kō-trō′pin) SYN β-corticotropin. [G. *tropē*, a turning]

**cor·ti·co·tro·pin-re·leas·ing fac·tor (CRF)** (kōr′ti-kō-trō′pin-rĕ-lēs′ing fak′tŏr) SYN corticotropin-releasing hormone.

**cor·ti·co·tro·pin-re·leas·ing hor·mone (CRH)** (kōr′ti-kō-trō′pin-rĕ-lēs′ing hōr′mōn) Factor secreted by hypothalamus that stimulates pituitary to release adrenocorticotropic hormone. SYN corticotropin-releasing factor.

**cor·ti·sol** (kōr′ti-sol) Principal glucocorticoid produced by the zona fasciculata of the cortex of the suprarenal gland; promotes gluconeogenesis and lipolysis and inhibits inflammatory and immune responses.

**cor·ti·sone** (kōr′ti-sōn) *Avoid using this word as a synonym of adrenocortical steroid.* Biologically inactive adrenal corticosteroid produced by the reversible 11-hydroxylation of cortisol (17-hydroxycorticosterone).

**co·run·dum** (kŏ-rŭn′dŭm) Native crystalline aluminum oxide. [Hind. *kurand*]

**Cor·y·ne·bac·te·ri·um** (kŏ-rī′nē-bak-tēr′ē-ŭm) Genus of widely distributed aerobic to anaerobic bacteria containing irregularly staining, gram-positive, straight to slightly curved, often club-shaped rods; pathogenic in humans. [G. *coryne*, a club, + *bacterium*, a small rod]

**Cor·y·ne·bac·te·ri·um jei·kei·um** (kŏ-rī′nē-bak-tēr′ē-ŭm jī-kī′ŭm) Bacterial species associated with septicemia and skin lesions in immunocompromised patients.

**Cor·y·ne·bac·te·ri·um stri·a·tum** (kŏ-rī′nē-bak-tēr′ē-ŭm strī-ā′tŭm) Bacterial species found in nasal mucus and in the throat.

**co·ry·za** (kō-rī′ză) SYN acute rhinitis. [G.]

**cos·me·ceu·ti·cal** (koz′mĕ-sū′ti-kăl) Substance combining cosmetic and pharmaceutical properties, including topical preparations as well as agents such as botulinum toxin. [*cos-me*tic + pharmac*eutical*]

**cos·met·ic or·tho·don·tics** (koz-met′ik ōr′thŏ-don′tiks) Orthodontia limited to the improvement of cosmesis and aesthetics.

**cos·met·ic sur·ge·ry** (koz-met′ik sŭr′jĕr-ē) Operative procedure in which the principal purpose is to improve the appearance, usually with the connotation that the improvement sought is beyond the normal appearance, and its acceptable variations, for the age and physical state of the patient.

**Cos·ten syn·drome** (kos′tĕn sin′drōm) Symptom complex of loss of hearing; otalgia; tinnitus; dizziness; headache; and burning sensation of the throat, tongue, and side of the nose;

originally attributed to temporomandibular joint dysfunction resulting from occlusal disharmony, but currently recognized as not being well founded on anatomic and physiologic principles.

**co·ti·nine** (kō′ti-nēn) One of the major detoxication products of nicotine; eliminated rapidly and completely by the kidneys.

**cot·ton** (kot′ŏn) The white, fluffy, fibrous covering of the seeds of a plant of the genus *Gossypium;* used extensively in surgical dressings. [Ar. *qùtun*]

**cot·ton pel·let** (kot′ŏn pel′ĕt) Small rolled ball commonly used in dental procedures to dry cavity preparations and apply medications.

**cot·ton pli·ers** (kot′ŏn plī′ĕrz) Device resembling tweezers used to grasp small objects.

**cot·y·le** (kot′i-lē) Any cup-shaped structure. [G. *kotylē,* anything hollow, the cup or socket of a joint]

**cot·y·loid cav·i·ty** (kot′i-loyd kav′i-tē) SYN acetabulum.

**cough** (kawf) Sudden explosive forcing of air through the glottis, occurring immediately on opening the previously closed glottis, excited by irritation of the trachea or bronchi or by pressure from adjacent structures.

**cou·ma·rin** (kū′mă-rin) A general descriptive term applied to anticoagulants and other drugs derived from dicumarol.

**Coun·cil on Den·tal Ther·a·peu·tics** (kown′sil den′tăl thār′ă-pyū′tiks) Committee advisory to American Dental Association on therapeutic agents and materials.

**coun·sel·ing** (kown′sĕl-ing) A professional relationship and activity in which one person endeavors to help another to understand and to solve his or her adjustment problems. SYN counselling. [L. *consilium,* deliberation]

**counselling** [Br.] SYN counseling.

**count·er·die** (kown′tĕr-dī) The reverse image of a die, usually made of a softer and lower fusing metal than the die itself.

**count·er·ir·ri·tant** (kown′tĕr-ir′i-tănt) **1.** An agent that causes irritation or a mild inflammation of the skin to relieve symptoms of a deep-seated inflammatory process. **2.** An agent used to enhance blood flow to affected area.

**coup·ling a·gent** (kŭp′ling ā′jĕnt) A gel or lotion used to improve contact and reduce friction between transducer and skin during ultrasound examinations and treatmnts.

**cov·er·age** (kŏv′ĕr-ăj) A measure of the extent to which the services rendered cover the potential need for these services in a community.

**cov·er·ing** (kŭv′ĕr-ing) In dentistry, agreement by a dentist or oral health care provider to see to the needs of patients of a practitioner when she is unavailable due to unexpected absence or prior commitment (e.g., vacation).

**Cow·den dis·ease** (kow′dĕn di-zēz′) Hypertrichosis and gingival fibromatosis from infancy, accompanied by postpubertal fibroadenomatous breast enlargement; papules of the face are characteristic of multiple trichilemmomas.

**COX-2 in·hib·i·tor** (in-hib′i-tŏr) A drug class that relieves inflammation and pain by inhibiting the action of cyclooxygenase-2.

**CPITN** Abbreviation for Community Periodontal Index of Treatment Needs.

**CPT** Abbreviation for *Current Procedural Terminology.*

**Cr** Abbreviation for creatinine.

**Cr** Abbreviation for crown-rump length.

**crack** (krak) A fissure.

**crack co·caine** (krak kō-kān′) Derivative of cocaine, usually smoked, resulting in a brief, intense high. It is relatively inexpensive and extremely addictive.

**crack·ed tooth syn·drome** (krakt tūth sin′drōm) Transient acute dental pain that is difficult to locate and is experienced occasionally while chewing. Usually a vertical crack or split in the tooth extends across a marginal ridge through the crown and into the root, involving the pulp. Cracked teeth may be identified by clinicians by using transilluminated light or disclosing dyes. Pain is usually perceived when palpated; under pressure the tooth segments move independently.

**crack·ling jaw** (krak′ling jaw) Chronic subluxation with clicking on motion.

**cramp** (kramp) A painful muscle spasm caused by prolonged tetanic contraction. [M.E. *crampe,* fr. O.Fr., fr. Germanic]

**cra·ni·ad** (krā′nē-ad) Situated nearer the head in relation to a specific reference point.

**cra·ni·al** (krā′nē-ăl) Relating to the cranium or head. SEE ALSO cephalad. SYN cephalic.

**cra·ni·al a·rach·noid ma·ter** (krā′nē-ăl ă-rak′noyd mā′tĕr) [TA] Portion of arachnoid that lies within cranial cavity and surrounds brain and cranial portion of subarachnoid space. In several sites, it is relatively widely separated from the pia mater, creating the cranial subarachnoid cisterns.

**cra·ni·al base** (krā′nē-ăl bās) [TA] Sloping floor of cranial cavity; comprises both external base of cranium and internal base of cranium. SYN base of cranium, basicranium.

**cra·ni·al cav·i·ty** (krā'nē-ăl kav'i-tē) [TA] Space within cranium occupied by brain, its coverings, and cerebrospinal fluid.

**cra·ni·al du·ra ma·ter** (krā'nē-ăl dur'ă mā'tĕr) [TA] Intracranial dura mater, consisting of two layers: the outer *periosteal layer* that normally always adheres to the periosteum of the bones of the cranial vault; and the inner *meningeal layer* that in most places is fused with the outer.

**(cra·ni·al) ex·tra·du·ral space** (krā'nē-ăl eks'tră-dur'ăl spās) [TA] Area between cranial bones and external periosteal layer of the dura; becomes an actual space only pathologically, as when as extradural or epidural hemorrhage occurs forming a hematoma.

**cra·ni·al fi·brous joints** (krā'nē-ăl fī'brŭs joynts) [TA] Articulations of the cranium, including the cranial syndesmoses, cranial sutures, and dentoalveolar syndesmoses (gomphoses).

**cra·ni·al in·dex** (krā'nē-ăl in'deks) Ratio of maximal breadth to maximal length of the cranium, obtained by the formula: (breadth × 100)/length.

**cra·ni·al nerves** (krā'nē-ăl nĕrvz) [TA] Nerves that emerge from, or enter, the cranium. The 12 paired cranial nerves are the olfactory [CN I], optic [CN II], oculomotor [CN III], trochlear [CN IV], trigeminal [CN V], abducent [CN VI], facial [CN VII], vestibulocochlear [CN VIII], glossopharyngeal [CN IX], vagal [CN X], accessory [CN XI], and hypoglossal [CN XII].

**cra·ni·al pros·the·sis** (krā'nē-ăl pros-thē'sis) Permanently implanted artificial biocompatible replacement for bones of the craniofacial skeleton. SYN skull plate.

**cra·ni·al root of ac·ces·so·ry nerve** (krā'nē-ăl rūt ak-ses'ŏr-ē nĕrv) [TA] Roots of accessory nerve that arise from medulla. Recent studies indicate that the cranial root should be considered a root of the vagus nerve.

**cra·ni·al su·tures** (krā'nē-ăl sū'chŭrz) [TA] Sutures between the bones of the cranium.

**cra·ni·al syn·chon·dro·ses** (krā'nē-ăl syn'kon-drō'sēz) [TA] Cartilaginous joints of cranium.

**cra·ni·al syn·des·mo·ses** (krā'nē-ăl sin'dez-mō'sēz) [TA] Fibrous joints of cranium collectively.

**cra·ni·al sy·no·vi·al joints** (krā'nē-ăl si-nō'vē-ăl joynts) [TA] Those of the head, composed of the temporomandibular joint (TMJ) and atlanto occipital joint.

**cra·ni·al ver·te·bra** (krā'nē-ăl vĕr'tĕ-bră) Segment of cranium regarded as homologous with a segment of the vertebral column.

**cra·ni·o·au·ral** (krā'nē-ō-aw'răl) Relating to cranium and the ear.

**cra·ni·o·car·di·ac re·flex** (krā'nē-ō-kahr' dē-ak rē'fleks) Stimulation of nerve endings of some cranial nerves (e.g., olfactory, ophthalmic branch of trigeminal), with resultant cardiac depressor reflex, manifested by bradycardia and hypotension, through cardiac branch of vagus.

**cra·ni·o·ce·re·bral** (krā'nē-ō-ser'ĕ-brăl) Relating to cranium and brain.

**cra·ni·o·di·a·phys·i·al dys·pla·si·a** (krā'nē-ō-dī-ă-fiz'ē-ăl dis-plā'zhē-ă) Syndrome involving small stature, sclerosis of cranial bones, and diaphysial widening of tubular bones.

**cra·ni·o·fa·cial** (krā'nē-ō-fā'shăl) Relating to both face and cranium.

**cra·ni·o·fa·cial an·gle** (krā'nē-ō-fā'shăl ang'gĕl) Area formed by basifacial and basicranial axes at midpoint of the sphenoethmoidal suture.

**cra·ni·o·fa·cial a·nom·a·ly** (krā'nē-ō-fā'shăl ă-nom'ă-lē) Deviation from average or norm of the structures of head and face.

**cra·ni·o·fa·cial ap·pli·ance** (krā'nē-ō-fā'shăl ă-plī'ăns) Device used to immobilize and/or reduce mandibular or midfacial fractures. SEE ALSO fixation.

**cra·ni·o·fa·cial ax·is** (krā'nē-ō-fā'shăl ak' sis) Straight line passing through mesethmoid, presphenoid, basisphenoid, and basioccipital bones.

**cra·ni·o·fa·ci·al com·plex** (krā'nē-ō-fā' shăl kom'pleks) In aggregate, bones and soft tissues of face and cranium.

**cra·ni·o·fa·cial fix·a·tion** (krā'nē-ō-fā' shăl fik-sā'shŭn) Stabilization of facial fractures to the cranial base by direct wiring or by external skeletal pin fixation.

**cra·ni·o·fa·cial sur·ge·ry** (krā'nē-ō-fā' shăl sŭr'jĕr-ē) General term for procedures performed separately or in combined fashion on the cranium and facial bones.

**cra·ni·o·fa·cial sus·pen·sion wir·ing** (krā'nē-ō-fā'shăl sŭs-pen'shŭn wīr'ing) Method of wiring using areas of bones not contiguous with the oral cavity for the support of fractured jaw segments.

**cra·ni·o·graph** (krā'nē-ō-graf) An instrument for making drawings to scale of the diameters and general configuration of the skull.

**cra·ni·og·ra·phy** (krā'nē-og'ră-fē) Art of representing, by drawings made from measurements, the configuration of the cranium and relations of its angles and craniometric points. [*cranio-* + G. *graphō*, to write]

**cra·ni·ol·o·gy** (krā′nē-ol′ŏ-jē) The science concerned with variations in size, shape, and proportion of the cranium.

**cra·ni·o·met·a·phys·i·al dys·pla·si·a** (krā′nē-ō-met′ă-fiz′ē-ăl dis-plā′zhē-ă) Syndrome of metaphysial dysplasia associated with severe sclerosis and overgrowth of bones of cranium and with hypertelorism.

**cra·ni·om·e·ter** (krā′nē-om′ĕ-tĕr) An instrument for measuring skull diameters.

**cra·ni·o·met·ric points** (krā′nē-ō-met′rik poynts) Fixed points on cranium used as landmarks in craniometry.

**cra·ni·om·e·try** (krā′nē-om′ĕ-trē) Measurement of the dry skull after removal of the soft parts and study of its topography. [*cranio-* + G. *metron,* measure]

**cra·ni·op·a·thy** (krā′nē-op′ă-thē) Any pathologic condition of the cranial bones. [*cranio-* + G. *pathos,* suffering]

**cra·ni·o·pha·ryn·ge·al** (krā′nē-ō-făr-in′jē-ăl) Relating to cranium and pharynx.

**cra·ni·o·pha·ryn·ge·al duct** (krā′nē-ō-fă-rin′jē-ăl dŭkt) Slender tubular part of the pituitary diverticulum.

**cra·ni·o·pha·ryn·gi·o·ma** (krā′nē-ō-făr-in′jē-ō′mă) A suprasellar neoplasm that develops from the Rathke pouch. SYN Rathke pouch tumor. [*cranio-* + *pharyngio-* + *-oma*]

**cra·ni·o·sa·cral** (krā′nē-ō-sā′krăl) Denoting cranial and sacral origins of parasympathetic division of the autonomic nervous system.

**cra·ni·o·spi·nal** (krā′nē-ō-spī′năl) Relating to cranium and spinal column.

**cra·ni·o·syn·os·to·sis** (krā′nē-ō-sin′os-tō′sis) Premature ossification of cranium and obliteration of sutures.

**cra·ni·o·ta·bes** (krā′nē-ō-tā′bēz) A disease marked by areas of thinning and softening in skull bones and widening of the sutures and fontanelles. [*cranio-* + L. *tabes,* a wasting]

**cra·ni·ot·o·my** (krā′nē-ot′ŏ-mē) Opening into the skull, either by attached or detached craniotomy or by trephination. [*cranio-* + G. *tomē,* incision]

**cra·ni·o·tym·pan·ic** (krā′nē-ō-tim-pan′ik) Relating to both cranium and middle ear.

**cra·ni·o·ver·te·bral joints** (krā′nē-ō-vĕr′tĕ-brăl joynts) Collective term for articulations permitting movement between cranium and cervical vertebrae.

**cra·ni·um,** pl. **cra·ni·a** (krā′nē-ŭm, -ă) [TA] The bones of the head collectively. SYN skull. [Mediev. L. fr. G. *kranion* ]

**cra·ter·i·form** (krā-ter′i-fōrm) Hollowed out

like a bowl or a saucer. [L. *crater,* bowl, + *forma,* shape]

**craz·ing** (krāz′ing) In dentistry, appearance of minute cracks on surface of plastic restorations such as filling materials, denture teeth, or denture bases.

**C-re·ac·tive pro·tein** (rē-ak′tiv prō′tēn) β-globulin found in serum of people with some inflammatory, degenerative, and neoplastic diseases.

**crease** (krēs) A line or linear depression as produced by a fold. SEE ALSO fold, groove, line.

**cre·a·tine ki·nase (CK)** (krē′ă-tin kī′nās) An enzyme catalyzing the reversible transfer of phosphate from phosphocreatine to adenosine diphosphate, forming creatine and adenosine triphosphate.

**cre·at·i·nine (Cr)** (krē-at′i-nin) A component of urine and the final product of creatine catabolism; formed by the nonenzymatic dephosphorylative cyclization of phosphocreatine to form the internal anhydride of creatine.

**creep** (krēp) Any time-dependent strain developing in a material or an object in response to the application of a force or stress.

**creep re·cov·e·ry** (krēp rĕ-kŭv′ĕr-ē) Time-dependent portion of decrease in strain in a material or object following removal of the stress that has deformed it.

**cre·o·sote** (krē′ŏ-sōt) A mixture of phenols obtained during distillation of wood-tar; used as a disinfectant. [G. *kreas,* flesh, + *sōtēr,* preserver]

**crep·i·ta·tion** (krep′i-tā′shŭn) **1.** Crackling; the quality of a fine bubbling sound (rale) that resembles noise heard on rubbing hair between the fingers. **2.** Sensation palpated over seat of fracture when broken ends of bone are moved, or over tissue, in which gas gangrene is present. **3.** Noise or vibration produced by rubbing bone or irregular degenerated cartilage surfaces together as in arthritis and other conditions. SYN crepitus (1).

**crep·i·tus** (krep′i-tŭs) **1.** SYN crepitation. **2.** A noisy discharge of gas from the intestine. **3.** The grating of a joint, often in association with osteoarthritis. [L. fr. *crepo,* to rattle]

***m*-cre·sol** (krē′sol) A local antiseptic with a higher germicidal power than phenol and less toxicity to tissues; used in disinfectants and fumigants.

**crest** (krest) [TA] A ridge, especially a bony ridge. SYN crista [TA]. [L. *crista*]

**crest·al re·sorp·tion** (krest′ăl rē-sōrp′shŭn) Resorption of the crestal bone of the alveolar ridge.

**crest of al·ve·o·lar ridge** (krest al-vē′ŏ-lăr rij) Highest continuous surface of the ridge, but not necessarily its center.

**CREST syn·drome** (krest sin′drōm) Acronym for variant of systemic sclerosis characterized by *c*alcinosis, *R*aynaud phenomenon, *e*sophageal motility disorders, *s*clerodactyly, and *t*elangiectasia.

**cre·tin** (kret′in) **1.** Obsolete term for a patient exhibiting cretinism. **2.** Obsolete term for anyone exhibiting congenital hypothyroidism. *This offensive term should be avoided.* [Fr. *crétin*]

**cre·tin·ism** (kret′in-izm) Obsolete term for congenital hypothyroidism. *This offensive term should be avoided.*

**cre·tin·ous** (kret′in-ŭs) Relating to cretinism or a cretin; affected with cretinism. *This offensive term should be avoided.*

**crev·ice** (krev′is) A crack or small fissure, especially in a solid substance. [Fr. *crevasse*]

**cre·vic·u·lar** (krĕ-vik′yū-lăr) **1.** Relating to any crevice. **2.** In dentistry, relating especially to the gingival crevice or sulcus.

**cre·vic·u·lar ep·i·the·li·um** (krĕ-vik′yū-lăr ep′i-thē′lē-ŭm) Stratified squamous epithelium lining inner aspect of soft tissue wall of gingival sulcus.

**cre·vic·u·lar fluid** (krĕ-vik′yū-lăr flū′id) SYN gingival fluid.

**CRF** Abbreviation for corticotropin-releasing factor.

**CRH** Abbreviation for corticotropin-releasing hormone.

**crib death** (krib deth) SYN sudden infant death syndrome.

**cri·bra·tion** (kri-brā′shŭn) **1.** Sifting; passing through a sieve. **2.** The condition of being cribrate or numerously pitted or punctured.

**crib·ri·form** (krib′ri-fōrm) [TA] Sievelike; containing many perforations. [L. *cribrum,* a sieve, + *forma,* form]

**crib·ri·form plate of eth·moid bone** (krib′ri-fōrm plāt eth′moyd bōn) [TA] Horizontal plate from which are suspended the labyrinth and the lamina perpendicularis.

**crib splint** (krib splint) A resin-metallic device to immobilize teeth temporarily; covers facial and lingual surfaces of the teeth.

**cri·coid car·ti·lage** (krī′koyd kahr′ti-lăj) [TA] The lowermost of the laryngeal cartilages. It is shaped like a signet ring.

**cri·coi·dyn·i·a** (krī′koy-din′ē-ă) Pain in the cricoid. [*cricoid* + G. *odynē,* pain]

**cri·co·thy·rot·o·my, cri·co·thy·roid·ot·o·my** (krī′kō-thī-rot′ŏ-mē, -thī′royd-ot′ŏ-mē) Incision through the skin and cricothyroid membrane for relief of respiratory obstruction; used before or in place of tracheotomy in certain emergency respiratory obstructions. SYN intercricothyrotomy. [*cricoid* + *thyroid* + G. *tomē,* incision]

**cri-du-chat syn·drome** (krē-dū-shah′ sin′drōm) Disorder characterized by microcephaly, hypertelorism, antimongoloid palpebral fissures, epicanthal folds, micrognathia, strabismus, mental and physical retardation, and a characteristic high-pitched catlike whine.

**crin·o·gen·ic** (krin′ō-jen′ik) Causing secretion; stimulating a gland to increased function. [G. *krinō,* to separate, + *-gen,* to produce]

**cri·sis** (krī′sis) A sudden change, usually for the better, in the course of an acute disease. [G. *krisis,* a separation, crisis]

**cris·pa·tion** (kris-pā′shŭn) A ''creepy'' sensation due to slight, fibrillary muscular contractions. [L. *crispo,* pp. *-atus,* to curl]

**cris·ta,** pl. **cris·tae** (kris′tă, -tē) [TA] SYN crest. [L. crest]

**cris·ta den·ta·lis** (kris′tă den-tā′lis) SYN dental crest.

**cris·ta mar·gi·na·lis den·tis** (kris′tă mahr′ji-nā′lis den′tis) [TA] SYN marginal ridge.

**cris·ta pa·la·ti·na** (kris′tă pal′ă-tī′nă) SYN palatine crest of horizontal process of palatine bone.

**cris·ta pal·a·to·phar·yn·ge·a** (kris′tă pal′ă-tō-fă-rin′jē-ă) [TA] SYN palatopharyngeal ridge.

**cris·ta su·pra·mas·toi·de·a** (kris′tă sū′pră-mas-toy′dē-ă) [TA] SYN supramastoid crest.

**cris·ta trans·ver·sa·lis** (kris′tă tranz′vĕr-sā′lis) [TA] Crest or ridge on occlusal surface of a tooth formed by union of two triangular crests. SYN transverse ridge [TA].

**cris·ta tri·an·gu·la·ris** (kris′tă trī-ang′gyū-lā′ris) [TA] Crest or ridge that extends from apex of a cusp of a premolar or molar tooth toward central part of occlusal surface. SYN triangular ridge [TA], triangular crest.

**cris·to·ba·lite** (kris-tō′bă-līt) Form of crystalline silica used in casting investments.

**cri·te·ri·on,** pl. **cri·te·ri·a** (krī-tēr′ē-ŏn, -ă) Standard or rule for judging; usually plural (i.e., criteria) to denote a set of standards or rules applicable to dentistry and dental procedures. [G. *kritērion,* a standard]

**cri·te·ri·on-re·lat·ed va·lid·i·ty** (krī-tēr′-ŏn rĕ-lā′tĕd vă-lid′i-tē) Degree of effectiveness with which performance on a test or procedure predicts performance in real life.

**crit·i·cal** (krit′ĭ-kăl) **1.** Denoting or of the nature of a crisis. **2.** Denoting a morbid condition in which death is possible. **3.** In sufficient quantity as to constitute a turning point.

**crit·i·cal pH** (krit′ĭ-kăl) The pH range, about 5.5, at which saliva ceases to be saturated with respect to calcium and phosphate, and below which tooth mineral and other hard tissues lose calcium.

**CRL** Abbreviation for crown-rump length.

**CRNA** Abbreviation for certified registered nurse anesthetist.

**croc·o·dile tears syn·drome** (krok′ŏ-dīl tērz sin′drōm) Lacrimation, usually unilateral, on eating or anticipation of eating.

**Crohn co·li·tis** (krōn kŏ-lī′tis) Regional enteritis affecting the colon; characterized by mucosal skip ulcers and transmural inflammation of the bowel wall. See this page.

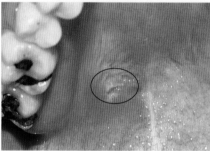

**pseudoaphthae:** corrugated ulcers due to Crohn disease

**cross-arch bar splint** (kraws ahrch bahr splint) Splint that uses a metal bar that unites teeth of one side of the dental arch with those of the other side.

**cross-arch bar splint con·nec·tor** (kraws ahrch bahr splint kŏ-nek′tŏr) Removable connector that crosses to the opposite side of the dental arch to stabilize weakened abutment teeth of a fixed prosthesis.

**cross-arch ful·crum** (kraws ahrch ful′krŭm) Advanced intraoral fulcrum in which the finger rest is established on the side of the arch opposite the treatment area.

**cross-bite** (kraws′bīt) Abnormal relationship of one or more teeth of one arch to opposing tooth or teeth of other arch due to labial, buccal, or lingual deviation of tooth position, or to abnormal jaw position. SYN reverse articulation.

**cross-bite tooth** (kraws′bīt tūth) Posterior tooth designed to permit modified cusp of maxillary tooth to be positioned in fossae of mandibular tooth.

**cross-con·tam·i·na·tion** (kraws kŏn-tam′i-nă′shŭn) Transfer of infectious agent or matter from one person or site to another.

**cross-cut bur** (kraws kŭt bŭr) Dental instrument with blades located at right angles to its long axis.

**cross·ed eyes, cross-eye** (krawst īz, kraws′ī) SYN strabismus.

**cross·ed lat·er·al·i·ty** (krawst lat′ĕr-al′ĭ-tē) Right dominance of some members' functions (e.g., use of upper limb or sighting with eye) and left dominance of others.

**cross·ed re·flex** (krawst rē′fleks) Reflex movement on one side of the body in response to a stimulus applied to the opposite side.

**cross-link·ed pol·y·mer** (kraws lingkt pol′i-měr) Material used in dental appliances in which long-chain molecules are attached to each other, forming a dimensional network.

**cross-re·sis·tance** (kraws rĕ-zis′tăns) Resistance to one agent or drug that confers resistance to another, usually similar agent.

**cross-sec·tion** (kraws′sek′shŭn) **1.** Planar or two-dimensional view, diagram, or image of internal structure of the body, part of the body, or any anatomic structure afforded by slicing, actually or through imaging. **2.** Slice of a given thickness created by actual serial parallel cuts through a structure or by application of imaging technique.

**cross-sec·tion·al** (kraws sek′shŭn-ăl) Relating to planar sections of an anatomic or other structure.

**cross-sec·tion·al stud·y** (kraws′sek-shŭn-ăl stŭd′ē) **1.** Study in which groups of individuals of different types are composed into one large sample and studied at only a single timepoint. **2.** Analysis of anatomic or other structure(s) by series of planar sections or radiographic images through the structure(s) and surrounding environment.

**cross-tol·er·ance** (kraws tol′ĕr-ăns) Resistance to one or several effects of a compound as a result of tolerance developed to a pharmacologically similar compound.

**cro·taph·i·on** (krō-taf′ē-on) Tip of the greater wing of the sphenoid bone. [G. *krotaphos,* the temple of the head]

**Crou·zon syn·drome** (krū-zōn[h]′ sin′drōm) Craniosynostosis with broad forehead, ocular hypertelorism, exophthalmos, beaked nose, and hypoplasia of the maxilla.

**crowd·ing** (krowd′ing) A condition in which the teeth are too close, assuming altered positions such as bunching, overlapping, displacement in various directions, and torsiversion.

**crown** (krown) **1.** [TA] In dentistry, that part

of a tooth that is covered with enamel. **2.** An artificial substitute for the part of a tooth that is normally covered with enamel. See this page. [L. *corona*]

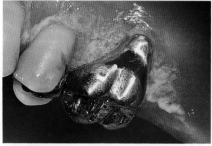

**gold crown**

**crown and bridge pros·tho·don·tics** (krown brij pros´thŏ-don´tiks) Therapy encompassing dental treatment that employs crowns and partial dentures cemented into place so as to be not readily removable.

**crown cav·i·ty** (krown kav´i-tē) SYN pulp cavity of crown.

**crown flask** (krown flask) SYN denture flask.

**crown-heel length** (krown-hēl length) Length of an outstretched 8-week embryo or fetus from the vertex of the cranium to the heel. SEE ALSO crown-rump length.

▪**crown·ing** (krown´ing) Preparation of natural crown of tooth by removal of part or all of the natural structure and replacement of prepared surfaces with a veneer of suitable dental material (gold or nonprecious metal casting, porcelain, plastic, or combinations). See page 151.

**crown leng·then·ing** (krown leng´thĕn-ing) Surgical procedure that apically repositions the gingiva and possibly the alveolar bone so as to expose more tooth structure; may be done to facilitate restorative procedures or enhance aesthetics.

**crown of tooth** (krown tūth) SYN anatomic crown.

**crown pulp** (krown pŭlp) [TA] Portion of dental pulp contained within the pulp chamber or crown cavity of tooth. SYN coronal pulp.

**crown:root ra·ti·o** (krown-rūt´ rā´shē-ō) Relative length of the crown of a tooth to the length of its root; may be specified on basis of anatomic crown and root or to that of the clinical crown and root.

**crown-rump length (CRL)** (krown-rŭmp length) A measurement from the vertex of the cranium to the midpoint between the apices of the buttocks of an embryo or fetus to assess of embryonic or fetal age.

**crown tu·ber·cle** (krown tū´bĕr-kĕl) SYN dental tubercle.

**Cro·zat ap·pli·ance** (krō´zat ă-plī´ăns) A wrought-wire removable orthodontic device.

**crus of he·lix** (krūs hē´liks) [TA] Transverse ridge continuing backward from helix of auricle, dividing the concha into an upper portion (cymba) and a lower (cavity of concha).

**crust** (krŭst) **1.** A hard outer layer or covering; cutaneous crusts are often formed by dried serum or pus on the surface of a ruptured blister or pustule. **2.** A scab. [L. *crusta*]

**cryanaesthesia** [Br.] SYN cryanesthesia.

**cry·an·es·the·si·a** (krī´an-es-thē´zē-ă) Inability to perceive cold. SYN cryanaesthesia. [G. *kryos*, cold, + *an-* priv. + *aisthēsis*, sensation]

**cry·o·an·es·the·si·a** (krī´ō-an-es-thē´zē-ă) Localized application of cold to elicit regional anesthesia.

**cry·o·sur·gery** (krī´ō-sŭr´jĕr-ē) An operation using freezing temperature (achieved by liquid nitrogen or carbon dioxide) to destroy tissue.

**cry·o·ther·a·py** (krī´ō-thār´ă-pē) SYN cold therapy.

**crypt** (kript) [TA] A pitlike depression or tubular recess.

**cryp·tic** (krip´tik) Hidden; occult; larvate. [G. *kryptikos*]

**cryp·to·coc·co·sis** (krip´tō-kok-ō´sis) An acute, subacute, or chronic infection by *Cryptococcus neoformans*.

**cryp·to·gen·ic** (krip´tō-jen´ik) Of obscure, indeterminate etiology or origin.

**cryp·to·gen·ic py·e·mi·a** (krip´tō-jen´ik pī-ē´mē-ă) Infection with source that is not evident.

**cryp·toz·y·gous** (krip-toz´i-gŭs) Having a narrow face compared with the width of the cranium, so that, when the skull is viewed from above, the zygomatic arches are not visible. [*crypto-* + G. *zygon*, yoke]

**crys·tal** (kris´tăl) A solid of regular shape and, for a given compound, characteristic angles, formed when an element or compound solidifies slowly enough, as a result either of freezing from the liquid form or of precipitating out of solution, to allow the individual molecules to take up regular positions with respect to one another. [G. *krystallos*, clear ice, crystal]

**crys·tal·line in·ter·face** (kris´tă-lēn in´tĕr-fās) In dentistry, boundary between adjacent crystals.

**crys·tal·li·za·tion** (kris´tăl-ī-zā´shŭn) Assumption of a crystalline form when a vapor or

cd

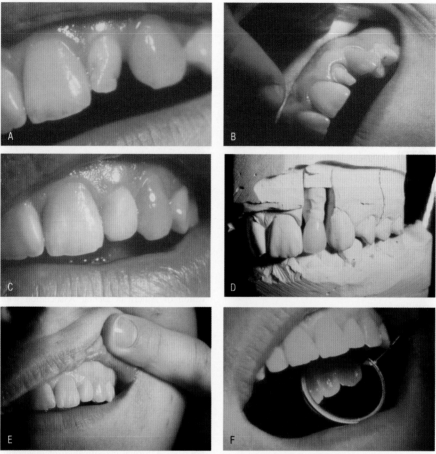

**restoration:** (A) preoperative peg-shaped lateral incisor; (B) crown preparation; (C) temporary crown; (D) articulated casts with permanent all-ceramic crown; (E, F) cemented crown in place

liquid becomes solidified, or a solute precipitates from solution.

**Cs** Symbol for cesium.

**CSD** Abbreviation for catscratch disease.

**CSF** Abbreviation for cerebrospinal fluid.

**CSI** Abbreviation for Calculus Surface Index.

**"C" slid·ing os·te·ot·o·my** (slīd´ing os´tē-ot´ŏ-mē) Extraoral osteotomy in the shape of a "C" performed bilaterally in the mandibular rami to correct retrognathia or apertognathia.

**CT** Abbreviation for computed tomography.

**CTD** Abbreviation for cumulative trauma disorder.

**cu·bi·tal** (kyū´bi-tăl) Relating to the elbow or to the ulna.

**cu·bi·tus,** pl. **cu·bi·ti** (kyū´bi-tŭs, -tī) [TA] **1.** SYN elbow (2). **2.** SYN ulna. [L. elbow]

**cu·boid, cu·boi·dal** (kyū´boyd, -boy´dăl) [TA] **1.** Resembling a cube. **2.** Relating to the os cuboideum. [G. *kybos,* cube, + *eidos,* resemblance]

**cue** (kyū) In conditioning and learning theory, a pattern of stimuli to which an individual has learned or is learning to respond.

**cuff** (kŭf) Any structure with a gap that nearly encircles some extension or outgrowth, thus, anything shaped like a cuff.

**cul-de-sac,** pl. **culs-de-sac** (kul-dĕ-sahk´) *This word is correctly spelled with two hyphens.* A blind pouch or tubular cavity closed at one end; e.g., diverticulum.

**cul·ture** (kŭl´chŭr) Propagation of microorganisms on or in any media. [L. *cultura,* tillage, fr. *colo,* pp. *cultus,* to till]

**cul·ture me·di·um** (kŭl´chŭr mē´dē-ŭm) A substance, either solid or liquid, used for the cultivation, isolation, identification, or storage of microorganisms. SYN medium (3).

**Cum·mer clas·si·fi·ca·tion** (kŭm′ĕr klas′ i-fi-kā′shŭn) Listing of several types of removable partial dentures in accordance with distribution of direct retainers.

**cu·mu·la·tive dose** (kyūm′yŭ-lă-tiv dōs) Total dose resulting from repeated exposures to radiation or chemotherapy of the same part of the body or of the whole body.

**cu·mu·la·tive trau·ma dis·or·der (CTD)** (kyūm′yŭ-lă-tiv traw′mă dis-ōr′dĕr) Any of the chronic disorders involving tendon, muscle, joint, and nerve damage, often resulting from work-related physical activities. SYN microtrauma, repetitive strain disorder.

**cu·ne·ate** (kyū′nē-āt) Wedge-shaped. [L. *cuneus,* wedge]

**cup** (kŭp) An excavated or hollowed structure, either anatomic or pathologic. [A.S. *cuppe*]

**cu·pric** (kyū′prik) Pertaining to copper, particularly to copper in the form of a doubly charged positive ion.

**cu·pu·la** (kŭp′ū-lă) [TA] A cup-shaped or domelike structure. [L. dim. of *cupa,* a tub]

**cu·ra·re** (kyū-rah′rē) An extract of various plants that produces nondepolarizing paralysis of skeletal muscle after intravenous injection by blocking transmission at the myoneuronal junction; used clinically to relax muscles during surgery.

**cur·a·tive** (kyūr′ă-tiv) 1. That which heals or cures. 2. Tending to heal or cure.

**cur·a·tive dose** (kyūr′ă-tiv dōs) 1. Quantity of substance required to effect cure of a disease or correct manifestations of a deficiency of a particular factor in the diet. 2. Effective dose used with therapeutically applied compounds.

**curd·y pus** (kŭr′dē pŭs) Pus containing flakes of caseous matter.

**cure** (kyūr) 1. To heal; to make well. 2. A restoration to health. 3. A special method or course of treatment. [L. *curo,* to care for]

**cu·ret·tage** (kyūr-e-tahzh′) A scraping, usually of the interior of a cavity or tract, for the removal of new growths or other abnormal tissues, or to obtain material for tissue diagnosis.

🔲**cu·rette, cu·ret** (kyūr-et′) Instrument in the form of a loop, ring, or scoop with sharpened edges, attached to a rod-shaped handle, used for curettage. See this page. [Fr.]

**cu·rie (C)** (kyūr′ē) A unit of measurement of radioactivity superseded by the S.I. unit, the becquerel (1 disintegration per second).

**cur·ing** (kyūr′ing) 1. The act of accomplishing

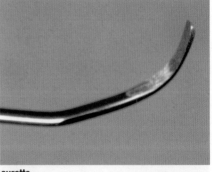

curette

a cure. 2. A process by which something is prepared for use, as by heating or aging.

**cur·rent** (kŭr′rĕnt) A stream or flow of fluid, air, or electricity. [L. *currens,* pres. p. of *curro,* to run]

**Cur·rent Den·tal Ter·mi·nol·o·gy (CDT)** (kŭr′ĕnt den′tăl tĕr′mi-nol′ŏ-jē) Publication of American Dental Association with glossary of dental terms, codes for dental procedures and nomenclature, and other information about dental care; mainly useful for record-keeping, billing, and similar information.

**cur·rent of in·ju·ry** (kŭr′ĕnt in′jūr-ē) Current generated when an injured part of a nerve, muscle, or other excitable tissue is connected through a conductor with the uninjured region; the injured tissue is negative to the uninjured.

**Cur·rent Pro·ce·dur·al Ter·mi·nol·o·gy (CPT)** (kŭr′ĕnt prŏ-sē′dyŭr-ăl tĕr′mi-nol′ŏ-jē) A formal classification of diagnostic and therapeutic procedures performed by physicians and other health care providers, published in annual revisions since 1996 by the American Medical Association (AMA). Each procedure is assigned a 5-digit code.

**curve** (kŭrv) 1. A nonangular continuous bend or line. 2. A chart or graphic representation, by means of a continuous line connecting individual observations, of the course of a physiologic activity, of the number of cases of a disease in a given period, or of any entity that might be otherwise presented by a table of figures. [L. *curvo,* to bend]

**curve of oc·clu·sion** (kŭrv ŏ-klū′zhŭn) 1. Curved surface that makes simultaneous contact with major portion of the incisal and occlusal prominences of existing teeth. 2. Curve of dentition on which occlusal surfaces lie. SYN occlusal curvature.

**curve of Spee** (kŭrv shpā) Anatomic curvature of the mandibular occlusal plane beginning at the tip of the lower cuspid and following the buccal cusps of the posterior teeth, continuing to the terminal molar. SYN von Spee curve.

**curve of Wil·son** (kŭrv wil′sŏn) Curvature in a frontal plane through the cusp tips of both the right and left molars.

**Cush·ing dis·ease** (kush′ing di-zēz′) Adrenal hyperplasia (Cushing syndrome) caused by an adrenocorticotropic hormone–secreting basophil adenoma of the pituitary.

**cush·ing·oid** (kush′ing-oyd) Resembling the signs and symptoms of Cushing disease or syndrome: moon facies, buffalo hump obesity, striations, adiposity, hypertension, diabetes, and osteoporosis.

**Cush·ing syn·drome** (kush′ing sin′drōm) Disorder resulting from increased adrenocortical secretion of cortisol.

**cush·ion** (kush′ŭn) In anatomy, any structure resembling a pad or cushion.

**cusp** (kŭsp) [TA] In dentistry, a conic elevation arising on the surface of a tooth from an independent calcification center. SEE ALSO dental tubercle. SYN cuspis [TA]. [L. *cuspis,* point]

**cus·pad** (kŭsp′ad) In a direction toward the cusp of a tooth. [L. *ad,* to]

**cus·pal in·ter·fe·rence** (kŭsp′ăl in′tĕr-fĕr′ĕns) SYN deflective occlusal contact.

**cusp-and-groove pat·tern** (kŭsp grūv pat′ĕrn) Arrangement of cusps and grooves on molars; in the lower molars, there are four principal ones, Y-5, Y-4, +5, and +4

**cusp an·gle** (kŭsp ang′gĕl) **1.** Angle made by slopes (i.e., incline) of a cusp (mesiodistally or buccolingually) with plane that passes through tip of cusp and is perpendicular to a line bisecting the cusp, measured mesiodistally or buccolingually. **2.** Angle made by the slopes of a cusp with a perpendicular line bisecting the cusp, measured mesiodistally or buccolingually. **3.** Half the angle included between the buccal and lingual or mesial and distal cusp inclines.

**cusp-fos·sa re·la·tion** (kŭsp fos′ă rĕ-lā′shŭn) Interocclusal arrangement by which maxillary and mandibular centric cusps articulate with opposing fossae.

**cusp height** (kŭsp hīt) **1.** Shortest distance between tip of cusp and its base plane. **2.** Shortest distance between deepest part of central fossa of posterior tooth and line connecting points of cusps of tooth.

**cus·pid** (kŭs′pid) **1.** Having but one cusp. SYN cuspidate. **2.** SYN canine tooth. [L. *cuspis,* point]

**cus·pi·date** (kŭs′pi-dāt) SYN cuspid (1).

**cus·pid tooth, cus·pi·date tooth** (kŭs′pid tūth, kŭs′pi-dāt) SYN canine tooth.

**cus·pis,** pl. **cus·pi·des** (kŭs′pis, -pi-dēz) [TA] SYN cusp. [L. a point]

**cus·pis den·tis** (kŭs′pis den′tis) [TA] SYN cusp of tooth.

**cusp·less tooth** (kŭsp′lĕs tūth) **1.** Tooth devoid of cusp formation. **2.** Severe abrasion of an occlusal surface. **3.** Type of artificial denture tooth.

**cusp of Ca·ra·bel·li** (kŭsp kah-ră-bel′lē) Fifth cusp found on maxillary first molars, usually located lingual to the mesiolingual cusp.

**cusp of tooth** (kŭsp tūth) [TA] Elevation or mound on crown of a tooth making up a part of the occlusal surface. SYN cuspis dentis [TA].

**cusp ridge** (kŭsp rij) An elevation extending both mesially and distally from cusp tip of molars and premolars, thus forming lingual and buccal boundaries of occlusal surface.

**cut** (kŭt) **1.** To sever or divide. **2.** To separate into fractions.

**cu·ta·ne·ous** (kyū-tā′nē-ŭs) Relating to the skin. [L. *cutis,* skin]

**cu·ta·ne·ous re·flex** (kyū-tā′nē-ŭs rē′fleks) Wrinkling of skin, caused by cutaneous stimulus, due to contraction of arrectores pilorum muscles.

**cu·ti·cle** (kyū′ti-kĕl) An outer thin layer, usually horny. [L. *cuticula,* dim. of *cutis,* skin]

**cu·tic·u·la,** pl. **cu·tic·u·lae** (kyū-tik′yū-lă, -lē) SYN epidermis. [L. cuticle]

**cu·tic·u·la den·tis** (kyū-tik′yū-lă den′tis) SYN enamel cuticle.

**cu·tis** (kyū′tis) [TA] SYN skin. [L.]

**cu·tis plate** (kyū′tis plāt) SYN dermatome (2).

**cut·ting edge** (kŭt′ing ej) **1.** Line formed where face and lateral edges of the working-end of an instrument meet at an angle forming a sharp cutting surface. **2.** SYN incisal margin.

**cut·ting teeth** (kŭt′ing tēth) The maxillary and mandibular anterior teeth.

**cut·tle·fish disc** (kŭt′ĕl-fish disk) Circle of paper or thin plastic coated with ground cuttlefish bone; used for fine smoothing and finishing of dental materials and teeth.

**CV** Abbreviation for cardiovascular.

**CVA** Abbreviation for cerebrovascular accident.

**CVS** Abbreviation for cardiovascular system.

**cy·a·no·co·bal·a·min** (sī′ă-nō-kō-bal′ă-min) A complex of cyanide and cobalamin, as in vitamin B12.

**cy·a·no·sis** (sī′ă-nō′sis) A dark bluish or purplish discoloration of the skin and mucous membrane due to deficient oxygenation of the blood.

**cy·cla·mate** (sī'klă-māt) A salt or ester of cyclamic acid; the calcium and sodium are non-caloric artificial sweetening agents.

**cy·cle** (sī'kĕl) **1.** A recurrent series of events. **2.** A recurring period of time. [G. *kyklos*, circle]

**cy·clic, cy·cli·cal** (sik'lik, -li-kăl) Pertaining to, or characteristic of, a cycle; occurring periodically, denoting the course of the symptoms in certain diseases or disorders.

**⊟cy·clic neu·tro·pe·ni·a** (sik'lik nū'trō-pē'nē-ă) See page A5. SYN periodic neutropenia.

**cy·clo·phos·pha·mide** (sī'klō-fos'fă-mīd) Alkylating agent with antitumor activity and uses similar to those of its parent compound, nitrogen mustard.

**cy·clo·ser·ine** (sī'klō-ser'ēn) An antibiotic produced by strains of *Streptomyces orchidaceus* or *S. garyphalus* with a wide spectrum of antibacterial activity.

**cy·clo·spor·ine** (sī'klō-spōr'ēn) A cyclic oligopeptide immunosuppressant used to inhibit organ transplant rejection.

**cy·clo·thy·mic dis·or·der** (sī'klō-thī'mik dis-ōr'dĕr) Mental disorder characterized by noticeable, clinically significant swings of mood, largely unrelated to life events, from depression to hypomania, though of lesser magnitude than in bipolar disorder.

**cy·clo·tron** (sī'klō-tron) A particle accelerator that speeds up particles in a spiral pattern to produce protons for nuclear research or radiation treatment.

**cyl·in·dro·ma** (sil'in-drō'mă) Slow growing, infiltrative tumor frequently found in submaxillary and parotid salivary glands and accessory glands of the palate. Chief histologic feature is presence of uniform, small dark-staining basal cells in anastomosing cords, with acellular areas between. [G. *kulindros*, roller, cylinder, fr. *kulindō*, to roll, + *-oma*, growth, neoplasm]

**cym·ba con·chae** (sim'bă kong'kē) [TA] Upper, smaller part of external ear lying above the crus helicis. [G. *kymbē*, the hollow of a vessel, a cup, a bowl, a boat]

**cyn·o·dont** (sī'nō-dont) **1.** A canine tooth. **2.** A tooth having one cusp or point. [G. *kyōn*, dog, + *odous* (*odont-*), tooth]

**cyst** (sist) An abnormal sac containing gas, fluid, or a semisolid material, with a membranous lining. [G. *kystis*, bladder]

**cyst·ad·e·no·ma** (sist'ad-ĕ-nō'mă) A histologically benign neoplasm derived from glandular epithelium.

**cys·te·ine (C)** (sis-tē'in) *Do not confuse this word with cystine.* L-isomer of this acid is found in most proteins; especially abundant in keratin.

**cys·ti·cer·co·sis** (sis'ti-sĕr-kō'sis) Disease caused by encystment of cysticercus larvae of some tapeworms (e.g., *Taenia solium* or *T. saginata*) in subcutaneous, muscle, or central nervous system tissue; encystment in the eye (usually the rear chamber) may cause ophthalmic damage.

**cys·tic fi·bro·sis, cys·tic fi·bro·sis of the pan·cre·as** (sis'tik fī-brō'sis, pan'krē-ăs) Congenital metabolic disorder in which secretions of exocrine glands are abnormal; excessively viscid mucus obstructs passageways; the sodium and chloride content of sweat is increased throughout the patient's life.

**⊟cys·tic hy·gro·ma** (sis'tik hī-grō'mă) Lymphangioma hygroma, poorly encapsulated tumor composed of lymph-filled endothelial-lined cysts, usually found around the neck, but may occur in the axilla, groin, or elsewhere. See this page.

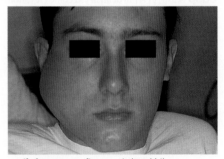

**cystic hygroma:** soft, present since birth

**cys·ti·nu·ri·a** (sis'ti-nyūr'ē-ă) Excessive urinary excretion of cystine, along with lysine, arginine, and ornithine. [*cystine* + G. *ouron*, urine]

**cys·tos·to·my** (sis-tos'tŏ-mē) Creation of an opening into the urinary bladder. SYN vesicostomy.

**cy·to·chrome** (sī'tō-krōm) A class of hemoprotein the principal biologic function of which is electron or hydrogen transport. [*cyto-* + G. *chrōma*, color]

**cy·to·chrome P-450 sys·tem** (sī'tō-krōm sis'tĕm) A heterogeneous group of enzymes that catalyzes various oxidative reactions in the human liver, intestines, kidneys, lungs, and central nervous system.

**cy·to·kine** (sī'tō-kīn) Any of numerous hormonelike, low-molecular-weight proteins, secreted by various cell types, which regulate the intensity and duration of immune response and mediate cell-to-cell communication. SEE interferon, interleukin. [*cyto-* + G. *kinēsis*, movement]

**cy·to·log·ic smear** (sī'tō-loj'ik smēr) A type of cytologic specimen made by smearing a sample before fixing it and staining it.

**cy·tol·o·gy** (sī-tol'ŏ-jē) The study of the anatomy, physiology, pathology, and chemistry of the cell. [*cyto-* + G. *logos,* study]

**cy·to·meg·a·lic in·clu·sion dis·ease** (sī'tō-mĕ-gă'lik in-klū'zhŭn di-zēz') The presence of inclusion bodies within the cytoplasm and nuclei of enlarged cells of various organs of newborn infants dying because of jaundice, hepatomegaly, and other symptoms; also has been found incidentally in salivary gland epithelium, apparently as a localized or mild infection (salivary gland virus disease). SYN inclusion body disease.

**cy·to·skel·e·ton** (sī'tō-skel'ĕ-tŏn) The tonofilaments, keratin, desmin, neurofilaments, or other intermediate filaments serving as supportive cytoplasmic elements to stiffen cells or to organize intracellular organelles.

**cy·to·tox·ic** (sī'tō-tok'sik) Detrimental or destructive to cells.

**cy·to·tox·ic·i·ty** (sī'tō-tok-sis'i-tē) The quality or state of being cytotoxic.

cd

# D

**Δ, δ 1.** Fourth letter of the Greek alphabet, delta. **2.** ANATOMY a triangular surface.

**D** Abbreviation for deciduous; dexter.

**D-** Abbreviation for dextro-.

**dac·ry·on** (dak'rē-on) Junction point of frontomaxillary and lacrimomaxillary sutures on medial wall of orbit. [G. a tear]

**dac·ti·no·my·cin** (dak'ti-nō-mī'sin) An antineoplastic antibiotic produced by several species of *Streptomyces* (e.g., *S. parvulus*).

**dai·ly dose** (dā'lē dōs) Total amount of a therapeutic substance to be taken within 24 hours.

**Dal·ton law** (dawl'tŏn law) Each gas in a mixture of gases exerts a pressure proportionate to the percentage of the gas and independent of the presence of the other gases present. SYN law of partial pressures. [John *Dalton*]

**dam** (dam) **1.** Any barrier to the flow of fluid. **2.** In surgery and dentistry, sheet of thin rubber arranged to shut off operative site from the access of fluid. [A.S. *fordemman,* to stop up]

**da·na·zol** (dā'nă-zol) A synthetic steroid used to treat endometriosis, fibrocystic breast disease, and angioedema.

**dap·sone** (dap'sōn) Antibiotic used to treat leprosy; active against the tubercle bacillus; used as a second-line agent in *Pneumocystis jiroveci (carinii)* pneumonia.

**d'Ar·cet met·al** (dahr-sā' met'ăl) Alloy of lead, bismuth, and tin; used in dentistry.

**Da·ri·er dis·ease** (dah-rē-ā' di-zēz') SYN keratosis follicularis.

**dark-field mi·cro·scope** (dahrk-fēld mī'krō-skōp) A microscope that has a special condenser and objective with a diaphragm that scatters light from the object observed, so the object appears bright on a dark background.

**dark·room** (dahrk'rūm) Enclosed area or chamber dimly lit by safelight (usually red) but otherwise intentionally lightproof room where films are handled and processed.

**da·ta** (dā'tă) **1.** Facts (usually established by observation, measurement, or experiment) used as a basis for inference, testing, or models. **2.** Information collected about a patient, family, or community. USAGE NOTE the word is plural and takes a plural verb.

**da·ta·base** (dā'tă-bās) A collection of information on a given topic, stored digitally for rapid search and retrieval.

**date of birth (DOB)** (dāt bǐrth) The day of birth of a patient or the insured party; often essential in determining eligibility.

**daugh·ter isotope** (daw'těr ī'sŏ-tōp) An element produced by radioactive decay of another. [O.E. *dohtor*]

**dau·no·ru·bi·cin** (daw'nō-rū'bi-sin) An anti-neoplastic antibiotic of the rhodomycin group, obtained from *Streptomyces peucetius.*

**day hos·pi·tal** (dā hos'pi-tăl) Special facility or within a hospital setting, which enables the patient to come to the hospital for daily treatment and return home at night.

**dB** Abbreviation for decibel.

**DC** Abbreviation for direct current.

**dead** (ded) **1.** Without life. **2.** Numb.

**dead nerve** (ded něrv) Colloq. misnomer for nonvital dental pulp.

**dead on ar·ri·val (DOA)** (ded ă-rī'văl) Charting notation used in the emergency department stating the patient has not survived the trip to the hospital.

**dead pulp** (ded pŭlp) SYN necrotic pulp.

**dead space** (ded spās) A cavity, potential or real, remaining after the closure of a wound that is not obliterated by the operative technique.

**dead tooth** (ded tūth) Colloq. misnomer for pulpless tooth.

**dead tracts** (ded trakts) Dentin areas characterized by degenerated odontoblastic processes; may result from injury caused by caries, attrition, erosion, or cavity preparation.

**deaf** (def) Unable to hear; hearing indistinctly; hard of hearing. [A.S. *deáf*]

**de·af·fer·en·ta·tion** (dē-af'ĕr-ĕn-tā'shŭn) Loss of sensory input from portion of the body. [L. *de,* from, + *afferent*]

**deaf·ness** (def'nĕs) General term for inability to hear.

**de·am·i·na·tion, de·am·i·ni·za·tion** (dē'am-i-nā'shŭn, dē-am'i-nī-zā'shŭn) Removal, usually by hydrolysis, of the NH$_2$ group from an amino compound.

**Dean fluor·o·sis in·dex** (dēn flūr-ō'sis in' deks) Measurement of degree of mottled enamel (fluorosis) in teeth; used most often in epidemiologic field studies.

**death** (deth) The cessation of life. In humans, manifested by loss of heartbeat, lack of breathing, and cerebral death. SYN mors.

**de·band·ing** (dē-band'ing) Removal of fixed orthodontic appliances. See page 157.

**de·bil·i·tat·ing** (dĕ-bil'i-tāt-ing) Denoting or characteristic of a morbid process that causes weakness.

**de·bil·i·ty** (dĕ-bil'i-tē) Weakness. [L. *debilitas,* fr. *debilis,* weak, fr. *de-* priv. + *habilis,* able]

**de·bond** (dē-bond') To separate a dental appli-

cd

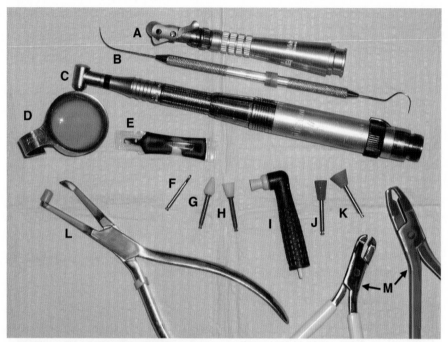

**debanding and debonding armamentarium:** (A) latch-type prophy angle; (B) explorer; (C) slow-speed handpiece with screw-type prophy angle; (D) pumice slurry; (E) disclosing solution; (F) tapered tungsten-carbide finishing bur; (G) aluminum finishing point; (H) aluminum oxide finishing cup; (I) disposable prophy angel and rubber cup; (J) brown polishing cup; (K) green polishing cup; (L) debanding pliers; (M) debonding pliers

ance such as an orthodontic band from the tooth to which it has been attached or bonded by a resin cement.

**de·bond·ing** (dē-bond´ing) Removal of orthodontic brackets and residual adhesive, after which the tooth surface is returned to its normal contour.

**dé·bride·ment** (dā-brēd-mawn[h]´) 1. Removal of foreign matter and devitalized tissue from a wound. 2. In dentistry, scaling, root planing, and ultrasonic instrumentation of root surfaces subgingivally to attain healthy gingival tissue. [Fr. unbridle]

**de·bris** (dĕ-brē´) A useless accumulation of miscellaneous particles; waste in the form of fragments. [Fr. *débris,* fr. O.Fr. *desbrisier,* to break apart, (fr. *des-* down, away + *brisier* to break) rubble, rubbish]

**debt** (det) A deficit, a liability, or obligation. [L. *debitum,* debt]

**de·cal·ci·fi·ca·tion** (dē-kal´si-fi-kā´shŭn) Removal of calcium salts from bones and teeth. [L. *de-,* away, + *calx* (*calc-*), lime, + *facio,* to make]

**de·cal·ci·fy·ing** (dē-kal´si-fī-ing) Denoting an agent, measure, or process that causes decalcification.

**de·car·box·yl·a·tion** (dē´kahr-bok-sil-ā´shŭn) Reaction involving removal of a molecule of carbon dioxide from a carboxylic acid.

**de·cay** (dĕ-kā´) 1. In dentistry, caries. 2. Destruction of an organic substance by slow combustion or gradual oxidation. 3. SYN putrefaction. 4. To deteriorate; to undergo slow combustion or putrefaction. [L. *de,* down, + *cado,* to fall]

**de·cel·er·a·tion** (dē-sel´ĕr-ā´shŭn) A slowing of contractions during the first stage of labor. [*de-* + as*celeration*]

**de·chlo·ri·da·tion** (dē-klōr´i-dā´shŭn) Reduction of sodium chloride in the body by reducing intake or increasing excretion.

**de·cho·les·ter·ol·i·za·tion** (dē´kō-les´tĕr-ol-ī-zā´shŭn) Therapeutic reduction of the cholesterol concentration of the blood.

**dec·i·bel (dB)** (des´i-bĕl) One tenth of a bel. [L. *decimus,* tenth, + *bel*]

**de·cid·u·al** (dĕ-sij´ū-ăl) Relating to the decidua.

**de·cid·u·ous (D)** (dĕ-sij´ū-ŭs) 1. Not permanent; denoting that which eventually falls off. 2. In dentistry, the first or primary dentition. [L. *deciduus,* falling off]

deciduous tooth 158 defibrillation

**de·cid·u·ous tooth** (dĕ-sij′ū-ŭs tūth) [TA] Tooth of the first set of teeth, comprising 20 in all, which erupts between 6–24 months of life. SYN dens deciduus [TA], baby tooth, dens lacteus, first dentition, milk dentition, milk tooth, primary dentition, temporary tooth.

**de·ci·sion tree** (dĕ-sizh′ŭn trē) A graphic construct showing available choices at each decision node of managing a clinical problem along with probabilities (if known) of possible outcomes for patient's freedom from disability, life expectancy, and mortality.

**de·coc·tion** (dē-kok′shŭn) 1. The process of boiling. 2. The pharmacopeial name for preparations made by boiling crude vegetable drugs, and then straining them, in the proportion of 50 g of the drug to 1000 mL of water.

**de·com·pres·sion** (dē-kŏm-presh′ŭn) Removal of pressure. [L. de-, from, down, + comprimo, pp. -pressus, to press together]

**de·con·ges·tive** (dē′kon-jes′tiv) Reducing tissue swelling or pathogens.

**de·con·tam·i·na·tion** (dē-kŏn-tam′i-nā′shŭn) Removal or neutralization of poisonous gas or other injurious agents.

**de·cor·ti·ca·tion** (dē-kōr′ti-kā′shŭn) Removal of the cortex, or external layer, beneath the capsule from any organ or structure. [L. decortico, pp. -atus, to deprive of bark, fr. de, from, + cortex, rind, bark]

**de·cru·des·cence** (dē-krū-des′ĕns) Abatement of the symptoms of disease. [L. de, from, + crudesco, to become worse, fr. crudus, crude]

**de·cu·bi·tus** (dē-kyū′bi-tŭs) 1. The position of the patient in bed; e.g., dorsal decubitus. 2. Sometimes refers to a decubitus ulcer. [L. decumbo, to lie down]

**de·cu·bi·tus ul·cer** (dē-kyū′bi-tŭs ŭl′sĕr) Focal ischemic necrosis of skin and underlying tissues at sites of pressure or friction in patients confined to bed or immobilized by illness; malnutrition worsens prognosis. SYN bedsore, bed sore, pressure sore, pressure ulcer.

**de·cur·rent** (dē-kŭr′ĕnt) Extending downward. [L. de-curro, pp. -cursus, to run down]

**de·duc·ti·ble** (dē-dŭk′ti-bĕl) The amount for which the insured is responsible before the health care plan pays; amount usually set on an annual basis. SYN annual deductible.

**deep bite** (dēp bīt) Abnormally large vertical overlap of anterior teeth in centric occlusion. Cf. closed bite.

**deep fa·cial vein** (dēp fā′shăl vān) [TA] Communicating vein that passes from pterygoid venous plexus of infratemporal fossa to facial vein.

**defaecation** [Br.] SYN defecation.

**def car·ies in·dex, DEF car·ies in·dex** (def kar′ēz in′deks) Index of past caries experience based on number of decayed, extracted, and filled deciduous (indicated by lower case letters) or permanent (indicated by CAPITAL LETTERS) teeth.

**def·e·ca·tion** (def′ĕ-kā′shŭn) The discharge of feces from the rectum. SYN defaecation. [L. defaeco, pp. -atus, to remove the dregs, purify]

**◨de·fect** (dē′fekt) An imperfection, malformation, dysfunction, or absence; an attribute of quality, in contrast with deficiency, which is an attribute of quantity. See this page and page A2. [L. deficio, pp. -fectus, to fail, to lack]

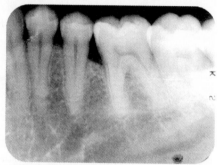
vertical one-wall defect: distal to premolar

**de·fec·tive** (dĕ-fek′tiv) Denoting or exhibiting a defect; imperfect; a failure of quality.

**defence** [Br.] SYN defense.

**de·fense** (dĕ-fens′) 1. The psychological mechanisms used to control anxiety. 2. Any protective posture, drug, or device. SYN defence. [L. defendo, to ward off]

**de·fense mech·a·nism** (dĕ-fens′ mek′ănizm) 1. Psychological means of coping with conflict or anxiety, e.g., conversion, denial, dissociation, rationalization, repression, sublimation. 2. Immunologic mechanism vs. nonspecific defense mechanism.

**de·fen·sive med·i·cine** (dĕ-fen′siv med′isin) Diagnostic or therapeutic measures conducted primarily as a safeguard against possible subsequent malpractice liability.

**def·er·ent** (def′ĕr-ĕnt) Carrying away. [L. deferens, pres. p. of defero, to carry away]

**def·er·ves·cence** (def′ĕr-ves′ĕns) Falling of an elevated temperature; abatement of fever. [L. de-fervesco, to cease boiling, fr. de- neg. + fervesco, to begin to boil]

**de·fib·ril·la·tion** (dē-fib′ri-lā′shŭn) The arrest of fibrillation of the cardiac muscle (atrial or ventricular) with restoration of the normal rhythm.

**de·fi·cien·cy** (dĕ-fish′ĕn-sē) An insufficient quantity of some substance, or organizational activity of which the amount present is of normal quality. [L. *deficio*, to fail, fr. *facio*, to do]

**de·fi·cien·cy dis·ease** (dĕ-fish′ĕn-sē di-zēz′) Disease resulting from undernutrition or an inadequacy of calories, proteins, or other needed elements.

**de·fi·cien·cy symp·tom** (dĕ-fish′ĕn-sē simp′tŏm) Manifestation of a lack, in varying degrees, of a substance necessary for normal structure and/or function of an organism.

**de·fin·i·tive care** (dĕ-fin′i-tiv kār) Completed therapy; end point at which all treatment required at the time has occurred.

**de·fin·i·tive pros·the·sis** (dĕ-fin′i-tiv pros-thē′sis) Dental appliance to be used over a prescribed period of time, usually long term.

**de·flec·tion** (dĕ-flek′shŭn) *Do not confuse this word with deflexion.* **1.** A moving to one side. **2.** In the electrocardiogram, a deviation of the curve from the isoelectric base line. [L. *deflecto*, pp. *-flexus*, to bend aside]

**de·flec·tive oc·clu·sal con·tact** (dĕ-flek′tiv ŏ-klū′zăl kon′takt) Condition of tooth contacts that diverts the mandible from a normal path of closure to centric jaw relation or displaces a removable denture from its seat. SYN cuspal interference, interceptive occlusal contact, premature contact.

**de·flu·o·ri·da·tion** (dē-flōr′i-dā′shŭn) Removal of excess fluoride from a community water supply.

**de·for·ma·tion** (dē-fōr-mā′shŭn) Deviation of form from normal; specifically, an alteration in shape and/or structure of a body part. [L. *deformo*, pp. *-atus*, to deform, fr. *forma*, form]

**de·for·mi·ty** (dĕ-fōrm′i-tē) A permanent structural deviation from the normal shape, size, or alignment, resulting in disfigurement; may be congenital or acquired.

**de·gen·er·a·cy** (dĕ-jen′ĕr-ă-sē) A condition marked by deterioration of mental or physical processes.

**de·gen·er·a·tive** (dĕ-jen′ĕr-ă-tiv) *Negative or pejorative connotations of this word may render it offensive in some contexts.* Relating to degeneration.

**de·gen·er·a·tive joint dis·ease (DJD)** (dĕ-jen′ĕr-ă-tiv joynt di-zēz′) SYN osteoarthritis.

**de·glov·ing** (dē-glŏv′ing) **1.** Intraoral surgical exposure of anterior mandible used in various orthognathic surgical operations. **2.** Intraoral exposure of the midfacial skeleton used in operations on the nose and paranasal sinuses.

**deglut.** (dē-glūt′) Abbreviation for L. *deglutiatur*, swallow.

**de·glu·ti·tion** (dē-glū-tish′ŭn) The act of swallowing. [L. *de-glutio*, to swallow]

**deg·ra·da·tion** (deg′ră-dā′shŭn) The change of a chemical compound into a less complex compound. [L. *degradatus*, degrade]

**de·gree** (dĕ-grē′) **1.** One of the divisions on the scale of a measuring instrument such as a thermometer or barometer. **2.** The 360th part of the circumference of a circle. **3.** A position or rank within a graded series. **4.** A measure of damage to tissue. [Fr. *degré*; L. *gradus*, a step]

**de·grees of free·dom** (dĕ-grēz′ frē′dŏm) In statistics, number of independent comparisons that can be made between the members of a sample.

**de·gus·ta·tion** (dē-gŭs-tā′shŭn) Sense of taste. [L. *de-gusto*, pp. *-atus*, to taste]

**de·his·cence** (dē-his′ĕns) A bursting open, splitting, or gaping along natural or sutured lines. [L. *dehisco*, to split apart or open]

**de·hy·drate** (dē-hī′drāt) **1.** To extract water from. **2.** To lose water. [L. *de*, from + G. *hydōr* (*hydr-*), water]

**de·hy·dra·tion** (dē-hī-drā′shŭn) *Avoid the jargonistic use of this word as a synonym of thirst.* **1.** Deprivation of water. **2.** Reduction of water content. **3.** SYN exsiccation. **4.** Used in emergency departments to describe a state of water loss sufficient to cause intravascular volume deficits leading to orthostatic symptoms.

**de·hy·dro·gen·ase** (dē′hī-droj′ĕ-nās) Class name for those enzymes that oxidize substrates by catalyzing removal of hydrogen from metabolites (hydrogen donors) and transferring it to other substances (hydrogen acceptors).

**de·hy·dro·ret·i·nol** (dē-hī′drō-ret′i-nol) Retinol with an additional double bond in the 3-4 position of the cyclohexane ring. SYN vitamin A2.

**de·i·on·iz·ed wa·ter** (dē-ī′ŏ-nīzd waw′tĕr) Water purified by passing through ion-exchange columns.

**DEJ** Abbreviation for dentinoenamel junction.

**de·jec·tion** (dĕ-jek′shŭn) **1.** The discharge of excrementitious matter. **2.** The matter so discharged. [L. *dejectio*, fr. *de-jicio*, pp. *-jectus*, to cast down]

**de·lam·i·na·tion** (dē-lam′i-nā′shŭn) Division into separate layers. [L. *de*, from, + *lamina*, a thin plate]

**de·layed al·ler·gy** (dĕ-lād′ al′ĕr-jē, dĕ-lād′ al′ĕr-jē) A type IV hypersensitivity allergic reaction; in a sensitized patient, the reaction becomes evident hours after contact with the allergen, reaches a peak after 24 to 48 hours, then slowly recedes.

**de·layed den·ti·tion** (dĕ-lād′ den-tish′ŭn) Late eruption of teeth.

**de·lay·ed e·rup·tion** (dĕ-lād′ ē-rŭp′shŭn) Dental eruption pattern chronologically later than normal; first tooth erupts at a later age than average, and intervals between subsequent dental eruptions are longer than average.

**de·layed hy·per·sen·si·ti·vi·ty** (dĕ-lād′ hī′pĕr-sen′si-tiv′i-tē) A cell-mediated response that occurs in immune people peaking at 24–48 hours after challenge with the same antigen used in an initial challenge.

**de·lir·i·ous** (dĕ-lir′ē-ŭs) In a state of delirium.

**de·lir·i·um,** pl. **de·lir·i·a** (dĕ-lir′ē-ŭm, dĕ-lir′ē-ŭm, -ă) An altered state of consciousness, consisting of confusion, distractibility, disorientation, disordered thinking and memory and other signs; caused by illness, medication, or toxic, structural, and metabolic disorders. [L. fr. *deliro,* to be crazy]

**de·lir·i·um tre·mens** (dĕ-lir′ē-ŭm trēm′ enz) Severe, sometimes fatal, form of delirium due to alcohol withdrawal following a period of sustained intoxication.

**del·ta hep·a·ti·tis** (del′tă hep′ă-tī′tis) SYN viral hepatitis type D.

**de·lu·sion** (dĕ-lū′zhŭn) *Do not confuse this word with hallucination or illusion.* A false belief or wrong judgment, sometimes associated with hallucinations, held with conviction despite evidence to the contrary. [L. *de-ludo,* pp. *-lusus,* to play false, deceive, fr. *ludo,* to play]

**de·mand** (dĕ-mand′) To ask, claim, or require with urgency or authority. [Med. L. *demandare*]

**de·mar·ca·tion** (dē′mahr-kā′shŭn) A setting of limits; a boundary. [Fr. fr. L. *de,* from, + Mediev. L. *marco,* to mark]

**de·men·ti·a** (dĕ-men′shē-ă) The loss, usually progressive, of cognitive and intellectual functions, without impairment of perception or consciousness; most commonly associated with structural brain disease. [L. fr. *de-* priv. + *mens,* mind]

**de·min·er·al·i·za·tion** (dē-min′ĕr-ăl-ī-zā′ shŭn) Loss or decrease of mineral constituents of body or individual tissues, especially bone.

**de·mog·ra·phy** (dĕ-mog′ră-fē) Study of populations, especially with reference to size, density, fertility, mortality, growth rate, age distribution, migration, and vital statistics. [G. *demos,* people, + *graphō,* to write]

**de·mul·cent** (dĕ-mŭl′sĕnt) **1.** Soothing; relieving irritation. **2.** An agent that relieves irrita-

tion. [L. *de-mulceo,* pp. *-mulctus,* to stroke lightly, to soften]

**de·my·e·li·na·tion, de·my·e·lin·i·za·tion** (dē-mī′e-lin-ā′shŭn, -ī-zā′shŭn, dē-mī′ē-li-nā′shŭn, -lin-ī-zā′shŭn) Loss of myelin with preservation of the axons or fiber tracts.

**de·na·tured** (dē-nā′chŭrd) **1.** Made unnatural or changed from the normal in any of its characteristics. **2.** Adulterated, as by addition of methanol to ethanol.

**de·na·tured al·co·hol** (dē-nā′chŭrd al′kŏ-hol) Ethyl alcohol rendered unfit for consumption as a beverage by the addition of one or several chemicals for commercial purposes.

**den·drite** (den′drīt) **1.** One of the two types of branching protoplasmic processes of the nerve cell. SYN neurodendrite. **2.** A crystalline treelike structure formed during the freezing of an alloy. [G. *dendritēs,* relating to a tree]

**den·drit·ic cell** (den-drit′ik sel) Cell of neural crest origin with extensive processes; they develop melanin early.

**de·ner·va·tion** (dē′nĕr-vā′shŭn) Loss of nerve supply.

**de·ni·al** (dĕ-nī′ăl) An unconscious defense mechanism used to allay anxiety by denying the existence of important conflicts, troublesome impulses, events, actions, or illness. [M.E., fr, O.Fr., fr. L. *denegare,* to say no]

**dens,** pl. **den·tes** (denz, den′tēz) **1.** [TA] SYN tooth. **2.** A strong toothlike process projecting upward from body of axis (second cervical vertebra), or epistropheus, around which the atlas rotates. See page 161. SYN odontoid process of epistropheus, odontoid process. [L.]

**dens an·gu·la·ris** (denz ang′gyū-lā′ris) SYN canine tooth.

**dens bi·cus·pi·dus,** pl. **den·tes bi·cus·pi·di** (denz bī-kŭs′pi-dŭs, den′tēz bī-kŭs′pi-dī) SYN premolar tooth.

**dens ca·ni·nus,** pl. **den·tes ca·ni·ni** (denz kā-nī′nŭs, den′tēz kā-nī′nē) [TA] SYN canine tooth.

**dens cus·pi·da·tus,** pl. **den·tes cus·pi·da·ti** (denz kŭs′pi-dā′tŭs, den′tēz kŭs′pi-dā′tī) SYN canine tooth.

**dens de·ci·d·u·us,** pl. **den·tes de·ci·du·i** (denz dē-sid′yū-ŭs, den′tēz dē-sid′yū-ī) [TA] SYN deciduous tooth.

**dens e·vag·i·na·tus** (denz ē-vaj′i-nā′tŭs) Anomaly wherein an extra cusp or tubercle protrudes from the occlusal surface of a tooth. SYN accessory tubercle (2).

**den·si·me·ter** (den-sim′e-tĕr) SYN densitometer.

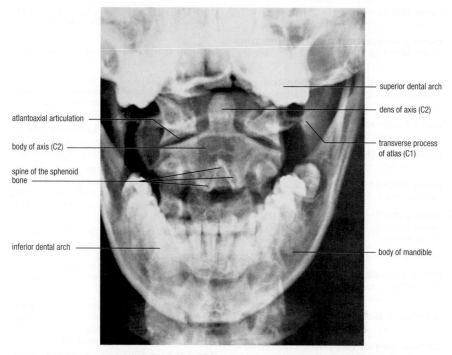

superior dental arch

dens of axis (C2)

atlantoaxial articulation

body of axis (C2)

transverse process
of atlas (C1)

spine of the sphenoid
bone

inferior dental arch

body of mandible

**dens:** radiograph taken through open mouth in anteroposterior projection; observe dens, a strong toothlike process projecting upward from body of axis (C2) around which atlas (C1) rotates

**dens in·ci·si·vus,** pl. **den·tes in·ci·si·vi** (denz in-si-sī'vŭs, den'tēz in-si-sī'vī) [TA] SYN incisor tooth.

**dens in den·te** (denz den'tē) Developmental disturbance in tooth formation due to invagination of the epithelium associated with crown development into area destined to become pulp space; after calcification, enamel and dentin invaginate the pulp space, giving the radiographic appearance of a "tooth within a tooth," the translation of this term's Latin. SYN dens invaginatus.

**⬛dens in·va·gi·na·tus** (denz in-vaj´i-nā´tŭs) See this page. SYN dens in dente. [Mediev. L. folded inward, fr. L. *vagina*, sheath]

**den·si·tom·e·ter** (dens'i-tom'ĕ-tĕr) **1.** An instrument for measuring the density of a fluid. **2.** An instrument for measuring the growth of bacteria in broth. **3.** An instrument for measuring the density of components separated by electrophoresis or chromatography, using light absorption or reflection. **4.** An electronic instrument for measuring the blackening of radiographic film by x-ray exposure; used for film densitometry and bone densitometry. [L. *densitas,* density, + G. *metron,* measure]

**den·si·ty,** pl. **den·si·ties** (dens'i-tē, -tēz) **1.** Compactness of a substance. **2.** Quantity of electricity on a given surface or in a given time

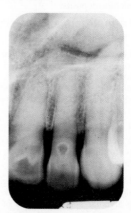

**dens invaginatus:** tear- or bulb-shaped type

per unit of volume. **3.** RADIOLOGIC PHYSICS opacity to light of an exposed radiographic or photographic film; the darker the film, the greater the measured density. **4.** CLINICAL RADIOLOGY a less exposed area on a film, corresponding to a region of greater x-ray attenuation (radiopacity) in the subject. [L. *densitas,* fr. *densus,* thick]

**dens lac·te·us** (denz lak'tē-ŭs) SYN deciduous tooth.

**dens mo·la·ris,** pl. **den·tes mo·la·res** (denz mō-lā'ris, den'tēz mō-lā'rēz) [TA] SEE ALSO molar. SYN molar tooth.

**dens mo·la·ris ter·ti·us** (denz mō-lā´ris tĕr´shē-ŭs) [TA] SYN third molar tooth.

**dens per·ma·nens,** pl. **den·tes per·ma·nen·tes** (denz pĕr´mă-nenz, den-tēz´ pĕr-mă-nen´tēz) [TA] SYN permanent tooth.

**dens pre·mo·la·ris,** pl. **den·tes pre·mo·la·res** (denz prē-mō-lā´ris, den-tez´ prē-mō-lā´rēz) [TA] SYN premolar tooth.

**dens sa·pi·en·ti·ae** (denz sā´pē-en´shē-ē) SYN third molar tooth. [L. *sapientia,* wisdom]

**dens se·ro·ti·nus** (denz sē-rō-tī´nŭs) [TA] SYN third molar tooth.

**dens suc·ce·da·ne·us** (denz sŭk´sĕ-dā´ nē-ŭs) SYN permanent tooth.

♻ **dent-, denti-, dento-** Combining forms meaning teeth; dental. SEE ALSO odonto-. [L. *dens,* tooth]

**den·tal** (den´tăl) Relating to the teeth.

**den·tal ab·scess, den·to·al·ve·o·lar ab·scess** (den´tăl ab´ses, den´to-al-vē´ō-lăr) SYN alveolar abscess.

**den·tal a·but·ment** (den´tăl ă-bŭt´mĕnt) SYN abutment.

**den·tal ac·qui·red pel·li·cle** (den´tăl ă-kwīrd´ pel´i-kĕl) Thin membranous layer, amorphous, acellular, and organic, which forms on exposed tooth surfaces, dental restorations, and dental calculus deposits.

**den·tal a·mal·gam al·loy** (den´tăl ă-mal´ găm al´oy) SYN amalgam.

**den·tal a·nat·o·my** (den´tăl ă-nat´ŏ-mē) 1. Branch of gross anatomy concerned with the morphology of teeth, their location, position, and relationships. 2. Anatomy course specifically designed to meet the needs of the curriculum of a school of dentistry.

**den·tal an·es·the·si·a** (den´tăl an-es-thē´zē-ă) General, conduction, local, or topical anesthesia for operations on the teeth, gingivae, or associated structures.

**den·tal an·ky·lo·sis** (den´tăl ang´ki-lō´sis) Bony union of radicular surface of tooth to surrounding alveolar bone in an area of previous partial root resorption.

**den·tal a·nom·a·ly** (den´tăl ă-nom´ă-lē) Abnormality or deviation from the average norm of anatomy, function, or position of teeth.

**den·tal an·thro·po·lo·gy** (den´tăl an´thrŏ-pol´ŏ-jē) Branch of physical anthropology concerned with the origin, evolution, and development of dentition of primates, especially humans, and to the relationship between primates' dentition and their physical and social relationships.

**den·tal an·xi·e·ty** (den´tăl ang-zī´ĕ-tē) Fear related to seeking or receiving dental care.

**den·tal a·pla·si·a** (den´tăl ă-plā´zē-ă) Defective development or congenital absence of teeth.

**den·tal ap·pa·ra·tus** (den´tăl ap´ă-rat´ŭs) SYN masticatory system.

**den·tal arch** (den´tăl ahrch) Curved composite structure of the natural dentition and residual ridge, or the remains thereof after the loss of some or all natural teeth. SEE ALSO arch.

**den·tal ar·ma·men·ta·ri·um** (den´tăl ahr´mă-men-tar´ē-ŭm) The equipment and instruments used in the delivery of dental care.

**den·tal ar·ti·cu·la·tion** (den´tăl ahr-tik´ yū-lā´shŭn) Contact relationship of occlusal surfaces of upper and lower teeth when moving into and away from centric occlusion. SYN gliding occlusion.

**den·tal as·sis·tant** (den´tăl ă-sis´tănt) A person trained to provide support to a dentist with general tasks ranging from clerical work and assistance at chairside to laboratory, infection control, dental laboratory, and exposure of radiographic images.

**den·tal aux·i·li·ary** (den´tăl awg-zil´yĕr-ē) Employees or staff involved in provision of dental care (e.g., dental assistant, dental hygienist, office manager). SEE ALSO auxiliary.

**den·tal bi·o·film** (den´tăl bī´ō-film) An organized community of microorganisms that attaches to the teeth; may contribute to oral disease; dental plaque is a biofilm.

**den·tal bi·o·mech·a·nics** (den´tăl bī´ō-mē-kan´iks) SYN dental biophysics.

**den·tal bi·o·phys·ics** (den´tăl bī´ō-fiz´iks) Relationship between biologic behavior of oral structures and the physical influence of a dental restoration. SYN dental biomechanics.

**den·tal branch·es** (den´tăl branch´ĕz) [TA] Branches to the teeth. *Terminologica Anatomica* lists dental branches of the following: 1) anterior superior alveolar artery (rami dentales arteriarum alveolarium superiorum anteriorum [TA]); 2) inferior alveolar artery (rami dentales arteriae alveolaris inferioris [TA]); and 3) posterior superior alveolar artery (rami dentales arteriae alveolaris posterioris [TA]). SYN dental rami.

**den·tal bulb** (den´tăl bŭlb) Papilla, which forms part of primordium of a tooth situated within the cup-shaped enamel organ.

**den·tal cal·cu·lus** (den´tăl kal´kyū-lŭs) 1. Calcified deposits formed around the teeth; may appear as subgingival or supragingival calculus. 2. SYN tartar (1). SYN calculus (1).

**den·tal ca·nals** (den´tăl kă-nalz´) SYN alveolar canals of maxilla.

**den·tal car·ies** (den´tăl kar´ēz) Localized, progressively destructive disease of the teeth that starts at external surface (usually enamel) with the apparent dissolution of inorganic components by organic acids produced in immediate proximity to tooth by enzymatic action of masses of microorganisms (in the bacterial plaque) on carbohydrates; initial demineralization is followed by an enzymatic destruction of the protein matrix with subsequent cavitation and direct bacterial invasion; in the dentin, demineralization of the walls of the tubules is followed by bacterial invasion and destruction of the organic matrix. SYN saprodontia.

**den·tal cast** (den´tăl kast) Positive likeness of a part or parts of the oral cavity. See this page.

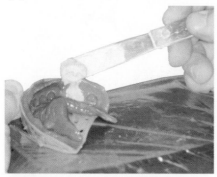

**fabrication of dental cast by pouring dental stone into impression**

**den·tal cast·ing in·vest·ment** (den´tăl kas´ting in-vest´mĕnt) Combination of silica phosphate and gypsum bonding materials used in dentistry to enclose wax or plastic patterns during the casting process in the laboratory fabrication of dental crowns and bridges.

**den·tal ce·ment** (den´tăl sĕ-ment´) SEE cement (1).

**den·tal chart** (den´tăl chahrt) Dental record containing patient information, medical and dental histories, illustrative and written description of existing conditions, treatment needed and provided, radiographs, and other material.

**den·tal clin·ic** (den´tăl klin´ik) A facility where dental services are rendered.

**den·tal con·tin·u·ing care** (den´tăl kŏn-tin´yū-ing kār) A term referring to dental or dental hygiene care rendered to patients of record. It encompases recall examinations, treatments, and maintenance procedures.

**den·tal cord** (den´tăl kōrd) Aggregation of epithelial cells forming rudimentary enamel organ.

**den·tal crest** (den´tăl krest) Maxillary ridge on alveolar processes of maxillary bones in the fetus. SYN crista dentalis.

**den·tal crypt** (den´tăl kript) Space filled by dental follicle.

**den·tal cur·ing** (den´tăl kyūr´ing) Process by which plastic materials become rigid to form

a denture base, filling, impression tray, or other appliance.

**den·tal cu·ti·cle** (den´tăl kyū´ti-kĕl) SYN enamel cuticle.

**den·tal cyst** (den´tăl sist) SYN periodontal cyst.

**den·tal dam clamp** (den´tăl dam klamp) Springlike metal piece encircling or grasping cervix of a tooth and shaped so as to prevent a rubber dam from coming off the tooth. See this page. SYN rubber dam clamp.

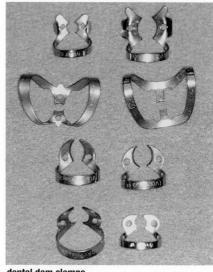

**dental dam clamps**

**den·tal de·cay** (den´tăl dĕ-kā´) SEE ALSO decay. SYN dental caries.

**den·tal de·pos·it** (den´tăl dĕ-poz´it) Any soft or hard substance attached to tooth surfaces; often associated with dental diseases such as caries or periodontal disease (e.g., dental plaque or calculus).

**den·tal drill** (den´tăl dril) Rotary power-driven instrument into which cutting points may be inserted. SEE ALSO handpiece.

**den·tal dys·func·tion** (den´tăl dis-fŭngk´shŭn) Abnormal function of dental structures.

**den·tal e·nam·el** (den´tăl ĕ-nam´ĕl) SYN enamel.

**den·tal en·do·scope** (den´tăl en´dō-skōp) An illuminated optic instrument inserted into the periodontal pocket to provide the clinician with direct vision of subgingival root conditions.

**den·tal en·gine** (den´tăl en´jin) Motive power of a dental handpiece that causes it to rotate.

**den·tal en·gi·neer·ing** (den´tăl en´ji-nēr´ing) Application of engineering principles to dentistry.

**den·tal eth·ics** (den´tăl eth´iks) Ethical principles that relate to the dental profession (e.g., beneficence, nonmaleficence, autonomy).

**den·tal fis·tu·la** (den´tăl fis´tyū-lă) SYN gingival fistula.

**den·tal floss** (den´tăl flaws) Untwisted thread made of fine, short, silk or synthetic fibers, frequently waxed; used for cleansing interproximal spaces and between contact areas of the teeth. SYN floss silk, floss (1).

**den·tal flu·or·o·sis** (den´tăl flōr-ō´sis) SYN fluorosis.

**den·tal fol·li·cle** (den´tăl fol´i-kĕl) Fibrous sac that encloses odontogenic organ and developing tooth. SEE ALSO dental sac.

**den·tal for·ceps** (den´tăl fōr´seps) Device used to luxate teeth and remove them from the alveolus. SYN extracting forceps.

**den·tal fur·nace** (den´tăl fŭr´năs) **1.** Furnace used to eliminate wax pattern from investment mold before to casting in metal. **2.** Furnace used to fuse and glaze dental porcelains.

**den·tal ger·i·at·rics** (den´tăl jer´ē-at´riks) SEE geriatric dentistry.

**den·tal germ** (den´tăl jĕrm) SYN tooth bud.

**den·tal·gi·a** (den-tal´jē-ă) SYN toothache. [L. *dens*, tooth, + G. *algos*, pain]

**den·tal gran·u·lo·ma** (den´tăl gran´yū-lō´mă) SYN periapical granuloma.

**den·tal groove** (den´tăl grūv) Transitory depression in gingival surface of embryonic jaw along line of ingrowth of dental lamina.

**den·tal health ed·u·ca·tion** (den´tăl helth ed-yū-kā´shŭn) Provision of oral health information to patients in such a way that they can apply it in everyday living.

**den·tal his·to·ry** (den´tăl his´tŏr-ē) A written documentation of a patient's oral health covering all particulars of disease and therapy.

**den·tal hy·giene ar·ma·men·ta·ri·um** (den´tăl hī´jēn ahr´mă-men-tar´ē-ŭm) A variety of equipment used by dental hygienist in the delivery of dental hygiene services.

**den·tal hy·giene care plan** (den´tăl hī´jēn kār plan) Services within the framework of the total dental treatment plan to be carried out by a dental hygienist.

**den·tal hy·giene di·ag·no·sis** (den´tăl hī´jēn dī´ăg-nō´sis) The determination of the oral health conditions presented in patients with the intent of formulating dental hygiene intervention plan.

**den·tal hy·gien·ist (DH)** (den´tăl hī-jē´nist) Licensed, professional auxiliary in dentistry who is both an oral health educator and clinician, and who uses preventive, therapeutic, and educational methods for the control of oral diseases.

**den·tal im·pac·tion** (den´tăl im-pak´shŭn) Confinement of a tooth in alveolus and prevention of its eruption into normal position. SEE ALSO impacted tooth. See this page.

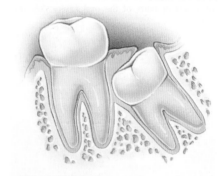

**mesioangular impaction**

**den·tal im·plant** (den´tăl im´plant) The artificial replacement for a tooth root SEE ALSO dental implants, endosseous dental implant. See this page.

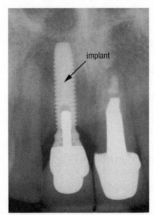

**radiographic image of dental implant:** titanium implant screw supporting a single crown

**den·tal im·plant a·but·ment** (den´tăl im´plant ă-bŭt´ment) SYN implant superstructure.

**den·tal im·plants** (den´tăl im´plants) Metal anchors, most frequently titanium posts, permanently attached to the jaw bone to which crowns, bridges, or dentures are attached. See page 165. SYN endosseous dental implant.

**den·tal in·dex (DI)** (den´tăl in´deks) **1.** Rela-

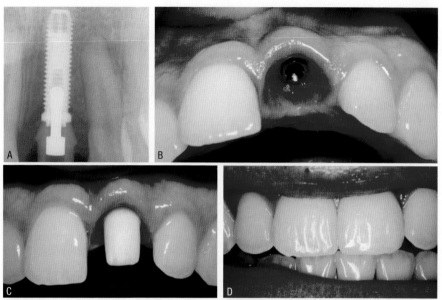

**endosseous single-tooth implant restored with crown:** (A) radiograph of implant, abutment, abutment screw; (B) clinical photograph of implant; (C) esthetic abutment and cylinder; (D) crown supported by implant

tion of the dental length (distance from the mesial surface of the first premolar to the distal surface of the third molar) to the basinasal (basion to nasion) length: (dental length × 100)/ basinasal length. **2.** System of numbers for indicating comparative size of teeth. SYN Flower dental index.

**den·tal in·stru·ment** (den´tăl in´strŭ-mĕnt) The tools or implements used for the diagnosis and treatment of dental disease. SEE ALSO instrument.

**den·tal ju·ris·pru·dence** (den´tăl jŭr´is-prū´dĕns) SYN forensic dentistry.

**den·tal lab·o·ra·tory** (den´tăl lab´ŏ-ră-tō-rē, lab´ră-, lă-bōr´ă-) A facility equipped for fabrication of dental models and appliances (e.g., dentures, partial dentures, crowns, fixed bridges).

**den·tal lam·i·na** (den´tăl lam´i-nă) SYN dental ledge.

**den·tal ledge** (den´tăl lej) Band of ectodermal cells growing from epithelium of the embryonic jaws into underlying mesenchyme; local buds from the ledge give rise to the primordia of the enamel organs of the teeth. SYN dental lamina, dental shelf, dentogingival lamina, enamel ledge, primary dental lamina.

**den·tal le·ver** (den´tăl lev´ĕr) SYN elevator (1).

**dental li·cen·sure** (den´tăl lī´sĕns-shŭr) Legal credential signifying the right to practice dentistry.

**den·tal lit·er·a·ture** (den´tăl lit´ĕr-ă-chŭr)

Written books or journals related to the art and science of dentistry.

**den·tal·ly dys·func·tional** (den´tăl-ē dis-fŭngk´shŭn-ăl) Denotes abnormal functioning of dental structures.

**den·tal lymph** (den´tăl limf) SYN dentinal fluid.

**den·tal mir·ror** (den´tăl mir´ŏr) Device that has a reflecting mirrored surface at its working end to view tooth surfaces that cannot be directly visualized.

**den·tal neck** (den´tăl nek) SYN neck of tooth.

**den·tal ne·glect** (den´tăl nĕg-lekt´) The term describing the decision to not obtain dental care.

**den·tal nerve** (den´tăl nĕrv) **1.** Colloquial term for dental pulp. **2.** Branches of the inferior and superior alveolar nerves to the teeth.

**den·tal or·gan** (den´tăl ōr´găn) SYN enamel organ.

**den·tal or·tho·pe·dics** (den´tăl ōr´thŏ-pē´diks) SYN orthodontics.

**den·tal os·te·o·ma** (den´tăl os´tē-ō´mă) Exostosis arising from a tooth root.

**den·tal pa·pil·la** (den´tăl pă-pil´ă) [TA] Projection of the mesenchymal tissue of the developing jaw into the cup of the enamel organ; its outer layer becomes a layer of specialized columnar cells, the odontoblasts, which form the dentin of the tooth. SYN dentinal papilla.

**den·tal path·ol·ogy** (den′tăl pă-thol′ŏ-jē) SYN oral pathology.

**den·tal per·cus·sion** (den′tăl pĕr-kŭsh′ŏn) Method of examining a tooth by tapping the dentition with a solid object, such as the handle of an intraoral mirror, to evaluate tooth vitality and presence of periapical pathology.

**∎ den·tal plaque** (den′tăl plak) **1.** Noncalcified accumulation mainly of oral microorganisms and their products that adheres tenaciously to the teeth and is not readily dislodged. See this page. **2.** SYN bacterial plaque.

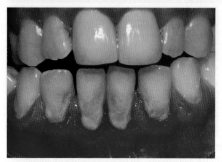

**plaque:** gingival margins affected

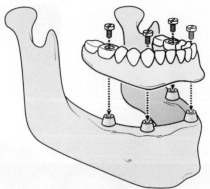

dentist-retrievable prosthesis: prosthesis shown here is similar to a full denture except it is attached by screws to tops of abutment posts; this restorative option is now rarely used because patient cannot remove it thus making plaque removal difficult and time consuming

**den·tal plas·ter** (den′tăl plas′tĕr) Beta form of calcium sulfate hemihydrate; a fibrous aggregate of fine crystals with capillary pores that are irregular in shape and porous in character; also referred to as plaster of Paris.

**den·tal pol·yp** (den′tăl pol′ip) SYN hyperplastic pulpitis.

**den·tal prac·tice man·age·ment** (den′tăl prak′tis man′ăj-mĕnt) The business principles utilized in the formation, operation, or management of a dental facility or office.

**den·tal pro·cess** (den′tăl pro′ses) SYN alveolar process of maxilla.

**den·tal proph·y·lax·is** (den′tăl prō′fi-lak′sis) Procedures whereby calculus, stains, and other accretions are removed from the crowns and roots of the teeth and the enamel surfaces are polished. SYN cleaning.

**∎ den·tal pros·the·sis** (den′tăl pros-thē′sis) Artificial replacement of teeth and associated dental or alveolar structures. See this page.

**den·tal pros·thet·ics** (den′tăl pros-thet′iks) SYN prosthodontics.

**den·tal pub·lic health** (den′tăl pŭb′lik helth) Preventing and controlling dental diseases and promoting dental health through organized community efforts.

**den·tal pulp** (den′tăl pŭlp) [TA] Soft tissue within pulp cavity, consisting of connective tissue containing blood vessels, nerves, and lymphatics, and at the periphery, layer of odontoblasts capable of internal deposition and repair of the dentin. SYN dentinal pulp, tooth pulp.

**dental pump** (den′tăl pŭmp) SYN saliva ejector.

**den·tal rami** (den′tăl rā′mī) SYN dental branches.

**den·tal rec·ord** (den′tăl rek′ŏrd) Electronic or hard copy of all patient information and documentation kept on dental patients.

**den·tal re·search** (den′tăl rĕ-sĕrch′) Formalized acquisition and investigation of subject matter related to the dental profession.

**den·tal ridge** (den′tăl rij) Prominent border of a cusp or margin of a tooth.

**den·tal root cyst** (den′tăl rūt sist) SYN periodontal cyst.

**den·tal sac** (den′tăl sak) Outer investment of ectomesenchymal tissue surrounding a developing tooth; involved in formation of periodontal ligament, alveolus, and cementum.

**den·tal scal·ing** (den′tăl skāl′ing) SYN scaling.

**den·tal seal·ant** (den′tăl sēl′ănt) SYN fissure sealant.

**den·tal se·nes·cence** (den′tăl sĕ-nes′ĕns) Condition of the teeth and associated structures with deterioration due to normal or premature aging.

**den·tal shelf** (den′tăl shelf) SYN dental ledge.

**den·tal splint** (den′tăl splint) Device used to fasten teeth in the same dental arch to support them or to prevent or minimize movement; may connect natural teeth either directly or to a prosthesis (e.g., artificial crown).

**den·tal staff** (den′tăl staf) Health care personnel employed to render dental services.

**den·tal stone** (den′tăl stōn) Alpha form of calcium sulfate semihydrate with physical properties superior to those of the beta form (dental plaster); consists of cleavage fragments and crystals in the form of rods and prisms and is thereby denser than the beta form; can form a dense stonelike material when mixed with water; used to pour models (casts) of dental structures.

**den·tal sur·geon** (den′tăl sŭr′jŏn) General practitioner of dentistry; a dentist with the D.D.S. or D.M.D. degree.

**den·tal sy·ringe** (den′tăl sir-inj′) Breech-loading metal cartridge syringe into which fits a hermetically sealed glass cartridge containing the anesthetic solution.

**den·tal tape** (den′tăl tāp) A wide thread similar to dental floss composed of fine, short, silk or synthetic fibers; used for clean interproximal spaces and between contact areas of the teeth.

**den·tal tech·ni·ci·an** (den′tăl tek-nish′ăn) The dental professional who fabricates crowns, bridges, and prosthetic devices under supervision of or following a prescription by a dentist.

**den·tal tu·ber·cle** (den′tăl tū′bĕr-kĕl) [TA] Small elevation on some portions of a crown produced by an extra formation of enamel. SYN crown tubercle, tubercle of tooth.

**den·tal tu·bules** (den′tăl tū′byūlz) SYN dentinal tubules.

**den·tal ul·cer** (den′tăl ŭl′sĕr) Lesion on oral mucuous membranes due to biting friction.

**den·tal unit** (den′tăl yū′nit) Mobile or fixed equipment used by dentists and dental hygienists to provide dental care.

**den·tal var·nish** (den′tăl vahr′nish) Solutions of natural resins and gums in a suitable solvent, of which a thin coating is applied over surfaces of cavity preparations before placement of restorations, used to protect tooth from restorative materials. SYN cavity liner, vernix.

**den·tal wedge** (den′tăl wej) Double inclined plane used to separate teeth, maintain separation obtained, or hold matrix in place.

**den·ta·ry cen·ter** (den′tăr-ē sen′tĕr) Specific ossification center of mandible that gives rise to lower border of its outer plate.

**den·tate** (den′tāt) Notched; toothed; cogged. [L. *dentatus,* toothed]

**den·tate line** (den′tāt līn) SYN pectinate line.

**den·tate su·ture** (den′tāt sū′chŭr) SYN serrate suture.

**den·tes a·cus·ti·ci** (den′tēz ă-kūs′ti-sī) [TA] SYN acoustic teeth.

**den·ti·a** (den′shē-ă) The process of tooth development or eruption.

**den·ti·a prae·cox** (den′shē-ă prē′koks) Premature tooth eruption.

**den·ti·a tar·da** (den′shē-ă tahr′dă) Delayed tooth eruption. Delayed tooth eruption.

**den·ti·cle** (den′ti-kĕl) **1.** SYN endolith. **2.** A toothlike projection from a hard surface. [L. *denticulus,* a small tooth]

**den·tic·u·late, den·tic·u·lat·ed** (den-tik′yū-lăt, -lāt-ed, den-tik′yū-lăt, -lā-tĕd) **1.** Finely dentated, notched, or serrated. **2.** Having small teeth.

**den·ti·form** (den′ti-fōrm) Tooth-shaped.

**den·ti·frice** (den′ti-fris) Any preparation used to cleanse teeth, e.g., a tooth powder, toothpaste, or tooth wash.

**den·ti·frice a·bra·sion** (den′ti-fris ă-brā′zhŭn) The frictional removal of the tooth surface by a dentifrice.

**den·tig·er·ous** (den-tij′ĕr-ŭs) Arising from or associated with teeth, as a dentigerous cyst. [*denti-* + L. *gero,* to bear]

**den·tig·er·ous cyst** (den-tij′ĕr-ŭs sist) Odontogenic cyst derived from the reduced enamel epithelium surrounding crown of impacted tooth. See this page. SYN follicular cyst (2).

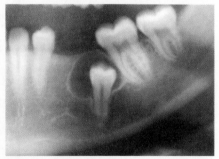

**dentigerous cyst:** mandibular premolar

**den·ti·la·bi·al** (den′ti-lā′bē-ăl) Relating to the teeth and lips. [*denti-* + L. *labium,* lip]

**den·ti·lin·gual** (den′ti-ling′gwăl) Relating to teeth and tongue. [*denti-* + L. *lingua,* tongue]

**den·tin** (den′tin) [TA] Ivory forming mass of tooth. SYN dentinum [TA], ebur dentis. [L. *dens,* tooth]

**den·ti·nal** (den′ti-năl) Relating to dentin.

**den·ti·nal ca·nals** (den′ti-năl kă-nalz′) SYN dentinal tubules.

**den·ti·nal fibers, den·tal fi·bers** (den′ti-năl fī′běrz, den′tăl) Processes of pulpal cells, the odontoblasts, which extend in radial fashion through dentin toward dentoenamel junction and are contained within dentinal tubules. SYN odontoblastic processes, Tomes fibers.

**den·ti·nal flu·id** (den′ti-năl flū′id) Lymph of dentin, which appears on surface of freshly cut dentin, especially in young teeth; a transudate of extracellular fluid, mainly cytoplasm of odontoblastic processes, from dental pulp via dentinal tubules. SYN dental lymph.

**den·ti·nal·gi·a** (den′ti-nal′jē-ă) Dentinal sensitivity or pain.

**den·ti·nal la·mi·na cyst** (den′ti-năl lam′i-nă sist) A small keratin-filled cyst, usually multiple, on the alveolar ridge of newborn infants; it is derived from remnants of the dental lamina.

**den·ti·nal pa·pil·la** (den′ti-năl pă-pil′ă) SYN dental papilla.

**den·ti·nal pulp** (den′ti-năl pŭlp) SYN dental pulp.

**den·ti·nal tu·bules** (den′ti-năl tū′byūlz) Minute, wavy, branching tubes or canals in the dentin; they contain the long cytoplasmic pro-cesses of odontoblasts and extend radially from the pulp to the dentoenamel and dentocemental junctions. See this page. SYN dental tubules, dentinal canals.

**den·tin bridge** (den′tin brij) A deposit of reparative dentin or other substances that forms across and reseals exposed tooth pulp tissue.

**den·tin ca·ries** (den′tin kar′ēz) Decay involving the dentin of a tooth. SEE ALSO caries.

**den·tin (den·ti·nal) hy·per·sen·si·tiv·i·ty** (den′tin den′tĭ-năl hī-pĕr-sen-sĭ-tiv′ĭ-tē) Short, sharp transient painful reaction (possibly related to loss of cementum) that occurs when some areas of exposed dentin are subjected to a mechanical stimulus, thermal stimulus, or chemical stimulus; cannot be explained as arising from any other form of dental defect or pathology and subsides quickly when stimulus ceases.

**den·tin dys·pla·si·a** (den′tin dis-plā′zē-ă) Hereditary tooth disorder involving both primary and permanent dentition, in which the clinical morphology and color of the teeth are normal, but the teeth radiographically exhibit short roots, obliteration of the pulp chambers and canals, mobility, and premature exfoliation. See page 169.

**den·tin glob·ules** (den′tin glob′yūlz) Calcospherites formed by calcification or mineral-

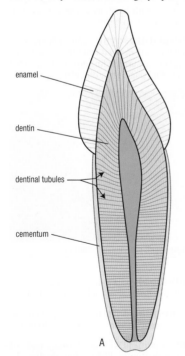
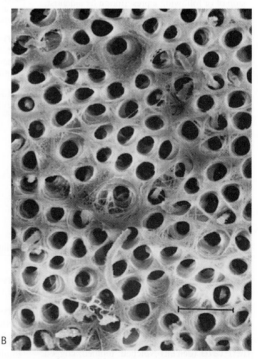

enamel

dentin

dentinal tubules

cementum

A      B

**dentinal tubules:** (A) schematic of dentinal tubules that penetrate dentin; (B) scanning electron micrograph of dentinal tubules of a human tooth

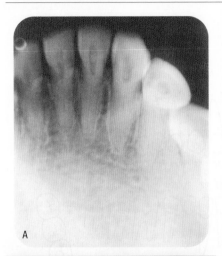

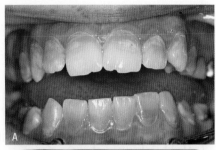

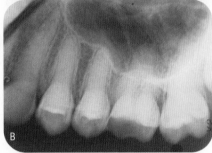

**dentinogenesis imperfecta:** (A) Shields type I, enamel chipping; (B) radiograph showing obliterated pulps

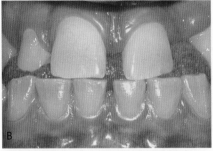

**dentin dysplasia:** (A) radiograph; (B) frontal view

ization of the coronal dentin matrix occurring in globular areas.

**den·tin·o·ce·ment·al** (den′ti-nō-sĕ-men′tăl) Relating to dentin and cementum of teeth. SYN cementodentinal.

**den·tin·o·e·nam·el** (den′ti-nō-ĕ-nam′ĕl) Relating to dentin and enamel of teeth. SYN amelodentinal.

**den·tin·o·e·nam·el junc·tion (DEJ)** (den′ti-nō-ĕ-nam′ĕl jŭngk′shŭn) Surface at which the enamel and the dentin of the crown of a tooth are joined.

**den·tin·o·gen·e·sis** (den′ti-nō-jen′ĕ-sis) Process of dentin formation in development of teeth. [*dentin* + G. *genesis,* production]

**⬛den·tin·o·gen·e·sis im·per·fec·ta** (den′ti-nō-jen′ĕ-sis im-pĕr-fek′tă) Dental disorder characterized clinically by translucent gray to yellow-brown teeth involving both primary and permanent dentition; such enamel fractures easily, leaving exposed dentin, which undergoes rapid attrition. See this page and page A4. SYN hereditary opalescent dentin (1).

**den·ti·noid** (den′ti-noyd) **1.** Resembling dentin. **2.** SYN dentinoma.

**den·ti·no·ma** (den′ti-nō′mă) Rare benign odontogenic tumor consisting microscopically of dysplastic dentin and strands of epithelium within a fibrous stroma. SYN dentinoid (2).

**den·ti·num** (den-ti′nŭm) [TA] *Avoid the mispronunciation den′tinum.* SYN dentin.

**den·tip·a·rous** (den-tip′ă-rŭs) Tooth-bearing.

**den·tist** (den′tist) A legally qualified practitioner of dentistry.

**den·tis·try** (den′tis-trē) The healing science and art concerned with structure and function of the orofacial complex, and with the prevention, diagnosis, and treatment of deformities, pathoses, and traumatic injuries thereof. SYN odontology, odontonosology.

**⬛den·ti·tion** (den-tish′ŭn) Natural teeth, considered collectively, in dental arch; may be deciduous, permanent, or mixed. See page 170. [L. *dentitio,* teething]

**den·to·al·ve·o·lar** (den′tō-al-vē′ŏ-lăr) Usually, denoting that portion of the alveolar bone immediately about teeth; used also to denote the functional unity of teeth and alveolar bone.

**den·to·al·ve·o·lar cyst** (den′tō-al-vē′ŏ-lăr sist) SYN periodontal cyst.

**den·to·al·ve·o·lar syn·des·mo·sis** (den′tō-al-vē′ŏ-lăr sin-dez-mō′sĭs) [TA] Fibrous joint by which the root of a tooth is fixed into the dental alveoli or sockets of the alveolar part of

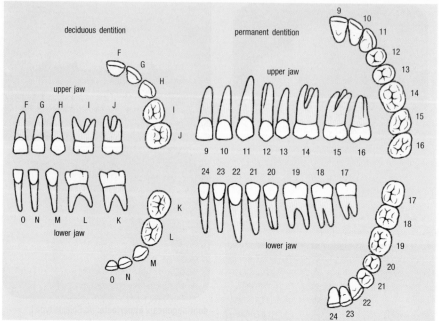

**deciduous dentition, half view, left side** (lettering code, universal system of deciduous teeth): central incisor F, O; lateral incisor G, N; canine H, M; first molar J, K

**permanent dentition, half view, left side** (numbering code, universal system of permanent teeth): central incisor 9, 24; lateral incisor 10, 23; canine 11, 22; first bicuspid 12, 21; second bicuspid 13, 20; first molar 14, 19; second molar 15, 18; third molar 16, 17

the mandible by the periodontium. SYN gompholic joint.

**den·tode** (den'tōd) An exact reproduction of a tooth on a gnathographically mounted cast.

**den·to·fa·cial com·plex** (den'tō-fā'shăl kom'pleks) Dentition, its surrounding and supporting structures, and those of the facial region.

**den·to·gin·gi·val junc·tion** (den'tō-jin'ji-văl jŭngk'shŭn) Area of epithelial attachment between the gingiva and the enamel or cementum of the tooth.

**den·to·gin·gi·val lam·i·na** (den'tō-jin'ji-văl lam'i-nă) SYN dental ledge.

**den·toid** (den'toyd) SYN odontoid (1).

**den·to·le·gal** (den'tō-lē'găl) Relating to both dentistry and the law. SEE forensic dentistry.

**den·tu·lous** (den'tyū-lŭs) Having natural teeth present in the mouth.

**den·ture** (den'chŭr) An artificial substitute for missing natural teeth and adjacent tissues. SYN artificial dentition.

**den·ture ad·he·sive** (den'chŭr ad-hē'siv) Soft material used to affix a denture to the oral mucosa.

**den·ture ba·sal sur·face** (den'chŭr bā'săl sŭr'făs) SYN denture foundation surface.

**den·ture base** (den'chŭr bās) 1. Denture part that rests on oral mucosa (i.e., supporting tissue) and to which teeth are attached. 2. Part of complete or partial denture that rests on basal seat and to which teeth are attached. SYN saddle (1).

**den·ture-bear·ing a·re·a** (den'chŭr ber'ing ar'ē-ă) SYN denture foundation area.

**den·ture bor·der** (den'chŭr bōr'dĕr) 1. Limit or boundary or circumferential margin of a denture base. 2. Margin of denture base at junction of polished surface with impression (tissue) surface. 3. Extreme edges of denture base at the buccolabial, lingual, and posterior limits. SYN denture edge, denture periphery, periphery (1).

**den·ture brush** (den'chŭr brŭsh) Brush used to clean removable dentures.

**den·ture char·ac·ter·i·za·tion** (den'chŭr kar'ăk-tĕr-ī-zā'shŭn) Modification of form and color of denture base or teeth to produce a more lifelike appearance.

**den·ture clean·ser** (den'chŭr klen'zĕr) Any product used to effectively clean dentures.

**den·ture edge** (den'chŭr ej) SYN denture border.

**den·ture es·thet·ics** (den´chŭr es-thet´iks) **1.** Cosmetic effect produced by dental prosthesis. **2.** Qualities involved in the appearance of a given restoration.

**den·ture flange** (den´chŭr flanj) **1.** Essentially vertical extension from body of denture into vestibule of oral cavity; also, on lower denture, essentially vertical extension along lingual side of alveololingual sulcus. **2.** Buccal and labial vertical extension of the upper or lower denture base and lingual vertical extension of lower; buccal, and labial denture flanges have two surfaces: buccal or labial surface and the basal seat surface; the lower lingual flange also has two surfaces: basal seat surface and lingual surface.

**den·ture flask** (den´chŭr flask) Sectional metal boxlike case in which a sectional mold is made of plaster of Paris or artificial stone to compress and cure dentures or other resinous restorations. SYN crown flask.

**den·ture foun·da·tion** (den´chŭr fowndā´shŭn) Portion of oral structures available to support a denture.

**den·ture foun·da·tion a·re·a** (den´chŭr fown-dā´shŭn ar´ē-ă) Portion of basal seat area that supports the complete or partial denture base under occlusal load. SYN basal seat area, basal seat, denture-bearing area, denture-supporting area, saddle area, stress-bearing area (1), supporting area (2), tissue-bearing area.

**den·ture foun·da·tion sur·face** (den´chŭr fown-dā´shŭn sŭr´făs) Portion of surface of a denture that has its contour determined by the impression and bears the greater part of the occlusal load. SYN denture basal surface.

**den·ture im·pres·sion sur·face** (den´chŭr im-presh´ŭn sŭr´făs) Portion of denture surface that has its contour determined by the impression; includes denture borders and extends to polished surface.

**den·ture oc·clu·sal sur·face** (den´chŭr ŏ-klū´zăl sŭr´făs) [TA] Portion of denture surface that makes contact with corresponding surface of an opposing denture or tooth. SYN occlusal surface of tooth (2) [TA], facies masticatoria, facies occlusalis dentis, grinding surface, masticating surface, masticatory surface.

**den·ture pack·ing** (den´chŭr pak´ing) Filling and compressing a denture base material into a mold in a flask.

**den·ture pe·riph·er·y** (den´chŭr pĕr-if´ĕr-ē) SYN denture border.

**den·ture pol·ished sur·face** (den´chŭr pol´isht sŭr´făs) Part of denture that extends in occlusal direction from denture border and includes palatal surface; part of denture base that is usually polished and includes buccal and lingual surfaces of teeth.

**den·ture prog·no·sis** (den´chŭr prog-nō´sis) Opinion given in advance of treatment, of prospects for success in construction and usefulness of a denture or restoration.

**den·ture re·ten·tion** (den´chŭr rĕ-ten´shŭn) Means by which dentures are held in position in the mouth.

**den·ture ser·vice** (den´chŭr ser´vis) Those procedures performed in diagnosis, construction, and maintenance of artificial substitutes for missing natural teeth.

**den·ture sore** (den´chŭr sōr) Wearing away of oral mucosa by a denture that creates an area of discomfort. SEE ALSO sore (1).

**den·ture sore mouth** (den´chŭr sōr mowth) Mucosal erythema underlying a denture base, usually representing inflammation caused by ill-fitting dentures, poor oral hygiene, or *Candida albicans* infection.

**den·ture space** (den´chŭr spās) **1.** Portion of oral cavity available to maxillary and/or mandibular denture(s). **2.** Space between residual ridges available for dentures. SEE ALSO interarch distance.

**den·ture sta·bil·ity** (den´chŭr stă-bil´i-tē) Quality of a denture to be firm, steady, constant, and resistant to change of position when functional forces are applied. SYN stabilization (2).

**den·ture-sup·port·ing a·re·a** (den´chŭr sŭ-pōrt´ing ar´ē-ă) SYN denture foundation area.

**den·ture-sup·port·ing struc·tures** (den´chŭr sŭ-pōrt´ing strŭk´shŭrz) Tissues, teeth, and residual ridges, which may serve as the foundation for removable partial or complete dentures.

**den·tur·ist** (den´chŭr-ist) Dental technician who fabricates and fits dentures without supervision of a dentist.

**den·u·da·tion** (dē´nū-dā´shŭn) Depriving of a covering or protecting layer.

**de·os·si·fi·ca·tion** (dē-os´i-fi-kā´shŭn) Removal of the mineral constituents of bone.

**de·ox·y·cor·ti·co·ster·one** (dē-oks´ē-kōr-ti-kos´tĕr-ōn) Potent mineralocorticoid with no appreciable glucocorticoid activity.

**de·ox·y·ri·bo·nu·cle·ic ac·id (DNA)** (dē-oks´ē-rī´bō-nū-klē´ik as´id) The type of nucleic acid containing deoxyribose as the sugar component; found principally in the nuclei (chromatin, chromosomes) and mitochondria of animal and plant cells, usually loosely bound to protein (hence the term deoxyribonucleoprotein).

**de·pen·dence** (dĕ-pen´dĕns) *Avoid the misspelling dependance.* The quality or condition of relying on, being influenced by, or being subservient to a person, object, or substance. [L. *dependeo,* to hang from]

cd

**de·pen·dent e·de·ma** (dĕ-pen'dĕnt ĕ-dē' mă) A clinically detectable increase in extracellular fluid volume localized in a dependent area, as of a limb, characterized by swelling.

**de·plaq·u·ing** (dē-plak'ing) Disruption or removal of the subgingival plaque biofilm and its byproducts from root surfaces and pocket spaces.

**de·ple·tion** (dĕ-plē'shŭn) 1. Removal of accumulated fluids or solids. 2. Excessive loss of a constituent, usually essential, of the body.

**de·ple·tion·al hy·po·na·tre·mi·a** (dĕ-plē'shŭn-ăl hī'pō-nă-trē'mē-ă) Decreased serum sodium concentration associated with loss of sodium from circulating blood through gastrointestinal tract, kidney, or skin.

**de·po·lar·i·za·tion** (dē-pō'lăr-ī-zā'shŭn) Destruction, neutralization, or change in direction of polarity.

**de·pos·it** (dĕ-poz'it) 1. Sediment or precipitate. 2. Pathologic accumulation of inorganic material in a tissue. [L. *de- pono,* pp. *-positus,* to lay down]

**dep·o·si·tion** (dep'ŏ-zish'ŭn) A sworn pretrial testimony given by a witness in response to oral and written questions and cross examination.

**de·pot in·jec·tion** (dē'pō in-jek'shŭn) Injection of substance in a vehicle that tends to keep it at site so absorption is prolonged.

**de·pres·sant** (dĕ-pres'ănt) An agent to reduce nervous or functional activity. [L. *de-primo,* pp. *-pressus,* to press down]

**de·pres·sion** (dĕ-presh'ŭn) [TA] 1. Opening or indentation on an oral cavity surface. 2. Reduction of the level of functioning.

**de·pres·sive psy·cho·sis** (dĕ-pres'iv sī-kō'sis) Major mood disorder in which biologic factors are believed to play a prominent role.

**de·pres·sor** (dĕ-pres'ŏr) 1. Instrument or device used to push structures out of the way during an operation or anatomic examination. 2. A muscle that flattens or lowers a part. [L. *de-primo,* pp. *-pressus,* to press down]

**depth** (depth) 1. Distance from the surface downward. 2. Degree (of understanding of a concept or ability to reason, i.e., depth of comprehension).

**de·riv·a·tive** (dĕ-riv'ă-tiv) Chemical compound that may be produced from another compound of similar structure in one or more steps.

✪ **derm-** SEE dermato. [G. *derma,* skin]

**der·ma·tal·gi·a** (der'mă-tăl'jē-ă) Localized pain, usually to the skin. [*dermat-* + G. *algos,* pain]

**der·ma·tan sul·fate** (der'mă-tan sŭl'fāt) Anticoagulant with properties similar to those of heparin.

**der·ma·ti·tis,** pl. **der·ma·tit·i·des** (der' mă-tī'tis, -tit'i-dēz) Inflammation of the skin. [*derm-* + G. *-itis,* inflammation]

**der·ma·ti·tis her·pet·i·for·mis** (der'mă-tī'tis her-pet-i-fōr'mis) Chronic skin disease marked by a symmetric itching eruption of vesicles and papules that occur in groups; relapses are common.

✪ **dermato-** Combining form denoting skin. [G. *derma,* skin]

**der·mat·o·gen·ic tor·ti·col·lis** (der'mă-tō-jen'ik tōr'ti-kol'is) Painful stiff neck with limitation of motion due to skin lesions.

**der·ma·to·glyph·ics** (der'mă-tō-glif'iks) Configurations of the characteristic ridge patterns of the volar surfaces of the skin; in the human hand, the distal segment of each digit has three types of configurations: whorl, loop, and arch.

**der·mat·o·log·ic paste** (der'mă-tŏ-loj'ik pāst) Class of preparations consisting of starch, dextrin, sulfur, calcium carbonate, or zinc oxide made into a paste with glycerin or other substance.

**der·ma·tol·o·gy** (der'mă-tol'ŏ-jē) Medical branch concerned with the study and diseases of the skin.

**der·ma·to·ma** (der'mă-tō'mă) A circumscribed thickening or hypertrophy of the skin. [*dermato-* + G. *-oma,* tumor]

**der·ma·tome** (der'mă-tōm) 1. An instrument for cutting thin slices of skin for grafting, or excising small lesions. 2. The dorsolateral part of an embryonic somite. SYN cutis plate. 3. Skin supplied by cutaneous branches from a single spinal nerve.

**der·ma·to·my·o·si·tis** (der'mă-tō-mī'ō-sī'tis) A progressive condition characterized by symmetric proximal muscular weakness with elevated muscle enzyme levels and a rash, typically a purplish-red or heliotrope erythema on the face, and edema of the eyelids and periorbital tissue; affected muscle tissue shows degeneration of fibers with a chronic inflammatory reaction; occurs in children and adults, and in the latter may be associated with visceral cancer. [*dermato-* + G. *mys,* muscle, + *-itis,* inflammation]

**der·ma·to·phyte** (der'mă-tŏ-fīt) Fungus that causes superficial infections of the skin, hair, and nails.

**der·mat·o·scle·ro·sis** (der'mă-tō-skler-ō'sis) SYN scleroderma. [*dermato-* + G. *sklēroō,* to harden]

**der·ma·to·sis,** pl. **der·ma·to·ses** (der'

mă-tō´sis, -sēz) Nonspecific term denoting cutaneous abnormality or eruption. [*dermato-* + G. *-osis*, condition]

**der·mis** (děr´mis) [TA] Two-zone skin layer: a superficial stratum that interdigitates with the epidermis, the stratum papillare, and the deeper and coarser stratum reticulare. [G. *derma*, skin]

🔲**der·moid cyst** (děr´moyd sist) A tumor consisting of displaced ectodermal structures along lines of embryonic fusion, the wall being formed of epithelium-lined connective tissue, including skin appendages and spaces containing keratin, sebum, and hair. See this page and page A5.

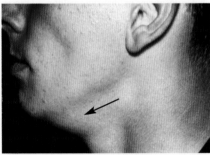

**dermoid cyst:** below mylohyoid muscle

**DES** Abbreviation for diethylstilbestrol.

**de·sat·u·ra·tion** (dē-sat´yūr-ā´shŭn) The act, or the result of the act, of making something less completely saturated.

**de·scend·ing neu·ri·tis** (dě-send´ing nūr-ī´tis) Inflammation progressing along a nerve trunk toward the periphery.

**de·scrip·tive sta·tis·tics** (dě-skrip´tiv stă-tis´tiks) Data deductively derived from nonparametric measures.

**desensitisation** [Br.] SYN desensitization.

**de·sen·si·tiz·a·tion** (dē-sen´si-tī-zā´shŭn) **1.** The reduction or abolition of allergic sensitivity or reactions to the specific antigen (allergen). SYN desensitisation. **2.** The act of removing an emotional complex.

**de·sen·si·tize** (dē-sen´si-tīz) In dentistry, to eliminate or subdue the painful response of exposed, vital dentin to irritative agents or thermal changes.

**de·sen·si·tiz·ing paste** (dē-sen´si-tīz-ing pāst) Ointment applied to tooth cervix to diminish pain due to sensitive exposed cementum or dentin.

**des·ic·cant** (des´i-kǎnt) Agent that absorbs moisture; a drying agent. SYN exsiccant. [L. *de-sicco*, pp. *-siccatus*, to dry up]

**des·ic·cate** (des´i-kāt) To dry thoroughly; to render free from moisture. SYN exsiccate.

**des·ic·ca·tion** (des´i-kā´shŭn) The process of being desiccated. SYN dehydration (4), exsiccation (1).

**de·sign den·ture** (dě-zīn´ den´chŭr) Planned visualization of the form of a dental prosthesis, made after a study of all factors involved.

**des·mins** (dez´minz) Proteins found in intermediate filaments that copolymerize with vimentin to form constituents of structural elements (e.g. connective tissue).

**des·mo·den·ti·um, des·mo·don·ti·um** (des´mō-den´tē-ŭm, -don´tē-ŭm) [TA] Collagen fibers, running from cementum to alveolar bone, which suspend a tooth in its socket; include apical, oblique, horizontal, and alveolar crest fibers. SYN periodontal fiber.

**des·mog·e·nous** (des-moj´ě-nŭs) Denoting connective tissue or ligamentous origin or causation.

**des·mop·a·thy** (des-mop´ă-thē) Any disease of the ligaments.

🔲**des·mo·plas·tic fi·bro·ma** (des´mō-plas´ tik fī-brō´mă) A benign fibrous tumor of bone affecting children and young adults; cortical destruction may result. See page A15.

**des·qua·ma·tion** (des´kwă-mā´shŭn) The shedding of the cuticle in scales or of the outer layer of any surface.

**de·ter·gent** (dě-těr´jěnt) A cleansing or purging agent that provides cleansing (i.e., oil-dissolving) and antibacterial effects. [L. *de-tergeo*, pp. *-tersus*, to wipe off]

**de·tox·i·fi·ca·tion** (dē-tok´si-fi-kā´shŭn) **1.** Recovery from toxic effects of a drug. **2.** Removal of toxic properties from a poison.

**de·tox·i·fy** (dē-tok´si-fī) To diminish or remove the poisonous quality of any substance; to lessen the virulence of any pathogenic organism. [L. *de*, from, + *toxicum*, poison]

**de·tri·tus** (dě-trī´tŭs) Any broken-down material, carious or gangrenous matter, or gravel.

**deu·te·ri·um** (dū-tēr´ē-ŭm) SYN hydrogen (2). [G. *deuteros*, second]

**de·vel·op** (dē-vel´ŏp, dě-vel´ŏp) To process an exposed photographic or radiographic film to render a latent image permanent. [O.Fr. *desveloper*, to unwrap, fr. *voloper*, to wrap]

**de·vel·op·er** (dě-vel´ŏp-ěr) **1.** SYN eluent. **2.** The chemicals used to develop film by reducing the light-activated silver halide molecules to atomic silver.

**de·vel·op·ment** (dě-vel´ŏp-měnt) The act or process of natural progression in physical and psychological maturation from a previous, lower, or embryonic stage to a later, more complex, or adult stage.

**de·vel·op·men·tal a·nom·a·ly** (dĕ-vel′ŏp-men′tăl ă-nom′ă-lē) Anomaly established during intrauterine life; a congenital anomaly.

**de·vel·op·men·tal cyst** (dĕ-vel′ŏp-men′tăl sist) Lesion formed when epithelium becomes included within connective tissue. SYN inclusion cyst.

**de·vel·op·men·tal dis·a·bil·ity** (dĕ-vel′ŏp-men′tăl dis′ă-bil′i-tē) Loss of function brought on by prenatal and postnatal events in which the predominant disturbance is in the acquisition of cognitive, language, motor, or social skills.

**de·vel·op·men·tal grooves** (dĕ-vel′ŏp-men′tăl grūvz) Fine lines in tooth enamel that mark junction of lobes of crown in its development.

**de·vi·a·tion** (dē′vē-ā′shŭn) **1.** A turning away or aside from the normal point or course. **2.** An abnormality. [L. *devio*, to turn from the straight path, fr. *de*, from, + *via*, way]

**de·vice** (dĕ-vīs′) An appliance, usually mechanical, designed to perform a specific function.

**de·vi·tal·i·za·tion** (dē-vī′tăl-ī-zā′shŭn) **1.** In dentistry, process by which tooth pulp is destroyed; e.g., by chemical means, by infection, or by extirpation. **2.** Deprivation of vitality or of vital properties.

**de·vi·tal·ize** (dē-vī′tăl-īz) To deprive of vitality or of vital properties.

**de·vi·tal·ized tooth** (dē-vī′tăl-īzd tūth) Misnomer for pulpless tooth.

**de·vi·tal tooth** (dē-vī′tăl tūth) A misnomer for a pulpless tooth.

**dex·a·meth·a·sone** (dek′să-meth′ă-sōn) Potent synthetic analogue of cortisol, with similar action; used as an antiinflammatory and to test for adrenal cortical function.

**dex·ter (D)** (deks′tĕr) Latin meaning located on or relating to the right side. [L. fr. *dextra*, neut. *dextrum*]

**dex·tran** (deks′tran) Any of several water-soluble high molecular weight glucose polymers; used in isotonic sodium chloride solution to treat shock and to relieve edema of nephrosis.

**dex·tro·am·phet·a·mine sul·fate** (deks′trō-am-fet′ă-mēn sul′făt) A sympathomimetic and appetite depressant.

**dex·tro·ro·ta·to·ry** (deks′trō-rō′tă-tōr-ē) Denoting dextrorotation, or certain crystals or solutions capable of such action; as a chemical prefix, usually abbreviated D. Cf. levorotatory.

**dex·trose** (deks′trōs) SEE d-glucose.

**DF, df** Abbreviation for df caries index.

**df car·ies in·dex, DF car·ies in·dex (df, DF)** (kar′ēz in′deks) Record of past caries experience based on the number of decayed and filled deciduous (indicated by lower case letters) or permanent (indicated by CAPITAL LETTERS) teeth. SYN df, DF.

**DH** Abbreviation for dental hygienist.

**DI** Abbreviation for dental index; diabetes insipidus.

**di·a·be·tes** (dī-ă-bē′tēz) *Avoid using the simple word diabetes for diabetes mellitus unless the sense is clear from the context.* Either diabetes insipidus or diabetes mellitus, diseases having in common the triad of symptoms polyuria, weight loss, and significant glucosuria. [G. *diabētēs*, a compass, a siphon, diabetes]

**di·a·be·tes in·sip·i·dus (DI)** (dī-ă-bē′tēz in-sip′i-dŭs) Chronic excretion of very large amounts of pale urine of low specific gravity, causing dehydration and extreme thirst.

**di·a·be·tes mel·li·tus** (dī-ă-bē′tēz mel′i-tŭs) A chronic metabolic disorder in which the use of carbohydrate is impaired and that of lipid and protein is enhanced. It is caused by an absolute or relative deficiency of insulin and is characterized, in more severe cases, by chronic hyperglycemia, glycosuria, water and electrolyte loss, ketoacidosis, and coma. Long-term complications include neuropathy, retinopathy, nephropathy, generalized degenerative changes in large and small blood vessels, and increased susceptibility to infection. [L. sweetened with honey]

**di·a·bet·ic** (dī-ă-bet′ik) Relating to or suffering from diabetes.

**di·a·bet·ic a·ci·do·sis** (dī-ă-bet′ik as-i-dō′sis) Metabolic acidosis caused by accumulation of ketone bodies and loss of fixed base in diabetes mellitus.

**di·a·bet·ic co·ma** (dī-ă-bet′ik kō′mă) Coma in severe and inadequately treated cases of diabetes mellitus; commonly fatal, unless appropriate therapy is instituted promptly; results from reduced oxidative metabolism of the central nervous system that, in turn, stems from severe ketoacidosis and possibly also from the histotoxic action of the ketone bodies and disturbances in water and electrolyte balance.

**di·a·bet·ic di·et** (dī-ă-bet′ik dī′ĕt) Adjustment in eating habits for patients with diabetes mellitus intended to decrease the need for insulin or oral diabetic agents and control weight by adjusting caloric and carbohydrate intake.

**di·a·bet·ic gin·gi·vi·tis** (dī′ă-bet′ik jin′ji-vī′tis) Gum disease in which the host response to bacterial plaque is presumably modified by metabolic alterations encountered in patients with uncontrolled diabetes.

**di·a·betic ke·to·a·ci·do·sis (DKA)** (dī-ă-bet′ik kē′tō-as′i-dō′sis) Buildup of ketones in blood due to breakdown of stored fats for energy; a complication of diabetes mellitus. Untreated, can lead to coma and death.

**di·a·bet·ic ne·phrop·a·thy** (dī-ă-bet′ik nĕ-frop′ă-thē) Syndrome characterized by albuminuria, hypertension, and progressive renal insufficiency.

**di·a·bet·ic neu·ro·path·ic ca·chex·i·a** (dī′ă-bet′ik nŭr′ō-path′ik kă-kek′sē-ă) Syndrome seen in old men with diabetes, consisting of the sudden onset of severe limb pain, marked weight loss, depression, and impotence.

**di·a·bet·ic neu·rop·a·thy** (dī-ă-bet′ik nŭr-op′ă-thē) Generic term for any diabetes mellitus–related disorder of the peripheral nervous system, autonomic nervous system, and particular cranial nerves.

**di·a·bet·ic ret·i·nop·a·thy** (dī-ă-bet′ik ret′i-nop′ă-thē) Retinal changes occurring in diabetes of long duration, marked by hemorrhages, microaneurysms, sharply defined waxy deposits, or proliferative retinopathy.

**di·ad·o·cho·ki·ne·si·a, di·ad·o·cho·ki·ne·sis, di·ad·o·cho·ci·ne·si·a** (dī-ad′ŏ-kō-ki-nē′zē-ă, -ki-nē′sis, -si-nē′sē-ă) The normal power of alternately bringing a limb into opposite positions. [G. *diadochos*, working in turn, + *kinēsis*, movement]

**di·ag·nose** (dī-ăg-nōs′) To make a diagnosis.

**di·ag·no·sis (Dx)** (dī-ăg-nō′sis) The determination of the nature of a disease, injury, or congenital defect. [G. *diagnōsis*, a deciding]

**di·ag·no·sis by ex·clu·sion** (dī-ăg-nō′sis eks-klū′zhŭn) Diagnosis made by excluding diseases to which only some of the patient's symptoms might belong, leaving one disease as the most likely diagnosis, although no definitive tests or findings establish that diagnosis.

**di·ag·no·sis-re·lat·ed group (DRG)** (dī-ăg-nō′sis-rĕ-lā′tĕd grŭp) U.S. billing program for medical and especially hospital services by combining diseases into groups according to the resources needed for care, arranged by diagnostic category.

**di·ag·nos·tic** (dī-ăg-nos′tik) 1. Relating to or aiding in diagnosis. 2. Establishing or confirming a diagnosis.

***Di·ag·nos·tic and Sta·tis·ti·cal Man·u·al of Men·tal Dis·or·ders*** (dī-ăg-nos′tik stă-tis′ti-kăl man′yū-ăl men′tăl dis-ōr′dĕrz) A system of classification, published by the American Psychiatric Association, which divides recognized mental disorders into clearly defined categories.

**di·ag·nos·tic an·es·the·si·a** (dī′ăg-nos′tik an-es-thē′zē-ă) Anesthesia induced for evaluation of mechanism responsible for a painful condition.

**di·ag·nos·tic cast** (dī′ăg-nos′tik kast) Positive replica of form of the teeth and tissues made from an impression.

**di·ag·nos·ti·cian** (dī′ăg-nos-tish′ăn) One who is skilled in making diagnoses.

**di·ag·nos·tic ra·di·ol·ogy** (dī-ăg-nos′tik rā′dē-ol′ŏ-jē) SYN radiology (2).

**di·ag·nos·tic ul·tra·sound** (dī-ăg-nos′ tik ŭl′tră-sownd) Ultrasound used to obtain images for medical diagnostic purposes.

**di·al·y·sis** (dī-al′i-sis) 1. Filtration to separate crystalloid from colloid substances (or smaller molecules from larger ones) in a solution by interposing a semipermeable membrane between solution and dialyzing fluid; crystalloid (smaller) substances pass through membrane into dialyzing fluid on other side, colloids do not. 2. Separation of substances across a semipermeable membrane on basis of particle size or concentration gradients. 3. Method of artificial kidney function. [G. a separation, fr. *dialyo*, to separate]

**di·a·mond cut·ting ins·tru·ments** (dī′ mŏnd kŭt′ing in′strŭ-mĕnts) In dentistry, cylinders, discs, and instruments to which numerous small diamond pyramids have been attached by a plating of metal.

**di·a·mond disc** (dī′mŏnd disk) Steel disc with cutting surface(s) covered with fine diamond chips, for use in a dental handpiece.

**di·a·mond stone** (dī′mŏnd stōn) SEE diamond cutting instruments.

**di·a·pho·re·sis** (dī′ă-fŏr-ē′sis) SYN perspiration (1). [G. *diaphorēsis*, fr. *dia*, through, + *phoreō*, to carry]

**di·a·phragm** (dī′ă-fram) [TA] 1. [TA] Musculomembranous partition between abdominal thoracic cavities. 2. In radiography, a grid (2) or a lead sheet with an aperture. SEE collimator. 3. A thin disc pierced with an opening, used in a microscope, camera, or other optic instrument to shut out the marginal rays of light, thus giving a more direct illumination. [G. *diaphragma*]

**di·a·phragm of mouth** (dī′ă-fram mowth) SYN mylohyoid (muscle).

**di·aph·y·sis,** pl. **di·aph·y·ses** (dī-af′i-sis, -sēz) [TA] SYN shaft. [G. a growing between]

**di·ar·rhe·a** (dī′ă-rē′ă) Abnormally frequent discharge of semisolid or fluid fecal matter from the bowel. SYN diarrhoea. [G. *diarrhoia*, fr. *dia*, through, + *rhoia*, a flow, a flux]

**diarrhoea** [Br.] SYN diarrhea.

**di·ar·thro·di·al joint** (dī′ahr-thrō′dē-ăl joynt) SYN synovial joint.

**di·ar·thro·sis**, pl. **di·ar·thro·ses** (dī'ahr-thrō'sis, -sēz) SYN synovial joint. [G. articulation]

**di·a·ste·ma**, pl. **di·a·ste·ma·ta** (dī'ă-stē'mă, -tă) **1.** [TA] Space between two adjacent teeth in the same dental arch. SEE ALSO gap. **2.** Cleft or space between the maxillary lateral incisor and canine teeth, into which the lower canine is received when the jaws are closed; abnormal in humans. See this page. [G. *diastēma,* an interval]

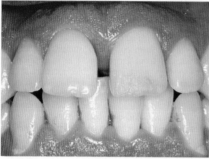

diastema

**di·as·to·le** (dī-as'tŏ-lē) Normal postsystolic dilation of the heart cavities, during which they fill with blood. [G. *diastolē,* dilation]

**di·a·stol·ic pres·sure** (dī'ă-stol'ik presh'ŭr) Intracardiac pressure during or resulting from diastolic relaxation of a cardiac chamber.

**di·a·tax·i·a** (dī'ă-tak'sē-ă) Ataxia affecting both sides of the body.

**di·a·ther·my** (dī'ă-thĕr-mē) Local elevation of temperature within tissues, produced by high-frequency current or other means.

**di·ath·e·sis**, pl. **di·ath·e·ses** (dī-ath'ĕ-sis, -sēz) Constitutional or inborn state disposing to disease, group of diseases, or metabolic or structural anomaly. [G. arrangement, condition]

**di·a·tor·ic** (dī'ă-tōr'ik) **1.** Vertical cylindric aperture formed in the base of artificial porcelain teeth and extending into body of tooth, serving as a mechanical means of attaching the tooth to the denture base. **2.** Denoting teeth that contain a diatoric. [G. *diatoros,* pierced]

**di·bu·caine** (dib'yū-kān) Potent local anesthetic with long action used by injection or topically on skin or mucous membranes.

**DIC** Abbreviation for disseminated intravascular coagulation.

**di·chei·li·a, di·chi·li·a** (dī-kī'lē-ă) A lip that appears to be double because of the presence of an abnormal fold of mucosa. [G. *di-,* two, + *cheilos,* lip]

**Dick test** (dik test) An intracutaneous test of

susceptibility to the erythrogenic toxin of *Streptococcus pyogenes* responsible for the rash and other manifestations of scarlet fever.

**di·cy·clo·mine hy·dro·chlor·ide** (dī-sī'klŏ-mēn hī'drŏ-klōr'īd) An anticholinergic agent.

**die** (dī) **1.** In dentistry, positive reproduction of form of a prepared tooth in any suitable hard substance, usually metal or specially prepared artificial stone. **2.** To cease to exist.

**di·et** (dī'ĕt) **1.** Food and drink in general. **2.** Prescribed course of eating and drinking in which amount and kind of food, as well as times consumed, are regulated for therapeutic purposes. **3.** Reduction of intake to lose weight. **4.** To carry out any prescribed or specific diet. [G. *diaita,* a way of life; a diet]

**di·e·tar·y as·sess·ment** (dī'ĕ-tar-ē ă-ses'mĕnt) Division of a dietary food record into individual components of the Food Guide Pyramid; assessment of quality, of whether the patient has an adequate diet, and of where modifications in that diet may be needed.

**di·e·tar·y fi·ber** (dī'ĕ-tar-ē fī'bĕr) Plant polysaccharides and lignin that are resistant to hydrolysis by the digestive enzymes in humans.

**di·e·tar·y his·to·ry** (dī'ĕ-tar-ē his'tŏr-ē) Narration or documentation of any and all food and drink consumed in a set time period.

**di·e·tet·ic** (dī'ĕ-tet'ik) **1.** Relating to diet. **2.** Descriptive of food that, naturally or through processing, has a low caloric content.

**di·e·tet·ics** (dī'ĕ-tet'iks) Practical application of diet in prophylaxis and treatment of disease.

**di·e·tet·ic treat·ment** (dī'ĕ-tet'ik trēt'mĕnt) Therapy for a clinical condition that involves a specific diet.

**di·eth·yl·ene·di·a·mine** (dī-eth'il-ēn-dī'ă-mēn) SYN piperazine.

**di·eth·yl·stil·bes·trol (DES)** (dī-eth'il-stil-bes'trol) A synthetic nonsteroidal estrogenic compound; formerly used as a postcoital antipregnancy agent to prevent implantation of the fertilized oocyte. SYN stilboestrol.

**di·et qual·i·ty in·dex** (dī'ĕt kwahl'i-tē in' deks) Measure of quality of diet using a composite of eight recommendations regarding the consumption of foods and nutrients from the U.S. National Academy of Sciences (NAS).

**dif·fer·en·tial di·ag·no·sis** (dif'ĕr-en'shăl dī-ăg-nō'sis) Determination of which of two or more diseases with similar symptoms is the one with which the patient is afflicted, by a systematic comparison and contrasting of the clinical findings. SYN differentiation (2).

**dif·fer·en·tial white blood cell count** (dif'ĕr-en'shăl wīt blŭd sel kownt) An estimate of the percentage of each white blood cell type making up the total white blood cell count.

**dif·fer·en·ti·a·tion** (dif'ĕr-en-shē-ā'shŭn) **1.** The acquisition or possession of one or more characteristics or functions different from that of the original type. SYN specialization (2). **2.** SYN differential diagnosis.

**dif·fuse e·soph·a·ge·al spasm** (di-fyūs´ ĕ-sof´ă-jē´ăl spazm) Abnormal contraction of muscular wall of the esophagus causing pain and dysphagia, often in response to regurgitation of acid gastric contents.

**dif·fu·sion** (di-fyū'zhŭn) **1.** The random movement of molecules or ions or small particles in solution or suspension toward a uniform distribution throughout the available volume. **2.** SYN dialysis (1).

**dif·fu·sion hy·pox·ia** (di-fyū'zhŭn hī-pok' sē-ă) Abrupt transient decrease in alveolar oxygen tension when room air is inhaled at the conclusion of nitrous oxide anesthesia.

**di·gas·tric branch of fa·cial nerve** (dī-gas´trik branch fā´shăl nĕrv) [TA] Branch of facial nerve, arising as nerve exits facial canal, proximal to parotid plexus, innervating the posterior belly of the digastric muscle.

**di·gas·tric fos·sa** (dī-gas'trik fos'ă) [TA] Hollow on posterior surface of base of mandible, on either side of median plane, giving attachment to the anterior belly of digastric muscle.

**di·gas·tric (mus·cle)** (dī-gas´trik mŭs´ĕl) [TA] One of suprahyoid group of muscles consisting of two bellies united by a central tendon that passes through a fascial loop connected to the body of the hyoid bone; elevates the hyoid when mandible is fixed; depresses the mandible when hyoid is fixed. SYN musculus digastricus.

**di·ges·tion** (di-jes'chŭn) Mechanical, chemical, and enzymatic process whereby ingested food is converted into material suitable for assimilation for synthesis of tissues.

**di·ges·tive tract** (di-jes'tiv trakt) Passage from mouth to anus through pharynx, esophagus, stomach, and intestine. SYN alimentary tract.

**dig·it** (dij'it) [TA] A finger or toe. [L. *digitus*]

**dig·i·tal** (dij'i-tăl) Relating to or resembling a digit or digits or an impression made by them.

**dig·i·tal di·la·tion** Use of the finger or finger-tip to enlarge an orifice or opening.

**Dig·i·tal·is** (dij´i-tal´is, -tā´lis) A genus of perennial flowering plants; *D. lanata*, a European species, and *D. purpurea*, purple foxglove, are the main sources of cardioactive steroid glycosides used to treat some heart diseases, especially congestive heart failure. [L. *digitalis*, re-

lating to the fingers; in allusion to the fingerlike flowers]

**digitalisation** [Br.] SYN digitalization.

**dig·i·tal·is tinc·ture** (dij´i-tal´is tingk´shŭr) An hydroalcoholic solution containing the glycosides of the leaves of the foxglove (digitalis) plant *Digitalis purpurea* or *D. lanata*. Although digitalis preparations are used extensively, they are currently used as the pure glycosides, digoxin and digitoxin.

**dig·i·tal·i·za·tion** (dij'i-tăl-ī-zā'shŭn) Administration of digitalis until sufficient amounts are present in the body to produce the desired therapeutic effects. SYN digitalisation.

**dig·i·tal meth·od** (dij´i-tăl meth´ŏd) SYN bisecting angle technique.

**dig·i·tal mo·tion ac·ti·va·tion** (dij´i-tăl mō´shŭn ak´ti-vā´shŭn) Moving the dental instrument by flexing the thumb, index, and middle fingers.

**dig·i·tal ra·di·og·ra·phy (DR)** (dij´i-tăl rā´dē-og´ră-fē) A filmless imaging system wherein a radiographic image is captured using nonfilm, solid-state detectors. The signal so captured is sent to a computer where it is digitized so the image may be displayed in multiple gray levels on a monitor. SEE ALSO storage phosphor imaging. See page 178.

**digit suck·ing** (dij´it sŭk´ing) Sucking fingers, thumbs, or toes.

**di·glos·si·a** (dī-glos´ē-ă) A developmental condition that results in a longitudinal split in tongue. [G. *di-*, two, + *glōssa*, tongue]

**di·gox·in** (dī-gok'sin) A cardioactive steroid glycoside obtained from *Digitalis lanata*.

**2,6-di·i·so·pro·pyl phe·nol** (dī-ī'sō-prō' pil fē'nol) SYN propofol.

**dil.** Abbreviation for dilute.

**di·lac·er·a·tion** (dī-las'ĕr-ā'shŭn) Displacement of some portion of a developing tooth, which is then further developed in its new relation. See page 178.

**di·lan·tin gin·gi·vit·is** (dī-lan´tin jin´ji-vī´tis) SYN diphenylhydantoin gingivitis.

**dil·a·ta·tor** (dil'ă-tā-tŏr) **1.** Instrument designed to enlarge a hollow structure or opening. **2.** Muscle that pulls open an orifice. **3.** Substance that causes dilation or enlargement of an opening or the lumen of a hollow structure.

**di·la·tion, dil·a·ta·tion** (dī-lā'shŭn, dil'ă-tā'shŭn) **1.** Physiologic or artificial enlargement of a hollow structure or opening. **2.** Stretching an opening of a hollow structure.

**di·la·tor** (dī'lā-tŏr) SEE dilatator.

**dil·u·ent** (dil'yū'ĕnt, dil'yĕ-wĕnt) *Avoid the in-*

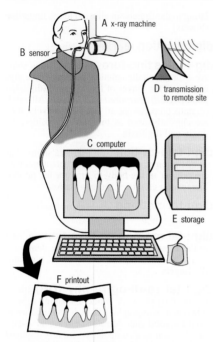

**direct digital imaging system:** (A) image is exposed by x-ray machine; (B) captured on a CCD (charge-coupled device) or CMOS (complementary-metal-oxide semiconductor) sensor in patient's mouth; (C) signal is transmitted via cable to computer, where it is digitized into 256 gray levels and displayed on the computer monitor; (D) image is transmitted electronically to a remote site; (E) or stored on file server; (F) or printed on paper

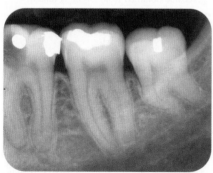

**dilaceration of third molar:** bulbous root of first molar

---

*correct forms dilutent and dilutant.* Ingredient in a medicinal preparation that lacks pharmacologic activity but is pharmaceutically necessary or desirable.

**di·lute (dil.)** (di-lūt′) **1.** To reduce a solution or mixture in concentration, strength, quality, or

purity. **2.** Diluted; denoting a solution or mixture so effected. [L. *di-luo,* to wash away, dilute]

**di·men·sion** (di-men′shŭn) Scope, size, magnitude; denoting, in the plural, linear measurements of length, width, and height.

**di·men·sion·al sta·bil·ity** (di-men′shŭn-ăl stă-bil′i-tē) Property of a material to retain its size and form.

**di·meth·yl·ben·zene** (dī-meth′il-ben′zēn) SYN xylol.

**di·meth·yl sul·fox·ide (DMSO)** (dī-meth′il sŭl-foks′īd) A penetrating solvent, enhancing absorption of therapeutic agents from the skin; an industrial solvent proposed as a useful analgesic and antiinflammatory agent. SYN dimethyl sulphoxide.

**dimethyl sulphoxide** [Br.] SYN dimethyl sulfoxide.

**dim·ple** (dim′pĕl) A natural indentation, usually circular and of small area, in the chin, cheek, or sacral region.

**di·phen·yl·hy·dan·to·in gin·gi·vi·tis** (dī-fē′nil-hī-dan′tō-in jin′ji-vī′tis) Gingivitis exacerbated by long-term therapy with diphenylhydantoin; host response to bacterial plaque is characterized by marked hyperplasia of fibrous connective tissue and, to a lesser degree, of surface epithelium, resulting in gross enlargement of interdental papillae that may coalesce and obscure crowns of teeth. SYN dilantin gingivitis.

**di·phos·pha·tase** (dī-fos′fă-tās) SYN pyrophosphatase.

**diph·the·ri·a** (dif-thēr′ē-ă) *Avoid the misspelling/mispronunciation dipheria.* A specific infectious disease due to infection by the bacterium *Corynebacterium diphtheriae* and its highly potent toxin. [G. *diphthera,* leather]

**diph·the·roid** (dif′thĕ-royd) One of a group of local infections suggesting diphtheria, but caused by microorganisms other than *Corynebacterium diphtheriae.* SYN Epstein disease. [*diphtheria* + G. *eidos,* resemblance]

**di·phy·o·dont** (dī-fī′ō-dont) Possessing two sets of teeth, as occurs in humans and most other mammals. [G. *di-,* two, + *phyō,* to produce, + *odous (odont-),* tooth]

**di·ple·gi·a** (dī-plē′jē-ă) Paralysis of corresponding parts on both sides of the body. [G. *di-,* two, + *plēgē,* a stroke]

**dip·lo·ë** (dip′lŏ-wē) [TA] The central layer of spongy bone between the two layers of compact bone, outer and inner plates, or tables, of the flat cranial bones. [G. *diploē,* fem. of *diplous,* double]

**di·plo·ic ca·nals** (dip-lō′ik kă-nalz′) [TA] Channels in the diploë that accommodate diploic veins.

**di·plo·ic vein** (dip-lō'ik vān) [TA] Veins in the diploë of the cranial bones, connected with the cerebral sinuses by emissary veins.

**di·plo·pi·a** (dip-lō'pē-ă) The condition in which a single object is perceived as two objects. SYN double vision. [G. *diplous*, double + G. *ōps*, eye]

**dip·se·sis, dip·so·sis** (dip-sē'sis, -sō'sis) An abnormal or excessive thirst, or a craving for unusual forms of drink. [G. *dipseō*, to thirst]

**di·rect a·cryl·ic res·tor·a·tion** (di-rekt' ă-kril'ik res'tŏr-ā'shŭn) Direct resin restoration of autopolymerizing acrylic material.

**di·rect bond·ing** (di-rekt' bond'ing) Single-step intraoral procedure in which orthodontic attachments are bonded to teeth with resin.

**di·rect bone im·pres·sion** (di-rekt' bōn im-presh'ŭn) Impression of denuded bone, used to make subperiosteal denture implants.

**di·rect com·pos·ite res·in res·tor·a·tion** (di-rekt' kŏm-poz'it rez'in res'tŏr-ā'shŭn) SYN direct resin restoration.

**di·rect cur·rent (DC)** (di-rekt' kŭr'ĕnt) An electrical current that flows only in one direction; also referred to as galvanic current.

**di·rect fill·ing res·in** (di-rekt' fil'ing rez'in) Autopolymerizing resin especially designed for use as a dental restorative material.

**di·rec·tion** (di-rek'shŭn) 1. Order for procedure in health care according to mandate of supervisory personnel or dictates of other prevailing authority. 2. Alignment of movement from one bodily locus to another. [L. *directione*]

**di·rec·tive psy·cho·ther·a·py** (di-rek' tiv sī'kō-thār'ă-pē) Psychotherapy involving the authority of the therapist to direct the course of the patient's therapy.

**di·rect meth·od for mak·ing in·lays** (di-rekt' meth'ŏd māk'ing in'lāz) In dentistry, an inlay technique in which wax pattern is made directly in a cavity prepared in the tooth.

**di·rec·tor** (di-rek'tŏr) 1. A smoothly grooved instrument used with a knife to limit the incision of tissues. SYN staff (2). 2. The head of a service or specialty division in a large dental or other health care facility. [L. *dirigo*, pp. *-rectus*, to arrange, set in order]

**di·rect pulp cap·ping** (di-rekt' pŭlp kap' ing) Procedure for covering and protecting exposed vital pulp by placing dental material directly on exposed pulp tissue to stimulate formation of a dentinal bridge.

**di·rect res·in res·tor·a·tion** (di-rekt' rez'in res'tŏr-ā'shŭn) Direct restoration made by inserting a plastic mix of auto- or light-polymerized resins in a cavity prepared in a tooth. SYN direct composite resin restoration.

**di·rect res·tor·a·tion** (di-rekt' res'tŏr-ā' shŭn) Reconstruction placed and formed in the cavity preparation; includes types using gold, amalgam, composite resin, and glass ionomer cement restorations.

**di·rect re·tain·er** (di-rekt' rĕ-tā'nĕr) Clasp or attachment applied to an abutment tooth to keep a removable appliance in position.

**di·rect re·ten·tion** (di-rekt' rĕ-ten'shŭn) Retention obtained in a removable partial denture by use of attachments or clasps that resist their removal from abutment teeth.

**di·rect vi·sion** (di-rekt' vizh'ŭn) SYN central vision.

**dis·a·bil·i·ty** (dis'ă-bil'i-tē) According to the International Classification of Impairments, Disabilities and Handicaps (World Health Organization), any restriction or lack of ability to perform an activity in a manner or within the range considered normal for a human being.

**dis·ac·cha·ride** (dī-sak'ă-rīd) A condensation product of two monosaccharides by elimination of water.

**dis·ar·tic·u·la·tion** (dis'ahr-tik'yū-lā'shŭn) Amputation of a limb through a joint, without cutting of bone. SYN exarticulation. [L. *dis-*, apart, + *articulus*, joint]

**disc, disk** (disk) DENTISTRY a circular piece of thin paper or other material, coated with an abrasive substance, used for cutting and polishing teeth and fillings. [L. *discus*; G. *diskos*, a quoit, disc]

**dis·charge** (dis'chahrj) That which is emitted or evacuated, as an excretion or a secretion.

**dis·clos·ing a·gent** (dis-klōz'ing ā'jĕnt) Selective dye in solution or tablet form used to visualize and identify soft debris, pellicle, and bacterial plaque on the surfaces of the teeth; in dental offices, a solution is most commonly used; chewable tablets are available for use in home dental care.

**dis·clo·sure** (dis-klō'zhŭr) Communicating confidential patient information to others in accordance with legal guidelines. SYN release of information.

**dis·coid** (dis'koyd) 1. In dentistry, an excavating or carving instrument with a circular blade with a cutting edge around its periphery. 2. Resembling a disc. [*disco-* + G. *eidos*, appearance]

▌**dis·coid lu·pus er·y·the·ma·to·sus** (dis'koyd lū'pŭs er'ă-thē-mă-tō'sŭs) Form of lupus erythematosus in which cutaneous lesions are present. See page 180.

**dis·crim·i·na·tion** (dis-krim'i-nā'shŭn) In conditioning, responding differentially, as when an organism makes one response to a reinforced stimulus and a different response to an unrein-

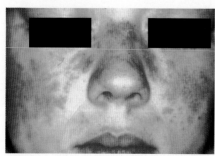

**discoid lupus erythematosus:** butterfly rash

forced stimulus. [L. *discrimino,* pp. *-atus,* to separate]

**dis·ease** (di-zēz) **1.** An interruption, cessation, or disorder of a body, system, or organ structure or function. **2.** A morbid entity ordinarily characterized by two or more of the following criteria: recognized etiologic agent(s), identifiable group of signs and symptoms, or consistent anatomic alterations. [Eng. *dis-* priv. + *ease*]

**dis·ease de·ter·mi·nants** (di-zēz′ dĕ-tĕr′ mi-nănts) Variables that directly or indirectly influence frequency of occurrence and/or distribution of any given disease; they include specific disease agents, host characteristics, and environmental factors.

**dis·ease-mod·i·fy·ing an·ti·rheu·ma·tic drugs (DMARD)** (di-zēz′mod′i-fī-ing an′ tē-rū-mat′ik drŭgz) Agents that alter the course and progression of rheumatoid arthritis.

**dis·ease sus·cep·ti·bil·i·ty** (di-zēz′ sŭ-sep′ti-bil′i-tē) Predisposal to or having a risk of a disease.

**dis·ease trans·mis·sion** (di-zēz′ trans-mish′ŭn) The spread or transfer of a disease from one individual to another.

**dis·e·qui·lib·ri·um, dys·e·quil·i·bri·um** (dis-ē-kwi-lib′rē-ŭm) A disturbance or absence of equilibrium.

**dis·har·mo·ny** (dis-har′mŏ-nē) Being deranged or lacking in orderliness.

**dis·in·fect** (dis-in-fekt′) To destroy pathogenic microorganisms in or on any substance or to inhibit their growth and vital activity.

**dis·in·fec·tant** (dis-in-fek′tănt) Agent capable of destroying pathogenic microorganisms or inhibiting their growth activity.

**dis·in·fec·tion** (dis-in-fek′shŭn) Destruction of pathogenic microorganisms or their toxins or vectors by direct exposure to chemical or physical agents.

**dis·in·te·gra·tion** (dis-in′tĕ-grā′shŭn) Loss or separation of component parts of substance. [*dis-* + L. *integer,* whole, intact]

🔲**dis·lo·ca·tion** (dis′lō-kā′shŭn) Displacement of an organ or any part; specifically disturbance or disarrangement of normal relation of bones at a joint in which there is complete loss of contact between two articular surfaces. See this page. SYN luxation (2). [L. *dislocatio,* fr. *dis-,* apart, + *locatio,* a placing]

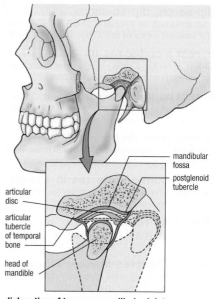

**dislocation of temporomandibular joint**

mandibular fossa

postglenoid tubercle

articular disc

articular tubercle of temporal bone

head of mandible

**dis·lo·ca·tion frac·ture** (dis′lō-kā′shŭn frak′shŭr) Fracture of bone near an articulation with dislocation of the adjacent joint.

**dis·or·der** (dis-ōr′dĕr) A disturbance of function, structure, or both, resulting from a genetic or embryonic failure in development or from exogenous factors such as poison, trauma or disease.

**dis·pen·sa·ry** (dis-pen′săr-ē) **1.** A physician's office, especially of one who dispenses medicines. **2.** The office of a hospital pharmacist, where medicines are given out on physicians' orders. [L. *dis-penso,* pp. *-atus,* to distribute by weight, fr. *penso,* to weigh]

*Dis·pen·sa·to·ry* (dis-pen′să-tōr-ē) A work originally intended as a commentary on the *Pharmacopeia,* but now more of a supplement to that work. [L. *dispensator,* a manager, steward]

**dis·per·sion** (dis-pĕr′zhŭn) **1.** Dispersing or being dispersed. **2.** Incorporation of the particles of one substance into the mass of another, including solutions, suspensions, and colloidal dispersions (solutions). **3.** Specifically, what is usually called a colloidal solution. [L. *dispersio*]

**dis·sect** (di-sekt') *Avoid the mispronunciation dī'sekt.* **1.** To cut apart or separate the tissues of the body for study. **2.** In an operation, to separate the different structures along natural lines by dividing the connective tissue framework. [L. *dis-seco,* pp. *-sectus,* to cut asunder]

**dis·sem·i·nat·ed in·tra·vas·cu·lar co·ag·u·la·tion (DIC)** (di-sem'i-nā'tĕd in'trăvas'kyū-lăr kō-ag'yū-lā'shŭn) A hemorrhagic syndrome that occurs following the uncontrolled activation of clotting factors and fibrinolytic enzymes throughout small blood vessels.

**dis·so·ci·at·ed an·es·the·si·a** (dis-sō' sē-ā-tĕd an'es-thē'zē-ă) Loss of some types of sensation with persistence of others; most often used in context of nerve blocks.

**dis·so·ci·a·tion, dis·as·so·ci·a·tion** (di-sō'sē-ā-'shŭn, dis'ă-) An unconscious separation of a group of mental processes from the rest, resulting in an independent functioning of these processes and a loss of usual associations.

**dis·so·ci·a·tion sen·si·bil·i·ty** (di-sō' sē-ā'shŭn sens'i-bil'i-tē) Loss of pain and thermal senses with preservation of tactile sensibility or vice versa.

**dis·so·ci·a·tive an·es·the·si·a** (di-sō' sē-ă-tiv an'es-thē'zē-ă) Form of general anesthesia, but not necessarily complete unconsciousness, characterized by catalepsy, catatonia, and amnesia.

**dis·solve** (di-zolv') To change or cause to change from a solid to a dispersed form by immersion in a fluid of suitable properties. [L. *dissolvo,* pp. *-solutus,* to loose asunder, to dissolve]

**dis·tad** (dis'tad) Toward the periphery.

**dis·tal** (dis'tăl) **1.** In dentistry, away from the median sagittal plane of the face, following curvature of dental arch. **2.** [TA] Situated away from center of the body or point of origin; specifically applied to extremity or distant part of a limb or organ. SYN distalis [TA]. [L. *distalis*]

**dis·tal an·gle** (dis'tăl ang'gĕl) Angle formed by meeting of distal with labial, buccal, or lingual surface of a tooth.

**dis·tal ca·ries** (dis'tal kar'ēz) Loss of structure on tooth surface directed away from median plane of dental arch.

**dis·tal cusp** (dis'tal kŭsp) SYN hypoconulid.

**dis·tal end** (dis'tăl end) Posterior extremity of a dental instrument or appliance. SYN heel (3).

**dis·tal fo·ve·a of tooth** (dis'tal fō'vē-ă tūth) [TA] Shallow depression related to the cusps on posterior aspect of a molar.

**dis·tal in·tes·ti·nal ob·struc·tive syn·drome** (dis'tăl in-tes'ti-năl ŏb-strŭk'tiv sin' drōm) A syndrome seen in cystic fibrosis secondary to impaction with feces and mucus.

**dis·ta·lis** (dis-tā'lis) [TA] SYN distal (2).

**dis·tal my·op·a·thy** (dis'tăl mī-op'ă-thē) Muscular disorder affecting predominantly the distal portions of the limbs; onset is usually after age 40 years.

**dis·tal oc·clu·sion** (dis'tăl ŏ-klū'zhŭn) **1.** Tooth occluding in a position more distal than normal. SYN retrusive occlusion (2). **2.** SYN distoclusion.

**dis·tal root of tooth** (dis'tal rūt tūth) [TA] Root of a multirooted tooth located toward distal side of the tooth.

**dis·tal step** (dis'tăl step) Projection of a cavity prepared in a tooth into the distal surface perpendicular to the main part of the cavity to prevent displacement of the restoration (i.e., filling) by forces of mastication.

**dis·tal sur·face of tooth** (dis'tal sŭr'făs tūth) [TA] Contact surface of tooth that is directed away from the median plane of the dental arch; opposite to the mesial surface of a tooth. SYN facies distalis dentis.

**dis·tal tongue bud** (dis'tăl tŭng bŭd) SYN lateral lingual swelling.

**dis·tance** (dis'tăns) Measure of space between two objects.

**dis·ten·tion, dis·ten·sion** (dis-ten'shŭn) The act or state of being distended or stretched. SEE ALSO dilation. [L. *dis-tendo,* to stretch apart]

**dis·til·la·tion** (dis'ti-lā'shŭn) Volatilization of a liquid by heat and subsequent condensation of the vapor. [L. *de-(di-)stillo,* pp. *-atus,* to drop down]

**dis·to·buc·cal** (dis'tō-bŭk'ăl) Relating to distal and buccal surfaces of tooth; denoting angle formed by their junction.

**dis·to·buc·co·oc·clu·sal** (dis'tō-bŭk'ō-ŏ-klū'zăl) Relating to the distal, buccal, and occlusal surfaces of a premolar or molar tooth; denoting especially the angle formed by the junction of these surfaces.

**dis·to·buc·co·pul·pal** (dis'tō-bŭk'ō-pŭl' păl) Relating to the point (trihedral) angle formed by the junction of distal, buccal, and pulpal walls of a cavity.

**dis·to·cer·vi·cal** (dis'tō-sĕr'vi-kăl) Relating to line angle formed by junction of distal and cervical (gingival) walls of a class V cavity.

**dis·to·clu·sal, dis·to·oc·clu·sal** (dis' tō-klū'zăl, ŏ-klū'zăl) **1.** Relating to or characterized by distoclusion. **2.** Denoting compound cavity or restoration involving tooth's distal and occlusal surfaces. **3.** Denoting line angle formed by distal and occlusal walls of a class V cavity.

**dis·to·clu·sion, dis·to·oc·clu·sion** (dis' tō-klū'zhŭn, dis'tō-ŏ-klū'zhŭn) Malocclusion in

cd

which the mandibular arch articulates with the maxillary arch in a position distal to normal; in Angle classification, a class II malocclusion. SYN distal occlusion (2).

**dis·to·gin·gi·val** (dis′tō-jin′ji-văl) Relating to junction of distal surface with tooth's gingival line.

**dis·to·in·ci·sal** (dis′tō-in-sī′zăl) Relating to line (dihedral) angle formed by junction of distal and incisal walls of a class V cavity in an anterior tooth.

**dis·to·la·bi·al** (dis′tō-lā′bē-ăl) Relating to distal and labial surfaces of teeth; denoting angle formed by their junction.

**dis·to·la·bi·o·pul·pal** (dis′tō-lā′bē-ō-pŭl′păl) Relating to point (trihedral) angle formed by junction of distal, labial, and pulpal walls of incisal part of class IV (mesioincisal) cavity.

**dis·to·lin·gual** (dis′tō-ling′gwăl) Relating to distal and lingual surfaces of tooth; denoting angle formed by their junction.

**dis·to·lin·guo·oc·clu·sal** (dis′tō-ling′gwŏ-ŏ-klū′zăl) Relating to the distal, lingual, and occlusal surfaces of a premolar or molar tooth; denoting especially the angle formed by the junction of these surfaces.

**dis·to·mo·lar** (dis′tō-mō′lăr) Supernumerary tooth located in region posterior to third molar tooth.

**dis·to·place·ment** (dis′tō-plās′mĕnt) SYN distoversion.

**dis·to·pul·pal** (dis′tō-pŭl′păl) Relating to line (dihedral) angle formed by junction of distal and pulpal walls of cavity.

**dis·tor·tion** (dis-tōr′shŭn) 1. In dentistry, permanent deformation of the impression material after the registration of an imprint. 2. A twisting out of normal shape or form. [L. *distortio,* fr. *dis-torqueo,* to wrench apart]

**dis·to·ver·sion** (dis′tō-vĕr-zhŭn) Malposition of a tooth distal to normal, in a posterior direction following curvature of dental arch. SYN distoplacement.

**dis·trac·tion** (dis-trak′shŭn) 1. Difficulty or impossibility of concentration or fixation of the mind. 2. A force applied to a body part to separate bony fragments or joint surfaces. [L. *dis-traho,* pp. *-tractus,* to pull in different directions]

**dis·tri·bu·tion** (dis′tri-byū′shŭn) 1. Passage of branches of arteries or nerves to tissues and organs. 2. Area in which branches of an artery or a nerve terminate or area supplied by such artery or nerve. [L. *dis-tribuo,* pp. *-tributus,* to distribute, fr. *tribus,* a tribe]

**ditch·ing** (dich′ing) Formation of a gap or groove between the cavity preparation margin and the restorative material.

**Ditt·rich plugs** (dit′rik plŭgz) Minute, dirty-grayish, foul-smelling masses of bacteria and fatty acid crystals in sputum.

**di·u·ret·ic** (dī-yūr-et′ik) *Do not confuse this word with dieretic.* 1. Promoting excretion of urine. 2. An agent that increases amount of urine excreted.

**di·ur·nal** (dī-ŭr′năl) 1. Pertaining to the daylight hours. 2. Repeating once each 24 hours. [L. *diurnus,* of the day]

**di·ver·tic·u·lar dis·ease** (dī-vĕr-tik′yū-lăr di-zēz′) Symptomatic congenital or acquired diverticula of any portion of gastrointestinal tract.

**di·ver·tic·u·li·tis** (dī′vĕr-tik′yū-lī′tis) Inflammation of a diverticulum, especially of the small pockets in the wall of the colon that fill with stagnant fecal material and become inflamed.

**di·vid·ed dose** (di-vīd′ĕd dōs) Definite fraction of a full dose; given repeatedly at short intervals so that the full dose is taken within a specified period, usually 1 day. SYN fractional dose.

**div. in p. aeq.** Abbreviation for L. *divide in partes aequales,* divide into equal parts.

**di·vi·sion** (di-vizh′ŭn) A separating into two or more parts. SEE ALSO ramus.

**diz·zi·ness** (diz′ē-nĕs) Imprecise term commonly used to describe various symptoms such as faintness, giddiness and imbalance. [A.S. *dyzig,* foolish]

**DJD** Abbreviation for degenerative joint disease.

**DKA** Abbreviation for diabetic ketoacidosis.

**DMARD** Abbreviation for disease-modifying antirheumatic drugs.

**DMD** Abbreviation for doctor of dental medicine.

**dmf, DMF** Abbreviation for decayed, missing, and filled teeth. SEE ALSO dmfs caries index.

**dmfs, DMFS** Abbreviation for decayed, missing, and filled surfaces. SEE ALSO dmfs caries index.

**dmfs car·ies in·dex, DMFS car·ies in·dex** (kar′ēz in′deks) Record of past caries experience based on number of decayed, missing, and filled surfaces of deciduous (indicated by lower-case letters) or permanent (indicated by CAPITAL LETTERS) teeth. The abbreviation DMFT is used when ''complete'' permanent teeth are referred to; DMFS is the abbreviation for the index that includes only the surfaces of permanent teeth.

**DMSO** Abbreviation for dimethyl sulfoxide.

**DNA** Abbreviation for deoxyribonucleic acid.

**DNA fin·ger·print·ing** (fing'gĕr-print'ing) A technique used to compare people using molecular genotyping.

**DNAR** Abbreviation for do not attempt resuscitation.

**DNR** Abbreviation for do not resuscitate. SEE do not attempt resuscitation.

**DOA** Abbreviation for dead on arrival.

**DOB** Abbreviation for date of birth.

**DO cavity** (kav'i-tē) The presence of a carious lesion involving the distal (D) and occlusal (O) surfaces of a tooth.

**doc·tor** (dok'tŏr) **1.** A title conferred by a university on one who has followed a prescribed course of study, or given as a title of distinction, such as doctor of dentistry, medicine, laws, philosophy. **2.** A physician, especially one on whom has been conferred the degree of M.D. [L. a teacher, fr. *doceo,* pp. *doctus,* to teach]

**doctor of den·tal med·i·cine (DMD)** (dok'tŏr den'tăl med'i-sin) The holder of a doctoral degree denoting a high level of proficiency in the study of oral diseases and functions.

**doc·u·men·ta·tion** (dok'yū-mĕn-tā'shŭn) A written record of information.

**DOE** Abbreviation for dyspnea on exertion.

**dol** (dōl) A unit measure of pain. [L. *dolor,* pain]

**dol·i·cho·ce·phal·ic, dol·i·cho·ceph· a·lous** (dol'i-kō-sĕ-fal'ik, -sef'ă-lŭs) Having a disproportionately long head. [*dolicho-* + G. *kephalē,* head]

**dol·i·cho·u·ran·ic, dol·i·chu·ran·ic** (dol'i-kō-yūr-an'ik, dol'i-yūr-) Having a long palate. [*dolicho-* + G. *ouranos,* vault of the palate]

**do·lor** (dō'lŏr) Pain, as one of the four signs of inflammation (the others are calor, rubor, tumor). [L.]

**do·mes·tic vi·o·lence** (dŏ-mĕs'tik vī'ŏ-lĕns) Intentionally inflicted injury perpetrated by and on family member(s); varieties include spousal abuse, child abuse, and sexual abuse, including incest.

**dom·i·nant fre·quen·cy** (dom'i-nănt frē'kwĕn-sē) The frequency occurring most often in an electroencephalogram.

**dom·i·nant hand** (dom'i-nănt hand) Operant hand generally used for performing fine motor-skills tasks (e.g., writing, holding dental instruments). SYN writing hand.

**dom·i·nant hem·i·sphere** (dom'i-nănt hem'is-fēr') Cerebral hemisphere containing representation of speech and controlling arms and legs used preferentially in skilled movements; usually the left.

**do not at·tempt re·sus·ci·ta·tion (DNAR)** (dū not ă-tempt' rē-sus'i-tā'shŭn) Directive to health care workers from a patient who has expressed in writing a wish not to be resuscitated in cardiac or respiratory arrest.

**don·o·va·no·sis** (don'ō-vă-nō'sis) SYN granuloma inguinale.

**do·pa, DOPA** (dō'pă) Intermediate in catabolism of L-phenylalanine and L-tyrosine and in biosynthesis of norepinephrine, epinephrine, and melanin.

**do·pa·mine** (dō'pă-mēn) An intermediate in tyrosine metabolism and precursor of norepinephrine and epinephrine.

**do·pa·mine hy·dro·chlor·ide** (dō'pă-mēn hīdrŏ-klōr'īd) Biogenic amine and neural transmitter substance, used as vasopressor agent to treat shock.

**dope** (dōp) *Colloq.* Any drug, either stimulating or depressing, administered for its temporary effect, or taken habitually or addictively. [Dutch, *doop,* sauce]

**Do·rel·lo ca·nal** (dōr-el'lō kă-nal') Bony canal sometimes found at the tip of the temporal bone enclosing the abducent nerve and inferior petrosal sinus where these two structures enter the cavernous sinus.

**dor·sad** (dōr'sad) Toward or in the direction of the back. [L. *dorsum,* back, + *ad,* to]

**dor·sal** (dōr'săl) Pertaining to the back or any dorsum. [Mediev. L. *dorsalis,* fr. *dorsum,* back]

**dor·sal na·sal ar·te·ry** (dōr'săl nā'zăl ahr'tĕr-ē) [TA] *Origin,* supratrochlear artery (derivative of ophthalmic artery); *distribution,* penetrates orbicularis oculi to supply skin of side of root of nose; *anastomosis,* angular (facial) artery. SYN external artery of nose.

**dor·sum,** pl. **dor·sa** (dōr'sŭm, -să) [TA] **1.** Back of body. **2.** Upper or posterior surface, or back, of any part, especially in the quadrupedal position. [L. back]

**dor·sum of nose** (dōr'sŭm nōz) [TA] External ridge of nose, directed forward and upward.

**dor·sum of tongue** (dōr'sŭm tŭng) [TA] Superior lingual surface divided by the sulcus terminalis into an anterior two thirds, the presulcal part (pars presulcalis), and posterior third, the postsulcal part (pars postsulcalis).

**dos·age** (dō'săj) *Do not confuse this word with dose.* **1.** The giving of medicine or another therapeutic agent in prescribed amounts. **2.** The determination of the proper dose of a remedy.

**dose** (dōs) *Do not confuse this word with dosage.* Quantity of drug or other remedy to be taken or applied at once or in fractional amounts within a given period. [G. *dosis*, a giving]

**do·sim·e·ter** (dō-sim′ĕ-tĕr) SYN film badge. [G. *dosis*, dose, + *metron*, measure]

**do·sim·e·try** (dō-sim′ĕ-trē) Measurement of radiation exposure, especially x-rays or gamma rays.

**dot** (dot) A small spot. SEE identification dot.

**dou·ble-blind stud·y** (dŭb′ĕl-blind stŭd′ē) Study in which neither the patients, the experimenter, nor any other assessor of the results, knows which participants are subject to which procedure, thus helping to ensure that any biases or expectations will not influence results.

**dou·ble chin** (dŭb′ĕl chin) SYN buccula.

**dou·ble-end·ed in·stru·ment** (dŭb′ĕl-en′dĕd in′strŭ-mĕnt) An instrument with a handle and two working ends. SEE ALSO instrument.

**dou·ble lip** (dŭb′ĕl lip) Redundant congenital or acquired fold of tissue on the mucosal surface of the upper lip.

**dou·ble-point thresh·old** (dŭb′ĕl-poynt thresh′ōld) The least degree of separation of two tactile stimuli applied simultaneously to the body surface that permits their being perceived as two.

**dou·ble pro·tru·sion** (dŭb′ĕl prō-trū′zhŭn) SYN bimaxillary protrusion.

**dou·ble vi·sion** (dŭb′ĕl vizh′ŭn) SYN diplopia.

**doub·ling dose** (dŭb′ling dōs) Amount of radiation that doubles the incidence of stochastic effects.

**douche** (dūsh) 1. Current of water, gas, or vapor directed against surface or projected into a cavity. 2. An instrument for giving a douche. 3. To apply a douche. [Fr. fr. *doucher*, to wash off]

**dove·tail** (dŭv′tāl) Widened portion of cavity preparation usually established to increase retention and resistance form.

**dove·tail stress-bro·ken a·but·ment** (dŭv′tāl stres′brō-kĕn ă-bŭt′mĕnt) Abutment connected to a fixed partial denture by a nonrigid connector.

**dow·el** (dow′ĕl) 1. Cast gold or preformed metal pin placed into root canal to provide retention for a crown. 2. Preformed metal pin placed in a copper-plated die to provide a die stem. 3. Pin or rod that aligns or joins two structures by fitting into holes in both; dowels of various materials are used in orthopedic surgery and dentistry.

**dow·el crown** (dow′ĕl krown) SYN post-crown.

**Dow·ney cell** (dow′nē sel) The atypical lymphocyte of infectious mononucleosis.

**Downs a·nal·y·sis** (downz ă-nal′i-sis) Cephalometric criteria used to aid orthodontic diagnosis.

**Down syn·drome** (down sin′drōm) A chromosomal dysgenesis syndrome consisting of a variable constellation of abnormalities caused by triplication or translocation of chromosome 21. The abnormalities include mental retardation, retarded growth, flat hypoplastic face with short nose, prominent epicanthic skin folds, small low-set ears with prominent antihelix, fissured and thickened tongue, laxness of joint ligaments, pelvic dysplasia, broad hands and feet, stubby fingers, and transverse palmar crease.

**down·time** (down′tīm) As used in emergency medical service parlance, temporal duration from cardiac arrest until beginning cardiopulmonary resuscitation or advanced cardiac life support.

**dox·y·cy·cline** (doks′ē-sī′klēn) A broad-spectrum antibiotic.

**DR** Abbreviation for digital radiography.

**dr** Abbreviation for dram.

**drachm** (dram) SYN dram. [G. *drachmē*, an ancient Greek weight, equivalent to about 60 gr.]

**draft** (draft) 1. A current of air in a confined space. 2. A quantity of liquid medicine ordered as a single dose. Also spelled draught.

**drag** (drag) 1. The lower or cast side of a denture flask. 2. Any tendency for one moving thing to pull something else along with it.

**drain** (drān) 1. To remove fluid from a cavity as it forms. 2. A device, usually in the shape of a tube or wick, for removing fluid as it collects in a cavity.

**drain·age** (drān′ăj) Continuous flow or withdrawal of fluids from a wound or other cavity.

**drain·age tube** (drān′ăj tūb) Tube put in wound or cavity to facilitate removal of fluid.

**dram (dr)** (dram) A unit of weight: 1/8 oz.; 60 gr., apothecaries' weight; 1/16 oz., avoirdupois weight. SYN drachm.

**drape** (drāp) 1. To cover parts of the body other than those to be examined or on which to be operated. 2. The cloth or materials used for such cover. [M.E., fr. L.L. *drappus*, cloth]

**draught** (draft) SEE draft.

**draw** (draw) To extract blood from a vein for various diagnostic purposes or in the process of blood donation and collection. [O.E. *dragan*]

**dress·ing** (dres′ing) The material applied, or the application of material, to a wound for protection, absorbance, drainage, or other uses.

**DRG** Abbreviation for diagnosis-related group.

**drib·ble** (dri′bĕl) To drool, slobber, drivel.

**drift** (drift) In dentistry, movement of teeth usually medially due to loss of adjacent teeth or wear of proximal surfaces. See this page. SYN mesial drift, migrating teeth.

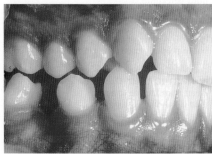

**distal drift of mandibular premolars and canine**

**drift·ing** (drift′ing) Random movement of tooth to position of greater stability.

**drift·ing tooth** (drift′ing tūth) A tooth that has moved from its normal anatomic position to an adjacent vacant space. SEE ALSO drift.

**drill** (dril) **1.** To make a hole in bone or other hard substance. **2.** An instrument for making or enlarging a hole in bone or in a tooth.

**drip** (drip) **1.** To flow one drop at a time. **2.** A flowing in drops.

**drive fin·ger** (drīv fing′gĕr) Finger used to turn the instrument handle while holding the instrument in a modified pen grasp. Either the index finger or the thumb turns the instrument. The digit used to roll the handle determines the direction in which the working-end will turn.

**drop** (drop) **1.** To fall, or to be dispensed or poured in globules. **2.** A liquid globule. **3.** A volume of liquid regarded as unit of dosage, equivalent in case of water to about 1 minim. **4.** A solid confection in globular form, usually intended to be allowed to dissolve in the mouth. [A.S. *droppan*]

**drop·let** (drop′lĕt) A small drop, such as a particle of moisture discharged from the mouth during coughing, sneezing, or speaking. [*drop* + -*let*, dim. suffix]

**drown·ing** (drow′ning) Death within 24 hours of immersion in liquid, either due to anoxia or cardiac arrest. [M.E. *drounen*]

**drug** (drŭg) **1.** Therapeutic agent; any substance, other than food, used in the prevention, diagnosis, alleviation, treatment, or cure of dis-

ease. SEE ALSO agent. **2.** To administer or take a drug, usually implying an overly large quantity or a narcotic. **3.** General term for any substance, stimulating or depressing, which can be habituating or addictive, especially a narcotic.

**drug a·buse** (drŭg ă-byūs′) Habitual use of drugs not needed for therapeutic purposes, solely to alter one's mood, affect, or state of consciousness, or to affect a body function unnecessarily (e.g., laxative abuse).

**drug al·ler·gy** (drŭg al′ĕr-jē) Sensitivity (hypersensitivity) to a drug or other chemical.

**drug e·rup·tion** (drŭg ē-rŭp′shŭn) Dermatologic reaction caused by ingestion, injection, or inhalation of a drug, most often the result of allergic sensitization. See page A13.

**drug-fast** (drŭg-fast) Pertaining to microorganisms that resist or become tolerant to antibacterial agents.

**drug fe·ver** (drŭg fē′vĕr) Pyrexia due to allergic reaction to a drug that clears rapidly on discontinuation of the drug.

**drug hol·i·day** (drŭg hol′i-dā) Interval of time when a patient on long-term medication temporarily stops taking the medication; used to allow some recuperation of normal functions.

**drug-in·duced dis·ease** (drŭg-in-dūst′ di-zēz′) Toxic reaction or morbid condition due to administration of a drug.

**drug-in·duced gin·gi·val hy·per·pla·sia** (drŭg′in-dūst′ jin′ji-văl hī′pĕr-plā′zē-ă) Increased gingival growth in response to medication.

**drug in·ter·ac·tions** (drŭg in-tĕr-ak′shŭnz) Pharmacologic result, either desirable or undesirable, of drugs interacting with other drugs.

**drug o·ver·dose (OD)** (drŭg ō′vĕr-dōs) The ingestion, accidentally or intentionally, of sufficient drug or drugs to cause injury or death.

**drug path·o·gen·e·sis** (drŭg path′ŏ-jen′i-sis) Production of morbid symptoms by drugs.

**drug re·sis·tance** (drŭg rĕ-zis′tăns) Capacity of disease-causing microorganisms to withstand exposure to drugs previously toxic to them.

**dry·clave** (drī′klāv) Colloq. usage for dry heat sterilization (q.v.)

**dry eye syn·drome** (drī ī sin′drōm) SYN keratoconjunctivitis sicca.

**dry gan·grene** (drī gang′grēn) A form of gangrene in which the involved part is dry and shriveled. SYN mummification (1).

**dry-heat ov·en** (drī-hēt ŏv′ĕn) SYN dry heat sterilization.

**dry heat ster·il·i·za·tion** (drī hēt ster′i-lī-zā´shŭn) Disinfection in an ovenlike device at about 160°C. SYN dry-heat oven.

**Dry·o·pi·the·cus pat·tern** (drī-ō-pith´ĕ-kŭs pat´ĕrn) 1. Ancestral pattern of cusps and grooves in humans. 2. A Y-5 cusp and groove. [*Dryopithecus*, a genus of anthropoid apes of the Miocene epoch]

**dry rale** (drī rahl) Harsh or musical breath sound produced by constriction in a bronchial tube or presence of a viscid secretion that narrows the lumen.

**dry soc·ket** (drī sok´ĕt) SYN alveoalgia.

**dual-cure res·in** (dū´ăl-kyŭr´ rez´in) Resin that uses both light and chemical initiation to activate polymerization.

**du·al re·la·tion·ships** (dū´ăl rĕ-lā´shŭn-ships) Relationships in which a health service provider is concurrently participating in two or more role categories with a patient.

**Du·breuil-Cham·bar·del syn·drome** (dū-broy´ shahm-bahr-del´ sin´drōm) Simultaneous caries of upper incisor teeth occurring in either sex between the ages of 14 and 17; after an interval of varying length, other teeth also become involved.

**duct** (dŭkt) [TA] Tubular structure giving exit to secretion of a gland or organ. SEE ALSO canal. SYN ductus. [L. *duco,* pp. *ductus,* to lead]

**duc·tule** (dŭk´tūl) A minute duct. SYN ductulus.

**duc·tu·lus,** pl. **duc·tu·li** (dŭk´tyū-lŭs, -lī) [TA] SYN ductule. [Mod. L. dim. of L. *ductus,* duct]

**duc·tus,** pl. **duc·tus** (dŭk´tŭs) [TA] SYN duct. [L. a leading, fr. *duco,* pp. *ductus,* to lead]

**duc·tus co·chle·a·ris** (dŭk´tūs kok´lē-ā´ris) [TA] SYN cochlear duct.

**duc·tus lin·gua·lis** (dŭk´tūs ling-gwā´lis) SYN foramen cecum of tongue.

**duc·tus sub·man·di·bu·la·ris** (dŭk´tūs sŭb´man-dib´yū-lā´ris) [TA] SYN submandibular duct.

**duc·tus sub·max·il·la·ris** (dŭk´tūs sŭb-mak´si-lā´ris) SYN submandibular duct.

**Duke test** (dūk test) Procedure to measure bleeding time.

**dull** (dŭl) Not sharp or acute, in any sense.

**du·o·de·num,** pl. **du·o·de·na** (dū´ō-dē´nŭm, -nă) [TA] The first division of the small intestine, about 25 cm in length, extending from the pylorus to the junction with the jejunum at the level of the first or second lumbar vertebra on the left side. [Mediev. L. fr. L. *duodeni,* twelve]

**du·pli·ca·tion** (dū´pli-kā´shŭn) 1. A doubling. [L. *duplicatio,* a doubling, fr. *duplico,* to double]

**dwarf** (dwōrf) An abnormally undersized person with disproportion among the body parts.

**dwarf·ed e·nam·el** (dwōrft ĕ-nam´ĕl) SYN nanoid enamel.

**dwarf·ism** (dwōrf´izm) A condition in which the standing height of the subject is below the third percentile.

**Dx** Abbreviation for diagnosis.

**dye** (dī) A stain or coloring matter. Commonly but improperly used to mean radiographic contrast medium. [A.S. *deah, deag*]

**dy·nam·ic mur·mur** (dī-nam´ik mŭr´mŭr) Heart murmur due to anemia or any cause other than a valvular lesion.

**dy·nam·ic re·la·tions** (dī-nam´ik rĕ-lā´shŭnz) Relative movements between two objects, e.g., the relationship of the mandible to the maxillae.

**dy·nam·ics** (dī-nam´iks) Science of motion in response to forces. [G. *dynamis,* force]

**dysaesthesia** [Br.] SYN dysesthesia.

**dys·a·phi·a** (dis-ā´fē-ă) Impairment of the sense of touch. [*dys-* + G. *haphē,* touch]

**dys·ar·thri·a** (dis-ahr´thrē-ă) A disturbance of speech due to emotional stress or other causes. [*dys-* + G. *arthroō,* to articulate]

**dys·ar·thro·sis** (dis´ahr-thrō´sis) 1. Malformation of a joint. 2. A false joint. [*dys-* + G. *arthrōsis,* joint]

**dys·au·to·no·mi·a** (dis´aw-tō-nō´mē-ă) Abnormal functioning of autonomic nervous system. [*dys-* + G. *autonomia,* self-government]

**dys·ce·pha·li·a man·di·bu·lo·oc·u·lo·fa·ci·a·lis** (dis´sĕ-fā´lē-ă man-dib´yū-lō-ok´yū-lō-fā´shē-ā´lis) Syndrome of bony anomalies of the calvaria, face, and jaw, with brachygnathia, narrow curved nose, and multiple ocular defects including microphthalmia, microcornea, and cataracts. SYN oculomandibulodyscephaly, oculomandibulofacial syndrome.

**dys·chei·ri·a, dys·chi·ri·a** (dis-kī´rē-ă) A disorder of sensibility in which, although there is no apparent loss of sensation, the patient is unable to tell which side of the body has been touched, or refers it to the wrong side, or to both.

**dys·cra·si·a** (dis-krā´zē-ă) Morbid general state resulting from presence of abnormal material in blood. [G. bad temperament, fr. *dys-* + *krasis,* a mixing]

**dys·di·ad·o·cho·ki·ne·si·a, dys·di·ad·o·cho·ci·ne·si·a** (dis´dī-ad´ō-kō-ki-nē´zē-ă, -si-nē′zē-ă) Impairment of the ability to perform rapidly alternating movements. [*dys-* + G. *diadochos,* working in turn, + *kinēsis,* movement]

**dys·en·ter·y** (dis′ĕn-ter′ē) Disease marked by frequent watery stools, often with blood and mucus, and characterized clinically by pain and fever.

**dys·er·e·thism** (dis-er′ĕ-thizm) A condition of slow response to stimuli. [*dys-* + G. *erethismos,* irritation]

**dys·er·gi·a** (dis-ĕr′jē-ă) Lack of harmonious action between the muscles concerned in executing any definite voluntary movement. [*dys-* + G. *ergon,* work]

**dys·es·the·si·a** (dis′es-thē′zē-ă) **1.** Impairment of sensation short of anesthesia. **2.** A condition in which a disagreeable sensation is produced by ordinary stimuli; caused by lesions of the sensory pathways, peripheral or central. SYN dysaesthesia.

**dys·func·tion** (dis-fŭngk′shŭn) Abnormal or difficult function.

**dys·gen·e·sis, dys·ge·ne·si·a** (dis-jen′ĕ-sis, -jĕ-nē′zē-ă) Defective development. [*dys-* + G. *genesis,* generation]

**dys·geu·si·a** (dis-gū′sē-ă) Distortion or perversion in the perception of a tastant. [*dys-* + G. *geusis,* taste]

**dys·gnath·i·a** (dis-gnath′ē-ă) Any abnormality that extends beyond the teeth and includes maxilla, mandible, or both. [*dys-* + G. *gnathos,* jaw]

**dys·gno·si·a** (dis-gnō′zē-ă) Any cognitive disorder, i.e., any mental illness. [G. *dysgnōsia,* difficulty of knowing]

**dys·junc·tion** (dis-jŭngk′shŭn) A separation of parts or structures normally joined; cleavage.

**dys·ker·a·to·sis** (dis-ker′ă-tō′sis) Premature keratinization in individual epithelial cells that have not reached the keratinizing surface layer. [*dys-* + G. *keras,* horn, + *-osis,* condition]

**dys·ki·ne·si·a** (dis′ki-nē′zē-ă) Difficulty in performing voluntary movements; usually in relation to various extrapyramidal disorders. [*dys-* + G. *kinēsis,* movement]

**dys·ki·net·ic** (dis′ki-net′ik) Denoting or characteristic of dyskinesia.

**dys·lex·i·a** (dis-lek′sē-ă) Impaired reading ability with a competence level below that expected on the basis of the person's level of intelligence, and in the presence of normal vision, letter recognition, and recognition of the meaning of pictures and objects. [*dys-* + G. *lexis,* word, phrase]

**dys·lo·gi·a** (dis-lō′jē-ă) Impairment of speech and reasoning as the result of a mental disorder. [*dys-* + G. *logos,* speaking, reason]

**dys·ma·se·sis** (dis′mă-sē′sis) Difficulty in chewing. [*dys-* + G. *masēsis,* chewing]

**dys·men·or·rhe·a** (dis-men′ōr-ē′ă) Difficult and painful menstruation. SYN menorrhalgia, dysmenorrhoea. [*dys-* + G. *mēn,* month, + *rhoia,* a flow]

**dysmenorrhoea** [Br.] SYN dysmenorrhea.

**dys·met·ri·a** (dis-mē′trē-ă) An aspect of ataxia, in which the ability to control the distance, power, and speed of an act is impaired. [*dys-* + G. *metron,* measure]

**dys·mor·phism, dys·mor·phi·a** (dismōr′fizm, -fē-ă) Abnormality of shape. [G. *dysmorphia,* badness of form]

**dys·mor·phol·o·gy** (dis′mōr-fol′ŏ-jē) The study of developmental structural defects; a branch of clinical genetics. [*dys-* + G. *morphē,* form, + *logos,* study]

**dys·my·e·li·na·tion** (dis′mī-ĕ-li-nā′shŭn) Improper laying down or breakdown of a myelin sheath of a nerve fiber, caused by abnormal myelin metabolism.

**dys·my·o·to·ni·a** (dis′mī-ō-tō′nē-ă) Abnormal muscular tonicity (either hyper- or hypo-).

**dys·nys·tax·is** (dis′nis-tak′sis) A condition of half sleep. [*dys-* + G. *nystaxis,* drowsiness]

**dys·o·don·ti·a·sis** (dis′ō-don-tī′ă-sis) Difficulty or irregularity in eruption of teeth. [*dys-* + G. *odous,* tooth, + *-iasis,* condition]

**dys·o·rex·i·a** (dis′ōr-ek′sē-ă) Diminished or disordered appetite. [*dys-* + G. *orexis,* appetite]

**dys·os·te·o·gen·e·sis** (dis-os′tē-ō-jen′ĕ-sis) Defective bone formation. SYN dysostosis. [*dys-* + G. *osteon,* bone, + *genesis,* production]

**dys·os·to·sis** (dis′os-tō′sis) SYN dysosteogenesis. [*dys-* + G. *osteon,* bone, + *-osis,* condition]

**dys·os·to·sis mul·ti·plex** (dis-ŏs-tō′sis mul′tē-pleks) Specific pattern of radiographic changes observed in many lysosomal storage disorders.

**dys·pep·si·a** (dis-pep′sē-ă) Impaired gastric function or "upset stomach" due to some disorder of the stomach. [*dys-* + G. *pepsis,* digestion]

**dys·pha·gi·a, dys·pha·gy** (dis-fā′jē-ă, dis′fā-jē) Difficulty in swallowing. SYN aglutition. [*dys-* + G. *phagō,* to eat]

**dys·pha·si·a** (dis-fā′zē-ă) Impairment in the production of speech and failure to arrange words in an understandable way. [*dys-* + G. *phasis,* speaking]

**dys·phe·mi·a** (dis-fē′mē-ă) Disordered phonation, articulation, or hearing due to emotional or mental deficits. [*dys-* + G. *phēmē,* speech]

**dys·pho·ri·a** (dis-fōr′ē-ă) Mood of general dissatisfaction, restlessness, depression, and anxiety; a feeling of unpleasantness or discomfort. [*dys-* + G. *phora,* a bearing]

**dys·pi·tu·i·tar·ism** (dis′pi-tū′i-tĕr-izm) The complex of phenomena due to excessive or deficient secretion by the pituitary gland.

**dys·pla·si·a** (dis-plā′zē-ă, dis-plā′zē-ă) Abnormal tissue development.

**dysp·ne·a** (disp-nē′ă) *In the diphthong pn, the p is silent only at the beginning of a word.* Shortness of breath, a subjective difficulty or distress in breathing, usually associated with disease of the heart or lungs; occurs normally during intense physical exertion or at high altitude. SYN dyspnoea. [G. *dyspnoia,* fr. *dys-,* bad, + *pnoē,* breathing]

**dysp·ne·a on ex·er·tion (DOE)** (disp-nē′ă eg-zĕr′shŭn) Shortness of breath (due to cardiovascular and respiratory disorders) elicited by physical activity.

**dyspnoea** [Br.] SYN dyspnea.

**dys·prax·i·a** (dis-prak′sē-ă) Impaired or painful functioning in any organ. [*dys-* + G. *praxis,* a doing]

**dys·rhyth·mi·a** (dis-ridh′mē-ă) Defective rhythm. [*dys-* + G. *rhythmos,* rhythm]

**dys·to·ni·a** (dis-tō′nē-ă) A syndrome of abnormal muscle contraction that produces repetitive involuntary twisting movements and abnormal posturing of the neck, trunk, face, and extremities. [*dys-* + G. *tonos,* tension]

**dys·tro·phi·a ad·i·po·so·ge·ni·ta·lis** (dis-trō′fē-ă ad-i-pō′sō-jen-i-tā′lis) Disorder characterized primarily by obesity and hypogonadotrophic hypogonadism in adolescent boys. SYN adiposogenital dystrophy, Fröhlich syndrome, hypophysial syndrome.

**dys·tro·phic cal·ci·fi·ca·tion** (dis-trō′fik kal′si-fi-kā′shŭn) Calcification occurring in degenerated or necrotic tissue, as in hyalinized scars, degenerated foci in leiomyomas, and caseous nodules.

**dys·tro·phy, dys·tro·phi·a** (dis′trŏ-fē, dis-trō′fē-ă) Progressive changes that may result from defective nutrition of a tissue or organ. [*dys-* + G. *trophē,* nourishment]

# E

**Ea·gle syn·drome** (ē′gĕl sin′drōm) Pain (usually pharyngeal) and inflammation (usually tonsillar) due to overlong styloid process or calcification.

**EAHF com·plex** (kom′pleks) Combination of allergies consisting of *e*czema, *a*sthma and *ha*y *f*ever.

**Eames tech·nique** (ēmz tek-nēk′) A procedure for mixing dental amalgam in approximately a 1:1 ratio of mercury and alloy to minimize free mercury in the unset mix.

**EAR** Abbreviation for estimated average requirement.

**ear** (ēr) [TA] Organ of hearing and equilibrium, composed of **external ear,** consisting of auricle, external acoustic meatus, and tympanic membrane; **middle ear,** or tympanic cavity, with its auditory ossicles and associated muscles; and **internal ear,** the vestibulocochlear organ, which includes the bony labyrinth (of semicircular canals, vestibule, and cochlea), and vestibular and cochlear labyrinths. SYN auris.

**ear bones** (ēr bōnz) SYN auditory ossicles.

**ear·drum** (ēr′drŭm) SYN tympanic membrane.

**ear·ly-on·set per·i·o·don·ti·tis (EOP)** (ēr′lē-on′set per′ē-ō-don-tī′tis) SEE aggressive periodontal disease.

**ear·ly post·trau·mat·ic ep·i·lep·sy** (ĕr′lē pōst′traw-mat′ik ep′i-lep-sē) Seizures beginning within 1 week after craniocerebral trauma.

**ear·ly syph·i·lis** (ĕr′lē sif′i-lis) Primary, secondary, or early latent syphilis, before any tertiary manifestations have appeared.

**earth wax** (ĕrth waks) SYN ceresin.

**eat** (ēt) **1.** To take solid food. **2.** To chew and swallow any substance as one would food. **3.** To corrode. [A.S. *etan*]

**eat·ing dis·or·ders (ED)** (ēt′ing dis-ōr′dĕrz) Mental disorders including anorexia nervosa, bulimia nervosa and pica.

**eat·ing ep·i·lep·sy** (ēt′ing ep′i-lep′sē) Epileptic, often generalized, seizures provoked by eating; a type of reflex epilepsy.

**e·bur** (ē′bŭr) Tissue resembling ivory in outward appearance or structure. [L. ivory]

**e·bur den·tis** (ē′bŭr den′tis) SYN dentin.

**e·bur·na·tion** (ē-bŭr-nā′shŭn) A change in exposed subchondral bone in degenerative joint disease in which it is converted into a dense substance with a smooth surface like ivory. [L. *eburneus*, of ivory]

**e·bur·na·tion of den·tin** (ē′bŭr-nā′shŭn den′tin) Condition in arrested dental caries wherein decalcified dentin is burnished and a polished with a brown stain.

**e·bur·ni·tis** (ē-bŭr-nī′tis) Increased density and hardness of dentin, which may occur after dentin is exposed. [L. *eburneus*, of ivory, + G. *-itis*, inflammation]

**EBV** Abbreviation for Epstein-Barr virus.

**ec·cen·tric** (ek-sen′trik) *Do not confuse this word with acentric.* **1.** Abnormal or peculiar in ideas or behavior. SYN erratic (1). **2.** Proceeding from a center.

**ec·cen·tric check·bite** (ek-sen′trik chek′ bīt) Colloq. for eccentric interocclusal record. SEE interocclusal record.

**ec·cen·tric mus·cle con·trac·tion** (ek-sen′trik mŭs′ĕl kŏn-trak′shŭn) Increase in muscle tone during lengthening of the muscle such that the muscle opposes, but does not stop, movement. Movement is controlled, as in the opening of the jaw.

**ec·cen·tric oc·clu·sion** (ek-sen′trik ŏ-klū′zhŭn) Any occlusion other than centric.

**ec·cen·tric po·si·tion** (ek-sen′trik pŏ-zish′ŏn) SYN eccentric relationship.

**ec·cen·tric re·la·tion·ship** (ek-sen′trik rē-lā′shŭn-ship) Any maxillary-mandibular relationship that is not centric. SYN acentric relation, eccentric position.

**ec·chy·mo·sis** (ek-i-mō′sis) Purplish patch due to blood extravasation into the skin, differing from petechiae only in size. See this page. [G. *ekchymōsis*, ecchymosis, fr. *ek,* out, + *chymos,* juice]

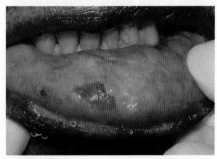

ecchymosis

**ec·dem·ic** (ek-dem′ik) Denoting a disease brought into a geographic region from without.

**e·chi·no·sto·mi·a·sis** (ē-kī′nō-stō-mī′ă-sis) Infection of humans with trematodes of the genus *Echinostoma*.

**ech·o** (ek′ō) **1.** Reverberating sound sometimes heard during chest auscultation. **2.** In ultrasonography, acoustic signal received from scattering or reflecting structures or corresponding pattern of light on a cathose ray tube or ultrasonogram. **3.** In magnetic resonance imaging, signal detected following an inverting pulse. [G.]

**ech·o·a·cou·si·a** (ek′ō-ă-kyū′zē-ă) Subjective hearing disturbance in which a sound repeats. [*echo* + G. *akouō,* to hear]

**ech·o·car·di·o·gram** (ek′ō-kahr′dē-ō-gram) Ultrasonic record by echocardiography.

**ech·o·car·di·og·ra·phy** (ek′ō-kahr-dē-og′ră-fē) The use of ultrasound in the investigation of the heart and great vessels and diagnosis of cardiovascular lesions. [*echo* + *cardiography*]

**ech·o·en·ceph·a·log·ra·phy** (ek′ō-en-sef-ă-log′ră-fē) Use of reflected ultrasound in diagnosis of intracranial processes. [*echo* + *encephalography*]

**ech·og·ra·phy** (e-kog′ră-fē) SYN ultrasonography. [*echo* + G. *graphō,* to write]

**ech·o·la·li·a** (ek′ō-lā′lē-ă) Involuntary parrotlike repetition of something just spoken by another person. [*echo* + G. *lalia,* a form of speech]

**ech·o·mo·tism** (ek′ō-mō′tizm) SYN echopraxia. [*echo* + L. *motio,* motion]

**e·chop·a·thy** (e-kop′ă-thē) Form of psychopathology, usually associated with schizophrenia, in which words or actions of another are imitated. [*echo* + G. *pathos,* suffering]

**ech·o·prax·i·a, ech·o·prax·is** (ek′ō-prak′sē-ă, -prak′sis) Involuntary imitation of movements made by another. SEE echopathy. SYN echomotism. [*echo* + G. *praxis,* action]

**ECHO vi·rus, ech·o·vi·rus** (ek′ō vī′rŭs, ek′ō-vī-rŭs) Enterovirus isolated from humans; although there are many inapparent infections, some serotypes are associated with fever, aseptic meningitis, and other mild respiratory disease.

**ec·la·bi·um** (ek-lā′bē-ŭm) Eversion of a lip. [G. *ek,* out, + L. *labium,* lip]

**ec·lec·tic** (ek-lek′tik) Picking out from different sources what seems most desirable. [G. *eklektikos,* selecting, fr. *ek,* out, + *lego,* to select]

**ECoG** Abbreviation for electrocorticography.

**e·col·o·gy** (ē-kol′ŏ-jē) Branch of biology concerned with total complex of interrelationships among living organisms, encompassing relations of organisms to each other, the environment, and entire energy balance within a given ecosystem.

**e·co·sys·tem** (ē′kō-sis-tĕm) Fundamental unit in ecology, comprising living and nonliving elements that interact in a defined region.

**é·cou·vil·lon** (ā-kū-vē-yon[h]′) Brush with firm bristles for freshening sores or abrading interior of a cavity. [Fr., cleaning brush]

**ec·sta·sy** (ek′stă-sē) A drug of abuse, used at clubs, raves, and rock concerts.

**ECT** Abbreviation for electroconvulsive therapy; electroshock therapy.

**ec·tad** (ek′tad) Outward. [G. *ektos,* outside, + L. *ad,* to]

**ec·tal** (ek′tăl) Outer; external. [G. *ektos,* outside]

**ec·tat·ic em·phy·se·ma** (ek-tat′ik em′fi-sē′mă) Obstructive airway disease with areas of dilation of alveoli (acini). Associated with inherited deficiency of α-1-antitrypsin.

**ec·to·derm** (ek′tō-dĕrm) Outer layer of cells in the embryo, after establishment of the three primary germ layers (ectoderm, mesoderm, endoderm). [*ecto-* + G. *derma,* skin]

🔲**ec·to·der·mal dys·pla·si·a** (ek′tō-dĕr′măl dis-plā′zē-ă) A congenital defect of the ectodermal tissues, including the skin and its appendages; associated with tooth dysplasia. See page A4.

**ec·to·en·tad** (ek′tō-en′tad) From without inward.

**ec·tog·e·nous** (ek-toj′ĕ-nŭs) SYN exogenous. [*ecto-* + G. *-gen,* producing]

**ec·to·mes·en·chyme** (ek′tō-mes′en-kīm) SYN mesectoderm (2). [*ecto-* + G. *mesos,* middle, + *enkyma,* infusion]

**ec·to·morph** (ek′tō-mōrf) A constitutional body type or build (biotype or somatotype) in which tissues originating from the ectoderm predominate; limbs predominate over trunk. [*ecto-* + G. *morphē,* form]

**ec·to·pi·a, ec·to·py** (ek-tō′pē-ă, ek′tō-pē) Congenital displacement of any organ or body part of the body. [G. *ektopos,* out of place]

**ec·to·pi·a len·tis** (ek-tō′pē-ă len′tis) Displacement of the lens of the eye.

🔲**ec·top·ic** (ek-top′ik) Out of place; said of an organ not in its proper position, or of a pregnancy outside the cavity of the uterus. See this page.

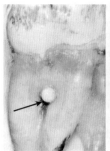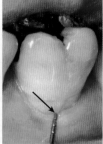

**ectopic enamel:** enamel pearls (enamelomas) at furcations of multirooted teeth

**ec·top·ic cal·ci·fi·ca·tion** (ek-top´ik kal´ si-fi-kā´shŭn) Calcification that occurs at an abnormal site (e.g., pulp stones, salivary calculi).

**ec·top·ic e·rup·tion** (ek-top´ik ē-rŭp´ shŭn) Tooth eruption in an abnormal location. See this page.

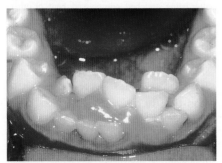

**ectopic eruption:** axial tilting and rotated teeth

**ec·top·ic hor·mone** (ek-top´ik hōr´mōn) Hormone formed by tissue outside normal endocrine site of production.

**ec·tos·te·al** (ek-tos´tē-ăl) Relating to the external surface of a bone. [*ecto-* + G. *osteon,* bone]

**ec·tro·pi·on, ec·tro·pi·um** (ek-trō´pē-on) A rolling outward of the margin of a part, e.g., of an eyelid. [G. *ek,* out, + *tropē,* a turning]

**ECVT** Abbreviation for electroconvulsive therapy.

**ec·ze·ma** (ek´sĕ-mă) Generic term for inflammatory skin conditions, particularly with vesiculation in acute stage, typically erythematous, edematous, papular, and crusting; followed often by lichenification and scaling and occasionally by dusky erythema; often hereditary and associated with allergic rhinitis and asthma. [G. fr. *ekzeō,* to boil over]

**ec·ze·ma mar·gi·na·tum** (ek´sĕ-mă mar-ji-nā´tŭm) SYN tinea cruris.

**ED** Abbreviation for eating disorders; effective dose.

**ED₅₀** Abbreviation for median effective dose.

**e·de·ma** (ĕ-dē´mă) **1.** Excessive fluid in cells or intercellular tissues. **2.** At the gross level, used to describe physical sign commonly likened to swelling or increased girth that often accompanies fluid accumulation in a limb. [G. *oidēma,* a swelling]

**e·den·tate** (ē-den´tāt) SYN edentulous. [L. *edentatus*]

**e·den·tul·ism** (ē-den´tyū-lizm) State of being partially or completely without teeth.

**e·den·tu·lous** (ē-den´tyū-lŭs) Toothless, having lost the natural teeth. SYN agomphious, edentate. [L. *edentulus,* toothless]

**edge** (ej) Line at which surface terminates. SEE ALSO border, margin.

**edge-to-edge bite** (ej ej bīt) SYN edge-to-edge occlusion.

**edge-to-edge oc·clu·sion** (ej ej ŏ-klū´ zhŭn) Occlusion in which anterior teeth of both jaws meet along their incisal edges when teeth are in centric occlusion. SYN edge-to-edge bite, end-to-end bite, end-to-end occlusion.

**edge·wise ap·pli·ance** (ej´wīz ă-plī´ăns) A fixed, multibanded orthodontic appliance using an attachment bracket the slot of which receives a rectangular archwire horizontally, which gives precise control of tooth movement in all three planes of space.

**EDRF** Abbreviation for endothelium-derived relaxing factor.

**EDTA** Abbreviation for ethylenediaminetetraacetic acid.

**ed·u·ca·tion** (ed´yū-kā´shŭn) NURSING teaching patient, family, community members, staff, and others by implementing learning activities to meet intended outcomes.

**EEG** Abbreviation for electroencephalogram; electroencephalograph; electroencephalography.

**EEG ac·ti·va·tion** The fast low-voltage pattern of attentive wakefulness measured by electroencephalography.

**ef·fect** (e-fekt´) The result of therapy. [L. *efficio,* pp. *effectus,* to accomplish, fr. *facio,* to do]

**ef·fec·tive dose (ED)** (e-fek´tiv dōs) Dose that produces a specific result; when followed by a subscript (generally ''$ED_{50}$''), it denotes the dose having such an effect on a given percentage (e.g., 50%) of the test animals; $ED_{50}$ is the median effective dose.

**ef·fec·tive·ness** (e-fek´tiv-nĕs) Measure of accuracy of diagnostic or therapeutic technique when carried out in an average clinical environment.

**ef·fec·tor** (e-fek´tŏr) **1.** Peripheral tissue that receives nerve impulses and reacts by muscular contraction, glandular secretion, or electric discharge (from an electric organ, as in the case of certain bony fishes such as the electric eel). **2.** Small metabolic molecule that, by combining with a repressor gene, depresses the operon activity. [L. producer]

**ef·fer·ent** (ef´ĕr-ĕnt) Conducting fluid or nerve impulse outward from a given organ, cell, or part thereof. [L. *efferens,* fr. *effero,* to bring out]

**ef·fer·ves·cent mag·ne·si·um sul·fate** (ef´ĕr-ves´ĕnt mag-nē´zē-ŭm sŭl´fāt) Effervescent Epsom salt; magnesium sulfate, sodium bicarbonate, tartaric acid, and citric acid, moistened, passed through a sieve, and dried to a coarse granular powder; a purgative.

**ef·fi·ca·cy** (ef´i-kă-sē) Extent to which a specific intervention, procedure, regimen, or service produces a beneficial result under ideal conditions. Cf. effectiveness. [L. *efficacia*, fr, *ef-ficio*, to perform, accomplish]

**ef·fi·cien·cy** (ĕ-fish´ĕn-sē) 1. Production of desired effects or results with minimum waste of time, money, effort, or skill. 2. Measure of effectiveness; specifically, useful work output divided by the energy input.

**ef·flu·vi·um,** pl. **ef·flu·vi·a** (ĕ-flū´vē-ŭm, -ă) *Do not confuse this word with defluvium.* Shedding of hair. [L. a flowing out, fr. *ef-fluo*, to flow out]

**ef·fu·sion** (e-fyu´zhŭn) 1. Escape of fluid from blood vessels or lymphatics into tissues or cavity. 2. Collection of effused fluid. [L. *effusio*, a pouring out]

**e·ges·ta** (ē-jes´tă) Unabsorbed food residues discharged from digestive tract. [L. *e-gero*, pp. *-gestus*, to carry out, discharge]

**egg-white syn·drome** (eg´wīt sin´drōm) Dermatitis, loss of hair, and loss of muscle coordination.

**e·go·cen·tric** (ē´gō-sen´trik) Marked by extreme self-concentration.

**Ehl·ers-Dan·los syn·drome** (ā´lerz dahn´lōs sin´drōm) Connective tissue disorders characterized by hyperelasticity and fragility of skin, hypermobility of joints, and fragility of cutaneous blood vessels.

**ehr·lich·i·o·sis** (er-lik´ē-ō´sis) Infection with leukocytic rickettsiae of the genus *Ehrlichia;* in humans, especially by *E. sennetsu,* which produces manifestations similar to those of Rocky Mountain spotted fever.

**eighth cra·ni·al nerve [CN VIII]** (ātth krā´nē-ăl nĕrv) SYN vestibulocochlear nerve [CN VIII].

**Ei·ken·el·la cor·ro·dens** (ī-kĕ-nel´ă kō-rō´denz) A species of nonmotile, rod-shaped, gram-negative, facultatively anaerobic bacteria; part of normal flora of adult human oral cavity but may be an opportunistic pathogen, in immunocompromised people.

**e·jac·u·late** (ē-jak´yū-lāt, ē-jak-yū-lăt) 1. To expel suddenly. 2. Semen expelled in ejaculation.

**e·jec·tion** (ē-jek´shŭn) 1. Driving or throwing out by physical force from within. 2. That which is ejected. [L. *ejectio*, from *ejicio*, to cast out]

**e·jec·tor** (ē-jek´tŏr, -tōr) A device used for forcibly expelling (ejecting) a substance.

**e·las·tic** (ĕ-las´tik) 1. Rubber or plastic band used in orthodontics as either a primary or adjunctive source of force to move teeth. 2. Having the property of returning to original shape after being stretched, compressed, bent, or otherwise distorted. [G. *elastreō,* epic form of *elaunō,* drive, push]

**e·las·tic band fix·a·tion** (ĕ-las´tik band fik-sā´shŭn) Stabilization of fractured segments of the jaws with intermaxillary elastics applied to splints or appliances.

**e·las·tic·i·ty** (ĕ-las-tis´i-tē) Quality of being able to expand and contract.

**e·las·tic lig·a·ture** (ĕ-las´tik lig´ă-chŭr) 1. Rubber ligature that slowly constricts. 2. In orthodontics, stretchable threadlike material that may be tied from a tooth to an archwire or from tooth to tooth to gain movement.

**e·las·to·mer** (ĕ-las´tŏ-mĕr) Elastoplastic ring or latex ring used to hold an arch wire in a bracket ring.

**e·las·to·sis** (ĕ-las-tō´sis) 1. Degenerative change in elastic tissue. 2. Degeneration of collagen fibers, with altered staining properties resembling elastic tissue.

**e·la·tion** (ē-lā´shŭn) The feeling or expression of excitement or gaiety; if prolonged and inappropriate, a characteristic of mania. [L. *elatio*, fr. *ef-fero*, pp. *e-latus*, to lift up]

**el·bow** (el´bō) [TA] 1. The region of the upper limb between arm and forearm surrounding the elbow joint, especially posteriorly. 2. SYN elbow joint. 3. An angular body resembling a flexed elbow. [A.S. *elnboga*]

**el·bow joint** (el´bō joynt) [TA] A compound hinge synovial joint between the humerus and the bones of the forearm. SYN elbow (2) [TA].

**el·der a·buse** (el´dĕr ă-byūs´) Physical or emotional maltreatment, including financial exploitation, of an elderly person.

**e·lec·tive mut·ism** (ĕ-lek´tiv myū´tizm) Mutism due to psychogenic causes. SYN voluntary mutism.

**e·lec·tric bath, e·lec·tro·ther·a·peu·tic bath** (ĕ-lek´trik bath, ĕ-lek´trō-thār´ă-pyū´tik) 1. Bath in which the medium is charged with electricity. 2. Therapeutic application of static electricity, with patient placed on an insulated platform.

**e·lec·tric shock** (ĕ-lek´trik shok) Sum of immediate and delayed pathophysiologic responses of living tissue to electrical current of sufficient magnitude to induce abnormal sensations or objective changes.

**electroanaesthesia** [Br.] SYN electroanesthesia.

**e·lec·tro·an·al·ge·si·a** (ē-lek′trō-an-ăl-jē′zē-ă) Analgesia induced by electric current.

**e·lec·tro·an·es·the·si·a** (ē-lek′trō-an-esthē′zē-ă) Anesthesia produced by an electric current. SYN electroanaesthesia.

**e·lec·tro·car·di·og·ra·phy** (ĕ-lek′trō-kahrdē-og′ră-fē) **1.** A method of recording the electrical activity of the heart: impulse formation, conduction, depolarization, and repolarization of atria and ventricles. **2.** The study and interpretation of electrocardiograms.

**e·lec·tro·cau·ter·i·za·tion** (ĕ-lek′trō-kaw′tĕr-ī-zā′shŭn) Cauterization by passage of high-frequency current through tissue or a metal device that has been electrically heated.

**e·lec·tro·cau·ter·y** (ĕ-lek′trō-kaw′tĕr-ē) An instrument for directing a high frequency current through a local area of tissue.

**e·lec·tro·co·ag·u·la·tion** (ĕ-lek′trō-kōag′yū-lā′shŭn) Coagulation produced by an electrocautery.

**e·lec·tro·con·vul·sive** (ĕ-lek′trō-kŏn-vŭl′siv) Denoting a convulsive response to electrical stimulus. SEE electroshock therapy.

**e·lec·tro·con·vul·sive ther·a·py (ECT, ECVT)** (ĕ-lek′trō-kŏn-vŭl′siv thār′ă-pē) SYN electroshock therapy.

**e·lec·tro·cor·ti·co·gram** (ĕ-lek′trō-kōr′ti-kō-gram) Record of electrical activity derived directly from the cerebral cortex.

**e·lec·tro·cor·ti·cog·ra·phy (ECoG)** (ĕ-lek′trō-kōr′ti-kog′ră-fē) Recording technique of electrical activity of cerebral cortex with electrodes placed directly on it.

**e·lec·trode** (ĕ-lek′trōd) Device to record one of two extremities of an electric circuit; one of two poles of an electric battery or of the end of the conductors connected thereto. [*electro-* + G. *hodos,* way]

**e·lec·tro·di·ag·no·sis** (ĕ-lek′trō-dī-ăg-nō′sis) **1.** Use of electronic devices for diagnostic purposes. **2.** By convention, studies performed in the electromyographic (EMG) laboratory, i.e., nerve conduction studies and needle electrode examination (EMG proper).

**e·lec·tro·di·ag·nos·tic med·i·cine** (ĕ-lek′trō-dī-ăg-nos′tik med′i-sin) Specific area of medical practice in which recording and analyzing biologic electrical potentials are used to diagnose and treat neuromuscular disorders.

**e·lec·tro·en·ceph·a·lo·gram (EEG)** (ĕ-lek′trō-en-sef′ă-lō-gram) Record obtained by an electroencephalograph.

**e·lec·tro·en·ceph·a·lo·graph (EEG)** (ĕ-lek′trō-en-sef′ă-lō-graf) System for recording electric brain potentials derived from electrodes attached to the scalp.

**e·lec·tro·en·ceph·a·log·ra·phy (EEG)** (ĕ-lek′trō-en-sef′ă-log′ră-fē) Registration of electrical potentials recorded by an electroencephalograph.

**e·lec·tro·gas·trog·ra·phy** (ĕ-lek′trō-gastrog′ră-fē) Recording of electrical phenomena associated with gastric secretion and motility.

**electrohaemostasis** [Br.] SYN electrohemostasis.

**e·lec·tro·he·mo·sta·sis** (ĕ-lek′trō-hē-mos′tă-sis) Arrest of hemorrhage by electrocautery. SYN electrohaemostasis. [*electro-* + G. *haima,* blood, + *stasis,* halt]

**e·lec·tro·lyte** (ĕ-lek′trō-līt) Any compound that, in solution, conducts electricity and is decomposed (electrolyzed) by it.

**e·lec·tro·mag·net·ic ra·di·a·tion, elec·tro·mag·ne·tic spec·trum** (ĕ-lek′trō-mag-net′ik rā′dē-ā′shŭn, spek′trŭm) Wavelike energy propagated through matter or space; varies widely in wavelength, frequency, photon energy, and properties; may be natural or artificial and includes x-rays, gamma rays, and other forms.

**e·lec·tro·mal·let** (ĕ-lek′trō-mal′ĕt) An electromechanical device for compacting direct-filling gold.

**e·lec·trom·e·ter** (ĕ-lek-trom′ĕ-tĕr) A device for measuring the electromotive force (voltage) of a source of electricity.

**e·lec·tro·mic·tu·ra·tion** (ĕ-lek′trō-mik′chŭr-ā′shŭn) Electrical stimulation of the conus medullaris to empty the urinary bladder of paraplegic patients.

**e·lec·tro·mo·tive force (EMF)** (ĕ-lek′trō-mō′tiv fōrs) The force (measured in volts) that causes electricity to flow.

**e·lec·tro·my·o·gram (EMG)** (ĕ-lek′trō-mī′ō-gram) A graphic representation of the electric currents associated with muscular action.

**e·lec·tro·my·o·graph (EMG)** (ĕ-lek′trō-mī′ō-graf) An instrument for recording electrical currents generated in an active muscle.

**elec·tro·my·o·graph·ic (EMG) bi·o·feed·back** (ĕ-lek′trō-mī′ō-graf′ik bī′ō-fēd′bak) Biofeedback that uses an electromyographic measure of muscle tension as the physical symptom to be deconditioned.

**e·lec·tro·my·o·graph·ic ex·am·i·na·tion** (ĕ-lek′trō-mī-ō-graf′ik eg-zam′i-nā′shŭn) **1.** Needle electrode examination portion of electrodiagnostic examination. **2.** SYN electromyography (2).

**e·lec·tro·my·og·ra·phy (EMG)** (ĕ-lek′trō-mī-og′ră-fē) **1.** Recording of electrical activ-

ef

ity generated in muscle for diagnostic purposes. **2.** Umbrella term for the entire electrodiagnostic study performed in the EMG laboratory, including not only needle electrode examination, but also nerve conduction studies. [*electro-* + G. *mys,* muscle, + *graphō,* to write]

**e·lec·tron** (ĕ-lek′tron) Negatively charged subatomic particles that orbit the positive nucleus, in one of several energy levels called shells. A nucleus and its electrons constitute an atom. [*electro-* + *-on*]

**e·lec·tron beam** (ĕ-lek′tron bēm) Form of radiation used principally in superficial radiotherapy.

**e·lec·tro·neu·rol·y·sis** (ĕ-lek′trō-nū-rol′i-sis) Destruction of nerve tissue by electricity.

**e·lec·tron·ic** (ĕ-lek-tron′ik) **1.** Pertaining to electrons. **2.** Denoting devices or systems utilizing the flow of electrons in a vacuum, gas, or semiconductor.

**e·lec·tron·ic·al·ly pow·er·ed in·stru·men·ta·tion** (ĕ-lek-tron′ik-lē pow′ĕrd in′strŭ-men-tā′shŭn) Use of devices involving rapid energy vibrations to detach calculus from the tooth surface and clean the environment of the periodontal pocket.

**e·lec·tron mi·cro·graph** (ĕ-lek′tron mī′krŏ-graf) Image produced by electron beam of an electron microscope, recorded on an electron-sensitive plate or film.

**e·lec·tron mi·cro·scope** (ĕ-lek′tron mī′krŏ-skōp) Visual and photographic microscope in which electron beams with wavelengths thousands of times shorter than visible light are used instead of light, thereby allowing much greater resolution and magnification.

**e·lec·tro·pher·o·gram** (ĕ-lek′trō-fer′ŏ-gram) Densitometric or colorimetric pattern obtained from filter paper or other strips on which substances have been separated by electrophoresis; may also refer to the strips themselves.

**e·lec·tro·pho·re·sis** (ĕ-lek′trō-fŏr-ē′sis) The movement of particles in an electric field toward anode or cathode. SYN ionophoresis, phoresis (1).

**elec·tro·pho·reto·gram** SYN electropherogram.

**e·lec·tro·sec·tion** (ĕ-lek′trō-sek′shŭn) Use of electrical current for surgically cutting tissue.

**e·lec·tro·shock ther·a·py (ECT)** (ĕ-lek′trō-shok′ thār′ă-pē) Form of treatment of mental disorders in which convulsions are produced by passage of an electric current through the brain. SYN electroconvulsive therapy.

**e·lec·tro·spec·trog·ra·phy** (ĕ-lek′trō-spek-trog′ră-fē) Recording and interpretation of electroencephalographic wave patterns.

**e·lec·tro·spi·nog·ra·phy** (ĕ-lek′trō-spī-nog′ră-fē) The recording of spontaneous electrical activity of the spinal cord.

**e·lec·tro·steth·o·graph** (ĕ-lek′trō-steth′ŏ-graf) Electrical instrument that amplifies or records chest respiratory and cardiac sounds. [*electro-* + G. *stēthos,* chest, + *graphō,* to record]

**e·lec·tro·sur·ger·y** (ĕ-lek′trō-sŭr′jĕr-ē) Division of tissues by high frequency current applied locally with a metal instrument or needle.

**e·lec·tro·ther·a·peu·tics, e·lec·tro·ther·a·py** (ĕ-lek′trō-thār′ă-pyū′tiks, -ă-pē) Use of electricity in treatment of disease.

**e·lec·tro·therm** (ĕ-lek′trō-thĕrm) Flexible sheet of resistance coils to apply heat to body surface. [*electro-* + G. *thermē,* heat]

**e·le·i·din** (ĕ-lē′i-din) Refractile and weakly staining keratin in cells of the stratum lucidum of palmar and plantar epidermis.

**el·e·ment** (el′ĕ-mĕnt) Substance composed of atoms of only one kind that therefore cannot be decomposed into two or more elements and can lose its chemical properties only by union with another element or by nuclear reaction changing the proton number. [L. *elementum,* a rudiment, beginning]

**el·e·men·ta·ry par·ti·cle** (el′ĕ-men′tar-ē pahr′ti-kĕl) **1.** SYN platelet. **2.** A unit on the matrical surface of mitochondrial cristae.

**el·e·phan·ti·a·sis** (el′ĕ-fan-tī′ă-sis) Hypertrophy, edema, and fibrosis of the skin and subcutaneous tissue.

**el·e·va·tor** (el′ĕ-vā-tŏr) Surgical instrument used to luxate and remove teeth and roots that cannot be engaged by the beaks of forceps, or to loosen teeth and roots before forceps application. SYN dental lever. [L. fr. *e-levo,* pp. *-atus,* to lift up]

**el·ev·enth cra·ni·al nerve [CN XI]** (ĕ-lev′ĕnth krā′nē-ăl nĕrv) SYN accessory nerve [CN XI].

**elf·in facies** (el′fin fā′shē-ez) Facies characterized by a short, upturned nose, wide mouth, widely spaced eyes, and full cheeks.

**e·lim·i·na·tion** (ĕ-lim′i-nā′shŭn) Expulsion; removal of waste material from the body; the getting rid of anything. [L. *elimino,* pp. *-atus,* to turn out of doors, fr. *limen,* threshold]

**e·lim·i·na·tion di·et** (ĕ-lim′i-nā′shŭn dī′ĕt) Diet designed to detect which food causes allergic manifestations in the patient; food items to which the patient may be sensitive are withdrawn separately and successively until that item that causes symptoms is discovered.

**e·lix·ir** (ĕ-lik′sĭr) Clear, sweetened, flavored, hydroalcoholic liquid intended for oral use either as vehicle or for therapeutic effect of active medicinal agents. [Mediev. L., fr. Ar. *al-iksir,* the philosopher's stone]

**el·lip·soid, el·lip·soid·al** (ē-lip'soyd, -al) Spheric or spindle-shaped condensation of phagocytic macrophages in a reticular stroma investing wall of splenic arterial capillaries shortly before they release their blood in red pulp cords. [G. *ellips,* oval, + *eidos,* form]

**el·lip·ti·cal re·cess of bon·y lab·y·rinth** (ē-lip'ti-kăl rē'ses bōn'ē lab'i-rinth) [TA] Oval depression in the roof and inner wall of vestibule of the labyrinth, lodging the utriculus.

**el·lip·to·cy·to·sis** (ē-lip'tō-sī-tō'sis) A hereditary abnormality of hemopoiesis in which 50–90% of the red blood cells consist of rod forms and elliptocytes. SYN ovalocytosis.

**El·lis-van Cre·veld syn·drome** (el'is van-krev'ĕlt sin'drōm) SYN chondroectodermal dysplasia.

**e·lon·ga·tion** (ē-lawng-gā'shŭn) Stretching lengthwise or result of such action.

**el·u·ant** (el'yū-ănt) A material that has undergone elution.

**el·u·ate** (el'yū-āt) The solution emerging from a column or paper in chromatography.

**el·u·ent** (el'yū-ĕnt) The mobile phase in chromatography. SYN developer (1).

**e·lu·tion** (ē-lū'shŭn) 1. Separation, by washing, of one solid from another. 2. Removal, with a suitable solvent, of one material from another that is insoluble in that solvent. 3. Removal of antibodies absorbed onto the erythrocyte surface.

**e·ma·ci·a·tion** (ĕ-mā'shē-ā'shŭn) Becoming abnormally thin due to extreme loss of flesh. SYN wasting (1). [L. *e-macio,* pp. *-atus,* to make thin]

**e·mar·gi·nate** (ē-mahr'ji-năt) Nicked; with a broken margin. [L. *emargino,* to deprive of its edge, fr. *e-* priv. + *margo (margin-),* edge]

**em·bed** (em-bed') To surround a pathologic or histologic specimen with a medium such as paraffin or wax, to facilitate cutting thin sections for microscopic examination.

**em·bo·le·mi·a** (em'bō-lē'mē-ă) Presence of emboli in circulating blood. [G. *embolos,* a plug (embolus), + *haima,* blood]

**em·bol·i·form nu·cle·us** (em-bol'i-fōrm nū'klē-ŭs) A small wedge-shaped nucleus in the central white substance of the cerebellum just internal to the hilus of the dentate nucleus. SYN embolus (2).

**em·bo·lism** (em'bŏ-lizm) 1. Obstruction or occlusion of a vessel by an embolus. 2. In approximate common usage, any foreign substance that enters and is carried off in the vasculature by flowing blood. [G. *embolisma,* a piece or patch; literally something thrust in]

**em·bo·lus,** pl. **em·bo·li** (em'bō-lŭs, -lī) 1. A plug, composed of a detached thrombus or vegetation, mass of bacteria, quantity of air or gas or foreign body, which occludes a vessel. 2. SYN emboliform nucleus. [G. *embolos,* a plug, wedge or stopper]

**em·bos·sed dot** (em-bawst' dot) SYN identification dot.

**em·bra·sure** (em-brā'shŭr) In dentistry, an opening that widens outwardly or inwardly; specifically, that space adjacent to the interproximal contact area that spreads toward facial, gingival, lingual, occlusal, or incisal aspect. [Fr. an opening in a wall for cannon]

**em·bra·sure clasp** (em-brā'shŭr klasp) Removable partial denture clasp with circumferential arms and adjacent occlusal rests attached to a common body; passes through embrasure where no edentulous space exists between two adjacent teeth occlusal to contact area; employs two occlusal rests.

**em·bra·sure hook** (em-brā'shŭr huk) Hook-shaped extension of a removable partial denture that extends into occlusal embrasure between adjacent teeth; prevents cervical movement of appliance.

**em·bry·o** (em'brē-ō) In humans, developing organism from conception until end of the eighth week; developmental stages from this time to birth are commonly designated as fetal. [G. *embryon,* fr. *en,* in, + *bryō,* to be full, swell]

**em·bry·ol·o·gy** (em'brē-ol'ŏ-jē) Science of the origin and development of the organism from fertilization of the oocyte to the end of the eighth week. [*embryo-* + G. *logos,* study]

**EMD** Abbreviation for emergency medical dispatcher.

**e·mer·gence** (ē-mĕr'jĕns) Stage in recovery from general anesthesia that includes return to spontaneous breathing, voluntary swallowing, and normal consciousness. [L. *emergo,* arise, come forth]

**e·mer·gen·cy** (ē-mĕr'jĕn-sē) A patient's condition requiring immediate treatment. [L. *e-mergo,* pp. *-mersus,* to rise up, emerge, fr. *mergo,* to plunge into, dip]

**e·mer·gen·cy doc·trine** (ē-mĕr'jĕn-sē dok'trin) In medical jurisprudence, an assumption that a disabled or nonresponsive patient will agree to life-saving measures. SYN implied consent (1).

**e·mer·gen·cy med·i·cine** (ē-mĕr'jĕn-sē med'i-sin) That branch of health care involved with remediation or therapy of patients who are acutely ill or traumatized.

ef

**e·mer·gent** (ē-mĕr′jĕnt) **1.** Arising suddenly, calling for prompt action. **2.** Coming out; leaving a cavity or other part.

**em·er·y** (em′ĕr-ē) An abrasive containing aluminum oxide and iron. [O.Fr. *emeri,* fr. L.L. *smericulum,* fr. G. *smiris*]

**em·er·y discs** (em′ĕr-ē disks) Discs coated with emery powder used to abrade or smooth the surface of teeth or fillings.

**em·e·sis** (em′ĕ-sis) **1.** SYN vomiting. **2.** Combining form, used as a suffix, for vomiting. [G. fr. *emeō,* to vomit]

**em·e·sis ba·sin, kid·ney ba·sin** (em′ĕ-sis bā′sin, kid′nē) *Avoid the incorrect form Emerson* (or *Emerson's*) *basin.* Shallow basin of curved, kidney-shaped design, used to collect body fluids.

**e·met·ic** (ĕ-met′ik) **1.** Relating to or causing vomiting. **2.** An agent that causes vomiting, e.g., ipecac syrup. [G. *emetikos,* producing vomiting, fr. *emeō,* to vomit]

**em·e·tine** (em′ĕ-tēn) The principal alkaloid of ipecac, used as an emetic.

**em·e·to·ca·thar·tic** (em′ĕ-tō-kă-thahr′tik) **1.** Both emetic and cathartic. **2.** An agent that causes vomiting and purging of the lower intestines.

**em·e·to·gen·ic** (em′ĕ-tō-jen′ik) Having the capacity to induce emesis (vomiting), a common property of some drugs.

**e·me·to·ge·nic·i·ty** (em′ĕ-tō-jĕ-nis′i-tē) The property of being emetogenic.

**EMF** Abbreviation for electromotive force.

**EMG** Abbreviation for electromyogram; electromyograph; electromyography.

**em·i·gra·tion** (em-i-grā′shŭn) The passage of white blood cells through the endothelium and wall of small blood vessels. [L. *e-migro,* pp. *-atus,* to emigrate]

**em·i·nec·tomy** (em′i-nek′tŏ-mē) Operative removal of the anterior articular surface of the glenoid fossa.

**em·i·nence** (em′i-nĕns) [TA] Circumscribed area raised above general level of surrounding surface, particularly in bone. [L. *eminentia*]

**em·i·nence of con·cha** (em′i-nĕns kong′kă) [TA] Prominence on cranial surface of auricle corresponding to the concha.

**em·i·nence of sca·pha** (em′i-nĕns skaf′ă, skā′fă) [TA] Prominence on cranial surface of auricle corresponding to the scapha.

**em·i·nence of tri·an·gu·lar fos·sa of aur·i·cle** (em′i-nĕns trī-ang′gyū-lăr fos′ă awr′I-kĕl) [TA] Prominence on cranial surface of auricle corresponding to triangular fossa. SYN agger perpendicularis.

**em·is·sa·ry vein** (em′i-sar-ē vān) [TA] A communicating channel between venous sinuses of dura mater and veins of diploë and scalp.

**em·men·i·a** (ĕ-men′ē-ă) SYN menses. [G. *emmēnos,* monthly]

**e·mol·li·ent** (ĕ-mol′ē-ĕnt) An agent that softens the skin or soothes irritation.

**e·mo·tion** (ē-mō′shŭn) A strong feeling, aroused mental state, or intense state of drive or unrest, which may be directed toward a definite object. [L. *e-moveo,* pp. *-motus,* to move out, agitate]

**e·mo·tion·al** (ē-mō′shŭn-ăl) Relating to or marked by an emotion.

**e·mo·ti·o·vas·cu·lar** (ē-mō′shē-ō-vas′kyū-lăr) Relating to vascular changes (e.g., pallor and blushing) caused by emotions.

**em·path·ic** (em-path′ik) *Avoid the incorrect form empathetic.* Relating to or marked by empathy.

**em·path·ic in·dex** (em-path′ik in′deks) Degree of emotional understanding or empathy experienced by a health care provider or other person concerning another person.

**em·pa·thize** (em′pă-thīz) To put oneself in another's place.

**em·pa·thy** (em′pă-the) Ability to sense intellectually and emotionally emotions, feelings, and reactions that another person is experiencing and it communicate.

**em·phy·se·ma** (em′fi-sē′mă) **1.** Presence of air in the interstices of the connective tissue of a part. **2.** A condition of the lung characterized by increase beyond the normal in the size of air spaces distal to the terminal bronchiole (those parts containing alveoli), with destructive changes in their walls and reduction in their number. Clinical manifestation is breathlessness on exertion. [G. inflation of stomach. fr. *en,* in, + *physēma,* a blowing, fr. *physa,* bellows]

**em·pir·ic** (em-pir′ik) Founded on practical experience, rather than on reasoning alone, but not established scientifically, in contrast to rational.

**em·pir·i·cism** (em-pir′i-sizm) Using experience as a guide to practice or use of any remedy.

**em·pir·ic treat·ment** (em-pir′ik trēt′mĕnt) Therapy based on experience, usually without adequate data to support its use.

**em·py·e·ma,** pl. **em·py·e·ma·ta** (em′pī-ē′mă, -tă) Pus in a body cavity. [G. *empyēma,* suppuration, fr. *en,* in, + *pyon,* pus]

**emul·si·fi·er** (ē-mŭl′si-fī-ĕr) An agent (e.g., gum arabic, yolk of an egg) used to make an emulsion of a fixed oil. Soaps, detergents, steroids, and proteins can act as emulsifiers.

**e·mul·sion** (ē-mŭl′shŭn) A system containing two immiscible liquids in which one is dispersed, in the form of small globules, throughout the other. [Mod. L. fr. *e- mulgeo,* pp. *-mulsus,* to milk or drain out]

**e·nam·el** (ĕ-nam′ĕl) [TA] Hard, glistening substance covering coronal dentin of tooth. In its mature form, composed of an inorganic portion made up of 90% hydroxyapatite and about 6% calcium carbonate, calcium fluoride, and magnesium carbonate, with the remainder (4%) being an organic matrix of protein and glycoprotein. See this page. SYN enamelum [TA]. [M.E., fr. Fr. *enamailer,* to apply enamel, fr. *en,* on, + *amail,* enamel, fr. Germanic]

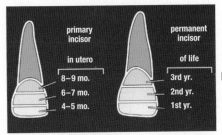

**enamel formation in teeth**

**e·nam·el cap** (ĕ-nam′ĕl kap) Enamel covering tooth crown.

**e·nam·el ca·ries** (ĕ-nam′ĕl kar′ēz) Decay of tooth enamel. SEE ALSO caries.

**e·nam·el cell** (ĕ-nam′ĕl sel) SYN ameloblast.

**e·nam·el cleav·age** (ĕ-nam′ĕl klē′văj) Splitting of enamel in a plane parallel to direction of enamel rods.

**e·nam·el cleav·er** (ĕ-nam′ĕl klē′vĕr) Instrument with a heavy shank and short blade at about 90 degrees to the axis of the handle; used with a hoeing motion to strip enamel from the axial tooth surfaces in preparation for a crown.

**e·nam·el crypt** (ĕ-nam′ĕl kript) Narrow, ectomesenchyme-filled space between dental ledge and an enamel organ. SYN enamel niche.

**e·nam·el cu·ti·cle** (ĕ-nam′ĕl kyū′ti-kĕl) Primary enamel cuticle, consisting of two extremely thin layers (the inner clear and structureless, the outer cellular), covering entire crown of newly erupted teeth and subsequently abraded by mastication; evident microscopically as an amorphous material between the attachment epithelium and the tooth. SYN adamantine membrane, cuticula dentis, dental cuticle, membrana adamantina, primary cuticle, skin of teeth.

**e·nam·el drop** (ĕ-nam′ĕl drop) SYN enameloma.

**e·nam·el dys·pla·si·a** (ĕ-nam′ĕl dis-plā′zē-ă) SYN amelogenesis imperfecta.

**e·nam·el ep·i·the·li·um** (ĕ-nam′ĕl ep′i-thē′lē-ŭm) Several layers of enamel organ remaining on enamel surface after formation of enamel is completed.

**e·nam·el fi·bers** (ĕ-nam′ĕl fī′bĕrz) SYN prismata adamantina.

**e·nam·el fis·sure** (ĕ-nam′ĕl fish′ŭr) Deep cleft between adjoining cusps affording retention to cariogenic agents.

**e·nam·el germ** (ĕ-nam′ĕl jĕrm) Enamel organ of developing tooth; one of a series of knoblike projections from dental lamina, later becoming bell shaped and receiving in its hollow the dental papilla.

**e·nam·el hy·po·cal·ci·fi·ca·tion** (ĕ-nam′ĕl hī′pō-kal′si-fi-kā′shŭn) Defect of enamel maturation, characterized by soft opaque or yellowish white lusterless enamel.

**e·nam·el hy·po·pla·si·a** (ĕ-nam′ĕl hī′pō-plā′zē-ă) Developmental disturbance of teeth characterized by deficient or defective enamel matrix formation. See this page.

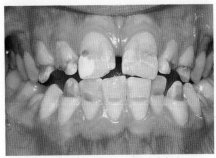

**enamel hypoplasia:** white and brown defects

**e·nam·el·ins** (ĕ-nam′ĕl-inz) Proteins that form organic matrix of mature tooth enamel. [*enamel + -in*]

**e·nam·el la·mel·la** (ĕ-nam′ĕl lă-mel′ă) Organic defect in enamel; thin, leaflike structure that extends from enamel surface toward dentinoenamel junction.

**e·nam·el lay·er** (ĕ-nam′ĕl lā′ĕr) SYN ameloblastic layer.

**e·nam·el ledge** (ĕ-nam′ĕl lej) SYN dental ledge.

**e·nam·el mem·brane** (ĕ-nam′ĕl mem′brān) Internal layer of enamel organ formed by ameloblasts.

**e·nam·el niche** (ĕ-nam′ĕl nich, nēsh) SYN enamel crypt.

**e·nam·el nodule** (ĕ-nam´ĕl nod´yūl) SYN en-ameloma.

**e·nam·el·o·blast** (ĕ-nam´ĕ-lō-blast) SYN ameloblast.

**e·nam·el·o·gen·e·sis** (ĕ-nam´ĕ-lō-jen´ĕ-sis) SYN amelogenesis.

**e·nam·el·o·ma** (ĕ-nam´ĕl-ō´mă) Developmental anomaly with small nodule of enamel below cementoenamel junction, usually at bifurcation of molar teeth. See this page. SYN enamel drop, enamel nodule, enamel pearl, pearl.

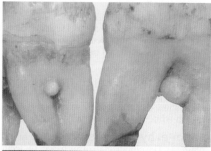
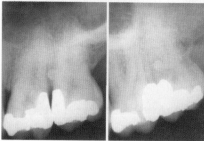

**enameloma**

**e·nam·el or·gan** (ĕ-nam´ĕl ōr´găn) Circumscribed mass of ectodermal cells budded off from dental lamina; becomes cup shaped and develops on its internal face the ameloblast layer of cells that produce enamel cap of developing tooth. It has three layers in the cap stage and four in bell stage of tooth development. SYN dental organ.

**e·nam·el pearl** (ĕ-nam´ĕl pĕrl) SYN enameloma.

**e·nam·el prisms** (ĕ-nam´ĕl prizmz) SYN prismata adamantina.

**e·nam·el pro·jec·tion** (ĕ-nam´ĕl prŏ-jek´shŭn) Extension of enamel into furcation.

**e·nam·el pulp** (ĕ-nam´ĕl pŭlp) Layer of stellate cells in enamel organ.

**e·nam·el re·tic·u·lum** (ĕ-nam´ĕl rĕ-tik´yŭ-lŭm) Central core of loosely arranged tissue in enamel organ between inner and outer layers of enamel epithelium of developing tooth. SYN stellate reticulum.

**e·nam·el rod in·clin·a·tion** (ĕ-nam´ĕl rod in´kli-nā´shŭn) Direction of the enamel rods with reference to outer surface tooth enamel.

**e·nam·el rods** (ē-nam´ĕl rodz) See this page. SYN prismata adamantina.

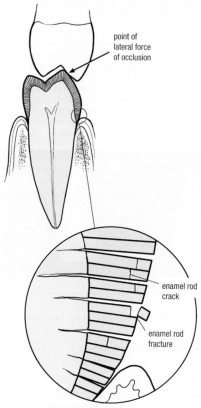

point of lateral force of occlusion

enamel rod crack

enamel rod fracture

**process of abfraction:** lateral occlusal forces stress enamel rods at cervical area, causing enamel rod fracture over time; although minute cracks in enamel rods may not be clinically evident, tooth can exhibit hypersensitivity; in advanced stage, wedge- or V-shaped cervical lesion is visible

**e·nam·el tuft** (ĕ-nam´ĕl tŭft) Structure represents defects in tooth mineralization that extend from dentinoenamel junction into enamel to about half its thickness.

**e·nam·e·lum** (ĕ-nam´ĕ-lŭm) [TA] SYN enamel.

**e·nam·el wall** (ĕ-nam´ĕl wawl) In dentistry, part of wall of cavity consisting of enamel.

**en·ce·phal·ic** (en´se-fal´ik) Relating to the brain, or to the structures within the cranium.

**en·ceph·a·lit·ic** (en-sef´ă-lit´ik) Relating to encephalitis.

**en·ceph·a·li·tis,** pl. **en·ceph·a·lit·i·des** (en-sef'ă-lī'tis, -lit'i-dēz) Inflammation of the brain. [G. *enkephalos,* brain, + *-itis,* inflammation]

**En·ceph·a·li·to·zo·on hel·lem** (en-sef' ă-lit-ō-zō'on hel'ĕm) Pathogen described in human ophthalmic infections.

**en·ceph·a·lo·cele** (en-sef'ă-lō-sēl) Congenital cranial gap with herniation of brain substance. [*encephalo-* + G. *kēlē,* hernia]

**en·ceph·a·lo·lith** (en-sef'ă-lō-lith) Concretion in brain or one of its ventricles. [*encephalo-* + G. *lithos,* stone]

**en·ceph·a·lo·my·e·li·tis** (en-sef'a-lō-mī'ĕ-lī'tis) Inflammation of brain and spinal cord. [*encephalo-* + G. *myelon,* marrow, + *-itis,* inflammation]

**en·ceph·a·lo·my·e·lop·a·thy** (en-sef'ă-lō-mī'ĕ-lop'ă-thē) Any disease of both brain and spinal cord. [G. *enkephalos,* brain, + *myelon,* marrow, + *pathos,* suffering]

**en·ceph·a·lop·a·thy, en·ceph·a·lo·path·i·a** (en-sef'ă-lop'ă-thē, -lō-path'ē-ă) Any disorder of the brain.

**en·ceph·a·lo·scle·ro·sis** (en-sef'ă-lō-skler-ō'sis) A sclerosis, or hardening, of the brain. [*encephalo-* + G. *sklērōsis,* hardening]

**en·coun·ter form** (en-kown'tĕr fōrm) A service form also called a superbill that lists codes for health care procedures.

**end bulb** (end bŭlb) One of the oval or rounded bodies in which the sensory nerve fibers terminate in mucous membrane.

**end-cut·ting bur** (end'kŭt-ing bŭr) Bur with blades only on its end.

**en·dem·ic** (en-dem'ik) Denoting a temporal pattern of disease occurrence in a population in which disease occurs with predictable regularity with only relatively minor fluctations. [G. *endēmos,* native, fr. *en,* in, + *dēmos,* the people]

**en·dem·ic in·flu·en·za** (en-dem'ik in'flū-en'ză) Influenza occurring with some degree of regularity during the winter. SYN influenza nostras.

**en·dem·ic sta·bil·i·ty** (en-dem'ik stă-bil'i-tē) Situation in which all factors influencing disease occurrence are relatively stable, resulting in little fluctuation in disease incidence over time.

**en·der·mic, en·der·mat·ic** (en-dĕr'mik, en'dĕr-mat'ik) In or through skin; denoting a method of treatment, as by inunction; the remedy produces its constitutional effect when absorbed through the skin surface to which it is applied. [G. *en,* in, + *derma* (*dermat-*), skin]

**en·der·mo·sis** (en'dĕr-mō'sis) Eruptive disease of mucous membrane.

**end-feet** (end'fēt) SYN axon terminals.

**end·ing** (end'ing) 1. A termination or conclusion. 2. A nerve ending.

**en·do·ba·si·on** (en'dō-bā'sē-on) Cephalometric and craniometric point located in midline at most posterior point of anterior border of foramen magnum on contour of the foramen; it is slightly posterior and internal to the basion.

**en·do·car·di·tis** (en'dō-kahr-dī'tis) Inflammation of the endocardium.

**en·do·car·di·um,** pl. **en·do·car·di·a** (en'dō-kahr'dē-ŭm, -ă) [TA] The innermost tunic of the heart. [*endo-* + G. *kardia,* heart]

**en·do·chon·dral bone** (en'dō-kon'drăl bōn) A bone that develops in a cartilaginous environment after the latter is partially or entirely destroyed by calcification and subsequent resorption. SYN cartilage bone.

**en·do·chon·dral os·si·fi·ca·tion** (en' dō-kon'drăl os'i-fi-kā'shŭn) Formation of osseous tissue by replacement of calcified cartilage.

**en·do·cra·ni·al** (en'dō-krā'nē-ăl) 1. Within the cranium. 2. Relating to the endocranium.

**en·do·cra·ni·um** (en'dō-krā'nē-ŭm) Lining membrane of cranium or dura mater of brain.

**en·do·crine** (en'dō-krin) Secreting internally, most commonly into the systemic circulation; of or pertaining to such secretion.

**en·do·crine glands** (en'dō-krin glandz) [TA] Glands that have no ducts, their secretions being absorbed directly into the blood.

**en·do·cri·nol·o·gy** (en'dō-kri-nol'ŏ-jē) Medical specialty concerned with internal or hormonal secretions and their physiologic and pathologic relations. [*endocrine* + G. *logos,* study]

**en·do·cri·nop·a·thy** (en'dō-kri-nop'ă-thē) Functional disorder of the endocrine gland.

**en·do·cri·no·ther·a·py** (en'dō-kri'nō-thār'ă-pē) Treatment of disease by administration of extracts of endocrine glands. [*endocrine* + G. *therapeia,* medical treatment]

**en·do·don·ti·a** (en'dō-don'shē-ă) SYN endodontics.

**en·do·don·tic cul·ture** (en'dō-don'tik kŭl'chŭr) Procedure wherein contents of a root canal are cultured to determine the presence of viable bacteria; usually done after canal has been cleaned and treated but before sealing.

**en·do·don·tic plug·ger** (en'dō-don'tik plŭg'ĕr) SYN condenser.

ef

**en·do·don·tics** (en′dō-don′tiks) Field of dentistry concerned with biology and pathology of dental pulp and periapical tissues, and with prevention, diagnosis, and treatment of diseases and injuries in these tissues. SYN endodontia, endodontology. [*endo-* + G. *odous,* tooth]

**en·do·don·tic sta·bi·li·zer** (en′dō-don′tik stā′bi-lī-zĕr) Pin implant passing through tooth apex from its root canal and extending well into the underlying bone to provide immobilization of periodontally involved teeth.

**en·do·don·tic treat·ment** (en′dō-don′tik trēt′mĕnt) See this page. SYN root canal treatment.

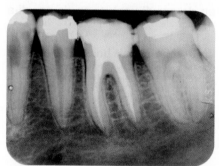

**radiograph of completed endodontic treatment:** root canals of left mandibular first molar have been filled with gutta percha and sealer; crown has been restored with temporary filling; both gutta percha and temporary filling appear whiter than enamel or dentin on the radiograph

**en·do·don·tist** (en′dō-don′tist) One who specializes in the practice of endodontics. SYN endodontologist.

**en·do·don·tol·o·gist** (en′dō-don-tol′ŏ-jist) SYN endodontist.

**en·do·don·tol·o·gy** (en′dō-don-tol′ŏ-jē) SYN endodontics.

**en·dog·e·nous, en·do·gen·ic** (en-doj′ĕ-nŭs, en′dō-jen′ik ) Originating or produced within the organism or one of its parts. [*endo-* + G. *-gen,* production]

**en·dog·e·nous py·ro·gen** (en-doj′ĕ-nŭs pī′rō-jen) Protein that induces fever.

**en·do·in·tox·i·ca·tion** (en′dō-in-tok′si-kā′shŭn) Poisoning by an endogenous toxin.

**en·do·lith** (en′dō-lith) Calcified body in pulp chamber of tooth; may be composed of irregular dentin or due to ectopic calcification of pulp tissue. SYN denticle (1), pulp calcification, pulp calculus, pulp nodule.

**en·do·lymph** (en′dō-limf) [TA] Fluid membranous labyrinth of inner ear.

**en·do·lym·phat·ic duct** (en′dō-lim-fat′ik dŭkt) [TA] Small membranous tube, connecting with both saccule and utricle of the membranous labyrinth, passing through the aqueduct of vestibule, and terminating in a dilated blind extremity, the endolymphatic sac, located on the posterior surface of the petrous portion of the temporal bone beneath the dura mater.

**en·do·lym·phat·ic sac** (en′dō-lim-fat′ik sak) [TA] Dilated blind extremity of endolymphatic duct, which lies external to the dura on posterior aspect of petrous part of temporal bone.

**en·do·lym·phat·ic space** [TA] Endolymph-filled space contained by the membranous labyrinth.

**en·do·me·tri·um,** pl. **en·do·me·tri·a** (endō-mē′trē-ŭm, -ă) [TA] The mucous membrane forming the inner layer of the uterine wall. [*endo-* + G. *mētra,* uterus]

**en·do·nu·cle·ase** (en′dō-nū′klē-ās) A nuclease (phosphodiesterase) that cleaves polynucleotides (nucleic acids) at interior bonds.

**en·do·os·se·ous im·plant** Implant into alveolar bone inserted through the prepared root canal of a tooth to increase effective root length.

**en·doph·thal·mi·tis, en·doph·thal·mi·a** (en′dof-thal-mī′tis, -thal′mē-ă) Inflammation of the tissues within the eyeball. [*endo-* + G. *ophthalmos,* eye, + *-itis,* inflammation]

**en·do·phyt·ic** (en′dō-fit′ik) Denotes an infiltrative, invasive tumor.

**en·do·plas·mic re·tic·u·lum (ER)** (en′dō-plas′mik rĕ-tik′yū-lŭm) The network of cytoplasmic tubules or flattened sacs with or without ribosomes on the surface of their membranes.

**end or·gan** (end ōr′găn) The special structure containing the terminal of a nerve fiber in peripheral tissue.

**en·dor·phins** (en-dōr′finz) Opioid peptides originally isolated from the brain but now found in many parts of the body.

**en·dos·co·py** (en-dos′kŏ-pē) Examination of the interior of a hollow structure with a special instrument.

**end·os·se·ous den·tal im·plants** (en-dos′ē-ŭs den′tal im′plants) SEE dental implants. See page 201.

**en·dos·te·al** (en-dos′tē-ăl) Relating to the endosteum.

**en·dos·te·al im·plants** (en-dos′tē-ăl im′plants) Devices inserted into alveolar and/or basal bone that protrude through the mucoperiosteum. See page 201.

**en·do·steth·o·scope** (en′dō-steth′ŏ-skōp) A stethoscopic tube used in endoauscultation. [*endo-* + G. *stēthos,* chest, + *skopeō,* to examine]

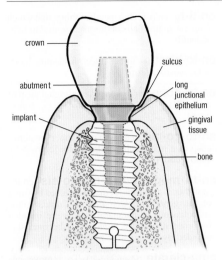

crown

sulcus

abutment

long
junctional
epithelium

implant

gingival
tissue

bone

**parts of endosseous implant with crown**

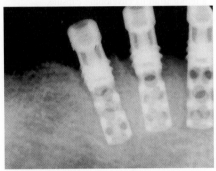

**endosteal implants in alveolar bone:** crowns
not yet in place

**en·dos·te·um** (en-dos′tē-ŭm) [TA] A layer
of cells lining the inner surface of bone in the
central medullary cavity. SYN medullary membrane. [*endo-* + G. *osteon,* bone]

**en·do·the·li·o·ma** (en′dō-thē-lē-ō′mă) Generic term for a group of neoplasms, particularly
benign tumors, derived from the endothelial tissue of blood vessels or lymphatic channels; en-
dotheliomas may be benign or malignant. [*endothelium* + *-oma,* tumor]

**en·do·the·li·um**, pl. **en·do·the·li·a** (en′-
dō-thē′lē-ŭm, -ă) [TA] A layer of flat cells that
line the blood vessels, lymphatic vessels, and
the heart. [*endo-* + G. *thēlē,* nipple]

**en·do·the·li·um-de·riv·ed re·lax·ing**
**fac·tor (EDRF)** (en′dō-thē′lē-ŭm-dĕ-rīvd′
rē-laks′ing fak′tŏr) Diffusible substance produced by endothelial cells that causes vascular
smooth muscle relaxation; nitric oxide (NO).

**en·do·tox·in** (en′dō-tok′sin) **1.** A bacterial
toxin not freely liberated into the surrounding medium. **2.** The complex phospholipid-

polysaccharide macromolecules that form an integral part of the cell wall of strains of gram-
negative bacteria; may cause shock, severe diarrhea, and fever. SYN intracellular toxin.

**en·do·tra·che·al** (en′dō-trā′kē-ăl) Within
the trachea.

**en·do·tra·che·al an·es·the·si·a** (en′dō-
trā′kē-ăl an′es-thē′zē-ă) Inhalation anesthesia in
which anesthetic and respiratory gases pass
through a tracheal tube.

**en·do·tra·che·al in·tu·ba·tion** (en′
dō-trā′kē-ăl in′tū-bā′shŭn) Passage of a tube
into trachea to maintain airway during anesthesia.

**en·do·vac·ci·na·tion** (en′dō-vak′si-nā′shŭn)
Oral administration of vaccines.

**end-round·ed fil·a·ment** (end-rown′dĕd
fil′ă-mĕnt) The form of the tip of the filament
or bristle of a toothbrush that is curved or
rounded; said to produce a safer and more effective removal of soft deposits from the teeth.

**end stage, end·stage** (end stāj) The late,
fully developed phase of a disease.

**end-to-end bite** (end end bīt) SYN edge-to-
edge occlusion. [end [O.E. *ende*] bite [O.E.
*bitan*]

**end-to-end oc·clu·sion** (end end ŏ-klū′
zhŭn) SYN edge-to-edge occlusion.

**end-tuft tooth·brush** (end-tŭft′ tūth′brŭsh)
An adjunct toothbrush designed with a small,
compact head of bristles that can access diffi-
cult-to-reach areas in the oral cavity.

**en·e·ma** (en′ĕ-mă) A rectal injection for clearing the bowel or administering drugs or food.

**en·er·gy** (en′ĕr-jē) Exertion of power; capacity to do work. [G. *energeia,* fr. *en,* in, + *ergon,*
work]

**en·gi·neer·ing** (en′jin-ēr′ing) The practical
application of physical, mechanical, and mathematical principles.

**en·gine ream·er** (en′jin rē′mĕr) Engine-
mounted spirally bladed instrument, used to enlarge root canals of teeth.

**en·gorged** (en-gōrjd′) Absolutely filled; distended with fluid.

**en·keph·a·lins** (en-kef′ă-linz) Pentapeptide
endorphins, found in many parts of the brain.

**en·large·ment** (en-lahrj′mĕnt) [TA] An increase in size; anatomic swelling or prominence.

**e·no·lase** (ē′nō-lās) An enzyme catalyzing the
reversible dehydration of 2-phospho-D-glycerate
to phospho*enol*pyruvate and water.

**en·os·to·sis** (en′os-tō′sis) A mass of proliferating bone tissue within a bone. [G. *en*, in, + *osteon*, bone, + *-osis*, condition]

**en·tad** (en'tad) Toward the interior.

**en·tal** (en'tăl) Relating to the interior; inside.

**Ent·a·moe·ba gin·gi·va·lis** (ent'ă-mē'bă jin-ji-vā'lis) Species of ameba found in human oral cavity; frequently associated with poor oral hygiene and its resultant diseases.

**en·ter·al, en·ter·ic** (en'tĕr-ăl, -ter'ik) Within, or by way of, the intestine or gastrointestinal tract. [G. *enteron*, intestine]

**en·ter·ic coat·ed tab·let** (en-ter'ik kō'tĕd tab'lĕt) Oral dosage form in which a tablet is coated with a material to prevent or minimize dissolution in the stomach but allow dissolution in the small intestine.

**en·ter·i·tis** (en'tĕr-ī'tis) Inflammation of the intestine. [*entero-* + G. *-itis*, inflammation]

**en·ter·o·coc·cus**, pl. **en·ter·o·coc·ci** (en'tĕr-ō-kok'ŭs, -sī) *Avoid the mispronunciation en-ter-ō-kok'ī of the plural of this word.* A streptococcus that inhabits the intestinal tract. [*entero-* + G. *kokkos*, a berry]

**en·ter·o·co·li·tis** (en'tĕr-ō-kŏ-lī'tis) Inflammation of mucous membrane of both small and large intestines.

**En·ter·o·cy·to·zo·on bi·e·neu·si** (en'tĕr-ō-sī'tō-zō'on bī'ĕ-nyū'sī) Pathogen of microsporidian infection, primarily infecting the small intestine, especially in immunocompromised patients.

**en·ter·og·e·nous** (en'tĕr-oj'ĕ-nŭs) Of intestinal origin. [*entero-* + G. *-gen*, producing]

**en·ter·og·ra·phy** (en'tĕr-og'ră-fē) Making a graphic record delineating intestinal muscular activity. [*entero-* + G. *graphō*, to write]

**en·ter·oi·de·a** (en'tĕr-oy'dē-ă) Fevers due to infection caused by any intestinal bacteria, including enteric and parenteric fevers. [*entero-* + G. *eidos*, resemblance]

**en·ter·o·my·co·sis** (en'tĕr-ō-mī-kō'sis) Intestinal disease of fungal origin. [*entero-* + G. *mykēs*, fungus, + *-osis*, condition]

**en·ter·o·path·o·gen·ic** (en'tĕr-ō-path'ŏ-jen'ik) Capable of producing disease in the intestinal tract.

**en·ter·op·a·thy** (en'tĕr-op'ă-thē) An intestinal disease. [*entero-* + G. *pathos*, suffering]

**en·ter·o·sta·sis** (en'tĕr-ō-stā'sis) Intestinal stasis; a retardation or arrest of the passage of the intestinal contents.

**en·ter·o·tro·pic** (en'tĕr-ō-trō'pik) Attracted by or affecting the intestine. [*entero-* + G. *tropikos*, turning]

**en·ti·ty** (en'ti-tē) Independent thing; that which contains in itself all conditions essential to individuality.

**en·to·blast** (en'tō-blast) Cell nucleolus. [*ento-* + G. *blastos*, germ]

**en·to·cone** (en'tō-kōn) Mesiolingual cusp of a maxillary molar tooth. [*ento-* + G. *kōnos*, cone]

**en·to·co·nid** (en'tō-kō'nid) Inner posterior cusp of a mandibular molar tooth. [*ento-* + G. *kōnos*, cone]

**en·to·moph·tho·ra·my·co·sis** (en'tō-mof-thōr'ă-mī-kō'sis) A disease caused by fungi of the genera *Basidiobolus* or *Conidiobolus;* subcutaneous or paranasal tissues are invaded by broad nonseptate hyphae that become surrounded by eosinophilic material.

**e·nu·cle·ate** (ē-nū'klē-āt) To remove entirely; to shell like a nut, as in the removal of a tumor from its enveloping capsule.

**en·u·re·sis** (en-yūr-ē'sis) *Do not confuse this word with emuresis.* Involuntary discharge or leakage of urine. [G. *en-oureō*, to urinate in]

**en·ve·lope** (en'vĕ-lōp) In anatomy, a structure that encloses or covers.

**en·ve·lope flap** (en'vĕ-lōp flap) Mucoperiosteal flap developed through a horizontal incision along free gingival margin.

**en·vi·ron·ment** (en-vī'rŏn-mĕnt) The milieu; aggregate of all external conditions and influences affecting life and development of an organism. [Fr. *environ*, around]

**en·zyme** (en'zīm) A macromolecule that acts as a catalyst to induce chemical changes in other substances, while itself remaining apparently unchanged by the process.

**en·zy·mop·a·thy** (en'zi-mop'ă-thē) Any disturbance of enzyme function, including genetic deficiency or defect in specific enzymes. [*enzyme* + G. *pathos*, disease]

**EOB** Abbreviation for explanation of benefits.

**EOP** Abbreviation for early-onset periodontitis

**e·o·sin** (ē'ō-sin) Fluorescent acid dye used for cytoplasmic stains and counterstains in histology. [G. *ēōs*, dawn]

**e·o·sin·o·phil ad·e·no·ma** (ē'ō-sin'ō-fil ad'ĕ-nō'mă, ē'ō-sin'ŏ-fil ad'ĕ-nō'mă) SYN acidophil adenoma.

**e·o·sin·o·phil·ic gran·u·lo·ma** (ē'ō-sin-ō-fil'ik gran'yū-lō'mă) A lesion observed more frequently in children and adolescents, occasionally in young adults, which occurs chiefly as a solitary focus in one bone, although multiple involvement is sometimes observed and similar foci may develop in the lung.

**e·o·sin·o·phil·ic leu·ko·cyte** (ē′ō-sin-ō-fil′ik lū′kŏ-sīt) A polymorphonuclear white blood cell characterized by prominent cytoplasmic granules that are bright yellow-red or orange when treated with Wright stain motile phagocyte with distinctive antiparasitic functions. SYN oxyphil (2), oxyphilic leukocyte.

**e·o·sin·o·phil·ic leu·ko·cy·to·sis** (ē′ō-sin-ō-fil′ik lū′kŏ-sī-tō′sis) A form of relative leukocytosis in which the greatest proportionate increase is in the eosinophils.

**e·o·sin·o·phil·ic pus·tu·lar fol·lic·u·li·tis** (ē′ō-sin-ō-fil′ik pŭs′chŭ-lăr fŏ-lik′yū-lī′tis) Dermatosis characterized by sterile pruritic papules and pustules that coalesce to form plaques with papulovesicular borders.

**e·pac·tal** (ē-pak′tăl) SYN supernumerary. [G. epaktos, imported, fr. epagō, to bring on or in]

**e·pen·dy·mo·ma** (ĕ-pen′di-mō′mă) Glioma derived from relatively undifferentiated ependymal cells, comprising approximately 1–3% of all intracranial neoplasms; occurs in all age groups and may originate from the lining of any of the ventricles or, more commonly, from the central canal of the spinal cord.

**e·phed·ra** (e-fed′ră) Ephedra equisetina; Ma huang; the plant source for the alkaloid ephedrine. Indigenous to China and India, it also contains some pseudoephedrine. [L., horsetail, fr. G. ephedros, sitting on]

**e·phed·rine** (ĕ-fed′rin, ef′ĕ-drin) Alkaloid from the leaves of Ephedra equisetina, and other species, or produced synthetically; an adrenergic (sympathomimetic) agent with actions similar to those of epinephrine; a bronchodilator, and topical vasoconstrictor.

**e·phe·lis,** pl. **e·phe·li·des** (ĕ-fē′lis, -li-dēz) SYN freckles. [G.]

**e·phem·er·al fe·ver** (e-fem′ŏr-ăl fē′vĕr) Febrile episode lasting no more than a day or two.

**e·pib·o·ly, e·pib·o·le** (ē-pib′ŏ-lē) Growth of epithelium in an organ culture to surround the underlying mesenchymal tissue. [G. epibolē, a throwing or laying on]

**ep·i·con·dy·li·tis** (ep′i-kon-di-lī′tis) Infection or inflammation of an epicondyle, or of associated tendons and other soft tissues.

**ep·i·cri·sis** (ep′i-krī-sis) A secondary crisis; a crisis terminating a recrudescence of morbid symptoms following a primary crisis.

**ep·i·dem·ic** (ep′i-dem′ik) Occurrence in a community or region of cases of an illness, specific health-related behavior, or other health-related events clearly in excess of normal expectancy. [epi- + G. dēmos, the people]

**ep·i·dem·ic hep·a·ti·tis** (ep′i-dem′ik hep′ă-tī′tis) SYN viral hepatitis type A.

**ep·i·dem·ic neu·ro·my·as·the·ni·a** (ep′i-dem′ik nūr′ō-mī-ăs-thē′nē-ă) Disease characterized by stiffness of the neck and back, headache, diarrhea, fever, and localized muscular weakness; probably viral in origin.

**ep·i·dem·ic non·bac·te·ri·al gas·tro·en·ter·i·tis** (ep′i-dem′ik non′bak-tēr′ē-ăl gas′trō-en′tĕr-ī′tis) Highly communicable but rather mild disease of sudden onset, caused by the epidemic gastroenteritis virus; infection is associated with some fever, abdominal cramps, nausea, vomiting, diarrhea, and headache.

**ep·i·dem·ic par·o·ti·tis** (ep′i-dem′ik par′ō-tī′tis) SYN mumps.

**ep·i·dem·ic sto·ma·ti·tis** (ep′i-dem′ik stō′mă-tī′tis) Contagious mouth infection, usually due to Group A coxsackievirus. SEE ALSO herpangina.

**ep·i·dem·ic ty·phus** (ep′i-dem′ik tī′fŭs) Typhus caused by Rickettsia prowazekii spread by body lice; marked by high fever, mental and physical depression, and a macular and papular eruption. SYN prison fever typhus.

**ep·i·de·mi·ol·o·gist** (ep′i-dē′mē-ol′ŏ-jist) An investigator who studies occurrence of disease or other health-related conditions, states, or events in specified populations.

**ep·i·de·mi·ol·o·gy** (ep′i-dē′mē-ol′ŏ-jē) Study of distribution and determinants of health-related states or events in specified populations and application of results to control health problems. [G. epidēmios, epidemic, + logos, study]

**ep·i·der·mal cyst** (ep′i-dĕr′măl sist) Lesion made of a mass of epidermal cells that, as a result of trauma, has been pushed beneath epidermis; the cyst is lined with stratified squamous epithelium and contains concentric layers of keratin. See this page.

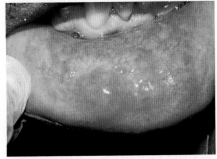

**epidermal cyst:** due to trauma

**ep·i·der·mis,** pl. **ep·i·derm·i·des** (ep′i-dĕr′mis, -mi-dēz) [TA] The superficial epithelial portion of the skin (cutis). [G. epidermis, the outer skin, fr. epi, on, + derma, skin]

**ep·i·der·moid car·ci·no·ma** (ep′i-děr′moyd kahr′si-nō′mă) Squamous cell carcinoma of the skin.

**ep·i·der·moid cyst** (ep′i-děr′moyd sist) A spheric, unilocular cyst of the dermis, composed of encysted keratin and sebum; the cyst is lined by a keratinizing epithelium resembling the epidermis derived from the follicular infundibulum.

**ep·i·der·mol·y·sis** (ep′i-děr-mol′i-sis) *Avoid the mispronunciation epidermoly′sis.* A condition in which the epidermis is loosely attached to the corium, readily exfoliating or forming blisters. [*epidermis* + G. *lysis,* loosening]

**ep·i·der·mol·y·sis bul·lo·sa** (ep′i-děr-mol′i-sis bul-ō′să) Group of inherited chronic noninflammatory skin diseases in which large bullae and erosions result from slight mechanical trauma.

**ep·i·der·mol·y·sis bul·lo·sa dys·tro·phi·ca** (ep′i-děr-mol′i-sis bu-lō′să dis-trō′fi-kă) Form in which scarring develops after separation of the entire epidermis with blistering.

**ep·i·der·mol·y·sis bul·lo·sa le·tha·lis** (ep′i-děr-mol′i-sis bu-lō′să lē-thā′lis) Form of epidermolysis bullosa characterized by persistent and nonhealing perioral and perinasal crusted lesions with bullae often present in the oral mucosa and trachea.

**ep·i·der·mol·y·sis bul·lo·sa sim·plex** (ep′i-děr-mol′i-sis bu-lō′să sim′pleks) Disorder in which lesions heal rapidly without scarring; bulla formation is intraepidermal and microscopy reveals basal cell vacuolation and dissolution of tonofibrils.

**ep·i·du·ral block** (ep′i-dūr′ăl blok) Obstruction in epidural space; used inaccurately to refer to epidural anesthesia.

**ep·i·fas·ci·al** (ep′i-fash′ē-ăl) On the surface of a fascia, denoting a method of injecting drugs in which the solution is put on the fascia lata instead of injected into the substance of the muscle.

**ep·i·fas·cic·u·lar ep·i·neu·ri·um** (ep′i-fă-sik′yū-lăr ep′i-nūr′ē-ŭm) Portion of epineurium that surrounds whole nerve trunk.

**ep·i·gas·tral·gi·a** (ep′i-gas-tral′jē-ă) Pain in the epigastric region. [*epigastrium* + G. *algos,* pain]

**ep·i·glot·tis** (ep′i-glot′is) [TA] A leaf-shaped plate of elastic cartilage, covered with mucous membrane, at the root of the tongue, which serves as a diverter valve over the superior aperture of the larynx during the act of swallowing; it stands erect when liquids are being swallowed but is passively bent over the aperture by solid foods that are being swallowed. [G. *epiglōttis,* fr. *epi,* on, + *glōttis,* the mouth of the windpipe]

**e·pil·a·to·ry** (e-pil′ă-tōr-ē) Having the property of removing hair; relating to epilation.

**ep·i·lep·sy** (ep′i-lep′sē) A chronic disorder characterized by paroxysmal brain dysfunction due to excessive neuronal discharge, and usually associated with some alteration of consciousness. The clinical manifestations of the attack may vary from complex abnormalities of behavior including generalized or focal convulsions to momentary spells of impaired consciousness. [G. *epilēpsia,* seizure]

**ep·i·lep·tic spasm** (ep′i-lep′tik spazm) Spasm characterized by a sudden flexion-extension, or mixed extension-flexion, predominantly proximal (including truncal muscles), which is usually more sustained than a myoclonic movement but not as sustained as a tonic seizure. Occurs frequently in clusters.

**ep·i·lep·to·gen·ic zone** (ep′i-lep-tō-jen′ik zōn) Cortical region that on stimulation reproduces the patient's spontaneous seizure or aura.

**ep·i·loi·a** (ep′i-loy′ă) SYN tuberous sclerosis.

**ep·i·man·dib·u·lar** (ep′i-man-dib′yū-lăr) On the lower jaw. [*epi-* + L. *mandibulum,* mandible]

**ep·i·mas·ti·cal** (ep′i-mast′i-kăl) Increasing steadily until an acme is reached, then declining; usually describing fever. [G. *epakmastikos,* coming to a height]

**ep·i·mas·ti·cal fe·ver** A fever increasing steadily until its acme is reached, then declining by crisis or lysis.

**ep·i·my·o·ep·i·the·li·al is·lands** (ep′i-mī′ō-ep′i-thē′lē-ăl ī′lăndz) Proliferation of salivary gland ductal epithelium and myoepithelium. Characteristic of benign lymphoepithelial lesions and Sjögren syndrome.

**ep·i·neph·rine** (ep′i-nef′rin) A catecholamine that is the chief neurohormone of the adrenal medulla of most species; also secreted by some neurons; used to treat bronchial asthma, acute allergic disorders, open-angle glaucoma, cardiac arrest, and heart block, and as a topical and local vasoconstrictor. SYN adrenaline. [*epi-* + G. *nephros,* kidney, + *-ine*]

**ep·i·neph·rine re·ver·sal** (ep′i-nef′rin rĕ-věr′săl) The fall in blood pressure produced by epinephrine when given following blockage of α-adrenergic receptors by an appropriate drug such as phenoxybenzamine; the vasodilation reflects the ability of epinephrine to activate β-adrenergic receptors that, in vascular smooth muscle, are inhibitory.

**ep·i·neu·ri·um** (ep′i-nūr′ē-ŭm) [TA] The outermost supporting structure of peripheral nerve trunks, consisting of a condensation of areolar connective tissue; subdivided into those layers that surround the whole nerve trunk (epifascicular epineurium), and those layers that extend between the nerve fascicles (interfascicular epineurium). With the endoneurium and perineurium, the epineurium comprises the peripheral nerve stroma. [*epi-* + G. *neuron,* nerve]

**ep·i·phe·nom·e·non** (ep'i-fĕ-nom'ĕ-non) Symptom appearing during disease course, not of usual occurrence, and not necessarily associated with the disease.

**ep·i·phys·i·al line** (ep'i-fiz'ē-ăl līn) [TA] Line of junction of epiphysis and diaphysis of a long bone where lengthening occurs.

**e·piph·y·sis,** pl. **e·piph·y·ses** (e-pif'i-sis, -sēz) [TA] Part of long bone developed from secondary center of ossification, distinct from that of the shaft, and separated at first from the latter by a layer of cartilage. [G. an excrescence, fr. *epi,* upon, + *physis,* growth]

**ep·i·sode** (ep'i-sōd) An important event or series of events taking place in the course of continuous events e.g., an episode of depression.

**ep·i·sode of care** (ep'i-sōd kăr) All services provided to a patient with a medical problem within a specific period of time across a continuum of care in an integrated system.

**ep·i·so·dic hy·per·ten·sion** (ep'i-sod'ik hī'pĕr-ten'shŭn) Hypertension that occurs intermittently, triggered by anxiety or emotional factors.

**ep·i·spi·nal** (ep'i-spī'năl) On the vertebral column or spinal cord, or on any structure resembling a spine.

**e·pis·ta·sis** (e-pis'tă-sis) Formation of a pellicle or scum on the surface of a liquid, especially as on standing urine. [G. scum; *epi-* + G. *stasis,* a standing]

**ep·i·stax·is** (ep'i-stak'sis) Bleeding from the nose. [G. fr. *epistazō,* to bleed at the nose, fr. *epi,* on, + *stazō,* to fall in drops]

**ep·i·the·li·al** (ep'i-thē'lē-ăl) Relating to or consisting of epithelium.

**ep·i·the·li·al at·tach·ment** (ep'i-thē'lē-ăl ă-tach'mĕnt) Junctional epithelial cells attaching the tooth to subepithelial tissues at base of gingival crevice.

**ep·i·the·li·al cell** (ep'i-thē'lē-ăl sel) One of the many varieties of cells that form epithelium.

**ep·i·the·li·al·i·za·tion, ep·i·the·li·za·tion** (ep'i-thē'lē-ăl-ī-zā'shŭn, -thē'li-zā'shŭn) Formation of epithelium over a denuded surface.

**ep·i·the·li·al mi·gra·tion** (ep'i-thē'lē-ăl mī-grā'shŭn) Apical shift of epithelial attachment, exposing more of the tooth crown.

**ep·i·the·li·al my·o·ep·i·the·li·al car·ci·no·ma** (ep'i-thē'lē-ăl mī'ō-ep'i-thē'lē-ăl kahr'si-nō'mă) Salivary gland malignancy composed of an inner layer of ductal cells surrounded by a layer of clear myoepithelial cells.

**ep·i·the·li·al tis·sue** (ep'i-thē'lē-ăl tish'ū) SEE epithelium.

**ep·i·the·li·o·ma** (ep'i-thē'lē-ō'mă) **1.** An epithelial neoplasm or hamartoma of the skin, especially of skin appendage origin. **2.** A carcinoma of the skin derived from squamous, basal, or adnexal cells. [*epithelium* + G. *-ōma,* tumor]

**ep·i·the·li·um,** pl. **ep·i·the·li·a** (ep'i-thē'lē-ŭm, -ă) [TA] The purely cellular avascular layer covering all free surfaces, cutaneous, mucous, and serous, including the glands and other structures derived therefrom. [G. *epi,* upon, + *thēlē,* nipple, a term applied originally to the thin skin covering the nipples and the papillary layer of the border of the lips]

**EPO** Abbreviation for exclusive provider organization.

**e·po·e·tin al·fa** (ē-pō'ĕ-tin al'fă) Recombinant human erythropoietin, a powerful stimulator of red blood cell synthesis. Often used in patients with anemia and in those undergoing organ transplantation or cancer chemotherapy.

**e·pox·y res·in** (ē-pok'sē rez'in) Any thermosetting resin based on the reactivity of epoxy; used as adhesives, protective coatings, and embedding media for electron microscopy.

**Ep·som salts** SYN magnesium sulfate.

**Ep·stein-Barr vi·rus (EBV)** (ep'stīn bahr vī'rŭs) A herpesvirus that causes infectious mononucleosis and is also found in cell cultures of Burkitt lymphoma; associated with nasopharyngeal carcinoma. SYN human herpesvirus 4.

**Ep·stein dis·ease** (ep'stīn di-zēz') SYN diphtheroid (1).

**Ep·stein pearls** (ep'stīn pĕrlz) Multiple small white epithelial inclusion cysts found in the midline of the palate in newborn infants. See this page.

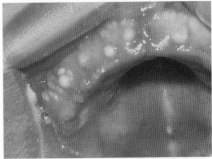

**dental lamina cysts and Epstein pearl**

**ep·u·lis** (ep-yū′lis) A nonspecific exophytic gingival mass. See page A15. [G. *epoulis*, a gumboil]

**ep·u·loid** (ep′yū-loyd) A gingival mass that resembles an epulis.

**e·qua·tion** (ĕ-kwā′zhŭn) A statement expressing the equality of two things, usually with the use of mathematical or chemical symbols. [L. *aequare*, to make equal]

**e·qui·an·al·ge·sic dose** (ēk′wē-an″ăl-jē′zik dōs) Qualitative ratio between actual milligram potency of comparable analgesics required to achieve the equivalent therapeutic effect.

**e·quil·i·bra·tion** (ē′kwi-li-brā′shŭn) **1.** In dentistry, modification of occlusal forms of teeth by grinding, with intent of equalizing occlusal stress, producing simultaneous occlusal contacts, or harmonizing cuspal relations. **2.** The act of maintaining an equilibrium or balance.

**e·qui·lib·ri·um** (ē′kwi-lib′rē-ŭm) Condition of being evenly balanced; a state of repose between two or more antagonistic forces that exactly counteract each other. [L. *aequilibrium*, a horizontal position, fr. *aequus*, equal, + *libra*, a balance]

**e·quip·ment** (ĕ-kwip′mĕnt) Supplies, tools, or other materials required to perform a specific task or function. [O.Fr. *equiper*, to equip, fr. Germanic]

**e·quiv·a·lent** (ē-kwiv′ă-lĕnt) **1.** Equal in any respect. **2.** That which is equal in size, weight, force, or any other quality to something else. **3.** Having the capability to counterbalance or neutralize each other. **4.** Used to describe a symptom complex less commonly associated with a syndrome than the usual classic symptoms.

**e·quiv·o·cal symp·tom** (ē-kwiv′ŏ-kăl simp′tŏm) Symptom that points definitely to no particular disease, being associated with any one of a number of morbid states, or one with a presence that remains uncertain or indefinite.

**ER** Abbreviation for endoplasmic reticulum; evoked response.

**Er** Symbol for erbium.

**er·bi·um (Er)** (ĕr′bē-ŭm) A rare earth element. [from Ytterby, a village in Sweden]

**erg** (ĕrg) Unit of work in the CGS system; amount of work done by 1 dyne acting through 1 cm, $1\ g\ cm^2\ s^{-2}$; in the SI, 1 erg equals $10^{-7}$ J. [G. *ergon*, work]

**er·go·cal·cif·er·ol** (ĕr′gō-kal-sif′ĕr-ol) Activated ergosterol, the vitamin D of plant origin; used in prophylaxis and treatment of vitamin D deficiency. SYN calciferol, vitamin D2.

**er·go·nom·ics** (ĕr′gŏ-nom′iks) The science of workplace, tools, and equipment designed to reduce worker discomfort, strain, and fatigue and to prevent work-related injuries. [*ergo-* + G. *nomos*, law]

**er·got** (ĕr′got) Resistant, overwintering stage of the parasitic ascomycetous fungus *Claviceps purpurea*. [O. Fr. *argot*, cock's spur]

**er·got al·ka·loids** (ĕr′got al′kă-loydz) Those obtained from the ergot fungus *Claviceps purpurea* or semisynthetically derived; e.g., ergotamine, lysergic acid diethylamide (LSD).

**er·got·a·mine** (er-got′ă-mēn) An alkaloid from ergot, used to relieve migraine.

**er·go·tox·ine** (er′gŏ-tok′sēn, -sin) A mixture of alkaloids obtained from ergot; potent stimulant of smooth muscle.

**er·got poi·son·ing** (ĕr′got poy′zŏn-ing) Syndrome brought on by consumption of bread (notably rye) contaminated by the ergot fungus, *Claviceps purpurea* (rye smut). Effects observed include peripheral vascular constriction leading to gangrene, partial paralysis with numbing and others; can be fatal.

**e·rode** (e-rōd′) **1.** To cause, or to be affected by, erosion. **2.** To remove by ulceration. [L. *erodo*, to gnaw away]

**e·ro·sion** (e-rō′zhŭn) **1.** Chemically induced tooth loss, occurring mainly through acid dissolution. When the cause is unknown, it is referred to as idiopathic erosion. SYN odontolysis. **2.** A wearing away or a state of being worn away, as by friction or pressure. Cf. corrosion. See this page and page A4. [L. *erosio*, fr. *erodo*, to gnaw away]

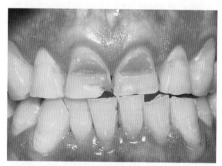

**erosion:** due to lemon sucking

**er·rat·ic** (ĕ-rat′ik) **1.** SYN eccentric (1). **2.** Denoting symptoms that vary in intensity, frequency, or location. [L. *erro*, pp. *erratus*, to wander]

**er·ror** (er′ŏr) A defect in structure or function; a false or mistaken belief; in biomedical and other sciences, there are many varieties of error, for example, due to bias, inaccurate measurements, or faulty instruments.

**e·ruc·ta·tion** (ē-rŭk-tā′shŭn) Voiding of gas

or of a small quantity of acidic fluid from the stomach through the mouth. SYN belching. [L. *eructo,* pp. *-atus,* to belch]

**e·rup·tion** (ē-rŭp´shŭn) 1. Passage of a tooth through the alveolar process and perforation of the gingiva. 2. A breaking out, especially the appearance of lesions on the skin. [L. *e-rumpo,* pp. *-ruptus,* to break out]

**e·rup·tion cyst** (ē-rŭp´shŭn sist) Dentigerous lesion in the soft tissues in conjunction with an erupting tooth; seen on the alveolar ridge of children. See this page.

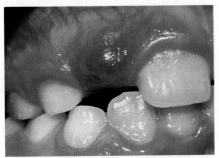

eruption cyst: blue, dome-shaped cyst nodule

**e·rup·tion se·ques·trum** (ē-rŭp´shŭn sĕ-kwes´trŭm) Spicule of bone overlying the central occlusal fossa of an erupting permanent molar.

**e·rup·tive** (ē-rŭp´tiv) Characterized by eruption.

**e·rup·tive phase** (ē-rŭp´tiv fāz) Period in tooth formation that includes the development of the roots, periodontal ligament, and dentogingival junction of the tooth.

**e·rup·tive xan·tho·ma** (ē-rŭp´tiv zan-thō´mă) Sudden appearance of groups of 1–4 mm waxy yellow or yellowish-brown papules with an erythematous halo, especially over extensors of the elbows and knees, and on the back and buttocks of patients with severe hyperlipemia, often familial or, more rarely, in cases of severe diabetes.

**ERV** Abbreviation for expiratory reserve volume.

**er·y·sip·e·las** (er´i-sip´ĕ-lăs) A specific, acute, cutaneous inflammatory disease caused by β-hemolytic streptococci and characterized by hot, red, edematous, brawny, and sharply defined eruptions. [G., fr. *erythros,* red + *pella,* skin]

**er·y·the·ma** (er´i-thē´mă) Redness due to capillary dilation, usually signaling a pathologic condition (e.g., inflammation, infection). Cf. telangiectasia. [G. *erythēma,* flush]

**er·y·the·ma in·fec·ti·o·sum** (er´i-thē´mă in-fek-shē-ō´sŭm) Mild infectious exanthema of childhood characterized by an erythematous maculopapular eruption, resulting in a lacelike rash on the extremities and a ''slapped cheek'' appearance on the face. Fever and arthritis may also accompany infection. SYN fifth disease. See page A5.

**erythraemia** [Br.] SYN erythremia.

**er·y·thral·gi·a** (er´i-thral´jē-ă) Painful redness of the skin. [erythro- + G. *algos,* pain]

**er·y·thre·mi·a** (er´i-thrē´mē-ă) SYN polycythemia vera, erythraemia. [erythro- + G. *haima,* blood]

**e·ryth·ri·tol** (ĕ-rith´ri-tol) Four-carbon sugar alcohol obtained by the reduction of erythrose, notable for its sweetness (twice that of sucrose); found in lichens, algae, and fungi.

**e·ryth·ro·blast** (ĕ-rith´rō-blast) The first generation of cells in the red blood cell series that can be distinguished from precursor endothelial cells. [erythro- + G. *blastos,* germ]

**e·ryth·ro·blas·tic a·ne·mi·a** (ĕ-rith´rō-blas´tik ă-nē´mē-ă) Anemia characterized by presence of large numbers of nucleated red blood cells (normoblasts and erythroblasts) in peripheral blood.

**e·ryth·ro·blas·to·sis** (ĕ-rith´rō-blas-tō´sis) Presence of erythroblasts in considerable numbers in the blood. [erythroblast + -osis, condition]

**e·ryth·ro·blas·to·sis fe·ta·lis** (ĕ-rith´rō-blas-tō´sis fē-tā´lis) Grave hemolytic anemia that, in most instances, results from development in an Rh-negative mother of anti-Rh antibody in response to the Rh factor in the (Rh-positive) fetal blood.

**e·ryth·ro·cyte** (ĕ-rith´rō-sīt) A mature red blood cell. SYN hemacyte, red blood cell, red cell, red corpuscle. [erythro- + G. *kytos,* cell]

**e·ryth·ro·cyte count** (ĕ-rith´rō-sīt kownt) SYN red blood cell count.

**e·ryth·ro·cyte in·di·ces** (ĕ-rith´rō-sīt in´di-sēz) Calculations for determining the average size, hemoglobin content, and concentration of hemoglobin in red blood cells, specifically mean cell volume, mean cell hemoglobin, and mean cell hemoglobin concentration.

**e·ryth·ro·cyte sed·i·men·ta·tion rate (ESR)** (ĕ-rith´rō-sīt sed´i-mĕn-tā´shŭn rāt) The rate of settling of red blood cells in anticoagulated blood; increased rates are often associated with anemia or inflammatory states.

**e·ryth·ro·cy·to·sis** (ĕ-rith´rō-sī-tō´sis) Polycythemia, especially that which occurs in response to some known stimulus.

**e·ryth·ro·don·ti·a** (ĕ-rith´rō-don´shē-ă) Reddish discoloration of the teeth, as may occur in porphyria. [erythro- + G. *odous,* tooth]

ef

**e·ryth·ro·my·cin** (ĕ-rith′rō-mī′sin) *Avoid the mispronunciation ĕ-rith-rō-mī′ă-sin.* Macrolide antibiotic agent obtained from cultures of a strain of *Streptomyces erythraeus* found in soil; active against *Corynebacterium diphtheriae* and several other species of *Corynebacterium*, Group A hemolytic streptococci, *Streptococcus pneumoniae*, *Legionella*, *Mycoplasma pneumoniae*, and *Bordetella pertussis*.

**e·ryth·ro·pla·ki·a** (ĕ-rith′rō-plā′kē-ă) A red, velvety plaquelike lesion of mucous membrane that often represents malignant change. See this page and page A9. [*erythro-* + G. *plax*, plate]

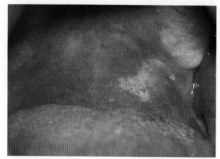

**erythroplakia:** tongue depressed to allow proper visualization

**e·ryth·ro·poi·e·sis** (ĕ-rith′rō-poy-ē′sis) Formation of red blood cells. [*erythrocyte* + G. *poiēsis*, a making]

**e·ryth·ro·poi·et·ic** (ĕ-rith′rō-poy-et′ik) Pertaining to or characterized by erythropoiesis.

**e·ryth·ro·poi·et·ic por·phy·ria** (ĕ-rith′rō-poy-et′ik pōr-fir′ē-ă) Classification of porphyria that includes congenital erythropoietic porphyria and erythropoietic protoporphyria.

**e·ryth·ro·pros·o·pal·gi·a** (ĕ-rith′rō-pros-ō-pal′jē-ă) A disorder similar to erythromelalgia, but with facial pain and redness. [*erythro-* + G. *prosōpon*, face, + *algos*, pain]

**es·cha·rot·ic** (es′kă-rot′ik) Caustic or corrosive. [G. *escharōtikos*]

***Esch·e·rich·i·a*** (esh-ĕ-rik′ē-ă) Genus of aerobic, facultatively anaerobic bacteria containing short, motile or nonmotile, gram-negative rods; found in feces; some are pathogenic to humans, causing enteritis, peritonitis, cystitis, and other disorders; type species is *E. coli*. [T. *Escherich*, German pediatrician and bacteriologist, 1857–1911]

**e·soph·a·ge·al** (ĕ-sof′ă-jē′ăl) *Although this word is more correctly pronounced esopha′-geal,* the pronunciation *esophage′al* is almost universally heard in the U.S. Relating to the esophagus.

**e·soph·a·ge·al a·cha·la·si·a** (ĕ-sof′ă-jē′ăl ak′ă-lā′zē-ă) Failure of normal relaxation of lower esophageal sphincter associated with uncoordinated contractions of thoracic esophagus, resulting in functional obstruction and difficulty swallowing.

**e·soph·a·ge·al a·tre·si·a** (ĕ-sof′ă-jē′ăl ă-trē′zē-ă) Neonatal condition in which the proximal end of the esophagus ends in a blind pouch such that food cannot enter the stomach through the esophagus.

**e·soph·a·ge·al dys·rhyth·mia** (ĕ-sof′ă-jē′ăl dis-ridh′mē-ă) Abnormal motility of muscular layers of esophageal wall, such as occurs in esophageal spasm.

**e·soph·a·ge·al re·flux, gas·tro·e·soph·a·ge·al re·flux** (ĕ-sof′ă-jē′ăl rē′flŭks, gas′trō-ĕ-sof′ă-jē-ăl) Regurgitation of stomach contents into esophagus, possibly into pharynx where they can be aspirated between vocal cords and into trachea; symptoms of burning pain and acid taste result; pulmonary complications of aspiration depend on the amount, content, and acidity of aspirate.

**e·soph·a·ge·al spasm** (ĕ-sof′ă-jē′ăl spazm) Disorder of motility of esophagus characterized by pain or belching after swallowing.

**e·soph·a·ge·al va·ri·ces** (ĕ-sof′ă-jē′ăl var′i-sēz) Longitudinal venous varices at lower end of esophagus as a result of portal hypertension; superficial and liable to ulceration and massive bleeding.

**e·soph·a·gi·tis** (ĕ-sof′ă-jī′tis) Inflammation of the esophagus.

**e·soph·a·go·gas·tric junc·tion** (ĕ-sof′ă-gō-gas′trik jŭngk′shŭn) Terminal end of esophagus and beginning of stomach at cardiac orifice; site of physiologic inferior esophageal sphincter.

**e·soph·a·go·sal·i·var·y re·flex** Salivation caused by irritation at lower end of esophagus, due to carcinoma.

**e·soph·a·go·spasm** (ĕ-sof′ă-gō-spazm) Spasm of the walls of the esophagus.

**e·soph·a·gus,** pl. **e·soph·a·gi** (ĕ-sof′ă-gŭs, -jī) [TA] Portion of alimentary canal between pharynx and stomach. It is about 25-cm long and consists of three parts: the cervical part, from the cricoid cartilage to the thoracic inlet; the thoracic part, from the thoracic inlet to the diaphragm; and the abdominal part, below the diaphragm to the cardiac opening of the stomach. [G. *oisophagos*, gullet]

**ESR** Abbreviation for erythrocyte sedimentation rate.

**es·sence** (es′ĕns) **1.** The true characteristic or substance of a body. **2.** An element. **3.** A fluidextract. **4.** An alcoholic solution, or spirit, of the volatile oil of a plant. **5.** Any volatile substance responsible for odor or taste of the

ef

organism producing it. [L. *essentia,* fr. *esse,* to be]

**es·sen·tial** (ĕ-sen′shăl) **1.** Necessary, indispensable, (e.g., essential amino acids, essential fatty acids). **2.** Characteristic of. **3.** Determining. **4.** SYN intrinsic.

**es·sen·tial hy·per·ten·sion** (ĕ-sen′shăl hī′pĕr-ten′shŭn) Hypertension with no known cause; accounts for between 90% and 95% of patients. SYN primary hypertension.

**es·sen·tial nu·tri·ents** (ĕ-sen′shăl nū′trē-ĕnts) Dietary substances required for optimal health that must be consumed because they are not provided by the body.

**es·sen·tial oil** (ĕ-sen′shăl oyl) A plant product, usually somewhat volatile, giving the odors and tastes characteristic of the particular plant.

**es·sen·tial trem·or** (ĕ-sen′shăl trem′ŏr) Action tremor of 4–8 Hz frequency that usually begins in early adult life and is limited to upper limbs and head.

**Es·sig splint** (es′ig splint) Stainless steel wire passed labially and lingually around segment of dental arch and held in position by individual ligature wires around contact areas of teeth; used to stabilize fractured or repositioned teeth and involved alveolar bone.

**es·ter** (es′tĕr) An organic compound containing the grouping, –X(O)–O–R (X = carbon, sulfur, phosphorus; R = radical of an alcohol), formed by the elimination of $H_2O$ between the –OH of an acid group and the –OH of an alcohol group.

**es·ter·ase** (es′tĕr-ās) A generic term for enzymes that catalyze the hydrolysis of esters.

**es·them·a·tol·o·gy** (es′thĕm-ă-tol′ŏ-jē) The science concerned with the senses and sense organs. [G. *aisthēma,* perception, + *logos,* study]

**es·the·si·a** (es-thē′zē-ă) SYN sensitivity (2), aesthesia. [G. *aisthēsis,* sensation]

**es·the·si·og·ra·phy** (es-thē′zē-og′ră-fē) **1.** Description of organs of sense and mechanism of sensation. **2.** Mapping out on skin areas of tactile and other forms of sensibility. [*esthesio-* + G. *graphē,* a writing]

**es·the·si·ol·o·gy** (es-thē′zē-ol′ŏ-jē) The science concerned with sensory phenomena. [*esthesio-* + G. *logos,* study]

**es·the·si·o·phys·i·ol·o·gy** (es-thē′zē-ō-fiz-ē-ol′ŏ-jē) Physiology of sensation and the sense organs.

**es·thet·ic** (es-thet′ik) **1.** Pertaining to the sensations. **2.** Pertaining to esthetics (i.e., beauty). [G. *aisthēsis,* sensation]

**es·the·tic den·tis·try** (es-thet′ik den′tis-trē) Dental field especially concerned with the appearance of dentition as achieved through its arrangement, form, and color.

**es·the·tic fac·tors** (es-thet′ik fak′tŏrz) Elements such as size, shape, color, position, and texture that influence the perception of beauty in oral facial structures and dental restorations.

**es·thet·ics** (es-thet′iks) The branch of philosophy concerned with art and beauty, especially with the components thereof. SYN aesthetics.

**es·ti·mate** (es′ti-măt) **1.** A measurement or a statement about the value of some quantity that is known, believed, or suspected to incorporate some degree of error. **2.** The result of applying any estimator to a random sample of data. [L. *aestimo,* pp. *aestimatum,* to appraise]

**es·ti·ma·ted av·er·age re·quire·ment (EAR)** (es′ti-mā′ted av′răj rĕ-kwīr′mĕnt) The daily intake of a specific nutrient estimated to meet the requirement in 50% of healthy people in an age- and gender-specific group.

**Est·land·er flap** (est′lahn-dĕr flap) A full-thickness flap of the lip, transferred from the side of one lip to the same side of the other lip and vascularized by the labial artery.

**es·tra·di·ol** (es-tră-dī′ol) Most potent naturally occurring estrogen in mammals, formed by the ovary, placenta, testis, and possibly the cortex of the suprarenal gland.

**es·tro·gen** (es′trŏ-jen) Generic term for any substance, natural or synthetic, which exerts biologic effects characteristic of estrogenic hormones; formed by the ovary, placenta, testes, and possibly the cortex of the suprarenal gland, as well as by some plants; stimulates secondary sexual characteristics and exerts systemic effects, such as growth and maturation of long bones; also used to prevent or stop lactation, suppress ovulation, and palliate carcinoma of the breast and prostate. SYN oestrogen. [G. *oistrus,* -heat, estrus, + *-gen,* producing]

**eth·a·cryn·ic ac·id** (eth′ă-krin′ik as′id) Unsaturated ketone derivative of aryloxyacetic acid; a potent loop diuretic and a weak antihypertensive;

**eth·ane** (eth′ān) Constituent of natural and "bottled" gases.

**eth·a·no·ic ac·id** (eth′ă-nō′ik as′id) SYN acetic acid.

**eth·a·nol** (eth′ăn-ol) Clear, colorless liquid with a faint ethereal odor and a burning taste; consumed in beer, wine, and distilled liquor; is made by fermentation of sugars obtained from natural sources (grain, grapes, potatoes, sugar cane). Toxic effects of ethanol can be modified or aggravatd by other substances (medicines, drugs of abuse) consumed along with it. About 25% of swallowed alcohol is absorbed through the gastric mucosa, and most of the rest from the duodenum. Regular heavy alcohol consumption is an established cause of cancers of the oral cavity, pharynx, larynx, esophagus, liver, and breast.

**e·ther** (ē'thĕr) Any organic compound in which two carbon atoms are independently linked to a common oxygen atom, but commonly used to refer to diethyl ether or an anesthetic ether, although a large number of ethers have anesthetic properties. [G. *aithēr,* the pure upper air]

**e·ther·i·za·tion** (ē'thĕr-ī-zā'shŭn) Administration of diethyl ether to produce anesthesia.

**eth·i·cal** (eth'i-kăl) Relating to ethics; in conformity with the rules governing personal and professional conduct.

**eth·ics** (eth'iks) The branch of philosophy that deals with the distinction between right and wrong and with the moral consequences of human actions. [G. *ethikos,* arising from custom, fr. *ethos,* custom]

**eth·mo·cra·ni·al** (eth'mō-krā'nē-ăl) Relating to the ethmoid bone and the cranium as a whole.

**eth·mo·fron·tal** (eth'mō-frŏn'tăl) Relating to ethmoid and frontal bones.

**eth·moi·dal** (eth-moy'dăl) Resembling a sieve.

**eth·moi·dal bul·la** (eth-moy'dăl bul'ă) [TA] Bulging of inner wall of the ethmoidal labyrinth in middle meatus of nose, just below middle nasal concha.

**eth·moi·dal crest** (eth-moy'dăl krest) [TA] Bony ridge that articulates with, or provides attachment for, any part of ethmoid bone, especially middle nasal concha.

**eth·moi·dal crest of max·il·la** (eth-moy'dăl krest mak-sil'ă) [TA] Ridge on upper part of nasal surface of frontal process of maxilla that gives attachment to anterior portion of middle nasal concha.

**eth·moi·dal crest of pal·a·tine bone** (eth-moy'dăl krest pal'ă-tīn bōn) [TA] Ridge on medial surface of perpendicular part of palatine bone to which middle nasal concha attaches posteriorly.

**eth·moi·da·le** (eth'moy-dā'lē) Cephalometric point in anterior cranial fossa located at lowest sagittal point of cribriform plate of ethmoid bone.

**eth·moi·dal for·a·men** (eth-moy'dăl fōr-ā'mĕn) [TA] Either of two foramina formed in the medial wall of the orbit by grooves on either edge of ethmoidal notch of frontal bone, and completed by similar grooves on ethmoid bone.

**eth·moi·dal groove** (eth-moy'dăl grūv) [TA] Groove on inner surface of each nasal bone, lodging external nasal branch of anterior ethmoid nerve.

**eth·moi·dal in·fun·dib·u·lum** (eth-moy' dăl in-fŭn-dib'yū-lŭm) [TA] Passage from middle meatus of nose communicating with anterior ethmoidal cells and frontal sinus.

**eth·moi·dal lab·y·rinth** (eth-moy'dăl lab' i-rinth) [TA] Mass of air cells with thin bony walls forming part of lateral wall of nasal cavity. SYN ectoethmoid.

**eth·moi·dal notch** (eth-moy'dăl noch) [TA] Oblong gap between orbital parts of frontal bone in which ethmoid bone is lodged.

**eth·moi·dal pro·cess of in·fe·ri·or na·sal con·cha** (eth-moy'dăl pro'ses in-fĕr'ē-ŏr nā'zăl kong'kă) [TA] Projection of inferior concha, situated behind lacrimal process and articulating with uncinate process of the ethmoid.

**eth·moi·dal si·nus·es** (eth-moy'dăl sī'nŭs-ĕz) SYN ethmoid cells.

**eth·moi·dal veins** (eth-moy'dăl vānz) [TA] Veins that accompany anterior and posterior ethmoidal arteries and pass into superior ophthalmic vein; drain the ethmoidal sinuses.

**eth·moid an·gle** (eth'moyd ang'gĕl) Area made by plane of cribriform plate of ethmoid bone extended to meet basicranial axis.

**eth·moid bone** (eth'moyd bōn) [TA] Irregularly shaped bone lying between orbital plates of frontal bone and anterior to the sphenoid bone of the cranium.

**eth·moid cells** (eth'moyd selz) Ethmoidal air cells; evaginations of mucous membrane of middle and superior meatus of nasal cavity into ethmoidal labyrinth forming multiple small paranasal sinuses; subdivided into anterior, middle and posterior ethmoidal sinuses. SEE anterior ethmoidal cells. SYN ethmoidal sinuses.

**eth·moi·do·lac·ri·mal su·ture** (eth-moy' dō-lak'ri-măl sū'chŭr) [TA] Line of union of orbital plate of ethmoid bone and posterior margin of lacrimal bone.

**eth·moi·do·max·il·lar·y su·ture** (eth-moy'dō-mak'si-lar-ē sū'chŭr) [TA] Line of apposition of orbital surface of body of maxilla with orbital plate of ethmoid bone.

**eth·mo·lac·ri·mal** (eth'mō-lak'ri-măl) Relating to the ethmoid and lacrimal bones.

**eth·mo·max·il·lar·y** (eth'mō-mak'si-lar-ē) Relating to ethmoid and maxillary bones.

**eth·mo·na·sal** (eth'mō-nā'zăl) Relating to ethmoid and nasal bones.

**eth·mo·pal·a·tal** (eth'mō-pal'ă-tăl) Relating to ethmoid and palate bones.

**eth·mo·sphe·noid** (eth'mō-sfē'noyd) Relating to the ethmoid and sphenoid bones.

**eth·mo·tur·bi·nals** (eth′mō-tŭr′bi-nălz) Collective term for conchae of ethmoid bone; superior and middle nasal conchae; occasionally a third, supreme concha, exists. SEE middle nasal concha, supreme nasal concha.

**eth·mo·vo·mer·ine** (eth′mō-vō′mĕr-in) Relating to ethmoid bone and vomer.

**eth·nic group** (eth′nik grūp) Social group characterized by distinctive social and cultural tradition maintained from generation to generation, common history and origin, and sense of identification with group; may be reflected in experience of health and disease.

**eth·no·cen·trism** (eth′nō-sen′trizm) Tendency to evaluate other ethnic groups according to values and standards of one's own, especially with conviction that one's own is superior to others. [G. *ethnos*, race, tribe, + *kentron*, center of a circle]

**eth·no·phar·ma·col·o·gy** (eth′nō-fahrm′ă-kol′ŏ-jē) Study of differences in response to drugs based on varied ethnicity; also called pharmacogenetics.

**eth·o·phar·ma·col·o·gy** (eth′ō-fahr-mă-kol′ŏ-jē) Study of drug effects on behavior, relying on observation and description of species-specific elements (e.g., acts and postures during social encounters). [G. *ethos*, character, habit, + *pharmacology*]

**eth·yl chlo·ride** (eth′il klōr′īd) Volatile explosive liquid; when sprayed on skin, produces local anesthesia by superficial freezing but also is a potent inhalation anesthetic.

**eth·yl·ene** (eth′il-ēn) An explosive constituent of ordinary illuminating gas.

**eth·yl·ene·di·a·mine** (eth′il-ēn-dī′ă-mēn) A volatile colorless liquid of ammoniac odor and caustic taste; the dihydrochloride is used as a urinary acidifier.

**eth·yl·ene·di·a·mine·tet·ra·a·ce·tic ac·id (EDTA)** (eth′i-lēn-dī′ă-mēn-tet′ră-ă-sē′tik as′id) Chelating agent; as the sodium salt, used as a water softener, to stabilize drugs rapidly decomposed in the presence of traces of metal ions, and as an anticoagulant; as the sodium calcium salt, used to remove radium and other metals from hard tissue.

**eth·yl·ene ox·ide** (eth′i-lēn ok′sīd) Fumigant, used for cold sterilization of surgical instruments.

**eth·yl for·mate** (eth′il fōr′māt) Volatile, flammable liquid used as a fumigant and flavoring agent.

**eth·yl·par·a·ben** (eth′il-par′ă-ben) An antifungal preservative.

**e·ti·o·gen·ic** (ē′tē-ō-jen′ik) Of a causal nature. [G. *aitia*, cause, + *genesis*, production]

**e·ti·ol·o·gy** (ē′tē-ol′ŏ-jē) **1.** Science and study of causes of disease and their mode of operation. **2.** The science of causes, causality; in common, but to some, incorrect, usage, the cause itself. [G. *aitia*, cause, + *logos*, treatise, discourse]

**e·ti·o·path·ic** (ē′tē-ō-path′ik) Relating to specific lesions concerned with the cause of a disease. [G. *aitia*, cause, + *pathos*, disease]

**e·ti·o·pa·thol·o·gy** (ē′tē-ō-pă-thol′ŏ-jē) Consideration of the cause of an abnormal state or finding. [G. *aitia*, cause, + pathology]

**e·ti·o·tro·pic** (ē′tē-ō-trō′pik) Directed against the cause; denoting a remedy that attenuates or destroys the causal factor of a disease. [G. *aitia*, cause, + *tropē*, a turning]

**Eu** Symbol for europium.

**Eu·bac·te·ri·um** (yū′bak-tēr′ē-ŭm) Genus containing more than 40 species of anaerobic, non-spore-forming, nonmotile bacteria containing straight or curved gram-positive rods that usually occur singly, in pairs, or in short chains. Usually these organisms attack carbohydrates; may be pathogenic, but rarely are associated with intraabdominal sepsis in humans.

**eu·bi·ot·ics** (yū′bī-ot′iks) The science of hygienic living. [*eu-* + G. *biotikos*, relating to life]

**eu·ca·lyp·tus oil** (yū′kă-lip′tŭs oyl) Volatile oil distilled with steam from the fresh leaf of *Eucalyptus globulus* or other species of *Eucalyptus;* used as an antiseptic and expectorant in cough lozenges and in vaporizer aromatics.

**eu·dip·si·a** (yū-dip′sē-ă) Ordinary mild thirst. [*eu-* + G. *dipsa*, thirst]

**eu·ge·nol** (yū′je-nol) Analgesic used in dentistry with zinc oxide; a base for impression materials.

**euglycaemia** [Br.] SYN euglycemia.

**eu·gly·ce·mi·a** (yū′glī-sē′mē-ă) Normal blood glucose concentration. SYN euglycaemia. [*eu-* + G. *glykys*, sweet, + *haima*, blood]

**eu·gna·thi·a** (yūg-nath′ē-ă) Abnormality limited to teeth and their immediate alveolar supports. [*eu-* + G. *gnathos*, jaw]

**eu·gno·si·a** (yūg-nō′sē-ă) Normal ability to synthesize sensory stimuli. [*eu-* + G. *gnōsis*, perception]

**eu·pho·ri·a** (yū-fōr′ē-ă) **1.** A feeling of well-being, not necessarily well founded. **2.** The pleasure state induced by a drug or substance of abuse. [*eu-* + G. *pherō*, to bear]

**eu·ploi·dy** (yū-ploy′dē) The state of a cell containing whole haploid sets. [*eu-* + G. *-ploos*, -fold]

**eup·ne·a** (yūp-nē′ă) Easy, free respiration; the

type observed in a normal person under resting conditions. [G. *eupnoia,* fr. *eu,* well, + *pnoia,* breath]

**eu·ro·pi·um (Eu)** (yū-rō′pē-ŭm) An element of the rare earth (lanthanide) group. [L. *Europa,* Europe]

**eu·ryg·na·thism** (yū-rig′nă-thizm) The condition of having a wide jaw. [*eury-* + G. *gnathos,* jaw]

**eu·sta·chian tube** (yū-stā′shăn tūb) SYN pharyngotympanic (auditory) tube.

**eu·tec·tic al·loy** (yū-tek′tik al′oy) Alloy, generally brittle and subject to tarnish and corrosion, with a fusion temperature lower than that of any of its components; used in dentistry mainly in soldering material.

**eu·tha·na·si·a** (yū′thă-nā′zē-ă) 1. A quiet, painless death. 2. The intentional putting to death of a person with an incurable or painful disease intended as an act of mercy. [*eu-* + G. *thanatos,* death]

**eu·ther·a·peu·tic** (yū′ther-ă-pyū′tik) Having excellent curative properties.

**eu·thy·mi·a** (yū-thī′mē-ă) 1. Joyfulness; mental peace and tranquility. 2. Moderation of mood. [*eu-* + G. *thymos,* mind]

**eu·thy·mic** (yū-thī′mik) Relating to, or characterized by, euthymia.

**eu·thy·roid hy·po·me·tab·o·lism** (yū-thī′royd hī′pō-mĕ-tab′ŏ-lizm) Unusual condition resembling myxedema but with an apparently normal thyroid gland.

**eu·thy·roid·ism** (yū-thī′royd-izm) A condition in which the thyroid gland is functioning normally, its secretion being of proper amount and constitution.

**e·vac·u·ate** (ē-vak′yū-āt) To empty out. [L. *e-vacuo,* pp. *-vacuatus,* to empty out]

**e·vac·u·a·tion** (ĕ-vak′yū-ā′shŭn) Removal of material or air from a closed vessel.

**e·vac·u·a·tion sys·tem** (ē-vak′yū-ā′shŭn sis′tĕm) In dentistry, a suction used to remove fluids such as saliva and blood from an area to provide a dry treatment field.

**e·val·u·a·tion** (ĕ-val′yū-ā′shŭn) Systematic, objective assessment of the relevance, effectiveness, and impact of activities in the light of specified objectives.

**ev·a·nes·cent** (ev′ă-nes′ĕnt) Of short duration. [L. *e,* out, + *vanesco,* to vanish]

**Ev·ans syn·drome** (ev′ănz sin′drōm) Acquired hemolytic anemia and thrombocytopenia.

**ev·i·dence-based med·i·cine** (ev′i-dĕns-bāst med′i-sin) Process and use of relevant information from peer-reviewed clinical and epidemiologic research to address a specific clinical issue, and thereby weighing the attendant risks and benefits of diagnostic tests and therapeutic measures; literature to address a specific clinical problem; application of simple rules of science and common sense to determine validity of information.

**e·voked re·sponse (ER)** (ē-vōkt′ rĕ-spons′) Alteration in electrical activity of a region of nervous system through which an incoming sensory stimulus is passing; may be somatosensory (SER), brainstem auditory (BAER), or visual (VER).

**e·vul·sion** (ē-vŭl′shŭn) A forcible pulling out or extraction. Cf. avulsion. [L. *evulsio,* fr. *e-vello,* pp. *-vulsus,* to pluck out]

**⊞Ew·ing tu·mor** (yū′ing tū′mŏr) Malignant neoplasm that occurs usually before the age of 20 years, about twice as frequently in males, and in about 75% of patients involves bones of the extremities, including the shoulder girdle, with a predilection for the metaphysis. See this page. Also called Ewing sarcoma.

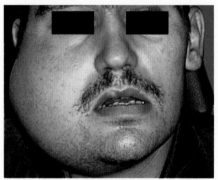

**Ewing tumor:** fast-growing malignancy

**ex·ac·er·ba·tion** (eg-zas′ĕr-bā′shŭn) Increased severity of a disease or any of its signs or symptoms. [L. *ex-acerbo,* pp. *-atus,* to exasperate, increase, fr. *acerbus,* sour]

**ex·am·i·na·tion** (eg-zam′i-nā′shŭn) 1. Any investigation or inspection made for the purpose of diagnosis; usually qualified by the method used. 2. A method of evaluation of skills after receiving instruction in a given field.

**ex·an·the·ma** (eg-zan′thĕ-mă) Skin eruption occurring as a symptom of an acute viral or coccal disease. [G. efflorescence, an eruption, fr. *anthos,* flower]

**ex·an·the·ma su·bi·tum** (eg′zan-thĕ′mă sū′bi-tŭm) Disease of infants and young children caused by human herpesvirus-6, marked by sudden onset with fever lasting several days and followed by a fine macular rash that appears within a few hours to a day after the fever has subsided.

**ex·an·the·sis** (ek′zan-thē′sis) **1.** A rash or exanthem. **2.** The coming out of a rash or eruption. [G.]

**ex·an·thrope** (ek′zan-thrōp) An external cause of disease, one not originating in the body. [G. *ex,* out of, + *anthrōpos,* man]

**ex·an·throp·ic** (ek′zan-throp′ik) Originating outside of the human body.

**ex·ar·tic·u·la·tion** (eks′ahr-tik-yū-lā′shŭn) SYN disarticulation. [L. *ex,* out, + *articulus,* joint]

**ex·ca·va·tor** (eks′kă-vā-tŏr) In dentistry, an instrument, generally a small spoon or curette, for cleaning out and shaping a carious cavity preparatory to filling.

**ex·ce·men·to·sis** (ek′sē-men-tō′sis) SYN hypercementosis.

**ex·cess (XS)** (ek′ses) That which is more than the usual or specified amount.

**ex·cip·i·ent** (ek-sip′ē-ĕnt) A more or less inert substance added in a prescription as a diluent or vehicle or to give form or consistency when the remedy is given in pill form; e.g., simple syrup, vegetable gums, aromatic powder, honey, and various elixirs. [L. *excipiens; pres. p. of ex-cipio,* to take out]

**ex·ci·sion** (ek-sizh′ŭn) *Avoid the misspelling exision.* Act of cutting out; surgical removal of part or all of a structure or organ. [L. *excido,* to cut out]

**ex·cit·a·ble** (ek-sī′tă-bĕl) **1.** Capable of quick response to a stimulus; having potentiality for emotional arousal. **2.** In neurophysiology, referring to a tissue, cell, or membrane capable of undergoing excitation in response to an adequate stimulus.

**ex·cit·ant** (ek-sī′tănt) SYN stimulant (2). [L. *excito,* pp. *-atus,* pres. p. *-ans,* to arouse]

**ex·ci·ta·tion** (ek′sī-tā′shŭn) Act of increasing the rapidity or intensity of the physical or mental processes.

**ex·cit·ing cause** (ek-sīt′ing kawz) Direct provoking cause of a condition.

**ex·clu·sive pro·vid·er or·gan·i·za·tion (EPO)** (eks-klū′siv prŏ-vī′dĕr ōr′găn-ī-zā′shŭn) A managed care plan in the U.S. in which enrollees *must* receive their care from affiliated providers; treatment provided outside the approved network must be paid for by the patients. SEE ALSO managed care.

**ex·co·ri·a·tion** (eks-kōr′ē-ā′shŭn) Scratch mark; linear break in skin surface, usually covered with blood or serous crusts. [L. *excorio,* to skin, strip, fr. *corium,* skin, hide]

**ex·cre·ment** (eks′krē-mĕnt) Waste matter cast out of the body; e.g., feces. [L. *ex-cerno,* pp. *-cretus,* to separate]

**ex·crete** (eks-krēt′) To separate from blood and cast out; to perform excretion.

**ex·cur·sion** (eks-kŭr′zhŭn) Any movement from one point to another, usually with the implied idea of returning again to the original position.

**ex·er·cise** (eks′ĕr-sīz) **1.** *Active:* Planned repetitive physical activity structured to improve and maintain physical fitness. **2.** *Passive:* motion of limbs without effort by the patient.

**ex·er·cise pros·the·sis** (eks′ĕr-sīz pros-thē′sis) Temporary, removable, edentulous device used to recondition supporting residual ridges. Intermittent pressure is applied by biting against interposed fingers.

**ex·fo·li·a·tion** (eks-fō′lē-ā′shŭn) **1.** Loss of deciduous teeth following physiologic loss of root structure. **2.** Detachment and shedding of superficial cells of an epithelium or from any tissue surface. **3.** Scaling or desquamation of the horny layer of epidermis. See this page. [Mod. L. fr. L. *ex,* out, + *folium,* leaf]

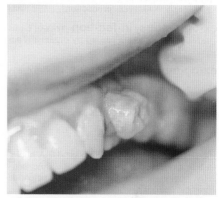

**exfoliating tooth:** 13-year-old child presented with tooth pain; permanent tooth visible behind exfoliating molar; gingival margin shows no sign of infection

**ex·ha·la·tion** (eks′hă-lā′shŭn) **1.** Breathing out. SYN expiration (1). **2.** The giving forth of gas or vapor. **3.** Any exhaled or emitted gas or vapor. [L. *ex-halo,* pp. *-halatus,* to breathe out]

**ex·hale** (eks-hāl′) **1.** To breathe out. **2.** To emit a gas or vapor or odor.

**ex·haus·tion** (eg-zaws′chŭn) **1.** Extreme fatigue; inability to respond to stimuli. **2.** Removal of contents; depletion of a supply of anything. **3.** Extraction of the active constituents of a drug by treating with water, alcohol, or other solvent. [L. *ex-haurio,* pp. *-haustus,* to draw out, empty]

**ex·hib·it** (eg-zib′it) To present or show up with, such as a sign or symptom.

**ex·it block** (eg′zit blok) Inability of an impulse to leave its point of origin, the mechanism for which is conceived as an encircling zone of refractory tissue denying passage to the emerging impulse.

**ex·o·crine** (ek'sō-krin) **1.** Denoting glandular secretion delivered onto the body surface. **2.** Denoting a gland that secretes outwardly through excretory ducts. [*exo-* + G. *krinō*, to separate]

**ex·o·cy·to·sis** (eks'ō-sī-tō'sis) Appearance of migrating inflammatory cells in the epidermis. [*exo-* + G. *kytos*, cell, + *-osis*, condition]

**ex·o·don·tics** (eks'ō-don'tiks) Branch area of dental care specializing in the surgical removal of teeth.

**ex·o·don·tist** (ek'sō-don'tist) Older term for clinician who specializes in the extraction of teeth.

**ex·o·gen·ic tox·i·co·sis** (eks'ō-jen'ik tok'si-kō'sis) Disease caused by a poison introduced from without and not generated within the body.

**ex·og·e·nous** (eks-oj'ĕ-nŭs) Originating or produced outside of the organism. SYN ectogenous. [*exo-* + G. *-gen*, production]

**ex·og·e·nous in·fec·tion** (eks-oj'ĕ-nŭs in-fek'shŭn) Infection caused by organisms acquired from outside the host.

**ex·og·e·nous py·ro·gens** (eks-oj'ĕ-nŭs pī'rō-jenz) Drugs or substances that are formed by microorganisms and induce fever.

**ex·o·lev·er** (ek'sō-lēv'ĕr) Modified elevator for extraction of tooth roots. [*exo-* + L. *levare*, to raise]

**ex·o·nu·cle·ase** (eks'ō-nū'klē-ās) A nuclease that releases one nucleotide at a time, serially, beginning at one end of a polynucleotide (nucleic acid). Cf. endonuclease.

**ex·oph·thal·mic oph·thal·mo·ple·gi·a** (eks'of-thal'mik of-thal'mō-plē'jē-ă) Ophthalmoplegia with protrusion of the eyeballs due to increased water content of orbital tissues incidental to thyroid disorders.

**ex·oph·thal·mos, ex·oph·thal·mus** (eks'of-thal'mos, -mŭs) Protrusion of one or both eyeballs; can be congenital and familial, or due to pathology. SYN proptosis. [G. *ex*, out, + *ophthalmos*, eye]

**ex·o·phyt·ic** (eks'ō-fit'ik) **1.** Pertaining to an exophyte. **2.** Denoting a neoplasm or lesion that grows outward from an epithelial surface.

**■ex·os·to·sis,** pl. **ex·os·to·ses** (eks'os-tō'sis, -sēz) Cartilage-capped bony projection arising from any bone that develops from cartilage. See this page. [*exo-* + G. *osteon*, bone, + *-osis*, condition]

**ex·o·tox·in** (eks'ō-tok'sin) A specific, soluble, antigenic, usually heat labile, injurious substance elaborated by certain gram-positive or gram-negative bacteria.

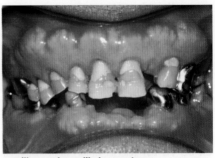

**maxillary and mandibular exostoses**

**ex·pan·sion** (eks-pan'shŭn) **1.** An increase in size as of chest or lungs. **2.** Spreading out of any structure (e.g., a tendon). [L. *ex-pando*, pp. *-pansus*, to spread out]

**ex·pan·sion arch** (eks-pan'shŭn ahrch) Orthodontic appliance that moves dental structures distally, bucally, or labially, creating increased molar-to-molar width and arch length.

**ex·pan·sion pros·the·sis** (eks-pan'shŭn pros-thē'sis) A prosthesis used to widen the lateral segment of the maxilla in cleft palate.

**ex·pec·to·rant** (eks-pek'tŏr-ănt) **1.** Promoting secretion from the mucous membrane of the air passages or facilitating its expulsion. **2.** An agent that increases bronchial secretion and facilitates its expulsion. [L. *ex*, out, + *pectus*, chest]

**ex·pec·to·rate** (eks-pek'tŏr-āt) To spit; to eject saliva, mucus, or other fluid from the mouth.

**ex·pec·to·ra·tion** (eks-pek'tŏr-ā'shŭn) **1.** Mucus and other fluids formed in the air passages and upper food passages of the mouth, expelled by coughing. SEE ALSO sputum (1). **2.** The act of spitting; expelling from the mouth saliva, mucus, and other material from airways or upper digestive passages.

**ex·per·i·ment** (eks-per'i-mĕnt) *Avoid the mispronunciations iks-per'i-ment and eks-pēr-i-ment.* Study in which investigator intentionally alters one or more factors under controlled conditions to study effects of doing so. [L. *experimentum*, fr. *experior*, to test, try]

**ex·per·i·men·tal group** (eks-per'i-men'tăl grŭp) Group of subjects exposed to variable of an experiment, vs. to control group.

**ex·per·i·men·tal med·i·cine** (eks-per'i-men'tăl med'i-sin) Scientific investigation of medical problems by experimentation on animals or by clinical research.

**ex·pert wit·ness** (eks'pĕrt wit'nĕs) In health care, someone with special training who testifies for the defense or prosecution in court.

**ex·pi·ra·tion** (eks'pir-ā'shŭn) **1.** SYN exhalation (1). **2.** A death. [L. *expiro* or *ex- spiro,* pp. *-atus,* to breathe out]

**ex·pi·ra·tion date** (eks′pir-ā′shŭn dāt) The date or time at which a product is no longer potent or of therapeutic value, determined by manufacturer.

**ex·pi·ra·to·ry** (eks-pī′ră-tōr-ē) *Avoid the mispronunciation with stress on the first syllable.* Relating to expiration.

**ex·pi·ra·to·ry re·serve vol·ume (ERV)** (eks-pī′ră-tōr-ē rē-zĕrv′ vol′yūm) The maximal volume of air (about 1000 mL) that can be expelled from the lungs after a normal expiration. SYN reserve air, supplemental air.

**ex·plan·a·tion of ben·e·fits (EOB)** (eks′plă-nā′shŭn ben′ĕ-fits) The report from an insurance carrier that explains benefits, deductibles, copayment responsibilities, and reasons for noncoverage of claims.

**ex·plo·ra·tion** (eks′plŏr-ā′shŭn) An active examination, usually involving a dental or surgical procedure, to ascertain conditions present within a body cavity as an aid in diagnosis.

**ex·plor·a·tor·y stroke ac·tion** (eks-plōr′ă-tōr′ē strōk ak′shŭn) Instrument movement used with a light grasp to evaluate tooth and root surfaces for deposits and other abnormalities.

**explore** (eks-plōr′) In dentistry, the use of an instrument and tactile skill to examine the surface texture of a tooth. [L. *ex-ploro,* to investigate, fr. *ex-,* out, + *ploro,* to deplore, weep over]

**ex·plor·er** (eks-plōr′ĕr) A sharp pointed instrument used to investigate natural or restored tooth surfaces to detect caries or other defects. Types include ODU 11/12 (to detect calculus) and 23 (to detect caries). See this page.

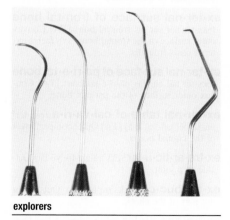

**explorers**

**ex·plor·er tip** (eks-plōr′ĕr tip) Area of 1–2 mm on the side of the explorer working-end that is used for calculus or caries detection.

**ex·plo·sion** (eks-plō′zhŭn) Sudden and violent increase in volume accompanied by noise and release of energy. [L. *explosio,* fr. *explodo,* to drive away by clapping]

**ex·pose** (eks-pōz′) To perform or undergo exposure. [O. Fr. *exposer,* fr. L. *ex-pono,* pp. *expositum,* to set out, expose]

**ex·pos·ed den·tin** (eks-pōsd′ den′tin) Dentin without the enamel or cementum that normally covers it.

**ex·pos·ed pulp** (eks-pōzd′ pŭlp) Pulp that has been laid bare by a pathologic process, trauma, or a dental instrument.

**ex·po·sure** (eks-pō′zhŭr) **1.** In dentistry, loss of hard tooth structure covering the dental pulp due to caries, dental instrumentation, or trauma. **2.** A condition of displaying, revealing, exhibiting, or making accessible. **3.** Proximity to contact with a source of a disease agent in such a manner that effective transmission of the agent or harmful effects of the agent may occur.

**ex·po·sure dose** (eks-pō′zhŭr dōs) Radiation dose, expressed in roentgens, delivered at a point in free air.

**ex·press** (eks-pres′) To press or squeeze out. [L. *ex-premo,* pp. *-pressus,* to press out]

**ex·press con·sent** (eks-pres′ kŏn-sent′) To convey in writing, by gesture, or verbally the agreement or permission of a patient to receive treatment.

**ex·pres·sion** (eks-presh′ŭn) **1.** Squeezing out; expelling by pressure. **2.** Mobility of the features giving a particular emotional significance to the face. SYN facies (4) [TA].

**ex·qui·site** (eks-kwiz′it) Extremely intense, sharp; said of pain in a part. [L. *exquiro,* pp. *exquisitus,* to search out]

**ex·san·gui·nate** (ek-sang′gwi-nāt) To remove or withdraw circulating blood. [L. *ex,* out, + *sanguis* (*-guin*), blood]

**ex·sic·cant** (ek-sik′ănt) SYN desiccant.

**ex·sic·cate** (ek′si-kāt) SYN desiccate.

**ex·sic·ca·tion** (ek′si-kā′shŭn) The removal of water of crystallization. SYN dehydration (3). [L. *ex sicco,* pp. *siccatus,* to dry up]

**ex·tend·ed clasp** (eks-ten′dĕd klasp) Clasp that extends from its minor connector along lingual or facial surface of two or more teeth.

**ex·tend·ed low·er shank** (eks-ten′dĕd lō′ĕr shank) Shank about 3 mm longer than a standard lower shank.

**ex·ten·sion** (eks-ten′shŭn) [TA] **1.** The act of bringing the distal portion of a joint in continuity with the long axis of the proximal portion. **2.** A pulling or dragging force exerted on a limb

**ef**

in a distal direction. **3.** To straighten a joint. [L. *extensus,* past part. of *extendere,* to stretch out, extend]

**ex·ten·sion bridge** (ek-sten´shŭn brij) SYN cantilever bridge.

**ex·ten·sion form** (eks-ten´shŭn fōrm) Extension of cavity preparation outline form to include areas of incipient carious lesions; provides a dental restoration with margins that are self-cleansing or easily cleaned.

**ex·ter·nal** (eks-tĕr´năl) [TA] *Do not confuse this word with lateral or outer.* On the outside or farther from the center; often incorrectly used to mean lateral. [L. *externus*]

**ex·ter·nal a·cous·tic me·a·tus** (eks-tĕr´năl ă-kūs´tik mē-ā´tŭs) [TA] The passage leading inward through the tympanic portion of the temporal bone, from the auricle to the tympanic membrane; it consists of a bony (inner) portion and a fibrocartilaginous (outer) portion, the cartilaginous external acoustic meatus. SYN acoustic meatus (1), antrum auris.

**ex·ter·nal a·cous·tic pore** (eks-tĕr´năl ă-kū´stik pōr) [TA] Orifice of external acoustic meatus in tympanic portion of temporal bone.

**ex·ter·nal ap·er·ture of ves·tib·u·lar aq·ue·duct** (eks-tĕr´năl ap´ĕr-chŭr ves-tib´ yū-lăr ahk´wĕ-dŭkt) SYN opening of vestibular canaliculus.

**ex·ter·nal ar·te·ry of nose** (eks-tĕr´năl ahr´tĕr-ē nōz) SYN dorsal nasal artery.

**ex·ter·nal au·di·to·ry ca·nal** (eks-tĕr´ năl aw´di-tōr-ē kă-nal´) The passage leading inward through the tympanic portion of the temporal bone, from the auricle to the tympanic membrane; it consists of fibrocartilaginous outer and bony inner portions lined with thin skin medially and thicker skin with ceruminous glands, hair follicles, and subcutaneous fat laterally. SYN acoustic meatus (2).

**ex·ter·nal branch of su·pe·ri·or la·ryn·ge·al nerve** (eks-tĕr´năl branch sŭ-pēr´ē-ŏr lă-rin´jē-ăl nĕrv) [TA] Terminal branch of superior laryngeal nerve (with internal laryngeal nerve) supplying motor innervation to cricothyroid muscle.

**ex·ter·nal den·tal ep·i·the·li·um, ex·ter·nal e·nam·el ep·i·the·li·um** (eks-tĕr´năl den´tăl ep´i-thē´lē-ŭm, ĕ-nam´ĕl) Cuboidal cells of outer layer of odontogenic organ (enamel organ) of a developing tooth.

**ex·ter·nal ear** (eks-tĕr´năl ēr) SEE ear.

**ex·ter·nal max·il·lar·y ar·te·ry** (eks-tĕr´năl mak´si-lar-ē ahr´tĕr-ē) SYN facial artery.

**ex·ter·nal na·sal veins** (eks-tĕr´năl nā´zăl vānz) [TA] Several vessels that drain the external nose, emptying into angular or facial vein.

**ex·ter·nal nose** (eks-tĕr´năl nōz) Visible portion of nose that forms a prominent feature of the face; it consists of a root, dorsum, and apex from above downward and is perforated inferiorly by two nostrils separated by a septum.

**ex·ter·nal ob·lique ridge** (eks-tĕr´năl ō-blēk´ rij) A line of bone located on the buccal side of the mandible extending from the anterior border of the ramus to the mandibular third molar area. Appears in x-rays as a radiopaque curved line ending in the mandibular molar area.

**ex·ter·nal open·ing of ca·rot·id ca·nal** (eks-tĕr´năl ō´pĕn-ing kă-rot´id kă-nal´) Roughly circular opening on the inferior surface of the petrous portion of the temporal bone by which the internal carotid artery enters the carotid canal.

**ex·ter·nal open·ing of co·chle·ar can·al·ic·u·lus** (eks-tĕr´năl ō´pĕn-ing kok´lē-ăr kan´ă-lik´yū-lŭs) [TA] External orifice of the cochlear aqueduct on the temporal bone medial to the jugular fossa.

**ex·ter·nal res·pi·ra·tion** (eks-tĕr´năl res´ pir-ā´shŭn) The exchange of respiratory gases in the lungs as distinguished from internal or tissue respiration.

**ex·ter·nal sal·i·var·y gland** (eks-tĕr´năl sal´i-var-ē gland) SYN parotid gland.

**ex·ter·nal se·cre·tion** (eks-tĕr´năl sĕ-krē´ shŭn) Substance formed by a cell and transported outside the cell's walls as a means of ridding the cell of the substance or as a messenger to affect the function of other cells.

**ex·ter·nal sur·face of co·chle·ar duct** (eks-tĕr´năl sŭr´făs kok´lē-ăr dŭkt) [TA] The aspect of the duct that faces the outer (spiral ligament) side of the cochlea.

**ex·ter·nal sur·face of fron·tal bone** (eks-tĕr´năl sŭr´făs frŏn´tăl bōn) [TA] Convex outer surface of the frontal bone. SYN facies externa ossis frontalis.

**ex·ter·nal sur·face of pa·ri·e·tal bone** (eks-tĕr´năl sŭr´făs pă-rī´ē-tăl bōn) [TA] Convex outer surface of the parietal bone.

**ex·ter·nal table of cal·va·ri·a** (eks-tĕr´ năl tā´bĕl kal-var´ē-ă) [TA] Outer compact layer of the cranial bones.

**ex·tra·ar·tic·u·lar** (eks´tră-ahr-tik´yū-lăr) Outside of a joint.

**ex·tra·buc·cal** (eks´tră-bŭk´ăl) Outside or not part of the cheek.

**ex·tra·cap·su·lar** (eks´tră-kap´sŭ-lăr) Outside of the capsule of a joint.

**ex·tra·cel·lu·lar** (eks´tră-sel´yŭ-lăr) Outside the cells.

**ex·tra·cor·o·nal re·tain·er** (ek´stră-kōr´ ŏ-năl rē-tā´nĕr) Retainer that depends on contact with the outer circumference of the crown of a tooth for its retentive qualities.

**ex·tra·cor·po·re·al** (eks´tră-kōr-pōr´ē-ăl) Outside of, or unrelated to, the body or any anatomic "corpus."

**ex·tra·cra·ni·al** (eks´tră-krā´nē-ăl) Outside of the cranial cavity.

**ex·tract** (eks-trakt´, eks´trakt) 1. To perform extraction. 2. A concentrated drug preparation obtained by removing active constituents of the drug with suitable solvents, evaporating all or nearly all solvent, and adjusting residual mass or powder to the prescribed standard. [L. *extraho*, pp. *-tractus*, to draw out]

**ex·tract·ant** (eks-trak´tănt) An agent used to isolate or extract a substance from a mixture or combination of substances, from the tissues, or from a crude drug.

**ex·tract·ing for·ceps** (eks-trak´ting fōr´ seps) SYN dental forceps.

**ex·trac·tion** (eks-trak´shŭn) 1. Luxation and removal of a tooth from its alveolus. 2. Surgical removal by pulling out. [L. *ex-traho*, pp. *-tractus*, to draw out]

**ex·trac·tor** (eks-trak´tŏr) Instrument for use in drawing or pulling out any natural part, as a tooth, or a foreign body.

**ex·tra·du·ral** (eks´tră-dū´răl) 1. On the outer side of the dura mater. 2. Unconnected with the dura mater.

**extradural haemorrhage** [Br.] SYN extradural hemorrhage.

**ex·tra·du·ral hem·or·rhage** (eks´trădūr´ăl hem´ŏr-äj) Extravasation of blood between cranium and dura mater. SYN extradural haemorrhage.

**ex·tra·me·dul·la·ry** (eks´tră-med´yū-lar-ē) Outside of, or unrelated to, any medulla, especially the medulla oblongata.

**ex·tra·o·ral** (eks´tră-ō´răl) Outside of the oral cavity; external to the oral cavity.

**ex·tra·o·ral an·chor·age** (eks´tră-ōr´ăl ang´kŏr-äj) Anchorage in which the resistance unit is outside the oral cavity.

**ex·tra·o·ral as·sess·ment** (eks´tră-ōr´ăl ă-ses´mĕnt) The evaluation of the health of the structures and tissues of the head and neck outside of the oral cavity.

**ex·tra·o·ral frac·ture ap·pli·ance** (eks´ tră-ōr´ăl frak´shŭr ă-plī´ăns) Device used for extraoral reduction and fixation of maxillary or mandibular fractures, in which pins, clamps, or screws interjoined with metal or acrylic connectors are used to align the fractured segments.

**ex·tra·o·ral ful·crum** (eks´tră-ōr´ăl ful´ krŭm) Stabilizing point outside the patient's mouth (e.g., against the patient's chin or cheek).

**ex·tra·o·ral trac·ing** (eks´tră-ōr´ăl trās´ ing) A drawing of mandibular movements using devices that are attached to the opposing arches and extend outside the mouth.

**ex·tra·py·ram·i·dal dis·ease** (eks´trăpir-am´i-dăl di-zēz´) General term for various disorders caused by abnormalities of the basal ganglia or certain brainstem or thalamic nuclei.

**ex·tra·sys·to·le** (eks´tră-sis´tŏ-lē) A nonspecific word for an ectopic beat from any source in the heart.

**ex·tra·tra·che·al** (eks´tră-trā´kē-ăl) Outside the trachea.

**ex·trav·a·sate** (eks-trav´ă-sāt) 1. To exude from or pass out of a vessel into tissues. 2. The substance thus exuded. [L. *extra*, out of, + *vas*, vessel]

**ex·trav·a·sa·tion** (eks-trav´ă-sā´shŭn) The act of extravasating. [*extra-* + L. *vas*, vessel]

**ex·tra·vas·cu·lar flu·id** (eks´tră-vas´kyŭlăr flū´id) All fluid outside the blood vessels; constitutes about 48–58% of the body weight.

**ex·trem·i·ty** (eks-trem´i-tē) [TA] One of the ends of an elongated or pointed structure. Incorrectly (but very commonly) used to mean limb.

**ex·trin·sic** (eks-trin´zik) Originating outside the part where found or on which it acts; denoting especially a muscle. [L. *extrinsecus*, from without]

**ex·trin·sic al·ler·gic al·ve·o·lit·is** (ekstrin´zik ă-lĕr´jik al-vē´ŏ-lī´tis) Pneumoconiosis resulting from hypersensitivity due to repeated inhalation of organic dust, usually specified according to occupational exposure; in the acute form, respiratory symptoms and fever start several hours after exposure to the dust; in the chronic form, there is eventual diffuse pulmonary fibrosis after exposure over several years.

**ex·trin·sic asth·ma** (eks-trin´zik az´mă) Bronchial asthma resulting from an allergic reaction to foreign substances.

**ex·trin·sic col·or** (eks-trin´zik kŭl´ŏr) Color applied to the external surface of a dental prosthesis.

**ex·trin·sic fac·tor** (eks-trin´zik fak´tŏr) Dietary vitamin B12.

**ex·trin·sic stain** (eks-trin´zik stān) Adherence of bacteria or discoloring agents to dental enamel that cause the tooth to assume an unusual color or tint. It varies in shade according to the agent: coffee, tea, and tobacco cause brownish-black stains; chromogenic bacteria green to brown; and leaks from amalgam restorations bluish-gray to black. See this page.

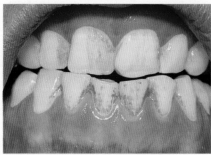

**extrinsic staining:** caused by chlorhexidine

**ex·tro·ver·sion** (eks'trō-vĕr'zhŭn) **1.** A turning outward. **2.** A personality patterned on the presence of others. Cf. introversion. [incorrectly formed fr. L. *extra,* outside, + *verto,* pp. *versus,* to turn]

**ex·trude** (eks-trūd') To thrust, force, or press out.

**ex·trud·ed teeth** (eks-trū'dĕd tēth) SEE extrusion of a tooth.

**ex·tru·sion** (eks-trū'zhŭn) **1.** A thrusting or forcing out of a normal position. **2.** The over-eruption or migration of a tooth beyond its normal occlusal position.

**ex·tru·sion of a tooth** (eks-trū'zhŭn tūth)

Elongation of a tooth; movement of a tooth in an occlusal or incisal direction.

**ex·tu·ba·tion** (eks'tū-bā'shŭn) Removal of a tube from an organ, structure, or orifice; specifically, removal of the endotracheal tube after intubation. [L. *ex,* out, + *tuba,* tube]

**ex·u·date** (eks'yū-dāt) Any fluid or semisolid that has oozed out of a tissue or its capillaries, more specifically because of injury or inflammation in which case it is characteristically high in protein and white blood cells. Cf. transudate. SYN exudation (2). [L. *ex,* out, + *sudo,* to sweat]

**ex·u·da·tion** (eks'yū-dā'shŭn) **1.** The act or process of exuding. **2.** SYN exudate.

**ex·ude** (eks-yūd') In general, to ooze or pass gradually out of a body structure or tissue. [L. *ex,* out, + *sudo,* to sweat]

**eye** (ī) [TA] **1.** The organ of vision comprising eyeball and optic nerve, **2.** Area of eye, including lids and other accessory organs; contents of orbit (common). [A.S. *eāge*]

**eye loupes** (ī lūps) SYN loupe.

**eye tooth** (ī tūth) SYN canine tooth.

**eye wash** (ī'wawsh) A soothing solution used for bathing the eye. [eye fr. O.E. *eage* + *wash,* fr. O.E. *waescan*]

**eye wash sta·tion** (ī wawsh stā'shŭn) A unit that attaches to a water supply and provides a gentle stream of water; used for emergency irrigation to remove contaminants from the ocular area.

# F

**F** Abbreviation for phenylalanine; fluorine.

**F.A.A.P.** Abbreviation for Fellow of the American Academy of Pediatrics.

**fab·ri·ca·tion** (fab′ri-kā′shŭn) **1.** Manufacture or crafting of dentures, appliances, and other forms of oral prostheses. **2.** Telling false tales as true; e.g., malingering of symptoms or illness calculation during examination.

**F.A.C.D.** Abbreviation for Fellow of the American College of Dentists.

**face** (fās) **1.** [TA] Surface between two lateral surfaces that converge to form a cutting edge; portion of dental instrument working-end opposite its back. On sickle scales and curettes, face is bounded by cutting edges. **2.** Front portion of head; visage, including eyes, nose, mouth, forehead, cheeks, and chin; excludes ears. SYN facies (1) [TA]. **3.** SYN surface.

**face-bow** (fās′bō) Caliperlike device used to record relationship of the jaws to temporomandibular joints; record may then be used to orient a cast or model of maxilla to the opening and closing axis of the articulator. SYN hinge-bow.

**face-bow fork** (fās bō fōrk) Section of face-bow assemblage used to attach maxillary trial base to face-bow proper. SYN bite fork.

**face-bow rec·ord** (fās bō rek′ŏrd) Registration with a face-bow of position of hinge axis and/or condyles; used to orient maxillary cast to opening and closing axes of articulator.

**face shield** (fās shēld) A type of personal protective equipment that is made of see-through material; prevents or reduces risk of transmitting substances to the face of the dental worker.

**fac·et** (fas′ĕt) **1.** [TA] A worn spot on a tooth, produced by chewing or grinding. **2.** [TA] Small smooth area on bone or other firm structure. SYN facies (3) [TA]. [Fr. *facette*]

**face va·lid·i·ty** (fās vă-lid′i-tē) Extent to which items used in a test or procedure appear superficially to sample that which is to be measured.

**fa·cial** (fā′shăl) Relating to the face.

**fa·cial an·gle** (fā′shăl ang′gĕl) **1.** Any of several variously named and variously defined anatomic angles that have been used to quantify facial protrusion. **2.** In dentistry, angle formed by intersection of orbitomeatal plane with nasion-pogonion line, which establishes anteroposterior relation of mandible to upper face at the orbitomeatal plane. SYN Frankfurt-mandibular incisor angle.

**fa·cial ar·te·ry** (fā′shăl ahr′tĕr-ē) [TA] *Origin*, anterior branch (typically, the third) of the external carotid; *branches*, ascending palatine, tonsillar and glandular branches, submental, inferior labial, superior labial, masseteric, buccal, lateral nasal branches, and angular. SYN external maxillary artery.

**fa·cial as·pect** (fā′shăl as′pekt) [TA] **1.** View of dental or oral surfaces directly from the front. **2.** Surface of cranium view from the front. See this page. SYN frontal aspect.

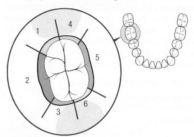

**facial and lingual aspects:** each tooth, sextant, quadrant, or dental arch is divided into two aspects, facial and lingual. A tooth's facial aspect is further subdivided into three areas: (1) distofacial, (2) facial, and (3) mesiofacial. The tooth's lingual aspect is also subdivided into three areas: (4) distolingual, (5) lingual, and (6) mesiolingual.

**fa·cial a·sym·me·try** (fā′shăl ā-sim′ĕ-trē) The condition that one half of the face is not equivalent or the same as the other half.

**fa·cial bones** (fā′shăl bōnz) Bones surrounding mouth and nose and contributing to orbits; made of paired maxillae, zygomatic, nasal, lacrimal, palatine, and inferior nasal conchae and unpaired ethmoid, vomer, mandible, and hyoid.

**fa·cial ca·nal** (fā′shăl kă-nal′) [TA] Bony passage in temporal bone through which facial nerve passes.

**fa·cial cleft** (fā′shăl kleft) Fissure resulting from incomplete merging or fusion of embryonic facial processes normally uniting in the formation of the face, e.g., cleft lip or cleft palate.

**fa·cial di·ple·gi·a** (fā′shăl dī-plē′jē-ă) Paralysis affecting both sides of the face.

**fa·cial height** (fā′shăl hīt) Linear dimension in midline from hairline to menton.

**fa·cial hem·i·at·ro·phy** (fā′shăl hem′ē-at′rŏ-fē) Atrophy, usually progressive, affecting tissues of one side of face.

**fa·cial hem·i·ple·gi·a** (fā′shăl hem′ē-plē′jē-ă) Paralysis of one side of the face; the muscles of the extremities are unaffected.

**fa·cial in·dex, su·pe·ri·or fa·cial in·dex, to·tal fa·cial in·dex** (fā′shăl in′deks, sŭ-pēr′ē-ŏr, tō′tăl) Relation of length of face to its maximal width between zygomatic prominences.

**fa·ci·a·lis phe·nom·e·non** (fā′shē-ā′lis fĕ-nom′ĕ-nŏn) Facial spasm produced by light rubbing of skin or tapping on the zygoma.

**fa·cial lymph nodes** (fā´shǎl limf nōdz) [TA] Chain of lymph nodes lying along the facial vein that receive afferent vessels from the eyelids, nose, cheek, lip, and gums, and send efferent vessels to the submandibular nodes.

🔳**fa·cial mus·cles** (fā´shǎl mǔs´ělz) [TA] Numerous muscles supplied by facial nerve that are attached to and move facial skin. *Terminologia Anatomica* includes the buccinator muscle in this group because of its innervation and embryonic origin, even though it functions primarily in mastication. See this page.

ă-kū´stik mē-ā´tǔs) [TA] Area of fundus of internal acoustic meatus superior to transverse crest through which facial nerve passes to enter facial canal.

🔳**fa·cial nerve [CN VII]** (fā´shǎl něrv) [TA] Nerve with origin in tegmentum of lower portion of pons; emerges from brain at posterior border of the pons; leaves the cranial cavity through internal acoustic meatus, where it is joined by intermediate nerve. See page 221. SYN motor nerve of face, nervus facialis [CN VII], seventh cranial nerve [CN VII].

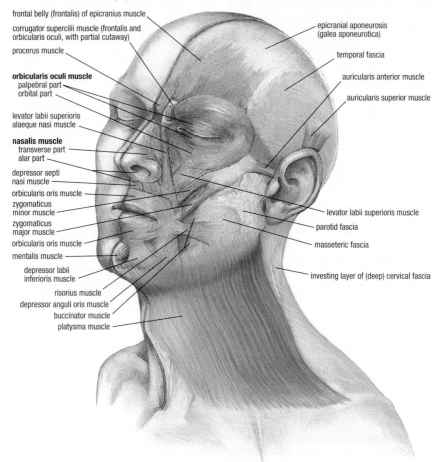

frontal belly (frontalis) of epicranius muscle

corrugator supercilii muscle (frontalis and orbicularis oculi, with partial cutaway)

procerus muscle

**orbicularis oculi muscle**
palpebral part
orbital part

levator labii superioris alaeque nasi muscle

**nasalis muscle**
transverse part
alar part

depressor septi nasi muscle

orbicularis oris muscle

zygomaticus minor muscle

zygomaticus major muscle

orbicularis oris muscle

mentalis muscle

depressor labii inferioris muscle

risorius muscle

depressor anguli oris muscle

buccinator muscle

platysma muscle

epicranial aponeurosis (galea aponeurotica)

temporal fascia

auricularis anterior muscle

auricularis superior muscle

levator labii superioris muscle

parotid fascia

masseteric fascia

investing layer of (deep) cervical fascia

**muscles controlling facial expression** (lateral view)

**fa·cial my·o·ky·mi·a** (fā´shǎl mī´ō-kī´mē-ă) Disorder that appears in the facial muscles, causing narrowing of the palpebral fissure and continuous undulation of the facial skin surface; the latter is colloquially referred to as ''bag of worms'' appearance.

**fa·cial nerve a·re·a of in·ter·nal a·cous·tic me·a·tus** (fā´shǎl něrv ar´ē-ă in-těr´nǎl

**fa·cial neu·ral·gi·a** (fā´shǎl nūr-al´jē-ă) SYN trigeminal neuralgia.

🔳**fa·cial pal·sy** (fā´shǎl pawl´zē) See page 222. SYN facial paralysis.

**fa·cial pa·ral·y·sis** (fā´shǎl păr-al´i-sis) Paresis or paralysis of facial muscles, usually unilateral, due to either a lesion involving either

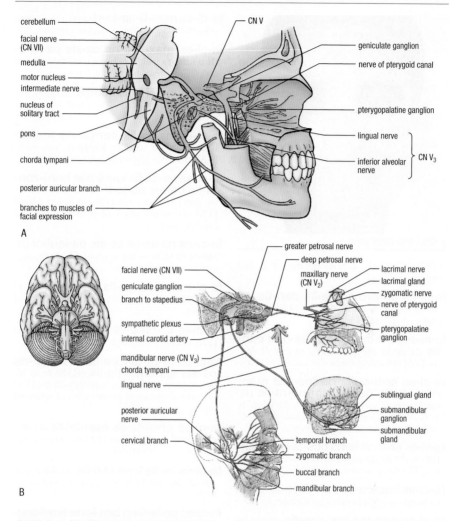

**distribution of facial nerve (cranial nerve VII):** (A) branches of facial nerve in situ; (B) schematic showing distribution of facial nerve fibers

nucleus or facial nerve peripheral to nucleus or supranuclear lesion in cerebrum or upper brainstem. Causes include Bell palsy, stroke, brain tumor, sarcoidosis, Lyme disease, infection, and birth trauma in affected newborns. SYN facial palsy, facioplegia.

**fa·cial plane** (fā′shăl plān) Measurement of bony profile of the face. SYN nasion-pogonion measurement.

**fa·cial pro·file** (fā′shăl prō′fīl) **1.** Outline form of face from a lateral view. **2.** Sagittal outline form of face.

**fa·cial skel·e·ton** (fā′shăl skel′ĕ-tŏn) SYN viscerocranium.

**fa·cial sur·face of tooth** (fā′shăl sŭr′făs tūth) SYN vestibular surface of tooth.

**fa·cial tic** (fā′shăl tik) Involuntary twitching of facial muscles, sometimes unilateral. SYN Bell spasm, palmus (1).

**fa·ci·al tri·an·gle** (fā′shăl trī′ang-gĕl) Angle formed by lines connecting basion, prosthion, and nasion.

**fa·cial vein** (fā′shăl vān) [TA] Continuation of angular vein at medial angle of eye; passes inferolaterally, uniting with retromandibular vein below border of lower jaw before emptying into internal jugular vein. SYN anterior facial vein.

**fa·cial vi·sion** (fā′shăl vizh′ŭn) Sensing proximity of objects by nerves of the face.

**fa·ci·es** (fash′ē-ēz) [TA] *This word is properly pronounced in 3 syllables, but U.S. usage often fuses the second and third syllables into one.* **1.**

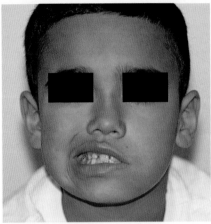

**patient with facial palsy**

[TA] SYN face (2). **2.** [TA] SYN surface. **3.** SYN expression (2). [L.]

**fa·ci·es ap·prox·i·ma·lis den·tis** (fā´shē-ēz ă-prok´si-mā´lis den´tis) [TA] SYN approximal surface of tooth.

**fa·ci·es ar·ti·cu·la·ris an·te·ri·or den·tis** (fā´shē-ēz ahr-tik´yū-lā´ris an-tēr´ē-ŏr den´tis) [TA] SYN anterior articular surface of dens.

**fa·ci·es ar·ti·cu·la·ris fos·sae man·dib·u·la·ris os·sis tem·po·ra·lis** (fā´shē-ēz ahr-tik´yū-lā´ris fos´ē man-dib´yū-lā´ris os´is tem´pō-rā´lis) [TA] SYN articular surface of mandibular fossa of temporal bone.

**fa·ci·es ar·ti·cu·la·ris pos·te·ri·or den·tis** (fā´shē-ēz ahr-tik´yū-lā´ris pos-tēr´ē-ŏr den´tis) [TA] SYN posterior articular facet of dens.

**fa·ci·es buc·ca·lis den·tis** (fā´shē-ēz bŭ-kā´lis den´tis) [TA] SYN buccal surface of tooth.

**fa·ci·es con·tac·tus den·tis** (fā´shē-ēz kon-tak´tŭs den´tis) SYN approximal surface of tooth.

**fa·ci·es dis·ta·lis den·tis** (fā´shē-ēz dis-tā´lis den´tis) [TA] SYN distal surface of tooth.

**fa·ci·es do·lo·ro·sa** (fā´shē-ēz dō´lō-rō´să) Facial expression of an unhappy or sick person.

**fa·ci·es ex·ter·na os·sis fron·ta·lis** (fā´shē-ēz eks-tĕr´nă os´is frŏn-tā´lis) [TA] SYN external surface of frontal bone.

**fa·ci·es fa·ci·a·lis den·tis** (fā´shē-ēz fā´shē-ā´lis den´tis) SYN vestibular surface of tooth.

**fa·ci·es la·bi·a·lis den·tis** (fā´shē-ēz lā´bē-ā´lis den´tis) [TA] SYN labial surface of tooth.

**fa·ci·es lin·gua·lis den·tis** (fā´shē-ēz linggwā´lis den´tis) [TA] SYN lingual surface of tooth.

**fa·ci·es mas·ti·ca·to·ri·a** (fā´shē-ēz mas´ti-kă-tō´rē-ă) SYN denture occlusal surface.

**fa·ci·es max·il·la·ris os·sis pa·la·ti·ni** (fā´shē-ēz mak´si-lā´ris os´is pal´ă-tē´nī) SYN maxillary surface of palatine bone.

**fa·ci·es me·si·a·lis den·tis** (fā´shē-ēz mē´sē-ā´lis den´tis) [TA] SYN mesial surface of tooth.

**fa·ci·es na·sa·lis cor·po·ris max·il·lae** (fā´shē-ēz nā-sā´lis kŏr-pō´ris mak-sil´ē) [TA] SYN nasal surface of body of maxilla.

**fa·ci·es na·sa·lis la·mi·nae hor·i·zon·ta·lis os·sis pa·la·ti·ni** (fā´shē-ēz nā-sā´lis lam´i-nē hōr´i-zon-tā´lis os´is pal´ă-tī´nī) [TA] SYN nasal surface of horizontal plate of palatine bone.

**fa·ci·es na·sa·lis os·sis pa·la·ti·ni** (fā´shē-ēz nā-sā´lis os´is pal´ă-tī´nī) [TA] SYN nasal surface of palatine bone.

**fa·ci·es oc·clu·sa·lis den·tis** (fā´shē-ēz ok´lū-sā´lis den´tis) [TA] SYN denture occlusal surface.

**fa·ci·es or·bi·ta·lis** (fā´shē-ēz ōr´bi-tā´lis) [TA] SYN orbital surface.

**fa·ci·es or·bi·ta·lis a·la·ris ma·jo·ris os·sis sphe·noi·da·lis** (fā´shē-ēz ōr´bi-tā´lis ă-lā´ris mā-jōr´is os´is sfē´nōy-dā´lis) [TA] SYN orbital surface of greater wing of sphenoid bone.

**fa·ci·es or·bi·ta·lis max·il·lae** (fā´shē-ēz ōr´bi-tā´lis mak-sil´ē) [TA] SYN orbital surface of body of maxilla.

**fa·ci·es pa·la·ti·na den·tis** (fā´shē-ēz pal´ă-tī´nă den´tis) [TA] SYN palatine surface of tooth.

**fa·ci·es pa·la·ti·na lam·i·nae hor·i·zon·ta·lis os·sis pa·la·ti·ni** (fā´shē-ēz pal´ă-tī´nă lam´i-nē hōr´i-zon-tā´lis os´is pal´ă-tī´nī) [TA] SYN palatine surface of horizontal plate of palatine bone.

**fa·ci·es sca·phoi·de·a** (fā´shē-ēz skaf-oy´dē-ă) Facial malformation characterized by protuberant forehead, depressed nose and maxilla, and prominent chin.

**fa·ci·es ves·ti·bu·la·ris den·tis** (fā´shē-ēz ves-tib´yū-lā´ris den´tis) [TA] SYN vestibular surface of tooth.

**fa·cil·i·ta·tion** (fă-sil´i-tā´shŭn) Enhancement or reinforcement of a reflex by arrival at the reflex center of other excitatory impulses. [L. *facilitas*, fr. *facilis*, easy]

**fac·ing** (fās´ing) A tooth-colored material (usually plastic or porcelain) used to hide buccal or labial surface of a metal crown to give outward appearance of a natural tooth.

**fa·ci·o·lin·gual** (fā′shē-ō-ling′gwăl) Relating to face and tongue, often denoting a paralysis affecting these parts.

**fa·ci·o·ple·gi·a** (fā′shē-ō-plē′jē-ă) SYN facial paralysis. [facio- + G. *plēgē,* a stroke]

**fa·ci·o·scap·u·lo·hu·mer·al mus·cu·lar dys·tro·phy** (fā′shē-ō-skap′yū-lō-hyū′měr-ăl mŭs′kyū-lăr dis′trŏ-fē) Highly variable hereditary disorder with onset in childhood or adolescence, characterized by muscular weakness and wasting.

**fac·ti·tious** (fak-tish′ŭs) Artificial; self-induced; not naturally occurring. [L. *factitius,* made by art, fr. *facio,* to make]

**fac·ti·tious dis·or·der** (fak-tish′ŭs dis-ŏr′děr) A mental condition in which the patient intentionally induces symptoms of illness for psychological reasons.

**fac·ti·tious ill·ness by prox·y** (fak-tish′ŭs il′něs prok′sē) SYN Munchausen by proxy syndrome.

**fac·tor** (fak′tŏr) A contributing cause in any action. [L. maker, causer, fr. *facio,* to make]

**fac·tor I** (fak′tŏr) In blood clotting, a factor converted to fibrin through thrombin action.

**fac·to·ri·al** (fak-tōr′ē-ăl) Pertaining to a statistical factor or factors.

**fac·tor II** (fak′tŏr) Glycoprotein converted in the clotting of blood to thrombin by factor Xa, platelets, calcium ions, and factor V.

**fac·tor IIa** (fak′tŏr) SYN thrombin.

**fac·tor III** (fak′tŏr) In the clotting of blood, tissue factor, or thromboplastin, initiates the extrinsic pathway by reacting with factor VII and calcium to form factor VIIa.

**fac·tor IV** (fak′tŏr) In the clotting of blood, calcium ions.

**fac·tor IX** (fak′tŏr) In blood clotting, also known as: Christmas factor and other designations; required for formation of intrinsic blood thromboplastin and affects the amount formed (rather than the rate).

**fac·tor P** (fak′tŏr) Chemical formed in ischemic skeletal or cardiac muscle, responsible for pain of intermittent claudication and angina pectoris.

**fac·tor V** (fak′tŏr) In blood clotting, it does not have enzymatic action itself but participates in the common pathway of coagulation by binding factor Xa to platelet surfaces.

**fac·tor VII** (fak′tŏr) In blood clotting, forms a complex with tissue thromboplastin and calcium to activate factor X. SYN prothrombinogen.

**fac·tor VIII** (fak′tŏr) In blood clotting, it participates in the clotting of the blood by forming a complex with factor IXa, platelets, and calcium and by enzymatically catalyzing the activation of factor X.

**fac·tor X** (fak′tŏr) A plasma coagulation factor that assists in the conversion of prothrombin to thrombin. SYN prothrombinase, Stuart factor, Stuart-Prower factor.

**fac·tor XI** (fak′tŏr) In blood clotting, a component of the contact system that is absorbed from plasma and serum by glass and similar surfaces.

**fac·tor XII** (fak′tŏr) In blood clotting, it activates factors VII and XI and converts factor XI to its active form, factor XIa.

**fac·tor XIII** (fak′tŏr) In blood clotting, it is catalyzed by thrombin into its active form, factor XIIIa, which cross-links subunits of the fibrin clot to form insoluble fibrin.

**fac·ul·ta·tive** (fak′ŭl-tā′tiv) Able to live under more than one specific set of environmental conditions; possessing an alternative pathway.

**fac·ul·ty** (fak′ŭl-tē) A natural or specialized power of a living organism.

**FAD** Abbreviation for flavin adenine dinucleotide.

**FAE** Abbreviation for fetal alcohol effects.

**faecal vomiting** [Br.] SYN fecal vomiting.

**faeces** [Br.] SYN feces.

**fail·ure** (fāl′yŭr) State of insufficiency or nonperformance.

**fail·ure to thrive** (fāl′yŭr thrīv) Condition in which an infant's weight gain and growth are far below usual levels for age.

**faint** (fānt) 1. Extremely weak; threatened with syncope. 2. An episode of syncope.

**faith heal·ing** (fāth hēl′ing) Sundry types of prayer-based efforts to alter the disease course.

**fal·ci·form** (fal′si-fōrm) Having a crescentic or sickle shape. [L. *falx,* sickle, + *forma,* form]

**fal·cu·lar** (fal′kyū-lăr) 1. Resembling a sickle or falx. 2. Relating to the falx cerebelli or cerebri.

**Fal·lot tri·ad** (fă-lō′ trī′ad) SYN trilogy of Fallot.

**false an·ky·lo·sis** (fawls ang′ki-lō′sis) SYN fibrous ankylosis.

**false cy·a·no·sis** (fawls sī′ă-nō′sis) Cyanosis due to presence of an abnormal pigment in blood, not oxygen deficiency.

**false joint** (fawls joynt) SYN pseudarthrosis.

**false mem·brane** (fawls mem′brăn) A thick, tough fibrinous exudate on the surface of a mucous membrane or the skin, as seen in diphthe-

ef

ria. SYN croupous membrane, neomembrane, plica (2), pseudomembrane.

**false neg·a·tive** (fawls neg'ă-tiv) **1.** A test result that erroneously excludes someone from a specific diagnostic or reference group. **2.** A patient whose test results exclude that person from a particular diagnostic group to which the person ought truly belong. **3.** Term commonly used to denote a false-negative reaction (q.v.).

**false-neg·a·tive re·ac·tion** (fawls-neg'ă-tiv rē-ak'shŭn) Erroneous or mistakenly negative response.

**false neu·ro·ma** (fawls nūr-ō'mă) SYN traumatic neuroma.

**false pos·i·tive** (fawls poz'i-tiv) **1.** A test result that erroneously assigns a patient to a specific diagnostic or reference group, due particularly to insufficiently exact methods of testing. **2.** A patient whose test results include that person in a particular diagnostic group to which the person may not truly belong. **3.** Term commonly used to denote a false-positive reaction (q.v.).

**false-pos·i·tive re·ac·tion** (fawls-poz'i-tiv rē-ak'shŭn) Erroneous positive response.

**false thirst** (fawls thĭrst) Thirst unsatisfied by drinking or taking water; thirst associated with a dry mouth but not with a bodily need for water.

**fal·si·fi·ca·tion** (fawl'si-fi-kā'shŭn) Deliberate act of misrepresentation so as to deceive. [L. *falsus*, false, + *facio*, to make]

**fal·si·fy** (fawl'si-fī) The deliberate action of telling, writing, or documenting information that is inaccurate or incomplete. SEE ALSO falsification.

**falx ce·re·bel·li** (fawlks ser'ĕ-bel'ī) [TA] Short process of dura mater projecting forward from internal occipital crest below tentorium.

**falx ce·re·bri** (fawlks ser'ĕ-brī) [TA] Scythe-shaped fold of dura mater in longitudinal fissure between two cerebral hemispheres; is attached anteriorly to crista galli of ethmoid bone and caudally to upper surface of tentorium. SYN cerebral falx.

**fa·mil·i·al** (fă-mil'ē-ăl) Affecting more members of the same family than can be accounted for by chance, usually within a single sibship; commonly but incorrectly used to mean genetic. [L. *familia*, family]

**fa·mil·i·al am·y·loid neu·rop·a·thy** (fă-mil'ē-ăl am'i-loyd nūr-op'ă-thē) Disorder in which various peripheral nerves are infiltrated with amyloid and their functions disturbed.

**fa·mil·i·al dys·au·to·no·mi·a** (fă-mil'ē-ăl dis'aw-tō-nō'mē-ă) Congenital syndrome with specific disturbances of nervous system and aberrations in autonomic nervous system function, such as indifference to pain, diminished lacrimation, and poor vasomotor homeostasis.

**fa·mil·i·al goi·ter** (fă-mil'ē-ăl goy'tĕr) Group of heritable thyroid disorders in which goiter is commonly apparent first during childhood; often associated with skeletal and/or mental retardation, and with other signs of hypothyroidism that may develop with age.

**fa·mil·i·al hy·per·lip·o·pro·tein·e·mi·a** (fă-mil'ē-ăl, hī'pĕr-lip'ō-prō-tēn-ē'mē-ă) Group of diseases characterized by changes in concentration of β-lipoproteins and pre-β-lipoproteins and the lipids associated with them.

**fa·mil·i·al hy·po·gon·a·do·trop·ic hy·po·go·nad·ism** (fă-mil'ē-ăl hī'pō-gon'ă-dō-trō'pik hī'pō-gon'ă-dizm) Disorders characterized by failure of sexual development, owing to inadequate secretion of pituitary gonadotropins.

**fa·mil·i·al hy·po·par·a·thy·roid·ism** (fă-mil'ē-ăl hī'pō-par'ă-thī'royd-izm) Inherited isolated hypoparathyroidism characterized by hypocalcemia, hyperphosphatemia, cataracts, intracerebral calcifications, and tetany.

**fa·mil·i·al neph·ro·sis** (fă-mil'ē-ăl ne-frō'sis) Nephrotic syndrome appearing in sibs in infancy, without nerve deafness.

**fa·mil·i·al non·he·mo·lyt·ic jaun·dice** (fă-mil'ē-ăl non'hē-mō-lit'ik jawn'dis) Mild icterus due to increased amounts of unconjugated bilirubin in the plasma without evidence of liver damage, biliary obstruction, or hemolysis.

**fa·mil·i·al screen·ing** (fă-mil'ē-ăl skrēn'ing) Testing directed at close relatives of probands with diseases that may lie latent, as in age-dependent dominant traits, or that may involve risk to progeny, as X-linked traits.

**fam·i·ly** (fam'i-lē) **1.** Group of two or more people united by blood, adoptive, or marital ties, or the common law equivalent. **2.** In biologic classification, taxonomic grouping at level intermediate between order and tribe or genus. **3.** Substances closely related structurally. [L. *familia*]

**fam·i·ly his·to·ry** (fam'i-lē his'tŏr-ē) A written documentation made after questioning the patient about the presence or absence of diseases or conditions that might have an effect on the health of the patient.

**fam·i·ly med·i·cine** (fam'i-lē med'i-sin) Medical specialty concerned with providing continuous comprehensive care to all age groups, from first patient contact to terminal care, with special emphasis on care of the family as a unit.

**Fan·co·ni syn·drome** (fahn-kō'nē sin'drōm) **1.** Type of idiopathic refractory anemia characterized by pancytopenia, hypoplasia of the bone marrow, and congenital anomalies, occurring in members of the same family. **2.** A group of conditions with characteristic disorders of renal tubular function.

**Far·a·beuf tri·an·gle** (fahr′ă-buf trī′ang-gĕl) Area formed by internal jugular and facial veins and hypoglossal nerve.

**far·a·do·ther·a·py** (fa′ră-dō-thār′ă-pē) Treatment of disorder with faradic (induced) electric current.

**farm·er's lung** (fahr′mĕrz lŭng) Hypersensitivity pneumonitis characterized by fever and dyspnea, caused by inhalation of organic dust from moldy hay containing spores of thermophilic actinomycetes such as *Micromonospora vulgaris*, *M. faeni*, and *Thermopolyspora polyspora*, which thrive in the elevated temperatures of hay lofts and silos.

**far·sight·ed·ness** (fahr′sīt′ĕd-nĕs) SYN hyperopia.

**fas·ci·a,** pl. **fas·ci·ae** (fash′ē-ă, -ē) [TA] Sheet of fibrous tissue that envelops body beneath the skin; also encloses muscles and groups of muscles and separates their several layers or groups. [L. a band or fillet]

**fas·ci·al** (fash′ē-ăl) *Do not confuse this word with facial or faucial.* Relating to any fascia.

⊞**fas·ci·a of head and neck** (fash′ē-ă hed nek) [TA] Sheaths, sheets, or other dissectible connective tissue aggregation of head and neck, collectively. See this page.

**fas·cic·u·lar de·gen·er·a·tion** (fă-sik′yū-lăr dĕ-jen′ĕr-ā′shŭn) Degeneration restricted to certain fascicles of nerves or muscles.

**fas·cic·u·lar oph·thal·mo·ple·gi·a** (fă-sik′yū-lăr of-thal′mō-plē′jē-ă) Ophthalmoplegia due to a lesion within the brainstem.

**fas·ci·i·tis** (fash′ē-ī′tis) **1.** Inflammation in fascia. **2.** Reactive proliferation of fibroblasts in fascia.

**fast** (fast) **1.** Durable; resistant to change; applied to stained microorganisms that cannot be decolorized. SEE ALSO acid-fast. **2.** Abstinence from ingesting food. [A.S. *foest,* firm, fixed]

**fas·ti·gi·um** (fas-tij′ē-ŭm) **1.** [TA] Apex of roof of fourth ventricle of brain, an angle formed by the anterior and posterior medullary vela extending into substance of vermis. **2.** The acme or period of full development of a disease. [L. top, as of a gable; a pointed extremity]

ef

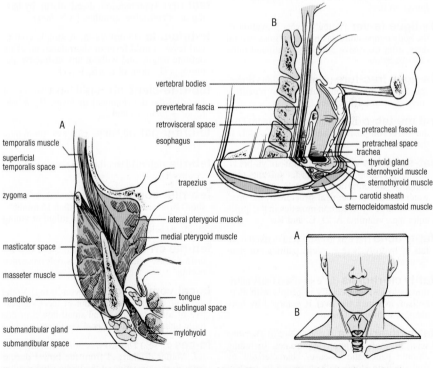

vertebral bodies
prevertebral fascia
retrovisceral space
esophagus

B

pretracheal fascia
pretracheal space
trachea
thyroid gland
sternohyoid muscle
sternothyroid muscle
carotid sheath
sternocleidomastoid muscle

A

temporalis muscle
superficial temporalis space
zygoma

trapezius

lateral pterygoid muscle
medial pterygoid muscle

masticator space

masseter muscle

mandible

tongue
sublingual space

submandibular gland
submandibular space

mylohyoid

A

B

**fascial planes of head and neck:** (A) coronal section of head; (B) cross-section of fascial planes of neck

**fast·ing hy·po·gly·ce·mi·a** (fast'ing hī'pō-glī-sē'mē-ă) Excessively low blood glucose in association with fasting.

**fast·ing plas·ma glu·cose (FPG)** (fast' ing plaz'mă glū'kōs) Blood levels of the substance measured after patient has not eaten for a given duration; generally assessed by phlebotomy first thing in the morning.

**fat** (fat) **1.** SYN adipose tissue. **2.** Common term for obese. **3.** A greasy, soft-solid material, found in animal tissues and many plants, composed of a mixture of glycerol esters; together with oils, fats comprise the homolipids. **4.** A triacylglycerol or a mixture of triacylglycerols. [A.S. *faet*]

**fa·tal·i·ty rate** (fă-tal'i-tē rāt) Death rate observed in a designated series of people affected by a simultaneous event such as a disaster.

**fate** (fāt) The ultimate outcome.

**fat em·bo·lism** (fat em'bŏ-lizm) The occurrence of fat globules in the circulation following fractures of a long bone, in burns, in parturition, and in association with fatty degeneration of the liver.

**fa·tigue** (fă-tēg') That state, following a period of mental or bodily activity, characterized by a lessened capacity or motivation for work and reduced efficiency of accomplishment, usually accompanied by a feeling of weariness, sleepiness, irritability, or loss of ambition. [Fr., fr. L. *fatigo*, to tire]

**fa·tigue fe·ver** (fă-tēg' fē'vĕr) Elevation of the body temperature, lasting sometimes several days, after excessive and long-continued muscular exertion.

**fa·tigue frac·ture** (fă-tēg' frak'shŭr) Breakage that occurs in bone subjected to repetitive stress. SYN stress fracture.

**fat me·tab·o·lism** (fat mĕ-tab'ŏ-lizm) Oxidation, decomposition, and synthesis of fats in the tissues.

**fat-sol·u·ble vi·ta·mins** (fat-sol'yū-bĕl vī'tă-minz) Vitamins, soluble in fat solvents (i.e., nonpolar solvents) and relatively insoluble in water, marked in chemical structure by the presence of large hydrocarbon moieties in the molecule; e.g., vitamins A, D, E, and K.

**fat·ty ac·id** (fat'ē as'id) Any acid derived from fats by hydrolysis (e.g., oleic, palmitic, or stearic acids).

**fat·ty cir·rho·sis** (fat'ē sir-ō'sis) Early nutritional cirrhosis, especially in people with alcoholism, in which the liver is enlarged by fatty change, with mild fibrosis.

**fat·ty di·ar·rhe·a** (fat'ē dī'ă-rē'ă) Diarrhea seen in malabsorption syndromes including chronic pancreatic disease, characterized by foul-smelling stools with increased fat content that usually float in water.

**fau·ces,** pl. **fau·ces** (faw'sēz) [TA] Area between oral cavity and pharynx, bounded by soft palate and lingual base.

**fau·cial diph·the·ri·a** (faw'shăl dif-thēr'ē-ă) Severe pharyngitis affecting the fauces.

**fau·cial re·flex** (faw'shăl rē'fleks) SYN gag reflex.

**faul·ty res·to·ra·tion** (fawl'tē res'tŏr-ā'shŭn) A restoration or replacement of tooth structure that does not adequately restore health or function to that tooth.

**faul·ty tooth·brush·ing** (fawl'tē tūth'brŭsh-ing) Inaccurate or inefficient technique of toothbrushing that results in retained deposits on tooth structures.

**FBS** Abbreviation for fasting blood sugar.

**F.D.A.** Abbreviation for Food and Drug Administration.

**F.D.I. den·tal no·men·cla·ture** (den'tăl nō'mĕn-klā-chŭr) A system of identifying teeth; used worldwide, which identifies each dental quadrant (1–4 for the permanent teeth and 5–8 for the deciduous teeth) and each tooth with a number indicating its location from the midline; e.g., 36 is the lower left first permanent molar and 62 is the upper left deciduous lateral incisor; devised by Fédération Dentaire Internationale.

**fear** (fēr) Apprehension; dread; alarm; by having an identifiable stimulus. [A.S. *faer*]

**fe·bric·u·la** (fĕ-brik'yū-lă) A simple continued fever; a mild fever of short duration, of indefinite origin, and without any distinctive pathology. [L. dim. of *febris,* fever]

**feb·ri·fa·cient** (feb'ri-fā'shĕnt) Causing or favoring the development of fever. [L. *febris,* fever, + *facio,* to make]

**fe·brif·u·gal** (fĕ-brif'yŭ-găl) SYN antipyretic (1).

**feb·rile** (feb'ril) Denoting or relating to fever. SYN pyretic.

**feb·rile con·vul·sion** (feb'ril kŏn-vŭl'shŭn) Brief seizure, lasting less than 15 minutes, seen in a neurologically normal infant or young child, associated with fever.

**feb·rile cri·sis** (feb'ril krī'sis) Stage in a febrile disease when spontaneous defervescence occurs.

**fe·cal vom·it·ing** (fē'kăl vom'it-ing) Vomitus with appearance and odor of feces suggestive of long-standing distal small bowel or colonic obstruction. SYN faecal vomiting.

**fe·ces** (fē'sēz) *This word is grammatically plural.* Matter discharged from the bowel during defecation, consisting of the undigested residue of food, epithelium, intestinal mucus, bacteria, and waste material. [L., pl. of *faex* (*faec-*), dregs]

**fec·u·lent** (fek′yū-lĕnt) Foul. [L. *faeculentus*, full of excrement, fr. *faeces*, dregs, feces]

**feed·back** (fēd′bak) **1.** In a given system, the return, as input, of some of the output, as a regulatory mechanism; e.g., regulation of a furnace by a thermostat. **2.** An explanation for the learning of motor skills: sensory stimuli set up by muscle contractions modulate the activity of the motor system. **3.** The feeling evoked by another person's reaction to oneself. SEE biofeedback.

**feed·ing** (fēd′ing) Giving food or nourishment.

**fee-for-ser·vice in·sur·ance** (fē sĕr′vis in-shŭr′ăns) Insurance coverage that reimburses participants and providers following submission of claim. Participants have few if any restrictions on which hospitals or doctors to use.

**fee-for-ser·vice plan** (fē sĕr′vis plan) A mechanism of reimbursement for services rendered; in dentistry, the agreement of patients to pay money for dental treatment as it is rendered; sometimes called indemnity insurance.

**feel·ing** (fēl′ing) **1.** Conscious experience of sensation. **2.** Mental perception of a sensory stimulus. **3.** Quality of any mental state or mood, whereby it is recognized as pleasurable or not. **4.** Bodily sensation correlated with a given emotion.

**Feer dis·ease** (fār di-zēz′) SYN acrodynia (2).

**fee sched·ule** (fē sked′jūl) A listing of the fees normally charged by a given health care provider for specific therapies and procedures.

**fel·low** (fel′ō) A board-qualified specialist pursuing subspecialty training.

**Fel·low of the A·mer·i·can A·cad·e·my of Pe·di·atrics (F.A.A.P.)** (fel′ō ă-mer′i-kăn ă-kad′ĕ-mē pē′dē-at′riks) Member of the U.S. professional organization based in Illinois; devoted to the health care needs of children.

**Fel·low of the A·mer·i·can Col·lege of Den·tists (F.A.C.D.)** (fel′ō ă-mer′i-kăn kol′ĕj den′tists) Member of a U.S. professional organization (based in Maryland) that seeks to levate and expand the profession and ethical standards of dentists.

**Fel·low of the Roy·al So·ci·ety (Can·a·da) (F.R.S.C.)** (fel′ō roy′ăl sŏ-sī′ĕ-tē kan′ă-dă) An elected member the the learned organization dedication to the promulgation of science and the humanities in Canada.

**fel·y·pres·sin** (fel′i-pres′in) Lysine vasopressin with L-phenylalanine 2. SYN octapressin.

**fe·male ath·lete tri·ad** (fē′māl ath′lĕt trī′ad)

Syndrome comprising eating disorders, amenorrhea, and osteoporosis; results from excessive physical training.

**fe·nes·tra,** pl. **fe·nes·trae** (fĕ-nes′tră, -trē) **1.** [TA] An anatomic aperture, often closed by a membrane. **2.** An opening left in a plaster of Paris cast or other form of fixed dressing to permit access to a wound or inspection of the part. **3.** Openings in the wall of a tube, catheter, or trocar designed to promote better flow of air or fluids. SYN window (1). [L. window]

**fe·nes·tra of the co·chle·a** (fĕ-nes′tră kok′lē-ă) SYN round window.

**fen·es·trat·ed** (fen′ĕs-trāt-ĕd) Having fenestrae or windowlike openings.

**fen·es·tra·tion** (fen′ĕs-trā′shŭn) **1.** In dentistry, a surgical perforation of the mucoperiosteum and alveolar process to expose the root tip of a tooth to permit drainage of tissue exudate. **2.** The presence of openings or fenestrae in a part. **3.** Making openings in a dressing to allow inspection of the parts. See this page.

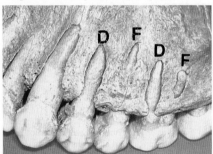

dehiscences (D) and fenestrations (F)

**fer·ment·a·ble** (fĕr-ment′ă-bĕl) Capable of undergoing fermentation.

**fer·men·ta·tion** (fĕr′mĕn-tā′shŭn) **1.** A chemical change induced in a complex organic compound by enzyme action, whereby a substance is split into simpler compounds. **2.** In bacteriology, anaerobic dissimilation of substrates with production of energy and reduced compounds. [L. *fermento*, pp. *-atus*, to ferment, from L. *fermentum*, yeast]

**fer·ment·a·tive dys·pep·si·a** (fĕr-men′tă-tiv dis-pep′sē-ă) Dyspepsia accompanied by fermentation of stomach contents.

**fer·ric** (fer′ik) Relating to iron, especially denoting a salt containing iron in its higher (triad) valence, $Fe^{3+}$. Many ferric salts are used as hematinics and supplements.

**fer·ri·tin** (fer′i-tin) An iron protein complex, containing up to 23% iron, formed by the union of ferric iron with apoferritin; it is found in the intestinal mucosa, spleen, bone marrow, reticulocytes, and liver.

**fer·rous** (fer′ŭs) Relating to iron. [L. *ferreus*, made of iron]

**fer·rule** (fer'ūl) Metal band or ring fitted a-round the crown or root of a tooth for strength. [corrupted through O. Fr. and Medieval L., fr. L. *viriola,* a small bracelet]

**fer·til·i·ty** (fĕr-til'i-tē) The actual production of live offspring.

**fer·til·i·za·tion** (fĕr'til-ī-zā'shŭn) Process beginning with penetration of secondary oocyte by one or more sperm(s) and completed by fusion of the male and female pronuclei.

**fer·ves·cence** (fer-ves'ĕns) An increase of fever. [L. *fervesco,* to begin to boil, fr. *ferveo,* to boil]

**fes·ti·nant** (fes'ti-nănt) Rapid; hastening; accelerating. [L. *festino,* to hasten]

**fes·ti·nat·ing gait** (fes'ti-nā'ting gāt) Gait in which trunk is flexed, legs are flexed at the knees and hips, but stiff; steps are short and progressively more rapid; characteristically seen with parkinsonism (1).

**fes·toon** (fes-tūn') Sculpting of denture base material to simulate natural contours of tissue, including the free and attached gingiva replaced by the appliance.

**fes·toon·ing** (fes-tūn'ing) Undulating.

**fe·tal** (fē'tăl) 1. Relating to a fetus. 2. In utero development after the eighth week.

**fe·tal al·co·hol ef·fects (FAE)** (fē'tăl al'kŏ-hol e-fekts') Physical appearance of the child of a mother with alcoholism who does not meet all the criteria for fetal alcohol syndrome (q.v.).

**fe·tal al·co·hol syn·drome** (fē'tăl al'kŏ-hol sin'drōm) Pattern of malformation with growth deficiency, craniofacial anomalies, and functional deficits including mental retardation that can result when a woman drinks alcohol during pregnancy.

**fe·tal hy·dan·to·in syn·drome** (fē'tăl hī-dan'tō-in sin'drōm) Syndrome resulting from maternal ingestion of a hydantoin analogue; involves growth deficiency, mental deficiency, dysmorphic facies, cleft palate and/or lip, and cardiac defects.

**fe·tal war·fa·rin syn·drome** (fē'tăl wōr'făr-in sin'drōm) Fetal bleeding, nasal hypoplasia, optic atrophy, and death resulting from ingestion of warfarin by the pregnant patient.

**fet·id** (fet'id) Foul-smelling. [L. *foetidus*]

**fe·tor** (fē'tōr) A very offensive odor. [L. an offensive smell, fr. *feteo,* to stink]

**fe·tor he·pat·i·cus** (fē'tōr hē-pat'i-kŭs) Peculiar breath odor in people with severe liver disease. SYN liver breath.

**fe·tor o·ris** (fē'tōr ōr'is) SYN halitosis.

**fe·tus,** pl. **fe·tus·es** (fē'tŭs, -ĕz) *Avoid the*

*incorrect plural feti.* In humans, product of conception from the end of the eighth week of gestation to the moment of birth. [L. offspring]

**FEV** Abbreviation for forced expiratory volume.

**fe·ver** (fē'vĕr) A complex physiologic response to disease mediated by pyrogenic cytokines and characterized by a rise in core temperature, generation of acute phase reactants, and activation of immune systems. SYN pyrexia. [A.S. *fefer*]

**fe·ver blis·ter** (fē'vĕr blis'tĕr) SYN herpes labialis.

**fe·ver of un·known or·i·gin** (fē'vĕr ŭn'nōn ōr'i-jin) Presence of fever (temperature >101°F or 38.3°C) of unknown cause after intensive investigation. Exact criteria for use of term vary, especially regarding duration of fever and extent of clinical investigation; generally a duration of longer than 1 week (some authors require 2–3 weeks) and thorough inpatient investigation or at least three outpatient visits, including a careful history, physical examination, and laboratory tests. SYN pyrexia of unknown origin.

**FFD** Abbreviation for focal-film distance.

**fi·ber** (fī'bĕr) 1. [TA] Extracellular filamentous structures such as collagenous elastic connective tissue fibers. See this page. 2. Nutrients in the diet that are not digested by gastrointestinal enzymes. SYN fibre. [L. *fibra*]

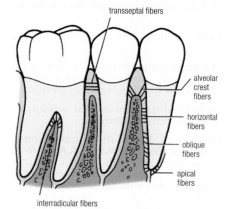

transseptal fibers

alveolar crest fibers

horizontal fibers

oblique fibers

apical fibers

interradicular fibers

**principal fiber groups of the periodontium:** five principal groups (apical, obliques, horizontal, alveolar crest, interradicular) are shown; transseptal fibers of the gingival fiber groups are also shown as they span from cervical area of one tooth to neighboring tooth

**fi·ber·op·tic gas·tro·scope** (fī'bĕr-op'tik gas'trŏ-skōp) Instrument using fiberoptics to inspect interior of stomach.

**fi·ber·op·tics** (fī'bĕr-op'tiks) An optic system in which flexible glass or plastic fibers are used to transmit light around curves and corners. SYN fibre-optics.

**fibre** [Br.] SYN fiber.

**fibre-optics** [Br.] SYN fiberoptics.

**fi·bril·lar, fi·bril·lar·y** (fī′bri-lăr, -lar-ē) **1.** Relating to a fibril. **2.** Denoting the fine rapid contractions or twitchings of fibers or of small groups of fibers in skeletal or cardiac muscle.

**fi·bril·lar·y con·trac·tions** (fī′bri-lar-ē kŏn-trak′shŭnz) Contractions occurring spontaneously in individual muscle fibers; commonly seen a few days after damage to the motor nerves supplying the muscle.

**fi·bril·lar·y my·o·clo·ni·a** (fī′bri-lar-ē mī′ō-klō′nē-ă) Twitching of a limited part or group of muscle fibers.

**fi·bril·la·tion** (fib′ri-lā′shŭn) **1.** The condition of being fibrillated. **2.** The formation of fibrils. **3.** Exceedingly rapid contractions or twitching of muscular fibrils.

**fi·brin·ase** (fī′brin-ās) **1.** Former term for factor XIII. **2.** SYN plasmin.

**fi·brin·o·gen** (fī-brin′ō-jen) A globulin of blood plasma converted into fibrin by action of thrombin in presence of ionized calcium to coagulate blood; the only coagulable protein in the blood plasma of vertebrates; it is absent in afibrinogenemia and defective in dysfibrinogenemia.

**fi·bri·nol·y·sin** (fī′bri-nol′i-sin) SYN plasmin.

**fi·bri·nol·y·sis** (fī′bri-nol′i-sis) Hydrolysis of fibrin. [*fibrino-* + G. *lysis,* dissolution]

**fi·brin·ous bron·chi·tis** (fī′brin-ŭs brong-kī′tis) Inflammation of bronchial mucous membrane, accompanied by fibrinous exudation, which often forms a cast of bronchial tree with severe obstruction of air flow.

**fi·bro·blast** (fī′brō-blast) Stellate or spindle-shaped cell with cytoplasmic processes present in connective tissue, capable of forming collagen fibers.

■**fi·bro·ma** (fī-brō′mă) A benign neoplasm derived from fibrous connective tissue. See page A15. [*fibro-* + G. *-oma,* tumor]

**fi·bro·ma·to·sis** (fī-brō′mă-tō′sis) **1.** A condition characterized by multiple fibromas, with relatively widespread distribution. **2.** Abnormal hyperplasia of fibrous tissue.

**fi·bro·my·al·gi·a, fi·bro·my·al·gi·a syn·drome** (fī′brō-mī-al′jē-ă, sin′drōm) A common syndrome of unknown cause of chronic widespread soft-tissue pain accompanied by weakness, fatigue, and sleep disturbances; characterized by chronic widespread aching and stiffness, involving particularly the neck, shoulders, back, and hips, which is aggravated by use of the affected muscles. Fibromyalgia frequently occurs in conjunction with migraine headaches, temporomandibular joint dysfunction, irritable

bowel syndrome, restless legs syndrome, chronic fatigue, and depression; symptoms are typically exacerbated by emotional stress.

**fi·bro·myx·o·ma** (fī′brō-mik-sō′mă) A myxoma that contains a relatively abundant amount of mature fibroblasts and connective tissue. [*fibro-* + G. *myxa,* mucus, + *-ōma,* tumor]

**fi·bro·nec·tins** (fī′brō-nek′tinz) High molecular weight multifunctional glycoproteins found on cell surface membranes and in blood plasma and other body fluids. [L. *fibra,* fiber, + *nexus,* interconnection]

**fi·bro·pap·il·lo·ma** (fī′brō-pap-i-lō′mă) A papilloma characterized by a conspicuous amount of fibrous connective tissue at the base and forming the cores on which the neoplastic epithelial cells are massed.

**fi·bro·sar·co·ma** (fī′brō-sahr-kō′mă) A malignant neoplasm derived from deep fibrous tissue.

**fi·bro·sis** (fī-brō′sis) Formation of fibrous tissue as a reparative or reactive process, as opposed to formation of fibrous tissue as a normal constituent of an organ or tissue.

**fi·bro·sit·ic head·ache** (fī′brō-sit′ik hed′āk) Headache centered in occipital region due to fibrositis of occipital muscles; tender areas are present and, commonly, tender nodules are found in scalp in lower occipital region.

**fi·bro·si·tis** (fī′brō-sī′tis) Inflammation of fibrous tissue. [fibro- + G. *-itis,* inflammation]

**fi·brous an·ky·lo·sis** (fī′brŭs ang′ki-lō′sis) Stiffening of a joint due to the presence of fibrous bands between and about the bones forming the joint. SYN false ankylosis, pseudankylosis.

**fi·brous dys·pla·si·a of jaws** (fī′brŭs dis-plā′zē-ă jawz) SYN cherubism.

**fi·brous in·teg·ra·tion** (fī′brŭs in′tĕ-grā′shŭn) Healing and fusing of a dental implant with a layer of such tissue between implant surface and bone; usually denotes failed osseointegration.

**fi·brous lay·er** (fī′brŭs lā′ĕr) Outer dense connective tissue layer of periosteum and perichondrium.

**fi·brous pneu·mo·ni·a** (fī′brŭs nū-mō′nē-ă) Process affecting pulmonary tissue and leading to deposition of collagen.

**field** (fēld) A definite area of plane surface, considered in relation to some specific object.

**field block** (fēld blok) Regional anesthesia produced by infiltration of local anesthetic solution into tissues surrounding an operative field.

**field block an·es·the·si·a** (fēld blok an′es-thē′zē-ă) Conduction anesthesia in which small nerves are not anesthetized individually but instead are blocked en masse by local anesthetic solution injected to form a barrier proximal to the operative site.

**fifth cra·ni·al nerve [CN V]** (fifth krā′nē-ăl nĕrv) SYN trigeminal nerve [CN V].

**fifth dis·ease** (fifth di-zēz′) SYN erythema infectiosum. [the others are measles, scarlet fever, rubella, and Filatov-Dukes diseases.]

**fil·a·ment** (fil′ă-mĕnt) **1.** SYN filamentum. **2.** BACTERIOLOGY a fine threadlike form, unsegmented or segmented without constrictions. [L. *filamentum,* fr. *filum,* a thread]

**fil·a·men·tum,** pl. **fil·a·men·ta** (fil-ă-men′tŭm, -tă) A fibril, fine fiber, or threadlike structure. SYN filament (1). [L.]

**fil·a·ri·a·sis** (fil′ă-rī′ă-sis) Presence of filariae in the tissues of the body or in blood or tissue fluids; occurring in tropic and subtropic regions.

**Fi·la·tov-Dukes dis·ease** (fē′lah-tof dūks di-zēz′) Exanthem-producing infectious childhood disease of unknown etiology. SYN fourth disease.

**file** (fīl) Dental instrument used to crush large calculus deposits and to smooth, grind, and cut. Its working-end has several cutting edges.

**fi·li·form pa·pil·lae** (fil′i-fōrm pă-pil′ē) [TA] Numerous elongated conic keratinized projections on dorsum of tongue. See this page.

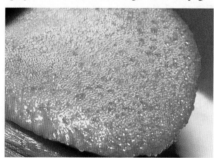

filiform and fungiform papillae of tongue

**fill·ed com·po·site** (fild kŏm-poz′it) Colloq. for fine particle composite resin (q.v.).

**fill·ed seal·ant** (fild sē′lănt) Adhesive agent that contains, in addition to Bis-GMA, microparticles of glass, quartz, silica, and other fillers used in composite restorations; fillers make the sealant more resistant to abrasion.

**fill·er** (fil′ĕr) In dentistry, glass or silicate particles used to occupy space in any resin composite restorative material.

**fill·er res·in** (fil′ĕr rez′in) SYN fine particle composite resin.

**fill·ing** (fil′ing) Lay term for a dental restoration. See this page.

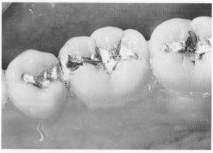

amalgam fillings in teeth

**film** (film) **1.** Thin sheet of flexible material coated with a light-sensitive or x-ray-sensitive substance used for radiographs. **2.** A radiograph (colloq.). See page 231.

**film badge** (film baj) Device consisting of a strip of photographic film in a lightproof envelope, worn by dentists and ancillary personnel to monitor occupational exposure to x-rays. SYN radiation dosimeter.

**film hang·er** (film hang′ĕr) A device with clamps that secures radiographic film(s).

**film mount·ing** (film mownt′ing) The procedure of systematically securing radiographs to a device for evaluation.

**film place·ment** (film plās′mĕnt) Putting radiographic film on an area or site.

**film plas·tic** (film plas′tik) Outer protective covering on dental radiographic film.

**film speed** (film spēd) Relative sensitivity of film emulsion to light or radiation exposure; is inversely related to detail resolution.

**Fi·lo·vi·ri·dae** (fī′lō-vī′ri-dē) A family of filamentous, single-stranded, negative sense RNA viruses with an enveloped nucleocapsid. [L. *filum,* thread, + virus]

**fil·ter** (fil′tĕr) **1.** A porous substance through which a liquid or gas is passed to separate it from contained particulate matter or impurities to sterilize. **2.** In diagnostic or therapeutic radiology, a plate made of one or more metals such as aluminum and copper that, placed in the x- or gamma ray beam, permits passage of a greater proportion of higher-energy radiation and attenuation of lower-energy and less desirable radiation. [Mediev. L. *filtro,* pp. -atus, to strain through felt, fr. *filtrum,* felt]

**fil·ter pa·per** (fil′tĕr pā′pĕr) Paper used in pharmacy and chemistry to filter solutions.

**fil·tra·tion** (fil-trā′shŭn) **1.** Process of passing liquid or gas through a filter. **2.** In radiology, process of attenuating and hardening a beam of x- or gamma rays by interposing a filter between radiation source and the object being irradiated. SYN percolation (2).

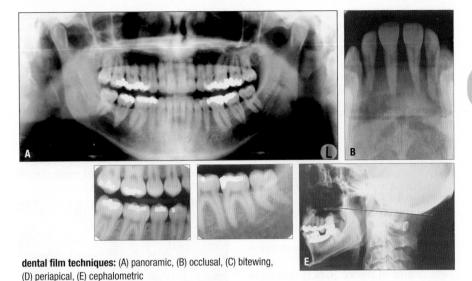

**dental film techniques:** (A) panoramic, (B) occlusal, (C) bitewing, (D) periapical, (E) cephalometric

**fim·bri·at·ed fold of in·fe·ri·or sur·face of tongue** (fim´brē-ā-tĕd fōld in-fēr´ē-ŏr sŭr´făs tŭng) [TA] One of several folds running outward from the frenulum on the lingual undersurface. See this page.

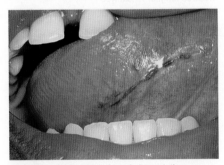

**fimbriated fold:** note darkened pigmentation

**fi·nal im·pres·sion** (fī´năl im-presh´ŭn) In dentistry, impression to make master cast.

**find·ing** (fīnd´ing) A clinically significant observation, usually used in relation to one found on physical examination or laboratory test.

**fine·ness** (fīn´nĕs) A designator used to indicate the precious metal content of an alloy, 1000 fine being 24-carat or pure gold.

**fine par·ti·cle com·pos·ite res·in** (fīn pahr´ti-kĕl kŏm-poz´it rez´in) Restorative material that contains irregularly shaped glass or quartz filler particles of more or less uniform size. SYN filler resin.

**fine trem·or** (fīn trem´ŏr) Tremor in which amplitude is small and frequency usually exceeds 12 Hz.

**fin·ger** (fing´gĕr) [TA] One of the digits of the hand. [A.S.]

**fin·ger as·sist ful·crum** (fing´gĕr ă-sist´ ful´krŭm) Advanced stabilizing point in which a finger of the nondominant hand is used to concentrate lateral pressure against the tooth surface and help control the instrument stroke.

**fin·ger grasp** (fing´gĕr grasp) The use of the digits of the hand to secure an instrument.

**fin·ger·like for·ma·tion** (fing´gĕr-līk fōr-mā´shŭn) Long narrow deposit of calculus running parallel or at an oblique angle to the long axis of the tooth.

**fin·ger-on-fin·ger ful·crum** (fing´gĕr fing´gĕr ful´krŭm) Advanced intraoral stabilizing point in which finger of the nondominant hand serves as a rest for the dominant.

**fin·ger per·cus·sion** (fing´gĕr pĕr-kŭsh´ŭn) Percussion in which a finger of one hand is used as a plessimeter and one of the other hand as a plessor.

**fin·ger po·si·tion** (fing´gĕr pŏ-zish´ŭn) Indication of where to place individual fingers on dental tools or structures.

**fin·ger·print** (fing´gĕr-print´) **1.** An impression of the inked bulb of the distal phalanx of a finger, showing the configuration of the surface ridges, used as a means of identification. **2.** Term for any analytic method capable of making fine distinctions between similar compounds or gel patterns.

**fin·ger rest** (fing´gĕr rest) The place on a structure (e.g., tooth) where the finger of the hand holding the instrument (i.e., fulcrum finger) is placed to provide stabilization and control during use of the instrument.

ef

**fin·ger·spell·ing** (fing′gĕr-spel′ing) Method of communication using specific finger and hand movements.

**fin·ish·ing bur** (fin′ish-ing bŭr) Bur with numerous fine cutting blades placed close together; used to contour restorations.

**fire** (fīr) **1.** In dentistry, the fusing of water and a powder containing kaolin, feldspar, and other substances to produce porcelain used in restorations and artificial teeth. **2.** One of five elements balanced by acupuncture treatments (the others are water, metal, earth, and wood).

**first aid** (fĭrst ād) Immediate assistance administered in the case of injury or sudden illness by a bystander or other layperson, before the arrival of trained medical personnel.

**first arch syn·drome** (fĭrst ahrch sin′drōm) Generic term that includes syndromes of malformations involving derivatives of the first branchial (pharyngeal) arch, with or without associated malformations.

**first cra·ni·al nerve [CN I]** (fĭrst krā′nē-ăl nĕrv) SYN olfactory nerve [CN I].

**first-de·gree burn** (fĭrst-dĕ-grē′ bŭrn) SYN superficial burn.

**first den·ti·tion** (fĭrst den-tish′ŭn) SYN deciduous tooth.

**first mes·sen·ger** (fĭrst mes′ĕn-jĕr) Hormone that binds to a receptor on cell surface and, in so doing, communicates with intracellular metabolic processes.

**first mo·lar, first per·ma·nent mo·lar** (fĭrst mō′lăr, pĕr′mă-nĕnt) Sixth permanent tooth or fourth deciduous tooth in the maxilla and mandible on either side of the midsagittal plane of the head following the arch form.

**first phar·yn·ge·al arch** (fĭrst fă-rin′jē-ăl ahrch) First postural arch in the branchial arch series. SYN mandibular arch.

**first phar·yn·ge·al groove** (fĭrst fă-rin′ jē-ăl grūv) SYN hyomandibular cleft.

**first vis·cer·al cleft** (fĭrst vis′ĕr-ăl kleft) SYN hyomandibular cleft.

**Fish·er syn·drome** (fish′ĕr sin′drōm) Syndrome characterized by ophthalmoplegia, ataxia, and areflexia.

**fis·sion** (fish′ŭn) **1.** The act of splitting, e.g., a mitotic division of a cell or its nucleus. **2.** Splitting of the nucleus of an atom. [L. *fissio*, a cleaving, fr. *findo*, pp. *fissus*, to cleave]

**fis·su·ra an·ti·tra·go·he·li·ci·na** (fi-sūr′ă an′tē-trā′gō-hel-i-sē′nă) [TA] A fissure in the auricular cartilage between the tail of the helix and the antitragus. SYN antitragohelicine fissure.

**fis·sur·al cyst** (fish′ŭr-ăl sist) Lesion derived from epithelial remnants entrapped along the fusion line of embryonal processes.

**fis·sure** (fish′ŭr) In dentistry, developmental break or fault in tooth enamel.

**fis·sure bur** (fish′ŭr bŭr) Cylindric or tapered rotary cutting tool used to extend or widen fissures in a tooth, as for general surface reduction of tooth substance.

**fis·sure ca·ries** (fish′ŭr kar′ēz) Caries beginning in a fissure on occlusal surfaces of posterior teeth.

**fis·sured frac·ture** (fish′ŭrd frak′chŭr) SYN linear fracture.

**fis·sured tongue** (fish′ŭrd tŭng) Painless lingual condition characterized by presence of numerous grooves or furrows on the dorsal surface. See this page. SYN grooved tongue, lingua fissurata, lingua plicata.

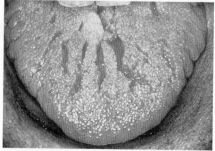

**fissured tongue:** variant type

**fis·sure seal·ant** (fish′ŭr sēl′ănt) Dental material used to seal nonfused, noncarious pits and fissures on surfaces of teeth. See this page. SYN dental sealant.

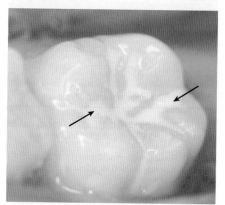

**fissure sealant:** tooth with opaque sealant

**fis·tu·la,** pl. **fis·tu·lae,** pl. **fis·tu·las** (fis′ tyū-lă, -lē, -lăz) An abnormal passage from one epithelial surface to another. See page 233. [L. a pipe, a tube]

**fit** (fit) **1.** In dentistry, adaptation of any dental restoration, e.g., of an inlay to the cavity preparation in a tooth, or of a denture to its basal seat. **2.** A convulsion. **3.** Epileptic seizure. [A.S. *fitt*]

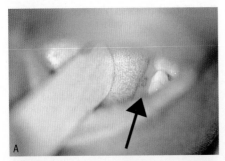

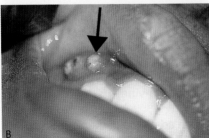

**fistula:** presence of lesion may be suggested by small red papule (arrow, A) or by large fluctuant swelling (arrow, B)

**fit·ness** (fit′nĕs) **1.** Well-being. **2.** Suitability.

**fix·a·tion** (fik-sā′shŭn) The condition of being firmly attached or set. [L. *figo*, pp. *fixus*, to fix, fasten]

**fix·a·tive** (fik′să-tiv) **1.** Serving to fix, bind, or make firm or stable. **2.** A substance used for the preservation of gross and histologic specimens.

◾**fix·ed ap·pli·ance** (fikst ă-plī′ăns) Bonded or banded device affixed to individual teeth or groups of teeth. See this page.

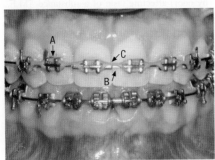

**fixed appliance system:** bonded brackets (A) with arch wire (B) held in place by elastomers (C)

**fix·ed bridge** (fikst brij) SYN fixed partial denture.

◾**fix·ed par·tial den·ture** (fikst pahr′shăl den′chŭr) Restoration of one or more missing teeth that cannot be readily removed by patient or dentist; permanently attached to natural teeth or roots that furnish the primary support to the appliance. See this page. SYN bridge (3), fixed bridge.

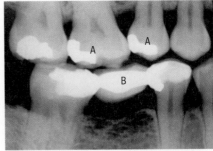

**amalgam restorations (A) and fixed bridge (B):** bitewing radiograph

**fix·ed space main·tain·er** (fikst spās mān-tā′nĕr) Any such dental device not removable by the patient.

**fix·ed splint** (fixt splint) A permanently affixed dental support.

**fix·er** (fiks′ĕr) In photography and radiography, a solution that removes both the unexposed and undeveloped silver halide crystals from the film emulsion and hardens the gelatin.

**flac·cid** (flak′sid) *Avoid the mispronunciation flas′id.* Relaxed, flabby, or without tone. [L. *flaccidus*]

**flac·cid part of tym·pan·ic mem·brane** (flak′sid pahrt tim-pan′ik mem′brān) [TA] Triangular loose part of tympanic membrane between malleolar folds.

**flag** (flag) MEDICAL TRANSCRIPTION warning or caution by the transcriptionist to the author of a report, pointing out problems (e.g., missing date, dictation errors, equipment problems, or potentially inflammatory remarks).

**fla·gel·lum,** pl. **fla·gel·la** (flă-jel′ŭm, -ă) Whiplike locomotory organelle of constant structural arrangement consisting of nine double peripheral microtubules and two single central microtubules. [L. dim. of *flagrum*, a whip]

**flange** (flanj) That part of denture base that extends from cervical ends of teeth to border of the denture.

**flange con·tour** (flanj kon′tūr) Design of a denture flange.

**flap** (flap) **1.** Tissue for transplantation, vascularized by a pedicle flap. **2.** An uncontrolled movement, as of the hands. [M.E. *flappe*]

**flap op·er·a·tion** (flap op-ĕr-ā′shŭn) In dental surgery, operation in which a portion of the mucoperiosteal tissues is surgically detached from the underlying bone for better access and visibility.

**flap sur·ge·ry** (flap sŭr′jĕr-ē) SEE flap operation.

**flash** (flash) Excess material extruded between the sections of a flask in the process of molding denture bases or other dental restorations. See this page.

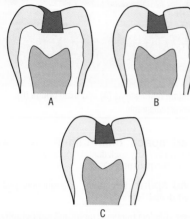

A        B

C

**defects due to poor carving:** (A) overextension or flash; (B) submarginal area (deficient margin); (C) open margin

**flash dis·per·sal** (flash dis-pĕr′săl) Rapid disintegration of a tablet lingually.

**flash·ing pain syn·drome** (flash′ing pān sin′drōm) Sudden, intermittent, and severe brief episodes of pain, without apparent cause in the distribution of a spinal dermatome; resembles pain of tic douloureux.

**flash ster·il·i·za·tion** (flash ster′i-lī-zā′shŭn) Method for sterilizing unwrapped patient-care items to be used immediately.

**flask** (flask) Small receptacle, usually glass, used for holding liquids, powder, or gases. [M.E. keg, fr. Fr. *flasque,* fr. Germanic]

**flask clo·sure** (flask klō′zhŭr) In dentistry, procedure of bringing two halves or parts of a flask together; trial flask closures are preliminary closures made to eliminate excess denture-base material and to ensure mold is completely filled; final flask closure is the last closure of a flask before curing, following trial packing of the mold with denture-base material.

**flask·ing** (flask′ing) Process of investing cast and a wax denture in a flask preparatory to molding the denture-base material into the form of the denture.

**flat af·fect** (flat a′fekt) Absence of emotional tone or reaction typically shown by oneself or others under similar circumstances.

**flat o·ral le·sion** (flat ō′răl lē′zhŭn) Abnormal tissue occurring on oral mucosa that is level with the surface of the tissue.

**flat tongue** (flat tŭng) A condition of the tongue wherein its borders cannot be rolled.

**flat·u·lence** (flat′yū-lĕns) Presence of an excessive amount of gas in the stomach and intestines.

**flat·u·lent dys·pep·si·a** (flat′yū-lĕnt dis-pep′sē-ă) Stomach upset with frequent eructations of swallowed air.

**fla·tus** (flā′tŭs) Gas or air in the gastrointestinal tract that may be expelled through the anus. [L. a blowing]

**fla·vin, fla·vine** (flā′vin, -vēn) SYN riboflavin. [L. *flavus,* yellow]

**fla·vin ad·e·nine di·nu·cle·o·tide (FAD)** (flā′vin ad′ĕ-nēn dī-nū′klē-ō-tīd) A condensation product of riboflavin and adenosine 5′-diphosphate.

*Fla·vo·bac·te·ri·um* (flā′vō-bak-tēr′ē-ŭm) A genus of aerobic to facultatively anaerobic, non-spore-forming, motile and nonmotile bacteria containing gram-negative rods. Some species are pathogenic. [L. *flavus,* yellow]

**fla·vone** (flā′vōn) A plant pigment that is the basis of the flavonoids; it is a potent inhibitor of prostaglandin biosynthesis.

**fla·vo·noids** (flā′vŏ-noydz) Substances of plant origin containing flavone in various combinations.

**fla·vor** (flā′vŏr) The quality (influenced mainly by odor) affecting taste of a substance. [M.E., fr. O. Fr., fr. L.L. *flator,* aroma, fr. *flo,* to blow]

**Flet·cher fac·tor** (flech′ĕr fak′tōr) SYN prekallikrein.

**flex·i·bil·i·ty** (fleks′i-bil′i-tē) Joint range of motion dependent on condition of surrounding structures.

**flex·i·ble shank** (fleks′i-bĕl shank) Thin diameter shank that enhances the amount of tactile information transmitted to the clinicians fingers.

**flex·ion** (flek′shŭn) **1.** The act of flexing or bending. **2.** The condition of being flexed or bent. SYN open-packed position (2). [L. *flecto,* pp. *flexus,* to bend]

**flex·ure** (flek′shŭr) [TA] A bend, as in an organ or structure. [L. *flexura*]

**flip·per** (flip′ĕr) Colloq. usage for interim prosthesis.

**float·er** (flōt′ĕr) **1.** Colloquial term for a cadaver removed from a body of water. **2.** An object in the field of vision that originates in the vitreous body.

**floor of mouth** (flōr mowth) That area of the oral cavity beneath the tongue.

**flo·ra** (flō′ră) **1.** Plant life. **2.** The population of microorganisms inhabiting body surfaces of healthy conventional animals. [L. *Flora,* goddess of flowers, fr. *flos* (*flor-*), a flower]

**floss** (flaws ) **1.** SYN dental floss. **2.** To use dental floss in oral hygiene.

**floss cleft** (flaws kleft) A groove in the gingival margin usually at a mesial or distal line angle of a tooth where dental floss was repeatedly applied improperly. SYN floss cut.

**floss cut** (flaws kŭt) SYN floss cleft.

**floss·ing** (flaws′ing) The act of manipulating dental floss on the interproximal surfaces of teeth to remove soft deposits.

**floss·ing aid** (flaws′ing ād) Device designed to secure dental floss and assist in holding it in place.

**floss silk** (flaws silk) SYN dental floss.

**flow** (flō) Movement of a liquid or gas; [A.S. *flōwan*]

**flow·a·ble com·pos·ite** (flō′ă-bĕl kŏm-poz′it) Resin compound that is relatively fluid when placed in a cavity before polymerization.

**Flow·er den·tal in·dex** (flow′ĕr den′tăl in′ deks) SYN dental index.

**flow·me·ter, flow me·ter** (flō′mē-tĕr) A device for measuring velocity or volume of flow of liquids or gases.

**flu** (flū) SYN influenza.

**fluc·tu·ate** (flŭk′shū-āt) **1.** To move in waves. **2.** To vary, to change from time to time. [L. *fluctuo,* pp. *-atus,* to flow in waves]

**fluc·tu·a·tion** (flŭk′shū-ā′shŭn) **1.** The act of fluctuating. **2.** A wavelike motion felt on palpating a cavity with nonrigid walls.

**flu·id** (flū′id) A nonsolid substance (i.e., liquid or gas) that tends to flow or conform to the shape of the container in which it is kept. [L. *fluidus,* fr. *fluo,* to flow]

**flu·id la·vage** (flū′id lă-vahzh′) Action produced within the confined space of a periodontal pocket by the constant stream of fluid that exits near the point of an electronically powered instrument tip; produces a flushing action that washes debris, bacteria, and unattached plaque from the periodontal pocket.

**flu·id·ounce** (flū′id-owns′) A measure of capacity: 8 fluidrachms.

**flu·id·rachm, flu·i·dram** (flū′id-ram′) *Avoid the misspellings fluid dram and fluiddram.* A measure of capacity: 1/8 of a fluidounce; a teaspoonful.

**flu·ma·ze·nil** (flū′mă-zē′nil) Benzodiazepine with antagonist properties used to treat overdose with benzodiazepine-type central nervous system depressants, or for controlled reversal of anesthesia induced by such agents.

**flu·men,** pl. **flu·mi·na** (flū′mĕn, -mi-nă) A flowing, or stream. SYN stream. [L.]

**fluor·ap·a·tite** (flōr-ap′ă-tīt) Component of teeth, fluorapatite resists acids resulting from plaque-forming bacteria and high carbohydrate intake.

**fluor·es·ce·in** (flōr-es′ē-in) Nontoxic, water-soluble indicator used diagnostically to trace water flow and visualize corneal abrasions.

**fluor·es·cence** (flōr-es′ĕns) Emission of a longer wavelength radiation by a substance due to absorption of energy from a shorter wavelength radiation, continuing only as long as stimulus present. [*fluor*spar + *-escence*, formative suffix]

**fluor·es·cent screen** (flōr-es′ĕnt skrēn) A screen coated with fluorescent crystals.

**fluor·es·cent tre·po·ne·mal an·ti·bod·y ab·sorp·tion test (FTE-ABS)** (flōr-es′ĕnt trep′ō-nē′măl an′ti-bod-ē ăb-sōrp′ shŭn test) Sensitive specific test for syphilis in which cross-reacting anti-treponemal antibodies are absorbed from the patient's serum so as not to interfere with detection of antibodies to the disease-causing strain using immunofluorescence.

**fluor·i·dat·ed salt** (flōr′i-dā-tĕd sawlt) Sodium chloride with a fluoride additive.

**fluo·ri·dat·ed tooth** (flōr′i-dā-tĕd tūth) Tooth exposed to fluorine salts during odontogenesis.

**fluor·i·da·tion** (flōr′i-dā′shŭn) Addition of fluorides to a community water supply, usually about 1 ppm, to reduce incidence of dental decay.

**fluor·ide** (flōr′īd) **1.** A compound of fluorine with a metal, a nonmetal, or an organic radical. **2.** The anion of fluorine; inhibits enolase; found in bone and tooth apatite; fluoride has a cariostatic effect; high levels are toxic. See page 236.

**fluor·ide di·e·ta·ry sup·ple·ments** (flōr′d dī′ĕ-tar-ē sŭp′lĕ-mĕnts) Fluoride treatment in an orally administered form used by patients who have less than optimal exposure to fluoride or none at all.

ef

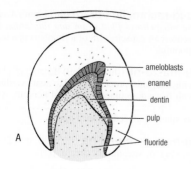

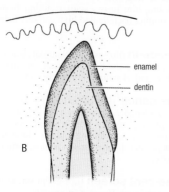

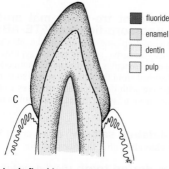

A — ameloblasts, enamel, dentin, pulp, fluoride

B — enamel, dentin

C — fluoride, enamel, dentin, pulp

**systemic fluoride:** green dots represent fluoride ions in tissues and as distributed throughout tooth; (A) developing tooth during mineralization shows fluoride from water and other systemic sources deposited in enamel and dentin; (B) maturation stage before eruption, when fluoride is taken up from tissue fluids around tooth crown; (C) erupted tooth continues to take up fluoride on surface from external sources. Note concentrated fluoride deposition on enamel surface and on pulpal surface of dentin

**fluor·ide drops** (flōr´ĭd drops) Liquid fluoride supplement solution sometimes given to children aged from 6 months to 3 years old who do not have adequate exposure to fluoride from other sources.

**fluor·ide loz·en·ges** (flōr´ĭd loz´ĕn-jĕz) SYN fluoride tablets.

**fluor·ide num·ber** (flōr´ĭd nŭm´bĕr) Percentage inhibition of pseudocholinesterase produced by fluorides; used to differentiate normal from atypical pseudocholinesterases.

**fluor·ide-re·leas·ing sea·lant** (flōr´ĭd-rĕ-lēs´ing sēl´ănt) A pit and fissure sealant that enhances caries resistance by facilitating remineralization of incipient carious lesions.

**fluor·ide tab·lets** (flōr´ĭd tab´lĕts) Supplement that may be chewed and swallowed to provide anticaries activity.

**fluor·ide tox·ic·i·ty** (flōr´ĭd tok-sis´i-tē) State in which the level of corporal fluoride absorption rises until it has become poisonous; symptoms of an acute toxic dose include: nausea, vomiting, diarrhea, abdominal pain, increased salivation, and thirst as a result of irritation to the stomach lining.

**fluor·ide var·nish** (flōr´ĭd vahr´nish) Clinically applied varnishlike coating with high concentrations of fluoride (20,000 ppm or greater) applied to the teeth every 3 to 6 months; intended to reduce tooth decay.

**fluor·i·di·za·tion** (flōr´i-dī-zā´shŭn) Therapeutic use of fluorides to reduce incidence of dental decay or topical application of fluoride agents to teeth.

**fluor·ine (F)** (flōr-ēn´) A gaseous chemical element used as a diagnostic aid in various tissue scans.

**fluor·o·scope** (flōr´ō-skōp) An apparatus for rendering visible the patterns of x-rays that have passed through a body under examination, by interposing a glass plate coated with fluorescent materials to examine a patient by fluoroscopy. [*fluorescence* + G. *skopeō*, to examine]

**fluor·o·sis** (flōr-ō´sis) Condition caused by an excessive fluoride intake (2 or more ppm in drinking water), characterized by mottling, staining, or hypoplasia of the tooth enamel. See this page.

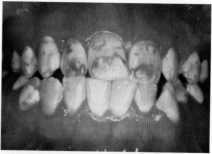

**intrinsic staining:** fluorosis

**flu·o·ro·u·ra·cil** (flōr'ō-yū'ră-sil) Antineoplastic effective in treatment of some carcinomas.

**flush** (flŭsh) **1.** To wash out with a full stream of fluid. **2.** A transient erythema due to heat, exertion, stress, or disease.

**flush ter·mi·nal plane** (flŭsh tĕr'mi-năl plān) The distal surfaces of maxillary and mandibular primary second molars that lie in the same vertical plane.

**flu·ta·mide** (flū'tă-mīd) A nonsteroidal anti-inflammatory drug used to treat arthritis.

**flu·tic·a·sone pro·pi·o·nate** (flū-tik'ă-sōn prō'pē-ŏ-nāt) Pharmaceutical corticosteroid treatment used to manage nasal symptoms of rhinitis.

**flut·ing** (flūt'ing) Stretched root branch depressions along the surface of the root. [flute, fr. O.Fr. *flaute,* + *-ing,* pr.p. suffix]]

**flut·ter** (flŭt'ĕr) Agitation; tremulousness. [A.S. *floterian,* to float about]

**flux** (flŭks) **1.** A material used to remove oxides from the surface of molten metal and to protect it when casting; serves a similar purpose in soldering operations. **2.** In diagnostic radiology, photon fluence per unit time. [L. *fluxus,* a flow]

**flux·ion·ar·y hy·per·e·mi·a** (flŭk'shŭn-ar-ē hī'pĕr-ē'mē-ă) SYN active hyperemia.

**Flynn-Aird syn·drome** (flin ārd sin'drōm) Familial syndrome characterized by muscle wasting, dementia, skin atrophy, dental caries, and other symptoms.

**foam** (fōm) **1.** Masses of small bubbles on the surface of a liquid. **2.** To produce such bubbles. **3.** Masses of air cells in a solid or semisolid, as in foam rubber.

**fo·cal** (fō'kăl) **1.** Denoting a focus. **2.** Relating to a localized area.

**fo·cal ap·pen·di·ci·tis** (fō'kăl ă-pen'di-sī'tis) Acute appendix pain involving only part of the appendix, sometimes at the site of, or distal to, an obstruction of the lumen.

**fo·cal ar·gy·ro·sis** (fō'kăl ahr'gir-ō'sis) See this page. SYN amalgam tattoo.

**fo·cal depth, depth of fo·cus** (fō'kăl depth, fō'kŭs) The greatest distance through which a point can move in focus.

**fo·cal ep·i·the·li·al hy·per·pla·si·a** (fō'kăl ep'i-thē'lē-ăl hī'pĕr-plā'zē-ă) Multiple soft nodular lesions of the lips, buccal mucosa,

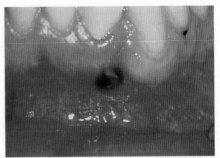
focal argyrosis: due to silver-point endodontics

tongue, and other oral sites in children and adolescents. See this page.

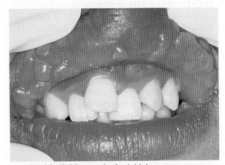
focal epithelial hyperplasia: labial mucosa

**fo·cal fi·brous hy·per·pla·si·a** (fō'kăl fī'brŭs hī'pĕr-plā'zē-ă) A small, solid mass on the tongue, lower lip, or the oral mucosa.

**fo·cal-film dis·tance (FFD)** (fō'kăl film dis'tăns) The distance from the source of radiation (the focal spot of the x-ray tube) to the film or other image-receptor. SYN source-to-image distance.

**fo·cal in·fec·tion** (fō'kăl in-fek'shŭn) Local infection that can serve as a source of disseminated or metastatic infection.

**fo·cal ker·a·to·sis** (fō'kăl ker'ă-tō'sis) Localized area of increased cornification usually confined to the lip. SEE keratosis.

**fo·cal met·a·stat·ic dis·ease** (fō'kăl met'ă-stat'ik di-zēz') Presence of a single area of metastasis of a malignant tumor or infection distant from primary lesion.

**fo·cal mo·tor sei·zure** (fō'kăl mō'tŏr sē'zhŭr) Simple partial seizure with localized motor activity.

**fo·cal spot** (fō'kăl spot) The area made of tungsten on the anode of a diagnostic x-ray tube. The electrons interact with it to produce x-rays.

**fo·cus,** pl. **fo·ci** (fō'kŭs, -sī) **1.** The point at which the light rays meet after passing through a convex lens. **2.** The center, or the starting point, of a disease process.

**fo·cused grid** (fō′kŭst grid) A term used in radiography; a grid type in which angled lead foils point toward a focus.

**fo·cus group** (fō′kŭs grūp) Small group of people gathered together to identify and discuss points of view; discussion led by outside facilitator.

**foetal** [Br.] SYN fetal.

**foetus** [Br.] SYN fetus.

**fog** (fawg) SYN light fog.

**Fo·gar·ty cath·e·ter, Fo·gar·ty em·bo· lec·to·my cath·e·ter** (fō′găr-tē kath′ĕ-tĕr, em′bō-lek′tŏ-mē) A catheter with an inflatable balloon at its tip. SYN balloon-tip catheter (3).

**fogg·ed film fault** (fawgd film vawlt) SYN artifact.

**fog·ging** (fawg′ing) A method of refraction in which accommodation is relaxed by overcorrection with a convex spheric lens.

**foil** (foyl) An extremely thin pliable sheet of metal.

**foil as·sis·tant** (foyl ă-sis′tănt) SYN foil holder.

**foil carrier** (foyl kar′ē-ĕr) SYN foil passer.

**foil con·den·ser** (foyl kŏn-dens′ĕr) Device used to impress soft gold directly into the cavity preparation of a tooth.

**foil cyl·in·der** (foyl sil′in-dĕr) One made of gold foil, usually cut into short pieces to facilitate placement in a cavity.

**foil hold·er** (foyl hōld′ĕr) Dental instrument designed to hold a pellet of gold foil in position in a cavity preparation prior to its condensation into the mass of filling material.

**foil pas·ser** (foyl pas′ĕr) A forklike instrument designed to hold and process foil being tempered for compaction into a prepared cavity. SYN foil carrier.

**foil pel·let** (foyl pel′ĕt) Small gold rounded mass used in dentistry.

**fo·late** (fō′lāt) A salt or ester of folic acid.

**fold** (fōld) A ridge or margin apparently formed by the doubling back of a lamina.

**fo·li·ate** (fō′lē-ăt) Pertaining to or resembling a leaf or leaflet.

**fo·li·ate pa·pil·lae** (fō′lē-ăt pă-pil′ē) [TA] Numerous projections arranged in several transverse folds on lateral lingual margins just anterior to the palatoglossal fold. See this page.

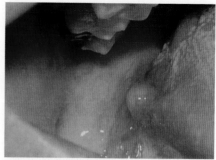

**foliate papilla:** posterolateral aspect of tongue

**fol·i·ate pa·pil·li·tis** (fō′lē-ăt pap′i-lī′tis) Inflamed vestigial foliate papillae on the posterior lateral tongue.

**fo·lic ac·id** (fō′lik as′id) The growth factor for *Lactobacillus casei*, and a member of the vitamin B complex necessary for the normal production of red blood cells. Natural sources of folic acid include whole-grain breads and cereals, orange juice, lentils, beans, yeast, liver, and green leafy vegetables such as broccoli, kale, and spinach. [L. *folium,* leaf, + -*ic*]

**fo·lic ac·id an·a·logue** (fō′lik as′id an′ă-lawg) A pharmaceutical substance that has similar, if not identical, properties to folic acid.

**folk med·i·cine** (fōk med′i-sin) Treatment of ailments outside clinical medicine using remedies and simple measures based on long experience.

**fol·li·cle** (fol′i-kĕl) [TA] **1.** A more or less spheric mass of cells usually containing a cavity. **2.** A crypt or minute cul-de-sac or lacuna, such as the depression in the skin from which the hair emerges.

**fol·lic·u·lar cyst** (fŏ-lik′yū-lăr sist) **1.** Cystic graafian follicle. **2.** SYN dentigerous cyst.

**fol·low-up, fol·low·up** (fol′ō-ŭp) Noun or adjective meaning the act of providing continuing or further attention to something.

**fo·men·ta·tion** (fō′men-tā′shŭn) **1.** A warm application. **2.** Application of warmth and moisture to treat disease.

**Fones meth·od** (fōnz meth′ŏd) A toothbrushing procedure in which occlusal surfaces are brushed in an anterior-posterior direction, the lingual and palatal surfaces are brushed in small circles, and the facial surfaces are brushed in sweeping circles with the teeth in occlusion.

**food** (fūd) That which is eaten to supply necessary nutritive elements. [A.S. *fōda*]

**Food and Drug Ad·min·i·stra·tion (F.D.A.)** (fūd drŭg ad-min′i-strā′shŭn) The U.S. federal agency charged with oversight of all issues related to the safety of pharmaceuticals and alimentation.

**food asth·ma** (fūd az′mă) Disorder caused by allergic reaction to a dietary item.

**food fe·ver** (fūd fē′vĕr) Disorder seen primarily in childhood, consisting of a sudden rise of temperature accompanied by marked digestive disturbances, of days to weeks.

**food fre·quen·cy check·list** (fūd frēk′wĕn-sē chek′list) A written record of what is eaten to allow dietary recommendations.

**food gorg·ing** (fūd gōrj′ing) A sudden and rapid consumption of food; may be followed by an expulsion of it through vomiting.

**Food Guide Pyr·a·mid** (fūd gīd pir′ă-mid) U.S. Department of Agriculture guidelines for sound nutrition that emphasize grains, vegetables, and fruits and downplay food sources high in animal protein, lipids, and dairy products. SYN MyPyramid.

**food im·pac·tion** (fūd im-pak′shŭn) Forcible wedging of food between adjacent teeth during mastication, producing gingival recession and pocket formation.

**food poi·son·ing** (fūd poy′zŏn-ing) Poisoning in which the active agent is contained in ingested food.

**food re·cord** (fūd rek′ŏrd) SYN dietary assessment.

**foot**, pl. **feet** (fut, fēt) **1.** [TA] The distal part of the leg. **2.** A unit of length, containing 12 inches, equal to 30.48 cm. [A.S. *fōt*]

**foot con·den·ser** (fut kŏn-dens′ĕr) Device used in working with gold foil; has a foot-shaped nib.

**foot plug·ger** (fut plŭg′ĕr) Plugger shaped like a foot; used for condensing gold foil.

**foot tim·er** (fut tī′mĕr) Radiographic timer controlled by a pedal.

**fo·ra·men**, pl. **fo·ram·i·na** (fōr-ā′mĕn, mi-nă) [TA] An aperture or perforation through a bone or a membranous structure. [L. an aperture, fr. *foro*, to pierce]

**for·a·men ce·cum of tongue** (fōr-ā′mĕn sē′kŭm tŭng) [TA] Median pit on dorsum of posterior part of tongue, from which limbs of a V-shaped furrow run forward and outward. SYN ductus, lingualis, cecal foramen of tongue.

**fo·ra·men mag·num** (fōr-ā′mĕn mag′nŭm) [TA] The large opening in the basal part of the occipital bone through which the spinal cord becomes continuous with the medulla oblongata. SYN great foramen.

**force** (fōrs) The external factor that causes a change in the state of rest, motion, or direction (or both), or shape of a fixed body.

**forced-air ster·il·izer** (fōrst-ār′ ster′i-lī-zĕr) Dry-heat disinfection unit in which heated air is circulated at high velocity throughout the sterilizer chamber, shortening sterilization time. SYN rapid heat-transfer sterilizer.

**forced e·rup·tion** (fōrst ĕ-rŭp′shŭn) Assisted eruption of a tooth through covering tissues into the oral cavity. SEE eruption, extrusion.

**forced ex·pi·ra·to·ry vol·ume (FEV)** (fōrst eks-pī′ră-tōr-ē vol′yŭm) Maximal volume of air that can be expired in a specific time interval when starting from maximal inspiration.

**forced feed·ing, forc·i·ble feed·ing** (fōrst fēd′ing, fōr′si-bĕl) **1.** Giving liquid food through a nasal tube passed into the stomach. **2.** Forcing a person to eat more food than desired.

**force of mas·ti·ca·tion** (fōrs mas′ti-kā′shŭn) Motive force created by dynamic action of muscles during physiologic act of mastication. SYN biting strength, chewing force, masticatory force.

**for·ceps** (fōr′seps) An instrument to grasp a structure, for compression or traction.

**Forch·heim·er sign** (fōrk′hī-mer sīn) The presence, in rubella, of a reddish maculopapular eruption on the soft palate.

**For·dyce spots, For·dyce gran·ules, For·dyce dis·ease** (fōr′dīs spots, gran′yūlz, di-zēz′) Condition marked by the presence of numerous small, yellowish-white bodies or granules on the inner surface and vermilion border of the lips and elsewhere. See this page.

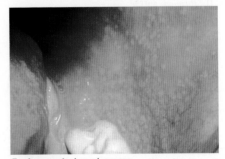
**Fordyce spots:** buccal mucosa

**fore·head** (fōr′hed) [TA] Area of face between eyebrows and hairy scalp.

**for·eign bod·y** (fōr′ĕn bod′ē) Anything in the tissues or cavities of the body that has been introduced there, is not present under normal circumstances, and is not rapidly absorbable.

**fo·ren·sic** (fōr-en′sik) Pertaining or applicable to personal injury, murder, and other legal proceedings. [L. *forensis,* of a forum]

**fo·ren·sic den·tis·try** (fŏr-en'sik den'tis-trē) **1.** Relation and application of dental facts to legal issues. **2.** Law in its bearing on the practice of dentistry. SYN dental jurisprudence, legal dentistry.

**fo·ren·sic med·i·cine** (fŏr-en'sik med'i-sin) **1.** Application of medical facts to legal matters. **2.** Law in its bearing on the practice of medicine. SYN medical jurisprudence.

**fore·shor·ten·ing** (fŏr'shŏrt-ĕn-ing) RADIOLOGY radiographic distortion occurring where the image appears shorter than the actual image.

**fork** (fōrk) **1.** A pronged instrument used for holding or lifting. **2.** An instrument resembling a fork in that it has tines or prongs.

**form** (fōrm) Shape; mold. [L. *forma*]

**for·mal·de·hyde** (fŏr-mal'dĕ-hīd) A pungent gas used as an antiseptic, disinfectant, and histologic fixative. [form(ic) + aldehyde]

**for·ma·lin** (fōr'mă-lin) A 37% aqueous solution of formaldehyde.

**for·ma·tion** (fōr-mā'shŭn) **1.** A structure of definite shape or cellular arrangement. **2.** That which is formed. **3.** The act of giving form and shape.

**forme fruste,** pl. **formes frustes** (fōrm früst) A partial, arrested, or inapparent form of disease. *The plural pronunciation is the same as the singular.* [Fr. unfinished form]

**for·mi·ca·tion** (fōr-mi-kā'shŭn) A form of paresthesia or tactile hallucination; a sensation as if small insects are creeping under the skin. [L. *formica,* ant]

**for·mo·cre·sol** (fōr'mō-krē'sol) An aqueous solution containing cresol, formaldehyde, and glycerine used in vital primary teeth needing coronal pulpotomy.

**for·mu·la,** pl. **for·mu·lae** (fōrm'yū-lă, -lē) **1.** A recipe or prescription containing directions for the compounding of a medicinal preparation. **2.** In chemistry, a symbol or collection of symbols expressing the number of atoms of the element or elements forming one molecule of a substance. [L. dim. of *forma,* form]

**for·mu·lar·y** (fōrm'yū-lar-ē) A collection of formulae for the compounding of medicinal preparations.

**for·ti·fied milk** (fōr'ti-fīd milk) Milk to which some essential nutrient, usually vitamin D, has been added.

**for·ward heart fail·ure** (fōr'wărd hahrt fāl'yŭr) A concept that maintains that the phenomena of congestive heart failure result from the inadequate cardiac output, and especially

from the consequent inadequacy of renal blood flow with resulting retention of sodium and water. Cf. backward heart failure.

**Fos·dick-Han·sen-Ep·ple test** (fos'dik hahn'sĕn ep'ĕl test) Assessment of dental caries activity based on a solution of powdered human enamel in a saliva-glucose-enamel mixture.

**fos·sa,** pl. **fos·sae** (fos'ă, -ē) [TA] Longitudinal depression below the level of the surface of a part.

**fos·sa an·ti·hel·ic·a** (fos'ă an'tē-hel'i-kă) [TA] The depression on the medial surface of the auricle that corresponds to the anthelix. SYN antihelical fossa.

**foun·da·tion** (fown-dā'shŭn) A base; a supporting structure.

**fourth cra·ni·al nerve [CN IV]** (fŏrth krā'nē-ăl nĕrv) SYN trochlear nerve [CN IV].

**fourth dis·ease** (fŏrth di-zēz') SYN Filatov-Dukes disease.

**fo·ve·a,** pl. **fo·ve·ae** (fō've-ă, -ē) [TA] Any natural depression on body surface or on surface of bone. SYN pit (2). [L. a pit]

**fo·ve·a pa·la·ti·nae** (fō've-ă pal'ă-tī'nē) Two small depressions in the posterior aspect of the palate, one on each side of the midline, at or near the attachment of the soft palate to the hard palate. See this page.

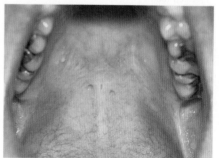

**soft palate:** fovea palatinae and median palatal raphe

**Fo·ville syn·drome** (fō-vēl' sin'drōm) Ipsilateral facial and abducens nerve paralysis, and contralateral hemiplegia, due to a lesion (usually infarction) within tegmentum of pons.

**FPG** Abbreviation for fasting plasma glucose.

**frac·tion** (frak'shŭn) **1.** The quotient of two quantities. **2.** An aliquot portion or any portion.

**frac·tion·al dose** (frak'shŭn-ăl dōs) SYN divided dose.

**frac·tion·a·tion** (frak'shŭn-ā'shŭn) **1.** Separation of the components of a mixture into its basic constituents. **2.** The administration of a course of therapeutic radiation of a neoplasm in a planned series of fractions of the total dose, most often once a day for several weeks, to minimize radiation damage.

**fracture** (frak′shŭr) A break, especially bone or cartilage. See this page. [L. *fractura,* a break]

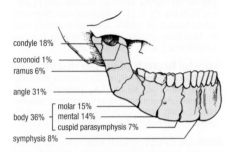

condyle 18%
coronoid 1%
ramus 6%
angle 31%
molar 15%
body 36% — mental 14%
cuspid parasymphysis 7%
symphysis 8%

**mandible:** sites and incidence of fractures

**frac·ture dis·lo·ca·tion** (frak′shŭr dis′lō-kā′shŭn) Dislocation associated with or accompanied by breakage of a bone of articulation.

**frac·ture tough·ness** (frak′shŭr tŭf′nĕs) Ability of material to resist breakage.

**fra·gile X syn·drome** (fraj′il sin′drōm) Syndrome consisting of mental retardation, characteristic facies, and macroorchidism.

**frag·ment** (frag′mĕnt) A small part broken from a larger entity.

**frame** (frām) A supporting or integrating structure made of parts fitted together.

**frame·work** (frām′wŏrk) In dentistry, skeletal prosthesis (usually metal) around which and to which are attached the remaining portions of the prosthesis to produce a partial denture.

**Fran·ci·sel·la** (fran-si-sel′lă) A genus of nonmotile, non-spore-forming, aerobic bacteria that are pathogenic and cause tularemia in humans.

**Frank·furt-man·dib·u·lar in·ci·sor an·gle** (frahngk′furt man-dib′yū-lăr in-sī′zŏr ang′gĕl) SYN facial angle (2).

**fraud** (frawd) An act of deliberate deception performed to acquire an unlawful benefit.

**FRC** Abbreviation for functional residual capacity.

**freck·le** (frek′ĕl) Yellowish or brownish macules developing on the exposed parts of the skin. SYN ephelis. [O. E. *freken*]

**free gin·gi·va** (frē jin′ji-vă) Portion of gingiva that surrounds a tooth and is not directly attached to tooth surface; outer wall of the gingival sulcus.

**free gin·gi·val groove** (frē jin′ji-văl grūv) Shallow linear notch that demarcates attached gingival tissue from free gingival tissue.

**free graft** (frē graft) Graft transplanted without normal attachments, from one site to another.

**free man·dib·u·lar move·ments** (frē man-dib′yū-lăr mūv′mĕnts) **1.** Any action made without tooth interference. **2.** Any uninhibited movements of mandible.

**free rad·i·cal** (frē rad′i-kăl) A radical in its (usually transient) uncombined state; an atom or atom group carrying an unpaired electron and no charge. SYN radical (4).

**free·way space** (frē′wā spās) Area between occluding surfaces of maxillary and mandibular teeth when mandible is in physiologic resting position. SYN interocclusal clearance, interocclusal distance (2), interocclusal gap, interocclusal rest space (2).

**frem·i·tus** (frem′i-tŭs) In dentistry, palpable vibrations or movement of a tooth, usually due to excessive contact with another tooth. [L. a dull roaring sound, fr. *fremo,* pp. *-itus,* to roar, resound]

**fre·nec·to·my** (frē-nek′tŏ-mē) Excision of frenum; usually done to reattach it to allow greater freedom of movement. [*frenum* + G. *ektomē,* excision]

**fre·no·plas·ty** (frē′nō-plas′tē) Correction of an abnormally attached frenum by surgically repositioning it. [*frenum* + G. *plastos,* formed]

**fre·not·o·my** (frē-not′ŏ-mē) Division of any frenum or frenulum. [*frenum* + G. *tomē,* a cutting]

**fren·u·lum,** pl. **fren·u·la** (fren′yū-lŭm, -lă) [TA] A small frenum or bridle. SEE ALSO frenum. [Mod. L. dim. of L. *frenum,* bridle]

**fren·u·lum at·tach·ment** (fren′yū-lŭm ă-tach′mĕnt) SEE ankyloglossia.

**fren·u·lum of low·er lip, fren·u·lum of up·per lip** (fren′yū-lŭm lō′ĕr lip, ŭp′ĕr) [TA] Folds of mucous membrane extending from gingiva to midline of lower and upper lips.

**fren·u·lum of tongue** (fren′yū-lŭm tŭng) [TA] Fold of mucous membrane extending from floor of mouth to midline of the undersurface of tongue. SYN lingual frenulum.

**fre·num,** pl. **fre·na,** pl. **fre·nums** (frē′nŭm, -nă, -nŭmz) Narrow reflection or fold of mucous membrane passing from a more fixed to a movable part, serving to check undue movement of the part. [L. a bridle, curb]

**fre·quen·cy** (frē′kwĕn-sē) The number of regular recurrences in a given time, e.g., heartbeats, sound vibrations. [L. *frequens,* repeated, often, constant]

ef

**fresh fro·zen plas·ma** (fresh frō´zĕn plaz´ mă) Separated plasma, frozen within 6 hours of collection, used in hypovolemia and coagulation factor deficiency.

**fress·re·flex** (fres´rē-fleks) Sucking and chewing movements elicited by stimulation of the face and lips. [Ger fr. *fressen,* to feed, said of animals]

**fre·tum,** pl. **fre·ta** (frē´tŭm, -tă) A strait; constriction. [L.]

**Frey hairs** (frī hārz) Short hairs of varying degrees of stiffness, set at right angles into the end of a light wooden handle; used for assessing sensation.

**Frey syn·drome** (frī sin´drōm) SYN auriculo-temporal nerve syndrome.

**fri·a·ble** (frī´ă-bĕl) **1.** Said of tissue that readily tears, fragments, or bleeds when gently palpated or manipulated. **2.** Easily reduced to powder.

**fric·a·tive** (frik´ă-tiv) Speech sound made by forcing the air stream through a narrow orifice, created by apposition of the teeth, tongue, or lips in producing consonantal phonemes such as f, v, s, and z.

**fric·tion** (frik´shŭn) **1.** The act of rubbing the surface of an object against that of another; especially rubbing the limbs of the body to aid the circulation. **2.** The force required for relative motion of two bodies that are in contact. [L. *frictio,* fr. *frico,* to rub]

**fric·tion-re·tain·ed pin** (frik´shŭn rē-tānd´ pin) Cylindric metal pin used for retention of a dental restoration and placed into a predrilled hole of a slightly smaller diameter.

**Fried·man splint** (frēd´măn splint) SYN cast bar splint.

**frit** (frit) **1.** Material from which glaze for artificial teeth is made. **2.** A powdered pigment material used in coloring the porcelain of artificial teeth. [Fr. *frit,* fried]

**Fröh·lich syn·drome** (froy´lik sin´drōm) SYN dystrophia adiposogenitalis.

**fron·tal** (frŏn´tăl) [TA] **1.** In front; relating to the anterior part of a body. **2.** Referring to the frontal plane or the frontal bone or forehead.

**fron·tal as·pect** (frŏn´tăl as´pekt) SYN facial aspect.

**fron·tal bone** (frŏn´tăl bōn) [TA] Large single bone forming forehead (anterior wall of neurocranium) and upper margin and roof of the orbit on either side.

**fron·tal bor·der** (frŏn´tăl bōr´dĕr) [TA] Edge of a bone that articulates with frontal bone. SEE frontal border of parietal bone.

**fron·tal bor·der of pa·ri·e·tal bone** (frŏn´tăl bōr´dĕr pă-rī´ĕ-tăl bōn) [TA] Margin of parietal bone that articulates with frontal bone.

**fron·tal branch of mid·dle me·nin·ge·al ar·te·ry** (frŏn´tăl branch mid´ĕl mĕ-nin´jē-ăl ahr´tĕr-ē) [TA] Anterior and larger terminal branch of middle meningeal artery; runs in deep bony groove, often perforating bone of lateralmost part of sphenoid ridge.

**fron·tal branch of su·per·fi·cial tem·po·ral ar·te·ry** (frŏn´tăl branch sū´pĕr-fish´ăl tem´pŏr-ăl ahr´tĕr-ē) [TA] Terminal branch of superficial temporal artery supplying anterolateral scalp and underlying musculature, periosteum, and outer table and diploë of cranium.

**fron·tal crest** (frŏn´tăl krest) [TA] Ridge ascending from foramen cecum to origin of sagittal sulcus on cerebral surface of frontal bone.

**fron·tal di·plo·ic vein** (frŏn´tăl dip-lō´ik vān) [TA] Vein with tributaries in spongy bone of anterior part of frontal bone that emerges through outer table of bone at or near the supraorbital notch to enter the supraorbital vein.

**fron·tal nerve** (frŏn´tăl nĕrv) [TA] Branch of ophthalmic nerve that divides within orbit into supratrochlear and the supraorbital nerves.

**fron·tal plane** (frŏn´tăl plān) [TA] Vertical plane at right angles to sagittal plane, dividing body into anterior and posterior portions, or any plane parallel to the central coronal plane.

**fron·tal pro·cess of max·il·la** (frŏn´tăl pro´ses mak-sil´ă) [TA] Upward extension from body of maxilla; articulates with frontal bone.

**fron·tal pro·cess of zy·go·mat·ic bone** (frŏn´tăl pro´ses zī´gō-mat´ik bōn) [TA] Process of zygomatic bone that extends upward to form lateral margin of orbit and articulates with frontal bone and greater wing of sphenoid bone.

**fron·tal re·gion of head** (frŏn´tăl rē´jŭn hed) [TA] Cranial surface corresponding to outlines of frontal bone.

**fron·tal si·nus** (frŏn´tăl sī´nŭs) [TA] Paranasal sinus formed on either side in lower part of squama of frontal bone.

**fron·tal squa·ma** (frŏn´tăl skwā´mă) SYN squamous part of occipital bone.

**fron·tal su·ture** (frŏn´tăl sū´chŭr) [TA] Suture between two halves of frontal bone, usually obliterated by about the sixth year.

**fron·tal tri·an·gle** (frŏn´tăl trī´ang-gĕl) Area bounded above by maximal frontal diameter and laterally by lines joining extremities of this diameter with the glabella.

**fron·tal tu·ber** (frŏn´tăl tū´bĕr) [TA] Most prominent portion of the frontal bone.

**fron·tal veins** (frŏn´tăl vānz) **1.** Superficial veins draining frontal cortex and emptying into the superior sagittal sinus. **2.** SYN supratrochlear veins.

**fron·to·eth·moi·dal su·ture** (frŏn´tō-eth-moyd´ăl sū´chŭr) [TA] Line of union between cribriform plate of the ethmoid and orbital plate and posterior margin of nasal process of the frontal bone.

**fron·to·lac·ri·mal su·ture** (frŏn´tō-lak´ri-măl sū´chŭr) [TA] Line of union between upper margin of lacrimal and orbital plate of frontal bone.

**fron·to·max·il·lar·y** (frŏn´tō-mak´si-lar-ē) Relating to frontal and maxillary bones.

**fron·to·max·il·lar·y su·ture** (frŏn´tō-mak´si-lar-ē sū´chŭr) [TA] Articulation of frontal process of maxilla with frontal bone.

**fron·to·na·sal** (frŏn´tō-nā´zăl) Relating to frontal and nasal bones.

**fron·to·na·sal duct** (frŏn´tō-nā´zăl dŭkt) Passage that leads downward from frontal sinus to open into ethmoidal infundibulum.

**fron·to·na·sal su·ture** (frŏn´tō-nā´zăl sū´chŭr) [TA] Line of union of frontal and of two nasal bones.

**fron·to·oc·cip·i·tal** (frŏn´tō-ok-sip´i-tăl) Relating to frontal and occipital bones, or to the forehead and the occiput.

**fron·to·pa·ri·e·tal** (frŏn´tō-păr-ī´ĕ-tăl) Relating to frontal and parietal bones.

**fron·to·tem·po·ral** (frŏn´tō-tem´pŏr-ăl) Relating to frontal and temporal bones.

**fron·to·zy·go·mat·ic** (frŏn´tō-zī-gō-mat´ik) Relating to frontal and zygomatic bones.

**fron·to·zy·go·mat·ic su·ture** (frŏn´tō-zī´gō-mat´ik sū´chŭr) [TA] Line of union between zygomatic process of the frontal bone and frontal process of zygomatic bone.

**F.R.S.C.** Abbreviation for Fellow of the Royal Society (Canada).

**Fru** Abbreviation for fructose.

**fruc·tose (Fru)** (fruk´tōs) A sugar that occurs naturally in fruits and honey; also called fruit sugar. [L. *fructus*, fruit, + *-ose*]

**fruc·tose mal·ab·sorp·tion** (fruk´tōs mal´ăb-sōrp´shŭn) Inborn error in metabolism in which oral D-fructose is incompletely absorbed; results in abdominal upset and diarrhea.

**FTE-ABS** Abbreviation for fluorescent treponemal antibody absorption test.

**fu·gu·tox·in** (fū´gū-tok´sin) A toxin, the roe and other parts of *Diodon*, *Triodon*, and *Tetradon*, fish found in waters of East Asia. [Japanese *fugu*, a poisonous fish]

**ful·crum,** pl. **ful·cra,** pl. **ful·crums** (ful´krŭm, -kră, -krŭmz) **1.** Point of stabilization for instrumentation with the ring finger. **2.** A support or the point thereon on which a lever turns.

**ful·crum line** (ful´krŭm līn) Imaginary line around which removable partial denture tends to rotate. SYN rotational axis.

**ful·gu·rant** (ful´gŭr-ănt) Sharp and piercing. Cf. fulminant. [L. *fulgur*, flashing lightning]

**ful·gu·rat·ing mi·graine** (ful´gŭr-āt-ing mī´grān) Headache characterized by its abrupt commencement and severity.

**ful·gu·ra·tion** (ful´gŭr-ā´shŭn) Destruction of tissue by means of a high-frequency electric current: **direct fulguration** uses an insulated electrode with a metal point, which is connected to the uniterminal of the high-frequency apparatus, from which a spark of electricity is allowed to impinge on the area to be treated; **indirect fulguration** involves directly connecting the patient by a metal contact to the uniterminal and utilizing an active electrode to complete an arc from the patient. [L. *fulgur*, lightning stroke]

**full crown** (ful krown) Artificial cap that covers the entire anatomic crown of a tooth. SYN complete crown.

**full den·ture** (ful den´chŭr) SYN complete denture.

**ful·ler's earth** (ful´ĕrz ĕrth) Amorphous variety of kaolin of varying composition, containing an aluminum magnesium silicate. [fr. *fulling*, an old process for cleaning wool, with earth or clay]

**full liq·uid di·et** (ful lik´wid dī´ĕt) Diet consisting only of liquids but including cream soups, ice cream, and milk.

**full mouth dé·bride·ment** (ful mowth dā-brēd-mon[h]´) Calculus removal completed in a single appointment or in two appointments within a 24-hour period.

**full-mouth dis·in·fec·tion** (ful mowth dis´in-fek´shŭn) Débridement of the entire oral cavity combined with the use of professionally applied topical antimicrobial therapy.

**full-thick·ness burn** (ful-thik´nĕs bŭrn) Burn involving destruction of entire skin; extend into subcutaneous tissue, muscle, or bone with scarring. SYN third-degree burn.

**full-thick·ness graft** (ful-thik´nĕs graft) A graft of the full thickness of mucosa and submucosa or of skin and subcutaneous tissue.

**ful·mi·nant** (ful´mi-nănt) Occurring suddenly, with lightninglike rapidity, and with great

ef

intensity or severity. [L. *fulmino,* pp. *-atus,* to hurl lightning, fr. *fulmen,* lightning]

**fu·mi·gate** (fyū'mi-gāt) To expose to action of smoke or fumes of any kind to disinfect or eradicate. [L. *fumigo* pp. *-atus,* to fumigate, fr. *fumus,* smoke, + *ago,* to drive]

**fu·mi·ga·tion** (fyū'mi-gā'shŭn) The act of fumigating; the use of a fumigant.

**func·ti·o lae·sa** (fŭngk'shē-ō lē'să) Impaired function. [L.]

**func·tion** (fŭngk'shŭn) **1.** Special action or physiologic property of an organ or other body part. **2.** General properties of any substance, depending on its chemical character and relation to other substances.

**func·tion·al** (fŭngk'shŭn-ăl) **1.** Relating to a function. **2.** Not organic in origin; denoting a disorder with no known or detectable organic basis to explain the symptoms.

**func·tion·al chew-in re·cord** (fŭngk' shŭn-ăl chū'in rek'ŏrd) Record of natural chewing movements of the mandible made on an occlusion rim by teeth or scribing studs.

**func·tion·al con·trac·ture** (fŭngk'shŭn-ăl kŏn-trak'shŭr) Muscular shortening that ceases during sleep or general anesthesia, caused by prolonged active muscle contraction.

**func·tion·al cross·bite** (fŭngk'shŭn-ăl kraws'bīt) Abnormal displacement when an occlusal interference requires the mandible to shift either anteriorly and/or laterally to achieve maximal occlusion.

**func·tion·al dis·or·der, func·tion·al dis·ease** (fŭngk'shŭn-ăl dis-ōr'dĕr, di-zēz') Disease characterized by physical symptoms with no known or detectable organic basis.

**func·tion·al im·pres·sion** (fŭngk'shŭn-ăl im-presh'ŭn) Imprint of dental structures in an active state, such as under a load or pressure.

**func·tion·al jaw or·tho·pe·dics** (fŭngk' shŭn-ăl jaw ōr'thŏ-pē'diks) Use of muscle forces to effect changes in jaw position and tooth alignment by removable appliances.

**func·tion·al man·dib·u·lar move·ments** (fŭngk'shŭn-ăl man-dib'yū-lăr mūv'mĕnts) All natural or characteristic movements of mandible made during speech, mastication, yawning, swallowing, and other movements.

**func·tion·al mur·mur** (fŭngk'shŭn-ăl mŭr' mŭr) A cardiac murmur not associated with a significant heart lesion. SYN innocent murmur.

**func·tion·al neck dis·sec·tion** (fŭngk' shŭn-ăl nek di-sek'shŭn) Operation to remove metastases to the lymph nodes of the neck. SYN limited neck dissection.

**func·tion·al oc·clu·sal har·mo·ny** (fŭngk' shŭn-ăl ŏ-klū'zăl hahr'mŏ-nē) Occlusal relationship of opposing teeth in all functional ranges and movements as will provide the greatest masticatory efficiency without causing undue strain or trauma on the supporting tissues, teeth, and muscles.

**func·tion·al oc·clu·sion** (fŭngk'shŭn-ăl ŏ-klū'zhŭn) **1.** Any tooth contacts made within the functional range of the opposing teeth surfaces. **2.** Occlusion that occurs during function.

**func·tion·al path·ol·ogy** (fŭngk'shŭn-ăl pă-thol'ŏ-jē) Pathology pertaining to abnormalities in function of a tissue, organ, or part, with or without associated changes in structure.

**func·tion·al re·sid·u·al ca·pac·i·ty (FRC)** (fŭngk'shŭn-ăl rĕ-zid'yū-ăl kă-pas'i-tē) The volume of gas remaining in the lungs at the end of a normal expiration; it is the sum of expiratory reserve volume and residual volume.

**func·tion·al shank** (fŭngk'shŭn-ăl shangk) Portion of the instrument shank that allows the working-end to be adapted to the tooth surface; begins below the working-end and extends to the last bend in the shank nearest the handle.

**func·tion·al splint** (fŭngk'shŭn-ăl splint) Joining of two or more teeth into a rigid unit of fixed restorations that cover all or part of abutment teeth.

**func·tion cor·rec·tor** (fŭngk'shŭn kŏr-ek' tŏr) Removable orthodontic appliance using oral and facial muscle forces to move teeth and possibly change the relationship of the dental arches.

**fun·do·pli·ca·tion** (fŭn'dō-pli-kā'shŭn) Suture of the fundus of the stomach completely or partially around the gastroesophageal junction to treat gastroesophageal reflux disease.

**fun·dus** (fŭn'dŭs) [TA] The bottom or lowest part of a sac or hollow organ; that part farthest removed from the opening or exit. [L. bottom]

**fun·du·scope** (fŭn'dŭ-skōp) SYN ophthalmoscope. [L. *fundus,* bottom, + G. *skopeō,* to view]

**fun·dus of in·ter·nal a·cous·tic me·a·tus** (fŭn'dŭs in-tĕr'năl ă-kū'stik mē-ā'tŭs) [TA] Its lateral end, the wall of which is formed by the thin cribriform plate of bone separating the cochlea and vestibule from the internal acoustic meatus.

**fun·gate** (fŭng'gāt) To grow exuberantly, like a fungus.

**fun·gi·cide** (fŭn'ji-sīd) Any substance that has a destructive killing action on fungi.

**fun·gi·form** (fŭn'ji-fōrm) Shaped like a fungus or mushroom.

**fun·gi·form pa·pil·lae** (fŭn'ji-fōrm pă-pil'ē) [TA] Numerous minute elevations on lingual dorsum of tongue, the tip being broader than the base and resembling a mushroom; their epithelia contains taste buds.

**fun·gus,** pl. **fun·gi** (fŭng´gŭs, fŭn´jī) A general term used to encompass the diverse morphologic forms of yeasts and molds. Fungi share with bacteria the important ability to break down complex organic substances of almost every type; important as foods and to the fermentation process in the development of substances of industrial and medical importance, including alcohol, the antibiotics, other drugs, and foods. Relatively few types of fungus are pathogenic for humans. [L. *fungus,* a mushroom]

**fun·gus ball** (fŭng´gŭs bawl) Compact mass of fungal mycelium and cellular debris, residing within a lung cavity, paranasal sinus, or urinary tract.

**fur·ca·tion** (fŭr-kā´shŭn) In dental anatomy, the region of a multirooted tooth at which the roots divide. See this page. [L. *furca,* fork]

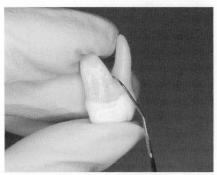

**mesial furcation of maxillary first molar probed by explorer tip**

**fur·ca·tion in·volve·ment** (fŭr-kā´shŭn in-volv´mĕnt) Extension of dental disease (involving pathologic resorption of alveolar bone and damage to periodontal ligament fibers) where roots of a multirooted tooth separate or divide.

**fur·ca·tion probe** (fŭr-kā´shŭn prōb) SYN Naber probe.

**fur·nace** (fŭr´năs) A stovelike apparatus containing a chamber for heating, melting, or fusing dental materials.

**fu·ro·se·mide** (fyū-rō´sĕ-mīd) A loop diuretic that acts by inhibiting reabsorption of sodium and chloride in the ascending loop of Henle.

**fur·red tongue** (fŭrd tŭng) SYN coated tongue.

**fur·row** (fŭr´rō) A groove or sulcus. [A.S. *furh*]

**fu·run·cle** (fŭr-ŭng´kĕl) A localized pyogenic infection, originating deep in a hair follicle. SYN boil.

**fus·ed teeth** (fyūzd tēth) Teeth joined by dentin as a result of embryologic fusion or juxtaposition of two adjacent tooth germs.

**fu·si·ble met·al** (fyū´zi-bĕl met´ăl) A metal with a low melting temperature.

**fus·ing point** (fyūz´ing poynt) SEE fusion temperature (wire method).

**fu·sion** (fyū´zhŭn) **1.** The joining of two or more adjacent teeth during their development by a dentinal union. **2.** Liquefaction, as by melting by heat. **3.** Union, as by joining together, e.g., bone fusion. **4.** Joining of two bones into a single unit, thereby obliterating motion between the two. See this page. [L. *fusio,* a pouring, fr. *fundo,* pp. *fusus,* to pour]

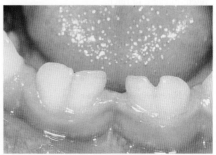

**fusion:** bilateral fusion of mandibular incisors

**fu·sion tem·per·a·ture (wire meth·od)** (fyū´zhŭn tem´pĕr-ă-chŭr) **1.** Recorded temperature at which a 20-gauge metal wire will collapse under a 3-ounce load. **2.** Recorded temperature at which porcelain becomes glazed.

*Fu·so·bac·te·ri·um* (fū´zō-bak-tēr´ē-ŭm) A genus of bacteria containing gram-negative, non-spore-forming, nonmotile, obligately anaerobic rods; found in oral cavities of humans and other animals; some species are pathogenic. [L. *fusus,* a spindle, + *bacterium*]

**fusospirochaetal** [Br.] SYN fusospirochetal.

**fu·so·spi·ro·chet·al** (fyū´zō-spī-rō-kē´tăl) Referring to the associated fusiform and spirochetal organisms such as those found in the lesions of Vincent angina. SYN fusospirochaetal.

**fu·so·spi·ro·chet·al dis·ease** (fyū´zō-spī-rō-kē´tăl di-zēz´) Infection of mouth and/or pharynx associated with fusiform bacilli and spirochetes, commonly part of the normal flora of the mouth.

**fu·so·spi·ro·chet·al gin·gi·vi·tis** (fyū´zō-spī-rō-kē´tăl jin´ji-vī´tis) SYN necrotizing ulcerative gingivitis.

**fu·so·spi·ro·chet·al sto·ma·ti·tis** (fyū´zō-spī-rō-kē´tăl stō´mă-tī´tis) Generalized infection of mouth with spirochetal organisms, usually in association with other anaerobes.

ef

# G

γ Third letter in the Greek alphabet, gamma; photon.

**G** Abbreviation for guanosine.

**Ga** Symbol for gallium.

**GAD** Abbreviation for generalized anxiety disorder.

**gad·o·lin·i·um (Gd)** (gad′ō-lin′ē-ŭm) An element of the lanthanide group; magnetic properties of this element are used in contrast media for magnetic resonance imaging.

**GAG** Abbreviation for glycosaminoglycan.

**gag** (gag) **1.** Device put in someone's mouth to prevent speech or closing of the mouth. **2.** To retch; to cause to retch.

**gag re·flex** (gag rē′fleks) Contact of a foreign body with the mucous membrane of the fauces thus causing retching or gagging. SYN faucial reflex.

**gait** (gāt) Manner of walking.

**Gal** Abbreviation for galactose.

**galactosaemia** [Br.] SYN galactosemia.

**ga·lac·tos·a·mine** (gă-lak-tō′să-mēn) The 2-amino-2-deoxy derivative of galactose.

**ga·lac·tose (Gal)** (gă-lak′tōs) An aldohexose constituent of lactose, cerebrosides, gangliosides, and mucoproteins.

**ga·lac·to·se·mi·a** (gă-lak′tō-sē′mē-ă) An inborn error of galactose metabolism due to congenital deficiency; of tissue accumulation of galactose 1-phosphate; manifested by nutritional failure, hepatosplenomegaly with cirrhosis, cataracts, mental retardation, galactosuria, aminoaciduria, and albuminuria. SYN galactosaemia. [galactose + G. haima, blood]

**ga·lac·to·su·ri·a** (gă-lak′tō-syūr′ē-ă) The excretion of galactose in the urine. [galactose + G. ouron, urine]

**ga·lac·to·ther·a·py** (gă-lak′tō-thār′ă-pē) Treatment of disease with a more or less exclusively milk diet.

**ga·le·a** (gā′lē-ă) **1.** A helmet-shaped structure. **2.** Form of head bandage. [L. a helmet]

**ga·len·i·cals** (gă-len′i-kălz) **1.** Herbs and other vegetable drugs. **2.** Crude drugs and the tinctures, decoctions, and other preparations made from them. **3.** Remedies prepared according to an official formula.

**gall** (gawl) **1.** SYN bile. **2.** An excoriation or erosion. [A.S. gealla]

**gal·lic ac·id** (gal′ik as′id) A topical astringent.

**gal·li·um (Ga)** (gal′ē-ŭm) A rare metal; atomic no. 31, atomic wt. 69.723. [L. Gallia, France]

**gal·lon** (gal′ŏn) A measure of U.S. liquid capacity containing 4 quarts. The British imperial gallon is larger by about 1 quart. [O.Fr. galon]

**gal·van·ic** (gal-van′ik) Pertaining to galvanism.

**gal·van·ic cur·rent** (gal-van′ik kŭr′rĕnt) Low-voltage direct current.

**gal·van·ic skin re·sponse (GSR)** (gal-van′ik skin rĕ-spons′) Measure of changes in emotional arousal recorded by attaching electrodes to any part of the skin and recording changes in moment-to-moment perspiration and related autonomic nervous system activity.

**gal·va·nism** (gal′vă-nizm) Oral manifestations of direct current electricity occurring when dental restorations with dissimilar electric potentials are placed in the mouth; characterized by pain or leukoplakia.

**gal·va·no·ther·a·py** (gal′vă-nō-thār′ă-pē) Treatment of disease by application of direct (galvanic) current.

**ga·me·to·cide** (gă-mē′tō-sīd) Agent destructive of gametes. [gameto- + L. caedo, to kill]

**Gam·ma Knife** (gam′ă nīf) Minimally invasive radiosurgical system used to treat benign and malignant intracranial neoplasms and arteriovenous malformations. [Gamma Knife is a registered trademark of Elekta Radiosurgery of Atlanta, Georgia.]

**gam·ma ra·di·a·tion** (gam′ă rā′dē-ā′shŭn) Ionizing electromagnetic radiation resulting from nuclear processes, such as radioactive decay or fission.

**gam·ma rays** (gam′ă rāz) Electromagnetic radiation emitted from radioactive substances; high-energy x-rays that originate from the nucleus rather than the orbital shell and are not deflected by a magnet.

**gan·gli·on,** pl. **gan·gli·a,** pl. **gan·gli·ons** (gang′glē-ŏn, -ă, -ŏnz) Originally, any group of nerve cell bodies in the central or peripheral nervous system; currently, an aggregation of nerve cell bodies located in the peripheral nervous system. [G. a swelling or knot]

**gan·gli·on·ec·to·my** (gang′glē-ŏ-nek′tŏ-mē) Excision of a ganglion.

**gan·gli·on·ic block·ade** (gang′glē-on′ik blok-ād′) Inhibition of nerve impulse transmission at autonomic ganglionic synapses by drugs.

**gan·gli·on·ic block·ing a·gent** (gang′glē-on′ik blok′ing ā′jĕnt) An agent that impairs the passage of impulses in autonomic ganglia.

**gan·gli·on·ic sa·li·va** (gang´lē-on´ik să-lī´vă) Submaxillary saliva obtained by direct irritation of the gland.

**gan·grene** (gang´grēn) *Avoid the mispronunciation gang-grēn´.* **1.** Necrosis due to obstruction, loss, or diminution of blood supply; may be localized or involve an entire extremity or organ; may be wet or dry. **2.** Extensive necrosis from any cause. [G. *gangraina,* an eating sore, fr. *graō,* to gnaw]

**gan·gre·nous cel·lu·li·tis** (gang´grĕ-nŭs sel´yū-lī´tis) Infection of soft tissue with organisms that produce extensive tissue necrosis and local vascular occlusions; streptococci, clostridia, and anaerobes are known causes, but most are polymicrobial.

**gan·gre·nous sto·ma·ti·tis** (gang´grĕ-nŭs stō´mă-tī´tis) Stomatitis characterized by necrosis of oral tissue. SEE noma.

**gap** (gap) **1.** Space created because two adjacent teeth in dental arch do not touch. **2.** A hiatus or opening in a structure.

**Gard·ner-Dia·mond syn·drome** (gahrd´nĕr dī´mŏnd sin´drōm) SYN autoerythrocyte sensitization syndrome.

**Gard·ner syn·drome** (gahrd´nĕr sin´drōm) Multiple polyposis predisposing to carcinoma of the colon. See page A6.

**gar·gle** (gahr´gĕl) **1.** To rinse the fauces with fluid in the mouth through which expired breath is forced to produce a bubbling effect while the head is held far back. It is therapeutically ineffective. **2.** A medicated fluid used for gargling. [O. Fr. fr. L. *gurgulio,* gullet, windpipe]

**gar·goyl·ism** (gahr´goyl-izm) A grossly offensive term describing appearance of patients suffering the constellation of symptoms and findings associated with Hurler syndrome.

**gar·lic oil** (gahr´lik oyl) Volatile oil from the bulb or entire plant of *Allium sativum;* contains diallyl disulfide and allyl propyl disulfide; has been used as an anthelmintic and rubefacient.

**Gar·ré os·te·o·my·e·li·tis** (gah-rā´ os´tē-ō-mī-ĕ-lī´tis) Chronic osteomyelitis with proliferative periostitis.

**gas** (gas) **1.** A thin fluid, such as air, capable of indefinite expansion but convertible by compression and cold into a liquid and, eventually, a solid. **2.** In clinical practice, a liquid entirely in its vapor phase at one atmosphere of pressure because ambient temperature is above its boiling point. [coined by J.B. van Helmont, Flemish chemist and physician, 1579–1644]

**gas·om·e·ter** (gas-om´ĕ-tĕr) A calibrated instrument used to measure volumes.

**gas ster·i·li·za·tion** (gas ster´i-lī-zā´shŭn) SYN low-temperature sterilization.

**gas·tric col·ic** (gas´trik kol´ik) Colicky pain associated with gastritis or peptic ulcer.

**gas·tric cri·sis** (gas´trik krī´sis) Attack, usually lasting several days, with severe pain in the abdomen or around the waist, accompanied by nausea and vomiting and occasionally diarrhea.

**gas·tric di·ges·tion** (gas´trik di-jes´chŭn) Stage of digestion, chiefly of proteins, carried on in the stomach by enzymes of gastric juice.

**gas·tric feed·ing** (gas´trik fēd´ing) Providing nutriment directly into the stomach with a tube inserted through nasopharynx and esophagus or more directly.

**gas·tric hy·per·se·cre·tion** (gas´trik hī´pĕr-sĕ-krē´shŭn) Excessive formation of gastric juice, especially its acidic component.

**gas·tric juice** (gas´trik jūs) Digestive fluid secreted by stomach glands; thin colorless liquid of acid reaction containing primarily hydrochloric acid.

**gas·tric tet·a·ny** (gas´trik tet´ă-nē) Tetany associated with gastric disorder.

**gas·tric va·ri·ces** (gas´trik var´i-sēz) Varices located in gastric mucosa, most commonly in the cardia and fundus, as a result of portal hypertension, which are prone to ulceration and massive bleeding.

**gas·trin·o·ma** (gas´tri-nō´mă) A gastrin-secreting tumor associated with the Zollinger-Ellison syndrome.

**gas·trins** (gas´trinz) Hormones secreted in the pyloric-antral mucosa of the mammalian stomach. [G. *gastēr,* stomach, + *-in*]

**gas·tri·tis** (gas-trī´tis) Inflammation, especially mucosal, of the stomach. [*gastr-* + G. *-itis,* inflammation]

**gas·tro·blen·nor·rhe·a** (gas´trō-blen´ŏ-rē´ă) Excessive proliferation of mucus by the stomach. [*gastro-* + *blennorrhea*]

**gas·tro·chron·or·rhe·a** (gas´trō-kron´ŏ-rē´ă) Excessive continuous gastric secretion. [*gastro-* + G. *chronos,* time (chronic), + *rhoia,* a flow]

**gas·tro·co·lic** (gas´trō-kol´ik) Relating to stomach and colon.

**gas·tro·co·lic re·flex** (gas´trō-kol´ik rē´fleks) Mass movement of colon contents, frequently preceded by a similar movement in small intestine, which sometimes occurs immediately after entrance of food into the stomach.

**gas·tro·co·li·tis** (gas´trō-kŏ-lī´tis) Inflammation of both stomach and colon.

**gas·tro·en·ter·ic** (gas´trō-en-ter´ik) SYN gastrointestinal.

**gas·tro·en·ter·i·tis** (gas´trō-en-tĕr-ī´tis) Inflammation of mucous membrane of both stomach and intestine. [*gastro-* + G. *enteron,* intestine, + *-itis,* inflammation]

**gas·tro·en·ter·i·tis vi·rus type B** (gas′ trō-en-tĕr-ī′tis vī′rŭs tīp) SYN Rotavirus.

**gas·tro·en·ter·o·co·li·tis** (gas′trō-en′tĕr-ō-kŏ-lī′tis) Inflammatory disease involving stomach and intestines. [*gastro-* + G. *enteron,* intestine, + *kōlon,* colon, + *-itis,* inflammation]

**gas·tro·en·ter·ol·o·gist** (gas′trō-en-tĕr-ol′ŏ-jist) A medical specialist in gastroenterology.

**gas·tro·en·ter·ol·o·gy** (gas′trō-en-tĕr-ol′ ŏ-jē) Medical specialty concerned with function and disorders of gastrointestinal tract, including stomach, intestines, and associated organs. [*gastro-* + G. *enteron,* intestine, + *logos,* study]

**gas·tro·en·ter·op·a·thy** (gas′trō-en-tĕr-op′ ă-thē) Any disorder of the alimentary canal.

**gas·tro·e·soph·a·ge·al** (gas′trō-ĕ-sof′ă-jē′ăl) Relating to both stomach and esophagus. [*gastro-* + G. *oisophagos,* gullet (esophagus)]

**gas·tro·e·soph·a·ge·al re·flux dis·ease (GERD)** (gas′trō-ĕ-sof′ă-jē′-ăl rē′flŭks di-zēz′) A syndrome of chronic or recurrent epigastric or retrosternal pain, accompanied by varying degrees of belching, nausea, cough, or hoarseness, due to reflux of acid gastric juice into the lower esophagus; results from malfunction of the lower esophageal sphincter (LES) and disordered gastric motility. SYN gastro-oesophageal reflux disease.

**gas·tro·e·soph·a·gi·tis** (gas′trō-ĕ-sof-ă-jī′tis) Inflammation of the stomach and esophagus. SYN gastro-esophagitis.

**gas·tro·gen·ic** (gas′trō-jen′ik) Deriving from or caused by the stomach.

**gas·trog·e·nous di·ar·rhe·a** (gas-troj′ ĕ-nŭs dī′ă-rē′ă) Diarrhea that may occur in achylia gastrica or may be caused by excess secretion of gastric and other intestinal juices.

**gas·tro·il·e·ac re·flex** (gas′trō-il′ē-ak rē′ fleks) Opening of ileocolic valve induced by entrance of food into stomach.

**gas·tro·in·tes·ti·nal (GI)** (gas′trō-in-tes′ ti-năl) Relating to stomach and intestines. SYN gastroenteric.

**gas·tro·in·tes·ti·nal hor·mone** (gas′trō-in-tes′ti-năl hōr′mōn) Any secretion of the gastrointestinal mucosa affecting the timing and quantity of various digestive secretions or causing enhanced motility of the target organ.

**gas·tro·li·thi·a·sis** (gas′trō-li-thī′ă-sis) Presence of one or more calculi in the stomach. [*gastro-* + G. *lithos,* stone + *-iasis,* condition]

**gas·trol·o·gy** (gas-trol′ŏ-jē) The branch of medicine concerned with the stomach and its diseases. [*gastro-* + G. *logos,* study]

**gas·tro·meg·a·ly** (gas′trō-meg′ă-lē) **1.** Enlargement of stomach. **2.** Enlargement of abdomen. [*gastro-* + G. *megas* (*megal-*), large]

**gas·tro·myx·or·rhe·a** (gas′trō-mik-sō-rē′ă) Excessive secretion of mucus in the stomach.

SYN gastromyxorrhoea. [*gastro-* + G. *myxa,* mucus, + *rhoia,* a flow]

**gastromyxorrhoea** [Br.] SYN gastromyxorrhea.

**gastro-oesophageal reflux disease** [Br.] SYN gastroesophageal reflux disease.

**gastro-oesophagitis** [Br.] SYN gastroesophagitis.

**gas·tro·pa·ral·y·sis** (gas′trō-păr-al′i-sis) Paralysis of muscular coat of stomach.

**gas·tro·pa·re·sis** (gas′trō-păr-ē′sis) Weakness of gastric peristalsis, resulting in delayed emptying of the bowels. [*gastro-* + G. *paresis,* a letting go, paralysis]

**gas·tro·pa·re·sis di·a·be·ti·co·rum** (gas′trō-păr-ē′sis dī′ă-bet-ti-kō′rŭm) Dilation of stomach with gastric retention in diabetic patients, commonly seen in association with severe acidosis or coma.

**gas·trop·a·thy** (gas-trop′ă-thē) Any disease of the stomach. [gastro- + G. *pathos,* disease]

**gas·tror·rhe·a** (gas′trōr-ē′ă) Excessive secretion of gastric juice or of mucus (gastromyxorrhea) by the stomach. SYN gastrorrhoea. [*gastro-* + G. *rhoia,* a flow]

**gastrorrhoea** [Br.] SYN gastrorrhea.

**gas·tro·scope** (gas′trō-skōp) An endoscope for inspecting the interior of the stomach. [*gastro-* + G. *skopeō,* to examine]

**gas·tros·co·py** (gas-tros′kŏ-pē) Inspection of the interior of the stomach through an endoscope.

**gas·tro·spasm** (gas′trō-spazm) Spasmodic contraction of the walls of the stomach.

**gas·tros·to·my** (gas-tros′tŏ-mē) Establishment of a new opening into the stomach. [*gastro-* + G. *stoma,* mouth]

**gas·tro·to·nom·e·try** (gas′trō-tō-nom′ĕ-trē) Measurement of intragastric pressure. [*gastro-* + G. *tonos,* tension, + *metron,* measure]

**gas·tro·tox·ic** (gas′trō-tok′sik) Poisonous to the stomach.

**gas·tro·tro·pic** (gas′trō-trō′pik) Affecting the stomach. [*gastro-* + G. *tropikos,* turning]

**gate-con·trol the·o·ry** (gāt′kŏn-trōl′ thē′ ŏr-ē) Proposition to explain mechanism of pain.

**gate·keep·er** (gāt′kēp-ĕr) A health care professional, typically a physician or nurse, who has the first encounter with a patient and who thus controls patient's entry into system.

**Gauch·er dis·ease** (gō-shā′ di-zēz′) Lysosomal storage disorder due to deficiency of glucocerebrosidase resulting in accumulation of glucocerebroside.

**gauge** (gāj) *Avoid the misspelling guage.* A measuring device.

**gauze** (gawz) Bleached cotton cloth of plain weave, used for dressings, bandages, and absorbent sponges. [Fr. *gaze*]

**ga·vage** (gă-vahzh′) **1.** Forced feeding by stomach tube. **2.** Therapeutic use of a high-potency diet administered by stomach tube. [Fr. *gaver,* to gorge fowls]

**Gay-Lus·sac law** (gā-lū-sahk law) SYN Charles law. [Joseph L. *Gay-Lussac*]

**Gd** Symbol for gadolinium.

**gel** (jel) **1.** A jelly, or the solid or semisolid phase of a colloidal solution. **2.** To form a gel or jelly; to convert a sol into a gel. See this page. [Mod. L. *gelatum*]

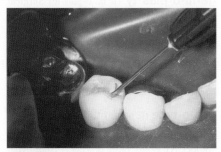

**gel etchant**

**gel·a·tin** (jel′ă-tin) Derived protein formed from collagen of tissues by boiling in water; it swells when put in cold water, but dissolves only in hot water; used as a hemostat. [L. *gelo,* pp. *gelatus,* to freeze, congeal]

**gel time** (jel tīm) Temporal duration required for a colloid solution to become a semisolid or solid gel; often refers to the setting time of hydrocolloid impression materials.

**gem·i·nate** (jem′i-năt) Occurring in pairs. [L. *gemino,* pp. *-atus,* to double, fr. *geminus,* twin]

**gem·i·nat·ed teeth** (jem′i-nā-těd tēth) Developmental anomaly arising from attempted division of one tooth bud, resulting in incomplete formation of two teeth and usually manifest as a bifid crown on a single root.

**gem·i·na·tion** (jem′i-nā′shŭn) Embryologic partial division of a primordium. For example, gemination of a single tooth germ results in two partially or completely separated crowns on a single root. See this page. [L. *geminatio,* a doubling]

**gene** (jēn) A functional unit of heredity that occupies a specific place (locus) on a chromosome, is capable of reproducing itself exactly at each cell division, and directs the formation of an enzyme or other protein. SYN factor (3). [G. *genos,* birth]

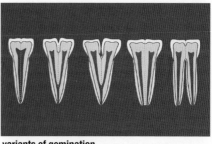

**variants of gemination**

**gen·er·al ad·ap·ta·tion syn·drome** (jen′ĕr-ăl ad′ap-tā′shŭn sin′drōm) Syndrome with single marked physiologic response in the pituitary-adrenal system, due to exposure to a variety of prolonged physical or psychological stressors. SYN adaptation syndrome of Selye.

**gen·er·al an·es·the·si·a** (jen′ĕr-ăl an′es-thē′zē-ă) Loss of ability to perceive pain associated with loss of consciousness produced by intravenous or inhalation anesthetic agents.

**gen·er·al an·es·thet·ics** (jen′ĕr-ăl an′es-thet′iks) Drugs used either intravenously or by inhalation that render patient unconscious and incapable of perceiving pain in surgery.

**gen·er·al·ized** (jen′ĕr-ă-līzd) Involving the whole organ.

**gen·er·al·ized anx·i·e·ty dis·or·der (GAD)** (jen′ĕr-ă-līzd ang-zī′ĕ-tē dis-ōr′dĕr) Chronic repeated episodes of anxiety reactions.

**gen·er·al·ized ep·i·lep·sy** (jen′ĕr-ă-līzd ep′i-lep-sē) Major category of epilepsy syndromes characterized by one or more types of generalized seizures.

**gen·er·al·ized my·o·ky·mi·a** (jen′ĕr-ăl-īzd mī′ō-kī′mē-ă) Widespread myokymia, present in multiple limbs and often the face.

**gen·er·al·ized tet·a·nus** (jen′ĕr-ăl-īzd tet′ă-nŭs) Most common type of tetanus, often with trismus as its initial manifestation; muscles of head, neck, trunk, and limbs become persistently contracted.

**gen·er·al·ized ton·ic-clo·nic sei·zure, gen·er·al·ized ton·ic-clo·nic ep·i·lep·sy** (jen′ĕr-ăl-īzd ton′ik-klon′ik sē′zhŭr, ep′i-lep′sē) Seizure characterized by sudden onset of tonic contraction of muscles often associated with a cry or moan, and frequently resulting in a fall.

**gen·er·al sen·sa·tion** (jen′ĕr-ăl sen-sā′shŭn) Sensation referred to the body as a whole rather than to any particular part.

**gen·er·at·ed oc·clu·sal path** (jen′ĕr-ā-těd ŏ-klū′zăl path) Registration of paths of movement of occlusal surfaces of mandibular teeth on a plastic or abrasive surface attached to the maxillary arch.

gh

**gen·er·a·tor** (jen′ĕr-ā-tŏr) An apparatus for conversion of chemical, or other forms of energy into electricity.

**ge·ner·ic name** (jĕ-ner′ik nām) **1.** In the pharmaceutical and commercial fields, a misnomer for nonproprietary name. **2.** BACTERIOLOGY the species name consists of two parts (comprising one name): the generic name and the specific epithet; in other biologic disciplines, the species name is regarded as being composed of two names: the generic name and the specific name.

**ge·ner·ic sub·sti·tu·tion** (jĕ-ner′ik sŭb′sti-tū′shŭn) Dispensing a chemically equivalent but less expensive drug in place of a brand-name product that has an expired patent.

**gene ther·a·py** (jēn thār′ă-pē) Inserting a gene into an organism to repair gene function to treat a disease or genetic defect.

**ge·net·ic coun·sel·ing** (jĕ-net′ik kown′sĕl-ing) The process whereby an expert in genetic disorders provides information about risk and clinical burden of a disorder or disorders to patients or relatives in families with genetic disorders.

**ge·net·ic de·ter·mi·nant** (jĕ-net′ik dĕ-tĕr′mi-nănt) Any antigenic identifying characteristic.

**ge·net·ic le·thal** (jĕ-net′ik lē′thăl) Denotes disorder that prevents effective reproduction by those affected; e.g., Klinefelter syndrome.

**ge·net·ics** (jĕ-net′iks) **1.** Branch of science concerned with means and consequences of transmission and generation of components of biologic inheritance. **2.** Genetic features and constitution of any single organism or set of organisms. [G. *genesis,* origin or production]

**ge·ni·al tu·ber·cle** (jĕ-nī′ăl tū′bĕr-kĕl) A small eminence of bone found on the lingual side of the mandible at the midline that serves as attachment site for the genioglossus and geniohyoid muscles. SYN mental spine.

**ge·nic·u·late neu·ral·gi·a** (jĕ-nik′yū-lăt nūr-al′jē-ă) Severe paroxysmal lancinating pain deep in the ear, on the anterior wall of the external meatus.

**ge·nic·u·lum,** pl. **ge·nic·u·la** (jĕ-nik′yū-lŭm, -lă) **1.** [TA] A small genu or angular kneelike structure. **2.** A knotlike structure. [L. dim. of *genu,* knee]

**ge·nic·u·lum of fa·cial ca·nal** (jĕ-nik′yū-lŭm fā′shăl kă-nal′) [TA] Bend in facial canal linking medial and lateral crura of horizontal port of canal.

**ge·nic·u·lum of fa·cial nerve** (jĕ-nik′yū-lŭm fā′shăl nĕrv) Sharp bend in facial nerve in facial canal where it turns posteriorly from its previously anterior course to run in the medial wall of middle ear (external geniculum).

**ge·ni·o·glos·sus (mus·cle)** (jē′nē-ō-glos′ŭs mŭs′ĕl) [TA] One of the paired lingual muscles; *origin,* mental spine of the mandible; *insertion,* lingual fascia beneath the mucous membrane and epiglottis; *action,* depresses and protrudes the tongue; *nerve supply,* hypoglossal. SYN musculus genioglossus [TA].

**ge·ni·o·hy·oid (mus·cle)** (jē′nē-ō-hī′oyd mŭs′ĕl) [TA] One of the suprahyoid muscles of the neck; *origin,* mental spine of mandible; *insertion,* body of hyoid bone; *action,* draws hyoid forward, or depresses jaw when hyoid is fixed; *nerve supply,* fibers from ventral primary rami of first and second cervical spinal nerves conveyed by hypoglossal nerve. SYN musculus geniohyoideus [TA].

**ge·ni·o·plas·ty** (jē′nē-ō-plas-tē) Surgical procedure performed extraorally or intraorally to reshape the bony contour of chin.

**gen·i·tal wart** (jen′i-tăl wŏrt) SYN condyloma acuminatum.

**ge·nome** (jē′nōm) Complete set of chromosomes derived from one parent; haploid number of a gamete.

**gen·o·type** (jē′nō-tīp) **1.** The genetic constitution of an individual. **2.** Gene combination at one specific locus or any specified combination of loci. [G. *genos,* birth, descent, + *typos,* type]

**gen·ta·mi·cin** (jen′tă-mī′sin) Broad spectrum aminoglycoside antibiotic that inhibits growth of both gram-positive and gram-negative bacteria.

**ge·nu,** pl. **gen·u·a** (jē′nyū, -ă) [TA] **1.** The joint between the thigh and the leg. SYN knee (1) [TA]. **2.** Any structure of angular shape resembling a flexed knee. [L.]

**gen·y·an·trum** (jen′ē-an′trŭm) SYN maxillary sinus. [G. *genys,* cheek, + *antron,* cave]

**▪ge·o·graph·ic tongue** (jē′ŏ-graf′ik tŭng) Idiopathic, asymptomatic erythematous circinate macules, due to atrophy of filiform papillae; with time, lesions resolve, coalesce, and change in distribution. See this page and page A7. SYN benign migratory glossitis, lingua geographica.

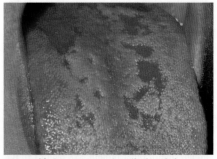

**geographic tongue:** asymptomatic denuded areas

**ge·o·met·ric un·sharp·ness** (jē'ō-met' rik ŭn-shahrp'nĕs) SYN penumbra.

**ge·o·pha·gi·a, ge·oph·a·gism, ge·oph· a·gy** (jē'ŏ-fā'jē-ă, jē-of'ă-jizm, -of'ă-jē) Eating dirt or clay. [*geo-* + G. *phagō*, to eat]

**ge·o·tri·cho·sis** (jē'ō-tri-kō'sis) An opportunistic systemic hyalohyphomycosis; diverse symptoms suggest mixed infections. [*geo-* + G. *thrix*, hair, + *-osis*, condition]

**GERD** Acronym for gastroesophageal reflux disease.

**ger·i·at·ric** (jer'ē-at'rik) Relating to old age or to geriatrics.

**ger·i·at·ric den·tis·try** (jer'ē-at'rik den' tis-trē) Dentistry that deals with the special knowledge and technical skills required to provide oral health care for older people.

**ger·i·at·ric med·i·cine** (jer'ē-at'rik med'i-sin) Medical specialty concerned with disease and health problems of older people.

**germ** (jĕrm) **1.** A microbe; a microorganism. **2.** A primordium; the earliest trace of a structure within an embryo. [L. *germen*, sprout, bud, germ]

**Ger·man mea·sles** (jĕr'măn mē'zĕlz) SYN rubella.

**germ cell** (jĕrm sel) SYN sex cell.

**ger·mi·cide** (jĕr'mi-sīd) Destructive to germs or microbes. [*germ* + L. *caedo*, to kill]

**germ lay·er** (jĕrm lā'ĕr) One of three primordial cell layers established in an embryo during gastrulation.

**ger·o·don·tics, ger·o·don·tol·o·gy** (jer'ō-don'tiks, -don-tol'ŏ-jē) SYN geriatric dentistry. [*gero-* + G. *odous*, tooth]

**ger·on·tol·o·gy** (jer'ŏn-tol'ŏ-jē) Scientific study of clinical, sociologic, biologic, and psychological phenomena related to aging. [*geronto-* + G. *logos*, study]

**ger·on·to·ther·a·peu·tics** (jer-on'tō-thār'ă-pyū'tiks) Science concerned with treatment of aged patients.

**Gerst·mann-Sträuss·ler-Schein·ker syn·drome** (gerst'mahn-stris'lĕr-shīn'kĕr sin' drōm) Chronic cerebellar form of spongiform encephalopathy.

**ges·ta·tion** (jes-tā'shŭn) SYN pregnancy. [L. *gestatio*, from *gesto*, pp. *gestatus*, to bear]

**ges·ta·tion·al age** (jes-tā'shŭn-ăl āj) In obstetrics, developmental age of a fetus, usually based on presumed first day of last normal menstrual period.

**G fac·tor** (fak'tŏr) Substance required for growth of a specific organism.

**GFR** Abbreviation for glomerular filtration rate.

**GH** Abbreviation for growth hormone.

**GHB** Abbreviation for γ-hydroxybutyrate.

**ghost tooth** (gōst tūth) SYN odontodysplasia.

**GI** Abbreviation for gastrointestinal; Gingival Index.

**gi·ant cell** (jī'ănt sel) A cell of large size, often with many nuclei.

▣**gi·ant cell fi·bro·ma** (jī'ănt sel fī-brō'mă) Tumor of oral mucosa composed of fibrous connective tissue with large stellate and multinucleate fibroblasts. See page A15.

**gi·ant cell gran·u·lo·ma** (jī'ănt sel gran'yū-lō'mă) Nonneoplastic lesion characterized by a proliferation of granulation tissue containing numerous multinucleated giant cells; occurs in gingiva and alveolar mucosa (occasionally in other soft tissues) where it presents as a soft red-blue hemorrhagic nodular swelling; also occurs within the mandible or maxilla as a unilocular or multilocular radiolucency.

**gi·ant cell hy·a·line an·gi·op·a·thy** (jī'ănt sel hī'ă-lin an'jē-op'ă-thē) Inflammatory infiltrate containing foreign body giant cells and eosinophilic material.

**gi·ant cell my·e·lo·ma** (jī'ănt sel mī'ĕ-lō'mă) SYN giant cell tumor of bone.

**gi·ant cell tu·mor of bone** (jī'ănt sel tū'mŏr bōn) A soft, reddish-brown, sometimes malignant, osteolytic tumor composed of multinucleated giant cells and ovoid or spindle-shaped cells; most frequent in young adults. SYN osteoclastoma.

**gi·ant ur·ti·car·i·a** (jī'ănt ŭr'ti-kar'ē-ă) SYN angioedema.

***Gi·ar·di·a*** (jē-ahr'dē-ă) A genus of flagellates that parasitizes the small intestine of human beings, domestic and wild mammals, and birds.

**gi·ar·di·a·sis** (jē'ahr-dī'ă-sis) Infection with the parasite *Giardia*; *G. lamblia* may cause diarrhea, dyspepsia, and malabsorption.

**gi·gan·ti·form ce·men·to·ma** (jī-gan'ti-fōrm sē'men-tō'mă) Familial occurrence of cemental masses in the jaws.

**gi·gan·tism** (jī-gant'izm) A condition of abnormal size or overgrowth of the entire body or of any of its parts. Also called giantism.

**Gil·lies op·er·a·tion** (gil'ēz op-ĕr-ā'shŭn) A technique for reducing fractures of the zygoma and the zygomatic arch through an incision in the temporal region above the hairline.

▣**Gill·more need·le** (gil'mōr nē'dĕl) Device

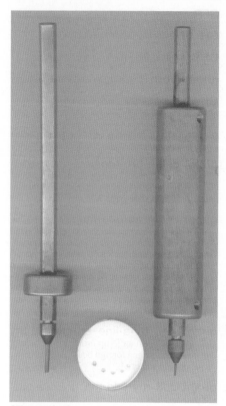

**Gillmore needles**

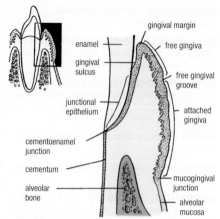

**parts of the gingiva:** cross-sectional diagram shows parts of gingiva and adjacent tissues of a partially erupted tooth. Note junctional epithelium on enamel

Labels in diagram: gingival margin, enamel, free gingiva, gingival sulcus, free gingival groove, junctional epithelium, attached gingiva, cementoenamel junction, cementum, alveolar bone, mucogingival junction, alveolar mucosa

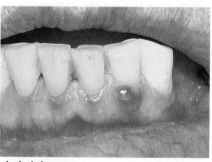

**gingival abscess**

for obtaining the setting time of dental cement. See this page.

**Gil·mer wir·ing** (gil′měr wīr′ing) Method of intermaxillary fixation in which single opposing teeth are wired circumferentially and the wires are twisted together.

**gin·gi·va,** pl. **gin·gi·vae** (jin′ji-vă, -vē) [TA] Dense fibrous tissue and overlying mucous membrane enveloping alveolar processes of upper and lower jaws and surrounding necks of teeth. See this page. SYN gum (1). [L.]

**gin·gi·val** (jin′ji-văl) Relating to the gums. See page A10.

**gin·gi·val ab·ra·sion** (jin′ji-văl ă-brā′zhŭn) Lesion of gingiva resulting from mechanical removal of a portion of the surface epithelium.

**gin·gi·val ab·scess** (jin′ji-văl ab′ses) Lesion confined to gingival soft tissue. See this page. SYN gumboil, parulis.

**gin·gi·val at·ro·phy** (jin′ji-văl at′rŏ-fē) SYN gingival recession.

**gin·gi·val at·tach·ment** (jin′ji-văl ă-tach′ment) SYN attached gingiva.

**gin·gi·val clamp** (jin′ji-văl klamp) Spring-like metal piece encircling cervix of a tooth and shaped to retract the gingival tissue.

**gin·gi·val cleft** (jin′ji-văl kleft) Fissure associated with pocket formation and lined by mixed gingival and pocket epithelium.

**gin·gi·val con·tour** (jin′ji-văl kon′tūr) Shape or form of the gingiva, either natural or artificial, around the necks of the teeth. SYN gum contour.

**gin·gi·val crest** (jin′ji-văl krest) SYN gingival margin.

**gin·gi·val crev·ice** (jin′ji-văl krev′is) SYN gingival sulcus.

**gin·gi·val cur·va·ture** (jin′ji-văl kŭrv′ă-chŭr) Rounding of gum along its line of attachment to neck of a tooth.

**gin·gi·val cyst** (jin′ji-văl sist) Lesion derived from remnants of dental lamina situated in attached gingiva, occasionally producing superficial erosion of cortical plate of bone.

**gin·gi·val el·e·phan·ti·a·sis** (jin′ji-văl

el´ĕ-făn-tī´ă-sis) Fibrous hyperplasia of gingiva.

**gin·gi·val em·bra·sure** (jin´ji-văl em-brā´shŭr) Space existing cervically to interproximal contact area between adjacent teeth.

**gin·gi·val en·large·ment** (jin´ji-văl en-lahrj´mĕnt) Overgrowth (localized or diffuse) of gingival tissue, nonspecific in nature.

**gin·gi·val ep·i·the·li·um** (jin´ji-văl ep´i-thē´lē-ŭm) Stratified squamous epithelium that undergoes some degree of keratinization and covers free and attached gingiva.

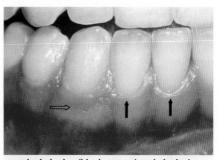
marginal gingiva (black arrows) and gingival groove (open arrow)

**gin·gi·val fes·toon** (jin´ji-văl fes-tūn´) Enlargement of margins of the gingival tissues occurring in early gingival disease.

**gin·gi·val fi·bers** (jin´ji-văl fī´bĕrz) Network of fibers that braces the free gingiva against the tooth and unites this free gingiva with the tooth root and alveolar bone.

◨**gin·gi·val fib·ro·ma·to·sis** (jin´ji-văl fī´brō-mă-tō´sis) Fibromatosis that may be associated with trichodiscomas. Several genetic forms are known. See this page.

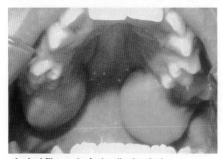
gingival fibromatosis: localized variant

**gin·gi·val fis·tu·la** (jin´ji-văl fis´tyū-lă) Sinus tract originating in a peripheral abscess and opening into the oral cavity on gingiva. SYN dental fistula.

**gin·gi·val flap** (jin´ji-văl flap) Portion of gingiva the coronal margin of which is surgically detached from the tooth and alveolar process.

**gin·gi·val fluid** (jin´ji-văl flū´id) Liquid containing plasma proteins, which is present in increasing amounts in association with gingival inflammation. SYN crevicular fluid.

◨**gin·gi·val groove** (jin´ji-văl grūv) See this page. SYN gingival sulcus.

**gin·gi·val hy·per·pla·si·a** (jin´ji-văl hī´pĕr-plā´zē-ă) Enlargement of gums due to proliferation of fibrous connective tissue. SYN gingival proliferation.

**Gin·gi·val In·dex (GI)** (jin´ji-văl in´deks) A

measure of periodontal disease based on severity and location of the lesion.

**gin·gi·val line** (jin´ji-văl līn) Position of margin of gingiva in relation to teeth in dental arch.

**gin·gi·val mar·gin** (jin´ji-văl mahr´jin) **1.** Most coronal portion of gingiva surrounding the tooth. **2.** Edge of free gingiva. SYN cervical margin (1), gingival crest.

**gin·gi·val mar·gin trim·mer** (jin´ji-văl mahr´jin trim´ĕr) Angulated chisellike instrument used to bevel gingival margin of a tooth in cavity preparation. SYN margin trimmer.

**gin·gi·val mas·sage** (jin´ji-văl mă-sahzh´) Mechanical stimulation of the gingiva by rubbing or pressure.

**gin·gi·val mu·co·sa** (jin´ji-văl myū-kō´să) Portion of oral mucous membrane that covers and is attached to necks of teeth and alveolar process of jaws; demarcated from lining mucosa on the facial aspect by a clearly defined line that marks mucogingival junction.

**gin·gi·val pa·pil·la** (jin´ji-văl pă-pil´ă) [TA] Thickening (seen as an elevation) of gingiva that fills interproximal space between two adjacent teeth. SYN gingival septum, interdental papilla, interproximal papilla.

**Gin·gi·val-Per·i·o·don·tal In·dex (GPI)** (jin´ji-văl per´ē-ō-don´tăl in´deks) Measure assessing gingivitis, gingival irritation, and advanced periodontal disease.

**gin·gi·val pig·men·ta·tion** (jin´ji-văl pig´mĕn-tā´shŭn) Coloration on gingiva that may be a variant of normal pigmentation; may be related to a patient's natural skin pigmentation or may be a sign of underlying disease.

**gin·gi·val pock·et** (jin´ji-văl pok´ĕt) Diseased gingival attachment in which increased sulcus depth is due to bulk of its gingival wall.

**gin·gi·val pro·lif·er·a·tion** (jin´ji-văl prō-lif´ĕr-ā´shŭn) SYN gingival hyperplasia.

◨**gin·gi·val re·ces·sion** (jin´ji-văl rĕ-sesh´

ŭn) Apical migration of the gingiva along the tooth surface, with exposure of the tooth surface. See this page. SYN gingival atrophy, gingival resorption.

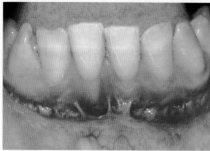

gingival recession due to frenal pull

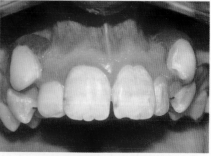

focal eruption gingivitis

**gin·gi·val re·po·si·tion·ing** (jin´ji-văl rē´pŏ-zish´ŭn-ing) Surgical relocation of attached gingiva to eliminate pathosis or to establish more acceptable form and function.

**gin·gi·val re·sorp·tion** (jin´ji-văl rē-sōrp´shŭn) SYN gingival recession.

**gin·gi·val re·trac·tion** (jin´ji-văl rĕ-trak´shŭn) **1.** Lateral movement of gingival margin away from tooth surface; may indicate underlying inflammation or pocket formation. **2.** Displacement of marginal gingivae away from the tooth by mechanical, chemical, or surgical means.

**gin·gi·val sep·tum** (jin´ji-văl sep´tŭm) SYN gingival papilla.

**gin·gi·val sul·cus** (jin´ji-văl sŭl´kŭs) [TA] Space between tooth surface and free gingiva. SYN gingival crevice, gingival groove.

**gin·gi·val trough** (jin´ji-văl trawf) Formation of a crater due to destruction of interdental tissues so that, in effect, there exists a labial and lingual curtain of gingiva with no interproximal connection at all.

**gin·gi·val zone** (jin´ji-văl zōn) Portion of oral mucosa that surrounds teeth and is firmly attached to underlying alveolar bone.

**gin·gi·vec·to·my** (jin´ji-vek´tŏ-mē) Surgical resection of unsupported gingival tissue. SYN gum resection. [gingiva + G. ektomē, excision]

🔲**gin·gi·vi·tis** (jin´ji-vī´tis) Inflammation of gingiva as a response to bacterial plaque on adjacent teeth; characterized by erythema, edema, and fibrous enlargement of the gingiva without resorption of the underlying alveolar bone. See this page. [gingiva + G. -itis, inflammation]

♻ **gingivo-** Combining form meaning the gingivae, the gums of the mouth. [L. gingiva]

**gin·gi·vo·ax·i·al** (jin´ji-vō-ak´sē-ăl) Pertain-

ing to line angle formed by gingival and axial walls of a cavity.

**gin·gi·vo·buc·cal groove** (jin´ji-vō-bŭk´ăl grŭv) SYN alveolobuccal groove.

**gin·gi·vo·buc·cal sul·cus** (jin´ji-vō-bŭk´ăl sŭl´kŭs) SYN alveolobuccal groove.

**gin·gi·vo·den·tal lig·a·ment** (jin´ji-vōden´tăl lig´ă-mĕnt) SYN periodontium.

**gin·gi·vo·glos·si·tis** (jin´ji-vō-glos-ī´tis) Inflammation of both gingival tissues and tongue.

**gin·gi·vo·la·bi·al** (jin´ji-vō-lā´bē-ăl) Referring to line angle formed by junction of gingival and labial walls of a (class III or IV) cavity.

**gin·gi·vo·la·bi·al groove** (jin´ji-vō-lā´bē-ăl grŭv) SYN alveololabial groove.

**gin·gi·vo·la·bi·al sul·cus** (jin´ji-vō-lā´bē-ăl sŭl´kŭs) SYN alveololabial groove.

**gin·gi·vo·lin·gual groove** (jin´ji-vō-ling´gwăl grŭv) SYN alveololingual groove.

**gin·gi·vo·lin·gual sul·cus** (jin´ji-vō-ling´gwăl sŭl´kŭs) SYN alveololingual groove.

**gin·gi·vo·lin·guo·ax·i·al** (jin´ji-vō-ling´gwŏak´sē-ăl) Referring to point angle formed by gingival, lingual, and axial walls of a cavity.

**gin·gi·vo·os·se·ous** (jin´ji-vō-os´ē-ŭs) Referring to gingiva and its underlying bone.

**gin·gi·vo·plas·ty** (jin´ji-vō-plas-tē) Surgical procedure that reshapes gingival tissue to attain esthetic and physiologic form.

**gin·gi·vo·sis** (jin´ji-vō´sis) SYN chronic desquamative gingivitis.

**gin·gi·vo·sto·ma·ti·tis** (jin´ji-vō-stō´mătī´tis) Inflammation of gingiva and other oral mucous membranes.

**gin·gly·moid joint** (jing´gli-moyd joynt) SYN hinge joint.

**gin·gly·mus** (jing´gli-mŭs) [TA] SYN hinge joint. [G. ginglymos]

**gir·dle** (gĭr'dĕl) [TA] Any structure that has the form of a belt or girdle. SYN cingulum [TA].

**gla·bel·la** (glă-bel'ă) A smooth prominence, more marked in the male, on the frontal bone above the root of the nose. SYN intercilium, mesophryon. [L. *glabellus,* hairless, smooth, dim. of *glaber*]

**gla·cial phos·phor·ic ac·id** (glā'shăl fos-fōr'ik as'id) Anhydride of phosphoric acid used to manufacture zinc oxyphosphate cement for dentistry.

**gland** (gland) [TA] Organized aggregation of cells functioning as a secretory or excretory organ. [L. *glans,* acorn]

**glan·dule** (glan'dyūl) A small gland. [L. *glandula*]

**glans,** pl. **glan·des** (glanz, glan'dēz) [TA] A conic or acorn-shaped structure. [L. acorn]

**glass** (glas) A transparent substance composed of silica and oxides of various bases. [A.S. *glaes*]

**glass bead ster·il·i·zer** (glas bēd ster'ĭ-lī'zĕr) Sterilizer for endodontic equipment; heat is transmitted to instruments, absorbent points, or cotton pellets by means of glass beads.

**glass i·o·no·mer ce·ment** (glas ī-on'ŏ-mĕr sĕ-ment') Dental fixative produced by mixing a powder prepared from a calcium aluminosilicate glass with an aqueous solution of polyacrylic acid. See this page.

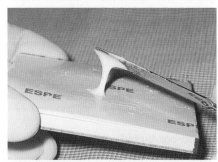

**glass ionomer cement:** consistency is correct when material assumes string formation

**glau·co·ma** (glaw-kō'mă) Eye disease associated with increased intraocular pressure and excavation and atrophy of the optic nerve; produces defects in the visual field and may result in blindness.

**gle·noid** (glē'noyd) Resembling a socket. [G. *glēnoeidēs,* fr. *glēnē,* pupil of eye, socket of joint, honeycomb, + *eidos,* appearance]

**gle·noid fos·sa** (glē'noyd fos'ă) 1. SYN mandibular fossa. 2. Glenoid cavity of the scapula.

**glide** (glīd) Smooth or effortless continuous movement.

**glid·ing oc·clu·sion** (glīd'ing ŏ-klū'zhŭn) SYN dental articulation.

**gli·o·ma** (glī-ō'mă) Neoplasm derived from cells that form interstitial tissue of the brain, spinal cord, pineal gland, posterior pituitary gland, and retina. [G. *glia,* glue, + *-oma,* tumor]

**glo·bal pa·ral·y·sis** (glō'băl pă-ral'i-sis) Complete paralysis of both sides of the body.

**glo·bin** (glō'bin) The protein of hemoglobin; α-globin and β-globin represent the two types of chains found in adult hemoglobin. SYN hematohiston.

**glob·ule** (glob'yūl) 1. A small spheric body of any kind. 2. A spheric drop of fluid. [L. *globulus,* dim. of *globus,* a ball]

**glob·u·lin** (glob'yū-lin) Name for a family of proteins precipitated from plasma (or serum) by half-saturation with ammonium sulfate. The main groups are α-, β-, and γ-globulin, which contain most antibodies.

**glob·u·lo·max·il·lar·y cyst** (glob'yū-lō-mak'si-lar-ē sist) Lesion of odontogenic origin found between roots of maxillary lateral incisors and canine teeth.

**glo·mer·u·lar fil·tra·tion rate (GFR)** (glō-mer'yū-lăr fil-trā'shŭn rāt) The volume of water filtered out of the plasma through glomerular capillary walls into Bowman capsules per unit of time.

**glo·mer·ule** (glō-mer'yūl) SYN glomerulus.

**glo·mer·u·lus,** pl. **glo·mer·u·li** (glō-mer'yū-lŭs, -lī) 1. A plexus of capillaries. 2. A tuft formed of capillary loops at the beginning of each nephric tubule in the kidney. 3. The twisted secretory portion of a sweat gland. SYN Bowman capsule. [Mod. L. dim. of L. *glomus,* a ball of yarn]

**glo·mus,** pl. **glo·mer·a** (glō'mŭs, glom'ĕr-ă) [TA] A small, globular body.

**glos·sec·to·my, glos·so·ster·e·sis** (glos-ek'tŏ-mē, glos'ō-ster-ē'sis) Resection or amputation of the tongue. SYN lingulectomy (1). [*gloss-* + G. *ektomē,* excision]

**glos·si·tis** (glos-ī'tis) Inflammation of the tongue. [*gloss-* + G. *-itis,* inflammation]

**glos·si·tis ar·e·a·ta ex·fo·li·a·ti·va** (glos-ī'tis ar-ē-ā'tă eks-fō-lē-ă-tī'vă) SYN geographic tongue.

**glosso-, gloss-** Combining forms indicating language; corresponds to L. *linguo-.* [G. *glōssa,* tongue]

**glos·so·cele** (glos'ō-sēl) Swelling and protrusion of the tongue from the mouth. SEE ALSO macroglossia. [*glosso-* + G. *kēlē,* tumor, hernia]

**glos·so·don·to·tro·pism** (glos'ō-don'tō-trŏ′pizm) Manifestation of tension or anxiety in which the tongue is attracted to the teeth or to dental faults.

**glos·so·dy·na·mom·e·ter** (glos′ō-dī′nă-mom′ĕ-tĕr) An apparatus to estimate contractile force of the tongue muscles. [*glosso-* + G. *dynamis*, power, + *metron*, measure]

**glos·so·dyn·i·a** (glos′ō-din′ē-ă) Burning or painful tongue. SYN burning tongue. [glosso- + G. *odynē*, pain]

**glos·so·dyn·i·o·tro·pism** (glos′ō-din′ē-ō-trō′pizm) Apparent satisfaction from subjecting the tongue to a pain-inducing dental fault. [*glosso-* + G. *odynē*, pain, + *tropē*, a turning]

**glos·so·ep·i·glot·tic, glos·so·ep·i·glot·tid·e·an** (glos′ō-ep-i-glot′ik, glos′ō-ep-i-glŏ-tid′ē-ăn) Relating to the tongue and epiglottis.

**glos·so·ep·i·glot·tic lig·a·ment** (glos′ō-ep′i-glot′ik lig′ă-mĕnt) Elastic ligamentous band passing from base of tongue to epiglottis in middle glossoepiglottic fold.

**glos·so·la·bi·o·la·ryn·ge·al pa·ral·y·sis, glos·so·la·bi·o·pha·ryn·ge·al pa·ral·y·sis** (glos′ō-lā′bē-ō-lă-rin′jē-ăl pă-ral′i-sis, -fă-rin′jē-ăl) SYN progressive bulbar palsy.

**glos·son·cus** (glos-ong′kŭs) Any swelling involving the tongue, including neoplasms. [*glosso-* + G. *onkos*, mass, tumor]

**glos·so·pha·ryn·ge·al breath·ing** (glos′ō-făr-in′jē-ăl brēdh′ing) Respiration unaided by usual primary muscles of respiration; air is forced into lungs by tongue and pharyngeal muscles.

**glos·so·pha·ryn·ge·al nerve [CN IX]** (glos′ō-făr-in′jē-ăl nĕrv) [TA] Ninth cranial nerve, which emerges from the rostral end of the medulla, through the retroolivary groove, and passes through jugular foramen to supply sensation (including taste) to pharynx and posterior third of tongue. SYN nervus glossopharyngeus [CN IX], ninth cranial nerve [CN IX].

**glos·so·pha·ryn·ge·al neu·ral·gi·a** (glos′ō-fă-rin′jē-ăl nūr-al′jē-ă) Paroxysmal lancinating pain in throat or palate.

**glos·so·pha·ryn·ge·o·la·bi·al pa·ral·y·sis** (glos′ō-fă-rin′jē-ō-lā′bē-ăl pă-ral′i-sis) SYN progressive bulbar palsy.

**glos·so·plas·ty** (glos′ō-plas-tē) Surgical repair of the tongue. [*glosso-* + G. *plastos*, formed]

**glos·so·ple·gi·a** (glos′ō-plē′jē-ă) Paralysis of the tongue. [*glosso-* + G. *plēgē*, stroke]

**glos·sop·to·sis, glos·sop·to·si·a** (glos′op-tō′sis, -op-tō′sē-ă) Displacement of tongue toward pharynx. [*glosso-* + G. *ptōsis*, a falling]

**glos·so·py·ro·sis** (glos′ō-pī-rō′sis) SYN burning tongue. [*glosso-* + G. *pyrōsis*, a burning]

**glos·sor·rha·phy** (glos-ōr′ă-fē) Suture of a wound of the tongue. [*glosso-* + G. *rhaphē*, suture]

**glos·sot·o·my** (glos-ot′ŏ-mē) Any cutting operation on the tongue, usually to obtain access to further reaches of the pharynx. [*glosso-* + G. *tomē*, incision]

**glos·so·trich·i·a** (glos′ō-trik′ē-ă) SYN hairy tongue. [*glosso-* + G. *thrix*, hair]

**gloss·y skin** (glaw′sē skin) Shiny dermal atrophy after nerve injury; type of neurotrophic atrophy.

**glot·tal** (glot′ăl) Relating to the glottis.

**glot·tic** (glot′ik) Relating to tongue or glottis.

**glot·tis,** pl. **glot·ti·des** (glot′is, -id′i-dēz) [TA] Vocal laryngeal apparatus, consisting of vocal folds of mucous membrane investing vocal ligament and vocal muscle on each side, free edges of which are the vocal cords, and of rima glottidis. [G. *glōttis*, aperture of the larynx]

**glove an·es·the·si·a** (glŏv an′es-thē′zē-ă) Loss of sensation in the distal upper limb, i.e., the hand and fingers.

■**gloves** (glŭvz) In dentistry, hand coverings intended to be discarded after a single use, which are worn to prevent transfer of infection between the patient and dental staff; many types available. See page 257.

**glu·ca·gon** (glū′kă-gon) A hormone consisting of a straight-chain polypeptide; activates hepatic phosphorylase, thereby increasing glycogenolysis, decreases gastric motility and gastric and pancreatic secretions. [*glucose* + G. *agō*, to lead]

**glu·ca·gon·o·ma syn·drome** (glū′kă-gon-ō′mă sin′drōm) Necrolytic migratory erythema or intertriginous and periorofacial dermatitis, due to glucagon-secreting pancreatic islet cell tumors.

**glu·co·cor·ti·coid** (glū′kō-kōr′ti-koyd) **1.** Any steroidlike compound capable of significantly influencing intermediary metabolism and exerting a clinically useful antiinflammatory effect. **2.** SYN corticoid.

**glu·co·cor·ti·co·tro·phic** (glū′kō-kōr′ti-kō-trōf′ik) Denoting a principle thought present in the anterior hypophysis that stimulates the production of glucocorticoid hormones of the cortex of the suprarenal gland.

**glu·co·ki·nase** (glū′kō-kī′nās) Phosphotransferase that catalyzes the conversion of D-glucose and adenosine triphosphate D-glucose 6-phosphate and adenosine diphosphate.

**glu·co·ne·o·gen·e·sis** (glū′kō-nē′ō-jen′ē-sis) The formation of glucose from noncarbohydrates, such as protein or fat.

gh

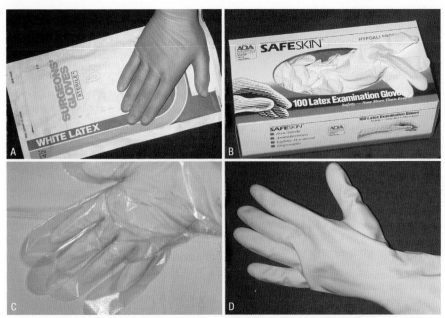

**gloves:** (A) sterile gloves for oral surgery; (B) nonsterile gloves for examination; (C) overglove; (D) utility glove

**glu·co·pe·ni·a** (glū′kō-pē′nē-ă) SYN hypoglycemia. [*gluco-* + G. *penia*, poverty]

**glu·cose** (glū′kōs) A dextrorotatory monosaccharide found in a free form in fruits and other parts of plants, and in combination in glucosides, glycogen, disaccharides, and polysaccharides; chief source of energy in human metabolism, the final product of carbohydrate digestion, and the principal sugar of the blood; insulin is required for the use of glucose by cells; in diabetes mellitus, the level of glucose in the blood is excessive, and it also appears in the urine. SYN d-glucose.

**gluc·ose-de·pen·dent in·su·lin·o·tro·pic pol·y·pep·tide** (glū′kōs-dĕ-pen′dĕnt in′sŭ-lin-ō-trō′pik pol′ē-pep′tīd) Insulinotropic substance originating in gastrointestinal tract and released into the circulation following ingestion of food containing glucose.

**glu·cose tol·er·ance test (GTT)** (glū′kōs tol′ĕr-ăns test) Assessment for diabetes or for hypoglycemic states. Following ingestion of 75-g glucose while the patient is fasting, blood sugar promptly rises and then falls to normal within 2 hours; in diabetic patients, increase is greater and return to normal unusually prolonged; in hypoglycemic patients, depressed glucose levels may be observed in 3-, 4-, or 5-hour measurements.

**α-glu·co·si·dase in·hib·i·tor** (glū-kō′si-dās in-hib′i-tŏr) Oral agent that aids control of diabetes mellitus by delaying absorption of glucose from digestive system.

**glu·co·si·dase in·hib·i·tors** (glū-kō′sid′

ās in-hib′i-tŏrz) Agents that reduce gastrointestinal absorption of carbohydrates; known popularly as "starch blockers." They lower plasma glucose levels and tend to cause weight loss but cause flatulence.

**glu·co·side, gly·co·side** (glū′kō-sīd, glī′) A compound of glucose with an alcohol or other R–OH compound.

**glu·co·su·ri·a, gly·co·su·ri·a** (glū′kō-syūr′ē-ă, glī-) Urinary excretion of glucose, usually in enhanced quantities. [*glucose* + G. *ouron*, urine]

**glue-sniff·ing** (glū′snif-ing) **1.** Intentional inhalation of fumes from plastic cements; the solvents, which include toluene, xylene, and benzene, induce central nervous system stimulation followed by depression. **2.** SYN huffing.

**glu·tam·ic acid** (glū-tam′ik as′id) An amino acid; the sodium salt is monosodium glutamate.

**glu·ta·ral·de·hyde** (glū′tăr-al′dĕ-hīd) A dialdehyde used as a fixative and germicidal agent for sterilization of instruments that cannot be heat sterilized.

**glu·ta·thi·one** (glū′tă-thī′ōn) A tripeptide of glycine, L-cysteine, and L-glutamate; essential for detoxification of acetaminophen.

**glu·ten** (glū′tĕn) Insoluble protein constituent of wheat and other grains; believed to be an agent in celiac disease. [L. *gluten*, glue]

**glu·ten a·tax·i·a** (glū′tĕn ă-tak′sē-ă) Ataxia resulting from immunologic damage to the cerebellum, posterior spinal columns, and peripheral nerves in people sensitive to gluten.

**glu·ten en·ter·o·pa·thy** (glū'tĕn en'tĕr-op'ă-thē) SYN celiac disease.

**glycaemia** [Br.] SYN glycemia.

**gly·can** (glī'kan) SYN polysaccharide.

**gly·ce·mi·a** (glī-sē'mē-ă) The presence of glucose in blood. SYN glycaemia.

**gly·ce·mic in·dex** (glī-sē'mik in'deks) Ranking of the rise in serum glucose from various foodstuffs.

**glyc·er·ide** (glis'ĕr-īd) An ester of glycerol.

**glyc·er·in** (glis'ĕr-in) SYN glycerol.

**glyc·er·in·at·ed tinc·ture** (glis'ĕr-i-nā'tĕd tingk'shŭr) Tincture made with diluted alcohol to which glycerin is added to facilitate extraction or to preserve preparation.

**glyc·er·ol, glyc·er·in** (glis'ĕr-ol, -in) A sweet viscous fluid obtained by the saponification of fats and fixed oils; used as a solvent, as a skin emollient, by injection or in the form of suppository for constipation, and as a sweetener.

**gly·cine** (glī'sēn) Simplest amino acid; used as a nutrient and dietary supplement.

**gly·ci·nu·ri·a** (glī'si-nyūr'ē-ă) Excretion of glycine in urine. [*glycine* + G. *ouron*, urine]

**gly·co·gen** (glī'kō-jen) A glucosan of high molecular weight, found in most of the tissues of the body, especially those of the liver and muscle; as principal carbohydrate reserve, readily converted into glucose. SYN animal starch.

**gly·co·gen·e·sis** (glī'kō-jen'ĕ-sis) Formation of glycogen from D-glucose by means of glycogen synthase and dextrin dextranase. [*glyco-* + G. *genesis*, production]

**gly·co·gen·ol·y·sis** (glī'kō-jĕ-nol'i-sis) The hydrolysis of glycogen to glucose.

**gly·co·ge·no·sis** (glī'kō-jĕ-nō'sis) A glycogen deposition disease characterized by accumulation of glycogen of normal or abnormal chemical structure in tissue; may be enlargement of the liver, heart, or striated muscle, including the tongue.

**gly·col·y·sis** (glī-kol'i-sis) The energy-yielding conversion of glucose to lactic acid in various tissues, notably muscle, when sufficient oxygen is not available. [*glyco-* + G. *lysis*, a loosening]

**gly·co·lyt·ic** (glī'kō-lit'ik) Relating to glycolysis.

**gly·co·ne·o·gen·e·sis** (glī'kō-nē'ō-jen'ĕ-sis) The formation of glycogen from noncarbohydrates by conversion of the latter to glucose. [*glyco-* + G. *neos*, new, + *genesis*, production]

**gly·co·pe·ni·a** (glī'kō-pē'nē-ă) Sugar deficiency in an organ or tissue. [*glyco-* + G. *penia*, poverty]

**gly·co·phil·i·a** (glī'kō-fil'ē-ă) Condition with

a distinct tendency to develop hyperglycemia. [*glyko-* + G. *phileō*, to love]

**gly·co·pro·tein** (glī'kō-prō'tēn) One of a group of proteins containing covalently linked carbohydrates, among which the most important are the mucins, mucoid, and amyloid.

**gly·co·se·cre·to·ry** (glī'kō-sĕ-krē'tŏr-ē) Causing or involved in the secretion of glycogen.

**gly·co·si·a·li·a** (glī'kō-sī-ā'lē-ă) Presence of sugar in saliva. [*glyco-* + G. *sialon*, saliva]

**gly·co·side** (glī'kō-sīd) Condensation product of a sugar with any other radical involving the loss of the OH of the hemiacetal or hemiketal of the sugar.

**gly·co·stat·ic** (glī'kō-stat'ik) Indicating the property of some extracts of the anterior hypophysis that permits the body to maintain its glycogen stores in muscle and other tissues.

**gly·co·sur·i·a** (glī'kō-syūr'ē-ă) Urinary excretion of carbohydrates. [*glyco-* + G. *ouron*, urine]

**gly·co·tro·pic, gly·co·tro·phic** (glī'kō-trō'pik, -fik) Pertaining to a principle in extracts of anterior lobe of pituitary that antagonizes action of insulin and causes hyperglycemia. [*glyco-* + G. *trophē*, nourishment; *tropē*, a turning]

**glyc·yr·rhi·za** (glis'i-rī'ză) Dried rhizome and root of *Glycyrrhiza glabra* and allied species; demulcent, mild laxative, and expectorant. SYN licorice. [G. fr. *glykys*, sweet, + *rhiza*, root]

**gnash·ing** (nash'ing) The grinding together of the teeth as a nonmasticatory function; sometimes associated with emotional tension.

**gnath·ic** (nath'ik) Relating to jaw or alveolar process. [G. *gnathos*, jaw]

**gnath·ic in·dex** (nath'ik in'deks) Relation between basialveolar and basinasal lengths. SYN alveolar index (1).

**gnath·i·on** (nath'ē-on) Most inferior point of mandible in midline. [G. *gnathos*, jaw]

**gnath·o·dy·nam·ics** (nath'ō-dī-nam'iks) Study of relationship of magnitude and direction of forces developed by and on components of the masticatory system during function. [*gnatho-* + G. *dynamis*, power]

**gnath·o·dy·na·mom·e·ter** (nath'ō-dī'nă-mom'ĕ-tĕr) Device for measuring biting pressure. SYN bite gauge. [*gnatho-* + *dynamometer*]

**gnath·og·ra·phy** (nath-og'ră-fē) Recording of action of masticatory apparatus in function.

**gnath·ol·o·gy** (nath-ol'ŏ-jē) Science of masticatory system, including physiology, functional disturbances, and treatment.

**gnath·o·plas·ty** (nath'ō-plas-tē) Plastic and reconstructive surgery of jaw. [*gnatho-* + G. *plastos*, formed]

**gnath·os·chi·sis** (nath-os′ki-sis) SYN cleft jaw. [*gnatho-* + G. *schisis,* a cleaving]

**gnath·o·stat·ics** (nath′ō-stat′iks) In orthodontic diagnosis, technical procedure for orienting dentition to certain cranial landmarks. [*gnatho-* + G. *statikos,* causing to stand]

**goi·ter** (goy′tĕr) Chronic enlargement of the thyroid gland, not due to a neoplasm, occurring endemically in certain localities, where soil is low in iodine. SYN struma (1). [Fr. from L. *guttur,* throat]

**goi·tro·gen** (goy′trō-jen) Any substance that induces goiter (e.g., cabbage, rapeseed).

**gold (Au)** (gōld) A yellow metallic element used in the treatment of tumors and in imaging. [L. *aurum*]

**gold al·loy** (gōld al′oy) Alloy with gold as principal ingredient; used in dentistry for restorations requiring considerable strength.

**gold cast·ing** (gōld kast′ing) Cast appliance made of gold, usually formed to represent and replace lost tooth structure.

🔲 **Gol·den·har syn·drome** (gōl′dĕn-hahr sin′drōm) See this page. SEE oculoauriculovertebral dysplasia.

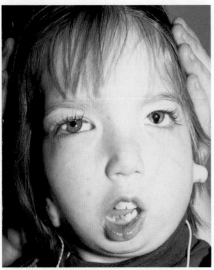

oculoauriculovertebral occlusion (Goldenhar syndrome): findings include right-sided limbal dermoid, right-sided inferotemporal lipodermoid, left iris coloboma, bilateral grade II microtia, and facial asymmetry with mandibular deficiency and dental malocclusion

**gold foil** (gōld foyl) Pure gold produced in extremely thin sheets that is then rolled for use in dentistry to restore carious or fractured teeth. SEE ALSO cohesive gold, noncohesive gold.

**gold in·lay** (gōld in′lā) Gold restoration fabricated by casting in a mold made from a wax pattern; restoration is sealed in the prepared cavity with dental cement.

**gold knife** (gōld nīf) Hand-held dental cutting device used infrequently to smooth and trim some types of gold restorations; no longer used in current general U.S. dental practice.

**Gold·man-Fox knife** (gōld′mǎn foks nīf) A flat-bladed surgical instrument used during gingivectomy and other periodontal procedures.

**Gol·gi ap·pa·ra·tus, Gol·gi bod·y, Gol·gi com·plex** (gol′jē ap′ǎ-rat′ŭs, bod′ē, kom′pleks) A membranous system of cisterns and vesicles located between the nucleus and the secretory pole or surface of a cell.

**gom·phol·ic joint** (gom-fō′lik joynt) SYN dentoalveolar syndesmosis.

**gom·pho·sis** (gom-fō′sis) [TA] 1. Form of fibrous joint in which a peglike process fits into a hole, as the root of a tooth into socket in alveolus. 2. Hollow part of a joint; excavation in one bone of a joint that receives the articular end of the other bone. [G. *gomphos,* bolt, nail, + *-osis,* condition]

**go·nad** (gō′nad) An organ that produces sex cells; a testis or an ovary. [Mod. L. fr. G. *gonē,* seed]

**gon·a·dop·ath·y** (gon′ǎ-dop′ǎ-thē) Disease affecting the gonads. [*gonado-* + G. *pathos,* suffering]

**go·nad·o·tro·pin, go·nad·o·tro·pic hor·mone** (gō-nad′ō-trō′pin, -pik hōr′mōn) 1. A hormone capable of promoting gonadal growth and function. 2. Any hormone that stimulates gonadal function.

**go·ni·o·cra·ni·om·e·try** (gō′nē-ō-krā′nē-om′ĕ-trē) Measurement of angles of cranium. [G. *gōnia,* angle, + *kranion,* skull, + *metron,* measure]

**go·ni·on,** pl. **go·ni·a** (gō′nē-on, -ǎ) [TA] Lowest posterior and most outward point of angle of mandible. In cephalometrics, it is measured by bisecting angle formed by tangents to lower and posterior borders of mandible; when angles of both sides of mandible appear on the lateral radiograph, a point midway between right and left sides is used. [G. *gōnia,* an angle]

**gon·o·coc·cal sto·ma·ti·tis** (gon′ŏ-kok′ǎl stō′mǎ-tī′tis) Inflammatory and ulcerative oral lesions resulting from infection with *Neisseria gonorrhoeae;* usually primary as a result of oral-genital contact, but occasionally is the result of gonococcemia.

**gon·or·rhe·a** (gon′ŏr-ē′ǎ) A contagious catarrhal inflammation of the genital mucous

gh

membrane, transmitted chiefly by coitus and due to *Neisseria gonorrhoeae;* may involve the lower or upper genital tract, especially urethra endocervix, and uterine tubes, or spread to the peritoneum and, rarely, to the heart, joints, or other structures by way of the bloodstream. SYN gonorrhoea. [G. *gonorrhoia,* fr. *gonē,* seed, + *rhoia,* a flow]

**gonorrhoea** [Br.] SYN gonorrhea.

**Good Sa·mar·i·tan leg·is·la·tion** (gud să-mar'i-tăn lej'is-lā'shŭn) State laws passed to protect suppliers of emergency medical assistance from litigation except in cases of gross malfeasance.

**Gor·lin cyst** (gōr'lin sist) SYN calcifying odontogenic cyst.

**Goth·ic arch** (goth'ik ahrch) SYN intraoral tracing.

vere recurrent acute arthritis of sudden onset resulting from deposition of crystals of sodium urate in connective tissues and articular cartilage. [L. *gutta,* drop]

**gout di·et** (gowt dī'ĕt) Diet containing a minimal quantity of purine bases (meats); liver, kidney, and sweetbreads are excluded and replaced by dairy products, fruits, and cereals.

**GPI** Abbreviation for Gingival-Periodontal Index.

**gr** Abbreviation for grain (abbrev. disallowed by order of JCAHO).

⬛**Gra·cey cu·rette** (grā'sē kyūr-et') A curved or hooked implement; its blade consists of a compound-curved bend at the end of the shank and two cutting edges formed by the junction of the outer and inner surfaces. See this page.

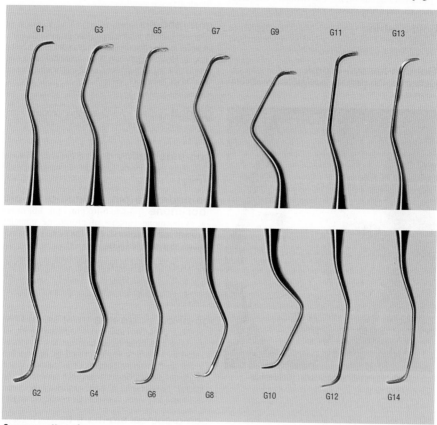

Gracey curette series

**Goth·ic arch trac·ing** (goth'ik ahrch trās'ing) SYN intraoral tracing.

**gout** (gowt) A disorder of purine metabolism, occurring especially in men, characterized by a raised but variable blood uric acid level and se-

**gra·di·ent** (grā'dē-ĕnt) Rate of change of temperature, pressure, magnetic field, or other variable as a function of distance, time, or other continuously changing influence.

**graft** (graft) **1.** Any free (unattached) tissue or

organ for transplantation. **2.** To transplant such structures. SEE ALSO flap, implant, transplant. [A.S. *graef* ]

**graft-ver·sus-host dis·ease (GVHD)** (graft vĕr′sŭs hōst di-zēz′) An incompatibility reaction (which may be fatal) in a subject (host) of low immunologic competence (deficient lymphoid tissue) who has been the recipient of immunologically competent lymphoid tissue from a donor who lacks at least one antigen possessed by the recipient host; the reaction, or disease, is the result of action of the transplanted cells against those host tissues that possess the antigen not possessed by the donor.

**grain (gr)** (grān) **1.** One of the cereal plants, or its seed. **2.** A hard, minute particle of any substance, e.g., sand. **3.** *The grain is obsolete as a unit in dentistry, medicine, pharmacy, and nursing. Avoid abbreviation gr, which is subject to frequent misinterpretation.* A unit of weight equivalent to 64.79 mg. **4.** A particle of a silver halide in a photographic emulsion. [L. *granum*]

**gram (g)** (gram) A unit of weight in the metric or centesimal system, the equivalent of 15.432358 gr or 0.03527 avoirdupois oz.

**gram·i·ci·din** (gram′i-sī′din) One of a group of polypeptide antibiotics produced by *Bacillus brevis* that are primarily bacteriostatic in action against gram-positive cocci and bacilli.

**gram-neg·a·tive** (gram-neg′ă-tiv) Refers to the inability of a type of bacterium to resist decolorization with alcohol after being treated with crystal violet.

**gram-pos·i·tive** (gram-poz′i-tiv) Refers to the ability of a type of bacterium to resist decolorization with alcohol after being treated with crystal violet stain, which imparts a violet color to the bacteria when viewed by light microscopy.

**Gram stain** (gram stān) Method for differential staining of bacteria; smears are fixed by flaming or methanol, stained in a solution of crystal violet, treated with iodine solution, rinsed, decolorized, and then counterstained with safranin O; gram-positive organisms stain purple-black and gram-negative organisms stain pink; useful in bacterial taxonomy and identification, and also in indicating fundamental differences in cell wall structure.

**grand mal sei·zure** (grŏn[h] mahl sē′zhŭr) SYN generalized tonic-clonic seizure.

**gran·u·lar cell tu·mor** (gran′yū-lăr sel tū′ mŏr) A microscopically specific, generally benign tumor, often involving peripheral nerves in skin, mucosa, or connective tissue, derived from Schwann cells.

**gran·u·la·tion** (gran′yū-lā′shŭn) **1.** Formation into grains or granules; state of being granular. **2.** Granular mass in or on surface of any organ or membrane; one of the individual gran-

ules that form the mass. **3.** Formation of minute, rounded, fleshy connective tissue projections on wound surface, ulcer, or inflamed tissue in process of healing; one of the fleshy granules composing this surface. **4.** In pharmacy, formation of crystals by constant agitation of a supersaturated solution of a salt; product used in the manufacture of tablets for oral use. [L. *granulatio*]

**gran·u·la·tion tis·sue** (gran′yū-lā′shŭn tish′ū) Vascular connective tissue forming granular projections on the surface of a healing wound, ulcer, or inflamed surface.

**gran·ule** (gran′yūl) **1.** Grainlike particle; a granulation; minute discrete mass. **2.** A small pill, usually gelatin or sugar coated, containing a drug to be given in a small dose. **3.** Colony of bacterium or fungus causing disease or simply colonizing tissues of patient. In immunocompromised patients, differentiation is difficult. **4.** Small particle that can be seen by electron microscopy; contains stored material. [L. *granulum,* dim. of *granum,* grain]

**gran·u·lo·cyte** (gran′yū-lō-sīt) A mature granular leukocyte, including neutrophilic, acidophilic, and basophilic types of polymorphonuclear leukocytes, i.e., respectively, neutrophils, eosinophils, and basophils. [*granulo-* + G. *kytos,* cell]

**gran·u·lo·cy·to·pe·ni·a** (gran′yū-lō-sī′tō-pē′nē-ă) Fewer than normal number of granular leukocytes in the blood. [*granulocyte* + G. *penia,* poverty]

**gran·u·lo·cy·to·sis** (gran′yū-lō-sī-tō′sis) A condition characterized by more than normal number of granulocytes in the circulating blood or in the tissues.

**gran·u·lo·ma,** pl. **gran·u·lo·ma·ta** (gran′ yū-lō′mă, -tă) Term applied to nodular inflammatory lesions, usually small or granular, firm, persistent, and containing compactly grouped modified phagocytes. [*granulo-* + G. *-oma,* tumor]

**gran·u·lo·ma grav·i·da·rum** (gran′yū-lō′mă grav′i-dā′rŭm) Pyogenic granuloma developing on gingiva during pregnancy. SYN pregnancy tumor.

**gran·u·lo·ma in·gui·na·le** (gran′yū-lō′ mă ing-gwi-nā′lē) A specific granuloma; lesions occur in the inguinal regions and on the genitalia. SYN donovanosis, ulcerating granuloma of pudenda.

**gran·u·lom·a·tous in·flam·ma·tion** (gran′yū-lom′ă-tŭs in′flă-mā′shŭn) A form of proliferative inflammation.

**graph** (graf) *Do not confuse this word with graft.* **1.** A line or tracing denoting varying values of commodities, temperatures, urinary output, and the like; more generally, any geometric or pictorial representation of measurements that might otherwise be expressed in tabular form. **2.** Visual display of the relationship between

**gh**

two variables, in which the values of one are plotted on the horizontal axis, the values of the other on the vertical axis; three-dimensional graphs that show relationships between three variables can be depicted and comprehended visually in two dimensions. [G. *graphō,* to write]

**graph·ite** (graf´īt) A crystallizable soft black form of carbon.

**grasp** (grasp) The act of taking securely and holding firmly. [M.E. *graspen*]

**grat·tage** (gră-tazh´) Scraping or brushing an ulcer or body surface covered with sluggish granulations to stimulate healing. [Fr. scraping]

**grave** (grāv) Denoting symptoms of a serious or dangerous character. [L. *gravis,* heavy, grave]

**Graves dis·ease** (grāvz di-zēz´) **1.** Toxic goiter characterized by diffuse hyperplasia of the thyroid gland, a form of hyperthyroidism. **2.** Thyroid dysfunction and all or any of its clinical associations. **3.** Organ-specific autoimmune disease of thyroid gland. SYN Basedow disease.

**Graves oph·thal·mop·a·thy** (grāvz of´thăl-mop´ă-thē) Exophthalmos caused by increased water content of retroocular orbital tissues; associated with thyroid disease, usually hyperthyroidism.

**gray (Gy)** (grā) The SI unit of absorbed dose of ionizing radiation, equivalent to 1 J/kg of tissue; 1 Gy = 100 rad. [Louis H. *Gray,* British radiologist, 1905–1965]

**great au·ric·u·lar nerve** (grāt awr-ik´yū-lăr nĕrv) [TA] Arises as branch of cervical plexus, conveying fibers from ventral primary rami of second and third cervical spinal nerves; supplies skin of part of auricle, adjacent portion of scalp, and that overlying angle of jaw; also innervates parotid sheath, conveying from it pain fibers stimulated by stretching of the sheath during parotitis (mumps).

**great·er oc·cip·i·tal nerve** (grā´tĕr ok-sip´i-tăl nĕrv) [TA] Medial branch of the dorsal primary ramus of the second cervical nerve; sends branches to the semispinalis capitis and multifidus cervicis but is mainly sensory, supplying back part of scalp, meningeal branches to the posterior cranial fossa, and pain and proprioceptive branches to first cervical nerve for the suboccipital muscles.

**great·er o·men·tum** (grā´tĕr ō-men´tŭm) [TA] A peritoneal fold passing from the greater curvature of the stomach to the transverse colon, hanging like an apron in front of the intestines. SYN caul (2), cowl, velum (3).

**great·er pal·a·tine ar·te·ry** (grā´tĕr pal´ă-tīn ahr´tĕr-ē) [TA] Anterior branch of descending palatine artery, supplying gingiva and mucous membrane of hard palate.

**great·er pal·a·tine ca·nal** (grā´tĕr pal´ă-tīn kă-nal´) [TA] That formed between maxilla and palatine bones; transmits the descending palatine artery and the greater palatine nerve from the pterygopalatine fossa to the oral mucosa of the hard palate.

**great·er pal·a·tine for·a·men** (grā´tĕr pal´ă-tīn fōr-ā´mĕn) [TA] Opening in the posterolateral corner of the hard palate opposite the last molar tooth, marking the lower end of the pterygopalatine canal. SYN anterior palatine foramen.

**great·er pal·a·tine groove** (grā´tĕr pal´ă-tīn grūv) [TA] Groove on both body of maxilla and perpendicular plate of palatine bone; when bones are articulated, grooves form the greater palatine canal.

**great·er pal·a·tine nerve** (grā´tĕr pal´ă-tīn nĕrv) [TA] Branch of pterygopalatine ganglion that passes inferiorly through greater palatine canal to supply mucosa and glands of hard palate and anterior part of the soft palate.

**great·er pe·tro·sal nerve** (grā´tĕr pĕ-trō´săl nĕrv) [TA] A branch from the genu of the facial nerve exiting by way of the hiatus of the facial canal and running in a groove on the anterior surface of the petrous part of the temporal bone beside the foramen lacerum to join the deep petrosal nerve, thus forming the nerve of the pterygoid canal, which passes through the pterygoid canal to reach the pterygopalatine ganglion. SYN greater superficial petrosal nerve, nervus petrosus major, parasympathetic root of pterygopalatine ganglion.

**great·er su·per·fi·cial pe·tro·sal nerve** (grā´tĕr sū´pĕr-fish´ăl pĕ-trō´săl nĕrv) SYN greater petrosal nerve.

**great·er wing of sphe·noid (bone)** (grā´tĕr wing sfē´noyd bōn) [TA] Strong squamous processes extending in a broad superolateral curve from the body of the sphenoid bone. SYN ala major ossis sphenoidalis.

**great for·a·men** (grāt fōr-ā´mĕn) SYN foramen magnum.

**green soap tinc·ture** (grēn sōp tingk´shŭr) Liquid preparation containing potassium soaps and alcohol; frequently used in skin cleansing.

**green spu·tum** (grēn spyū´tŭm) SYN sputum aeruginosum.

**green stain** (grēn stān) Such discoloration or deposit on the gingival half of the labial surfaces of the maxillary anterior teeth, usually in children. Caused by chromogenic bacteria or orally inhaling dust containing copper and nickel.

**green·stick frac·ture** (grēn´stik frak´shŭr) A fracture in which the bone is partially broken and partially bent; a type of incomplete fracture that occurs primarily in children.

**green tooth** (grēn tūth) Green to brown discoloration of primary teeth associated with erythroblastosis fetalis and hyperbilirubinemia; caused by deposition of hemoglobin pigments.

**Greig syn·drome** (greg sin'drōm) SYN ocular hypertelorism.

**grenz ray** (grenz rā) Very soft x-rays, closely allied to the ultraviolet rays in their long wavelength and in their biologic action on tissues. [Ger. *Grenze*, borderline, boundary]

**gres·sion** (gres'shŭn) Displacement of a tooth backward.

**grid** (grid) 1. A chart with horizontal and perpendicular lines for plotting curves. 2. In x-ray imaging, device formed of lead or aluminum strips for preventing scattered radiation from reaching the x-ray film. [M.E. *gridel*, fr. L. *craticula*, lattice]

**grind·ing** (grīnd'ing) SYN abrasion (1).

**grind·ing-in** (grīnd'ing-in') Term used to denote act of correcting occlusal disharmonies by grinding natural or artificial teeth.

**grind·ing sur·face** (grīnd'ing sŭr'făs) SYN denture occlusal surface.

**grippe** (grip) SYN influenza. [Fr. *gripper,* to seize]

**gris·e·o·ful·vin** (gris'ē-ō-ful'vin) A fungistatic antibiotic produced by *Penicillium* species; used in systemic treatment of superficial fungal infections.

**grit** (grit) Denotes the size of a particle found on the surface of abrasive materials.

**groin** (groyn) [TA] 1. SYN inguinal region. 2. Sometimes used to indicate just the crease in the junction of the thigh with the trunk.

**groove** (grūv) [TA] A narrow, elongated depression or furrow on any surface.

**grooved tongue** (grūvd tŭng) SYN fissured tongue.

**gross scal·ing** (grōs skā'ling) Older method of planning multiple calculus removal appointments that advocated removing only the largest-sized calculus deposits from the entire mouth at the first appointment; no longer recommended because of the undesirable consequences that can result from incomplete calculus removal. SYN circuit scaling.

**ground state** (grownd stāt) The normal, inactivated state of an atom from which, on activation, the singlet, triplet, and other excited states are derived.

**ground sub·stance** (grownd sub'stăns) The amorphous physiologic material in which structural element occur.

**group** (grūp) 1. A number of similar or related objects. 2. In chemistry, a radical.

**group A strep·to·coc·ci** (grūp strep'tō-kok'ī) Common bacteria that is the cause of strep throat, scarlet fever, impetigo, cellulitis-erysipelas, rheumatic fever, acute glomerular nephritis, endocarditis, and group A streptococcal necrotizing fasciitis. The prototype is *Streptococcus pyogenes.*

**group prac·tice** (grūp prak'tis) The cooperative practice of medicine by a group of dentists or physicians; such a group often shares a common suite of consulting rooms, laboratories, staff, and equipment.

**gh**

**growth** (grōth) Increase in size of a living being or any of its parts occurring in process of development.

**growth fac·tors** (grōth fak'tŏrz) Natural substances produced by the body (hormones) or obtained from food (vitamins, minerals) that promote growth and development by directing cell maturation and differentiation and by mediating maintenance and repair of tissues.

**growth hor·mone (GH)** (grōth hōr'mōn) SYN somatotropin.

**growth rate** (grōth rāt) Absolute or relative growth increase, expressed per unit of time.

**GSR** Abbreviation for galvanic skin response.

**GTT** Abbreviation for glucose tolerance test.

**guai·ac** (gwī'ak) The resin of *Guaiacum officinale* or *G. sanctum;* a nauseant, diaphoretic, stimulant, and reagent used in testing for occult blood.

**guai·fen·e·sin** (gwī-fen'ĕ-sin) An expectorant that allegedly reduces viscosity of sputum, thus facilitating its elimination.

**gua·no·sine (G, Guo)** (gwah'nō-sēn) A major constituent of RNA and of guanine nucleotides.

**guard·i·an** (gahr'dē-ăn) An adult considered legally responsible for the care and custody of a minor or another adult determined to be unable to provide self-care.

**guard·ing** (gahrd'ing) A spasm of muscles to minimize motion or agitation of sites affected by injury or disease.

**guar gum** (gwahr gŭm) Ground endosperms of *Cyamopsis tetragonolobus,* a legume; used in pharmaceutical jelly formulations.

**gu·ber·nac·u·lar ca·nal** (gū'bĕr-nak'yū-lăr kă-nal') Small canal located between permanent tooth germ and apex of deciduous tooth, containing remnants of dental lamina and connective tissue.

**gu·ber·nac·u·lar cord** (gū'bĕr-nak'yū-lăr

kōrd) Content of the gubernacular canal, usually composed of remnants of dental lamina and connective tissue.

**gu·ber·nac·u·lum** (gū'bĕr-nak'yū-lŭm) A fibrous cord connecting two structures (e.g., the testis and scrotum; the ovary and labium majus). The gubernaculum attaches to the uterus and becomes the ovarian ligament and the round ligament of the uterus. [L. a helm, rudder]

**gu·ber·nac·u·lum den·tis** (gū'bĕr-nak'yū-lŭm den'tis) Connective tissue band uniting tooth sac with overlying gum.

**Gue·del air·way** (gū-del' ār'wā) Oropharyngeal airway used to ensure airway patency during general anesthesia.

**Gué·rin frac·ture** (gā-rin[h]' frak'shŭr) Breakage of facial bones in which there is a horizontal fracture at base of maxillae above apices of the teeth. SYN Le Fort I fracture.

**guid·ance** (gī'dăns) **1.** The act of guiding. **2.** A guide.

**guide** (gīd) **1.** To lead in a set course. **2.** Any device or instrument by which another is led into its proper course, e.g., a grooved director, a catheter guide. [M.E., fr. O.Fr. *guier,* to show the way, fr. Germanic]

**guid·ed tis·sue re·gen·er·a·tion** (gīd'ĕd tish'ū rē-jen'ĕr-ā'shŭn) Regeneration of tissue directed by physical presence and/or chemical activities of a biomaterial; often involves placement of barriers to exclude one or more cell types during healing or regeneration of tissue.

**guide·line** (gīd'līn) Linear marking that serves as a guide or reference.

**guide plane** (gīd plān) A fixed or removable device used to displace a single tooth, an arch segment, or an entire arch toward an improved relationship.

**guid·ing plane** (gīd'ing plān) Parallel surfaces aligned superoinferiorly on dental or implant abutments that are oriented so as to contribute to the direction of the path of placement and removal of a removable dental prosthesis.

**Guil·lain-Bar·ré syn·drome** (gē-ahn[h]' bah-rā' sin'drōm) An acute, immune-mediated disorder of peripheral nerves, spinal roots, and cranial nerves, commonly presenting as a rapidly progressive, areflexive, relatively symmetric ascending weakness of the limb, truncal, respiratory, pharyngeal, and facial musculature, with variable sensory and autonomic dysfunction.

**gum** (gŭm) **1.** SYN gingiva. **2.** Dried exuded sap from various trees and shrubs, forming an amorphous brittle mass; usually forms a mucilaginous solution in water and is often used as a suspending agent in liquid preparations of insol-

uble drugs. **3.** Water-soluble glycans, often containing uronic acids, found in many plants. See this page. [L. *gummi*]

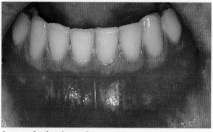

**lower gingiva (gums)**

**gum·boil** (gŭm'boyl) SYN gingival abscess.

**gum con·tour** (gŭm kon'tūr) SYN gingival contour.

**gum lan·cet** (gŭm lan'sĕt) Cutting tool used for incising gingiva over crown of an erupting tooth.

**gum line** (gŭm līn) Position of margin of gingiva in relation to teeth in dental arch.

**gum·ma,** pl. **gum·ma·ta** (gŭm'ă, -tă) An infectious granuloma that is characteristic of tertiary syphilis. Gummata are characterized by an irregular central portion that is firm, sometimes partially hyalinized, and consisting of coagulative necrosis. SYN syphiloma. [L. *gummi,* gum, fr. G. *kommi*]

**gum re·sec·tion** (gŭm rē-sek'shŭn) SYN gingivectomy.

**Gun·ning splint** (gŭn'ing splint) Prosthesis fabricated from models of edentulous maxillary and mandibular arches to aid in reduction and fixation of a fracture.

**Gunn phe·nom·e·non** (gŭn fĕ-nom'ĕ-non) SYN jaw-winking syndrome.

**Gunn syn·drome** (gŭn sin'drōm) SYN jaw-winking syndrome.

**Guo** Abbreviation for guanosine.

**gus·ta·tion** (gŭs-tā'shŭn) **1.** The act of tasting. **2.** The sense of taste. [L. *gustatio,* fr. *gusto,* pp. *-atus,* to taste]

**gus·ta·to·ry hy·per·hi·dro·sis** (gŭs'tă-tōr-ē hī'pĕr-hī-drō'sis) Excessive sweating of lips, nose, and forehead after eating certain foods; physiologic in many people, but sometimes occurs after parotid surgery or as a result of damage to the parasympathetic or sympathetic nerves of the head and neck.

**gus·ta·to·ry or·gan** (gŭs'tă-tōr-ē ōr'găn) [TA] Organ located in papillae of mucous membrane of tongue, chiefly in vallate papillae.

**gus·ta·to·ry sweat·ing** (gŭs´tă-tōr-ē swet´ing) SYN auriculotemporal nerve syndrome.

**gut·ta,** pl. **gut·tae** (gŭt´ă, -ē) **1.** A drop. (abbrev. gt, [sing.], gtt. [pl.]). **2.** A rubberlike polyterpene found in gutta-percha. Cf. chicle, guttapercha. [L.]

**gut·ta-per·cha** (gut´ă-pĕr´chă) The coagulated, dried, milky juice of trees of the genera *Palaquium*; polyterpene-containing a trans isomer of rubber used as a filling material in dentistry, and in the manufacture of splints and electrical insulators; a solution is used as a substitute for collodion, as a protective, and to seal incised wounds. [Malay *gatah,* gum, + *percha,* the name of a tree]

**gut·ta-per·cha cone** (gŭt´ă-pĕr´chă kōn) Conic, semirigid root canal filling material composed of gutta-percha and zinc oxide.

**gut·ta-per·cha points** (gut´ă-pĕr´chă poynts) Cones of gutta-percha compound used for filling root canals in conjunction with a cement, paste, or plastic.

**gut·ta-per·cha spread·er** (gŭt´ă-pĕr´chă spred´ĕr) Instrument used in dentistry for condensing gutta-percha laterally in a root canal.

**gut·ter** (gŭt´ĕr) [TA] Deep recess or groove.

**GVHD** Abbreviation for graft-versus-host disease.

**Gy** Abbreviation for gray.

**gynaecologist** [Br.] SYN gynecologist.

**gy·ne·col·o·gist** (gī´ně-kol´ŏ-jist) A physician specializing in gynecology. SYN gynaecologist.

**gyp·sum** (jip´sŭm) Natural hydrated form of calcium sulfate; component of stones, plasters, and investments used in dentistry. [L. fr. G. *gypsos*]

**gy·ro·spasm** (jī´rō-spazm) Spasmodic rotary movements of the head. [G. *gyros,* circle, + *spasmos,* spasm]

**gy·rus,** pl. **gy·ri** (jī´rŭs, -rī) [TA] One of the prominent rounded elevations or convolutions that form the cerebral hemispheres, each consisting of an exposed superficial portion and a portion hidden from view in the wall and floor of the sulcus (q.v.). [L. fr. G. *gyros,* circle]

**gh**

# H

**H** Abbreviation for histidine; hyperopia.

**hab·it** (hab′it) An act, behavioral response, practice, or custom established in one's repertoire by frequent repetition of the same activity. [L. *habeo*, pp. *habitus*, to have]

**hab·it cough** (hab′it kawf) Persistent cough due to tic or to psychological causes.

**hab·it tic** (hab′it tik) Habitual repetition of some grimace, shrug of the shoulder, twisting or jerking of the head, or the like.

**ha·bit·u·al cen·tric** (hă-bich′ū-ăl sen′trik) SYN centric occlusion.

**ha·bit·u·a·tion** (hă-bich′ū-ā′shŭn) **1.** Process of forming a habit, referring generally to psychological dependence on continued use of a drug to maintain a sense of well-being, which can result in drug addiction. **2.** Method by which nervous system reduces or inhibits responsiveness during repeated stimulation.

**hab·i·tus** (hab′i-tŭs) *The plural of this word is habitus, not habiti.* Physical characteristics of a person. [L. habit]

**Ha·der·up den·tal no·men·cla·ture** (hah′der-ŭp den′tăl nō′měn-klā-chŭr) **1.** European system of identifying teeth by use of a number for each permanent tooth and a + or − sign to indicate tooth position, e.g., 6 + is upper right first permanent molar. **2.** A system for primary teeth analogous to that for the permanent teeth in which a 0 is added before the tooth number, e.g., 03+ is the upper right deciduous canine.

**haem** [Br.] SYN heme.

**haemacyte** [Br.] SYN hemacyte.

**haemangioendothelioma** [Br.] SYN hemangioendothelioma.

**haemangiofibroma** [Br.] SYN hemangiofibroma.

**haemangioma** [Br.] SYN hemangioma.

**haemarthrosis** [Br.] SYN hemarthrosis.

**haemastatic** [Br.] SYN hemostatic.

**haematemesis** [Br.] SYN hematemesis.

**haematic** [Br.] SYN hematic.

**haematinic** [Br.] SYN hematinic.

**haematochezia** [Br.] SYN hematochezia.

**haematocrit** [Br.] SYN hematocrit.

**haematogenic** [Br.] SYN hematogenic.

**haematology** [Br.] SYN hematology.

**haematoma** [Br.] SYN hematoma.

**haematopoiesis** [Br.] SYN hematopoiesis.

**haematopoietic** [Br.] SYN hematopoietic.

**haematopoietic system** [Br.] SYN hematopoietic system.

**haematosis** [Br.] SYN hematosis.

**haematostatic** [Br.] SYN hematostatic.

**haematoxylin** [Br.] SYN hematoxylin.

**haematuria** [Br.] SYN hematuria.

**haemochromatosis** [Br.] SYN hemochromatosis.

**haemocyte** [Br.] SYN hemocyte.

**haemodialysis** [Br.] SYN hemodialysis.

**haemodynamics** [Br.] SYN hemodynamics.

**haemoglobin** [Br.] SYN hemoglobin.

**haemoglobin A** [Br.] SYN hemoglobin A.

**haemoglobinopathy** [Br.] SYN hemoglobinopathy.

**haemoglobinuria** [Br.] SYN hemoglobinuria.

**haemolysin** [Br.] SYN hemolysin.

**haemolysin unit** [Br.] SYN hemolysin unit.

**haemolysis** [Br.] SYN hemolysis.

**haemolytic anaemia** [Br.] SYN hemolytic anemia.

**haemolytic disease of newborn** [Br.] SYN hemolytic disease of newborn.

**haemolytic jaundice** [Br.] SYN hemolytic jaundice.

**haemolytic unit** [Br.] SYN hemolysin unit.

**haemophilia** [Br.] SYN hemophilia.

**haemophilia A** [Br.] SYN hemophilia A.

**haemophilia B** [Br.] SYN hemophilia B.

**haemophilia C** [Br.] SYN hemophilia C.

**haemophiliac** [Br.] SYN hemophiliac.

**Hae·moph·i·lus** (hē-mof′i-lŭs) A genus of aerobic to facultatively anaerobic, nonmotile, parasitic bacteria containing minute, gram-negative, rod-shaped cells; occur in various lesions and secretions, as well as in normal respiratory tracts, of vertebrates. [G. *haima*, blood, + *philos*, fond]

**Hae·moph·i·lus in·flu·en·zae** (hē-mof′ i-lŭs in-flū-en′zē) Bacterial species found in the respiratory tract that causes acute respiratory infections, including pneumonia and otitis.

**haemophoresis** [Br.] SYN hemophoresis.

**haemopoiesis** [Br.] SYN hemopoiesis.

**haemopoietic** [Br.] SYN hemopoietic.

**haemoptysis** [Br.] SYN hemoptysis.

**haemorrhage** [Br.] SYN hemorrhage.

**haemorrhagic cyst** [Br.] SYN hemorrhagic cyst.

**haemorrhagic shock** [Br.] SYN hemorrhagic shock.

**haemosiderin** [Br.] SYN hemosiderin.

**haemosiderosis** [Br.] SYN hemosiderosis.

**haemostasis** [Br.] SYN hemostasis.

**haemostat** [Br.] SYN hemostat.

**haemostatic** [Br.] SYN hemostatic.

**haemostatic forceps** [Br.] SYN hemostatic forceps.

**haemotoxin** [Br.] SYN hemotoxin.

**Hage·man fac·tor** (hāg′măn fak′tŏr) SYN factor XII.

**Hai·ley and Hai·ley dis·ease** (hā′lē di-zēz′) SYN keratosis follicularis. [Hugh *Hailey*, 1909–2008, American dermatologist, William *Hailey*, 1898–1967, American dermatologist]

**hair** (hār) [TA] **1.** One of the fine, keratinized filamentous epidermal growths arising from the skin of the body of mammals except the palms, soles, and flexor surfaces of the joints. **2.** One of the fine, hairlike processes of the auditory cells of the labyrinth, and of other sensory cells, called auditory or sensory hair. [A.S. *haer*]

**hair·y leu·ko·pla·ki·a** (hār′ē lū′kō-plā′kē-ă) White raised lesion seen on tongue, occasionally on buccal mucosa, in an immunocompromised host. See this page and page A10.

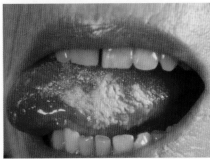
**hairy leukoplakia**

**hair·y tongue** (hār′ē tŭng) Tongue with abnormal elongation of filiform papillae, resulting in a thickened furry appearance. See page A7. SYN glossotrichia.

**hal·a·zone** (hal′ă-zōn) Chloramine used to sterilize drinking water.

**half-life** (haf′līf) **1.** The period in which the radioactivity or number of atoms of a radioactive substance decreases by half; similarly applied to any substance whose quantity decreases exponentially with time. Cf. half-time. **2.** Time required for the serum concentration of a drug to decline by 50%.

**half-time** (haf′tīm) The time, in a first-order chemical (or enzymic) reaction, for half of the substance to be converted or disappear.

**half-val·ue lay·er (HVL)** (haf-val′yū lā′ĕr) The thickness of a specific absorber (e.g., aluminum) that will reduce the intensity of a beam of radiation to one-half its initial value.

**hal·i·pha·gi·a** (hal′i-fā′jē-ă) Ingestion of an excessive quantity of a salt or salts. [G. *hals*, salt, + *phagō*, to eat]

**ha·lis·te·re·sis** (hă-lis′tĕr-ē′sis) Osseous deficiency of lime salts. [G. *hals*, salt, + *sterēsis*, privation, fr. *stereō*, to deprive]

**hal·i·to·pho·bi·a** (hal′i-tō-fō′bē-ă) An exaggerated fear of having bad breath. [*halitosis* + *phobia*]

**hal·i·to·sis** (hal-i-tō′sis) A foul odor from the mouth. SYN fetor oris, ozostomia. [L. *halitus*, breath, + G. *-osis*, condition]

**hal·i·tus** (hal′i-tŭs) Any exhalation, as of a breath or vapor. [L., fr. *halo*, to breathe]

**Hal·ler·vor·den-Spatz syn·drome** (hah′lĕr-fōr′den-shpahts sin′drōm) Disorder characterized by dystonia with other extrapyramidal dysfunctions appearing in the first two decades of life.

**hal·lu·ci·na·tion** (hă-lū′si-nā′shŭn) *Do not confuse this word with delusion or illusion.* Apparent, often strong subjective perception of an external object or event when no such stimulus or situation is present. [L. *alucinor*, to wander in mind]

**hal·lu·ci·no·gen** (hă-lū′si-nō-jen) A mind-altering chemical, drug, or agent, specifically a chemical the most prominent pharmacologic action of which is on the central nervous system; elicits optic or auditory hallucinations, depersonalization, and disturbances of thought processes. [L. *alucinor*, to wander in mind, + G. *-gen*, producing]

**hal·o·gen** (hal′ō-jen) One of the chlorine group of elements; forms monobasic acids with hydrogen, and their hydroxides. [G. *hals*, salt, + *-gen*, producing]

**ham·ar·to·ma** (ham′ahr-tō′mă) A developmental focal malformation that resembles a neoplasm, grossly and even microscopically. [G. *hamartion*, a bodily defect, + *-oma*, tumor]

gh

**Ham·bur·ger phe·nom·e·non** (hahm' būr-ger fĕ-nom'ĕ-non) SYN chloride shift.

**Ham·il·ton an·xi·e·ty rat·ing scale** (ham'il-tŏn ang-zī'ĕ-tē rāt'ing skāl) List of specific symptoms used as a measure of severity of anxiety.

**ham·mock lig·a·ment** (ham'ŏk lig'ă-mĕnt) Part of periodontium below growing end of tooth root.

**ham·u·lus,** gen. and pl. **ham·u·li** (ham'yū-lŭs, -lī) [TA] Any hooklike structure. SYN hook (2). [L. dim. of *hamus,* hook]

**hand-arm-vi·bra·tion syn·drome (HAVS)** (hand ahrm vī-brā'shŭn sin'drŏm) Disorder resulting from the use of hand-held vibration tools (e.g., pneumatic drills, electric polishers, gas-powered chainsaws). Symptoms consist of: a circulatory disturbance, specifically vasospasm with finger blanching (i.e., secondary Raynaud phenomenon); sensorineural changes (numbness and decreased sensitivity), principally limited to the fingers; and various skeletal abnormalities affecting the hand and forearm; may be unilateral or bilateral; initially episodic and triggered by cold exposure, but may ultimately progress and become constant; often carpal tunnel syndrome is associated.

**hand con·den·ser** (hand kŏn-den'sĕr) Dental instrument that compacts restorative material in a cavity by force applied manually or with the aid of a hand-held mallet.

**hand·ed·ness** (hand'ĕd-nĕs) Preference for the use of one hand, more commonly the right.

**hand-foot-and-mouth dis·ease** (hand-fut-mowth di-zēz') Exanthematous eruption of small, pearl-gray vesicles on fingers, toes, palms, and soles, accompanied by painful vesicles and ulceration of buccal mucous membrane and tongue and by slight fever; disease lasts 4–7 days, and is usually caused by Coxsackievirus type A-16; highly contagious and affects many children. See this page.

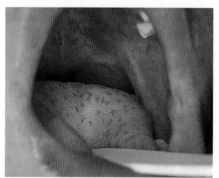

**Coxsackievirus hand-foot-and-mouth disease:** scattered petechiae present at center; note vesicle at juncture of hard and soft palates

**hand·i·cap** (hand'ē-kap) *Negative or pejorative connotations of this word may render it offensive in some contexts.* **1.** A physical, mental, or emotional condition that interferes with a person's normal functioning. **2.** Reduction in a person's capacity to fulfill a social role as a consequence of an impairment, inadequate role training or other circumstances. [fr. *hand in cap,* (game)]

**han·dle** (hand'ĕl) That part of a dental instrument that is gripped by the clinician.

**han·dle roll** (han'dĕl rōl) Act of turning the instrument handle slightly between the thumb and index finger to readapt the working-end to the next segment of the tooth.

**hand-o·ver-mouth ex·er·cise (H.O.M.E.)** (hand ō'vĕr mowth eks'ĕr-sīz) Patient-management technique for pedodontic dental patients where the dentist gently places his or her hand over the child's mouth and tells child that the hand will be removed as soon as the child is quiet and can listen without being loud and disruptive. **This method can only be employed by the dentist, not by dental auxiliaries, and must never include obstructing the nasal airway, which is illegal.**

**hand·piece** (hand'pēs) A hand-held powered dental instrument, used to hold rotary cutting, grinding, or polishing implements while they revolve.

**Hand-Schül·ler-Chris·tian dis·ease** (hand shē'lĕr kris'chăn di-zēz') Chronic disseminated form of Langerhans cell histiocytosis; triad of signs consists of diabetes insipidus, exophthalmos, and bony histiocytic lesions.

**hang·ing sep·tum** (hang'ing sep'tŭm) Deformity caused by abnormal width of septal portion of alar cartilages.

**Han·sen dis·ease** (hahn'sen di-zēz') SYN leprosy.

**hap·ten** (hap'tĕn) A molecule that is incapable, alone, of causing the production of antibodies but can, however, combine with a larger antigenic molecule called a carrier. SYN incomplete antigen, partial antigen. [G. *haptō,* to fasten, + -*en,* noun suffix]

**hap·tom·e·ter** (hap-tom'ĕ-tĕr) Instrument for measuring sensitivity to touch. [G. *haptō,* to touch, + *meter,* fr. M.E., fr. O.Fr., fr. L., fr. G. *metron,* measure]

**hard·en·ing** (hahrd'ĕn-ing) A condition of lessened reactions to allergens from repeated or prolonged nontherapeutic exposure, similar to hyposensitization.

**har·di·ness** (hahr'dē-nĕs) A health-enhancing behavior trait believed to increase one's resistance to illness, characterized by great personal control and commitment, in response to events of daily life. [M.E., fr. O.Fr. *hardi,* fr. Germanic]

**hard·ness** (hahrd′nĕs) **1.** The degree of firmness of a solid, as determined by its resistance to deformation, scratching, or abrasion. **2.** The relative penetrating power of a beam of x-rays.

**hard·ness test** (hahrd′nĕs test) Measurement of durability of a material, usually involving making and measuring an indentation in the material using a pressure device. SEE ALSO Brinell hardness test, Rockwell hardness test, Vickers hardness test, Knoop hardness test.

**hard pal·ate** (hahrd pal′ăt) [TA] Anterior part of palate, consisting of bony palate covered above by mucous membrane of the floor of the nasal cavity and below by the mucoperiosteum of the roof of the mouth, which contains the palatine vessels, nerves, and mucous glands. See this page.

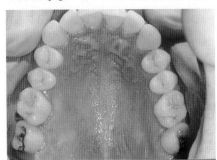

hard palate: incisive papilla and rugae in anterior fold

**hard par·af·fin** (hahrd par′ă-fin) Purified mixture of solid hydrocarbons derived from petroleum. SYN paraffin (2).

**hare·lip** (hār′lip) SYN cleft lip.

**Hart·man so·lu·tion** (hahrt′măn sŏ-lū′shŭn) Formulation used to desensitize dentin in dental operations; contains thymol, ethyl alcohol, and sulfuric ether.

**hash·ish** (hah-shēsh′) A form of cannabis that consists largely of resin from flowering tops and sprouts of cultivated female plants.

**Hatch clamp** (hach klamp) Adjustable device used with rubber dam in gingival procedures.

**hatch·et** (hach′ĕt) Dental instrument with an end cutting blade set at an angle to axis of handle and having one or two bevels; in the former case, made as right and left pairs called enamel hatchets; used to remove enamel and dentin. Also called hatchet excavator. See this page.

**haus·tus** (haw′stŭs) A potion or medicinal draft. [L. a drink, draft]

**ha·ver·si·an sys·tem** (ha-vĕr′zē-ăn sis′tĕm) SYN osteon.

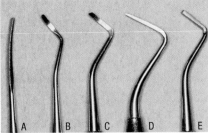

dental instruments for manual cutting procedures: (A) Wedelstadt chisel; (B) spoon excavator; (C) gingival margin trimmer; (D) hoe; (E) hatchet

**HAVS** Abbreviation for hand-arm-vibration syndrome.

**Haw·ley re·tain·er** (haw′lē rĕ-tā′nĕr) Removable wire and acrylic palatal appliance used to hold or stabilize teeth in their new position following orthodontic tooth movement; with modifications can be used to move teeth as an active orthodontic appliance. See this page.

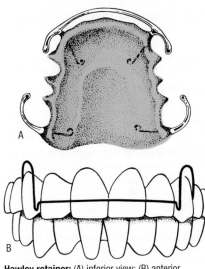

Hawley retainer: (A) inferior view; (B) anterior view, appliance in position

**hay fe·ver** (hā fē′vĕr) A form of atopy characterized by an acute irritative inflammation of the mucous membranes of the eyes and upper respiratory passages accompanied by itching and profuse watery secretion, followed occasionally by bronchitis and asthma.

**haz·ar·dous waste** (haz′ărd-ŭs wāst) Debris, trash, or byproducts from dental procedures that pose a risk.

**Hb** Abbreviation for hemoglobin.

**Hb A** Abbreviation for hemoglobin A.

gh

**HBO** Abbreviation for hyperbaric oxygen.

**HCl** Abbreviation for hydrochloric acid.

**Hct** Abbreviation for hematocrit.

**He** Symbol for helium.

**head** (hed) **1.** [TA] Upper or anterior extremity of animal body, containing brain and organs of sight, hearing, taste, and smell. **2.** [TA] Upper, anterior, or larger extremity, expanded or rounded, of any body, organ, or other anatomic structure. **3.** Rounded extremity of a bone. SYN caput.

**head·ache** (hed'āk) Pain in various cranial areas.

**Head ar·e·as** (hed ar'ē-ăz) Areas of skin exhibiting reflex hyperesthesia and hyperalgesia due to visceral disease.

**head-bob·bing doll syn·drome** (hed' bob-in dol sin'drōm) Congenital disorder manifested as intermittent flexion and extension movements of head, often accompanied by similar limb movements.

**head-drop·ping test** (hed'drop-ing test) Assessment used in diagnosis of disease of extrapyramidal or striatal system.

**head·gear** (hed'gēr) Removable extraoral appliance used to apply force to teeth and jaws.

**head mir·ror** (hed mir'ŏr) Circular concave mirror with a hole in its center to look through, attached to a head band, used to project a beam of light into a cavity, such as the mouth, nose or larynx, to examine and permit binocular vision.

**head of man·di·ble** (hed man'di-bĕl) [TA] Expanded articular portion of condylar process of mandible.

**head-tilt** (hed'tilt) An abnormal position of the head adopted to prevent double vision resulting from underaction of vertical ocular muscles.

**head-tilt/chin-lift ma·neu·ver** (hĕd'tilt-chin'lift mă-nū'vĕr) Basic procedure used in cardiopulmonary resuscitation to open the patient's airway. SYN manual airway maneuver, rescue breathing.

**heal** (hēl) To restore to health. [A.S. *haclan*]

**health** (helth) **1.** State of organism when it functions optimally without evidence of disease or abnormality. **2.** State of dynamic balance in which an individual's or a group's capacity to cope with all the circumstances of living is at an optimal level. [A.S. *health*]

**health care** (helth kār) Services provided to people or communities by agents of the health professions to promote, maintain, and restore health.

**health care–as·so·ci·a·ted in·fec·tion** (helth kār-ă-sō'sē-ā-tĕd in-fek'shŭn) Infection acquired in a health care-related setting other than a hospital (e.g., dialysis facility, provider of long-term care). SEE ALSO nosocomial.

**health care pro·vid·er** (helth kār prŏ-vī'dĕr) General term for any institution or member of the team providing health care.

**health ed·u·ca·tion** (helth ed'yū-kā'shŭn) NURSING education to gain knowledge, skills, values, and attitudes for maintaining and improving health in patients.

**health in·sur·ance** (helth in-shŭr'ăns) In the U.S., commercial product designed to protect consumers from the financial risks of illness and injury. SYN medical insurance.

**Health In·sur·ance Por·ta·bil·i·ty and Ac·count·a·bil·i·ty Act (HIPAA)** (helth in-shŭr'ăns pōr'tă-bil'i-tē ă-kownt'ă-bil'i-tē akt) U.S. federal legislation designed to preserve health insurance coverage for workers and their families when they change or lose their jobs. Includes security and privacy standards to protect personal health information and avoid misuse or inappropriate disclosure.

**health main·te·nance or·gan·i·za·tion (HMO)** (helth mān'tĕn-ăns ōr'găn-ī-zā' shŭn) Comprehensive prepaid system of health care intended to emphasize prevention and early detection of disease and continuity of care.

**health pro·mo·tion** (helth prŏ-mō'shŭn) Providing patients and clients with information to enhance health and prevent disease.

**health-re·lat·ed phys·i·cal fit·ness** (helth-rĕ-lā'tĕd fiz'i-kăl fit'nĕs) Components of physical fitness associated with some aspect of overall good health.

**health risk as·sess·ment (h.r.a.)** (helth risk ă-ses'mĕnt) Method of describing a person's chance of falling ill or dying of a specified condition, based on actuarial calculations and intended as a way to draw the person's attention to the probable health consequences of risky behavior.

**health·y** (hel'thē) Well; in a state of normal functioning; free from disease.

**hear·ing** (hēr'ing) The ability to perceive sound; sensation of sound not vibration.

**hear·ing aid** (hēr'ing ād) An electronic amplifying device designed to bring sound more effectively into the ear; it consists of a microphone, amplifier, and receiver.

**hear·ing im·pair·ment, hear·ing loss** (hēr'ing im-pār'mĕnt, laws) Reduction in ability to perceive sound; may range from slight inability to complete deafness. SEE ALSO deafness.

**heart** (hahrt) [TA] Hollow muscular organ that receives blood from veins and propels it into the arteries. In mammals, divided by a musculomembranous septum into two halves—right or venous and left or arterial—each of which consists of a receiving chamber (atrium) and an ejecting chamber (ventricle). [A.S. *heorte*]

**heart at·tack** (hahrt ă-tak´) SYN myocardial infarction.

**heart·burn** (hahrt´bŭrn) SYN pyrosis.

**heart fail·ure** (hahrt fāl´yŭr) **1.** Inadequacy of the heart so that as a pump it fails to maintain the circulation of blood, with the result that congestion and edema develop in the tissues. **2.** Resulting clinical syndromes including shortness of breath, pitting edema, enlarged tender liver, and pulmonary rales in various combinations.

**heart mas·sage** (hahrt mă-sahzh´) Rhythmic massage of the heart either in an open chest or through the chest wall to renew failed circulation during cardiac resuscitation. SYN cardiac massage.

**heart mur·mur** (hahrt mŭr´mŭr) A colloquialism for cardiac murmur (q.v.).

**heart rate** (hahrt rāt) Velocity of the heart's beat, in number of beats per minute.

**heart sounds** (hahrt sowndz) Noises made by muscle contraction and closure of heart valves during cardiac cycle.

**heat** (hēt) **1.** A high temperature; the sensation produced by proximity to fire or an incandescent object. **2.** The kinetic energy of atoms and molecules. [A.S. *haete*]

**heat-cur·ing res·in** (hēt´kyŭr-ing rez´in) Resin that requires elevated temperatures to initiate polymerization.

**heat treat·ment** (hēt trēt´mĕnt) In dentistry, method of controlled temperature handling of metals to change microscopic structure and thus physical properties. SEE ALSO temper, anneal.

**heav·y liq·uid pe·tro·la·tum** (hev´ē lik´ wid pet´rō-lā´tŭm) SYN mineral oil.

**heav·y met·al neur·op·a·thy** (hev´ē met´ăl nūr-op´ă-thē) Peripheral nervous system disorders attributed to intoxication due to one of the heavy metals (e.g., arsenic, gold, lead).

**he·be·phre·ni·a** (hē´bĕ-frē´nē-ă) Syndrome characterized by shallow and inappropriate affect, giggling, and silly regressive behavior and mannerisms. [G. *hēbē*, puberty, + *phrēn*, the mind]

**hec·tic flush** (hek´tik flŭsh) Redness of face associated with feverish rise of temperature.

**hec·to·gram** (hek´tō-gram) 100 grams.

**hec·to·li·ter** (hek´tō-lē-tĕr) 100 liters.

**Hed·ström file** (hed´strum fīl) Coarse dental root canal file similar to a rasp.

**heel** (hēl) **1.** Proximal portion of plantar surface of foot. **2.** SYN calx (2). **3.** SYN distal end. [A.S. *hēla*]

**Heer·fordt dis·ease** (hār´fōrt di-zēz´) SYN uveoparotid fever.

**height** (hīt) *Avoid the mispronunciation hīth.* Vertical measurement.

**height of con·tour** (hīt kon´tūr) Line encircling tooth or other structure at its greatest bulge or diameter, within a given or specified plane; relates to selected path of insertion of dental appliance or device.

**Heim·lich ma·neu·ver** (hīm´lik mă-nū´ vĕr) Action designed to expel an obstructing bolus of food from the throat by placing a fist on the abdomen between navel and costal margin, grasping fist from behind with other hand, and forcefully thrusting it inward and upward to force the diaphragm upward, thus forcing air up the trachea to dislodge obstruction.

**Hel·i·co·bac·ter** (hel´i-kō-bak´tĕr) Genus of helical, curved, or straight microaerophilic bacteria with rounded ends and multiple sheathed flagella with terminal bulbs. Found in gastric mucosa of primates, including human beings; some species are associated with gastric and peptic ulcers and predispose to gastric carcinoma. The type species is *H. pylori*.

**Hel·i·co·bac·ter py·lor·i** (hel´i-kō-bak´ter pī-lō´rī) Bacterial species that produces urease and causes gastritis and nearly all peptic ulcer disease of the stomach and duodenum. Infection with this organism also plays an etiologic role (probably along with dietary cofactors) in dysplasia and metaplasia of gastric mucosa, distal gastric adenocarcinoma, and non-Hodgkin lymphoma of the stomach. After infection occurs, typically lifelong without antibiotics.

**he·li·um (He)** (hē´lē-ŭm) A gaseous element present in minute amounts in the atmosphere used as a diluent of medicinal gases. [G. *hēlios*, the sun]

**hel·leb·o·rus** (he-leb´ŏ-rŭs) Black hellebore, dried rhizome and roots of *Helleborus niger;* used as a cardiac and arterial tonic, diuretic, and cathartic. [G. *helleboros*]

**hel·minth** (hel´minth) Intestinal vermiform parasite, primarily nematodes, cestodes, trematodes, and acanthocephalans.

**hel·min·tha·gogue** (hel-minth´ă-gog) SYN anthelmintic. [G. *helmins*, worm, + *agōgos*, leading]

**hel·min·thi·a·sis** (hel´min-thī´ă-sis) The condition of having intestinal vermiform parasites.

**he·ma·cyte** (hē´mă-sīt) SYN erythrocyte, haemacyte.

**he·man·gi·o·en·do·the·li·o·ma** (hē-

gh

man'jē-ō-en'dō-thē'lē-ō'mă) A neoplasm derived from blood vessels, characterized by numerous prominent endothelial cells that occur singly, in aggregates, and as the lining of congeries of vascular tubes or channels; in the elderly, may be malignant (angiosarcoma or hemangiosarcoma), but in children are benign. SYN haemangioendothelioma.

**he·man·gi·o·fi·bro·ma** (hē-man'jē-ō-fī-brō'mă) A hemangioma with an abundant fibrous tissue framework. SYN haemangiofibroma.

**he·man·gi·o·ma** (hē-man'jē-ō'mă) Vascular tumor, present at birth or developing during life, in which proliferation of blood vessels leads to a mass that resembles a neoplasm; can occur anywhere in the body but most frequently noticed in skin and subcutaneous tissues. See this page. SYN haemangioma. [*hemangio-* + G. *-oma*, tumor]

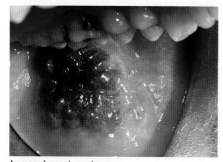

**hemangioma:** buccal mucosa

**he·mar·thro·sis** (hēm'ahr-thrō'sis) Blood in a joint. SYN haemarthrosis. [G. *haima*, blood, + *arthron*, joint]

**he·ma·tem·e·sis** (hē'mă-tem'ĕ-sis) Vomiting of blood. SYN haematemesis. [*hemat-* + G. *emesis*, vomiting]

**he·mat·ic** (hē-mat'ik) **1.** Relating to blood. **2.** SYN hematinic (2), haematic.

**he·ma·tin·ic** (hē'mă-tin'ik) **1.** Improving the condition of the blood. **2.** An agent that improves the quality of blood by increasing the number of erythrocytes and/or the hemoglobin concentration. SYN hematic (2), haematinic.

**he·ma·tin·ic prin·ci·ple** (hē'mă-tin'ik prin'si-pĕl) SEE vitamin B12.

**he·ma·to·che·zi·a** (hē'mă-tō-kē'zē-ă) Passage of bloody stools, in contradistinction to melena, or tarry stools. SYN haematochezia. [*hemato-* + G. *chezō*, to go to stool]

**he·mat·o·crit (Hct)** (hē-mat'ō-krit) Percentage of the volume of a blood sample occupied by cells. Cf. plasmacrit. SYN haematocrit. [*hemato-* + G. *krinō*, to separate]

**he·ma·to·gen·ic, he·ma·tog·e·nous** (hē'mă-tō-jen'ik, -toj'ĕ-nŭs) **1.** SYN hemopoietic, haematogenic. **2.** Pertaining to anything produced from, derived from, or transported by the blood.

**he·ma·to·his·ton** (hē'mă-tō-his'tŏn) SYN globin, haematohiston.

**he·ma·to·log·ic pro·file** (hē'mă-tō-loj'ik prō'fīl) Analysis of blood and blood-forming tissues.

**he·ma·tol·o·gy** (hē'mă-tol'ŏ-jē) The medical specialty that pertains to the anatomy, physiology, pathology, symptomatology, and therapeutics related to blood and blood-forming tissues. SYN haematology. [*hemato-* + G. *logos*, study]

**he·ma·to·ma** (hē'mă-tō'mă) Localized mass of extravasated blood relatively or completely confined within an organ or space; blood usually clots. SYN haematoma. See this page. [*hemato-* + G. *-oma*, tumor]

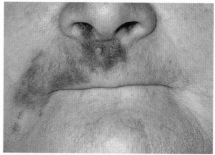

**hematoma:** trauma due to falling

**he·ma·to·poi·e·sis** (hē'mă-tō-poy-ē'sis) SYN hemopoiesis, haematopoiesis.

**he·ma·to·poi·et·ic** (hē'mă-tō-poy-et'ik) SYN hemopoietic, haematopoietic.

**he·ma·to·poi·et·ic sys·tem** (hē'mă-tō-poy-et'ik sis'tĕm) Blood-making organs. SYN haematopoietic system.

**he·ma·to·sis** (hē'mă-tō'sis) **1.** SYN hemopoiesis, haematosis. **2.** Oxygenation of the venous blood in the lungs.

**he·ma·to·stat·ic** (hē'mă-tō-stat'ik) Denotes something due to stagnation of blood in the vessels of the body part. SYN haematostatic.

**he·ma·tox·y·lin** (hē'mă-toks'i-lin) [CI 75290] A crystalline compound containing the coloring matter of *Haematoxylon campechianum* (logwood), from which it is obtained by extraction with ether. SYN haematoxylin.

**he·ma·tu·ri·a** (hē'mă-tyūr'ē-ă) Presence of blood or red blood cells in the urine. SYN haematuria. [*hemato-* + G. *ouron*, urine]

**heme** (hēm) **1.** The oxygen-carrying, color-furnishing, prosthetic group of hemoglobin. **2.** Iron complexed with nonporphyrins but related tetrapyrrole structures. SYN reduced hematin, haem. [G. *haima*, blood]

**hem·i·al·gi·a** (hem′ē-al′jē-ă) Pain affecting one entire half of the body. [*hemi-* + G. *algos*, pain]

**hemianaesthesia** [Br.] SYN hemianesthesia.

**hem·i·an·al·ge·si·a** (hem′ē-an-ăl-jē′zē-ă) Analgesia affecting one side of the body.

**hem·i·an·es·the·si·a** (hem′ē-an-es-thē′ zē-ă) Anesthesia on one side of the body. SYN hemianaesthesia.

**hem·i·at·ro·phy** (hem′ē-at′rŏ-fē) Atrophy of one lateral half of a part or of an organ, as in the face or tongue.

**hem·i·bal·lis·mus** (hem′ē-bal-iz′mŭs) Jerking movement involving one side of the body. [*hemi-* + G. *ballismos*, jumping about]

**hem·i·ceph·a·lal·gi·a** (hem′ē-sef-ă-lal′jē-ă) Unilateral headache characteristic of typical migraine. [*hemi-* + G. *kephalē*, head, + *algos*, pain]

**hemidysaesthesia** [Br.] SYN hemidysesthesia.

**hem·i·dys·es·the·si·a** (hem′ē-dis-es-thē′ zē-ă) Dysesthesia affecting one side of the body. SYN hemidysaesthesia.

**he·mi·fa·cial spasm** (hem′ē-fā′shăl spazm) Disorder of facial nerve characterized by unilateral involuntary paroxysmal contractions of facial muscles, caused by high-frequency bursts of motor units lasting from a few milliseconds to several seconds.

**he·mi·glo·bi·ne·mi·a** (hem′ē-glō-bi-nē′ mē-ă) SYN methemoglobinemia.

**hem·i·glos·sec·to·my** (hem′ē-glos-ek′tŏ-mē) Surgical removal of one half of the tongue. [*hemi-* + G. *glōssa*, tongue, + *ektomē*, excision]

**hem·i·gnath·i·a** (hem′ē-gnath′ē-ă) Defective development of one side of mandible. [*hemi-* + G. *gnathos*, jaw]

**hemihypaesthesia** [Br.] SYN hemihypesthesia.

**hem·i·hy·pal·ge·si·a** (hem′ē-hīp′al-je′zē-ă) Hypalgesia affecting one side of the body.

**hemihyperaesthesia** [Br.] SYN hemihyperesthesia.

**hem·i·hy·per·es·the·si·a** (hem′ē-hī′pĕr-es-thē′zē-ă) Hyperesthesia, or increased tactile and painful sensibility, affecting one side of the body. SYN hemihyperaesthesia.

**hem·i·hy·per·to·ni·a** (hem′ē-hī′pĕr-tō′nē-ă) Exaggerated muscular tonicity on one side of the body. [*hemi-* + G. *hyper*, over, + *tonos*, tone]

**hem·i·hy·per·tro·phy** (hem′ē-hī-pĕr′trŏ-fē) Muscular or osseous hypertrophy of one side of the face or body.

**hem·i·hyp·es·the·si·a** (hem′ē-hīp′es-thē′ zē-ă) Diminished sensibility involving only one side of the body. SYN hemihypaesthesia. [*hemi-* + G. *hypo*, under, + *aesthēses*, sensation]

**hem·i·hy·po·to·ni·a** (hem′ē-hī-pō-tō′nē-ă) Partial loss of muscular tonicity on one side of the body. [*hemi-* + G. *hypo*, under, + *tonos*, tone]

**hem·i·man·dib·u·lec·to·my** (hem′ē-man-dib′yū-lek′tŏ-mē) Resection of half the mandible.

**hem·i·o·pal·gi·a** (hem′ē-ō-pal′jē-ă) Pain in one eye. [*hemi-* + G. *ōps*, eye, + *algos*, pain]

**hem·i·pa·re·sis** (hem′ē-pă-rē′sis) Weakness affecting one side of the body.

**hem·i·ple·gi·a** (hem′ē-plē′jē-ă) Paralysis of one side of the body. [*hemi-* + G. *plēgē*, a stroke]

**hem·i·ple·gic gait** (hem′ē-plē′jik gāt) Gait in which the leg is stiff, without flexion at knee and ankle, and with each step is rotated away from the body, then toward it, forming a semicircle. SYN spastic gait.

**hem·i·sec·tion** (hem′ē-sek′shŭn) Surgical removal of tooth root and its related coronal portion of a multirooted tooth.

**hem·i·sen·so·ry** (hem′ē-sen′sŏr-ē) Loss of sensation on one side of the body.

**hem·i·sphere** (hem′is-fēr) [TA] Half a spheric structure. [*hemi-* + G. *sphaira*, ball, globe]

**he·mo·chro·ma·to·sis** (hē′mō-krō-mă-tō′ sis) Disorder of iron metabolism characterized by excessive absorption of ingested iron, saturation of iron-binding protein, and deposition of hemosiderin in tissue, particularly in the liver, pancreas, and skin; cirrhosis, diabetes (bronze diabetes), bronze pigmentation of the skin, and, eventually heart failure may occur; can also result from administration of large amounts of iron orally, by injection, or in forms of blood transfusion therapy. SYN haemochromatosis. [*hemo-* + G. *chrōma*, color, + *-osis*, condition]

**he·mo·cyte** (hē′mō-sīt) Any cell or formed element of the blood. SYN haemocyte. [*hemo-* + G. *kytos*, a hollow (cell)]

**he·mo·di·al·y·sis** (hē′mō-dī-al′i-sis) Dialysis of soluble substances and water from blood by diffusion through a semipermeable membrane. SYN haemodialysis.

**he·mo·dy·nam·ics** (hē′mō-dī-nam′iks) Study of physical dynamics of blood circulation. SYN haemodynamics. [*hemo-* + G. *dynamis, power*]

**he·mo·glo·bin (Hb)** (hē′mō-glō′bin) Red respiratory protein of erythrocytes. In humans, there are at least five kinds of normal Hb: two embryonic Hbs (Hb Gower-1, Hb Gower-2), fetal (Hb F), and two adult types (Hb A, Hb $A_2$). SYN haemoglobin.

**he·mo·glo·bin A (Hb A)** (hē′mō-glō′bin) Normal adult Hb A with formula $\alpha_2^A\beta_2^A$ or $\alpha_2\beta_2$. SYN haemoglobin A.

**he·mo·glo·bi·nop·a·thy** (hē′mō-glō′bi-nop′ă-thē) A disorder or disease caused by or associated with the presence of hemoglobins in the blood. SYN haemoglobinopathy. [*hemoglobin* + G. *pathos,* disease]

**he·mo·glo·bi·nu·ri·a** (hē′mō-glō′bi-nyūr′ē-ă) Presence of hemoglobin in urine; when present in sufficient quantities, they result in the urine's being colored in shades varying from light reddish-yellow to fairly dark red. SYN haemoglobinuria. [*hemoglobin* + G. *ouron,* urine]

**he·mol·y·sin** (hē-mol′i-sin) **1.** Any substance elaborated by a living agent and capable of lysing red blood cells and liberating their hemoglobin. SYN erythrocytolysin, erythrolysin, haemolysin. **2.** A sensitizing (complement-fixing) antibody that combines with red blood cells of the antigenic type that stimulated formation of the hemolysin. SYN haemolysin.

**he·mol·y·sin u·nit, he·mo·lyt·ic u·nit** (hē-mol′i-sin yū′nit, hē′mō-lit′ik) Smallest quantity (highest dilution) of inactivated immune serum (hemolysin) that will sensitize the standard suspension of erythrocytes so that the standard complement will cause complete hemolysis. SYN haemolysin unit, haemolytic unit.

**he·mol·y·sis** (hē-mol′i-sis) Alteration, dissolution, or destruction of red blood cells in such a manner that hemoglobin is liberated into the medium in which the cells are suspended. SYN haemolysis. [*hemo-* + G. *lysis,* destruction]

**he·mo·lyt·ic a·ne·mi·a** (hē′mō-lit′ik ă-nē′mē-ă) Anemia due to increased rate of erythrocyte destruction. SYN haemolytic anemia.

**he·mo·lyt·ic dis·ease of new·born** (hē′mō-lit′ik di-zēz′ nū′bōrn) SYN erythroblastosis fetalis, haemolytic disease of newborn.

**he·mo·lyt·ic jaun·dice** (hē′mō-lit′ik jawn′dis) Jaundice resulting from increased production of bilirubin from hemoglobin as a result of any process increasing destruction of erythrocytes. SYN haemolytic jaundice.

**he·mo·phil·i·a** (hē′mō-fil′ē-ă) Inherited disorder of blood coagulation characterized by a permanent tendency to hemorrhages, spontaneous or traumatic, because of a defect in the blood-coagulating mechanism. SYN haemophilia. [*hemo-* + G. *philos,* fond]

**he·mo·phil·i·a A** (hē′mō-fil′ē-ă) Blood disorder due to deficiency of factor VIII; occurring almost exclusively in male humans characterized by prolonged clotting time, decreased formation of thromboplastin, and diminished conversion of prothrombin. SYN classic hemophilia, haemophilia A.

**he·mo·phil·i·a B** (hē′mō-fil′ē-ă) Clotting disorder resembling hemophilia A, caused by hereditary deficiency of factor IX. SYN Christmas disease, haemophilia B.

**he·mo·phil·i·a C** (hē-mō-fil′ē-ă) Clotting disorder due to deficiency of factor XI; occurs primarily in people of Jewish ancestry. SYN haemophilia C.

**he·mo·phil·i·ac** (hē′mō-fil′ē-ak) A person suffering from hemophilia. SYN haemophiliac.

**he·mo·pho·re·sis** (hē′mō-fŏr-ē′sis) Blood convection or irrigation of tissues. SYN haemophoresis. [*hemo-* + G. *phoreō,* to bear]

**he·mo·poi·e·sis** (hē′mō-poy-ē′sis) Process of formation and development of various types of blood cells and other formed elements. SYN hematopoiesis, hematosis (1), haemopoiesis. [*hemo-* + G. *poiēsis,* a making]

**he·mo·poi·et·ic** (hē′mō-poy-et′ik) Pertaining to or related to the formation of blood cells. SYN hematogenic (1), hematopoietic.

**he·mop·ty·sis** (hē-mop′ti-sis) Spitting of blood derived from lungs or bronchial tubes as a result of pulmonary or bronchial hemorrhage. SYN haemoptysis. [*hemo-* + G. *ptysis,* a spitting]

**he·mo·re·pel·lant** (hē′mō-rĕ-pel′ănt) **1.** A substance or surface that discourages the adherence of blood. **2.** Having such an action.

**hem·or·rhage** (hem′ŏr-ăj) **1.** Escape of blood from the intravascular space. SYN haemorrhage. **2.** To bleed. [G. *haimorrhagia,* fr. *haima,* blood, + *rhēgnymi,* to burst forth]

**hem·or·rhag·ic a·ne·mi·a** (hem′ŏr-aj′ik ă-nē′mē-ă) Anemia resulting directly from loss of blood.

**hem·or·rhag·ic bron·chi·tis** (hem′ŏr-aj′ik brong-kī′tis) Chronic bronchitis due to infection with spirochetes characterized by cough and bloody sputum.

**hem·or·rhag·ic cyst** (hem′ŏr-aj′ik sist) A lesion containing blood or resulting from the encapsulation of a hematoma. SYN blood cyst, hematocele (1), hematocyst, haemorrhagic cyst.

**hem·or·rhag·ic shock** (hem′ŏr-aj′ik shok) Hypovolemic shock resulting from acute hemorrhage, characterized by hypotension; tachycardia; pale, cold, and clammy skin; and oliguria. SYN haemorrhagic shock.

**he·mo·si·al·em·e·sis** (hē′mō-sī′ăl-em′ĕ-sis) Vomiting of blood and saliva. [*hemo-* + G. *sialon,* saliva, + *emesis,* vomiting]

**he·mo·sid·er·in** (hē′mō-sid′ĕr-in) A yellow or brown protein produced by phagocytic digestion of hematin; found in most tissues, but especially in the liver. SYN haemosiderin. [*hemo-* + G. *sidēros,* iron, + *-in*]

**he·mo·sid·er·o·sis** (hē′mō-sid-ĕr-ō′sis) Accumulation of hemosiderin in tissue, particularly in liver and spleen. SYN haemosiderosis. [*hemosiderin* + *-osis,* condition]

**he·mo·sta·sis** (hē′mō-stā′sis) 1. Arrest of bleeding. 2. Arrest of circulation in a part. 3. Stagnation of blood. SYN haemostasis. [*hemo-* + G. *stasis,* a standing]

**he·mo·stat** (hē′mō-stat) 1. Any agent that arrests, chemically or mechanically, the flow of blood from an open vessel. 2. An instrument for arresting hemorrhage by compression of the bleeding vessel. SYN haemostat.

**he·mo·stat·ic** (hē′mō-stat′ik) 1. Arresting the flow of blood within the vessels. 2. SYN antihemorrhagic, haemastatic, haemostatic.

**he·mo·stat·ic for·ceps** (hē′mō-stat′ik fōr′seps) A forceps with a catch for locking the blades, used for seizing the end of a blood vessel to control hemorrhage. SYN artery forceps, haemostatic forceps.

**he·mo·tox·in** (hē′mō-tok′sin) Any substance that destroys red blood cells; used with reference to substances of biologic origin, in contrast to chemicals. SYN haemotoxin.

**He·noch-Schön·lein pur·pu·ra** (hen′awk shĕrn′līn pŭr′pyŭr-ă) Eruption of non-thrombocytopenic, palpable, purpuric lesions due to dermal leukocytoclastic vasculitis with IgA in vessel walls associated with joint pain and swelling, colic, and bloody stools; occurring characteristically in young children. SYN anaphylactoid purpura (2).

**He·pad·na·vi·ri·dae** (hē-pad′nă-vir′i-dē) A family of DNA-containing viruses. The principal genus *Hepadnavirus* is associated with hepatitis B. [*hep*atitis + *DNA* + *virus*]

**hep·a·rin·ize** (hep′ăr-in-īz) To perform therapeutic administration of heparin.

**hep·a·rin u·nit** (hep′ă-rin yū′nit) Quantity of heparin required to keep 1 mL of cat's blood fluid for 24 hours at 0°C; it is equivalent approximately to 0.002 mg of pure heparin.

**he·pa·tic in·suf·fi·cien·cy** (he-pat′ik in-sŭ-fish′ĕn-sē) Defective functional activity of the liver cells.

■**hep·a·ti·tis** (hep′ă-tī′tis) Inflammation of the liver, due usually to viral infection but some-

times to toxic agents. See page 276. [*hepat-* + *-itis*]

**hep·a·ti·tis G** (hep′ă-tī′tis) A disease caused by an RNA virus similar to hepatitis virus.

**hep·a·ti·tis, vi·ral, non-A, non-B (NANB)** (hep′ă-tī′tis, vī′răl) Disease due to viral agents other than hepatitis viruses A or B.

**he·pa·to·cel·lu·lar jaun·dice** (hep′ă-tō-sel′yū-lăr jawn′dis) Jaundice due to diffuse injury or inflammation or failure of function of the liver cells.

**hep·a·to·dys·en·ter·y** (hep′ă-tō-dis′ĕn-ter-ē) Dysentery associated with liver disease.

**hep·a·to·gen·ic, he·pa·tog·e·nous** (hep′ă-tō-jen′ik, -toj′ĕn-ŭs) Of hepatic origin; formed in the liver.

**he·pa·tog·e·nous jaun·dice** (hep-ă-toj′ĕn-ŭs jawn′dis) Jaundice due to liver disease.

**hep·a·to·meg·a·ly, he·pa·to·me·ga·li·a** (hep′ă-tō-meg′ă-lē, -mĕ-gā′lē-ă) Enlargement of the liver.

**hep·a·to·tox·ic·i·ty** (hep′ă-tō-tok-sis′i-tē) Capacity of a drug, chemical, or other exposure to injure the liver.

**he·red·i·tar·y** (hĕr-ed′i-tar-ē) Transmissible from parent to offspring by information encoded in the parental germ cell. [L. *hereditarius;* fr. *heres (hered-),* an heir]

**he·red·i·tar·y an·gi·o·e·de·ma** (hĕr-ed′i-tar-ē an′jē-ō-ĕ-dē′mă) Inherited disease characterized by episodic appearance of brawny nonpitting edema, most often affecting the limbs, but capable of involving other body parts, including mucosal surfaces of the intestine or respiratory tract.

**he·red·i·ta·ry brown o·pa·les·cent teeth** (hĕr-ed′i-tar-ē brown ō′pă-les′ĕnt tēth) SYN hereditary brown teeth.

**he·red·i·tar·y brown teeth** (hĕr-ed′i-tar-ē brown tēth) Dental manifestation of amelogenesis imperfecta. SYN hereditary brown opalescent teeth, hereditary dark teeth.

**he·red·i·tar·y dark teeth** (hĕr-ed′i-tar-ē dahrk tēth) SYN hereditary brown teeth.

■**he·red·i·tar·y hem·or·rhag·ic tel·an·gi·ec·ta·si·a** (hĕr-ed′i-tar-ē hem-ŏ-raj′ik tel-an′jē-ek-tā′zē-ă) Disease with onset usually after puberty, marked by multiple small telangiectases and dilated venules that develop slowly on the skin and mucous membranes; the face, lips, tongue, nasopharynx, and intestinal mucosa are frequent sites, and recurrent bleeding may occur. See page 277 and page A9.

**he·red·i·tar·y mul·ti·ple ex·os·to·ses** (hĕr-ed′i-tar-ē mŭl′ti-pĕl eks′os-tō′sēz)

| | nomenclature of viral hepatitis antigens and antibodies | |
|---|---|---|
| **disease** | **component of system** | **definition** |
| hepatitis A | HAV | hepatitis A virus–a picornavirus, the etiologic agent of hepatitis A |
| | anti-HAV/IgM | antibody to HAV–i ndicates recent infection; appears 3-4 weeks after exposure and remains positive for 4-6 months |
| | anti-HAV/IgG | antibody to HAV– detectable at onset of symptoms, persists throughout life |
| hepatitis B | HBV (Dane particle) | hepatitis B virus–a hepadnavirus, the etiologic agent of hepatitis B |
| | HB$_S$Ag | hepatitis B surface (capsule) antigen, detectable in serum before the onset of clinical symptoms and in acute and chronic infection and the carrier state |
| | anti-HB$_S$ | antibody to HB$_S$Ag–appears about 1 month after disappearance of HB$_S$Ag; indicates immunity to HBV from either past infection or vaccination (short-term immunity only after HBIG) |
| | HB$_C$Ag | hepatitis B core antigen |
| | anti-HB$_C$/IgG | antibody to HB$_C$Ag–appears just before onset of clinical symptoms and remains elevated for years, especially in chronic hepatitis; may be the only serologic marker of HBV infection between disappearance of HB$_S$Ag and anti-HB$_S$ |
| | anti-HB$_C$/IgM | antibody to Hb$_C$Ag–i ndicates recent infection with HBV; detectable for 4-6 months after infection; not useful to confirm immunity after vaccination |
| | HB$_e$Ag | hepatitis B envelope antigen–correlates with HBV replication and infectivity of serum; persistent elevation suggests chronic HBV infection |
| | anti-HB$_e$ | antibody to HB$_e$–presence in serum of an Hb$_S$Ag carrier indicates reduced risk of infectivity (low titer of HBV) in carriers |
| hepatitis C | HCV | hepatitis C virus–a flavivirus, the etiologic agent of hepatitis C; detection of viral RNA in plasma confirms presence of infection |
| | anti-HCV/IgM | antibody to HCV, a marker for acute infection |
| hepatitis D | HDV | hepatitis D virus–the etiologic agent of hepatitis D (delta hepatitis), a defective RNA virus that is able to replicate and cause disease only in the presence of hepatitis B virus infection; detectable by RIA within a few days after infection |
| | HDAg | delta antigen–detectable in early acute infection |
| | anti-HDV | antibody (IgG, IgM) to hepatitis D virus |
| hepatitis E | HEV | hepatitis E virus–a single-stranded RNA virus of unassigned genus, the etiologic agent of hepatitis E |
| | anti-HEV/IgM | antibody to HEV– elevated in acute infection |
| immune globulinsl | Gi | mmune globulin (USP)– contains antibodies to HAV; no antibodies to HB$_S$Ag, HCV, or HIV |
| | HBIG | hepatitis B immune globulin–contains high titer of antibody to HBV |

Disturbance of endochondral bone growth in which multiple, generally benign osteochondromas of long bones appear during childhood, commonly with shortening of the radius and fibula. Cranium is not involved.

**he·red·i·tar·y o·pa·les·cent den·tin** (hĕr-ed´i-tar-ē ō´pă-les´ĕnt den´tin) **1.** SYN dentinogenesis imperfecta. **2.** SYN opalescent dentin.

**he·red·i·tar·y spher·o·cy·to·sis** (hĕr-ed´i-tar-ē sfēr´ō-sī-tō´sis) Congenital defect of spectrin, the main component of the erythrocyte cell membrane; results in chronic anemia with reticulocytosis, episodes of mild jaundice due to hemolysis, and acute crises with gallstones, fever, and abdominal pain. SYN chronic familial icterus, chronic familial jaundice.

**he·red·i·ty** (hĕr-ed´i-tē) Transmission of char-

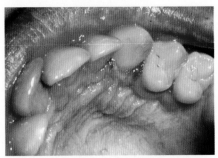

**hereditary hemorrhagic telangiectasia:** gingiva

acters from parent to offspring by information encoded in the parental germ cells. [L. *hereditas,* inheritance, fr. *heres* (*hered-*), heir]

**Her·ing-Breu·er re·flex** (her'ing broy'er rē'fleks) Effects of afferent impulses from pulmonary vagi in control of respiration.

**her·i·ta·bil·i·ty** (her'i-tă-bil'i-tē) In genetics, a statistical term used to denote the proportion of phenotypic variance due to variance in genotypes that is genetically determined, denoted by the traditional symbol $h^2$.

**her·ni·a,** pl. **her·ni·as,** pl. **her·ni·ae** (her' nē-ă, -ăz, -ē) Protrusion of a part or structure through the tissues normally containing it.

**her·ni·a·tion** (her'nē-ā'shŭn) Protrusion of an anatomic structure (e.g., intervertebral disc) from its normal anatomic position.

**he·ro·ic** (hēr-ō'ik) Denoting an aggressive, daring procedure in a dangerously ill patient that, in itself, may endanger the patient but also has a possibility of being successful, whereas lesser action would inevitably result in failure. [G. *hērōikos,* pertaining to a hero]

**her·o·in** (her'ō-in) An alkaloid, prepared from morphine by acetylation. Except for research, use in U.S. is prohibited by federal law because of its potential for abuse.

**her·pan·gi·na** (her-pan'ji-nă) Disease caused by *Coxsackievirus* marked by vesiculopapular lesions about 1–2 mm in diameter that are present around the fauces and soon break down to form grayish yellow ulcers.

**her·pes** (her'pēz) Inflammatory skin disease caused by herpes simplex virus or varicella-zoster virus; eruption of groups of deep-seated vesicles on erythematous bases. [G. *herpēs,* a spreading skin eruption, shingles, fr. *herpō,* to creep]

**her·pes la·bi·a·lis** (her'pēz lā-bē-ā'lis) Recurrent viral infection caused by herpesviruses types 1 and 2, producing lesions on the vermilion border of the lips. SYN fever blister.

**her·pes sim·plex** (her'pēz sim'pleks) Variety of infections caused by herpesvirus types 1

and 2; type 1 infections are marked most commonly by the eruption of one or more groups of vesicles on the vermilion border of the lips or at the external nares, type 2 by such lesions on the genitalia; both types often are recrudescent. See page A12.

**Her·pes·vir·i·dae** (her'pēz-vir'i-dē) A heterogeneous family of morphologically similar viruses, all of which contain double-stranded DNA and infect humans and a wide variety of other vertebrates. Infections produce type A inclusion bodies; in many instances, infection may remain latent for many years, even in the presence of specific circulating antibodies.

**her·pes·vi·rus, her·pes vi·rus** (her'pēz-vī'rŭs) Any virus belonging to the family Herpesviridae.

**her·pes zos·ter** (her'pēz zos'ter) An infection caused by varicella-zoster virus, characterized by an eruption of groups of vesicles on one side of the body along the course of a nerve, due to inflammation of ganglia and dorsal nerve roots; self-limited but may be accompanied by severe postherpetic pain. See page A12. SYN shingles, zona (2), zoster.

**her·pet·ic fe·ver** (her-pet'ik fē've̊r) Disease of short duration, apparently infectious, marked by chills, nausea, elevation of temperature, sore throat, and a herpetic eruption on face and other areas; primary infection is with herpes simplex virus.

**her·pet·ic le·sion** (her-pet'ik lē'zhŭn) Pathologic abnormality of tissue associated with or caused by the herpes virus.

**her·pet·ic me·nin·go·en·ceph·a·li·tis** (her-pet'ik mĕ-ning'gō-en-sef'ă-lī'tis) Severe form of meningoencephalitis due to herpesvirus type 1; high mortality rate.

**her·pet·ic whit·low** (her-pet'ik wit'lō) Painful herpes simplex virus infection of one or more fingers resulting from direct inoculation of the unprotected perionychial fold, often accompanied by lymphangitis and regional adenopathy; common in dentists, physicians, and nurses.

**her·pet·i·form aph·thae** (her-pet'i-fŏrm af'thē) Variant of oral aphthae, characterized by up to several dozen ulcers, 2–3 mm in diameter, organized in clusters.

**Hert·wig sheath** (hert'vig shēth) The merged outer and inner epithelial layers of the enamel organ that extend beyond the region of the anatomic crown and initiates formation of dentin in the root of a developing tooth; atrophies as the root is forms.

**Herx·hei·mer re·ac·tion** (herks'hīm-er rē-ak'shŭn) Inflammatory reaction in patients with syphilis induced in some cases by treatment with some drugs. SYN Jarisch-Herxheimer reaction.

gh

**hes·per·i·din** (hes-per′i-din) A flavone diglycoside obtained from unripe citrus fruit.

**heteraesthesia** [Br.] SYN heteresthesia.

**het·er·es·the·si·a** (het′ĕr-es-thē′zē-ă) A change occurring in the degree of sensory response to given cutaneous stimulus as the latter crosses a surface line. SYN heteraesthesia. [*heter-* + G. *aisthēsis*, sensation]

**het·er·o·cen·tric** (het′ĕr-ō-sen′trik) Having different centers. [*hetero-* + G. *kentron*, center]

**het·er·o·crine** (het′ĕr-ō-krin) Denoting the secretion of two or more kinds of material. [*hetero-* + G. *krinō*, to separate]

**het·er·o·dis·perse** (het′ĕr-ō-dis-pers′) Of varying size.

**het·er·o·dont** (het′ĕr-ō-dont) Having teeth of varying shapes, such as those of humans and most other mammals. [*hetero-* + G. *odous*, tooth]

**het·er·og·e·nous** (het′ĕr-oj′ĕ-nŭs) Of foreign origin.

**het·er·og·e·nous vac·cine** (het′ĕr-oj′ĕ-nŭs vak-sēn′) Vaccine that is not autogenous; may be prepared from other bacteria.

**het·er·o·ki·ne·si·a, het·er·o·ki·ne·sis** (het′ĕr-ō-ki-nē′zē-ă, -sis) Executing movements the reverse of those one is told to make. [*hetero-* + G. *kinēsis*, movement]

**het·er·on·o·mous** (het′ĕr-on′ŏ-mŭs) **1.** Different from the type; abnormal. **2.** Subject to direction or control of another. [*hetero-* + G. *nomos*, law]

**het·er·on·y·mous** (het′ĕr-on′i-mŭs) Having different names or expressed in different terms. [G. *heterōnymos*, having a different name, fr. *onyma*, or *onoma*, name]

**het·er·op·a·thy** (het′ĕr-op′ă-thē) Abnormal sensitivity to stimuli. [*hetero-* + G. *pathos*, suffering]

**het·er·o·phy·i·a·sis** (het′ĕr-ō-fī-ī′ă-sis) Infection with a heterophyid trematode, particularly *Heterophyes heterophyes*.

**het·er·o·re·cep·tor** (het′ĕr-ō-rĕ-sep′tŏr) A site on a neuron that binds a modulatory neuroregulator other than that released by the neuron. [*hetero-* + *receptor*]

**het·er·o·sex·u·al** (het′ĕr-ō-sek′shū-ăl) **1.** A person whose sexual orientation is toward people of the opposite sex. **2.** Relating to or characteristic of heterosexuality.

**het·er·o·tro·phic** (het′ĕr-ō-trō′fik) **1.** Relating to or exhibiting the properties of heterotrophy. **2.** Relating to a heterotroph.

**het·er·o·troph·ic or·al gas·tro·in·tes·tin·al cyst** (het′ĕr-ō-trō′fik ōr′ăl gas′trō-in-tes′ti-năl sist) Lesion of oral cavity lined by gastric or intestinal mucosa from misplaced embryonic rests.

**het·er·ot·ro·phy** (het′ĕr-ot′rŏ-fē) The ability or requirement to synthesize all metabolites from organic compounds.

**het·er·o·tro·pi·a, het·er·ot·ro·py** (het′ĕr-ō-trō′pē-ă, -ot′rŏ-pē) SYN strabismus. [*hetero-* + G. *tropē*, a turning]

**het·er·o·zy·gous** (het′ĕr-ō-zī′gŭs) Having different alleles at a given locus on the pair of chromosomes present in the diploid state.

**Heub·ner ar·te·ri·tis** (hoyb′ner ahr′tĕr-ī′tis) Inflammation of arteries within cerebral arterial circle secondary to chronic basal meningitis from a tubercle bacillus or fungi.

**hex·a·chlo·ro·phene** (hek′să-klō′rŏ-fēn) A topical antibacterial formerly widely used in wound care and as a surgical scrub. Use is currently restricted to disinfection of intact adult skin.

**hex·a·flu·o·ren·i·um bro·mide** (hek′să-flū-rēn′ē-ŭm brŏ′mīd) Potentiator for succinylcholine in anesthesia by producing a mild nondepolarizing neuromuscular blockade.

**hex·os·a·mine** (heks-ōs′ă-mēn) The amine derivative of a hexose.

**hex·yl·re·sor·ci·nol** (hek′sil-rē-zōr′si-nol) A broad-spectrum anthelmintic and antiseptic.

**hi·a·tal her·ni·a, hi·a·tus her·ni·a** (hī-ā′tăl hĕr′nē-ă, hī-ā′tŭs) Protrusion of a part of the stomach through the esophageal hiatus of the diaphragm.

**hi·a·tus**, pl. **hi·a·tus** (hī-ā′tŭs) [TA] An aperture, opening, or foramen. [L. an aperture, fr. *hio*, pp. *hiatus*, to yawn]

**hic·cup, hic·cough** (hik′ŭp) A diaphragmatic spasm causing a sudden inhalation interrupted by a spasmodic closure of the glottis.

**hi·drad·e·no·ma** (hī-drad′e-nō′mă) A benign neoplasm derived from epithelial cells of sweat glands. [G. *hidrōs*, sweat, + *adēn*, gland, + *-oma*, tumor]

**hi·dro·cys·to·ma** (hī′drō-sis-tō′mă) A cystic form of hidradenoma, usually apocrine. SYN syringocystoma. [G. *hidros*, sweat + G. *kystis*, bladder, + *-ōma*, tumor]

**hi·dro·poi·e·sis** (hī′drō-poy-ē′sis) Formation of sweat. [G. *hidros*, sweat + G. *poiēsis*, formation]

**hi·dros·che·sis** (hī-dros′kĕ-sis) Suppression of sweating. [G. *hidros*, sweat + G. *schesis*, a checking]

**hi·dro·sis** (hī-drō′sis) Production and excretion of sweat. [G. *hidrōs,* sweat, + *-osis,* condition]

**hi·er·ar·chy** (hī′ĕr-ahr-kē) Any system of people or things ranked one above the other. [G. *hierarchia,* rule or power of the high priest]

**hi·er·o·ther·a·py** (hī′ĕr-ō-thār′ă-pē) Treatment of disease by prayer and religious practices. [G. *hieros,* holy, + *therapeia,* therapy]

**high-cal·o·rie di·et** (hī-kal′ŏr-ē dī′ĕt) Diet containing more than 4,000 calories per day.

**high-fi·ber di·et** (hī-fī′bĕr dī′ĕt) Diet high in nondigestible part of plants, which is fiber. Fiber is found in fruits, vegetables, whole grains, and legumes. Insoluble fiber increases stool bulk, decreases transit time of food in the bowel, and decreases constipation and the risk of colon cancer.

**high lip line** (hī lip līn) Greatest height to which the lip is raised in normal function or during the act of smiling broadly.

**high·ly arch·ed pal·ate** (hī′lē ahrcht pal′ăt) SEE secondary palate.

**hi·lum,** pl. **hi·la** (hī′lŭm, -lă) [TA] **1.** The part of an organ where the nerves and vessels enter and leave. SYN porta (1). **2.** A depression or slit resembling the hilum in the olivary nucleus of the brain.

**hi·man·to·sis** (hī′man-tō′sis) Possessing an unusually long uvula. [G. *himas,* strap, + *-osis,* condition]

**hinge ax·is** (hinj ak′sis) SYN transverse horizontal axis.

**hinge ax·is points** (hinj ak′sis poyntz) Two posterior reference points located one on each side of the face in the area of the transverse horizontal axis, which, together with an anterior reference point, establish the horizontal reference plane.

**hinge-bow** (hinj′bō) SYN face-bow.

**hinge joint** (hinj joynt) [TA] A uniaxial joint in which a broad, transversely cylindric convexity on one bone fits into a corresponding concavity on the other, allowing of motion in one plane only. SYN ginglymoid joint, ginglymus.

**hinge move·ment** (hinj mūv′mĕnt) Movement of mandible on hinge axis.

**hinge-or·bi·tal ax·is** (hinj ōr′bi-tăl ak′sis) SYN condylar axis.

**hinge po·si·tion** (hinj pŏ-zish′ŏn) In dentistry, orientation of parts in a manner permitting hinge movement between them.

**HIPAA** Abbreviation for Health Insurance Portability and Accountability Act.

**hip·po·cam·pus,** pl. **hip·po·cam·pi** (hip′ō-kam′pŭs, -pī) [TA] The complex, inter-

nally convoluted structure that forms the medial margin of the cerebral hemisphere, bordering the choroid fissure of the lateral ventricle, and composed of two gyri (Ammon's horn and the dentate gyrus), together with their white matter, the alveus, and fimbria hippocampi. [G. *hippocampos,* seahorse]

**hip·po·crat·ic fa·ci·es** (hip′ō-krat′ik fash′ ē-ēz) Pinched facial expression, with sunken eyes, concavity of cheeks and temples, relaxed lips, and leaden complexion; observed in one close to death.

**hip·po·crat·ic nails** (hip′ō-krat′ik nālz) Coarse, curved nails capping clubbed digits.

**hir·cus,** pl. **hir·ci** (hir′kŭs, -sī) Underarm odor. [L. he-goat]

**Hirsch·feld ca·nals** (hĕrsh′feld kă-nalz′) SYN interdental canals.

**Hirsch·sprung dis·ease** (hĕrsh′sprŭng di-zēz′) SYN congenital megacolon.

**hir·sut·ism** (hir′sū-tizm) Presence of excessive bodily and facial hair, usually in a male pattern, especially in women; may be present in normal adults as an expression of an ethnic characteristic or may develop in children or adults as the result of androgen excess due to tumors. [L. *hirsutus,* shaggy]

**His** Abbreviation for histidine.

**His line** (hiz līn) Line extending from tip of the anterior nasal spine (acanthion) to hindmost point on posterior margin of foramen magnum (opisthion), dividing face into an upper and a lower, or dental, part.

**his·ta·mine** (his′tă-mēn) Vasodepressor amine present in ergot and in animal tissues. It is a powerful stimulant of gastric secretion, a constrictor of bronchial smooth muscle, and a vasodilator (capillaries and arterioles) that causes a fall in blood pressure.

**his·ta·mine flush** (his′tă-mēn flŭsh) Vasodilation and erythema due to release of histamine.

**his·ta·mine phos·phate** (his′tă-mēn fos′ fāt) Agent used to assess nonspecific bronchial hypersensitivity and as a positive control during skin testing for allergies.

**his·ti·dine (His, H)** (his′ti-dēn) The L-isomer is a basic amino acid found in most proteins.

✿ **histio-** Tissue, especially connective tissue. [G. *histion,* web (tissue)]

**his·ti·o·cyte** (his′tē-ō-sīt) A macrophage in connective tissue. [*histio-* + G. *kytos,* cell]

✿ **histo** Tissue. [G. *histos,* web (tissue)]

**his·to·com·pat·i·bil·i·ty** (his′tō-kŏm-pat′

i-bil′i-tē) State of immunologic similarity that permits successful homograft transplantation.

**his·to·com·pat·i·bil·i·ty test·ing** (his′ tō-kŏm-pat′i-bil′i-tē test′ing) A testing system for human leukocyte antigens, of major importance in transplantation.

**his·to·dif·fer·en·ti·a·tion** (his′tō-dif′ĕr-en-shē-ā′shŭn) The morphologic appearance of tissue characteristics during development.

**his·to·gen·e·sis** (his′tō-jen′ĕ-sis) Origin of a tissue; formation and development of tissues of the body. [*histo-* + G. *genesis*, origin]

**his·tog·e·nous** (his-toj′ĕ-nŭs) Formed by tissues. [*histo-* + G. *-gen*, producing]

**his·to·gram** (his′tō-gram) Graphic columnar or bar representation to compare magnitudes of frequencies or numbers of items. [*histo-* + G. *gramma*, a writing]

**his·tol·o·gy** (his-tol′ŏ-jē) Science concerned with minute structure of cells, tissues, and organs in relation to their function. [*histo-* + G. *logos*, study]

**his·to·mor·phom·e·try** (his′tō-mōr-fom′ ĕ-trē) The quantitative measurement and characterization of microscopic images using a computer; manual or automated digital image analysis typically involves measurements and comparisons of selected geometric areas, perimeters, length angle of orientation, form factors, center of gravity coordinates, as well as image enhancement. [*histo-* + G. *morphē*, shape, + *metron*, measure]

**his·to·pa·thol·o·gy** (his′tō-pă-thol′ŏ-jē) The science or study dealing with the cytologic and histologic structure of abnormal or diseased tissue.

**his·to·phys·i·ol·o·gy** (his′tō-fiz-ē-ol′ŏ-jē) Microscopic study of tissues in relation to their functions.

**his·to·plas·min** (his′tō-plaz′min) An antigenic extract of *Histoplasma capsulatum*; used in immunologic tests.

**his·to·plas·mo·sis** (his′tō-plaz-mō′sis) Widely distributed infectious disease caused by *Histoplasma capsulatum;* occasional outbreaks; usually acquired by inhalation of fungal spores in soil dust.

**his·to·tox·ic** (his′tō-tok′sik) Relating to poisoning of the respiratory enzyme system of the tissues.

**his·to·tro·phic** (his′tō-trō′fik) Providing-nourishment for or favoring formation of tissue. [*histo-* + G. *trophē*, nourishment]

**HIV** Abbreviation for human immunodeficiency virus.

**hives** (hīvz) **1.** SYN urticaria. **2.** SYN wheal.

**HLA** Abbreviation for human leukocyte antigen.

**HMG CoA-re·duc·tase in·hib·i·tors** (rĕ-dŭk′tās in-hib′i-tŏrz) Drugs used to treat hypercholesterolemia.

**HMO** Abbreviation for health maintenance organization.

**HNO₂** Abbreviation for nitrous acid.

**Hoag·land sign** (hōg′lănd sīn) Eyelid edema in infectious mononucleosis.

**hob·nail tongue** (hob′nāl tŭng) Interstitial glossitis with hypertrophy and verrucous changes in papillae; seen in some cases of late acquired syphilis.

**Hodg·kin dis·ease** (hoj′kin di-zēz′) Disease marked by chronic enlargement of the lymph nodes, often local at the onset and later generalized, together with enlargement of the spleen and often of the liver.

**hoe ex·ca·va·tor** (hō eks΄kă-vā-tŏr) Single-beveled dental excavator, with blade at an angle to axis of handle and cutting edge perpendicular to plane of angle.

**hoe scal·er** (hō skā′lĕr) Hoe-shaped dental instrument with a very short blade.

**ho·lis·tic med·i·cine** (hō-lis′tik med′i-sin) **1.** Approach to medical care that emphasizes study of aspects of a person's health, especially that a person should be considered as a unit, including psychological as well as social and economic influences on health status. **2.** SYN complementary and alternative medicine.

**hol·o·en·dem·ic dis·ease** (hol΄ō-en-dem΄ik di-zēz′) Disease for which a high prevalence of infection begins early in life and affects most or all children, leading to a state of equilibrium, such that the adult population evidences disease less frequently than children.

**hol·o·pros·en·ceph·a·ly** (hol′ō-pros-en-sef′ă-lē) Failure of the forebrain or prosencephalon to divide into hemispheres or lobes; cyclopia occurs in the severest form. [*holo-* + G. *prosō*, forward, + *enkephalos*, brain]

**H.O.M.E.** (hōm) Acronym for hand-over-mouth exercise.

**home health care** (hōm helth kār) Care of patients delivered within their residence rather than a clinical setting; usually provided by nurses, home health aides, and other professionals on a regularly scheduled visit.

**ho·me·o·path·ic** (hō′mē-ō-path′ik) **1.** Relating to homeopathy. **2.** Denoting an extremely small dose of a pharmacologic agent that theoretically mimics the symptoms produced by the condition being treated, such as might be used in homeopathy; more generally, a dose believed to be too small to produce the effect usually expected from that agent. A form of medicine alternative to allopathic, in which drugs antagonize the effects of the disease. [G. *homoios*, similar, + *pathos*, disease, + *-ic*, adj, suffix]

**ho·me·op·a·thy** (hŏ′mē-op′ă-thē) A system of therapy developed by Samuel Hahnemann based on the "law of similia," which holds that a medicinal substance that can evoke certain symptoms in healthy people may be effective in the treatment of illnesses having similar symptoms, if given in very small doses. [G. *homoios*, similar, + *pathos*, disease, + *-y*, noun suffix]

**ho·me·o·sta·sis** (hŏ′mē-ō-stā′sis) **1.** State of equilibrium in the body with respect to various functions and to the chemical compositions of fluids and tissues. **2.** Processes through which bodily equilibrium is maintained. [G. *homoios*, similar, + *stasis*, a standing, fr. *istēmi*, to stand]

**hom·i·cide** (hom′i-sīd) Murder of a human being. [L. *homo*, man, + *caedo*, to kill]

**☼ homo-** **1.** Prefix meaning the same, alike; opposite of hetero-. **2.** CHEMISTRY prefix used to indicate insertion of one more carbon atom in a chain (i.e., insertion of a methylene moiety). [G. *homos*, the same]

**ho·mo·cys·ti·nu·ri·a** (hŏ′mō-sis′ti-nyū′rē-ă) Metabolic disorder characterized by sparse blond hair, long limbs, pectus excavatum, dislocation of lens, failure to thrive, mental retardation, psychiatric disturbances, and thromboembolic episodes.

**ho·mo·cy·to·tro·pic an·ti·bod·y** (hŏ′mō-sī-tō-trŏ′pik an′ti-bod-ē) Antibody of the IgE class with an affinity for tissues of the same or a closely related species and that, on combining with specific antigen, triggers the release of pharmacologic mediators of anaphylaxis. SYN reaginic antibody.

**ho·mo·dont** (hŏ′mō-dont) Having teeth all alike in form, as those of the lower vertebrates, in contrast to heterodont. [*homo-* + G. *odous*, tooth]

**ho·mo·ge·ne·ous** (hŏ′mō-jē′nē-ŭs) *Do not confuse this word with homogenous* **1.** Of uniform structure or composition throughout. **2.** Consisting of a single phase. [*homo-* + G. *genos*, race]

**ho·mo·ge·ne·ous ra·di·a·tion** (hŏ′mō-jē′nē-ŭs rā′dē-ā′shŭn) Radiation consisting of a narrow band of frequencies, the same energy, or a single type of particle.

**ho·mo·gen·e·sis** (hŏ′mō-jen′ĕ-sis) Production of offspring similar to the parents, in contrast to heterogenesis. [*homo-* + G. *genesis*, production]

**ho·mog·e·nous** (hŏ-moj′ĕ-nŭs) Having a structural similarity because of descent from a common ancestor. [*homo-* + G. *genos*, family, kind]

**ho·mo·graft** (hŏ′mō-graft) Type of skin graft from another person or a cadaver used in the treatment of burns.

**ho·mo·plas·tic** (hŏ′mō-plas′tik) Similar in form and structure, but not in origin. [*homo-* + G. *plastos*, formed]

**ho·mo·sex·u·al** (hŏ′mō-sek′shū-ăl) **1.** Relating to or characteristic of homosexuality. **2.** One whose interests and behavior are characteristic of homosexuality with a sexual orientation to members of the same sex.

**ho·mo·va·nil·lic ac·id (HVA)** (hŏ′mō-vă-nil′ik as′id) A phenol found in human urine.

**ho·mo·zy·gous** (hŏ′mō-zī′gŭs) Having identical alleles at one or more loci.

**hone** (hōn) **1.** A sharpening stone. **2.** To sharpen the edge of a cutting device.

**hook** (huk) **1.** An instrument curved or bent near its tip, used for fixation of a part or traction. **2.** SYN hamulus. [A.S. *hōk*]

**hook·worm a·ne·mi·a** (huk′wŏrm ă-nē′mē-ă) Anemia associated with heavy infestation by *Ancylostoma duodenale* or *Necator americanus*.

**hor·i·zon·tal at·ro·phy** (hōr′i-zon′tăl at′rŏ-fē) Progressive loss of alveolar and supporting bone surrounding teeth, beginning at the most coronal level of bone.

**hor·i·zon·tal max·il·la·ry frac·ture** (hōr′i-zon′tăl mak′si-lar-ē frak′shŭr) Horizontal fracture at base of maxillae above apices of teeth.

**hor·i·zon·tal os·te·ot·o·my** (hōr′i-zon′tăl os′tē-ot′ŏ-mē) Osteotomy performed intraorally for genioplasty; inferior aspect of anterior mandible is advanced or retruded by movement of free segment.

**hor·i·zon·tal o·ver·lap** (hōr′i-zon′tăl ō′vĕr-lap) Projection of upper anterior and/or posterior teeth beyond their antagonists in a horizontal direction. SYN overjet.

**hor·i·zon·tal part of fa·cial ca·nal** (hōr′i-zon′tăl pahrt fā′shăl kă-nal′) First portion of facial canal, between beginning of canal (at the introitus of facial canal at end of internal auditory meatus) and point at which it turns to descend, beginning the descending part.

**hor·i·zon·tal plane** (hōr′i-zon′tăl plān) Surface parallel and relative to the horizon; in the anatomic position, horizontal planes are transverse planes; in the supine or prone positions, horizontal planes are frontal.

**hor·i·zon·tal stroke ac·tion** (hōr′i-zon′tăl strōk ak′shŭn) Circumferential movement of a dental instrument using a pulling action perpendicular to the long axis of the tooth.

gh

**hor·i·zon·tal strokes** (hōr-i-zon′tăl strōks) Instrumentation motions perpendicular to the long axis of the tooth; used at the line angles of posterior teeth, in furcation areas, and within pockets that are too narrow to permit vertical or oblique strokes.

**hor·i·zon·tal trans·mis·sion** (hōr′i-zon′tăl trans-mish′ŭn) Transmission of infectious agents from an infected individual to a susceptible contemporary.

**hor·me·sis** (hōr-mē′sis) The stimulating effect of subinhibitory concentrations of any toxic substance on any organism.

🄓**hor·mo·nal gin·gi·vi·tis** (hōr-mōn′ăl jin′ji-vī′tis) Gum disease in which host response to bacterial plaque is presumably exacerbated by hormonal alterations occurring during puberty, pregnancy, oral contraceptive use, or menopause. See this page. SYN pregnancy gingivitis.

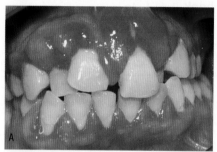

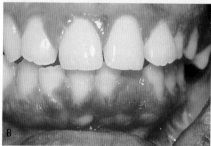

**hormonal gingivitis:** (A) during pregnancy; (B) 3-weeks postpartum

**hor·mone** (hōr′mōn) A chemical substance, formed in one organ or part of the body and carried in the blood to another organ or part where it produces functional effects; depending on the specificity of their effects, hormones can alter the functional activity, and sometimes the structure, of just one organ or tissue or various numbers of them. [G. *hormōn*, pres. part. of *hormaō*, to rouse or set in motion]

**horn** (hōrn) [TA] Any structure resembling a horn in shape. SYN cornu (1). [A.S.]

**Hor·ner syn·drome** (hōr′nĕr sin′drōm) Ipsilateral myosis, ptosis, and facial anhydrosis due to ipsilateral lesion of cervical sympathetic chain or its central pathway.

**Hor·ner teeth** (hōr′nĕr tēth) Incisor teeth with a horizontal, hypoplastic groove.

**hos·pice** (hos′pis) Institution that provides a centralized program of palliative and supportive services to dying people and their families, in the form of physical, psychological, social, and spiritual care. [L. *hospitium*, hospitality, lodging, fr. *hospes*, guest]

**hos·pi·tal** (hos′pi-tăl) Institution for treatment, care, and cure of the sick and wounded, for the study of disease, and for the training of physicians, nurses, and allied health care personnel. [L. *hospitalis*, for a guest, fr. *hospes* (*hospit-*), a host, a guest]

**hos·pi·tal for·mu·lar·y** (hos′pi-tăl fōrm′yū-lar-ē) Continually revised compilation of approved pharmaceuticals, plus important ancillary information, which reflects the current clinical judgment of the institution's medical staff.

**hospitalisation** [Br.] SYN hospitalization.

**hos·pi·tal·ist** (hos′pit-ăl-ist) **1.** Physician whose professional activities are performed chiefly within a hospital. **2.** Primary care physician who assumes responsibility for observation and treatment of hospitalized patients and returns them to the care of their private physicians when discharged from the hospital. [*hospital* + *-ist*]

**hos·pi·tal·i·za·tion** (hos′pi-tăl-ī-zā′shŭn) Confinement in a hospital as a patient for diagnostic study and treatment. SYN hospitalisation.

**hos·pi·tal rec·ord** (hos′pi-tăl rek′ŏrd) Medical record generated during a period of hospitalization, usually including written accounts of consultants' opinions, physicians' and nurses' observations, treatments, and results of all tests and procedures performed.

**host cell** (hōst sel) Cell (e.g., a bacterium) in which a vector can be propagated.

**hos·tile be·hav·ior** (hos′til bĕ-hāv′yŏr) Varying degrees of antagonistic action with malice to negate or destroy some aspects of another.

**hot nod·ule** (hot nod′yūl) Thyroid nodule with a much higher uptake of radioactive iodine than the surrounding parenchyma.

**hot pack** (hot pak) Pouch of cloth or other material soaked in hot water or producing moist heat by another means.

**hot salt ster·il·i·zer** (hot sawlt ster′i-lī-zĕr) Sterilizer for endodontic equipment in which table salt is heated in a container at 218–246°C; dry heat is transmitted to root canal instruments, absorbent points, or cotton pellets for their rapid (5–10 seconds) sterilization.

**house staff** (hows staf) Physicians and surgeons in specialty training at a hospital who care for the patients under the direction and supervision of the attending staff.

**Hous·say syn·drome** (ū´sā sin´drōm) The amelioration of diabetes mellitus by a destructive lesion in, or surgical removal of, the pituitary gland.

**How·ship la·cu·nae** (how´ship lă-kū´nē) Tiny depressions, pits, or irregular grooves in bone that is being resorbed by osteoclasts.

**HPA** Abbreviation for hypothalamic-pituitary-adrenal (axis).

**h.r.a.** Abbreviation for health risk assessment.

**5-HT** Abbreviation for 5-hydroxytryptamine.

**HTN** Abbreviation for hypertension.

**hub** (hŭb) The expanded portion of a hollow needle that serves as a handle for manipulation and as a site of attachment for a syringe, infusion tube, or some other appliance.

**huff·ing** (hŭf´ing) **1.** Colloquial but general term for the inhalation abuse of volatile solvents (e.g., gasoline) to achieve intoxication or alter consciousness. **2.** SYN glue-sniffing.

**hu·man bite** (hyū´măn bīt) A wound caused by human teeth; because the human oral cavity harbors multiple pathogens; must be thoroughly cleaned to prevent serious infection.

**hu·man fi·brin foam** (hyū´măn fī´brin fōm) Dry artificial sponge of human fibrin prepared by clotting with thrombin a foam of a solution of human fibrinogen.

**hu·man fi·brin·o·gen** (hyū´măn fī-brin´ō-jen) Fibrinogen prepared from normal human plasma; coagulant (clotting factor), used as an adjunct in management of acute, congenital, or acquired chronic hypofibrinogenemia.

**hu·man gam·ma glob·u·lin** (hyū´măn gam´ă glob´yū-lin) Preparation of the proteins of liquid human serum, containing the antibodies (primarily IgG) of normal adults.

**Hu·man Ge·nome Pro·ject** (hyū´măn jē´nōm proj´ekt) A comprehensive effort by molecular biologists worldwide to map the human genome, completed in 2003. The resulting projection reflects the 3 billion DNA letters of the human genome with 99.99% accuracy.

**hu·man her·pes·vi·rus 4** (hyū´măn hĕr´pēz-vī´rŭs) SYN Epstein-Barr virus.

**hu·man im·mu·no·de·fi·cien·cy vi·rus (HIV)** (hyū´măn im´yū-nō-dĕ-fish´ĕn-sē vī´rŭs) Human T-cell lymphotropic virus type III; a cytopathic retrovirus that is 100–120 nm in diameter, has a lipid envelope, and has a characteristic dense cylindric nucleoid containing core proteins and genomic RNA; two types

exist: HIV-1 infects only humans and chimpanzees and is more virulent than HIV-2, which is more closely related to Simian or monkey viruses. HIV-2 is found primarily in West Africa. It is the etiologic agent of acquired immunodeficiency syndrome (AIDS).

**hu·man in·su·lin** (hyū´măn in´sŭ-lin) Protein that has the normal structure of insulin produced by the human pancreas, prepared by recombinant DNA techniques and by semisynthetic processes.

**hu·man leu·ko·cyte an·ti·gen (HLA)** (hyū´măn lū´kō-sīt an´ti-jen) Any of several members of a system consisting of the gene products of at least four linked loci (A, B, C, and D) and a number of subloci on the sixth human chromosome that have been shown to have a strong influence on human allotransplantation, transfusions in refractory patients, and some disease associations.

**hu·mec·tant** (hyū-mek´tănt) Agent that promotes retention of moisture; added to prevent hardening. [L. *humectus*, moist, fr. *humor*, moisture]

**hu·mec·ta·tion** (hyū-mek-tā´shŭn) **1.** Therapeutic application of moisture. **2.** Serous infiltration of the tissues. **3.** Soaking of a crude drug in water preparatory to the making of an extract. [L. *humecto*, pp. *-mectus*, to moisten, fr. *humeo*, to be damp]

**hu·mid·i·fi·er** (hyū-mid´i-fī-ĕr) A device for increasing the water vapor content of a gas or of ambient air.

**hu·mid·i·ty** (hyū-mid´i-tē) Moisture or dampness, as of the air. [L. *humiditas*, dampness]

**hu·mor** (hyū´mŏr) [TA] **1.** Any clear fluid or semifluid hyaline anatomic substance. **2.** One of the elemental body fluids that were the basis of the physiologic and pathologic teachings of the hippocratic school: blood, yellow bile, black bile, and phlegm. SEE ALSO humoral doctrine. SYN humour. [L. correctly, *umor*, liquid]

**hu·mor·al doc·trine** (hyū´mŏr-ăl dok´trin) Ancient Greek theory of four body humors (blood, yellow bile, black bile, and phlegm) that determined health and disease.

**humour** [Br.] SYN humor.

**hun·ger** (hŭng´gĕr) **1.** A desire or need for food. **2.** Any appetite, strong desire, or craving. [M.E., fr. O.E. *hungor*]

**Hun·ter-Schre·ger bands** (hŭn´tĕr shrā´gĕr bandz) Alternating light and dark lines seen in tooth enamel that begin at the dentoenamel junction and end before they reach enamel surface; may represent areas of enamel rods cut in cross-sections dispersed between areas of rods cut longitudinally.

**Hunt·ing·ton cho·re·a** (hŭn´ting-tŏn kŏ-rē´ă) Neurodegenerative disorder, with onset

gh

usually in the third or fourth decade, characterized by chorea and dementia. [L. fr. G. *choreia,* a choral dance, fr. *choros,* a dance]

**Hunt syn·drome** (hŭnt sin′drōm) **1.** Intention tremor beginning in one extremity, gradually increasing in intensity, and subsequently involving other parts of the body. **2.** Facial paralysis, otalgia, and herpes zoster due to viral infection of the seventh cranial nerve and geniculate ganglion.

**Hur·ler-Scheie syn·drome** (hŭr′lĕr shā sin′drōm) Phenotypic intermediate between Hurler syndrome and Scheie syndrome. [Gertrud *Hurler,* Harold G. *Scheie*]

**Hürth·le cell car·ci·no·ma** (hērt′lĕ sel kahr′si-nō′mă) Salivary or thyroid carcinoma composed of cells with eosinophilic cytoplasm.

**Husch·ke au·di·to·ry teeth** (hūsh′kĕ aw′di-tōr-ē tēth) SYN acoustic teeth.

**Husch·ke car·ti·lag·es** (hūsh′kĕ kahr′ti-lăj-ĕz) Two horizontal cartilaginous rods at the edge of cartilaginous septum of the nose.

**Husch·ke for·a·men** (hūsh′kĕ fōr-ā′mĕn) Opening in floor of bony part of external acoustic meatus near tympanic membrane.

**Hutch·in·son cres·cen·tic notch** (hŭch′ in-sŏn krĕ-sent′ik noch) Semilunar notch on incisal edge of Hutchinson teeth (q. v.).

**Hutch·in·son fa·ci·es** (hŭch′in-sŏn fash′ ē-ēz) Peculiar facial expression produced by the drooping eyelids and motionless eyes in external ophthalmoplegia.

**Hutch·in·son in·ci·sors** (hŭch′in-sŏn in-sī′zŏrz) See this page. SYN Hutchinson teeth.

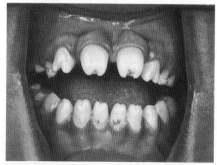

**Hutchinson incisors:** affected teeth are small and more widely spaced than normal; their sides taper toward the biting edges. Upper central incisors in permanent dentition are most often affected. Sign of congenital syphilis infection

**Hutch·in·son pu·pil** (hŭch′in-sŏn pyū′pil) Dilation of pupil on side of lesion as part of a palsy of third cranial nerve.

**Hutch·in·son teeth** (hŭch′in-sŏn tēth) Teeth seen in congenital syphilis in which the incisal edge is notched and narrower than the cervical area. SEE ALSO Hutchinson crescentic notch. See this page. SYN notched teeth, screwdriver teeth, syphilitic teeth, Hutchinson incisors.

**Hutch·in·son tri·ad** (hŭch′in-sŏn trī′ad) Parenchymatous keratitis, labyrinthine disease, and Hutchinson teeth, significant sign of congenital syphilis.

**HVA** Abbreviation for homovanillic acid.

**HVL** Abbreviation for half-value layer.

**hy·a·lin·i·za·tion** (hī′ă-lin-ī-zā′shŭn) The formation of hyalin.

**hy·a·lu·ron·ic ac·id** (hī′ă-lūr-on′ik as′id) A mucopolysaccharide forming a gelatinous material in the tissue spaces and acting as a lubricant and shock absorbant.

**hy·a·lu·ron·i·dase** (hī′ă-lū-ron′i-dās) Soluble enzyme product prepared from mammalian testes; used to increase the effect of local anesthetics and to permit wider infiltration of subcutaneously administered fluids, is suggested in the treatment of forms of arthritis to promote resolution of redundant tissue.

**hy·brid** (hī′brid) **1.** An individual (plant or animal) with parents that are different varieties of the same species or belong to different but closely allied species. **2.** Fused tissue culture cells, as in a hybridoma. [L. *hybrida,* offspring of a tame sow and a wild boar, fr. G. *hybris,* violation, wantonness]

**hy·brid com·pos·ite** (hī′brid kŏm-poz′it) Colloq. for hybrid composite resin (q.v.).

**hy·brid com·pos·ite res·in** (hī′brid kŏm-poz′it rez′in) Restorative compound that contains a blend of fine or microfine filler particles. The inorganic particles may comprise up to 70% of volume; the smaller particles fit into spaces among the larger. See page 285.

**hybridisation** [Br.] SYN hybridization.

**hy·brid·i·za·tion** (hī′brid-ī-zā′shŭn) **1.** The process of breeding a hybrid. **2.** Crossing over between related but nonallelic genes. SYN hybridisation.

**hy·brid pros·the·sis** (hī′brid pros-thē′sis) SYN overlay denture.

**hydraemia** [Br.] SYN hydremia.

**hy·dre·mi·a** (hī-drē′mē-ă) A condition in which the blood volume is increased due to increased water content of plasma, with or without a reduction in the concentration of protein. SYN hydraemia. [*hydr-* + G. *haima,* blood]

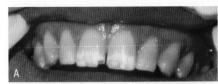

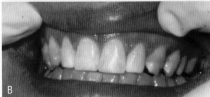

**hybrid composite resin:** (A) patient with chipped mesial of central incisor, small diastema, enamel discoloration; (B) both central incisors restored with hybrid composite resin bonded to mesial and facial surfaces, restoring the fracture, closing diastema, covering some of discolored enamel

⟡ **hydro-** *Do not confuse this combining form with hidro-. These are not merely spelling variants but are derived from different words.* **1.** Prefix denoting the presense of water or watery fluid or of hydrogen. **2.** A hydatid. [G. *hydōr,* water]

**hy·dro·cele** (hī′drō-sēl) A collection of serous fluid in a sacculated cavity. [*hydro-* + G. *kēlē,* hernia]

**hy·dro·ceph·a·lus** (hī′drō-sef′ă-lŭs) Excessive accumulation of cerebrospinal fluid resulting in dilation of the cerebral ventricles and raised intracranial pressure; may also result in cranial enlargement and brain atrophy. [*hydro-* + G. *kephalē,* head]

**hy·dro·chlor·ic ac·id (HCl)** (hī′drō-klōr′ik as′id) Acid of gastric juice; commercial product used as an escharotic. SYN muriatic acid.

**hy·dro·chlo·ro·thi·a·zide** (hī′drō-klōr′ō-thī′ă-zīd) A potent orally effective diuretic and antihypertensive agent related to chlorothiazide; can cause hypokalemia and hyperglycemia.

**hy·dro·cho·le·re·sis** (hī′drō-kō-lĕr-ē′sis) Increased output of watery bile of low specific gravity, viscosity, and solid content. [*hydro-* + G. *cholē,* bile, + *hairesis,* a taking]

**hy·dro·co·done** (hī′drō-kō′dōn) Potent analgesic derivative of codeine used as an antitussive and analgesic.

**hy·dro·col·loid** (hī′drō-kol′oyd) Gelatinous colloid in unstable equilibrium with its contained water; useful in dentistry for impressions because of its dimensional stability under controlled conditions.

**hy·dro·cor·ti·sone** (hī′drō-kōr′ti-sōn) Prin-

cipal glucocorticoid produced by the cortex of the suprarenal gland. Although synthetic products used medicinally are usually known by this name, the natural hormone is more often called cortisol (q.v.).

**hy·dro·dy·nam·ic the·o·ry** (hī′drō-dī-nam′ik thē′ŏr-ē) Widely accepted theory that explains pain impulse conduction to dental pulp resulting from fluid movement within the dentinal tubules, stimulating the nerve endings, which cause pain and hypersensitivity.

**hy·dro·dy·nam·ic the·or·y of tooth sen·si·tiv·i·ty** (hī′drō-dī-nam′ik thē′ŏr-ē tŭth sen′si-tiv′i-tē) Currently accepted mechanism explaining pain impulse transmission to the pulp resulting from fluid shifts within patent dentinal tubules occur with mechanical, osmotic, and evaporative stimuli (including air blasts).

**hy·dro·fluor·ic ac·id** (hī′drō-flōr′ik as′id) A solution of hydrogen fluoride gas in water.

**hy·dro·gen** (hī′drō-jen) **1.** Gaseous element, atomic no. 1, atomic wt. 1.00794. **2.** Molecular form ($H_2$) of the element. [*hydro-* + G. *-gen,* producing]

**hy·dro·gen·a·tion** (hī-droj′ĕ-nā′shŭn) Addition of hydrogen to a compound, especially to an unsaturated fat or fatty acid; thus, soft fats or oils are solidified or "hardened."

**hy·dro·gen per·ox·ide** (hī′drō-jen pĕr-ok′sīd) Unstable compound readily broken down to water and oxygen used as a mild antiseptic for skin and mucous membranes.

**hy·dro·gen sul·fide** (hī′drō-jen sŭl′fīd) Colorless, flammable, toxic gas with familiar "rotten egg" odor.

**hy·dro·ki·net·ic ac·tiv·i·ty** (hī′drō-ki-net′ik ak-tiv′i-tē) Action relating to motions of fluids or the forces that effect or affect such motions; opposite of hydrostatic.

**hy·drol·y·sis** (hī-drol′i-sis) **1.** Process by which water slowly penetrates suture filaments and breaks down the suture's polymer chain; hydroxylation produces less tissue reaction. **2.** Chemical process in which compound is cloven into two or more simpler compounds; effected by action of acids, alkalis, or enzymes. [*hydro-* + G. *lysis,* dissolution]

**hy·dro·ma** (hī-drō′mă) SYN hygroma.

**hy·dro·mor·phone hy·dro·chlor·ide** (hī′drō-mōr′fōn hī′drō-klōr′īd) Synthetic derivative of morphine, with analgesic potency about 10 times that of morphine.

**hy·dro·phil·ic** (hī′drō-fil′ik) Denoting the property of attracting or associating with water molecules, possessed by polar radicals or ions, as opposed to hydrophobic (2).

**hy·dro·pho·bic** (hī′drō-fō′bik) **1.** Relating to

or suffering from rabies. **2.** Lacking an affinity for water molecules.

**hy·drops** (hī′drops) Excessive clear, watery fluid in any body tissues or cavities. [G. *hydrōps*]

**hy·dro·ther·a·py** (hī′drō-thār′ă-pē) Therapeutic use of water by external application, either for its pressure effect or to apply physical energy to the tissues. [*hydro-* + G. *therapeia,* therapy]

**hy·drox·ide** (hī-drok′sīd) A compound containing a potentially ionizable hydroxyl group.

**hy·drox·y·ap·a·tite** (hī-drok′sē-ap′ă-tīt) A natural mineral structure that the crystal lattice of bones and teeth closely resembles; used in chromatography of nucleic acids; also found in pathologic calcifications.

**hy·drox·y·ap·a·tite cer·am·ic** (hī-drok′sē-ap′ă-tīt sĕr-am′ik) Composition of calcium and phosphate used to provide a dense, nonresorbable, biocompatible ceramic for dental implants; metal implants may be coated with tricalcium phosphate or hydroxyapatite.

**γ-hy·drox·y·bu·tyr·ate (GHB)** (hī-drok′sē-byū′tir-āt) Naturally occurring short-chain fatty acid, found in all body tissues, with the highest concentration in the brain. Synthetic GHB, formerly used in anesthesia and in the treatment of narcolepsy and alcohol withdrawal, has been banned by the U.S. Food and Drug Administration because of severe neurologic, cardiovascular, respiratory, and gastrointestinal side effects.

**5-hy·drox·y·tryp·ta·mine (5-HT)** (hī-drok-sē-trip′tă-mēn) SYN serotonin.

**hy·drox·y·u·re·a** (hī-drok′sē-yū-rē′ă) Oral antineoplastic agent that inhibits DNA synthesis; used to treat various malignancies including melanoma, chronic myelocytic leukemia, and carcinoma of the ovary.

**hy·drox·y·zine** (hī-drok′si-zēn) Mild sedative and minor tranquilizer used to treat neuroses.

**hy·giene** (hī′jēn) **1.** Science of health and its maintenance. **2.** Cleanliness that promotes health and well-being. [G. *hygieinos,* healthful, fr. *hygiēs,* healthy]

**hy·gien·ist** (hī-jē′nist) One skilled in the science of health and its maintenance.

**hygro-** Combining form meaning moisture, humidity; opposite of xero-. [G. *hygros,* moist]

**hy·gro·ma** (hī-grō′mă) A cystic swelling containing a serous fluid. SYN hydroma. [*hygro-* + G. *-oma,* tumor]

**hy·gro·scop·ic** (hī′grō-skop′ik) Denoting a substance capable of readily absorbing and retaining moisture; e.g., NaOH, CaCl₂.

**hy·gro·scop·ic ex·pan·sion** (hī′grō-skop′ik eks-pan′shŭn) **1.** Expansion due to absorption of moisture. **2.** In dental casting, addition of water to surface of casting investment during setting to increase the size of the mold.

**hy·o·bran·chi·al cleft** (hī′ō-brang′kē-ăl kleft) Cleft caudal to hyoid (second) pharyngeal arch of the embryo.

**hy·o·glos·sus mus·cle** (hī′ō-glos′ŭs mŭs′ĕl) *Origin,* body and greater horn of hyoid bone; *insertion,* side of the tongue; *action,* retracts and pulls down side of tongue; *nerve supply,* motor by hypoglossal, sensory by lingual. SYN musculus hyoglossus [TA].

**hy·oid bone** (hī′oyd bōn) U-shaped bone lying between the mandible and the larynx, suspended from styloid processes by slender stylohyoid ligaments. SYN lingual bone, tongue bone.

**hy·o·man·dib·u·lar cleft** (hī′ō-man-dib′yū-lăr kleft) Cleft between the hyoid (second) and mandibular (first) pharyngeal arches of the embryo; external acoustic meatus is developed from its dorsal portion. SYN first pharyngeal groove, first visceral cleft.

**hy·o·scine** (hī′ō-sēn) SYN scopolamine.

**hy·o·scy·a·mine** (hī′ō-sī′ă-mēn) Alkaloid; used as an antispasmodic, analgesic, and sedative.

**hy·o·scy·a·mine sul·fate** (hī′ō-sī′ă-mēn sŭl′fāt) Antispasmodic, hypnotic, and sedative, also used in parkinsonism to relieve tremor, rigidity, and excessive salivation.

**hypaesthesia** [Br.] SYN hypesthesia.

**hyp·al·ge·si·a** (hīp′al-jē′zē-ă) Decreased sensibility to pain. SYN hypoalgesia. [G. *hypo,* under, + *algēsis,* sense of pain]

**hyper-** Prefix meaning excessive, above normal; opposite of hypo-. [G. *hyper,* above, over]

**hy·per·a·cid·i·ty** (hī′pĕr-ă-sid′i-tē) Abnormally high degree of acidity, as in gastric juices.

**hy·per·ac·tiv·i·ty** (hī′pĕr-ak-tiv′i-tē) General restlessness or excessive movement such as that characterizing children with attention deficit disorder or hyperkinesis.

**hy·per·ad·e·no·sis** (hī′pĕr-ad′ĕ-nō′sis) Glandular enlargement, especially of the lymphatic glands. [*hyper-* + G. *adēn,* gland, + *-ōsis,* condition]

**hyperaesthesia** [Br.] SYN hyperesthesia.

**hyperaesthetic** [Br.] SYN hyperesthetic.

**hy·per·al·ge·sia** (hī′pĕr-al-jē′zē-ă) Increased response to pain exceeding that normally elicited by such pain. [*hyper-* + G. *algos,* pain]

**hy·per·bar·ic** (hī′pĕr-bar′ik) Concerning solutions, those that are denser than the diluent or medium; e.g., in spinal anesthesia, a hyperbaric solution has a density greater than that of spinal fluid. [*hyper-* + G. *baros,* weight]

**hy·per·bar·ic an·es·the·si·a** (hī´pĕr-bar´ ik an´es-thē´zē-ă) Inhalation of depressant gases or vapors at pressures greater than 1 atmosphere, especially as a means of producing general anesthesia with agents too weak to produce anesthesia at 1 atmosphere.

**hy·per·bar·ic ox·y·gen, high pres·sure ox·y·gen (HBO)** (hī´pĕr-bar´ik ok´si-jĕn, hī presh´ŭr) Oxygen at a pressure greater than 1 atmosphere. SEE ALSO hyperbaric oxygenation.

**hy·per·bar·ic ox·y·gen·a·tion** (hī´pĕr-bar´ik ok´si-jĕ-nā´shŭn) Increased amount of oxygen in organs and tissues due to administration of oxygen in a compression chamber at an ambient pressure greater than 1 atmosphere.

**hyperbilirubinaemia** [Br.] SYN hyperbilirubinemia.

**hy·per·bil·i·ru·bi·ne·mi·a** (hī´pĕr-bil´i-rū-bi-nē´mē-ă) Abnormally high level of bilirubin in circulating blood, resulting in clinically apparent icterus or jaundice when concentration is sufficient. SYN hyperbilirubinaemia.

**hypercalcaemia** [Br.] SYN hypercalcemia.

**hy·per·cal·ce·mi·a** (hī´pĕr-kal-sē´mē-ă) Abnormally high concentration of calcium compounds in circulating blood; commonly used to indicate an elevated concentration of calcium ions in the blood. SYN hypercalcaemia.

**hy·per·cal·ci·u·ri·a** (hī´pĕr-kal´sē-yūr´ē-ă) Excretion of abnormally large amounts of calcium in urine.

**hy·per·cap·ni·a** (hī´pĕr-kap´nē-ă) Abnormally increased arterial carbon dioxide tension. [*hyper-* + G. *kapnos,* smoke, vapor]

**hy·per·ca·tab·o·lism** (hī´pĕr-kă-tab´ŏ-lizm) Excessive metabolic breakdown of a specific substance or of body tissue in general, leading to weight loss and wasting.

▪**hy·per·ce·men·to·sis** (hī´pĕr-sē´mĕn-tō´ sis) Excessive deposition of secondary cementum on tooth root, which may be caused by localized trauma or inflammation, excessive tooth eruption, or osteitis deformans, or may occur idiopathically. See this page. SYN cementum hyperplasia, excementosis. [*hyper-* + L. *caementum,* a rough quarry stone, + *-osis,* condition]

**hyperchloraemia** [Br.] SYN hyperchloremia.

**hy·per·chlor·e·mi·a** (hī´pĕr-klōr-ē´mē-ă) Abnormally large amount of chloride ions in the circulating blood. SYN hyperchloraemia.

**hy·per·chlor·hy·dri·a** (hī´pĕr-klōr-hī´drē-ă) Presence of an excessive amount of hydro-

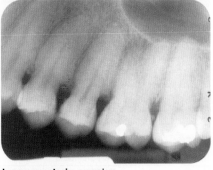

**hypercementosis:** premolars

chloric acid in the stomach. [*hyper-* + *chlorhydric* (acid)]

**hy·per·chlor·u·ri·a** (hī´pĕr-klōr-yū´rē-ă) Increased excretion of chloride ions in the urine.

**hypercholesterolaemia** [Br.] SYN hypercholesterolemia.

**hy·per·cho·les·ter·ol·e·mi·a** (hī´pĕr-kŏ-les´tĕr-ol-ē´mē-ă) The presence of an abnormally large amount of cholesterol in the blood. SYN hypercholesteremia, hypercholesterolaemia.

**hypercholestoremia** SYN hypercholesterolemia.

**hy·per·chro·mic a·ne·mi·a, hy·per·chro·mat·ic a·ne·mi·a** (hī´pĕr-krō´mik ă-nē´mē-ă, -krō-mat´ik) Hematologic disorder characterized by decreased ratio of the weight of hemoglobin to the volume of the erythrocyte.

**hy·per·cor·ti·coid·ism** (hī´pĕr-kōr´ti-koyd-izm) Excessive secretion of steroid hormones of the cortex of the suprarenal gland; sometimes used also to designate the state produced by therapeutic administration of large quantities of steroids having glucocorticoid activity. SYN adrenalism.

**hypercryaesthesia** [Br.] SYN hypercryesthesia.

**hy·per·cry·es·the·si·a** (hī´pĕr-krī´es-thē´zē-ă) Extreme sensibility to cold. SYN hypercryaesthesia. [*hyper-* + G. *kryos,* cold, + *aisthēsis,* sensation]

**hy·per·cy·a·not·ic** (hī´pĕr-sī´ă-not´ik) Marked by extreme cyanosis.

**hy·per·dip·si·a** (hī´pĕr-dip´sē-ă) Intense thirst that is relatively temporary. [*hyper-* + G. *dipsa,* thirst]

▪**hy·per·don·ti·a** (hī´pĕr-don´shē-ă) Having an excessive number of teeth. See page 288.

**hy·per·e·mi·a** (hī´pĕr-ē´mē-ă) Increased amount of bloodflow in a body part or organ. SEE ALSO congestion. [*hyper-* + G. *haima,* blood]

**hy·per·e·o·sin·o·phil·i·a** (hī´pĕr-ē´ō-sin-

gh

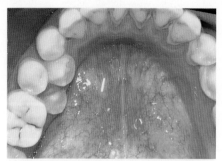

**hyperdontia:** supernumerary premolars

ō-fil′ē-ă) A greater degree of abnormal increase in the number of eosinophilic granulocytes in the circulating blood or the tissues.

**hy·per·e·o·sin·o·phil·ic syn·drome** (hī′pĕr-ē′ō-sin-ō-fil′ik sin′drōm) Persistent peripheral eosinophilia with eosinophilic infiltration into bone marrow, heart, and other organ systems; accompanied by nocturnal sweating, coughing, and anorexia and weight loss.

**hy·per·es·the·si·a** (hī′pĕr-es-thē′zē-ă) Abnormal acuteness of sensitivity to touch, pain, or other sensory stimuli. SYN hyperaesthesia. [*hyper-* + G. *aisthēsis*, sensation]

**hy·per·es·thet·ic** (hī′pĕr-es-thet′ik) Marked by hyperesthesia. SYN hyperaesthetic.

**hy·per·eu·ry·pro·so·pic** (hī′pĕr-yūr′i-prō-sop′ik) Pertaining to or characterized by a very low and wide face. [*hyper-* + G. *eurys*, wide, + *prosōpon*, face]

**hyperferraemia** [Br.] SYN hyperferremia.

**hy·per·fer·re·mi·a** (hī′pĕr-fĕr-ē′mē-ă) High serum iron level; found in hemochromatosis. SYN hyperferraemia.

**hy·per·fruc·to·se·mi·a** (hī′pĕr-fruk′tō-sē′mē-ă) Elevated serum fructose levels.

**hy·per·func·tion·al oc·clu·sion** (hī′pĕr-fŭngk′shŭn-ăl ŏ-klū′zhŭn) Occlusal stress of tooth or teeth exceeding normal physiologic demands.

**hypergammaglobulinaemia** [Br.] SYN hypergammaglobulinemia.

**hy·per·gam·ma·glob·u·lin·e·mi·a** (hī′pĕr-gam′ă-glob′yū-lin-ē′mē-ă) Increased γ-globulins in plasma, as in chronic infectious diseases. SYN hypergammaglobulinaemia.

**hy·per·geu·si·a** (hī′pĕr-gū′sē-ă) Abnormal acuity of the sense of taste. [*hyper-* + G. *geusis*, taste]

**hy·per·glan·du·lar** (hī′pĕr-glan′dyū-lăr) Characterized by overactivity or increased size of a gland.

**hyperglobulinaemia** [Br.] SYN hyperglobulinemia.

**hy·per·glob·u·lin·e·mi·a** (hī′pĕr-glob′yū-lin-ē′mē-ă) An abnormally high concentration of globulins in the circulating blood plasma. SYN hyperglobulinaemia.

**hyperglycaemia** [Br.] SYN hyperglycemia.

**hy·per·gly·ce·mi·a** (hī′pĕr-glī-sē′mē-ă) Abnormally high concentration of glucose in the circulating blood, seen in diabetes mellitus. SYN hyperglycaemia. [*hyper-* + G. *glykys*, sweet, + *haima*, blood]

**hyperglycinaemia** [Br.] SYN hyperglycinemia.

**hy·per·gly·ci·ne·mi·a** (hī′pĕr-glī′si-nē′mē-ă) Elevated plasma glycine concentration. SYN hyperglycinaemia.

**hy·per·gly·co·su·ri·a** (hī′pĕr-glī′kō-syūr′ē-ă) Persistent excretion of unusually large amounts of glucose in the urine.

**hy·per·go·nad·ism** (hī′pĕr-gō′nad-izm) A clinical state resulting from enhanced secretion of gonadal hormones.

**hy·per·go·nad·o·tro·pic** (hī′pĕr-gō-nad′ō-trō′pik) Indicating an increased production or excretion of gonadotropic hormones.

**hyperhaemoglobinaemia** [Br.] SYN hyperhemoglobinemia.

**hy·per·he·mo·glo·bi·ne·mi·a** (hī′pĕr-hē′mō-glō-bin-ē′mē-ă) Unusually large amount of hemoglobin in circulating blood plasma. SYN hyperhaemoglobinemia.

**hy·per·hi·dro·sis** (hī′pĕr-hi-drō′sis) Excessive or profuse sweating. [*hyper-* + *hidrosis*]

**hy·per·hy·dra·tion** (hī′pĕr-hī-drā′shŭn) Excess water content of the body; may result from the intravenous administration of unduly large amounts of glucose solution.

**hy·per·im·mune** (hī′pĕr-im-yūn′) Having large quantities of specific antibodies in the serum from repeated immunizations or infections.

**hy·per·im·mu·ni·za·tion** (hī′pĕr-im-yū′nī-zā′shŭn) Induction of a heightened state of immunity by administration of repeated doses of antigen; often used in allergy desensitization.

**hy·per·in·fec·tion** (hī′pĕr-in-fek′shŭn) Infection by large numbers of organisms as a result of immunologic deficiency.

**hy·per·in·fla·tion** (hī′pĕr-in-flā′shŭn) Overdistention of airways and alveoli, sometimes leading to emphysema, caused by obstructive lung disease. [*hyper-* + *inflation*]

**hyperinsulinaemia** [Br.] SYN hyperinsulinemia.

**hy·per·in·su·li·ne·mi·a** (hī'pĕr-in'sŭ-lin-ē'mē-ă) Increased levels of insulin in the plasma due to increased secretion of insulin by the beta cells of the islets of Langerhans. SYN hyperinsulinism, hyperinsulinaemia.

**hy·per·in·su·lin·ism** (hī'pĕr-in'sŭ-lin-izm) SYN hyperinsulinemia.

**hyperkalaemia** [Br.] SYN hyperkalemia.

**hy·per·ka·le·mi·a** (hī'pĕr-kă-lē'mē-ă) Higher than normal concentration of potassium ions in circulating blood. SYN hyperkalaemia. [hyper- + G. kalium, potash, + G. haima, blood]

**hy·per·ker·a·to·sis** (hī'pĕr-ker'ă-tō'sis) Thickening of the horny layer of the epidermis or mucous membrane.

**hy·per·ke·to·nu·ri·a** (hī'pĕr-kē'tō-nyūr'ē-ă) Increased urinary excretion of ketonic compounds.

**hy·per·ki·ne·sis, hy·per·ki·ne·si·a** (hī'pĕr-ki-nē'sis, -zē-ă) 1. Excessive motility. 2. Excessive muscular activity. [hyper- + G. kinēsis, motion]

**hyperlipidaemia** [Br.] SYN hyperlipidemia.

**hy·per·lip·id·e·mi·a** (hī'pĕr-lip'i-dē'mē-ă) Elevated levels of lipids in the blood plasma. SYN hyperlipidaemia.

**hyperlipoproteinaemia** [Br.] SYN hyperlipoproteinemia.

**hy·per·lip·o·pro·tein·e·mi·a** (hī'pĕr-lip'ō-prō-tēn-ē'mē-ă) An increase in the lipoprotein concentration of the blood. SYN hyperlipoproteinaemia.

**hy·per·lor·do·sis** (hī'pĕr-lōr-dō'sis) An abnormal anteriorly convex curvature of the spine, usually lumbar.

**hy·per·lor·dot·ic** (hī'pĕr-lōr-dot'ik) Having a pathologically exaggerated lordotic curve of the lumbar spine; colloquial term is "swayback."

**hyperlysinaemia** [Br.] SYN hyperlysinemia.

**hy·per·ly·si·ne·mi·a** (hī'pĕr-lī-si-nē'mē-ă) Metabolic disorder characterized by mental retardation, convulsions, anemia, and asthenia; associated with abnormal increase of amino acid lysine in the circulating blood due to a deficiency of lysine-ketoglutarate reductase. SYN hyperlysinaemia.

**hypermagnesaemia** [Br.] SYN hypermagnesemia.

**hy·per·mag·ne·se·mi·a** (hī'pĕr-mag'nĕ-sē'mē-ă) Excessive magnesium in blood; may be a result of chronic renal insufficiency, overuse of magnesium-containing laxatives or antacids, or severe dehydration. Signs include weakness, paralysis, drowsiness, confusion, bradycardia, hy-potension, nausea, and vomiting. SYN hypermagnesaemia.

**hy·per·men·or·rhe·a** (hī'pĕr-men-ŏr-ē'ă) Excessively prolonged or profuse menses. SYN menorrhagia, menostaxis, hypermenorrhoea. [hyper- + G. mēn, month, + rhoia, flow]

**hypermenorrhoea** [Br.] SYN hypermenorrhea.

**hy·per·me·tab·o·lism** (hī'pĕr-mĕ-tab'ŏ-lizm) Heat production by the body above normal levels, as in thyrotoxicosis.

**hy·per·me·tro·pi·a** (hī'pĕr-mē-trō'pē-ă) SYN hyperopia. [hyper- + G. metron, measure, + ōps, eye]

**hy·per·morph** (hī'pĕr-mōrf) Person whose sitting height is low in proportion to standing height, owing to excessive length of limb. Cf. ectomorph. [hyper- + G. morphē, form]

**hy·per·mo·tor sei·zure** (hī'pĕr-mō'tŏr sē'zhŭr) Seizure characterized by automatisms involving predominantly proximal limb muscles and producing marked limb displacement.

**hy·per·na·sal·i·ty** (hī'pĕr-nā-zal'i-tē) Speech produced with excessive resonance in the nasal cavity, often due to dysfunction of the soft palate. SYN hyperrhinophonia.

**hypernatraemia** [Br.] SYN hypernatremia.

**hy·per·na·tre·mi·a** (hī'pĕr-nă-trē'mē-ă, hī'pĕr-nā-trē'mē-ă) An abnormally high plasma concentration of sodium ions. SYN hypernatraemia. [hyper- + natrium, + G. haima, blood]

**hy·per·nom·ic** (hī'pĕr-nom'ik) Controlled to excess. [hyper- + G. nomos, law]

**hy·per·o·pi·a (H)** (hī'pĕr-ō'pē-ă) An ocular condition in which only convergent rays can be brought to focus on the retina. SYN farsightedness, hypermetropia. [hyper- + G. ōps, eye]

**hy·per·o·ral·i·ty** (hī'pĕr-ō-ral'i-tē) A condition characterized by insertion of inappropriate objects in the mouth. [hyper- + L. os (or-), mouth]

**hy·per·o·rex·i·a** (hī'pĕr-ō-rek'sē-ă) SYN bulimia nervosa. [hyper- + G. orexis, appetite]

**hy·per·os·mi·a** (hī'pĕr-oz'mē-ă) An exaggerated or abnormally acute sense of smell. [hyper- + G. osmē, sense of smell]

**hy·per·os·mo·lar (hy·per·gly·cem·ic) non·ke·tot·ic co·ma** (hī'pĕr-oz-mō'lăr hī'per-glī-sē'mik non'kē-tot'ik kō'mă) Complication seen in diabetes mellitus (q.v.) in which very marked hyperglycemia occurs; can be fatal or lead to permanent neurologic damage.

**hy·per·os·to·sis** (hī'pĕr-os-tō'sis) 1. Hypertrophy of bone. 2. SYN exostosis. [hyper- + G. osteon, bone, + -ōsis, condition]

gh

**hy·per·ox·a·lu·ri·a** (hī'pĕr-ok-să-lyūr'ē-ă) Presence of an unusually large amount of oxalic acid or oxalates in the urine. SYN oxaluria.

**hy·per·ox·i·a** (hī'pĕr-ok'sē-ă) **1.** An increased amount of oxygen in tissues and organs. **2.** A greater oxygen tension than normal.

**hy·per·pan·cre·a·tism** (hī'pĕr-pan'krē-ă-tizm) A condition of increased activity of the pancreas, trypsin being in excess among the enzymes.

**hy·per·par·a·thy·roid·ism** (hī'pĕr-par'ă-thī'royd-izm) Condition due to increased secretion of parathyroids, causing elevated serum calcium, decreased serum phosphorus, and increased excretion of both calcium and phosphorus, calcium stones, and sometimes generalized osteitis fibrosa cystica.

**hy·per·pa·rot·i·dism** (hī'pĕr-pa-rot'i-dizm) Increased activity of the parotid glands.

**hy·per·per·i·stal·sis** (hī'pĕr-per'i-stal'sis) Excessive rapidity of the passage of food through the stomach and intestine.

**hy·per·pha·gi·a** (hī'pĕr-fā'jē-ă) Gluttony; overeating. [*hyper-* + G. *phagein*, to eat]

**hyperphosphataemia** [Br.] SYN hyperphosphatemia.

**hy·per·phos·pha·ta·se·mi·a** (hī'pĕr-fos'fă-tă-sē'mē-ă) Abnormally high alkaline phosphatase in circulating blood. SYN hyperphosphataemia.

**hy·per·phos·pha·ta·si·a** (hī'pĕr-fos'fă-tā'zē-ă) A skeletal dysplasia characterized by dwarfism, macrocranium, expansion of the diaphyses of tubular bones with multiple fractures, and other findings.

**hy·per·phos·pha·te·mi·a** (hī'pĕr-fos'fă-tē'mē-ă) Abnormally high concentration of phosphates in the circulating blood. SYN hyperphosphataemia.

**hy·per·phos·pha·tu·ri·a** (hī'pĕr-fos'fă-tyūr'ē-ă) An increased excretion of phosphates in the urine.

**hy·per·pig·men·ta·tion** (hī'pĕr-pig-men-tā'shŭn) An excess of pigment in a tissue or part.

**hy·per·pi·tu·i·ta·rism** (hī'pĕr-pi-tū'i-tă-rizm) SYN acromegaly.

▣**hy·per·pla·si·a** (hī'pĕr-plā'zē-ă) Increased number of normal cells in tissue or organ, excluding tumor formation, whereby bulk of the part or organ may be increased. SEE ALSO hyper-

trophy. See this page. [*hyper-* + G. *plasis*, a molding]

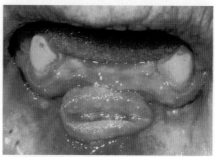

**inflammatory fibrous hyperplasia:** at location of contact of partial denture flange

**hy·per·plas·tic** (hī'pĕr-plas'tik) Relating to hyperplasia.

**hy·per·plas·tic gin·gi·vi·tis** (hī'pĕr-plas'tik jin'ji-vī'tis) Gingivitis of long-standing duration in which the gingiva becomes enlarged and firm due to proliferation of fibrous connective tissue.

▣**hy·per·plas·tic pulp·i·tis** (hī'pĕr-plas'tik pŭl-pī'tis) Hyperplastic granulation tissue growing out of the exposed pulp chamber of a grossly decayed tooth. See this page. SYN dental polyp, pulp polyp, tooth polyp.

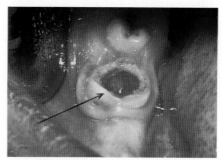

**hyperplastic pulpitis:** red exuberant mass arising from pulp

**hy·per·plas·tic tis·sue** (hī'pĕr-plas'tik tish'ū) In dentistry, excessively movable tissue about the maxilla or mandible.

**hy·per·pne·a** (hī'pĕrp-nē'ă) Breathing that is deeper and more rapid than normal. SYN hyperpnoea. [*hyper-* + G. *pnoē*, breathing]

**hyperpnoea** [Br.] SYN hyperpnea.

**hy·per·po·lar·i·za·tion** (hī'pĕr-pō'lăr-ī-zā'shŭn) Increased polarization of membranes of nerves or muscle cells.

**hyperpotassaemia** [Br.] SYN hyperpotassemia.

**hy·per·po·tas·se·mi·a** (hī′pĕr-pŏ-tas-ē′mē-ă)
SYN hyperkalemia, hyperpotassaemia.

**hyperprebetalipoproteinaemia** [Br.]
SYN hyperprebetalipoproteinemia.

**hy·per·pre·be·ta·lip·o·pro·tein·e·mi·a**
(hī′pĕr-prē′bā′tă-lip′ō-prō′tēn-ē′mē-ă) Increased
concentrations of pre-β-lipoproteins in the
blood. SYN hyperprebetalipoproteinaemia.

**hyperprolinaemia** [Br.] SYN hyperproli-
nemia.

**hy·per·pro·li·ne·mi·a** (hī′pĕr-prō′li-nē′mē-ă)
A metabolic disorder characterized by enhanced
plasma proline concentrations and urinary excretion of proline, hydroxyproline, and glycine.
SYN hyperprolinaemia.

**hyperproteinaemia** [Br.] SYN hyperpro-
teinemia.

**hy·per·pro·tein·e·mi·a** (hī′pĕr-prō′tēn-ē′
mē-ă) An abnormally large concentration of
protein in plasma. SYN hyperproteinaemia.

**hy·per·pro·te·o·sis** (hī′pĕr-prō′tē-ō′sis) A
condition resulting from excessive consumption
of protein in the diet.

**hy·per·re·ac·tive ma·lar·i·ous sple·
no·meg·a·ly** (hī′pĕr-ak′tiv mă-lar′ē-ŭs splē′
nō-meg′ă-lē) Syndrome characterized by persistent splenomegaly, exceptionally high serum
IgM and malaria antibody levels, and hepatic
sinusoidal lymphocytosis.

**hy·per·re·flex·i·a** (hī′pĕr-rē-flek′sē-ă) Exaggeration of the deep tendon reflexes; may be
generalized, regional, or focal.

**hy·per·res·o·nance** (hī′pĕr-rez′ŏ-năns) Resonance increased above normal, and often of
lower pitch, on percussion of body area; occurs
in chest as a result of overinflation of the lung
as in emphysema or pneumothorax and in abdomen over distended bowel.

**hy·per·rhi·no·pho·ni·a** (hī′pĕr-rī′nō-fō′nē-ă)
SYN hypernasality.

**hy·per·sal·i·va·tion** (hī′pĕr-sal′i-vā′shŭn)
Increased salivation.

**hy·per·se·cre·tion** (hī′pĕr-sĕ-krē′shŭn) Excessive secretion of any tissue or gland.

**hy·per·sen·si·tive den·tin** (hī′pĕr-sen′si-
tiv den′tin) Exposed dentin, usually at the cervical portion of a tooth, painful to touch, sweetness, or temperature changes.

**⊞hy·per·sen·si·tiv·i·ty** (hī′per-sen′si-tiv′i-
tē) In endocrinology, an excessive target tissue
response to a hormone. See page A14.

**hy·per·sen·si·tiv·i·ty re·ac·tion** (hī′pĕr-
sen′si-tiv′i-tē rē-ak′shŭn) SYN allergic reaction.

**hy·per·sen·si·ti·za·tion** (hī′pĕr-sen′si-tī-

zā′shŭn) The immunologic process by which
hypersensitivity is induced.

**hy·per·som·ni·a** (hī′pĕr-som′nē-ă) A condition in which sleep periods are excessively
long, but the person responds normally in the
intervals. [hyper- + L. somnus, sleep]

**hy·per·sphyx·i·a** (hī′pĕr-sfik′sē-ă) A condition of high blood pressure and increased circulatory activity. [hyper- + G. sphyxis, pulse]

**hy·per·splen·ism** (hī′pĕr-splēn′izm) Any
of a group of conditions in which cellular components of blood or platelets are removed at an
abnormally high rate by the spleen.

**hy·per·sthe·nu·ri·a** (hī′pĕr-sthĕ-nyū′rē-ă)
Excretion of urine with an unusually high specific gravity and concentration of solutes.
[hyper- + G. sthenos, strength, + ouron, urine]

**hy·per·sus·cep·ti·bil·i·ty** (hī′pĕr-sŭ-sep′ti-
bil′i-tē) Increased susceptibility or response to
an infective, chemical, or other agent.

**hy·per·tau·ro·dont** (hī′pĕr-tawr′ō-dont) Developmental anomaly in which pulp chamber is
elongated such that its floor nearly or completely
approximates root apices.

**hy·per·tel·or·ism** (hī′pĕr-tel′ŏr-izm) Abnormal distance between two paired organs.
[hyper- + G. tēle, far off, + horizō, to separate,
fr. horos, a boundary]

**hy·per·ten·sion (HTN)** (hī′pĕr-ten′shŭn)
Persisting high arterial blood pressure; generally established guidelines are values exceeding
140 mmHg systolic or exceeding 90 mmHg diastolic blood pressure. [hyper- + L. tensio, ten-
sion]

**hy·per·ther·mal·ge·si·a** (hī′pĕr-thĕrm′al-
jē′zē-ă) A distortion of sensation whereby
warmth is perceived as being painful. [hyper- +
G. thermē, heat, + algēsis, pain]

**hy·per·ther·mi·a** (hī′pĕr-thĕr′mē-ă) Therapeutically or iatrogenically induced hyperpy-
rexia. [hyper- + G. thermē, heat]

**hy·per·thy·mi·a** (hī′pĕr-thī′mē-ă) State of
overactivity, greater than average but less
than the overactivity of manic state of bipolar
disorder.

**hy·per·thy·mism** (hī′pĕr-thī′mizm) Excessive activity of the thymus gland; formerly postulated to be a causal factor in certain instances
of unexpected and sudden death.

**hy·per·thy·roid·ism** (hī′pĕr-thī′royd-izm)
An abnormality of the thyroid gland in which
secretion of thyroid hormone is usually increased and no longer under regulatory control
of hypothalamic-pituitary centers; characterized
by a hypermetabolic state, usually with weight
loss, tremulousness, elevated plasma levels of
thyroxin and/or triiodothyronine, and sometimes exophthalmos.

**hy·per·to·ni·a** (hī′pĕr-tō′nē-ă) Extreme tension of the muscles or arteries. [*hyper-* + G. *tonos*, tension]

**hy·per·ton·ic** (hī′pĕr-ton′ik) 1. Having a greater degree of tension. SYN spastic (1). 2. Having a greater osmotic pressure than a reference solution.

**hy·per·tri·cho·sis** (hī′pĕr-tri-kō′sis) Growth of hair in excess of the normal. SEE ALSO hirsutism. [*hyper-* + G. *trichōsis*, being hairy]

**hypertriglyceridaemia** [Br.] SYN hypertriglyceridemia.

**hy·per·tri·glyc·er·i·de·mi·a** (hī′pĕr-trī-glis′ĕr-i-dē′mē-ă) Elevated triglyceride concentration in the blood. SYN hypertriglyceridaemia.

**hy·per·tro·phic ar·thri·tis** (hī′pĕr-trō′fik ahr-thrī′tis) SYN osteoarthritis.

**hy·per·tro·phic car·di·o·my·op·a·thy** (hī′pĕr-trō′fik kahr′dē-ō-mī-op′ă-thē) Cardiac hypertrophy of unknown cause, with impairment of left ventricular filling, emptying, or both. Signs and symptoms include fatigue and syncope.

**hy·per·tro·phy** (hī-pĕr′trŏ-fē) General increase in bulk of a part or organ, not due to tumor formation. [*hyper-* + G. *trophē*, nourishment]

**hy·per·u·ri·cu·ri·a** (hī′pĕr-yūr′i-kyū′rē-ă) Increased urinary excretion of uric acid.

**hy·per·ven·ti·la·tion** (hī′pĕr-ven′ti-lā′shŭn) Increased alveolar ventilation relative to metabolic carbon dioxide production.

**hy·per·ven·ti·la·tion tet·a·ny** (hī′pĕr-ven′ti-lā′shŭn tet′ă-nē) A neurologic disorder caused by forced overbreathing, due to reduced levels of $CO_2$ in the blood.

**hy·per·vi·ta·min·o·sis** (hī′pĕr-vī′tă-mi-nō′sis) Condition due to ingestion of excessive vitamin preparations; serious effects may be caused by overdosage with fat-soluble vitamins, especially A or D.

**hypervolaemia** [Br.] SYN hypervolemia.

**hy·per·vo·le·mi·a** (hī′pĕr-vol-ē′mē-ă) Abnormally increased volume of blood. SYN circulatory overload, plethora (1), repletion (1), hypervolaemia. [*hyper-* + L. *volumen*, volume, + G. *haima*, blood]

**hyp·es·the·si·a** (hīp′es-thē′zē-ă) Diminished sensitivity to stimulation. SYN hypaesthesia. [G. *hypo*, under, + *aisthēsis*, feeling]

**hyp·he·do·ni·a** (hīp′hē-dō′nē-ă) Habitually lessened or attenuated degree of pleasure from something that should normally give great pleasure. [G. *hypo*, under, + *hēdonē*, pleasure]

**hyp·na·gog·ic** (hip′nă-goj′ik) Denoting a transitional state, related to the hypnoidal, preceding sleep; applied also to various hallucinations. [*hypno-* + G. *agōgos*, leading]

✪ **hypno-, hypn-** Combining forms meaning sleep, hypnosis. [G. *hypnos,* sleep]

**hyp·no·sis** (hip-nō′sis) Artificially induced trancelike state, resembling somnambulism, in which the subject is highly susceptible to suggestion, oblivious to all else, and responds readily to the commands of the hypnotist. [G. *hypnos,* sleep, + *-osis,* condition]

**hyp·no·ther·a·py** (hip′nō-thār′ă-pē) 1. Psychotherapeutic treatment by means of hypnotism. 2. Treatment of disease by inducing a trancelike sleep.

**hyp·not·ic** (hip-not′ik) 1. Causing sleep. 2. An agent that promotes sleep. 3. Relating to hypnotism. [G. *hypnōtikos,* causing one to sleep]

**hyp·no·tism** (hip′nŏ-tizm) SEE hypnosis. [G. *hypnos,* sleep]

**hyp·no·tize** (hip′nŏ-tīz) To induct someone into hypnosis.

✪ **hypo-** 1. Prefix meaning deficient, below normal. Cf. sub-. 2. CHEMISTRY denoting the lowest, or least rich in oxygen, of a series of chemical compounds. [G. *hypo,* under]

**hy·po·a·cid·i·ty** (hī′pō-ă-sid′i-tē) A lower than normal degree of acidity, as of the gastric juice.

**hy·po·a·de·ni·a** (hī′pō-ă-dē′nē-ă) Any deficiency in the function of a glandular organ or tissue. [*hypo-* + G. *adēn,* gland]

**hy·po·a·dre·nal·ism** (hī′pō-ă-drē′năl-izm) Reduced adrenocortical function.

**hypoaesthesia** [Br.] SYN hypoesthesia.

**hypoalbuminaemia** [Br.] SYN hypoalbuminemia.

**hy·po·al·bu·mi·ne·mi·a** (hī′pō-al-bū′mi-nē′mē-ă) An abnormally low concentration of albumin in the blood. SYN hypalbuminemia, hypoalbuminaemia.

**hy·po·al·dos·ter·on·ism** (hī′pō-al-dos′tĕr-on-izm) Condition due to deficient secretion of aldosterone.

**hy·po·al·ge·si·a** (hī′pō-al-jē′zē-ă) SYN hypalgesia. [*hypo-* + G. *algēsis,* a sense of pain]

**hy·po·al·ler·gen·ic** (hī′pō-al′ĕr-jen′ik) Property of a substance or material that indicates it does not elicit a hypersensitivity reaction; may also denote various chemicals in clinical use.

**hy·po·bar·ic** (hī′pō-bar′ik) 1. Pertaining to pressure of ambient gases below 1 atmosphere.

**2.** With respect to solutions, less dense than the diluent or medium. [*hypo-* + G. *baros,* weight]

**hy·po·bar·ism** (hī′pō-bar′izm) Dysbarism resulting from decreasing barometric pressure on the body without hypoxia; gas in body cavities tends to expand, and gases dissolved in body fluids tend to come out of solution as bubbles.

**hypobetalipoproteinaemia** [Br.] SYN hypobetalipoproteinemia.

**hy·po·be·ta·lip·o·pro·tein·e·mi·a** (hī′pō-bā′tă-lip′ō-prō-tēn-ē′mē-ă) Abnormally low levels of β-lipoproteins in plasma, occasionally with acanthocytosis and neurologic signs. SYN hypobetalipoproteinaemia.

**hy·po·be·ta·lip·o·pro·tein·e·mi·a with apo B-37** (hī′pō-bā′tă-lip′ō-prō-tē-nē′mē-ă) Disorder in which levels of low density lipoproteins are low, there is a mild fat malabsorption, and a truncated apolipoprotein B-37 is formed.

**hypocalcaemia** [Br.] SYN hypocalcemia.

**hy·po·cal·ce·mi·a** (hī′pō-kal-sē′mē-ă) Abnormally low levels of calcium in the circulating blood. SYN hypocalcaemia.

**hy·po·cal·ci·fi·ca·tion** (hī′pō-kal′si-fi-kā′shŭn) Deficient calcification of bone or teeth.

**hy·po·cap·ni·a** (hī′pō-kap′nē-ă) Abnormally decreased arterial carbon dioxide tension. SYN hypocarbia. [*hypo-* + G. *kapnos,* smoke, vapor]

**hy·po·car·bi·a** (hī′pō-kahr′bē-ă) SYN hypocapnia.

**hypochloraemia** [Br.] SYN hypochloremia.

**hy·po·chlor·e·mi·a** (hī′pō-klōr-ē′mē-ă) An abnormally low level of chloride ions in the circulating blood. SYN hypochloraemia.

**hy·po·chlor·hy·dri·a** (hī′pō-klōr-hī′drē-ă) Presence of an abnormally small amount of hydrochloric acid in the stomach.

**hy·po·chlor·ite** (hī′pō-klōr′īt) A salt of hypochlorous acid.

**hy·po·chlor·ous ac·id** (hī′pō-klōr′ŭs as′id) Acid with oxidizing and bleaching properties.

**hypocholesterolaemia** [Br.] SYN hypocholesterolemia.

**hy·po·cho·les·ter·ol·e·mi·a** (hī′pō-kŏles′tĕr-ol-ē′mē-ă) Presence of abnormally small amounts of cholesterol in circulating blood. SYN hypocholesterolaemia.

**hy·po·chon·dri·a** (hī′pō-kon′drē-ă) *Negative and pejorative connotations of this word may render it offensive in some contexts.* SYN hypochondriasis.

**hy·po·chon·dri·ac** (hī′pō-kon′drē-ak) *Negative and pejorative connotations of this word may render it offensive in some contexts.* **1.** A

person with a somatic overconcern, including morbid attention to the details of bodily functioning and exaggeration of any symptoms no matter how insignificant. **2.** Beneath the ribs.

**hy·po·chon·dri·a·cal** (hī′pō-kŏn-drī′ă-kăl) Relating to or suffering from hypochondriasis.

**hy·po·chon·dri·a·sis** (hī′pō-kŏn-drī′ă-sis) A morbid concern about one's own health and exaggerated attention to any unusual bodily or mental sensations; delusion one is suffering from some disease for which no physical basis is evident. SYN hypochondria. [fr. *hypochondrium,* regarded as the site of hypochondria, + G. *-iasis,* condition]

**hy·po·chon·dro·pla·si·a** (hī′pō-kon′drō-plā′zē-ă) Skeletal dysplasia characterized by dwarfism with features similar to but much milder than achondroplasia; cranium and facies are normal. [*hypo-* + G. *chondros,* cartilage, + *plasis,* a molding]

**hy·po·chro·ma·tism** (hī′pō-krō′mă-tizm) **1.** The condition of being hypochromatic. **2.** SYN hypochromia.

**hy·po·chro·mi·a** (hī′pō-krō′mē-ă) An anemic condition in which the percentage of hemoglobin in the red blood cells is less than the normal range. SYN hypochromatism (2). [*hypo-* + G. *chrōma,* color]

**hy·po·chro·mic a·ne·mi·a** (hī′pō-krō′mik ă-nē′mē-ă) Anemia characterized by decrease in ratio of weight of hemoglobin to volume of erythrocyte, i.e., the mean corpuscular hemoglobin concentration is less than normal.

**hy·po·chro·mic mi·cro·cyt·ic a·ne·mi·a** (hī′pō-krō′mik mī′krō-sit′ik ă-nē′mē-ă) Anemia due to iron deficiency or thalassemia; characterized by subnormal mean corpuscular volume, mean corpuscular hemoglobin, and mean corpuscular hemoglobin concentration.

**hy·po·cone** (hī′pō-kōn) Distolingual cusp of an upper molar tooth. [*hypo-* + G. *kōnos,* pine cone]

**hy·po·con·id** (hī′pō-kon′id) Distobuccal cusp of a mandibular molar tooth. [*hypocone* + *id*]

**hy·po·con·ule** (hī′pō-kon′yūl) Distal, or fifth, cusp of an maxillary molar tooth. [*hypo-* + Mod. L. dim. of L. *conus,* cone]

**hy·po·con·u·lid** (hī′pō-kon′yū-lid) [TA] Distal, or fifth, cusp of a mandibular molar tooth. SYN distal cusp. [*hypo-* + Mod. L. dim. of L. *conus,* cone]

**hy·po·der·mic** (hī′pō-dĕr′mik) **1.** SYN subcutaneous. **2.** SYN hypodermic syringe.

**hy·po·der·mic in·jec·tion** (hī′pō-dĕr′mik in-jek′shŭn) Administration of a remedy in liquid form by injection into subcutaneous tissues.

**hy·po·der·mic sy·ringe** (hī′pō-dĕr′mik sir-

gh

inj′) Small syringe with a barrel (which may be calibrated), perfectly matched plunger, and tip; used with a hollow needle for subcutaneous injections and for aspiration. SYN hypodermic (3).

**hy·po·der·mic tab·let** (hī′pō-dĕr′mik tab′lĕt) Compressed or molded tablet that dissolves completely in water to form an injectable solution.

**hy·po·der·mo·cly·sis** (hī′pō-dĕr-mok′li-sis) Subcutaneous injection of a saline or other solution. [*hypo-* + G. *derma*, skin, + *klysis*, a washing out]

**hy·po·dip·si·a** (hī′pō-dip′sē-ă) Physiologic condition, perhaps caused by hypertonicity of body fluids, insufficient to initiate drinking but at times sufficient to sustain drinking when started; loosely, oligodipsia. [*hypo-* + G. *dipsa*, thirst]

**⊞hy·po·don·ti·a** (hī′pō-don′shē-ă) Congenital or acquired condition of having fewer than the normal complement of teeth. See this page. [*hypo-* + G. *odous*, tooth]

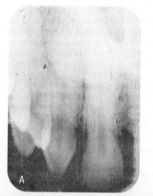

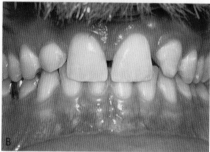

**hypodontia:** in same patient (A) congenitally absent lateral incisor; (B) missing maxillary lateral incisor

**hy·po·es·the·si·a** (hī′pō-es-thē′zē-ă) SYN hypesthesia, hypoaesthesia.

**hypogammaglobulinaemia** [Br.] SYN hypogammaglobulinemia.

**hy·po·gam·ma·glob·u·lin·e·mi·a** (hī′pō-

gam′ă-glob′yū-li-nē′mē-ă) Decreased gamma fraction of serum globulin; associated with increased susceptibility to pyogenic infections. SYN hypogammaglobulinaemia.

**hy·po·geu·si·a** (hī′pō-gū′sē-ă) Diminished sense of taste due to transport or sensorineural disorders; may be general to all tastants, partial to some tastants, or specific to one or more tastants. [*hypo-* + G. *geusis*, taste]

**hy·po·glos·sal** (hī′pō-glos′ăl) *Do not confuse this word with* hyoglossal. **1.** Below the tongue. **2.** Relating to the twelfth cranial nerve (nervus hypoglossus). [L. *hypoglossus* fr. hypo- + *glossus*, tongue]

**hy·po·glos·sal ca·nal** (hī′pō-glos′ăl kă-nal′) [TA] Canal through which the hypoglossal nerve emerges from the skull. SYN anterior condyloid foramen.

**hy·po·glos·sal nerve [CN XII]** (hī′pō-glos′ăl nĕrv) [TA] Arises from an oblong nucleus in the medulla and emerges by several root filaments between pyramid and olive via preolivary groove; passes through the hypoglossal canal, then courses downward and forward to supply the intrinsic and four of five extrinsic muscles of the tongue. SYN nervus hypoglossus [CN XII], twelfth cranial nerve [CN XII].

**hy·po·glot·tis** (hī′pō-glot′is) Undersurface of the tongue. [G. *hypoglōssis*, or -*glōttis*, undersurface of tongue, fr. hypo, under, + *glōssa*, tongue]

**hypoglycaemia** [Br.] SYN hypoglycemia.

**hypoglycaemic** [Br.] SYN hypoglycemic.

**hypoglycaemic coma** [Br.] SYN hypoglycemic coma.

**hy·po·gly·ce·mi·a** (hī′pō-glī-sē′mē-ă) Symptoms resulting from low blood glucose (normal glucose range 60–100 mg/dL [3.3–5.6 mmol/L]), which are either autonomic or neuroglycopenic. SYN glucopenia, hypoglycaemia.

**hy·po·gly·ce·mic** (hī′pō-glī-sē′mik) Pertaining to or characterized by hypoglycemia. SYN hypoglycaemic.

**hy·po·gly·ce·mic co·ma** (hī′pō-glī-sē′mik kō′mă) Metabolic encephalopathy caused by hypoglycemia; usually seen in diabetic patients, and due to exogenous insulin excess. SYN hypoglycaemic coma.

**hy·pog·na·thous** (hī-pog′nă-thŭs) *In the diphthong gn, the g is silent only at the beginning of a word.* Having a congenitally defectively developed small lower jaw. [*hypo-* + G. *gnathos*, jaw]

**hy·po·go·nad·ism** (hī′pō-gō′nad-izm) Inadequate gonadal function, as manifested by deficiencies in gametogenesis or secretion of gonadal hormones.

**hypokalaemia** [Br.] SYN hypokalemia.

**hy·po·ka·le·mi·a** (hī′pō-kă-lē′mē-ă) Presence of an abnormally low concentration of potassium ions in the circulating blood. SYN hypokalaemia. [*hypo-* + G. *kalion*, L. *kalium*, potassium, + G. *haima*, blood]

**hy·po·lo·gi·a** (hī′pō-lō′jē-ă) Lack of ability for speech. [*hypo-* + G. *logos*, word]

**hypomagnesaemia** [Br.] SYN hypomagnesemia.

**hy·po·mag·ne·se·mi·a** (hī′pō-mag′nĕ-sē′mē-ă) Subnormal blood serum concentration of magnesium; may cause convulsions and concurrent hypocalcemia. SYN hypomagnesaemia.

**hy·po·met·a·bol·ic state** (hī′pō-met″ă-bol′ik stāt) Rare state of reduced metabolism with symptoms resembling hypothyroidism but with some tests for thyroid gland function normal; also used to describe the reduced metabolic activity seen in true hypothyroidism.

**hy·po·met·a·bol·ic syn·drome** (hī′pō-met″ă-bol′ik sin′drōm) Clinical situation suggesting hypothyroidism or myxedema, in which some test results of thyroid function may be normal and the gland is not obviously atrophic or diseased; indicates a lack of sensitivity of peripheral tissues to thyroid hormone.

**hy·po·me·tab·o·lism** (hī′pō-mĕ-tab′ŏ-lizm) Reduced metabolism. SEE ALSO hypometabolic state.

**hy·po·mo·tor sei·zure** (hī′pō-mō′tŏr sē′zhŭr) Seizure characterized by complete or partial arrest of ongoing motor activity in a patient whose level of consciousness cannot be determined accurately (e.g., newborns, infants, mentally retarded patients).

**hy·po·myx·i·a** (hī′pō-mik′sē-ă) Condition in which mucus secretion is diminished. [*hypo-* + G. *myxa*, mucus]

**hy·po·na·sal·i·ty** (hī′pō-nā-zal′i-tē) Insufficient nasal resonance during speech, usually due to obstruction of the nasal tract. SYN hyporhinophonia.

**hyponatraemia** [Br.] SYN hyponatremia.

**hy·po·na·tre·mi·a** (hī′pō-nă-trē′mē-ă) Abnormally low concentrations of sodium ions in circulating blood. SYN hyponatraemia. [*hypo-* + *natrium*, + G. *haima*, blood]

**hy·po·ne·o·cy·to·sis** (hī′pō-nē′ō-sī-tō′sis) Leukopenia associated with the presence of immature and young leukocytes, i.e., a "shift to the left" in the hemogram. [*hypo-* + G. *neos*, new, + *kytos*, cell, + *-osis*, condition]

**hy·po·noi·a** (hī′pō-noy′ă) Deficient or sluggish mental activity. [*hypo-* + G. *noeō*, to think]

**hy·po·o·var·i·an·ism** (hī′pō-ō-vā′rē-ăn-izm) Inadequate ovarian function, commonly referring to reduced secretion of ovarian hormones.

**hy·po·pan·cre·a·tism** (hī′pō-pan′krē-ă-tizm) Disorder of diminished activity of digestive enzyme secretion by the pancreas.

**hy·po·pan·cre·or·rhe·a** (hī′pō-pan′krē-ō-rē′ă) Reduced delivery of pancreatic digestive enzyme secretions. [*hypo-* + *pancreas* + G. *rhoia*, flow]

**hy·po·par·a·thy·roid·ism** (hī′pō-par′ă-thī′royd-izm) Condition due to diminution or absence of secretion of parathyroid hormones, with low serum calcium and tetany, and sometimes with increased bone density.

**hy·po·par·a·thy·roid·ism syn·drome** (hī′pō-par″ă-thī′royd-izm sin′drōm) Syndrome characterized by fatigue, muscular weakness, paresthesia and cramps of the extremities, tetany, and laryngeal stridor.

**hy·po·pep·si·a** (hī′pō-pep′sē-ă) Impaired digestion, especially that due to a deficiency of pepsin. [*hypo-* + G. *pepsis*, digestion]

**hy·po·phar·ynx** (hī′pō-far′ingks) SYN laryngopharynx.

**hy·po·pho·ne·sis** (hī′pō-fō-nē′sis) In percussion or auscultation, a sound that is diminished or fainter than usual. [*hypo-* + G. *phōnēsis*, a sounding]

**hypophosphataemia** [Br.] SYN hypophosphatemia.

**hy·po·phos·pha·ta·si·a** (hī′pō-fos′fă-tā′zē-ă) An abnormally low content of alkaline phosphatase in circulating blood.

**hy·po·phos·pha·te·mi·a** (hī′pō-fos-fă-tē′mē-ă) Abnormally low concentrations of phosphates in circulating blood. SYN hypophosphataemia.

**hy·po·phy·si·al** (hī′pō-fiz′ē-ăl) Relating to a hypophysis.

**hy·po·phy·si·al ca·chex·i·a** (hī′pō-fiz′ē-ăl kă-kek′sē-ă) SYN panhypopituitarism.

**hy·po·phys·i·o·sphe·noi·dal syn·drome** (hī′pō-fiz′ē-ō-sfē-noy′dăl sin′drōm) Neoplastic invasion of cranial base in the region of the sphenoidal sinus.

**hy·po·phys·i·o·tro·pic** (hī′pō-fiz′ē-ō-trō′pik) Denoting a stimulatory hormone that acts on the pituitary gland (hypophysis).

**hy·po·phys·i·o·trop·ic hor·mone** (hī′pō-fiz′ē-ō-trō′pik hōr′mōn) Hormone that stimulates rate of secretion of hypophysial hormones.

**hy·poph·y·sis** (hī-pof′i-sis) [TA] SEE ALSO hypothalamus. SYN pituitary gland. [G. an undergrowth]

**hy·po·pi·tu·i·ta·rism** (hī′pō-pi-tū′i-tăr-izm)

A condition due to diminished activity of the anterior lobe of the hypophysis, with inadequate secretion, to varying degrees, of one or more anterior pituitary hormones.

**hy·po·pla·si·a** (hī′pō-plā′zē-ă) **1.** Underdevelopment of a tissue or organ, usually due to a deficiency in the number of cells. **2.** Atrophy due to destruction of some of the elements and not merely to their general reduction in size. [*hypo-* + G. *plasis,* a molding]

**hy·po·plas·tic** (hī′pō-plas′tik) Pertaining to or characterized by hypoplasia.

**hy·po·plas·tic a·ne·mi·a** (hī′pō-plas′tik ă-nē′mē-ă) Progressive nonregenerative anemia resulting from greatly depressed functioning of bone marrow; as the process persists, aplastic anemia may occur.

**hy·pop·ne·a** (hī-pop′nē-ă) Breathing that is shallower or slower than normal. SYN hypopnoea. [*hypo-* + G. *pnoē,* breathing]

**hypopnoea** [Br.] SYN hypopnea.

**hy·po·po·si·a** (hī′pō-pō′sē-ă) Hypodipsia, primarily due to reduced tendency to drink rather than the reduced sensation of thirst. [*hypo-* + G. *posis,* drinking]

**hypopotassaemia** [Br.] SYN hypopotassemia.

**hy·po·po·tas·se·mi·a** (hī′pō-pŏ-ta-sē′mē-ă) SYN hypokalemia, hypopotassaemia.

**hypoproteinaemia** [Br.] SYN hypoproteinemia.

**hy·po·pro·tein·e·mi·a** (hī′pō-prō′tēn-ē′mē-ă) Abnormally small amounts of total protein in the blood. SYN hypoproteinaemia.

**hy·po·pro·te·in·o·sis** (hī′pō-prō′tē-in-o′sis, -prō′tēn-) A condition, especially in children, due to a dietary deficiency of protein.

**hy·pop·ty·a·lism** (hī′pop-tī′ă-lizm) SYN hyposalivation. [*hypo-* + G. *ptyalon,* saliva]

**hy·po·py·on** (hī-pō′pē-on) The presence of leukocytes in the anterior chamber of the eye. [*hypo-* + G. *pyon,* pus]

**hy·po·re·flex·i·a** (hī′pō-rē-flek′sē-ă) A condition in which the reflexes are weakened. Reduction of the deep tendon reflexes may be generalized, regional, or focal.

**hyporeninaemia** [Br.] SYN hyporeninemia.

**hy·po·ren·i·ne·mi·a** (hī′pō-rē′ni-nē′mē-ă) Low levels of renin in the circulating blood. SYN hyporeninaemia., hyporeninaemia.

**hyporhinophonia** SYN hyponasality.

**hy·po·sal·i·va·tion** (hī′pō-sal′i-vā′shŭn) Reduced salivation. SYN hypoptyalism.

**hy·po·sen·si·tiv·i·ty** (hī′pō-sen′si-tiv′i-tē)

A condition of subnormal sensitivity, in which the response to a stimulus is unusually delayed or lessened in degree.

**hy·pos·mi·a** (hī-poz′mē-ă) Diminished sense of smell; may be both hereditary or acquired; may be general to all odorants, partial to some odorants, or more specific. [*hypo-* + G. *osmē,* smell]

**hy·po·so·ma·to·tro·pism** (hī′pō-sō-mat′ō-trō′pizm) A state characterized by deficient secretion of pituitary growth hormone (somatotropin).

**hy·pos·the·nu·ri·a** (hī′pos-thĕ-nyūr′ē-ă) The excretion of urine of low specific gravity, due to inability of the renal tubules to produce concentrated urine; also occurs following excessive water ingestion in association with diabetes insipidus. [*hypo-* + G. *sthenos,* strength, + *ouron,* urine]

**hy·po·sto·mi·a** (hī′pō-stō′mē-ă) A form of microstomia in which the oral opening is a small vertical slit. [*hypo-* + G. *stoma,* mouth]

**hy·po·ten·sion** (hī′pō-ten′shŭn) **1.** Subnormal arterial blood pressure. **2.** Reduced pressure or tension of any kind. [*hypo-* + L. *tensio,* a stretching]

**hy·po·thal·a·mus** (hī′pō-thal′ă-mŭs) [TA] Ventral and medial regions of diencephalon forming walls of approximately the ventral half of third ventricle; delineated from the thalamus by the hypothalamic sulcus, lying medial to the internal capsule and subthalamus, continuous with the precommissural septum anteriorly and with the mesencephalic tegmentum and central gray substance posteriorly. [*hypo-* + *thalamus*]

**hy·po·ther·mi·a** (hī′pō-thĕr′mē-ă) A body temperature significantly less than 98.6°F (37°C). [*hypo-* + G. *thermē,* heat]

**hy·po·ther·mic an·es·the·si·a** (hī′pō-thĕr′mik an′es-thē′zē-ă) General anesthesia administered in conjunction with artificial lowering of body temperature.

**hy·poth·e·sis,** pl. **hy·poth·e·ses** (hī-poth′ĕ-sis, -sēz) A conjecture advanced for heuristic purposes, cast in a form that is amenable to confirmation or refutation by conducting of definable experiments and the critical assembly of empiric data. SEE ALSO theory. [G. foundation, assumption fr. *hypotithenai,* to lay down]

**hy·po·thy·roid·ism** (hī′pō-thī′royd-izm) Diminished production of thyroid hormone, leading to clinical manifestations of thyroid insufficiency. See page 297. [*hypo-* + G. *thyreoeidēs,* thyroid]

**hy·po·to·ni·a** (hī′pō-tō′nē-ă) **1.** Reduced tension in any body part. **2.** Relaxation of the arteries. **3.** Diminution or loss of muscular tonicity. [*hypo-* + G. *tonos,* tone]

**hy·po·ton·ic** (hī′pō-ton′ik) **1.** Having a lesser

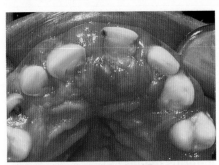

**gingival edema due to hypothyroidism:** severe case

degree of tension. **2.** Having a lesser osmotic-pressure than a reference solution, ordinarily plasma or interstitial fluid.

**hy·po·tri·cho·sis** (hī′pō-tri-kō′sis) A less than normal amount of hair on the head and/or body. [*hypo-* + G. *trichōsis,* hairiness]

**hy·po·u·re·sis** (hī′pō-yū-rē′sis) Reduced flow of urine.

**hy·po·ven·ti·la·tion** (hī′pō-ven-ti-lā′shŭn) Reduced alveolar ventilation relative to metabolic carbon dioxide production increases above.

**hy·po·ven·ti·la·tion co·ma** (hī′pō-ven′ti-lā′shŭn kō′mă) Coma seen with advanced lung failure and resultant hypoventilation. SYN CO$_2$ narcosis.

**hy·po·vi·ta·min·o·sis** (hī′pō-vī′tă-min-ō′sis) Nutritional deficiency state characterized by relative insufficiency of one or more vitamins in the diet; manifested first by depletion of tissue levels, then by functional changes, and finally by appearance of morphologic lesions. Cf. avitaminosis.

**hypoxaemia** [Br.] SYN hypoxemia.

**hy·po·xan·thine** (hī′pō-zan′thēn) A purine present in the muscles and other tissues.

**hy·pox·e·mi·a** (hī′pok-sē′mē-ă) Subnormal oxygenation of arterial blood, short of anoxia. SYN hypoxaemia. [*hypo-* + *oxygen,* + G. *haima,* blood]

**hy·pox·i·a** (hī-pok′sē-ă) Decreased below normal levels of oxygen in inspired gases, arterial blood, or tissue, without reaching anoxia. [*hypo-* + *oxygen*]

**hy·pox·ic hy·pox·i·a** (hī-pok′sik hī-pok′sē-ă) Hypoxia due to defective mechanism of oxygenation in the lungs; may be caused by a low tension of oxygen, abnormal pulmonary function or respiratory obstruction, or a right-to-left shunt in the heart.

♻ **hypso-** Combining form meaning high, height. [G. *hypsos,* height]

**hyp·so·dont** (hip′sŏ-dont) Having long teeth. [*hypso-* + G. *odous,* tooth]

**hys·ter·e·sis** (his′tĕr-ē′sis) Failure of either one of two related phenomena to keep pace with the other; or any situation in which the value of one depends on whether the other has been increasing or decreasing. [G. *hysterēsis,* a coming later]

**hys·te·ri·a** (his-ter′ē-ă) *Negative or pejorative connotations of this word may render it offensive in some contexts.* SEE psychosomatic. [G. *hystera,* womb, from the original notion of womb-related disturbances in women]

**hys·ter·ics** (his-ter′iks) *Negative or pejorative connotations of this word may render it offensive in some contexts.* An expression of emotion often accompanied by crying, laughing, and screaming.

gh

**I** Abbreviation for intensity; iodine; isoleucine.

**IA** Abbreviation for intraarterial.

**i·at·ro·gen·ic** (ī-at′rō-jen′ik) Denoting response to medical or surgical treatment. [*iatro-* + G. *-gen,* producing]

**i·at·ro·gen·ic trans·mis·sion** (ī-at′rō-jen′ik trans-mish′ŭn) Infectious agents transmitted to patients due to medical interference, such as transmission by contaminated needles.

**i·bu·pro·fen** (ī′byū-prō′fen) Nonsteroidal analgesic and antiinflammatory agent derived from propionic acid.

**IBW** Abbreviation for ideal body weight.

**ICD** Abbreviation for International Classification of Diseases.

**I-cell dis·ease** (sel di-zēz′) SYN mucolipidosis II.

**ice pack** (īs pak) A cold local application to limit or reduce swelling in recently traumatized tissues, usually in the form of a waterproof container for ice.

**i·chor** (ī′kōr) Thin watery discharge from an ulcer or unhealthy wound. [G. *ichōr,* serum]

**ichorhaemia** [Br.] SYN ichorrhemia.

**i·chor·ous pus** (ik′ŏr-ŭs pŭs) Thin fetid pus containing shreds of sloughing tissue.

**i·chor·rhe·a** (ī′kō-rē′ă) Profuse ichorous discharge. SYN ichorrhoea. [G. *ichōr,* serum, + *rhoia,* a flow]

**i·chor·rhe·mi·a, i·cho·re·mi·a** (ī′kō-rē′ mē-ă) Sepsis resulting from infection accompanied by an ichorous discharge. SYN ichorhaemia. [G. *ichōr,* serum, + *rhoia,* a flow, + *haima,* blood]

**ichorrhoea** [Br.] SYN ichorrhea.

**ich·thy·ism** (ik′thē-izm) Poisoning by eating stale or otherwise unfit fish. [G. *ichthys,* fish]

**ich·thy·o·he·mo·tox·ism** (ik′thē-ō-hē′mō-tok′sizm) Poisoning due to ingestion of fish containing toxic, ichthyohemotoxin.

**ICP** Abbreviation for intracranial pressure.

**ic·tal** (ik′tăl) Relating to or caused by a stroke or seizure. [L. *ictus,* a stroke]

**ic·ter·ic** (ik-ter′ik) Relating to or marked by jaundice. [G. *ikterikos,* jaundiced]

**ic·ter·o·gen·ic** (ik′tĕr-ō-jen′ik) Causing jaundice. [*ictero-* + G. *-gen,* producing]

**ic·ter·o·he·ma·tu·ric** (ik′tĕr-ō-hē′mă-tyūr′ ik) Denoting jaundice with the passage of blood in the urine.

**ic·ter·o·he·mo·glo·bi·nu·ri·a** (ik′tĕr-ō-hē′mō-glō′bi-nyūr′ē-ă) Jaundice with hemoglobin in the urine.

**ic·ter·oid** (ik′tĕr-oyd) Yellow or seemingly jaundiced. [*ictero-* + G. *eidos,* resemblance]

**ic·ter·us** (ik′tĕr-ŭs) SYN jaundice. [G. *ikteros*]

**ic·ter·us gra·vis** (ik′tĕr-ŭs grav′is) Jaundice associated with high fever and delirium; seen in severe hepatitis and other diseases of the liver with severe functional failure.

**ic·ter·us me·las** (ik′tĕr-ŭs mē′las) Jaundice that causes pale skin to darken to an unhealthy brownish tinge.

**ic·tus** (ik′tŭs) **1.** A stroke or attack. **2.** A beat. [L.]

**ICU** Abbreviation for intensive care unit.

**id** (id) In psychoanalysis, one of three components of the psychic apparatus in the freudian structural framework, the other two being the ego and superego. It is completely in the unconscious realm, is unorganized, is the reservoir of psychic energy or libido, and is under the influence of the primary processes. [L. *id,* that]

**IDC** Abbreviation for indwelling catheter.

**IDDM** Abbreviation for insulin-dependent diabetes mellitus. SEE Type 1 diabetes.

**i·de·a** (ī-dē′ă) Any mental image or concept. [G. form, appearance, fr. *idein,* to have seen, fr. obs. *eidō,* to see]

**i·deal bod·y weight (IBW)** (ī-dēl′ bod′ē wāt) Weight believed to be maximally healthful for a person, based chiefly on height but modified by factors such as gender, age, build, and degree of muscular development.

**i·den·ti·fi·ca·tion** (ī-den′ti-fi-kā′shŭn) **1.** Act or process of determining classification or nature of. **2.** A sense of oneness or psychic continuity with another person or group. [Mediev. L. *identicus,* fr. L. *idem,* the same, + *facio,* to make]

**i·den·ti·fi·ca·tion dot** (ī-den′ti-fi-ka′shŭn dot) Small raised indicator on an intraoral radiographic film; used to determine film orientation. SYN embossed dot.

**i·den·ti·ty** (ī-den′ti-tē) Summation of a person's internalized history of relationship with objects, his or her social role, and his or her perception of both; the experience of ''I.''

**i·den·ti·ty cri·sis** (ī-den′ti-tē krī′sis) Disorientation concerning one's sense of self, and role in society, often of acute onset.

**i·den·ti·ty dis·or·der** (ī-den′ti-tē dis-ōr′dĕr) Mental disorder in which one suffers severe distress regarding one's ability to reconcile aspects of the self into a coherent acceptable whole.

🜂 **idio-** Combining form meaning private, distinctive, peculiar to. [G. *idios*, one's own].

**id·i·o·gen·e·sis** (id′ē-ō-jen′ĕ-sis) Origin without evident cause. [*idio-* + G. *genesis*, production]

**id·i·o·gram** (id′ē-ō-gram) **1.** SYN karyotype. **2.** Diagrammatic representation of chromosome morphology characteristic of a species or population. [*idio-* + G. *gramma*, something written]

**id·i·o·path·ic** (id′ē-ō-path′ik) Denoting a disease of unknown cause. [*idio-* + G. *pathos*, suffering]

**id·i·o·path·ic al·dos·ter·on·ism** (id′ē-ō-path′ik al-dos′tĕr-ōn-izm) SYN primary aldosteronism.

**id·i·o·path·ic bi·lat·er·al ves·tibu·lop·a·thy** (id′ē-ō-path′ik bī-lat′ĕr-ăl ves-tib′yū-lop′ă-thē) Slowly progressive disorder affecting young to middle-aged adults, manifested by gait unsteadiness and oscillopsia.

**id·i·opath·ic stab·bing head·ache** (id′ē-ō-path′ik stab′ing hed′āk) Brief repetitive sharp pains in the temporoparietal area of the head.

**id·i·o·path·ic throm·bo·cy·to·pe·nic pur·pu·ra (ITP)** (id′ē-ō-path′ik throm′bō-sī-tō-pē′nik pŭr′pyŭr-ă) Systemic illness characterized by extensive ecchymoses and hemorrhages from mucous membranes and very low platelet counts; due to platelet destruction by macrophages due to an antiplatelet factor.

**id·i·op·a·thy** (id′ē-op′ă-thē) An idiopathic disease. [*idio-* + G. *pathos*, suffering]

**id·i·o·syn·cra·sy** (id′ē-ō-singk′ră-sē) **1.** Particular mental, behavioral, or physical characteristic or peculiarity. **2.** In pharmacology, abnormal reaction to a drug. [G. *idiosynkrasia*, fr. *idios*, one's own, + *synkrasis*, a mixing together]

**id·i·o·trop·ic** (id′ē-ō-trō′pik) Turning inward on one's self. [*idio-* + G. *tropē*, a turning]

**id·i·o·type** (id′ē-ō-tīp) Collection of idiotopes within the variable region that confers on an immunoglobulin molecule an antigenic specificity and is frequently a unique attribute of a given antibody in a given animal. It is the product of a limited number of B lymphocyte clones. [*idio-* + G. *typos*, model]

**i·dox·ur·i·dine** (ī′doks-yūr′i-dēn) Pyrimidine analogue that produces both antiviral and anticancer effects; topical agent used to treat viral keratitis.

**id re·ac·tion** (id rē-ak′shŭn) Allergic manifestation of candidiasis, the dermatophytoses, and other mycoses characterized by itching.

**IF** Abbreviation for intrinsic factor.

**IFDH** Abbreviation for International Federation of Dental Hygienists.

**IFN** Abbreviation for interferon.

**IGF** Abbreviation for insulinlike growth factor.

**IL** Abbreviation for interleukin.

**il·e·um** (il′ē-ŭm) [TA] The third and longest portion of the small intestine, about 12 feet in length in humans. [L.L. bowel, fr. L. *ilium*, groin, flank, hip]

**il·e·us** (il′ē-ŭs) Mechanical, dynamic, or adynamic obstruction of the intestines; may be accompanied by severe colicky pain, abdominal distention, vomiting, and absence of passage of stool. [L., fr. G. *eileos*, intestinal obstruction, fr. *eileō*, to roll up, + *-os*, noun suffix]

**il·i·um,** pl. **il·i·a** (il′ē-ŭm, -ă) [TA] The broad, flaring portion of the hip bone, distinct at birth but later becoming fused with the ischium and pubis. [L. groin, flank]

**il·lu·mi·na·tion** (i-lū′mi-nā′shŭn) Throwing light on the body part or into a cavity for diagnostic purposes. [L. *il-lumino*, pp. *-atus*, to light up]

**il·lu·sion** (i-lū′zhŭn) A false perception; the mistaking of something for what it is not. [L. *illusio*, fr. *il- ludo*, pp. *-lusus*, to play at, mock]

**IM** Abbreviation for internal medicine; intramuscular.

**im·age** (im′ăj) **1.** Representation of an object made by the rays of light emanating or reflected from it. **2.** Representation produced by x-rays, magnetic resonance imaging, tomography, ultrasound, thermography, radioisotopes, summated electrocardiograms, positron-emission tomography scans, detection of electron energy states, among others. [L. *imago*, likeness]

**i·mag·i·nar·y bi·sec·tor** (i-maj′i-nar-ē bī′sek-tŏr) Hypothetical plane that evenly subdivides angle formed where x-ray film and long axis of the tooth come in contact.

**im·ag·ing** (im′ăj-ing) Production of a clinical image using x-rays, ultrasound, computed tomography, magnetic resonance imaging, radionuclide scanning, and thermography. SEE image.

**im·bi·bi·tion** (im′bi-bish′ŭn) **1.** Absorption of fluid by a solid body without resultant chemical change in either. **2.** Taking up of water by a gel. [L. *im-bibo*, to drink in (*in* + *bibo*)]

**im·bri·ca·tion lines of von Eb·ner** (im′bri-kā′shŭn līnz von eb′nĕr) Incremental lines in peritubular dentin of the tooth that correspond to daily rate of dentin formation.

**im·i·pen·em** (im′i-pen′em) A β-lactam antibiotic with broad spectrum activity used to treat various infections.

**im·me·di·ate den·ture** (i-mē′dē-ăt den′ chŭr) Complete or partial denture inserted immediately after removal of natural teeth.

**im·me·di·ate hy·per·sen·si·tiv·i·ty** (i-mē′dē-ăt hī′pĕr-sen-si-tiv′ĭ-tē) An exaggerated immune response mediated by mast cell–bound IgE antibodies occurring within minutes after exposing a sensitized patient to the approximate antigen; also called Type I hypersensitivity.

**im·me·di·ate per·cus·sion** (i-mē′dē-ăt pĕr-kŭsh′ŭn) Striking of the body part under examination directly with finger or plessor, without the intervention of another finger or plessimeter.

**im·mer·sion** (i-mĕr′zhŭn) **1.** Placing a body under water or other liquid. **2.** MICROSCOPY filling space between objective lens and top of cover glass with a fluid, such as water or oil, to reduce spheric aberration and increase effective numeric aperture. [L. *immergo,* pp. *-mersus,* to dip in (*in + mergo*)]

**immobilisation** [Br.] SYN immobilization.

**im·mo·bi·li·za·tion** (i-mō′bi-lī-zā′shŭn) The act or process of fixing or rendering immobile. SYN immobilisation.

**im·mune** (i-myūn′) **1.** Free from possibility of acquiring a given infectious disease; resistant to an infectious disease. **2.** Pertaining to mechanism of sensitization in which the reactivity is so altered by previous contact with an antigen that the responsive tissues respond quickly on subsequent contact. [L. *immunis,* free from service, fr. *in,* neg., + *munus* (*muner-*), service]

**im·mune com·plex dis·ease** (i-myūn′ kom′pleks di-zēz′) Immunologic category of diseases evoked by the deposition of antigen-antibody in the microvasculature. Complement is frequently involved and the breakdown products of complement attract polymorphonuclear leukocytes to site of deposition. Damage to tissue is frequently caused by "frustrated" phagocytosis by polymorphonuclear cells. Immune complex diseases can also occur during a variety of diseases of known etiology, such as subacute bacterial endocarditis. SEE ALSO autoimmune disease.

**im·mune re·ac·tion** (i-myūn′ rē-ak′shŭn) Antigen-antibody reaction indicating a certain degree of resistance.

**im·mune se·rum glob·u·lin** (i-myūn′ sēr′ŭm glob′yū-lin) Sterile solution of globulins that contains many antibodies normally present in adult human blood; a passive immunizing agent frequently used for prophylaxis against hepatitis A virus and other disorders.

**im·mune sys·tem** (i-myūn′ sis′tĕm) Intricate complex of interrelated cellular, molecular, and genetic components that provides a defense, the immune response, against foreign organisms or substances and aberrant native cells.

**im·mu·ni·ty** (i-myū′ni-tē) Status or quality of being immune. [L. *immunitas*]

**im·mu·ni·za·tion** (im′yū-nī-zā′shŭn) Protection of susceptible patients from communicable diseases by administration of a living modified agent, suspension of killed organisms, a protein expressed in a heterologous organism, or an inactivated toxin.

☼ **immuno-** Combining form meaning immune, immunity. [L. *immunis,* immune]

**im·mu·no·as·say** (im′yū-nō-as′ā) Detection and assay of substances by serologic (immunologic) methods; in most applications substance in question serves as antigen, both in antibody production and in measurement of antibody by the test substance.

**im·mun·o·bi·ol·o·gy** (im′yū-nō-bī-ol′ŏ-jē) Study of immune factors that affect growth, development, and health of biologic organisms.

**im·mu·no·com·pro·mised** (im′yū-nō-kom′prŏ-mīzd) Denoting a person with an immunologic mechanism deficient either because of an immunodeficiency disorder or it made by immunosuppressive agents.

**im·mu·no·de·fi·cien·cy** (im′yū-nō-dĕ-fi sh′ĕn-sē) A condition resulting from a defective immune mechanism; may be *primary,* or *secondary, specific* or *nonspecific.*

**im·mu·no·de·fi·cien·cy syn·drome** (im′ yū-nō-dĕ-fish′ĕn-sē sin′drōm) Immunologic disorder, of which the chief symptom is an increased susceptibility to infection; pattern of susceptibility is dependent on the kind of deficiency. SEE ALSO immunodeficiency.

**im·mu·no·dif·fu·sion** (im′yū-nō-di-fyū′zhŭn) A technique of studying antigen-antibody reactions by observing precipitates formed by combination of specific antigen and antibodies that have diffused in a gel in which they have been separately placed.

**im·mu·no·e·lec·tro·pho·re·sis** (im′yū-nō-ĕ-lek′trō-fŏr-ē′sis) Precipitin test in which the components of one group of immunologic reactants are first separated on the basis of electrophoretic mobility.

**im·mu·no·glob·u·lin** (im′yū-nō-glob′yū-lin) One of a class of structurally related proteins. On the basis of the structural and antigenic properties of the H chains, immunoglobulins are classified (in order of relative amounts present in normal human serum) as IgG, IgA, IgM, IgD, and IgE.

**im·mu·no·his·to·chem·is·try** (im′yū-nō-his′tō-kem′is-trē) Demonstration of specific antigens in tissues by the use of markers that are either fluorescent dyes or enzymes.

**im·mu·nol·o·gy** (im′yū-nol′ŏ-jē) **1.** The science concerned with the various phenomena of immunity, induced sensitivity, and allergy. **2.** Study of the structure and function of the immune system. [*immuno-* + G. *logos,* study]

**im·mu·no·sup·pres·sant** (im′yū-nō-sŭ-pres′ănt) Agent that induces immunosuppression (e.g., cyclosporine, corticosteroids).

**im·mu·no·sup·pres·sion** (im′yū-nō-sŭ-presh′ŭn) Prevention or interference with the development of immunologic response; may reflect natural immunologic unresponsiveness, may be artificially induced by chemical, biologic, or physical agents, or caused by disease.

**im·mu·no·ther·a·py** (im′yū-nō-thār′ă-pē) Immunotherapy includes nonspecific systemic stimulation, adjuvant active specific immunotherapy, and adoptive immunotherapy.

**im·pact** (im′pakt, im-pakt′) **1.** The forcible striking of something against another. **2.** To press two bodies, parts, or fragments closely together. [L. *impingo,* pp. *-pactus,* to strike at (*in* + *pango*), fasten, drive in]

**im·pact·ed** (im-pak′tĕd) Wedged or pressed closely so as to move as a single unit.

**im·pact·ed frac·ture** (im-pak′tĕd frak′shŭr) A fracture in which one of the fragments is driven into the cancellous tissue of the other.

**im·pact·ed tooth** (im-pak′tĕd tūth) **1.** Tooth the normal eruption of which is prevented by adjacent teeth or bone. **2.** Tooth that has been driven into the alveolar process or surrounding tissue as a result of trauma. See this page.

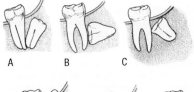
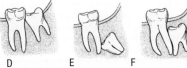

A     B     C

D     E     F

**impacted mandibular third molar:** (A) distoangular; (B) horizontal; (C) mesioangular; (D) high level; (E) low level; (F) vertical

**im·pac·tion** (im-pak′shŭn) The process or condition of being impacted.

**im·pair·ment** (im-pār′mĕnt) Physical or mental defect at the level of a body system or organ. The official World Health Organization definition reads any loss of psychological, physiologic, or anatomic structure or function.

**im·pe·tig·i·nous chei·li·tis** (im′pĕ-tij′i-nŭs kī-lī′tis) Pyoderma of the lips with yellow crusts due to *Staphylococcus aureus* or other streptococcal infection.

**im·pe·ti·go** (im′pĕ-tī′gō) Contagious dermatologic pyoderma, caused by *Staphylococcus aureus* and/or group A streptococci, which begins with a superficial flaccid vesicle that ruptures and forms a yellowish crust; most commonly occurs in children. [L. a scabby eruption, fr. *im-peto* (*inp-*), to rush on, attack]

**im·plant** (im-plant′) **1.** To graft or insert. **2.** (īm′plant) A surgically inserted or imbedded graft or device; also, a zone of cells or tissue transferred from another site through a developmental error or neoplastic process. SEE ALSO prosthesis. [L. *im-,* in, + *planto,* pp. *-atus,* to plant, fr. *planta,* a sprout, shoot]

**im·plant a·but·ment** (im′plant ă-bŭt′mĕnt) SYN abutment.

**im·plan·ta·tion** (im′plan-tā′shŭn) **1.** Insertion of a natural tooth into an artificially constructed alveolus. **2.** The process of placing a device or substance within the body. **3.** Tissue grafting.

**im·plant den·ture** (im′plant den′chŭr) Tooth substitute that receives its stability and retention from a substructure that is partially or wholly implanted under the soft tissues of the denture basal seat. SEE ALSO implant denture substructure, subperiosteal implant.

**im·plant den·ture sub·struc·ture** (im′plant den′chŭr sŭb′strŭk-shŭr) Metal framework that is placed beneath the soft tissues in contact with, or embedded into, bone for the purpose of supporting an implant denture superstructure.

**im·plant fix·ture** (im′plant fiks′chŭr) Portion of the implant surgically placed into the bone. The fixture will act as the ''root'' of the implant and needs a period of 3 to 6 months to be fully surrounded and supported by bone.

**im·plant pros·the·sis** (im′plant pros-thē′sis) Any prosthesis that uses dental implants in part or whole for retention, support, and stability. See page 302.

**im·plant sub·struc·ture** (im′plant sŭb′strŭk-chŭr) Metal framework placed beneath soft tissues in contact with bone and stabilized by screws into bone; supports prosthesis, usually with superstructure components.

**im·plant su·per·struc·ture** (im′plant sū′per-strŭk-chŭr) The portion of a dental implant that attaches to its implant substructure and to a fixed or removable dental prosthesis to support or retain that prosthesis. See page 302. SYN dental implant abutment.

**im·plied con·sent** (im-plīd′ kŏn-sent′) **1.** SYN emergency doctrine. **2.** Granting of permission for health care without formal agree-

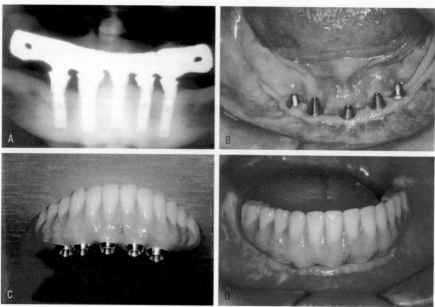

**implant-supported prosthesis:** (A) radiograph of implant-supported prosthesis in place; (B) atrophic mandible with five implants; (C) prosthesis showing attachments that will connect to implants; (D) implant-supported prosthesis in place

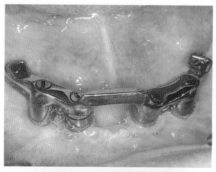

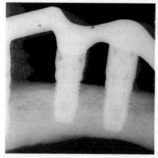

**implant superstructure:** on mandibular arch, patient has four titanium endosseous implants, abutment posts are linked together with a bar

ment, when a patient makes an appointment with a physician.

**im·plo·sion** (im-plō′zhŭn) Sudden collapse, as of an evacuated vessel, in which there is a bursting inward rather than outward as in an explosion.

**im·preg·nate** (im-preg′nāt) **1.** To diffuse or permeate with another substance. **2.** To fecundate or fertilize an oocyte; to cause to conceive. [L. *im-*, in, + *praegnans*, with child]

◨**im·pres·sion** (im-presh′ŭn) **1.** [TA] An imprint or negative likeness; especially, negative form of the teeth and/or other tissues of the oral cavity, made in a plastic material that becomes relatively hard or set while in contact with these tissues, made to reproduce a positive form or cast of the recorded tissues; classified, according to the materials of which they are made, as reversible and irreversible hydrocolloid impression, modeling plastic impression, plaster impression, and wax impression. **2.** [TA] Mark seemingly made by pressure of one structure or organ on another, seen especially during cadaveric dissections. **3.** Effect produced on the mind by some external objects acting through the organs of sense. See page 303. [L. *impressio,* fr. *im- primo,* pp. *-pressus,* to press upon]

**im·pres·sion a·re·a** (im-presh′ŭn ar′ē-ă) In dentistry, surface that is recorded in an impression.

**im·pres·sion com·pound** (im-presh′ŭn kom′pownd) SYN modeling plastic.

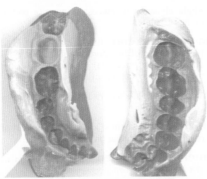

impression taken using triple tray, showing simultaneous capture of maxillary and mandibular teeth

**im·pres·sion ma·te·ri·al** (im-presh´ŭn mă-tēr´ē-ăl) Substance or combination of substances used to make a negative reproduction or impression.

**im·pres·sion plas·ter** (im-presh´ŭn plas´tĕr) Nonelastic impression material with excellent surface detail, but little expansion due to additives to plaster; must be broken to be removed from undercuts and then the pieces must be reattached before pouring the cast.

**im·pres·sion tray** (im-presh´ŭn trā) Receptacle used to carry and confine plastic impression material when making an impression of oral structures. See this page.

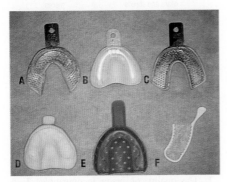

impression trays: (A) metal perforated tray for partially edentulous impressions; (B) solid metal tray for edentulous impressions; (C) metal tray for dentulous impressions; (D) custom tray; (E) plastic tray for dentulous impressions; and (F) bite registration tray

**im·prop·er dose quan·ti·ty** (im-prop´ĕr dōs kwahn´ti-tē) Drug error in which the health care provider gives the wrong dose or quantity.

**im·pulse** (im´pŭls) **1.** A sudden pushing or driving force. **2.** A sudden, often unreasoning, determination to perform some act. [L. *im-pello,* pp. *-pulsus,* to push against, impel (*inp*-)]

**in·ac·ti·vate** (in-ak´ti-vāt) To destroy the biologic activity or the effects of an agent.

**in·a·ni·tion** (in´ă-nish´ŭn) Severe weakness and wasting due to lack of food, defect or disease.

**in·breed·ing** (in´brēd-ing) Mating between organisms that are genetically more closely related than organisms selected at random from the population.

**in·ca·ri·al bone** (in-kar´ē-ăl bōn) SYN interparietal bone.

**in·ci·dence** (in´si-dĕns) *Do not confuse this word with prevalence.* Number of specified new events, during a specified period in a specified population.

**in·cip·i·ent car·ies** (in-sip´ē-ĕnt kar´ēz) Beginning caries; initiating decay.

**in·ci·sal** (in-sī´zăl) Cutting; relating to the cutting edges of the incisor and cuspid teeth. [L. *incido,* pp. *-cisus,* to cut into]

**in·ci·sal an·gle** (in-sī´zăl ang´gĕl) Angle formed by the incisal edge of a tooth with its interproximal surface.

**in·ci·sal edge** (in-sī´zăl ej) SYN incisal margin.

**in·ci·sal em·bra·sure** (in-sī´zăl em-brā´shŭr) Space existing on the incisal aspect of the interproximal contact area between adjacent anterior teeth.

**in·ci·sal guid·ance** (in-sī´zăl gīd´ăns) Influence on mandibular movements caused by contacting surfaces of mandibular and maxillary anterior teeth during eccentric excursions. SYN incisal path.

**in·ci·sal guide** (in-sī´zăl gīd) In dentistry, that part of an articulator on which anterior guide pin rests to maintain vertical dimension of occlusion and incisal guide angle as established by the incisal guidance; may be adjustable, with a changeable superior surface that may be changed to provide variations in the incisal guide angle, or customized, being individually formed in plastic to allow other than straight line incisal guidance in eccentric movements. SYN anterior guide.

**in·ci·sal guide an·gle** (in-sī´zăl gīd ang´gĕl) Area formed with the horizontal plane by drawing a line in the sagittal plane between incisal edges of maxillary and mandibular central incisors when teeth are in centric occlusion.

**in·ci·sal guide pin** (in-sī´zăl gīd pin) Component of an articulator that maintains vertical separation of casts and can provide guidance in articulator movements (together with the condylar components of the articulator); typically a rod attached to one member of the articulator that contacts the anterior guide table on the opposing member.

ij

**in·ci·sal mar·gin** (in-sī′zăl mahr′jin) [TA] Part of an anterior tooth farthest from the apex of the root. SYN cutting edge (2), incisal edge, incisal surface, margo incisalis, shearing edge.

**in·ci·sal path** (in-sī′zăl path) SYN incisal guidance.

**in·ci·sal point** (in-sī′zăl poynt) Point located between incisal edges of the mandibular central incisors; graphic projection of excursions of incisal point in certain planes is generally used to illustrate the envelope of motion of mandibular movement.

**in·ci·sal rest** (in-sī′zăl rest) Portion of removable partial denture supported by incisal edge.

**in·ci·sal sur·face** (in-sī′zăl sŭr′făs) SYN incisal margin.

**in·cis·ed wound** (in-sīzd′ wūnd) A clean cut, as by a sharp instrument.

**in·ci·sion** (in-sizh′ŭn) A cut; a surgical wound; a division of the body parts. [L. *incisio*]

**in·ci·sive** (in-sī′siv) **1.** Relating to the incisor teeth. **2.** Cutting; having the power to cut.

**in·ci·sive bone** (in-sī′siv bōn) [TA] Anterior and inner portion of maxilla, which is always in the fetus and sometimes in the adult a separate incisive suture that runs from incisive canal between lateral incisor and canine tooth; is further divided by a suture between two incisor teeth on each side into two bones: endognathion and mesognathion. SYN intermaxilla, intermaxillary bone, os intermaxillare, os premaxillare, premaxilla (1), premaxillary bone.

**in·ci·sive ca·nal cyst** (in-sī′siv kă-nal′ sist) Lesion in or near that area, arising from proliferation of epithelial remnants of nasopalatine duct; most common maxillary developmental cyst. SYN median anterior maxillary cyst.

**in·ci·sive ca·nals** (in-sī′siv kă-nalz′) [TA] Bony canals leading from floor of nasal cavity into incisive fossa on palatal surface of maxilla; convey nasopalatine nerves and branches of greater palatine arteries that anastomose with septal branch of sphenopalatine artery.

**in·ci·sive duct** (in-sī′siv dŭkt) [TA] Infrequent rudimentary duct, or protrusion of the mucous membrane into the incisive canal, on either side of the anterior extremity of the nasal crest.

**in·ci·sive for·a·men** (in-sī′siv fōr-ā′mĕn) [TA] One of several (usually four) openings of incisive canals into incisive fossa. SYN incisor foramen.

**in·ci·sive fos·sa** (in-sī′siv fos′ă) [TA] Depression in midline of bony palate behind central incisors into which the incisive canals open.

**in·ci·sive pa·pil·la** (in-sī′siv pă-pil′ă) [TA] Slight elevation of mucosa at anterior end of raphe of palate.

**in·ci·sive su·ture** (in-sī′siv sū′chŭr) [TA] Line of union of two portions of maxilla (premaxilla and postmaxilla); present at birth but may persist. SYN premaxillary suture.

**in·ci·sor** (in-sī′zŏr) SYN incisor tooth. [L. *incido*, to cut into]

**in·ci·sor crest** (in-sī′zŏr krest) Front part of nasal crest of palatine process of maxilla.

**in·ci·sor for·a·men** (in-sī′zŏr fōr-ā′mĕn) SYN incisive foramen.

**in·ci·sor tooth** (in-sī′zŏr tūth) [TA] Tooth with a chisel-shaped crown and a single conic tapering root; there are four of these teeth in anterior part of each jaw, in both deciduous and permanent dentitions. See this page. SYN dens incisivus; incisor. [TA].

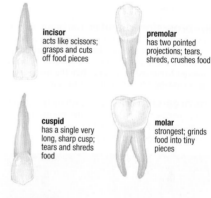

incisor
acts like scissors; grasps and cuts off food pieces

premolar
has two pointed projections; tears, shreds, crushes food

cuspid
has a single very long, sharp cusp; tears and shreds food

molar
strongest; grinds food into tiny pieces

**types of teeth**

**in·cli·na·tion** (in′kli-nā′shŭn) [TA] In dentistry, deviation of the long axis of a tooth from the perpendicular. [L. *inclinatio*, a leaning]

**in·clu·sion cyst** (in-klū′zhŭn sist) SYN developmental cyst.

**in·com·pat·i·bil·i·ty** (in′kŏm-pat′i-bil′i-tē) **1.** The quality of being incompatible. **2.** A means of classifying bacterial plasmids.

**in·com·pat·i·ble** (in-′kŏm-pat′i-bĕl) Not of suitable composition to be combined or mixed with another agent or substance, without resulting in an undesirable reaction (including chemical alteration or pharmacologic effect). [L. *in-* neg., + *con-*, with, + *patior*, pp. *passus*, to suffer, tolerate]

**in·com·pe·tence, in·com·pe·ten·cy** (in-kom′pĕ-tĕns, -tĕn-sē) The quality of being incapable of performing the allotted function, especially failure of cardiac or venous valves to close completely. [L. *in-*, neg. + *com-peto*, strive after together]

**in·com·plete an·ti·gen** (in´kŏm-plēt´ an´ti-jen) SYN hapten.

**in·com·plete dis·in·fec·tant** (in´kŏm-plēt´ dis´in-fek´tănt) Disinfectant that kills only vegetative forms of a potential pathogen.

**in·com·plete Hor·ner syn·drome** (in´kŏm-plēt´ hŏr´nĕr sin´drōm) SYN paratrigeminal syndrome.

**in·con·ti·nence** (in-kon´ti-nĕns) Inability to prevent the discharge of bodily excretions. [L. *incontinentia,* fr. *in-* neg. + *con-tineo,* to hold together, fr. *teneo,* to hold]

**in·cre·men·tal lines** (in´krĕ-men´tăl līnz) **1.** In dental enamel, calcification lines of Retzius. **2.** In dentin, Owen lines or imbrication lines of von Ebner.

**in·cre·tin** (in-krē´tin) Generic term for all insulinotropic substances originating in the gastrointestinal tract.

**in·cu·ba·tion** (in´kyū-bā´shŭn) **1.** Act of maintaining controlled environmental conditions to favor growth or development of microbial or tissue cultures or to maintain optimal conditions for a chemical or immunologic reaction. **2.** Development, without sign or symptom, of an infection. [L. *incubo,* to lie on]

**in·cu·ba·tion pe·ri·od** (in´kyū-bā´shŭn pēr´ē-ŏd) **1.** The interval between invasion of the body by an infecting organism and the appearance of the first sign or symptom it causes. SYN latent period (3), latent stage, prodromal stage. **2.** In a disease vector, the period between entry of the disease organism and the time at which the vector is capable of transmitting the disease to another human host.

**in·cu·ba·tor** (in´kyū-bā´tŏr) A container in which controlled environmental conditions can be maintained (e.g., for culturing microorganisms).

**in·cus** (ing´kŭs) [TA] Middle of the three ossicles in the middle ear; has a body and two limbs or processes; at tip of long crus is a small knob, the lenticular process, which articulates with head of the stapes. SYN anvil.

**in·dane·di·ones** (in´dān-dī´ōnz) Orally effective indirect-acting anticoagulants similar to warfarin in action.

**in·den·ta·tion hard·ness** (in´den-tā´shŭn hahrd´nĕs) Number related to size of impression made by an indenter (or tool) of specific size and shape under a known load.

**in·de·pen·dent var·i·a·ble** (in´dĕ-pen´dĕnt var´ē-ă-bĕl) Characteristic being measured or observed that is hypothesized to influence another event or manifestation within a defined area of relationships under study.

**in·dex,** pl. **in·di·ces,** pl. **in·dex·es** (in´deks, -di-sēz, -deks-ĕz) [TA] **1.** A core or mold used to record or maintain the relative position of a tooth or teeth to one another and/or to a cast. **2.** A guide, usually made of plaster, used to reposition teeth, casts, or parts.

**in·di·ca·tion** (in´di-kā´shŭn) The basis for initiation of a treatment for a disease or of a diagnostic test. [L. fr. *in-dico,* pp. *-atus,* to point out, fr. *dico,* to proclaim]

**in·di·ca·tor** (in´di-kā-tŏr) **1.** In chemical analysis, a substance that changes color within a certain definite range of pH or oxidation potential, or in any way renders visible the completion of a chemical reaction, e.g., litmus. **2.** An isotope that is used as a tracer. [L. one that points out]

**in·dif·fer·ence to pain syn·drome** (in-dif´ĕr-ĕns pān sin´drōm) Congenital insensitivity to pain, possibly due to an absence of organized nerve endings in the skin.

**in·di·ges·tion** (in´di-jes´chŭn) Nonspecific term for various symptoms resulting from a failure to digest and absorb food in the alimentary tract properly.

**in·di·rect bond·ing** (in´di-rekt´ bond´ing) Two-step process by which orthodontic attachments are affixed temporarily to teeth of a study cast from which they are transferred to the mouth at one time by means of a template or tray that preserves the predetermined orientation and permits them to be bonded simultaneously.

**in·di·rect frac·ture** (in´di-rekt´ frak´shŭr) A fracture, especially of the skull, which occurs at a point other than the site of impact.

**in·di·rect il·lu·mi·na·tion** (in´di-rekt´ i-lū´mi-nā´shŭn) Use of the mirror surface to reflect light onto a tooth surface in a darker area of the mouth.

**in·di·rect meth·od for mak·ing in·lays** (in´di-rekt´ meth´ŏd māk´ing in´lāz) Method whereby the inlay is constructed entirely on a model made from an impression of the prepared tooth or teeth in the mouth.

**in·di·rect pulp cap** (in´di-rekt´ pŭlp kap) Placement of a restorative covering or dressing material over a thin layer of remaining caries when removal of all would result in an exposure of the pulp, to promote healing and dentin formation.

**in·di·rect pulp cap·ping** (in´di-rekt´ pŭlp kap´ing) Application of a suspension of calcium hydroxide to a thin layer of dentin overlying pulp (near exposure) to stimulate secondary dentin formation and protect pulp.

**in·di·rect res·tor·a·tion** (in´di-rekt´ res´tŏr-ā´shŭn) Restoration formed on a die reproduction of a prepared tooth and then cemented into place; includes porcelain, gold inlays, and porcelain crowns.

**in·di·rect re·tain·er** (in-di-rekt´ rĕ-tā´nĕr)

**ij**

Part of a removable partial denture that assists the direct retainers in preventing occlusal displacement of distal extension bases by functioning through lever action on the opposite side of the fulcrum line.

**in·di·rect re·ten·tion** (in'di-rekt' rĕ-ten' shŭn) Retention obtained in a removable partial denture through use of indirect retainers.

**in·di·rect vi·sion** (in'di-rekt' vizh'ŭn) Visualization afforded by use of a mouth mirror for viewing intraoral structures during dental treatment. See this page.

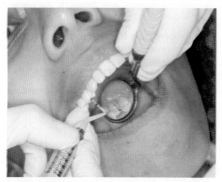

**indirect vision:** dental mirror allows view of lingual surfaces of maxillary premolar; note dental instrument is visible in mirror

**in·dis·po·si·tion** (in'dis-pŏ-zish'ŭn) Illness, usually slight; malaise.

**in·di·vid·u·al prac·tice as·so·ci·a·tion (IPA)** (in'di-vij'ū-ăl prak'tis ă-sō'sē-ā'shŭn) Form of health maintenance organization in which the patient does not need a referral or permission to see any participating physician.

**in·duced symp·tom** (in-dūst' simp'tŏm) Symptom elicited by a drug, or other means, often intentionally, for diagnostic purposes.

**in·duc·tance (L)** (in-dŭk'tăns) The coefficient of electromagnetic induction; the unit of inductance is the henry. SEE induction.

**in·duc·tion** (in-dŭk'shŭn) *Do not confuse this word with inducement.* **1.** Production or causation. **2.** The period from the start of anesthetization to the establishment of a depth of anesthesia adequate for a surgical procedure. [L. *inductio,* a leading in]

**in·duc·to·ther·my** (in-dŭk'tō-thĕr-mē) Artificial fever production by means of electromagnetic induction.

**in·du·ra·tion** (in'dūr-ā'shŭn) **1.** Process of becoming extremely firm or hard, or having such physical features. **2.** A focus or region of indurated tissue. SYN sclerosis (1). [L. *induratio*]

**in·dus·tri·al dis·ease** (in-dŭs'trē-ăl di-zēz')

Morbid condition resulting from environmental exposure to an agent discharged by a commercial enterprise.

**in·dwell·ing cath·e·ter (IDC)** (in'dwel-ing kath'ĕ-tĕr) A catheter left in place in the bladder, usually a balloon catheter.

**in·e·bri·a·tion** (in-ē'brē-ā'shŭn) Intoxication, especially by alcohol.

**in·e·bri·e·ty** (in'ē-brī'ĕ-tē) Habitual excessive indulgence in alcoholic beverages. [L. *in-* intensive + *ebrietas,* drunkenness]

**in·ert** (in-ĕrt') **1.** Slow in action; sluggish; inactive. **2.** Devoid of active chemical properties, as the inert gases.

**in·er·ti·a** (in-ĕr'shē-ă) **1.** Tendency of a physical body to oppose any force tending to move it from a position of rest or to change its uniform motion. **2.** Denoting inactivity or lack of force, lack of mental or physical vigor, or sluggishness of thought or action. [L. want of skill, laziness]

**in·er·ti·a time** (in-ĕr'shē-ă tīm) Interval elapsing between reception of stimulus from a nerve and contraction of the muscle.

**in ex·tre·mis** (in eks-trē'mis) At the point of death. [L. *extremus,* last]

**in·fant** (in'fănt) A child younger than 1 year old. [L. *infans,* not speaking]

**in·fan·tile** (in'făn-tīl) **1.** Relating to, or characteristic of, infants or infancy. **2.** Denoting childish behavior.

**in·fan·tile con·vul·sion** (in'făn-tīl kŏn-vŭl' shŭn) Convulsion occurring in infancy (ca. birth–2 years of age).

**in·fan·tile scur·vy** (in'făn-tīl skŭr'vē) Cachectic condition in infants, resulting from malnutrition and marked by pallor, fetid breath, coated tongue, diarrhea, and subperiosteal hemorrhages. SYN Barlow disease, Cheadle disease.

**in·fan·ti·lism** (in-fan'ti-lizm) A state marked by slow development of mind and body.

**in·farct** (in'fahrkt) SYN infarction.

**in·farc·tion** (in-fahrk'shŭn) Area of tissue necrosis caused by impaired arterial or venous blood supply due to mechanical factors (e.g., emboli, thrombi) or to blood pressure alterations. SYN infarct.

**in·farc·tus my·o·car·di·i** (in-fahrk'tŭs mī-ō-kahr'dē-ī) SYN myocardial infarction.

**in·fec·tion** (in-fek'shŭn) Invasion of the body with organisms that have the potential to cause disease. See page 307.

**in·fec·tious** (in-fek'shŭs) **1.** Disease capable of being transmitted from person to person, with or without actual contact. **2.** SYN infective.

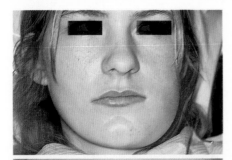

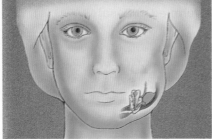

**masseteric space infection:** sited at tooth 19

**in·fec·tious a·ne·mi·a** (in-fek´shŭs ă-nē´ mē-ă) Blood disorder developing as a complication of infection; probably results from depressed formation and short survival of erythrocytes and abnormal iron metabolism.

**in·fec·tious dis·ease, in·fec·tive dis· ease** (in-fek´shŭs di-zēz´, in-fek´tiv) Disease resulting from the presence and activity of a microbial agent.

▣**in·fec·tious mon·o·nu·cle·o·sis** (in-fek´shŭs mon´ō-nū-klē-ō´sis) Acute febrile illness of young adults, caused by the Epstein-Barr virus; frequently spread by saliva transfer; characterized by fever, sore throat, enlargement of lymph nodes and spleen, and leukopenia that changes to lymphocytosis during the second week. See this page.

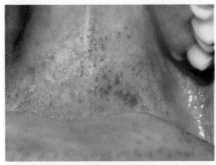

**infectious mononucleosis:** palatal petechiae

**in·fec·ti·ous waste** (in-fek´shŭs wāst) Refuse capable of causing infectious disease; items contaminated with blood, saliva, or other body substances, or those actually or potentially infected with pathogenic material.

**in·fec·tive** (in-fek´tiv) Capable of transmitting an infection. SYN infectious (2).

**in·fec·tiv·i·ty** (in´fek-tiv´i-tē) Characteristic of a disease agent that embodies capability of entering, surviving in, and multiplying and causing disease in a susceptible host.

**in·fer·i·or** (in-fēr´ē-ŏr) 1. Situated below or directed downward. 2. ANATOMY situated nearer the soles of the feet in relation to a specific reference point; opposite of superior. 3. Less useful or of poorer quality. [L. lower]

**in·fe·ri·or al·ve·o·lar nerve** (in-fēr´ē-ŏr al-vē´ŏ-lăr nĕrv) [TA] One of the terminal branches of the mandibular, it enters the mandibular canal to be distributed to the lower teeth, periosteum, and gingiva of the mandible. SYN nervus alveolaris inferior [TA].

**in·fe·ri·or bor·der of man·di·ble** (in-fēr´ē-ŏr bōr´dĕr man´di-bĕl) Linear undersurface of the lower jaw bone, made up of cortical bone. Viewed on a panoramic dental radiograph, it appears as a radiopaque band outlining the lower edge of the lower jaw. SYN mandibular border.

**in·fe·ri·or den·tal arch** (in-fēr´ē-ŏr den´tăl ahrch) SYN mandibular dental arcade.

**in·fe·ri·or den·tal branch·es of in· fe·ri·or den·tal plex·us** (in-fēr´ē-ŏr den´ tăl branch´ĕz in-fēr´ē-ŏr den´tăl plek´sŭs) [TA] Branches passing from inferior dental plexus to roots of teeth of lower jaw.

**in·fe·ri·or den·tal ca·nal** (in-fēr´ē-ŏr den´ tăl kă-nal´) SYN mandibular canal.

**in·fe·ri·or den·tal for·a·men** (in-fēr´ē-ŏr den´tăl fōr-ā´mĕn) SYN mandibular foramen.

**in·fe·ri·or max·il·lar·y nerve** (in-fēr´ē-ŏr mak´si-lar-ē nĕrv) SYN mandibular nerve [CN V3].

**in·fe·ri·or na·sal con·cha** (in-fēr´ē-ŏr nā´ zăl kong´kă) [TA] Thin, spongy, bony plate with curved margins, on lateral wall of nasal cavity; articulates with the maxillae and the ethmoid, lacrimal, and palatal bones.

**in·fe·ri·or or·bi·tal fis·sure** (in-fēr´ē-ŏr ōr´bi-tăl fish´ŭr) [TA] A gap or cleft between the greater wing of the sphenoid and the orbital plate of the maxilla, through which pass the maxillary nerve and the inferior ophthalmic vein or its communicating branches to the pterygoid venous plexus in the infratemporal fossa.

**in·fer·til·i·ty** (in´fĕr-til´i-tē) Diminished or absent ability to produce offspring. [L. in- neg. + fertilis, fruitful]

**in·fil·trate** (in´fil-trāt) To perform or undergo

infiltration. [L. *in* + Mediev. L. *filtro,* pp. *-atus,* to strain through felt, fr. *filtrum,* felt]

**in·fil·tra·tion** (in'fil-trā'shŭn) **1.** The act of permeating or penetrating into a substance, cell, or tissue. **2.** Injection of solution into tissues. **3.** Extravasation of solutions intended for intravascular injection.

**in·fil·tra·tion an·es·the·si·a** (in'fil-trā' shŭn an'es-thē'zē-ă) Anesthesia produced by injecting local anesthetic solution directly into a painful area or one to be operated on.

**in·firm** (in-fĭrm') Weak or feeble because of old age or disease.

**in·firm·i·ty** (in-fĭr'mi-tē) A weakness; an abnormal condition of mind or body.

**▣in·flam·ma·tion** (in'flă-mā'shŭn) *Avoid the misspelling inflamation.* Fundamental pathologic process consisting of a dynamic complex of histologically apparent cytologic changes, cellular infiltration, and mediator release that occurs in the affected blood vessels and adjacent tissues in response to an injury or abnormal stimulation caused by a physical, chemical, or biologic agent. See page A2. [L. *inflammo,* pp. *-atus,* fr. *in,* in, + *flamma,* flame]

**in·flam·ma·to·ry pap·il·lar·y hy·per· pla·si·a** (in-flam'ă-tōr-ē pap'i-lar-ē hī'pĕr-plā'zē-ă) Closely arranged papules of the palatal mucosa underlying an ill-fitting denture.

**in·fla·tion** (in-flā'shŭn) Distention by a fluid or gas. SYN vesiculation (2). [L. *inflatio,* fr. *in-flo,* pp. *-flatus,* to blow into, inflate]

**in·flu·en·za** (in'flū-en'ză) An acute infectious respiratory disease, caused by influenza viruses, in which inhaled virus attacks respiratory epithelial cells of susceptible people and produces a catarrhal inflammation; characterized by sudden onset, chills, and other symptoms. SYN flu, grippe. [It. influence (of planets or stars), fr. L. *influentia,* fr. *in-fluo,* to flow in]

**in·flu·en·za A** (in'flū-en'ză) Most common type of influenza, with a high propensity for antigenic change resulting in mutations, partly because they can infect various animals where dual infections can occur, giving rise to new hybrid strains. The infections occur in epidemics.

**in·flu·en·za B** (in'flū-en'ză) Influenza caused by strains of influenza virus type B; outbreaks are usually more limited than those due to influenza virus type A, although infections by the two types are clinically indistinguishable.

**in·flu·en·za C** (in'flū-en'ză) Influenza caused by strains of type C influenza virus; disease is milder than that caused by types A and B and has become uncommon in recent years.

**in·flu·en·zal vi·rus pneu·mo·ni·a** (in' flū-en'ză vī'rŭs nū-mō'ē-ă) Serious, often fatal, form of pneumonia caused by a virus of the influenzal type.

**in·flu·en·za nos·tras** (in'flū-en'ză nos'trăs) SYN endemic influenza.

**in·form·ed con·sent** (in-fōrmd' kŏn-sent') Voluntary agreement given by a patient or a patient's designated responsible proxy (e.g., a parent) for participation in a study, immunization program, treatment regimen, invasive procedure, or other medical or dental undertaking after being informed of the purpose, methods, procedures, benefits, and risks.

**in·form·ed re·fu·sal** (in-fōrmd' rĕ-fyū'zăl) Patient's decision to decline recommended treatment after all options, risks, and benefits have been thoroughly explained.

**in·fra·bon·y pock·et, in·tra·bon·y pock·et** (in'fră-bō'nē pok'ĕt, in'tră-) Pocket extending apically below the level of the adjacent alveolar crest. SYN subcrestal pocket.

**in·fra·bulge** (in'fră-bŭlj) **1.** Portion of crown of a tooth gingival to the height of contour. **2.** Area of tooth where retentive portion of a clasp of a removable partial denture is placed.

**in·fra·clu·sion** (in'fră-klū'zhŭn) State wherein a tooth fails to erupt to the maxillomandibular plane of interdigitation. SYN infraocclusion.

**in·fra·den·ta·le** (in'fră-den-tā'lē) In craniometrics, apex of septum between mandibular central incisors.

**in·fra·glot·tic cav·i·ty** (in'fră-glot'ik kav' i-tē) [TA] The part of the cavity of the larynx immediately below the glottis. SYN aditus glottidis inferior.

**in·fra·man·dib·u·lar** (in'fră-man-dib'yū-lăr) SYN submandibular.

**in·fra·max·il·lar·y** (in'fră-mak'si-lar-ē) SYN mandibular.

**in·fra·oc·clu·sion** (in'fră-ŏ-klū'zhŭn) SYN infraclusion.

**in·fra·or·bit·al** (in'fră-ōr'bi-tăl) Denotes below or beneath the orbit of the eye.

**in·fra·or·bit·al ar·te·ry** (in'fră-ōr'bi-tăl ahr'tĕr-ē) [TA] *Origin,* third part of maxillary artery; *distribution,* superior canine and incisor teeth, inferior rectus and inferior oblique muscles, inferior eyelid, lacrimal sac, maxillary sinus, and superior lip; *anastomoses,* branches of ophthalmic, facial, superior labial, transverse facial, and buccal.

**in·fra·or·bit·al ca·nal** (in'fră-ōr'bi-tăl kă-nal') [TA] Canal running beneath orbital margin of maxilla from infraorbital groove, in floor of orbit, to infraorbital foramen.

**in·fra·or·bit·al for·a·men** (in'fră-ōr'bi-tăl fōr-ā'mĕn) [TA] External opening of infraorbital canal on anterior surface of body of maxilla.

**in·fra·or·bit·al groove** (in´fră-ōr´bi-tăl grūv) [TA] Gradually deepening groove on orbital surface of maxilla.

**in·fra·or·bit·al mar·gin** (in´fră-ōr´bi-tăl mahr´jin) Inferior half of orbital rim, or the lower border of orbital opening, formed by maxilla medially and the zygomatic bone laterally.

**in·fra·or·bit·al nerve** (in´fră-ōr´bi-tăl nĕrv) [TA] Continuation of the maxillary nerve [CN V2] after it has traversed the pterygopalatine fossa and enters the orbit, via the infraorbital fissure; it is then transmitted by the infraorbital canal to reach the face; supplies mucosa of maxillary sinus; upper incisors, canine and premolar; upper gums; inferior eyelid and conjunctiva; part of the nose; and superior lip.

**in·fra·or·bit·al re·gi·on** (in´fră-ōr´bi-tăl rē´jŭn) [TA] Facial area below orbit of the eye and lateral to nose on each side.

**in·fra·or·bit·al su·ture** (in´fră-ōr´bi-tăl sū´chŭr) [TA] Inconstant suture running from infraorbital foramen to infraorbital groove.

**in·fra·tem·po·ral sur·face of (bod·y of) max·il·la** (in´fră-tem´pŏr-ăl sŭr´făs bod´ē mak-sil´ă) [TA] Convex posterolateral surface of body of maxilla that forms anterior wall of the infratemporal fossa.

**in·fra·troch·le·ar** (in´fră-trok´lē-ăr) Inferior to the trochlea or pulley of the superior oblique muscle of the eye.

**in·fra·troch·le·ar nerve** (in´fră-trok´lē-ăr nĕrv) [TA] Terminal branch of nasociliary nerve running beneath pulley of superior oblique muscle to the front of the orbit and supplying skin of eyelids and root of nose.

**in·fra·ver·sion** (in´fră-vĕr´zhŭn) 1. A turning (version) downward. 2. SYN infraclusion.

**in·fu·sion** (in-fyū´zhŭn) 1. The process of steeping a substance in water, either cold or hot (below the boiling point), to extract its soluble principles. 2. A medicinal preparation obtained by steeping the crude drug in water. [L. infusio, fr. in- fundo, pp. -fusus, to pour in]

**in·ges·ta** (in-jes´tă) Solid or liquid nutrients taken into the body. [pl. of L. ingestum, ntr. pp. of in-gero, -gestus, to carry in]

**in·gra·ves·cent** (in´gră-ves´ĕnt) Increasing in severity.

**in·gui·nal her·ni·a** (ing´gwi-năl hĕr´nē-ă) A hernia at the inguinal region.

**in·gui·nal re·gion** (ing´gwi-năl rē´jŭn) The topographic area of the inferior abdomen related to the inguinal canal, lateral to the pubic region. SYN groin (1).

**in·hal·ant** (in-hāl´ănt) A drug (or combination of drugs) with high vapor pressure, carried by an air current into the nasal passage, where it produces its effect.

**in·ha·la·tion** (in´hă-lā´shŭn) 1. The act of drawing in the breath. SYN inspiration. 2. Drawing in a medicated vapor with the breath. [L. inhalo, pp. -halatus, to breathe at or in]

**in·ha·la·tion an·al·ge·si·a** (in´hă-lā´shŭn an´ăl-jē´zē-ă) Analgesia produced by inhalation of a central nervous system–depressant gas (especially nitrous oxide) or vapor.

**in·ha·la·tion an·es·the·si·a** (in´hă-lā´shŭn an´es-thē´zē-ă) General anesthesia resulting from breathing of anesthetic gases.

**in·hal·er** (in-hāl´ĕr) 1. SYN respirator (2). 2. An apparatus for administering pharmacologically active agents by inhalation.

**in·hi·bi·tion** (in´hi-bish´ŭn) 1. Depression or arrest of a function. SEE ALSO inhibitor. 2. Reduction of rate of reaction or process. [L. in hibeo, pp. -hibitus, to keep back, fr. habeo, to have]

**in·hib·i·tor** (in-hib´i-tŏr) 1. An agent that restrains or retards physiologic, chemical, or enzymatic action. 2. A nervous system structure, stimulation of which represses activity.

**in·i·on** (in´ē-on) [TA] A point located on the external occipital protuberance at the intersection of the midline with a line drawn tangentially to the uppermost convexity of the right and left superior nuchal lines. [G. nape of the neck]

**in·i·tial con·tact** (i-nish´ăl kon´takt) 1. First meeting of opposing teeth on elevation of mandible toward maxillae. 2. First occlusal meeting of opposing teeth when the jaw is closed.

**in·i·tial dose** (i-nish´ăl dōs) SYN loading dose.

**in·ject** (in-jekt´) To introduce into the body; denoting a fluid forced beneath skin or into a blood vessel. [L. injicio, to throw in]

**in·jec·ta·ble** (in-jek´tă-bĕl) 1. Capable of being injected into anything. 2. Capable of receiving an injection.

**in·jec·tion** (in-jek´shŭn) 1. Introduction of a medicinal substance or nutrient material into subcutaneous tissue, muscular tissue, a vein, an artery, the rectum, or the other canals or cavities of the body. 2. An injectable pharmaceutical preparation. [L. injectio, a throwing in, fr. injicio, to throw in]

**in·jec·tion flask** (in-jek´shŭn flask) Denture flask designed so as to permit the forced flow of denture base material from a reservoir into the mold after flask is closed and during curing.

**in·jec·tion mold·ing** (in-jek´shŭn mōld´ing) Adaptation of a plastic material to negative

ij

form of closed mold by forcing material into mold through appropriate gateways.

**in·ju·ry** (in′jŭr-ē) Damage, harm, or loss, to a person. [L. *injuria,* fr. *in-* neg. + *jus (jur-),* right]

**in·lay** (in′lā) **1.** In dentistry, prefabricated restoration sealed into cavity with cement. **2.** Graft of bone into a bone cavity. **3.** A graft of skin into a wound cavity for epithelialization. See this page.

**e·nam·el ep·i·the·li·um** (in′ĕr den′tăl ep′i-thē′lē-ŭm, ĕ-nam′ĕl) Innermost layer of odontogenic organ, which develops into the enamel-producing ameloblasts.

**in·ner·va·tion** (in′ĕr-vā′shŭn) Supply of nerve fibers functionally connected with a part. See page 311.

**in·no·cent mur·mur** (in′ŏ-sĕnt mŭr′mŭr) SYN functional murmur.

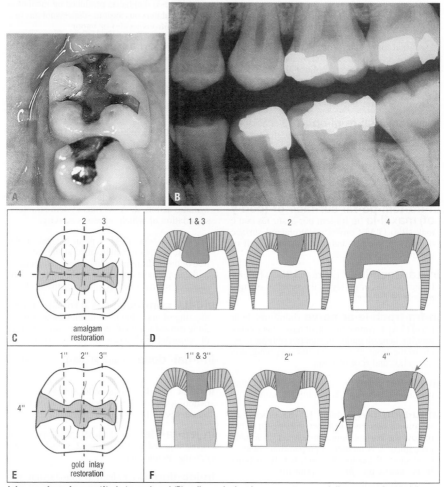

**inlays and amalgams:** (A) photograph and (B) radiograph showing convergence and divergence of materials. Amalgam (panels C, D) shows convergent wall at 1 and 3; inlay (panels E, F) has divergent walls at 1″, 2″, and 3″. Arrows = bevels of inlay

**in·lay wax** (in′lā waks) SYN casting wax.

**in·nate im·mu·ni·ty** (i-nāt′ i-myū′ni-tē) Resistance manifested by an organism that has not been sensitized by previous infection or vaccination; nonspecific and is not stimulated by specific antigens. SYN natural immunity, nonspecific immunity.

**in·ner den·tal ep·i·the·li·um, in·ner**

**in·oc·u·la·tion** (i-nok′yū-lā′shŭn) Introduction into the body of causative organism of a disease. Also used, incorrectly, to mean immunization with a vaccine.

**in·o·pex·i·a** (in′ŏ-pek′sē-ă) Tendency toward spontaneous coagulation of the blood. [*ino* + G. *pexis,* fixation, + *-ia*]

**in·or·gan·ic** (in′ōr-gan′ik) **1.** Not organic; not

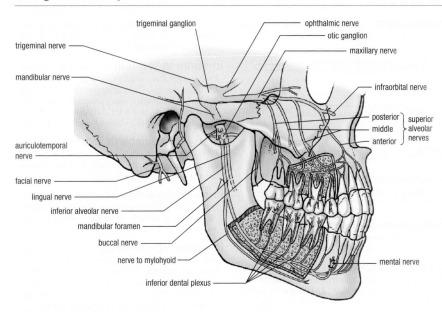

**innervation of teeth**

formed by living organisms. **3.** Not containing carbon.

**in·or·gan·ic com·pound** (in′ŏr-gan′ik kom′pownd) A compound in which the atoms or radicals consist of elements other than carbon.

**in·or·gan·ic den·tal ce·ment** (in′ŏr-gan′ik den′tăl sĕ-ment′) Fixative usually of metallic salts or oxides, which, when mixed with a specific liquid, forms a plastic mass that sets.

**in·o·si·tol** (in-ō′si-tol) A member of the vitamin B complex necessary for growth of yeast.

**in·o·tro·pic a·gents** (in′ō-trō′pik ā′jĕnts) Drugs that increase force of contraction cardiac muscle.

**in·scrip·tion, in·scrip·ti·o** (in-skrip′shŭn, -shē-ō) The main part of a prescription, which indicates drugs and amount of each to be used in the mixture.

**in·sen·si·ble** (in-sen′si-bĕl) **1.** SYN unconscious. **2.** Not appreciable by the senses.

**in·ser·tion** (in-sĕr′shŭn) **1.** In dentistry, the intraoral placing of a dental prosthesis. **2.** The usually more distal attachment of a muscle to the more movable part of the skeleton, as distinguished from origin. [L. *insertio*, a planting in, fr. *insero, -sertus*, to plant in]

**in·sid·i·ous** (in-sid′ē-ŭs) Treacherous; stealthy; denoting a disease that progresses gradually with inapparent symptoms.

**in si·tu** (in sit′ū) In position; not extending beyond the focus or level of origin. [L. *in*, in, + *situs*, site]

**in·sol·u·ble** (in-sol′yū-bĕl) Incapable of dissolving in solution.

**in·som·ni·a** (in-som′nē-ă) Inability to sleep, without external impediments when sleep should normally occur. [L. fr. *in-* priv. + *somnus*, sleep]

**in·spec·tion** (in-spek′shŭn) Close examination. [L. *inspectio*, fr. *in-*, into, + *specio*, to look]

**in·sper·sion** (in-spĕr′zhŭn) Sprinkling with a fluid or a powder.

**in·spi·ra·tion** (in′spir-ā′shŭn) SYN inhalation (1). [L. *inspiratio*, fr. *in- spiro*, pp. *-atus*, to breathe in]

**in·spi·ra·to·ry re·serve vol·ume (IRV)** (in′spir-ă-tōr-ē rĕ-zĕrv′ vol′yūm) The maximal volume of air that can be inspired after a normal inspiration. SYN complemental air.

**in·spi·ra·to·ry stri·dor** (in′spir-ă-tōr-ē strī′dŏr) A pathologic crowing sound during the inspiratory phase of respiration.

**in·spi·rom·e·ter** (in′spi-rom′ĕ-tĕr) An instrument for measuring force, frequency, or volume of inspirations. [L. *in-spiro*, to breathe in, + G. *metron*, measure]

**in·stil·la·tion** (in′sti-lā′shŭn) Dropping of a liquid on or into a body part.

**in·stinct** (in′stingkt) Enduring disposition or tendency of an organism to act in an organized and biologically adaptive manner characteristic of its species. [L. *instinctus*, impulse]

**in·stru·ment** (in′strŭ-mĕnt) A tool or implement. See this page. [L. *instrumentum*]

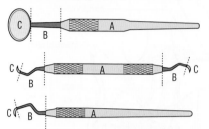

**parts of the mouth mirror and periodontal instrument:** (A) handle; (B) shank; (C) working-end

**in·stru·men·tar·i·um** (in′strŭ-mĕn-tar′ē-ŭm) A collection of instruments and other equipment for a dental procedure or operation.

**in·stru·men·ta·tion** (in′strŭ-mĕn-tā′shŭn) **1.** In dentistry, application of an armamentarium in a restorative procedure. **2.** The use of dental instruments.

**in·stru·men·ta·tion zones** (in′stru-men-tā′shŭn zōnz) Imaginary narrow tracts on the root surface (each only as wide as the toe-third of the instrument's cutting edge) used to help the clinician systematically remove calculus deposits from subgingival root surfaces.

**in·su·date** (in′sŭ-dāt) Fluid swelling within an arterial wall (ordinarily serous). [L. *in*, in, + *sudo*, pp. *-atus*, to sweat]

**in·suf·fi·cien·cy** (in′sŭ-fish′ĕn-sē) Lack of completeness of function or power.

**in·suf·flate** (in′sŭ-flāt) To deliver air or gas under pressure to a body cavity or chamber. [L. *in-sufflo*, to blow on or into]

**in·suf·fla·tion** (in′sŭ-flā′shŭn) **1.** The act or process of insufflating. **2.** SYN inhalant (3).

**in·suf·fla·tor** (in′sŭf-lā′tŏr) An instrument used in insufflation.

**in·su·lat·ing base** (in′sŭ-lā′ting bās) SYN liner.

**in·su·lin** (in′sŭ-lin) Polypeptide hormone, secreted by β cells in islets of Langerhans, which promotes glucose use, protein synthesis, and formation and storage of neutral lipids; available in various preparations including genetically engineered human insulin, which is currently favored; used parenterally to treat diabetes mellitus. [L. *insula*, island, + *-in*]

**in·su·lin an·tag·o·nist** (in′sŭ-lin an-tag′ŏ-nist) Substances that may induce a functional insulin deficiency; may include nonprecipitating antibodies against nonhuman insulin.

**in·su·lin-de·pen·dent di·a·be·tes mel·li·tus (IDDM)** (in′sŭ-lin-dĕ-pen′dĕnt dī′ă-bē′ tēz mel′i-tŭs) Former designation for Type 1 diabetes (q.v.); term declared obsolete by the American Diabetes Association.

**in·su·lin in·jec·tion** (in′sŭ-lin in-jek′shŭn) Preparation that usually contains 100 USP insulin units per mL; it is administered subcutaneously; occasionally intravenously; has rapid onset of action; and brief duration (5–7 hours). Used to treat diabetic acidosis and insulin coma.

**in·su·lin-like growth fac·tor (IGF)** (in′sŭ-lin grōth fak′tŏr) Most important somatomedin for postnatal growth; produced in the liver, kidney, and elsewhere.

**in·su·lin lip·o·dys·tro·phy** (in′sŭ-lin lip′ō-dis′trŏ-fē) Dystrophic atrophy of subcutaneous tissues in diabetic patients at site of frequent injections of insulin.

**in·su·lin re·sis·tance** (in′sŭ-lin rĕ-zis′tăns) Diminished effectiveness of insulin in lowering plasma glucose levels, arbitrarily defined as a daily requirement of at least 200 units to prevent hyperglycemia or ketosis; associated with obesity, ketoacidosis, and infection.

**in·su·lin shock** (in′sŭ-lin shok) Severe hypoglycemia produced by administration of insulin, manifested by sweating, tremor, anxiety, vertigo, and diplopia, followed by delirium, convulsions, and collapse.

**in·su·lin u·nit (in·ter·na·tion·al)** (in′sŭ-lin yū′nit in′tĕr-nash′ŏ-năl) Activity contained in 1/22 mg of the international standard of zinc-insulin crystals.

**in·su·li·tis** (in′sŭ-lī′itis) Inflammation of the islands of Langerhans that may be the initial lesion of Type 1 diabetes mellitus.

**in·sur·ance** (in-shŭr′ăns) Coverage against financial loss procured by contract from a company that provides such protection.

**in·sured** (in-shŭrd′) SYN beneficiary.

**in·take** (in′tāk) **1.** The act of consuming or absorbing anything. **2.** That which is taken in.

**in·te·gra·tion** (in′tĕ-grā′shŭn) **1.** In dentistry, attachment of tissue to an alloplastic material. **2.** Being combined, or the process of combining, into a complete and harmonious whole. **3.** In physiology, the process of building up.

**in·tel·li·gence** (in-tel′i-jĕns) A person's aggregate capacity to act purposefully, think rationally, and deal effectively with the environment.

**in·tel·li·gence quo·tient (IQ)** (in-tel′i-jĕns kwō′shĕnt) Psychologist's index of measured intelligence as one part of a two-part determination of intelligence, the other part being an index of adaptive behavior that includes such criteria as school grades or work performance.

**in·ten·si·ty (I)** (in-ten′si-tē) **1.** Marked tension; great activity; often used simply to denote a measure of the degree or amount of some quality. **2.** The magnitude of acoustic energy, energy flux, field strength, or force. [L. *in- tendo*, pp. *-tensus*, to stretch out]

**in·ten·sive care** (in-ten′siv kār) Management and care of critically ill patients.

**in·ten·sive care u·nit (ICU)** (in-ten′siv kār yū′nit) Hospital facility for provision of nursing and medical care of critically ill patients, characterized by the high quality and quantity of continuous nursing and medical supervision and by use of sophisticated monitoring and resuscitative equipment.

**in·ten·tion·al re·plan·ta·tion** (in-ten′shŭn-ăl rē′plan-tā′shŭn) Elective extraction of a tooth, obturation of the root canal(s), and replacement of tooth in alveolus.

**in·ten·tion trem·or** (in-ten′shŭn trem′ŏr) Tremor that occurs during performance of precise voluntary movements, caused by disorders of cerebellum or connections. SYN action tremor.

♻ **inter-** *Do not confuse this word with intra- or intro-.* Combining form meaning among, between. [L. *inter*, between]

**in·ter·ac·tion** (in′tĕr-ak′shŭn) **1.** The reciprocal action between two entities in a common environment as in chemical interaction, ecologic interaction, and social interaction. **2.** The effects when two entities concur that would not be observed with either in isolation.

**in·ter·al·ve·o·lar sep·tum** (in′tĕr-al-vē′ŏ-lăr sep′tŭm) [TA] **1.** The tissue intervening between two adjacent pulmonary alveoli; it consists of a close-meshed capillary network covered on both surfaces by thin alveolar epithelial cells. **2.** One of the bony partitions between the tooth sockets of the mandible and maxilla. SYN alveolar septum.

**in·ter·al·ve·o·lar space** (in′tĕr-al-vē′ŏ-lăr spās) SYN interarch distance.

**in·ter·arch dis·tance** (in′tĕr-ahrch dis′tăns) Vertical space between maxillary and mandibular arches under conditions of vertical dimensions that must be specified. SYN interalveolar space, interridge distance.

**in·ter·cel·lu·lar** (in′tĕr-sel′yū-lăr) Between or among cells.

**in·ter·cep·tive oc·clu·sal con·tact** (in′tĕr-sep′tiv ŏ-klū′zăl kon′takt) SYN deflective occlusal contact.

**in·ter·cep·tive/pre·ven·tive or·tho·don·tics** (in′tĕr-sep′tiv prĕ-ven′tiv ōr′thŏ-don′tiks) Dental services intended to prevent development of a malocclusion by maintaining the integrity of an otherwise normally developing dentition.

**in·ter·cil·i·um** (in′tĕr-sil′ē-ŭm) SYN glabella (2). [*inter-* + L. *cilium*, eyelid]

**in·ter·cos·tal neu·ral·gi·a** (in′tĕr-kos′tăl nūr-al′jē-ă) Pain in chest wall due to neuralgia of one or more intercostal nerves.

**in·ter·cri·co·thy·rot·o·my** (in′tĕr-krī′kō-thī-rot′ŏ-mē) SYN cricothyrotomy.

**in·ter·cur·rent** (in′tĕr-kŭr′ĕnt) Intervening; said of a disease attacking a person already ill of another malady. [*inter-* + L. *curro*, pr. p. *currens (-ent-)*, to run]

**in·ter·cus·pal po·si·tion** (in′tĕr-kŭs′păl pŏ-zish′ŏn) Placement of mandible when cusps and sulci of maxillary and mandibular teeth are in their greatest contact and mandible is in its most closed position.

**in·ter·cus·pa·tion** (in′tĕr-kŭs-pā′shŭn) **1.** Cusp-to-fossa relationship of maxillary and mandibular posterior teeth to each other. **2.** Interlocking or fitting together of cusps of opposing teeth. SYN interdigitation.

**in·ter·den·tal** (in′tĕr-den′tăl) **1.** Between teeth. **2.** Denoting the relationship between proximal surfaces of teeth of same arch. [*inter-* + L. *dens*, tooth]

**in·ter·den·tal ca·nals** (in′tĕr-den′tăl kă-nalz′) Canals that extend vertically through interdental alveolar bone between roots of mandibular and maxillary incisors and maxillary premolar teeth. SYN Hirschfeld canals.

**in·ter·den·tal car·ies** (in′tĕr-den′tăl kar′ēz) Caries occurring between teeth.

**in·ter·den·tal em·bra·sure** (in′tĕr-den′tăl em-brā′shŭr) SEE embrasure.

**in·ter·den·tal gin·gi·va** (in′tĕr-den′tăl jin′ji-vă) Triangular gingival tissue that fills the space between the proximal surfaces of adjacent teeth, apical to (i.e., beneath) the contact area.

**in·ter·den·tal pa·pil·la** (in′tĕr-den′tăl pă-pil′ă) SYN gingival papilla.

**in·ter·den·tal sep·tum** (in′tĕr-den′tăl sep′tŭm) Bony portion separating two adjacent teeth in a dental arch.

**in·ter·den·tal splint** (in′tĕr-den′tăl splint) For jaw fractures, splint consisting of two metal or acrylic resin bands wired to teeth of upper and lower jaws, respectively, and then attached to keep the jaws immovable.

**in·ter·den·tal tip** (in′tĕr-den′tăl tip) Flexible rubber cone used to remove plaque from between teeth.

**in·ter·den·tal tis·sues** (in′tĕr-den′tăl tish′ūz) The gingivae; those fibers of the periodontal ligament and the alveolar and supporting bone.

ij

**in·ter·den·ti·um** (in'tĕr-den'shē-ŭm) Interval between any two contiguous teeth.

**in·ter·dig·i·ta·tion** (in'tĕr-dij'i-tā'shŭn) SYN intercuspation (2). [*inter-* + L. *digitus,* finger]

**in·ter·dis·ci·pli·nar·y** (in'tĕr-dis'i-pli-nar-ē) Denoting the overlapping interests of different fields of dentistry, medicine, and science. [*inter-* + L. *disciplina,* instruction, teaching]

**in·ter·dis·ci·pli·nar·y team** (in'tĕr-dis'i-pli-nar-ē tēm) Group of dental professionals from various specialty disciplines who combine their expertise and resources to provide care.

**in·ter·face** (in'tĕr-fās) **1.** Surface that forms a common boundary of two bodies. **2.** Boundary between regions of different radiopacity, acoustic, or magnetic resonance properties.

**in·ter·fa·cial sur·face ten·sion** (in'tĕr-fā'shăl sŭr'făs ten'shŭn) Resistance to separation possessed by film of liquid between two well-adapted surfaces.

**in·ter·fer·ence** (in'tĕr-fēr'ĕns) **1.** The coming together of waves in various media in such a way that the crests of one series correspond to the hollows of the other, the two thus neutralizing each other; or so that the crests of the two series correspond, thus increasing the excursions of the waves. **2.** Condition in which infection of a cell by one virus prevents superinfection by another virus, or in which superinfection prevents effects that would result from infection by either virus alone, even though both viruses persist. [*inter-* + L. *ferio,* to strike]

**in·ter·fer·on (IFN)** (in'tĕr-fēr'on) A class of small protein and glycoprotein cytokines produced by T cells, fibroblasts, and other cells in response to viral infection and other biologic and synthetic stimuli.

**in·ter·fer·on al·pha** (in'tĕr-fēr'on al'fă) The major interferon made by virus-induced leukocytes; several subtypes exist that are elaborated by leukocytes in response to viral stimulation.

**in·ter·fer·on al·pha-2b** (in'tĕr-fēr'on al'fă) Water-soluble protein (MW 19,271) secreted by leukocytes infected by virus; used to treat cancer and other disorders.

**in·ter·fer·on be·ta** (in'tĕr-fēr'on bā'tă) Interferon elaborated by fibroblasts and microphages.

**in·ter·fer·on be·ta-1b** (in'tĕr-fēr'on bā'tă) Purified protein with antiviral and immunomodulatory effects.

**in·ter·fer·on gam·ma** (in'tĕr-fēr'on gam'ă) Interferon elaborated by T lymphocytes in response to either specific antigen or mitogenic stimulation.

**in·ter·glo·bu·lar den·tin** (in'tĕr-glob'yū-lăr den'tin) SYN interglobular space.

**in·ter·glob·u·lar space** (in'tĕr-glob'yū-lăr spās) Imperfectly calcified matrix of dentin situated between the calcified globules near the dentinal periphery; also called interglobular space of Owen. SYN interglobular dentin.

**in·ter·im den·ture** (in'tĕr-im den'chŭr) Dental prosthesis used briefly for esthetics, mastication, occlusal support, or convenience, or to condition the patient to accept an artificial substitute for missing natural teeth. SYN temporary denture.

**in·ter·im pros·the·sis** (in'tĕr-im pros-thē'sis) SYN provisional prosthesis.

**in·ter·leu·kin (IL)** (in'tĕr-lū'kin) Group of eight multifunctional cytokines designated after their amino acid structure is known. They are synthesized by lymphocytes, monocytes, macrophages, and some other cells. SEE cytokine. [*inter-* + *leuk*ocyte + *-in*]

**in·ter·leu·kin-1** (in'tĕr-lū'kin) A cytokine, derived primarily from mononuclear phagocytes, which enhances the proliferation of T-helper cells and growth and differentiation of B cells.

**in·ter·leu·kin-2** (in'tĕr-lū'kin) A cytokine derived from T-helper lymphocytes that causes proliferation of T lymphocytes and activated B lymphocytes.

**in·ter·max·il·la** (in'tĕr-mak-sil'ă) SYN incisive bone.

**in·ter·max·il·lar·y** (in'tĕr-mak'si-lar-ē) Between the maxillae, the upper jaw bones.

**in·ter·max·il·lar·y an·chor·age** (in'tĕr-mak'si-lar-ē ang'kŏr-ăj) Anchorage in which units in one jaw are used to effect tooth movement in the other.

**in·ter·max·il·lar·y bone** (in'tĕr-mak'si-lar-ē bōn) SYN incisive bone.

**in·ter·max·il·lar·y e·las·tics** (in'tĕr-mak'si-lar-ē ĕ-las'tiks) Elastic bands used to provide pulling forces between maxillary and mandibular teeth to move teeth into correct position.

**in·ter·max·il·lar·y fix·a·tion** (in'tĕr-mak'si-lar-ē fik-sā'shŭn) Fixation of fractures of mandible or maxilla by applying elastic bands or stainless steel wire between the maxillary and mandibular arch bars or other types of splint. SYN mandibulomaxillary fixation, maxillomandibular fixation.

**in·ter·max·il·lar·y re·la·tion** (in'tĕr-mak'si-lar-ē rĕ-lā'shŭn) SYN maxillomandibular relation.

**in·ter·max·il·lar·y seg·ment** (in'tĕr-mak'si-lar-ē seg'mĕnt) Primordial mass of tissue formed by merging of medial nasal prominences of embryo; contributes to intermaxillary portion of upper jaw, prolabial portion of upper lip, and primary palate.

**in·ter·max·il·lar·y trac·tion** (in′tĕr-mak′si-lar-ē trak′shŭn) SYN maxillomandibular traction.

**in·ter·me·di·ar·y move·ments** (in′tĕr-mē′dē-ar-ē mūv′mĕnts) In dentistry, all movements between extremes of mandibular excursions.

**in·ter·me·di·ar·y nerve** (in′tĕr-mē′dē-ar-ē nĕrv) SYN intermediate nerve.

**in·ter·me·di·ate** (in′tĕr-mē′dē-ăt) [TA] **1.** In dentistry, a cement base. **2.** Between two extremes; interposed; intervening.

**in·ter·me·di·ate a·but·ment** (in′tĕr-mē′dē-ăt ă-bŭt′mĕnt) Natural tooth, or an implanted tooth substitute, without other natural teeth in proximal contact, used with mesial and distal abutments to support a prosthesis; often also called a "pier."

**in·ter·me·di·ate la·ryn·ge·al cav·i·ty** (in′tĕr-mē′dē-ăt lă-rin′jē-ăl kav′i-tē) Portion of laryngeal cavity between vestibular and vocal folds. SYN aditus glottidis superior.

**in·ter·me·di·ate nerve** (in′tĕr-mē′dē-ăt nĕrv) [TA] Root of facial nerve containing sensory fibers for taste from anterior two thirds of the tongue with cell bodies located in geniculate ganglion and presynaptic parasympathetic autonomic fibers with cell bodies located in superior salivatory nucleus. SYN intermediary nerve.

**in·ter·me·din** (in′tĕr-mē′din) SYN melanotropin.

**in·ter·me·tal·lic com·pound** (in′tĕr-me-tal′ik kom′pownd) Phase formed on cooling of liquid metal solutions wherein the resulting phase has fixed chemical composition or narrow range of compositions.

**in·ter·mi·cro·bi·al ma·trix** (in′tĕr-mī-krō′bē-ăl mā′triks) Material present between bacteria in dental biofilm; derived from interactions of saliva, and microorganisms.

**in·ter·mit·tent ex·plo·sive dis·or·der** (in′tĕr-mit′ĕnt eks-plō′siv dis-ōr′dĕr) Disorder that may begin in early childhood, or following head injury at any age, characterized by repeated acts of violent, aggressive behavior in otherwise normal people.

**in·ter·nal at·tach·ment** (in-tĕr′năl ă-tach′mĕnt) SYN precision attachment.

**in·ter·nal cap·sule syn·drome** (in-tĕr′năl kap′sŭl sin′drōm) Hemianopia with contralateral facial hemianesthesia.

**in·ter·nal ear** (in-tĕr′năl ēr) SEE ear.

**in·ter·nal fix·a·tion** (in-tĕr′năl fik-sā′shŭn) Stabilization of fractured bony parts by direct fixation to one another with surgical wires, screws, pins, rods, or plates.

**in·ter·nal med·i·cine (IM)** (in-tĕr′năl med′i-sin) Branch of medicine concerned with nonsurgical diseases in adults, but not including diseases limited to skin or nervous system.

**in·ter·nal ob·lique ridge** (in-tĕr′năl ō-blēk′ rij) A bony linear projection found on inner surface of mandible extending downward from the ramus and ending near the apices of the mandibular molars; serves as a site of attachment for the mylohyoid muscle of the floor of the mouth. SYN mylohyoid ridge.

**in·ter·nal o·pen·ing of ca·rot·id ca·nal** (in-tĕr′năl ō′pĕn-ing kă-rot′id kă-nal′) An irregular opening on the floor of the middle cranial fossa in the petrous portion of the temporal bone. SYN apertura interna canalis carotici.

**in·ter·nal o·pen·ing of coch·le·ar can·a·lic·u·lus** (in-tĕr′năl ō′pĕn-ing kok′lē-ăr kan′ă-lik′yū-lŭs) Passage whereby canaliculus of the cochlea communicates with subarachnoid space. SYN apertura interna canaliculi cochleae.

**in·ter·nal o·pen·ing of ves·tib·u·lar can·a·lic·u·lus** (in-tĕr′năl ō′pĕn-ing vestib′yū-lăr kan′ă-lik′yū-lŭs) The opening on the posterior surface of the petrous portion of the temporal bone by which the endolymphatic duct communicates with the endolymphatic sac. SYN apertura interna canaliculi vestibuli.

**in·ter·nal re·sorp·tion** (in-tĕr′năl rē-sōrp′shŭn) Regressive alteration of tooth structure that occurs within the crown or root of a tooth.

**in·ter·nal res·pi·ra·tion** (in-tĕr′năl res′pir-ā′shŭn) SYN tissue respiration.

**in·ter·nal trac·tion** (in-tĕr′năl trak′shŭn) Pulling force created by using one of the cranial bones, above point of fracture, for anchorage.

**In·ter·na·tion·al Clas·si·fi·ca·tion of Dis·eas·es (ICD)** (in′tĕr-nash′ŭn-ăl klas′i-fi-kā′shŭn di-zēz′ĕz) The enumeration of specific conditions and groups of conditions determined by expert committee that advises the World Health Organization, which publishes the complete list in a periodically revised book, the *Manual of the International Statistical Classification of Diseases, Injuries and Causes of Death.*

**In·ter·na·tion·al Fed·er·a·tion of Den·tal Hy·gien·ists (IFDH)** (in′tĕr-nash′ŏ-năl fed′ĕr-ā′shŭn den′tăl hī-jēn′ists) International nonprofit organization uniting dental hygiene associations to promote dental health.

**In·ter·na·tion·al Pho·ne·tic Al·pha·bet (IPA)** (in′tĕr-nash′ŭn-ăl fŏ-net′ik al′fă-bet) System of orthographic symbols devised for representing speech sounds.

**In·ter·na·tion·al Sys·tem of U·nits (SI)** (in′tĕr-nash′ŭn-ăl sis′tĕm yū′nits) System of measurements, based on the metric, to cover both coherent units (basic, supplementary, and derived units) and the decimal multiples and submultiples of these units formed by use of prefixes proposed for general international scientific and technologic use. SI proposes seven basic units: meter (m), kilogram (kg), second (s), ampere (A), kelvin (K), candela (cd), and mole (mol) for the basic quantities of length, mass, time, electric current, temperature, luminous intensity, and amount of substance, respectively. Multiples (prefixes) in descending order are: exa- (E, $10^{18}$), peta- (P, $10^{15}$), tera- (T, $10^{12}$), giga- (G, $10^9$), mega- (M, $10^6$), kilo- (k, $10^3$), hecto- (h, $10^2$), deca- (da, $10^1$), deci- (d, $10^{-1}$), centi- (c, $10^{-2}$), milli- (m, $10^{-3}$), micro- ($\mu$, $10^{-6}$), nano- (n, $10^{-9}$), pico- (p, $10^{-12}$), femto- (f, $10^{-15}$), atto- (a, $10^{-18}$). Proposed prefixes are zetta- (Z, $10^{21}$), yotta- (Y, $10^{24}$), zepto- (z, $10^{-21}$), and yocto- (y, $10^{-24}$). [Fr. *Système International d'Unités*]

**in·ter·na·tion·al u·nit (IU)** (in'tĕr-nash'ŭn-ăl yū'nit) Amount of a substance (e.g., drug, hormone, vitamin, enzyme) that produces specific effect as defined and accepted internationally.

**in·ter·neu·rons** (in'tĕr-nūr'onz) Combinations or groups of neurons between sensory and motor neurons that govern coordinated activity.

**in·ter·oc·clu·sal** (in'tĕr-ŏ-klū'zăl) Between occlusal surfaces of opposing teeth.

**in·ter·oc·clu·sal clear·ance** (in'tĕr-ŏ-klū'zăl klēr'ăns) SYN freeway space.

**in·ter·oc·clu·sal con·tact** (in'tĕr-ŏ-klū'zăl kon'takt) Meeting of the chewing surfaces of the maxillary and mandibular teeth when the teeth close together in centric occlusion.

**in·ter·oc·clu·sal dis·tance** (in'tĕr-ŏ-klū'zăl dis'tăns) 1. Vertical distance between opposing occlusal surfaces, assuming rest relation unless otherwise designated. SYN interocclusal rest space (1). 2. SYN freeway space.

**in·ter·oc·clu·sal gap** (in'tĕr-ŏ-klū'zăl gap) SYN freeway space.

**in·ter·oc·clu·sal re·cord, cen·tric in·ter·oc·clu·sal re·cord, ec·cen·tric in·ter·oc·clu·sal re·cord, lat·er·al in·ter·oc·clu·sal re·cord, pro·tru·sive in·ter·oc·clu·sal re·cord** (in'tĕr-ŏ-klū'zăl rek'ŏrd, sen'trik, ek-sen'trik, lat'ĕr-ăl, prō-trū'siv) Record of positional relationship of teeth or jaws to each other, recorded by placing a plastic material that hardens (e.g., plaster of Paris, wax) between occlusal surfaces of rims or teeth; hardened material serves as the record; may be registered in centric or eccentric positions, as centric interocclusal record, a record of centric jaw relation; eccentric interocclusal record , a record of jaw position in other than centric relation; lateral interocclusal record, a record of a lateral eccentric jaw position; and protrusive interocclusal record, a record of a protruded eccentric jaw position. SYN checkbite.

**in·ter·oc·clu·sal rest space** (in'tĕr-ŏ-klū'zăl rest spās) 1. SYN interocclusal distance (1). 2. SYN freeway space.

**in·ter·pa·ri·e·tal bone** (in'tĕr-pă-rī'ĕ-tăl bōn) [TA] The upper part of the squama of the occipital bone. SYN incarial bone.

**in·ter·par·ox·ys·mal** (in'tĕr-par'ok-siz'măl) Occurring between successive paroxysms of a disease.

**in·ter·phase** (in'tĕr-fāz) The stage between two successive divisions of a cell nucleus in which the biochemical and physiologic functions of the cell are performed.

**in·ter·pleu·ral space** (in'tĕr-plūr'ăl spās) SYN mediastinum (2).

**in·ter·po·la·tion** (in-tĕr'pŏ-lā'shŭn) Surgical excision of tissue from one site for transfer to another site.

**in·ter·pre·ta·tion** (in-tĕr'prĕ-tā'shŭn) CLINICAL PSYCHOLOGY drawing inferences and formulating the meaning in terms of the psychological dynamics inherent in a person's responses in therapy.

**in·ter·prox·i·mal** (in'tĕr-prok'si-măl) Between adjoining surfaces.

**in·ter·prox·i·mal brush** (in'tĕr-prok'si-măl brŭsh) Thin tapered brush used to clean interproximal areas between teeth. SYN interdental brush.

**in·ter·prox·i·mal con·tact** (in'tĕr-proks'i-măl kon'takt) Area of a tooth that contacts, usually mesially or distally, an adjacent tooth in the same arch.

**in·ter·prox·i·mal gin·gi·va** (in'tĕr-prok'si-măl jin'ji-vă) Gingival tissues that fill the embrasure space between tooth contacts and alveolar bone and its covering mucosa. SEE ALSO gingival papilla. SYN interdental gingiva.

**in·ter·prox·i·mal pa·pil·la** (in'tĕr-prok'si-măl pă-pil'ă) SYN gingival papilla.

**in·ter·prox·i·mal space** (in'tĕr-prok'si-măl spās) Area between adjacent teeth in dental arch; divided into embrasure occlusal to contact area, and septal space gingival to contact area.

**in·ter·prox·i·mal sur·face of tooth** (in'tĕr-prok'si-măl sŭr'făs tūth) SYN approximal surface of tooth.

**in·ter·ra·dic·u·lar** (in'tĕr-ră-dik'yū-lăr) Denotes the bony area between the roots of multirooted teeth.

**in·ter·ra·dic·u·lar al·ve·o·lo·plas·ty, in·tra·sep·tal al·ve·o·lo·plas·ty** (in'tĕr-ră-dik'yū-lăr al-vē'ō-lō-plas'tē, in'tră-sep'tăl) Removal of interradicular bone and collapsing of cortical plates to a more desirable alveolar contour.

**in·ter·ra·dic·u·lar os·se·ous de·fect** (in´tĕr-ră-dik´yū-lăr os´ē-ŭs dē´fekt) Bony deformities resulting from periodontal disease seen in bone between root furcation areas of teeth.

**in·ter·ra·dic·u·lar sep·tum** (in´tĕr-ră-dik´yū-lăr sep´tŭm) A thin bony partition that projects into the alveoli between the roots of the molar teeth of the maxilla or mandible.

**in·ter·ra·dic·u·lar space** (in´tĕr-ră-dik´yū-lăr spās) Area between roots of multirooted teeth.

**in·ter·ridge dis·tance** (in´tĕr-rij´ dis´tăns) SYN interarch distance.

**in·ter·rupt·ed su·ture** (in´tĕr-ŭp´tĕd sū´chŭr) A single stitch with tied ends.

**in·ter·sti·tial** (in´tĕr-stish´ăl) Relating to spaces or interstices in any structure.

**in·ter·tu·bu·lar den·tin** (in´tĕr-tū´byū-lăr den´tin) Dentin located between the dentinal tubules.

**in·ter·tu·bu·lar zone** (in´tĕr-tū´byū-lăr zōn) Dentinal matrix that lies between zones of peritubular dentin.

**in·ter·val** (in´tĕr-văl) A time or space between two periods or objects; a break in continuity.

**in·ter·ven·tion stud·ies** (in´tĕr-ven´shŭn stŭd´ēz) Comparative and investigative case studies of epidemiologic testing of the occurrence and nonoccurrence of disease or findings in population groups to determine the cause-and-effect factors present in such groups.

**in·tes·ti·nal** (in-tes´ti-năl) Relating to the intestine.

**in·tes·ti·nal an·gi·na** (in-tes´ti-năl an´ji-nă) SYN abdominal angina.

**in·tes·ti·nal an·thrax** (in-tes´ti-năl an´thraks) Usually fatal form marked by chills, high fever, pain, vomiting, and other symptoms.

**in·tol·er·ance** (in-tol´ĕr-ăns) Abnormal metabolism, excretion, or other disposition of a given substance; term often used to indicate impaired use or disposal of dietary constituents.

✿ **intra-** *Do not confuse this word with inter- or intro-.* Combining form meaning inside, within; opposite of extra-. [L. within]

**in·tra·al·ve·o·lar pock·et** (in´tră-al-vē´ŏ-lăr pok´ĕt) Infraosseous or infrabony defects of alveolar bone with one, two or three walls. SEE infrabony pocket. SYN intraosseous defect.

**in·tra·ar·te·ri·al (IA)** (in´tră-ahr-tēr´ē-ăl) Route by which medications are administered directly into an artery.

**in·tra·ar·tic·u·lar frac·ture** (in´tră-ahr-tik´yū-lăr frak´shŭr) Fracture occurring through the articular surface into the joint.

**in·tra·au·ral** (in´tră-awr´ăl) Within the ear. [*intra-* + L. *auris,* ear]

**in·tra·au·ric·u·lar** (in´tră-awr-ik´yū-lăr) Within an auricle (e.g., of the ear).

**in·tra·buc·cal** (in´tră-bŭk´ăl) 1. Within the mouth. 2. Within the substance of the cheek. [*intra-* + L. *bucca,* cheek]

**in·tra·cap·su·lar frac·ture** (in´tră-kap´sŭ-lăr frak´shŭr) A fracture near a joint and within the line of insertion of the joint capsule.

**in·tra·cap·su·lar tem·po·ro·man·dib·u·lar joint ar·thro·plas·ty** (in´tră-kap´sŭ-lăr tem´pŏr-ō-man-dib´yū-lăr joynt ahr´thrō-plas´tē) Operative recontouring of articular surface of mandibular condyle without removal of articular disc.

**in·tra·cav·i·ta·ry** (in´tră-kav´i-tar-ē) Within an organ or body cavity.

**in·tra·cel·lu·lar** (in´tră-sel´yū-lăr) Within a cell or cells.

**in·tra·cer·e·bro·ven·tric·u·lar** (in´tră-ser-ē´brō-ven-trik´yū-lăr) The locus of administration of drugs or chemicals into the ventricular system of the brain. Often used in animal studies and occasionally for the introduction of antiinfectives or anticancer drugs that do not penetrate the blood-brain barrier into the brain in humans.

**in·tra·cor·o·nal** (in´tră-kōr´ŏ-năl) Within the crown portion of a tooth.

**in·tra·co·ro·nal at·tach·ment** (in´tră-kōr´ŏ-năl ă-tach´mĕnt) Precision fitting for a dental prosthesis of which one part is built into the crown of the tooth.

**in·tra·cor·o·nal re·tain·er** (in´tră-kōr´ŏ-năl rĕ-tā´nĕr) Retainer that depends on components placed within the crown portion of a tooth for its retentive qualities.

**in·tra·cra·ni·al** (in´tră-krā´nē-ăl) Within the cranium, usually meaning within the cranial cavity. See page 318.

**in·tra·cra·ni·al hem·or·rhage** (in´tră-krā´nē-ăl hem´ŏr-ăj) Bleeding within cranial vault.

**in·tra·cra·ni·al pres·sure (ICP)** (in´tră-krā´nē-ăl presh´ŭr) Pressure within the cranial cavity; may be due to pathogen, disease, or traumatic brain injury.

**in·tra·crine** (in´tră-krin) Denoting self-stimulation through cellular production of a factor that acts within the cell. [*intra-* + G. *krinō,* to separate, secrete]

**in·tra·der·mal test** (in´tră-dĕr´măl test) SYN skin test.

ij

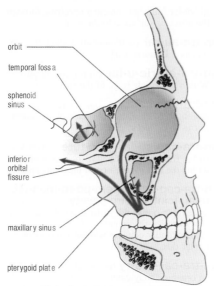

orbit

temporal fossa

sphenoid sinus

inferior orbital fissure

maxillary sinus

pterygoid plate

**routes of infection to intracranial cavity:** arrows indicate direction of spread from teeth to maxillary sinus and through inferior orbital fissure to orbit. A deeper route follows along lateral pterygoid lamina to base of cranium

**in·tra·ep·i·the·li·al dys·ker·a·to·sis** (in´tră-ep´i-thē´lē-ăl dis-ker´ă-tō´sis) White spongy lesions of buccal mucosa, floor of mouth, ventral lateral tongue, gingiva, and palate.

**in·tra·fe·brile** (in´tră-feb´ril, -fē´bril) Occurring during febrile stage of a disease. SYN intrapyretic.

**in·tra·le·sion·al ther·a·py** (in´tră-lē´zhŭn-ăl thār´ă-pē) Direct therapeutic injection into a lesion.

**in·tra·max·il·lar·y an·chor·age** (in´tră-mak´si-lar-ē ang´kŏr-ăj) A type in which resistance units are all situated within same jaw.

**in·tra·mem·bra·nous** (in´tră-mem´bră-nŭs) 1. Within, or between the layers of, a membrane. 2. Denoting a method of bone formation directly from mesenchymal cells without an intervening cartilage stage.

**in·tra·mus·cu·lar (IM)** (in´tră-mŭs´kyū-lăr) Within the substance of a muscle.

**in·tra·oc·u·lar pres·sure (IOP)** (in´tră-ok´yū-lăr presh´ŭr) The pressure of the intraocular fluid.

**in·tra·o·ral** (in´tră-ōr´ăl) Within the mouth. [*intra-* + L. *os,* mouth]

**in·tra·o·ral an·chor·age** (in´tră-ōr´ăl ang´kŏr-ăj) A type in which resistance units are all located within oral cavity.

**in·tra·o·ral an·es·the·si·a** (in´tră-ōr´ăl an´es-thē´zē-ă) 1. Insufflation anesthesia in which an inhalation anesthetic is added to inhaled air passing through mouth. 2. Regional anesthesia of mouth and associated structures with local anesthetic solutions used in oral cavity.

**in·tra·o·ral cam·er·a** (in´tră-ōr´ăl kam´ĕr-ă) Photographic device that uses a small wand to take digital pictures in the oral cavity for immediate viewing by dental staff and patient.

**in·tra·o·ral ex·am·i·na·tion** (in´tră-ōr´ăl eg-zam´i-nā´shŭn) Overall evaluation of the oral cavity to assess the status of the oral tissues and structures.

**in·tra·o·ral frac·ture ap·pli·ance** (in´tră-ōr´ăl frak´shŭr ă-plī´ăns) Metal or acrylic device attached to teeth with wire or cement; used to immobilize fractures of the maxilla and mandible.

**in·tra·o·ral ful·crum** (in´tră-ōr´ăl ful´krŭm) Stabilizing point inside the patient's mouth against a tooth surface.

**in·tra·o·ral trac·ing** (in´tră-ōr´ăl trās´ing) A drawing of mandibular movements using a device attached to the opposing arches; its shape resembles that of an arrowhead or a pointed (i.e., Gothic) arch; when the instrument's marking point is at the apex of the arch, the jaws are considered to be in centric relation. SYN arrow point tracing, Gothic arch tracing, Gothic arch, needlepoint tracing, stylus tracing.

**in·tra·or·bit·al** (in´tră-ōr´bi-tăl) Within the orbit.

**in·tra·os·se·ous** (in´tră-os´ē-ŭs) Within bone. [*intra-* + L. *os,* bone]

**in·tra·os·se·ous an·es·the·si·a** (in´tră-os´ē-ŭs an´es-thē´zē-ă) Injection of anesthetic into bone as a supplemental or primary technique in routine dental procedures.

**in·tra·os·se·ous in·jec·tion** (in´tră-os´ē-ŭs in-jek´shŭn) Injection of anesthetic into the intraradicular bone around a tooth. It is usually performed by penetrating the cortical bone with a dental bur, followed by injection of the anesthetic solution into the cancellous bone.

**in·tra·par·tum** (in´tră-pahr´tŭm) During labor and delivery or childbirth. Cf. antepartum, postpartum. [*intra-* + L. *partus,* childbirth]

**in·tra·per·i·to·ne·al (IP)** (in´tră-per´i-tō-nē´ăl) Within the peritoneal cavity.

**in·tra·pul·mo·nar·y** (in´tră-pul´mŏ-nar´ē) Within the lungs.

**in·tra·pul·pal** (in-tră-pŭl´păl) Within the pulp of a tooth.

**in·tra·pul·pal an·es·the·si·a** (in´tră-pŭlp´ăl an´es-thē´zē-ă) Injection of anesthetic solution directly into dental pulp chamber.

**in·tra·py·ret·ic** (in′tră-pī-ret′ik) SYN intrafe-brile. [*intra-* + L. *pyretos,* fever]

**in·tra·sep·tal in·jec·tion** (in′tră-sep′tăl in-jek′shŭn) Injection of local anesthetic to interdental papilla for anesthesia of terminal nerve endings at site and adjacent soft tissue.

**in·tra·the·cal (IT)** (in′tră-thē′kăl) Within a sheath.

**in·tra·the·cal in·jec·tion** (in′tră-thē′kăl in-jek′shŭn) Introduction of material for diffusion throughout subarachnoid space.

**in·tra·ton·sil·lar** (in′tră-ton′si-lăr) Within the substance of a tonsil.

**in·tra·tu·bu·lar/per·i·tu·bu·lar den·tin** (in′tră-tū′byū-lăr per′i-tū′byū-lăr den′tin) Lining of the dentinal tubules that becomes mineralized with increasing age of patients.

**in·tra·tym·pan·ic** (in′tră-tim-pan′ik) Within the middle ear or tympanic cavity.

**in·tra·vas·cu·lar (IV)** (in′tră-vas′kyū-lăr) Within the blood vessels or lymphatics.

**in·tra·ve·nous (IV)** (in′tră-vē′nŭs) Within a vein or veins.

**in·tra·ve·nous a·li·men·ta·tion** (in′tră-vē′nŭs al′i-měn-tā′shŭn) SYN parenteral nutrition.

**in·tra·ve·nous an·es·the·si·a** (in′tră-vē′nŭs an′es-thē′zē-ă) General anesthesia produced by injection of central nervous system depressants into venous circulation.

**in·tra·ve·nous drip** (in′tră-vē′nŭs drip) Slow but continuous introduction of solutions intravenously, a drop at a time.

**in·tra·ven·tric·u·lar (IV)** (in′tră-ven-trik′yū-lăr) Within a ventricle of the brain or heart.

**in·tra·ven·tric·u·lar hem·or·rhage** (in′tră-ven-trik′yū-lăr hem′ŏr-ăj) Extravasation of blood into ventricular system of brain.

**in·tra·ven·tric·u·lar in·jec·tion** (in′tră-ven-trik′yū-lăr in-jek′shŭn) Introduction of materials for diffusion throughout ventricular and subarachnoid space with ventricular puncture.

**in·tra vi·tam** (in′tră vī′tăm) During life. [L.]

**in·trin·sic** (in-trin′zik) 1. Pertaining to the essence or nature of a thing; inherent. 2. ANATOMY denoting those muscles with an origin and insertion that are both within structure under consideration. SYN essential (6). [L. *intrinsecus,* on the inside]

**in·trin·sic asth·ma** (in-trin′zik az′mă) Bronchial asthma in which no extrinsic causes can be identified.

**in·trin·sic col·or·ing** (in-trin′zik kŭl′ŏr-ing) Color pigment added within dental prosthesis material.

**in·trin·sic fac·tor (IF)** (in-trin′zik fak′tŏr) A relatively small mucoprotein secreted by the neck cell of the gastric glands and required for adequate absorption of vitamin B12; deficiency results in pernicious anemia.

**in·trin·sic stain·ing** (in-trin′zik stān′ing) Discoloration of internal tooth structure due to factors derived from within the body; an effect of substances such as the antibiotic tetracycline. Such stains are not usually removable but may be treated through cosmetic dental procedures. See this page and page A4.

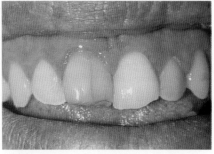

**intrinsic staining:** nonvital right central incisor

**in·tro·duc·er** (in′trō-dūs′ĕr) An instrument, such as a catheter, needle, or endotracheal tube, for introduction of a flexible device. [L. *introduco,* to lead into, introduce]

**in·tro·ver·sion** (in′trō-věr′zhŭn) The turning of a structure into itself. SEE ALSO invagination. [*intro-* + L. *verto,* pp. *versus,* to turn]

**in·tu·bate** (in′tū-bāt) To insert a tube.

**in·tu·ba·tion** (in′tū-bā′shŭn) Insertion of a tubular device into a canal, hollow organ, or cavity. [L. *in,* in, + *tuba,* tube]

**in·u·lin** (in′yū-lin) Fructose polysaccharide administered intravenously to determine rate of glomerular filtration.

**in·unc·tion** (in-ŭngk′shŭn) Administration of a drug in ointment form by rubbing to cause absorption. [L. *inunctio,* an anointing, fr. *inunguo,* pp. *-unctus,* to smear on]

**in u·ter·o** (in yū′těr-ō) Within the womb; not yet born. [L.]

**in·vag·i·na·tion** (in-vaj′i-nā′shŭn) Ensheathing, enfolding, or insertion of a structure within itself or another. See page 320.

**in·va·sion** (in-vă′zhŭn) 1. Beginning or incursion of disease. 2. Local spread of a malignant neoplasm by infiltration or destruction of adjacent tissue. 3. Entrance of foreign cells into tis-

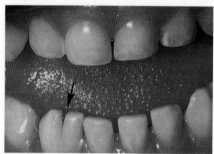

**gemination:** gemination of mandibular right lateral incisor caused by invagination of a single tooth germ, which produces a notched and grooved crown; note presence of six mandibular anterior teeth

sue. [L. *invasio,* fr. *in-vado,* pp. *-vasus,* to go into, attack]

**in·va·sion of pri·va·cy** (in-vā'zhŭn prī'vă-sē) In health care, illicit use of documentation related to treatment.

**in·va·sive** (in-vā'siv) Denoting a procedure requiring insertion of an instrument or device into the body through the skin or a body orifice for diagnosis or treatment.

**in·va·sive pro·ce·dure** (in-vā'siv prō-sē'jŭr) Therapy that involves entry into tissues during which bleeding occurs.

**in·ven·tor·y** (in'věn-tōr-ē) A detailed, often descriptive, list of items, tools, devices, dressings, or materials.

**in·verse jaw-wink·ing syn·drome** (in-věrs' jaw'wingk-ing sin'drōm) Condition with supranuclear lesions of trigeminal nerve, so that touching the cornea may produce a brisk movement of mandible to opposite side.

**in·verse-square law** (in-věrs' skwăr law) A rule relating to radiation stating that intensity of radiation is inversely proportional to the square of the distance from radiation source to irradiated surface.

**in·ver·sion** (in-věr'zhŭn) A turning inward, upside down, or in any direction contrary to the existing one. [L. *inverto,* pp. *-versus,* to turn upside down, to turn about]

**in·vert·ed cone bur** (in-věr'těd kōn bŭr) Rotary cutting instrument in the shape of a truncated cone with the smaller end attached to the shaft; generally used for entering carious pits or creating undercuts in cavity preparations.

**in·vest·ing** (in-vest'ing) In dentistry, covering or enveloping wholly or in part an object (e.g., denture, tooth, wax form, crown) with a refractory investment material before curing, soldering, or casting.

**in·vest·ment** (in-vest'měnt) In dentistry, any material used in investing.

**in·vest·ment cast** (in-vest'měnt kast) SYN refractory cast.

**in·vet·er·ate** (in-vet'ěr-ăt) Firmly established; said of a disease or of confirmed habits.

**in vi·tro** (in vē'trō) In an artificial environment, referring to a process or reaction occurring therein, as in a test tube. [L. in glass]

**in vi·vo** (in vē'vō) In the living body, referring to a process or reaction occurring therein. Cf. in vitro. [L. in the living being]

**in·vo·lu·crum,** pl. **in·vo·lu·cra** (in'vŏ-lū'-krŭm, -kră) **1.** An enveloping membrane. **2.** The sheath of new bone that forms around a sequestrum.

**in·vol·un·tar·y** (in-vol'ŭn-tar-ē) Independent of or contrary to the will.

**in·vo·lu·tion** (in'vŏ-lū'shŭn) **1.** Return of an enlarged organ to normal size. **2.** Turning inward of the edges of a part. [L. *in-volvo,* pp. *-volutus,* to roll up]

**io·dine (I)** (ī'ō-dīn, ī'ŏ-dēn) A nonmetallic chemical element, used in manufacture of iodine compounds and as a catalyst, reagent, or tracer among other purposes. [G. *iōdēs,* violet-like, fr. *ion,* a violet, + *eidos,* form]

**io·dine tinc·ture** (ī'ō-dīn tingk'shŭr) Hydroalcoholic solution used as an antiseptic/germicide on skin surfaces for cuts and scratches.

**io·dism** (ī'ō-dizm) Poisoning by iodine, a condition marked by severe coryza, an acneform eruption, weakness, salivation, and foul breath.

**io·do·phor** (ī-ō'dō-fōr) A combination of iodine with a surfactant carrier, usually polyvinylpyrrolidone. Used as skin disinfectants. [*iodine* + G. *phora,* a carrying]

**io·do·qui·nol** (ī-ō'dō-kwin'ol) An amebicide.

**ion** (ī'on) An atom or group of atoms carrying an electric charge by virtue of having gained or lost one or more electrons. Ions charged with negative electricity (anions) travel toward a positive pole (anode); those charged with positive electricity (cations) travel toward a negative pole (cathode). Ions may exist in solid, liquid, or gaseous environments, although those in liquid (electrolytes) are more common and familiar. [G. *iōn,* going]

**ion·i·za·tion** (ī'on-ī-zā'shŭn) Dissociation into ions, occurring when an electrolyte is dissolved in water or certain liquids or when molecules are subjected to electrical discharge or ionizing radiation.

**ion·i·za·tion cham·ber** (ī'on-ī-zā'shŭn chăm'běr) A chamber for detecting ionization of the enclosed gas.

**ion·iz·ing ra·di·a·tion** (ī'on-īz'ing rā'dē-ā'shŭn) Corpuscular or electromagnetic radiation of sufficient energy to ionize the irradiated material.

**ion·o·pho·re·sis** (ī-on'ō-fŏr-ē'sis) SYN electrophoresis. [*ion* + G. *phorēsis,* a carrying]

**ion·to·pho·re·sis** (ī-on'tō-fŏr-ē'sis) Introduction into tissues, by electric current, of ions of a medicament. [*ion* + G. *phorēsis,* a carrying]

**IOP** Abbreviation for intraocular pressure.

**IP** Abbreviation for intraperitoneal; interphalangeal; isoelectric point.

**IPA** Abbreviation for individual practice association; International Phonetic Alphabet.

**ip·e·cac sy·rup** (ip'ĕ-kak sir'ŭp) Sweetened liquid medicinal preparation containing powdered ipecac extract, which itself contains the alkaloids emetine and cephaline; used as an emetic in some cases of poisoning and (at lower doses) as an expectorant.

**ip·e·cac·uan·ha** (ip'ĕ-kak-wahn'ă) The dried root of *Uragoga (Cephaelis) ipecacuanha*; has expectorant, emetic, and antidysenteric properties.

**ip·si·lat·er·al** (ip'si-lat'ĕr-ăl) On the same side, with reference to a given point. [L. *ipse,* same, + *latus (later-),* side]

**IQ** Abbreviation for intelligence quotient.

**Ir** Symbol for iridium.

**ir·id·i·um (Ir)** (ī-rid'ē-ŭm) A white, silvery metallic element. [192]Ir is a radioisotope that has been used in the interstitial treatment of tumors. [L. *iris,* rainbow]

**ir·i·do·cy·cli·tis** (ir'i-dō-sī-klī'tis) Inflammation of both iris and ciliary body. [G. *iris,* rainbow, + *kyklos,* circle, + *-itis,* inflammation]

**i·ris,** pl. **ir·i·des** (ī'ris, ir'i-dēz) [TA] The anterior division of the vascular tunic of the eye, a diaphragm, perforated in the center (the pupil), attached peripherally to the scleral spur. [G. rainbow, the iris of the eye]

**iri·tis** (ī-rī'tis) Inflammation of the iris.

**iron** (ī'ŏrn) A metallic element that occurs in heme of hemoglobin, myoglobin, transferrin, ferritin, and iron-containing porphyrins and is an essential component of enzymes; its salts are used medicinally. [M.E. *iren,* fr. O.E. *īren*]

**iron-bind·ing ca·pac·i·ty** (ī'ŏrn bīnd'ing kă-pas'i-tē) Ability of iron-binding protein in serum (transferrin) to bind serum iron.

**iron de·fi·cien·cy a·ne·mia** (ī'ŏrn dĕ-fish'ĕn-sē ă-nē'mē-ă) Hypochromic microcytic anemia characterized by low serum iron, increased serum iron-binding capacity, decreased serum ferritin, and decreased marrow iron.

**iron sul·fate** (ī'ŏrn sŭl'fāt) Soluble iron salt frequently used as an iron supplement in tablets and liquid preparations as a hematinic.

**ir·ra·di·ate** (ir-rā'dē-āt) To apply radiation from a source to a structure or organism.

**ir·ra·di·at·ed vi·ta·min D milk** (ir-rā'dē-ā-tĕd vī'tă-min milk) Cow's milk exposed in a thin film to ultraviolet light and standardized to contain 400 USP units of vitamin D per quart.

**ir·ra·di·a·tion** (ir-rā'dē-ā'shŭn) **1.** The subjective enlargement of a bright object seen against a dark background. **2.** Exposure to the action of electromagnetic radiation. [L. *ir-radio, (in-r),* pp. *-radi-atus,* to beam forth]

**ir·reg·u·lar den·tin, ir·ri·ta·tion den·tin** (i-reg'yū-lăr den'tin, ir'i-tā'shŭn) SYN tertiary dentin.

**ir·re·spir·a·ble** (ir're-spīr'ă-bĕl) **1.** Incapable of being inhaled because of irritation to the airway, resulting in breath-holding. **2.** Denoting a gas or vapor either poisonous or containing insufficient oxygen.

**ir·re·vers·i·ble** (ir're-vĕr'si-bĕl) Incapable of being reversed; permanent. [L. *in- (ir-)* neg. + *re-verto,* pp. *-versus,* to turn back]

**ir·re·vers·i·ble col·loid** (ir're-vĕr'si-bĕl kol'oyd) Colloid that lacks capacity either to disassemble or resolubilize (or both).

**ir·re·vers·i·ble hy·dro·col·loid** (ir're-vĕr'si-bĕl hī'drō-kol'oyd) A hydrocolloid the physical state of which is changed by an irreversible chemical reaction when water is added to a powder and an insoluble substance is formed.

**ir·re·vers·i·ble pul·pi·tis** (ir're-vĕr'si-bĕl pŭl-pī'tis) Inflammation of dental pulp from which pulp is unable to recover; clinically, may be asymptomatic or characterized by pain that persists after thermal stimulation.

**ir·ri·ga·tion** (ir'i-gā'shŭn) Washing out a body cavity, space, or wound using a fluid.

**ir·ri·ga·tor** (ir'i-gā'tŏr) Device usually consisting of a reservoir with a flexible delivery tube that uses pressure to flush an area.

**ir·ri·ta·bil·i·ty** (ir'i-tă-bil'i-tē) The property inherent in protoplasm of reacting to a stimulus. [L. *irritabilitas,* fr. *irrito,* pp. *-atus,* to excite]

**ir·ri·ta·ble co·lon** (ir'i-tă-bĕl kō'lŏn) Tendency to colonic hyperperistalsis.

**ir·ri·tant** (ir'i-tănt) **1.** Irritating; causing irritation. **2.** Any agent with this action.

**ir·ri·ta·tion** (ir'i-tā'shŭn) **1.** Extreme incipient inflammatory reaction of tissues to injury. **2.** Normal response of nerve or muscle to stimulus. **3.** Evocation of normal or exaggerated reaction in tissues by application of stimulus. [L. *irritatio*]

ij

**ir·ri·ta·tion fi·bro·ma** (ir′i-tā′shŭn fī-brō′mă) Slow-growing nodule on oral mucosa, composed of fibrous tissue covered by epithelium, due to mechanical irritation by dentures, fillings, cheek biting, and other factors. See this page.

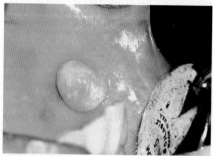

irritation fibroma: buccal mucosa

**ir·ri·ta·tion of gin·gi·val tis·sues** (ir′i-tā′shŭn jin′ji-văl tish′ūz) SYN gingivitis.

**IRV** Abbreviation for inspiratory reserve volume.

**ischaemia** [Br.] SYN ischemia.

**ischaemic heart disease** [Br.] SYN ischemic heart disease.

**ischaemic hypoxia** [Br.] SYN ischemic hypoxia.

**ischaemic necrosis** [Br.] SYN ischemic necrosis.

**is·che·mi·a** (is-kē′mē-ă) Local loss of blood supply due to mechanical vascular obstruction. SYN ischaemia.

**is·che·mic heart dis·ease** (is-kē′mik hahrt di-zēz′) A general term for diseases of the heart caused by insufficient blood supply to the myocardium. SYN ischaemic heart disease.

**is·che·mic hy·pox·i·a** (is-kē′mik hī-pok′sē-ă) Tissue hypoxia characterized by tissue oligemia and caused by obstruction or vasoconstriction. SYN ischaemic hypoxia.

**is·che·mic ne·cro·sis** (is-kē′mik nĕ-krō′sis) Cell death caused by hypoxia resulting from local deprivation of blood supply. SYN ischaemic necrosis, ischaemic necrosis.

**is·cho·chy·mi·a** (is′kō-kī′mē-ă) Retention of food in stomach due to dilation of that organ. [G. *ischō*, to keep back, + *chymos*, juice]

**is·chu·ri·a** (is-kyūr′ē-ă) Retention or suppression of urine. [G. *ischō*, to keep back, + *ouron*, urine]

**is·lets of Lan·ger·hans** (ī′lĕts lahng′er-hahnz) Cellular masses consisting of several to several hundred cells lying in interstitial pancreatic tissue.

**iso·bar** (ī′sō-bahr) One of two or more nuclides having the same total number of protons plus neutrons, but with different distribution. [*iso-* + G. *baros*, weight]

**iso-(i)** Prefix meaning equal, like. [G. *isos* equal]

**iso·e·lec·tric point (pI)** (ī′sō-ĕ-lek′trik poynt) The pH at which an amphoteric substance is electrically neutral.

**i·sog·na·thous** (ī-sog′nă-thŭs) Having jaws of approximately the same width. [*iso-* + G. *gnathos*, jaw]

**i·so·lat·ed a·but·ment** (ī′sō-lā-tĕd ă-bŭt′mĕnt) Lone-standing tooth, or tooth root, used as an abutment with edentulous areas mesial and distal to it.

**i·so·la·ted vi·ta·min E de·fi·cien·cy** (ī′sŏ-lā-tĕd vī′tă-min dĕ-fish′ĕn-sē) Ataxia due to a mutation in the gene coding for the α-tocopherol transfer protein, (α-TTP).

**iso·leu·cine (I)** (ī′sō-lū′sēn) An L-amino acid found in almost all proteins; an isomer of leucine and, like it, a dietary essential amino acid.

**iso·mer** (ī′sō-mĕr) 1. One of two or more substances displaying isomerism. 2. One of two or more nuclides having the same atomic and mass numbers but differing in energy states for a finite period of time. [*iso-* + G. *meros*, part]

**iso·met·ric** (ī′sō-met′rik) Of equal dimensions. [*iso-* + G. *metron*, measure]

**i·so·met·ric re·lax·a·tion** (ī′sō-met′rik rĕ-lak-sā′shŭn) Decrease in tension of a muscle while the length remains constant because of fixation of the ends.

**i·so·ni·a·zid** (ī′sō-nī′ă-zid) Isonicotinic acid hydrazide; first-line and probably most commonly used antituberculosis drug. Organisms rapidly develop resistance against this drug if it is used alone in the treatment of active disease.

**i·so·ni·a·zid neu·rop·a·thy** (ī′sō-nī′ă-zid nūr-op′ă-thē) Generalized polyneuropathy that occurs in some patients treated with isoniazid; its type involves axonal loss.

**i·so·phane in·su·lin** (ī′sō-fān in′sŭ-lin) SYN NPH insulin.

**i·so·pro·pyl al·co·hol** (ī′sō-prō′pil al′kŏ-hol) An isomer of propyl alcohol and a homologue of ethyl alcohol, similar in its properties, when used externally, to the latter, but more toxic when taken internally; used as an ingredient in medicinal preparations for external use.

**i·so·pro·te·re·nol** (ī′sō-prō-ter′ĕ-nol) Sympathomimetic β-receptor stimulant possessing cardiac excitatory, but not the vasoconstrictor, actions of epinephrine.

**i·sos·the·nu·ri·a** (ī-sos′thĕ-nyūr′ē-ă) A state in chronic renal disease in which kidney cannot form urine with a higher or a lower specific gravity than that of protein-free plasma. [*iso-* + G. *sthenos,* strength, + *ouron,* urine]

**i·so·tone** (ī'sō-tōn) One of several nuclides having the same number of neutrons in their nuclei. [*iso-* + G. *tonos,* stretching, tension]

**i·so·ton·ic** (ī'sō-ton'ik) **1.** Relating to isotonicity or isotonia. **2.** Having equal tension; denoting solutions possessing the same osmotic pressure. **3.** In physiology, denoting the condition when a contracting muscle shortens against a constant load.

**i·so·tope** (ī'sō-tōp) One of two or more nuclides that are chemically identical, having the same number of protons, yet differ in mass number, because their nuclei contain different numbers of neutrons. [*iso-* + G. *topos,* part, place]

**i·so·tret·i·no·in** (ī'sō-tret'i-nō'in) A retinoid used to treat severe recalcitrant cystic acne; known human teratogen.

**isth·mo·pa·ral·y·sis** (is'mō-păr-al'i-sis) Paralysis of velum pendulum palati and muscles forming anterior pillars of the fauces. [G. *isthmos,* isthmus, + *paralysis*]

**IT** Abbreviation for intrathecal.

**itch** (ich) An irritating skin sensation that arouses scratching. SYN pruritus. [A.S. *gikkan*]

**i·ter** (ī'tĕr) A passage leading from one anatomic part to another. SEE ALSO canaliculus. [L. *iter* (*itiner-*), a way, journey]

**i·ter den·tis** (ī'tĕr den'tis) Route(s) by which one or more teeth erupt.

**ITP** Abbreviation for idiopathic thrombocytopenic purpura.

**IU** Abbreviation for international unit.

**IV** Abbreviation for intravascular; intravenous, intraventricular.

**I·vy loop wir·ing** (ī'vē lūp wīr'ing) Placement of wire around two adjacent teeth to provide an attachment for intermaxillary elastics.

**Ix·o·des dam·mi·ni** (ik-sō'dēz dam'i-nī) Tick species that is a vector of Lyme disease (*Borrelia burgdorferi*) and human babesiosis (*Babesia microti*) in the U.S. Bites causing Lyme disease in humans are from nymphal ticks about the size of a pencil point, infected with *B. burgdorferi* from white-footed field mice. Adult ticks complete their 2-year life cycle feeding on deer. Also termed *I. scapularis.*

**ij**

# J

**jack·et** (jak'ĕt) In dentistry, term meaning an artificial crown composed of fired porcelain or acrylic resin.

**jack·et crown** (jak'ĕt krown) Hollow crown of acrylic resin, fused porcelain, cast gold, or combinations thereof; it fits over prepared stump of natural crown.

**jack·screw** (jak'skrū) Threaded device used in dental appliances for separation of approximated teeth or jaws.

**Jack·son crib clasp** (jak'sŏn krib klasp) One-piece clasp, usually wire, shaped to engage interproximal undercuts in adjacent natural teeth to retain a removable partial denture; also known as a Jackson crib.

**Jack·son sign** (jak'sŏn sīn) During quiet respiration the movement of the paralyzed side of the chest may be greater than that of the opposite side.

**JADA** Abbreviation for *Journal of the American Dental Association.*

**Ja·net test** (zhah-nā' test) Method to distinguish between functional or organic anesthesia.

**jar** (jahr) **1.** To jolt or shake. **2.** A jolting or shaking.

**jar·gon** (jahr'gŏn) Language or terminology peculiar to a specific field, profession, or group. [Fr. gibberish]

**Ja·risch-Herx·hei·mer re·ac·tion** (yah' rish herks'hīm-er rē-ak'shŭn) SYN Herxheimer reaction.

**jaun·dice** (jawn'dis) A yellowish staining of the integument, sclerae, deeper tissues, and excretions with bile pigments, due to increased plasma bile levels. SYN icterus.

**jaw** (jaw) **1.** One of the two bony structures in which teeth are set to form oral framework. **2.** Common name for either maxillae or mandible. [A.S. *ceōwan,* to chew]

**jaw·bone** (jaw'bōn) SYN mandible.

**jaw cyst** (jaw sist) Any epithelium-lined lesion involving the maxilla or mandible.

**jaw frac·ture** (jaw frak'shŭr) Osseous breakage or trauma to the maxilla or mandible.

**jaw gra·da·tion** (jaw grā-dā'shŭn) Controlled vertical mandibular movement during vocalization as a function of length, depth, and amount of muscular contraction.

**jaw joint** (jaw joynt) SYN temporomandibular joint.

**jaw re·flex** (jaw rē'fleks) Spasmodic contraction of temporal muscles following a downward tap on loosely hanging mandible. SYN mandibular reflex, masseter reflex.

**jaw re·la·tion rec·ord** (jaw rĕ-lā'shŭn rek' ŏrd) A registration of the positional relationship of the mandible in reference to the maxilla; relationships may be in horizontal, vertical, or other orientations.

**jaw re·po·si·tion·ing** (jaw rē'pŏ-zish'ŭn-ing) Changing of any relative position of mandible to maxillae, by altering occlusion of natural or artificial teeth or by surgical means.

**jaw sep·a·ra·tion** (jaw sep'ăr-ā'shŭn) Amount of space between jaws at any degree of opening.

**jaw skel·e·ton** (jaw skel'ĕ-tŏn) SYN viscerocranium.

**jaw-wink·ing syn·drome** (jaw'wingk'ing sin'drōm) Increased width of palpebral fissures during chewing, sometimes with a rhythmic elevation of upper lid when mouth is open and with ptosis when mouth is closed. SYN Gunn phenomenon, Marcus Gunn phenomenon.

**JCAHO** Abbreviation for Joint Commission on Accreditation of Healthcare Organizations.

**JCDA** Abbreviation for *Journal of the Canadian Dental Association.*

**je·ju·num** (je-jū'nŭm) [TA] The portion of small intestine, about 8 feet in length, between the duodenum and the ileum. [L. *jejunus,* empty]

**jerk** (jĕrk) A sudden pull.

**jerk nys·tag·mus** (jĕrk nis-tag'mŭs) Slow drift of eyes in one direction, followed by rapid recovery movement, always described in direction of recovery movement.

**jerks** (jĕrks) Chorea or any form of tic.

**jet in·jec·tor** (jet in-jek'tŏr) Device that employs high pressure to force liquid through a small orifice at a velocity sufficient to penetrate skin or mucous membrane without a needle.

**jet neb·u·li·zer** (jet neb'yū-lī-zĕr) Device that uses an air or gas stream to change a liquid into small particles.

**jew·el·er's rouge** (jū'ĕ-lĕrz rūzh) A ferric oxide compound used to impart a high luster to metals, usually gold.

**jock itch** (jok ich) SYN tinea cruris.

**jod-Ba·se·dow phe·nom·e·non** (yod-bah'zĕ-dō fĕ-nom'ĕ-non) Induction of thyrotoxicosis in patients previously euthyroid as a result of exposure to large quantities of iodine.

**John·son meth·od** (jon'sŏn meth'ŏd) SYN chloropercha method.

**joint** (joynt) [TA] ANATOMY Place of union, usually more or less movable, between two or more rigid skeletal components (bones, cartilage, or parts of a single bone). Joints between skeletal elements exhibit a great variety of form and function and are classified into three general morphologic types: fibrous, cartilaginous, and synovial. SYN articulation (2). [L. *junctura;* fr. *jungo,* pp. *junctus,* to join]

**joint cap·sule** (joynt kap′sŭl) [TA] SYN articular capsule.

**Joint Com·mis·sion on Ac·cre·di·ta·tion of Health·care Or·ga·ni·za·tions (JCAHO)** (joynt kŏ-mish′ŏn ă-kred′i-tā′shŭn helth′kār ōr′gǎn-ī-zā′shŭnz) A private, voluntary, not-for-profit group that provides accreditation to U.S. hospitals and other health care facilities.

**joint ef·fu·sion** (joynt ĕ-fyu′zhŭn) Increased fluid in synovial cavity of a joint.

**Jou·bert syn·drome** (zhū-bār′ sin′drōm) Agenesis of cerebellar vermis, characterized clinically by attacks of tachypnea or prolonged apnea, abnormal eye movements, and ataxia.

**Jour·nal of the A·mer·i·can Den·tal As·so·ci·a·tion (JADA)** (jŭr′năl ă-mer′ĭ-kăn den′tăl ă-sō′sē-ā′shŭn) Peer-reviewed journal that presents information of relevance to clinical and basic sciences related to dentistry. It is the official journal of the American Dental Association.

**Jour·nal of the Ca·na·di·an Den·tal As·so·ci·a·tion (JCDA)** (jŭr′năl kă-nā′dē-ăn den′tăl ă-sō′sē-ā′shŭn) Peer-reviewed Canadian journal that presents information of relevance to clinical and basic sciences related to dentistry. It is the authoritative voice of the Canadian Dental Association.

**judgement** [Br.] SYN judgment.

**judg·ment** (jŭj′mĕnt) Ability to evaluate aspects of a behavior or situation and act or react appropriately. SYN judgement.

**jug·u·lar wall of mid·dle ear** (jŭg′yū-lăr wawl mid′ĕl ēr) [TA] Floor of tympanic cavity.

**ju·gum,** pl. **ju·ga** (jū′gŭm, -gă) **1.** [TA] A ridge or furrow connecting two points. SYN yoke. **2.** A type of forceps. [L. a yoke]

**jump·ing dis·ease, jump·er dis·ease** (jŭmp′ing di-zēz′, jŭmp′ĕr) Pathologic startle syndromes found in isolated parts of the world, characterized by greatly exaggerated responses, such as jumping, flinging the arms, and yelling, due to minimal stimuli.

**jump·ing the bite** (jŭmp′ing bīt) Orthodontic technique for correcting a crossbite.

**junc·tion** (jŭngk′shŭn) [TA] The point, line, or surface of union of two parts, mainly bones or cartilages.

**junc·tion·al ep·i·the·li·um** (jŭngk′shŭn-ăl ep′i-thē′lē-ŭm) Wedge-shaped collar of epithelial cells attached to tooth surface and to gingival connective tissue; its coronal aspect forms base of the gingival crevice.

**jur·is·pru·dence** (jūr′is-prū′dĕns) Legal principles and concepts.

**jus·tice** (jŭs′tis) **1.** An ethical principle of fairness or equity, according equal rights to all and basing rewards on merit and punishments on guilt. **2.** NURSING ethical principle that individual people and groups with similar circumstances and conditions should be treated alike. [L. *justitia,* fr. *jus,* right, law]

**ju·ve·nile-on·set di·a·be·tes** (jū′vĕ-nil-on′set dī-ă-bē′tēz) SYN Type 1 diabetes.

**ju·ve·nile per·i·o·don·ti·tis** (jū′vĕ-nil per′ē-ō-don-tī′tis) Degenerative periodontal disease of adolescents in which periodontal destruction is out of proportion to local irritating factors present on adjacent teeth; inflammatory changes become superimposed, and bone loss, migration, and extrusion are observed. Two forms are recognized: localized, in which the destruction is limited to the incisors and first molars; and generalized, involving all teeth. SYN localized juvenile periodontitis, periodontosis.

**jux·ta·po·si·tion** (jŭks′tă-pŏ-zish′ŭn) Aggregate of several things placed side by side. [L. *juxta,* near to, + *positio,* a placing, fr. *pono,* pp. *positus,* to place]

**ij**

# K

**k** Abbreviation for kilo-.

**K1** Abbreviation for phytonadione.

**kal·li·kre·in** (kal'i-krē'in) A group of enzymes that can convert kininogen by proteolysis to bradykinin or kallidin.

**ka·o·lin** (kā'ō-lin) Hydrated aluminum silicate; when powdered and freed from gritty particles by elution, used as a demulcent and adsorbent. In dentistry, used to add toughness and opacity to porcelain teeth.

**Ka·po·si sar·co·ma (KS)** (kap'ŏ-zē sahr-kō'mă) Multifocal malignant neoplasm of primitive vasoformative tissue, occurring in skin and sometimes lymph nodes or viscera. Clinically manifested by cutaneous lesions consisting of reddish-purple to dark-blue macules, plaques, or nodules; seen most commonly in men older than 60 years of age and in AIDS patients.

**ka·rat** (kar'ăt) Measure of gold content of an alloy out of a possible 24 units (i.e., 24 units is pure gold). [Ar. *qirat*]

**Kar·ta·ge·ner syn·drome** (kahr-tag'ĕ-nĕr sin'drōm) Complete situs inversus associated with bronchiectasis and chronic sinusitis associated with ciliary dysmotility and impaired ciliary mucous transport in the respiratory epithelium.

♻ **karyo-** Combining form meaning nucleus. [G. *karyon*, nucleus]

**kar·y·o·type** (kar'ē-ō-tīp) The chromosome characteristics of an individual cell or of a cell line, usually presented as a systematized array of metaphase chromosomes from a photomicrograph of a single cell nucleus arranged in pairs in descending order of size and according to the position of the centromere. SYN idiogram (1). [*karyo-* + G. *typos*, model]

**Ka·wa·sa·ki dis·ease, Ka·wa·sa·ki syn·drome** (kah-wă-sah'kē di-zēz', sin' drōm) SYN mucocutaneous lymph node syndrome.

**Ka·zan·ji·an op·er·a·tion** (kah-zahn'jē-ăn op'ĕr-ā'shŭn) Surgical extension of vestibular sulcus of edentulous ridges to increase their height and improve denture retention.

**kcal** Abbreviation for kilocalorie; kilogram calorie.

**Kearns-Sayre syn·drome** (kĕrnz sār sin' drōm) Chronic progressive external ophthalmoplegia with associated cardiac conduction defects, short stature, and hearing loss.

**ke·loid** (kē'loyd) A nodular, firm, often linear mass of hyperplastic thickish scar tissue, consisting of irregularly distributed bands of collagen; occurs in the dermis. [G. *kēlē*, a tumor (or *kēlis*, a spot), + *eidos*, appearance]

**ke·lo·plas·ty** (kē'lō-plas'tē) Surgical removal of a scar or keloid. [*keloid* + G. *plastos*, formed]

**Ken·ne·dy bar** (ken'ĕ-dē bahr) SYN continuous bar connector.

**Ken·ne·dy clas·si·fi·ca·tion** (ken'ĕ-dē klas'i-fi-kā'shŭn) Listing of several forms of partially edentulous jaws depending on distribution of missing teeth.

**ker·a·tin** (ker'ă-tin) Collective name for a group of proteins that form intermediate filaments in epithelial cells. Keratins have a molecular weight of 40–68 kD and are either acidic or basic. Antibodies to keratin proteins are widely used for histologic typing of tumors and are especially useful for distinguishing carcinomas from sarcomas, lymphomas, and melanomas. [G. *keras (kerat-)*, horn, + *-in*]

**ker·a·tin·i·za·tion** (ker'ă-tin-ī-zā'shŭn) Keratin formation or development of a horny layer. SYN cornification.

**ker·at·i·niz·ed ep·i·the·li·um** (ker'i-tin-īzd ep'i-thē'lē-ŭm) Outer protective surface of stratified squamous epithelium.

**ker·a·tin lay·er** (ker'ă-tin lā'ĕr) Epithelial layer covered by keratinocytes protecting underlying tissues.

**ker·a·tin·o·cytes** (ker'ă-tin'ō-sīts) Cells that produce keratin. SEE ALSO keratin.

**ker·a·ti·tis** (ker'ă-tī'tis) Inflammation of the cornea. [*kerato-* + G. *-itis*, inflammation]

♻ **kerato-** 1. The cornea. 2. Horny tissue or cells. [G. *keras*, horn]

**ker·a·to·ac·an·tho·ma** (ker'ă-tō-ak'an-thō'mă) A rapidly growing, umbilicated tumor, usually occurring on exposed areas of the skin, which invades the dermis but remains localized and usually resolves spontaneously. [*kerato-* + G. *akantha*, thorn, +*-oma*, tumor]

**ker·a·to·con·junc·ti·vi·tis sic·ca** (ker' ă-tō-kŏn-jŭngk'ti-vī'tis sik'ă) A chronic mucopurulent conjunctivitis, sometimes leading to corneal ulceration and scarring. SYN dry eye syndrome.

**ker·a·to·cyst** (ker'ă-tō-sist) Odontogenic lesion derived from remnants of dental lamina and appearing as a unilocular or multilocular radiolucency that may produce jaw expansion; epithelial lining is characterized microscopically by a uniform thickness, a corrugated superficial layer of parakeratin, and a prominent basal layer composed of palisaded columnar cells.

**ker·a·to·der·ma** (ker'ă-tō-dĕr'mă) 1. Any horny superficial growth. 2. A generalized thickening of the horny layer of the epidermis. [*kerato-* + G. *derma*, skin]

**ker·a·to·der·ma blen·nor·rha·gi·cum** (ker′ă-tō-dĕr′mă blen′ō-raj′i-kŭm) Scattered, thickened, hyperkeratotic skin lesions (e.g., pustules, crusts) seen in Reiter syndrome.

**ker·a·tol·y·sis** (ker′ă-tol′i-sis) *Avoid the mispronunciation keratoly′sis.* **1.** Separation or loosening of horny epidermal layer. **2.** Specifically, disease characterized by shedding of epidermis recurring at more or less regular intervals. [*kerato-* + G. *lysis,* loosening]

**ker·a·to·plas·ty** (ker′ă-tō-plas′tē) Removal of a portion of the cornea and replacement with a piece of cornea of the same size and shape removed from elsewhere. SYN corneal graft. [*kerato-* + G. *plassō,* to form]

**ker·a·to·sis,** pl. **ker·a·to·ses** (ker′ă-tō′sis, -sēz) Any epidermal lesion marked by circumscribed overgrowths of horny layer. See this page and page A10. [*kerato-* + G. *-osis,* condition]

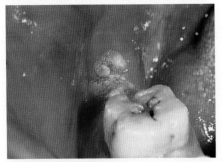
**frictional keratosis:** white lesion due to trauma

**ker·a·to·sis fol·lic·u·la·ris** (ker′ă-tō′sis fŏ-lik′yū-lā′ris) A familial eruption, beginning usually in childhood, in which keratotic papules originating from both follicles and interfollicular epidermis of the trunk, face, scalp, and axillae become crusted and verrucous; often intensely pruritic. SYN Darier disease, Hailey and Hailey disease.

**ker·nic·ter·us** (kĕr-nik′tĕr-ŭs) Yellow staining and degenerative lesions in basal ganglia associated with high levels of unconjugated bilirubin in infants; characterized by opisthotonos, high-pitched cry, lethargy and poor sucking, and loss of upward gaze; later consequences include deafness, cerebral palsy, other sensorineural deficits, and mental retardation. SYN bilirubin encephalopathy, nuclear jaundice. [Ger. *Kern,* kernel (nucleus), + *ikterus,* jaundice]

**ker·o·sene** (ker′ŏ-sēn) A mixture of petroleum hydrocarbons, chiefly of the methane series; used as fuel for lamps and stoves, as a degreaser and cleaner, and in insecticides. [G. *kēros,* wax, + *-ene*]

**ket·a·mine** (kēt′ă-mēn) A parenterally administered anesthetic that produces catatonia, profound analgesia, increased sympathetic activity, and little relaxation of skeletal muscles; side-effects include sialorrhea and occasional pronounced dysphoria.

**ke·to·ac·i·do·sis** (kē′tō-as-i-dō′sis) Acidosis, as in diabetes or starvation, caused by enhanced production of ketone bodies.

**ke·to·ac·i·du·ri·a** (kē′tō-as-i-dyūr′ē-ă) Excretion of urine with elevated content of keto acids.

**ke·to·gen·ic:an·ti·ke·to·gen·ic ra·ti·o** (kē′tō-jen′ik non′kē′tō-jen′ik rā′shē-ō) Proportion between substances that form ketones in the body and those that form D-glucose.

**ke·tone** (kē′tōn) A substance with the carbonyl group linking two carbon atoms; acetone is the most important in medicine and the simplest in chemistry.

**ke·tone bod·y** (kē′tōn bod′ē) One of a group of ketones that includes acetoacetate, its reduction product, β-hydroxybutyrate, and its decarboxylation product, acetone.

**ke·to·nu·ri·a** (kē′tō-nyūr′ē-ă) Enhanced urinary excretion of ketone bodies.

**ke·to·pro·fen** (kē′tō-prō′fĕn) Antiinflammatory drug given orally or rectally to treat vascular headache, dysmenorrhea, and rheumatic and nonrheumatic disorders.

**ke·to·sis** (kē-tō′sis) Condition characterized by enhanced production of ketone bodies, as in diabetes mellitus or starvation. [*ketone* + *-osis,* condition]

**ke·to·su·ri·a** (kē′tō-syū′rē-ă′) Presence of ketones in urine.

**ke·tot·ic hy·per·gly·ci·ne·mi·a** (kē-tot′ik hī′pĕr-glī-sē′mē-ă) Inherited metabolic disorder resulting from a deficiency of propionyl-CoA carboxylase PCC; clinical features are episodic vomiting and lethargy with hyperglycinemia and ketoacidosis; death may follow. SYN methylmalonic acidemia.

**key at·tach·ment** (kē ă-tach′mĕnt) SYN precision attachment.

**key·way** (kē′wā) In dentistry, the female portion of a precision attachment.

**key·way at·tach·ment** (kē′wā ă-tach′mĕnt) SYN precision attachment.

**kg** Abbreviation for kilogram.

**KHN** Abbreviation for Knoop hardness number.

**kHz** Abbreviation for kilohertz.

**kid·ney** (kid′nē) [TA] One of the paired organs that excrete urine, remove nitrogenous wastes of metabolism, reclaim important electrolytes and water, contribute to blood pressure control, and erythropoiesis.

kl

**kid·ney fail·ure** (kid'nē fāl'yŭr) SYN renal failure.

**Kies·sel·bach ar·e·a** (kē´sĕl-bahk ar´ē-ă) Anterior nasal septal region rich in capillaries that is frequently the site of epistaxis.

♻ **kilo- (k)** Prefix used in the SI and metric system to signify one thousand ($10^3$). [G. *chilioi,* one thousand]

**kil·o·cal·o·rie (kcal)** (kil'ŏ-kal'ŏr-ē) The quantity of energy required to raise the temperature of 1 kg of water from 14.5–15.5°C. SYN kilogram calorie, large calorie.

**kil·o·gram (kg)** (kil'ŏ-gram) The SI unit of mass, 1000 g.

**kil·o·gram cal·o·rie (kcal)** (kil'ŏ-gram kal'ŏr-ē) SYN kilocalorie.

**kil·o·hertz (kHz)** (kil´ŏ-hĕrts) A unit of frequency equal to $10^3$ hertz.

**kil·o·volt** (kil'ŏ-vōlt) A unit of electrical potential or potential difference equal to $10^3$ volts.

**kil·o·volt peak (kVp)** (kil'ŏ-vōlt pēk) Maximum voltage used in x-ray exposures.

**kinaesthesia** [Br.] SYN kinesthesia.

**kinaesthesiometer** [Br.] SYN kinesthesiometer.

**kinaesthesis** [Br.] SYN kinesthesia.

**kinaesthetic** [Br.] SYN kinesthetic.

**kinaesthetic sense** [Br.] SYN kinesthetic sense.

**kin·e·mat·ic face-bow** (kin´ĕ-mat´ik fās´ bō) SYN adjustable axis face-bow.

**ki·ne·sics** (ki-nē'siks) The study of nonverbal bodily motion in communication.

**ki·ne·si·ol·o·gy** (ki-nē'sē-ol'ŏ-jē) Science or the study of movement, and active and passive structures involved. [G. *kinēsis,* movement, + *-logos,* study]

**kin·es·the·si·a, kin·es·the·sis** (kin'es-thē'zē-ă, -sis) 1. Sense perception of movement; muscular sense. 2. Illusion of moving in space. SYN kinaesthesia, kinaesthesis. [G. *kinēsis,* motion, + *aisthēsis,* sensation]

**kin·es·the·si·om·e·ter** (kin'es-thē'zē-om' ĕ-tĕr) An instrument for determining the degree of muscular sensation. SYN kinaesthesiometer. [*kinesthesia,* + G. *metron,* measure]

**kin·es·thet·ic** (kin'es-thet'ik) 1. Relating to kinesthesia. 2. A person who preferentially uses mental imagery of sensate experience. SYN kinaesthetic.

**kin·es·thet·ic sense** (kin'es-thet'ik sens) Sensation of muscle contraction. SYN kinaesthetic sense.

**ki·net·ics** (ki-net'iks) The study of motion, acceleration, or rate of change.

**Kings·ley splint** (kingz'lē splint) Winged maxillary device used to apply traction to reduce maxillary fractures as well as immobilize them by having the wings attached to a head appliance by elastics.

**ki·nin** (kī'nin) Polypeptide hormones released from diffuse stores and not from specialized tissue, rapidly inactivated at the site of release. [G. *kineō,* to move, + *-in*]

**kink** (kingk) An angulation, bend, or twist.

**Kirk·land knife** (kĭrk´lănd nīf) Heart-shaped bladed device used in gingival surgery.

**Kirsch·ner wire (K-wire)** (kĭrsh'nĕr wīr) An apparatus for skeletal traction in long bone fracture fixation.

**Kisch re·flex** (kish rē'fleks) Closure of eye in response to stimulation of skin at depth of external auditory meatus.

**Kleine-Le·vin syn·drome** (klīn lĕ-vin´ sin´drōm) Periodic hypersomnia associated with bulimia, occurring in males aged 10–25 years.

**klep·to·ma·ni·a** (klep'tō-mā'nē-ă) A disorder of impulse control with a morbid tendency to steal. [G. *kleptō,* to steal, + *mania,* insanity]

**Kline·fel·ter syn·drome** (klīn'fel-tĕr sin' drōm) Chromosomal anomaly; buccal and other cells are usually sex chromatin positive; patients are male in development but have seminiferous tubule dysgenesis resulting in azospermia and infertility.

**Klip·pel-Feil syn·drome** (klip´ĕl fīl sin´ drōm) A congenital abnormality of the spine characterized by a reduction in the number of cervical vertebrae and their fusion.

**knee** (nē) [TA] 1. SYN genu (1). 2. Any structure of angular shape resembling a flexed knee. [A.S. *cneōw*]

**knife** (nīf) A cutting tool consisting of a relatively long, narrow blade with one edge sharpened and a handle. Various specialized types are used in surgery and dissection. [M.E. *knif,* fr. A.S. *cnif,* fr. O. Norse *knīfr*]

**knob** (nob) A protuberance; a mass; a nodule.

**Knoop hard·ness num·ber (KHN)** (nūp hahrd´nĕs nŭm´bĕr) Measure; used to measure hardness of any materials, especially very hard and brittle substances, such as tooth dentin and enamel.

**Knoop hard·ness test** (knūp hahrd´nĕs test) Dental measurement to determine hardness of brittle materials; uses a diamond or rhombic indenting tool; test result provides dental clinicians with the Knoop hardness number.

**knot** (not) **1.** Intertwining of ends of two cords, or sutures such that they cannot easily become separated. **2.** ANATOMY, PATHOLOGY a node, ganglion, or circumscribed swelling. [A.S. *cnotta*]

**knurl·ing** (nŭr′ling) Texturing of a knob or handle as by a continuous series of milled ridges to improve the clinician's grasp.

**Koe·nig syn·drome** (ker′nig sin′drōm) Alternating attacks of constipation and diarrhea, with colic, meteorism, and gurgling in the right iliac fossa.

**koi·lo·cyte** (koy′lō-sīt) A squamous cell, showing a perinuclear halo; characteristic of condyloma acuminatum.

**koi·lo·cy·to·sis** (koy′lō-sī-tō′sis) Perinuclear vacuolation.

**ko·lyt·ic** (kō-lit′ik) Denoting an inhibitory action. [G. *kolyō*, to hinder]

**ko·ni·o·cor·tex** (kō′nē-ō-kōr′teks) Regions of the cerebral cortex characterized by a particularly well-developed inner granular layer (layer 4); this type of cerebral cortex is represented by the primary sensory Brodmann area 17 of the visual cortex, Brodmann areas 1–3 of the somatic sensory cortex, and Brodmann area 41 of the auditory cortex.

**Kop·lik spots** (kop′lik spots) Small red lesions on buccal mucous membrane, in the center of each of which may be seen, with light, a minute bluish white speck; early in measles (morbilli), before skin eruption.

**Korff fi·bers** (kōrf fī′bĕrz) Fan-shaped arrangements of type I collagen fibers located in mantle dentin.

**ko·ro·ni·on** (kŏ-rō′nē-on) SYN coronion.

**Ko·rot·koff sounds** (kō-rot′kof sowndz) Characteristic noise heard over an artery when pressure over it is reduced below systolic arterial pressure.

**Kor·sa·koff syn·drome** (kor′sĕ-kawf sin′drōm) Alcohol amnestic syndrome characterized by confusion and severe impairment of memory, especially for recent events, for which the patient compensates by confabulation. Typically encountered in patients with long-term alcoholism, delirium tremens may precede syndrome, and Wernicke syndrome often coexists with it.

**Kr** Symbol for krypton.

**Krebs-Ring·er so·lu·tion** (krebz ring′ĕr sŏ-lū′shŭn) Modification of Ringer solution.

**Krue·ger in·stru·ment stop** (krū′gĕr in′strŭ-mĕnt stop) Mechanical device limiting insertion of a root canal instrument into a canal.

**kryp·ton (Kr)** (krip′ton) One of the inert gases, present in small amounts in the atmosphere; used in studies of cardiac abnormalities.

**KS** Abbreviation for Kaposi sarcoma.

**Kuss·maul res·pi·ra·tion** (kūs′mowl res′pir-ā′shŭn) Deep, rapid respiration characteristic of diabetic or other types of acidosis.

**kVp** Abbreviation for kilovolt peak.

**kVp se·lec·tor** (sĕ-lek′tŏr) An adjustable control on an x-ray unit that controls the kilovoltage setting.

**kwa·shi·or·kor** (kwah-shē-ōr′kōr) A dietary protein deficiency disease seen originally in African children; involving anemia, edema, pot belly, dermal depigmentation, loss of hair or change in hair color to red, and other signs.

**K-wire** Abbreviation for Kirschner wire.

**ky·pho·sco·li·o·sis** (kī′fō-skō-lē-ō′sis) Lateral and posterior curvature of spine. [G. *kyphōsis*, kyphosis, + *scoliosis*, curved]

**ky·pho·sis** (kī-fō′sis) **1.** An anteriorly concave curvature of the vertebral column; normal kyphoses of the thoracic and sacral regions are retained portions of the primary curvature of the vertebral column. **2.** Forward curvature of spine. [G. *kyphōsis*, hump-back, fr. *kyphos*, bent, hump-backed]

kl

# L

**L** Abbreviation for inductance; limes; liter.

**La·band syn·drome** (lă-band′ sin′drōm)
Fibromatosis of gingivae associated with hypoplasia of distal phalanges and nail dysplasia.

**la·bel (sig)** (lā′běl) To incorporate into a compound a substance that is readily detected, whereby its metabolism can be followed or its physical distribution detected.

**la belle in·dif·fér·ence** (lah bel an-dēf-ār-ahns′) Naive, inappropriate calmness or lack of concern in the face of perceptions by others of one's disability. [Fr.]

**la·bi·al** (lā′bē-ăl) **1.** Relating to lips or any labia. **2.** Toward a lip. **3.** A letter formed with lips. [L. *labium*, lip]

**la·bi·al arch** (lā′bē-ăl ahrch) Orthodontic arch wire that approximates labial surfaces of teeth.

**la·bi·al bar** (lā′bē-ăl bahr) Major connector located labially to dental arch joining two or more bilateral parts of a mandibular removable partial denture.

**la·bi·al com·mis·sure (of mouth)** (lā′bē-ăl kom′i-shŭr mowth) [TA] Junction of upper and lower lips lateral to mouth angle. SYN commissure of lips (of mouth).

**la·bi·al em·bra·sure** (lā′bē-ăl em-brā′shŭr) Space existing on facial aspect of interproximal contact area between adjacent anterior teeth.

**la·bi·al flange** (lā′bē-ăl flanj) Portion of flange of a denture that occupies the labial vestibule of mouth.

**la·bi·al fre·num** (lā′bē-ăl frē′nŭm) Folds of mucous membrane extending from gingiva to midline of lower and upper lips, respectively.

**la·bi·al gin·gi·va** (lā′bē-ăl jin′ji-vă) Portion of gingiva that covers labial surfaces of teeth and alveolar process.

**la·bi·al glands** (lā′bē-ăl glandz) [TA] Mucous glands in submucous tissue of lips.

**la·bi·al·ly** (lā′bē-ăl-ē) Toward the lips.

**la·bi·al mu·co·sa** (lā′bē-ăl myū-kō′să) The tissue lining that covers the inside of the lips. It consists mainly of the epithelium and subjacent connective tissue. See this page.

**la·bi·al notch** (lā′bē-ăl noch) An indentation placed in the flange of a denture base to accommodate the labial frenum.

**la·bi·al oc·clu·sion** (lā′bē-ăl ŏ-klū′zhŭn)

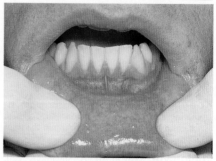
**labial mucosa:** inner lining of the lips

**1.** Malposition of tooth in a labial direction. **2.** Occlusion as seen from labial side of arches.

**la·bi·al splint** (lā′bē-ăl splint) Appliance of plastic, metal, or a combination, made to conform to outer aspect of dental arch and used to manage jaw and facial injuries.

**la·bi·al sul·cus** (lā′bē-ăl sŭl′kŭs) Furrow between developing lip and gingiva. SYN lip sulcus.

**la·bi·al sur·face of tooth** (lā′bē-ăl sŭr′făs tūth) [TA] Vestibular surface of anterior tooth that contacts vestibular surface of upper or lower lips. SYN facies labialis dentis.

**la·bi·al ves·ti·bule** (lā′bē-ăl ves′ti-byūl) That part of the oral vestibule related to the lips.

**la·bile** (lā′bīl) *Do not confuse this word with labial.* **1.** An adaptability to alteration or modification. **2.** Constituents of serum affected by increases in heat. **3.** Easily removable, e.g., a labile hydrogen atom. [L. *labilis*, liable to slip, fr. *labor*, pp. *lapsus*, to slip]

**labio-** Prefix meaning relating to lips. SEE ALSO cheilo-. [L. *labium*, lip]

**la·bi·o·cer·vi·cal** (lā′bē-ō-sěr′vi-kăl) Relating to lip and neck; specifically, to labial or buccal dental surfaces.

**la·bi·o·cli·na·tion** (lā′bē-ō-kli-nā′shŭn) Inclination of position more toward lips than normal; said of a tooth.

**la·bi·o·den·tal** (lā′bē-ō-den′tăl) **1.** Relating to lips and teeth. **2.** Letters the sound of which is formed by both lips and teeth.

**la·bi·o·gin·gi·val** (lā′bē-ō-jin′ji-văl) Relating to point of junction of labial border and gingival line on distal or mesial surface of an incisor tooth.

**la·bi·o·gin·gi·val lam·i·na** (lā′bē-ō-jin′ji-văl lam′i-nă) Band of ectodermal epithelial cells growing into mesenchyme of embryonic jaws between developing lip and the growing gingival elevation.

**la·bi·o·glos·so·la·ryn·ge·al** (lā′bē-ō-glos′ō-lă-rin′jē-ăl) Relating to lips, tongue, and larynx. [*labio-* + G. *glōssa,* tongue, + larynx]

**la·bi·o·glos·so·pha·ryn·ge·al** (lā′bē-ō-glos′ō-fă-rin′jē-ăl) Relating to lips, tongue, and pharynx. [*labio-* + G. *glōssa,* tongue, + pharynx]

**la·bi·o·lin·gual ap·pli·ance** (lā′bē-ō-ling′gwăl ă-plī′ăns) Orthodontic appliance with a maxillary labial and mandibular lingual arch wires.

**la·bi·o·lin·gual plane** (lā′bē-ō-ling′gwăl plān) Plane parallel to labial and lingual surfaces of teeth.

**la·bi·o·men·tal** (lā′bē-ō-men′tăl) Relating to lower lip and chin. [*labio-* + L. *mentum,* chin]

**la·bi·o·na·sal** (lā′bē-ō-nā′zăl) **1.** Relating to upper lip and the nose. **2.** Letter that is both labial and nasal in the production of its sound.

**la·bi·o·pal·a·tine** (lā′bē-ō-pal′ă-tīn) Relating to lips and palate.

**la·bi·o·place·ment** (lā′bē-ō-plās′mĕnt) Positioning a tooth more toward the lips than normal.

**la·bi·o·plas·ty** (lā′bē-ō-plas′tē) Plastic surgery of a lip. [*labio-* + G. *plastos,* formed]

**la·bi·o·ver·sion** (lā′bē-ō-vĕr′zhŭn) Malposition of anterior tooth from normal line of occlusion toward lips.

**la·bi·um,** pl. **la·bi·a** (lā′bē-ŭm, -ă) [TA] Any lip-shaped structure. [L.]

**la·bi·um su·pe·ri·us o·ris** (lā′bē-ŭm sū-pē′rē-ŭs ōr′is) [TA] The upper lip.

**lab·o·ra·to·ry** (lab′ŏ-ră-tōr-ē, lă-bōr′ă-trē) Place equipped for performance of tests, experiments, and procedures and for preparation of reagents and therapeutic chemical materials.

**lab·o·ra·to·ry di·ag·no·sis** (lab′ŏ-ră-tōr-ē dī-ăg-nō′sis) Diagnosis made by chemical, microscopic, microbiologic, immunologic, or pathologic study of secretions, discharges, blood, or tissue.

**la·bor·ed res·pi·ra·tion** (lā′bŏrd res′pir-ā′shŭn) Difficult, usually deep, breathing in patients with cardiac or pulmonary disease.

**la·bra·le in·fe·ri·us** (lă-brā′lē in-fē′rē-ŭs) Point where boundary of vermilion border of lower lip and the skin is intersected by median sagittal plane.

**la·bra·le su·pe·ri·us** (lă-brā′lē sū-pē′rē-ŭs) Point on upper lip lying in median sagittal plane on a line drawn across boundary of vermilion border and skin.

**la·brum,** pl. **la·bra** (lā′brŭm, -bră) [TA] **1.** A lip. **2.** A lip-shaped structure. **3.** A fibrocartilaginous lip around the margin of the concave portion of some joints. SYN articular lip. [L.]

**lab·y·rinth** (lab′i-rinth) [TA] Internal or inner ear, composed of the semicircular ducts, vestibule, and cochlea.

**lab·y·rin·thine a·po·plex·y** (lab′i-rin′thīn ap′ŏ-plek′sē) Clinical syndrome manifested as a single, abrupt attack of severe vertigo, nausea, and vomiting, with permanent loss of labyrinthine function on one side, but without associated hearing loss or tinnitus.

**lab·y·rin·thine ar·te·ry** (lab′i-rin′thīn ahr′tĕr-ē) [TA] Internal acoustic meatal branch; branch of basilar artery that enters bony labyrinth through internal acoustic meatus. SYN artery of labyrinth.

**lab·y·rin·thine re·flex·es** (lab′i-rin′thīn rē′fleks-ĕz) Reflexes initiated through stimulation of receptors in the utricle or semicircular canals. SEE ALSO statokinetic reflex.

**lab·y·rin·thine right·ing re·flex·es** (lab′i-rin′thīn rīt′ing rē′fleks-ĕz) Reflexes initiated through stimulation of receptors of labyrinth, causing changes in tone of neck muscles that bring head into appropriate position.

**lab·y·rin·thine veins** (lab′i-rin′thīn vānz) [TA] One or more veins accompanying the labyrinthine artery; drain internal ear, pass out through internal acoustic meatus, and empty into transverse sinus or the inferior petrosal sinus.

**lab·y·rin·thine wall of tym·pan·ic cav·i·ty** (lab′i-rin′thīn wawl tim-pan′ik kav′i-tē) [TA] Bony layer separating middle from internal ear or labyrinth.

**lac·er·a·tion** (las′ĕr-ā′shŭn) *Avoid using this term to describe all open wounds, including incised wounds.* **1.** Torn or jagged wound. **2.** Act of tearing tissues. See this page. [L. *lacero,* pp. *-atus,* to tear to pieces]

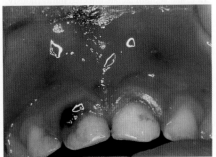

**oral trauma:** multiple injuries including lacerations of the upper lip and labial frenum and subluxation of right central incisor

kl

**lac·ri·mal ap·pa·ra·tus** (lak'ri-măl ap'ă-rat'ŭs) [TA] Consisting of the lacrimal gland, the lacrimal lake, the lacrimal canaliculi, the lacrimal sac, and the nasolacrimal duct.

**lac·ri·mal bone** (lak'ri-măl bōn) [TA] An irregularly rectangular thin plate, forming part of the medial wall of the orbit behind the frontal process of the maxilla; it articulates with the inferior nasal concha, ethmoid, frontal, and maxillary bones.

**lac·ri·mal flu·id** (lak'ri-măl flū'id) Watery physiologic saline that also contains the bacteriocidal enzyme lysozyme; it moistens the conjunctiva and cornea. SYN tears.

**lac·ri·mal nerve** (lak'ri-măl nĕrv) [TA] A branch of the ophthalmic nerve supplying sensory fibers to the lateral part of the upper eyelid, conjunctiva, and lacrimal gland. SYN nervus lacrimalis [TA].

**lac·ri·mal re·flex** (lak'ri-măl rē'fleks) Discharge of tears when conjunctiva is irritated.

**lac·ri·ma·tor** (lak'ri-mā-tŏr) An agent (e.g., tear gas) that irritates eyes and produces tears. [L. *lacrima,* tear]

**lac·ri·mo·gus·ta·to·ry re·flex** (lak'ri-mō-gŭs'tă-tōr-ē rē'fleks) Chewing of food that causes secretion of tears.

**lac·ri·mo·max·il·lar·y su·ture** (lak'ri-mō-mak'si-lar-ē sū'chŭr) [TA] Line of union, on medial wall of orbit, between anterior and inferior margins of lacrimal bone and maxilla.

**lact·ac·i·do·sis** (lakt-as'i-dō'sis) Acidosis due to increased lactic acid.

**lac·tal·bu·min** (lak'tal-bū'min) The albumin fraction of milk.

**lac·tate de·hy·dro·gen·ase (LDH)** (lak' tāt dē'hī-droj'ĕn-ās) Name for four enzymes; of diagnostic use in myocardial infarction.

**lac·tat·ed Ring·er in·jec·tion** (lak'tā-tĕd ring'ĕr sŏ-lū'shŭn) Sterile solution of calcium chloride, potassium chloride, sodium chloride, and sodium lactate injected intravenously.

**lac·tic** (lak'tik) Relating to milk. [L. *lac* (*lact-*), milk]

**lac·tic ac·id** (lak'tik as'id) Normal intermediate in the fermentation of sugar. In concentrated form, a caustic used internally to prevent gastrointestinal fermentation.

**lac·tic ac·i·do·sis** (lak'tik as'i-dō'sis) Metabolic acidosis caused by accumulation of lactic acid due to tissue hypoxia, drug effect, or unknown etiology.

*Lac·to·ba·cil·lus ac·i·doph·i·lus* (lak'tō-bă-sil'ŭs as'i-dof'i-lŭs) A bacterial species found in the feces of milk-fed infants and also in the feces of older people on a high milk-, lactose-, or dextrin-containing diet.

**lac·to·fer·rin** (lak'tō-fer'in) A transferrin found in the milk of several mammalian species.

**lac·tone** (lak'tōn) An intramolecular organic anhydride formed from a hydroxyacid by the loss of water between an –OH and a –COOH group; a cyclic ester.

**lac·to·per·ox·i·dase** (lak'tō-pĕr-ok'si-dās) A milk peroxidase that catalyzes oxidation of iodide to iodine.

**lac·tose** (lak'tōs) A disaccharide present in cow's milk and used in food for infants and convalescents and in pharmaceutical preparations. SYN milk sugar.

**lac·tose in·tol·er·ance** (lak'tōs in-tol' ĕr-ăns) Disorder characterized by abdominal cramps and diarrhea after consumption of food that contains lactose (e.g., milk, ice cream).

**lac·to·veg·e·tar·i·an** (lak'tō-vej-ĕ-tar'ē-ăn) One who lives on a mixed diet of milk and milk products, eggs, and vegetables, but avoids meat or seafood.

**la·cu·na,** pl. **la·cu·nae** (lă-kū'nă, -nē) 1. [TA] Small space, cavity, or depression. 2. Gap or defect. 3. Abnormal space between strata or between the cellular elements of the epidermis.

**Laën·nec cir·rho·sis** (lah-ĕ-nek' sir-ō'sis) Hepatic disorder in which normal liver lobules are replaced by small regeneration nodules, sometimes containing fat, separated by a fairly regular framework of fine fibrous tissue strands (hob-nail liver); usually due to chronic alcoholism.

**laevo-** [Br.] SYN levo-.

**laevodopa** [Br.] SYN levodopa.

**lake** (lāk) 1. Small collection of fluid. 2. To cause blood plasma to become red as a result of hemoglobin release from erythrocytes. [A.S. *lacu,* fr. L. *lacus,* lake]

**lamb·da** (lam'dă) 1. The 11th letter of the Greek alphabet. 2. Symbol (λ) for Avogadro number; wavelength; radioactive constant; Ostwald solubility coefficient; molar conductivity of an electrolyte (Λ). 3. The craniometric point at the junction of the sagittal and lambdoid sutures.

**la·mel·la,** pl. **la·mel·lae** (lă-mel'ă, -lē) 1. [TA] Thin sheet or layer or sublayer. 2. Medicated gelatin disc used to make local applications to conjunctiva. [L. dim. of *lamina,* plate, leaf]

**lam·i·na,** pl. **lam·i·nae** (lam'i-nă, -nē) [TA] SEE ALSO layer, stratum. SYN plate (1). [L]

**lam·i·na den·sa** (lam'i-nă den'să) 1. The electron-dense layer of the basal lamina as seen under the electron microscope. 2. The extraordinarily thick basal lamina of the renal glomerulus. SYN basal lamina (2).

**lam·i·na den·ta·ta** (lam´i-nă den-tā´tă) SYN vestibular lip of spiral limbus.

**lam·i·na du·ra** (lam´i-nă dūr´ă) The dense radioopaque layer of alveolar bone lining the tooth socket.

**lam·i·nag·ra·phy, lam·i·nog·ra·phy** (lam´i-nag´ră-fē, -nog´ră-fē) Radiographic technique in which the images of tissues above and below plane of interest are blurred out by reciprocal movement of x-ray tube and film holder, to clarify a specific area. [G. *lamina*, layer. + G. *graphē*, a writing]

**lam·i·na pro·pri·a** (lam´i-nă prō´prē-ă) [TA] Layer of connective tissue underlying mucous membrane epithelium.

**lam·i·nar, lam·i·nat·ed** (lam´i-năr, -nā´tĕd) 1. Arranged in plates or laminae. 2. Relating to any lamina.

**lam·i·nate ve·neer res·to·ra·tion** (lam´i-năt vĕ-nēr´ res´tŏr-ā´shŭn) A porcelain dental appliance bonded to the front surface of an anterior tooth to improve appearance, close up existing spaces, and improve alignment of the tooth.

**lam·i·nec·to·my** (lam´i-nek´tŏ-mē) Excision of a vertebral lamina; commonly used to denote removal of the posterior arch. [L. *lamina*, layer, + G. *ektomē*, excision]

**lam·i·nin (LN)** (lam´i-nin) A large, multimeric glycoprotein component of the basement membrane, particularly the lamina lucida; it has binding sites for integrins, type IV collagen, and heparan sulfate. It is a major protein component of the lamina lucida of the renal glomerulus.

**lamp** (lamp) Illuminating device; source of light. SEE ALSO light.

**lance** (lans) 1. To incise a body part, as an abscess or boil. 2. A lancet.

**lan·ci·nat·ing** (lan´si-nāt-ing) Denoting a sharp cutting or tearing pain. [L. *lancino*, pp. -atus, to tear]

**land·mark** (land´mahrk) Anatomic structure used in locating, identifying, referencing, and measurement.

**Lang·er·hans cell his·ti·o·cy·to·sis** (lahng´er-hahnz sel his´tē-ō-sī-tō´sis) Set of closely related disorders unified by a common proliferating element, the Langerhans cell. Three overlapping clinical syndromes are recognized: single site disease, multifocal unisystem process, and a multifocal, multisystem histiocytosis.

**Lan·ger·hans cells** (lahng´er-hahnz selz) Dendritic clear cells in epidermis, containing distinctive granules that appear rod- or racket-shaped in section, but lacking tonofilaments, melanosomes, and desmosomes.

**Lang·er lines** (lahng´ĕr līnz) SEE tension lines.

**lan·guage** (lang´gwăj) Use of spoken, manual, written, and other symbols to express, represent, or receive communication. [L. *lingua*]

**lan·guage zone** (lang´gwăj zōn) Large area of cerebral cortex on left side (in right-handed persons) considered by some to embrace all centers of memories and associations connected with language.

**lan·i·ar·y** (lan´ē-ar-ē) Adapted for tearing; in anatomy, sometimes applied to canine teeth (i.e., laniary teeth). [L. *lanio*, to tear to pieces]

**lap·a·rot·o·my** (lap´ă-rot´ŏ-mē) 1. Incision into the loin. 2. SYN celiotomy. [*laparo-* + G. *tomē*, incision]

**large cal·o·rie** (lahrj kal´ŏr-ē) SYN kilocalorie.

**large in·ter·arch dis·tance** (lahrj in´tĕr-ahrch´ dis´tăns) Space between maxillary and mandibular arches. SYN open bite (1).

**large in·tes·tine** (lahrj in-tes´tin) [TA] The portion of the digestive tube extending from the ileocecal valve to the anus; it comprises the cecum, colon, rectum, and anal canal.

**lar·va mi·grans** (lahr´vă mī´granz) Larval worm, typically a nematode, which wanders for a period in the host tissues but does not develop to the adult stage. [L. *larva*, mask, + *migro*, to transfer, migrate]

**la·ryn·ge·al cav·i·ty** (lă-rin´jē-ăl kav´i-tē) [TA] Cavity continuous above with the pharynx at the level of the aryepiglottic folds and extends downward through the rima glottidis to the infraglottic space. SYN cavity of larynx.

**la·ryn·ge·al cri·sis** (lă-rin´jē-ăl krī´sis) Attack of paralysis or spasm of laryngeal abductor muscles with dyspnea and noisy respiration.

**la·ryn·ge·al diph·the·ri·a** (lă-rin´jē-ăl dif-thĕr´ē-ă) Diphtheria affecting the larynx, usually with asphyxiation due to airway obstruction by membrane that forms, with fatal outcome.

**la·ryn·ge·al ep·i·lep·sy** (lă-rin´jē-ăl ep´i-lep-sē) Reflex epilepsy precipitated by coughing.

**la·ryn·ge·al in·let** (lă-rin´jē-ăl in´lĕt) [TA] The aperture between the pharynx and larynx, bounded by the superior edges of the epiglottis, the aryepiglottic folds, and the mucosa between the arytenoids. SYN aditus laryngis [TA].

**la·ryn·ge·al lym·phoid nod·ules** (lă-rin´jē-ăl lim´foyd nod´yūlz) Small follicles located on the posterior aspect of the epiglottis and laryngeal ventricle. SYN laryngeal tonsils.

**la·ryn·ge·al prom·i·nence** (lă-rin´jē-ăl

kl

prom′i-nĕns) [TA] The projection on the anterior portion of the neck formed by the thyroid cartilage of the larynx; serves as an external indication of the level of the fifth cervical vertebra. sᴜɴ Adam's apple.

**la·ryn·ge·al sac·cule** (lă-rin′jē-ăl sak′yūl) [TA] Small diverticulum provided with mucous glands extending upward from ventricle of larynx between vestibular fold and lamina of thyroid cartilage. sᴜɴ saccule of larynx.

**la·ryn·ge·al syn·co·pe** (lă-rin′jē-ăl sing′ kŏ-pē) Paroxysmal attacks of coughing, with unusual tickling in the throat, followed by brief unconsciousness.

**la·ryn·ge·al ton·sils** (lă-rin′jē-ăl ton′silz) sᴜɴ laryngeal lymphoid nodules.

**la·ryn·ge·al ven·tri·cle** (lă-rin′jē-ăl ven′ tri-kĕl) [TA] Recess in each lateral wall of larynx between vestibular and vocal folds and into which laryngeal sacculus opens.

**la·ryn·gec·to·my** (lar′in-jek′tŏ-mē) Excision of the larynx. [laryngo- + G. ektomē, excision]

**la·ryn·gi·tis** (lar′in-jī′tis) Inflammation of the mucous membrane of the larynx; accompanied by edema of the vocal cords, which produces hoarseness. [laryngo- + G. -itis, inflammation]

♻ **laryngo-** Avoid mispronouncing this combining form lar-in-jo.The larynx. [G. larynx]

**la·ryn·go·pa·ral·y·sis** (lă-ring′gō-păr-al′i-sis) Paralysis of laryngeal muscles.

**la·ryn·go·pha·ryn·ge·al** (lă-ring′gō-fă-rin′ jē-ăl) Relating to both larynx and pharynx or to the laryngopharynx.

**la·ryn·go·phar·ynx** (lă-ring′gō-far′ingks) [TA] The part of the pharynx lying below the aperture of the larynx and behind the larynx. sᴜɴ hypopharynx.

**la·ryn·go·scope** (lă-ring′gŏ-skōp) Any of several types of hollow tubes, equipped with electric lighting, used in examining or operating on the interior of the larynx through the mouth.

**lar·yn·gos·co·py** (lar′in-gos′kŏ-pē) Inspection of the larynx by means of the laryngoscope.

**la·ryn·go·spasm** (lă-ring′gō-spazm) Reflex closure of glottic aperture.

**la·ryn·go·tra·che·o·bron·chi·tis** (lă-ring′ gō-trā′kē-ō-brong-kī′tis) Acute respiratory infection involving larynx, trachea, and bronchi.

**la·ryn·go·tra·che·o·e·soph·a·ge·al cleft** (lă-ring′gō-trā′kē-ō-ĕ-sof′ă-jē′ăl kleft) Absence of fusion of interarytenoid musculature or cricoid cartilaginous laminae of varying severity. Symptoms of this anomaly are similar to those of tracheoesophageal fistula. sᴜɴ laryngotracheo-oesophageal cleft.

**laryngotracheo-oesophageal cleft** [Br.] sᴜɴ laryngotracheoesophageal cleft.

**lar·ynx,** pl. **la·ryn·ges** (lar′ingks, lă-rin′jēz) [TA] Organ of voice production; part of respiratory tract between pharynx and trachea. [Mod. L. fr. G.]

**la·ser** (lā′zĕr) A device that generates an intense, narrow beam of light created by bombarding an active medium (e.g., $CO_2$, Nd:YAG, argon), with energy in the form of high-voltage electricity, high-intensity light, or radio frequency waves. Lasers are used in microsurgery, for cauterization, excision, and for diagnostic purposes. [acronym coined from light amplification by stimulated emission of radiation]

**la·tent** (lā′tĕnt) Not manifest, dormant, but potentially discernible. [L. lateo, pres. p. latens (-ent-), to lie hidden]

**la·tent a·dre·no·cor·ti·cal in·suf·fi·cien·cy** (lā′tĕnt ă-drē′nō-kōr′ti-kăl in′sŭ-fish′ ĕn-sē) Disorder that is not clinically evident but can worsen if a sudden stress develops.

**la·tent di·a·be·tes** (lā′tĕnt dī′ă-bē′tēz) Prediabetic mild form of diabetes mellitus in which the patient displays no overt symptoms, but has abnormal responses to diagnostic procedures. Term declared obsolete by American Diabetes Association.

**la·tent gout** (lā′tĕnt gowt) Hyperuricemia without symptoms of gout. Often used synonymously with interval gout.

**la·tent im·age** (lā′tĕnt im′ăj) The undeveloped image on an exposed x-ray film; it becomes visible after chemical processing.

**la·tent in·fec·tion** (lā′tĕnt in-fek′shŭn) Asymptomatic infection capable of showing symptoms under some circumstances or if activated.

**la·tent pe·ri·od** (lā′tĕnt pēr′ē-ŏd) Duration between application of a stimulus and the response, e.g., contraction of a muscle.

**la·tent re·flex** (lā′tĕnt rē′fleks) Reflex that must be considered normal but usually appears only under some pathologic circumstance that lowers its threshold.

**la·tent stage** (lā′tĕnt stāj) sᴜɴ incubation period (1).

**la·tent syph·i·lis** (lā′tĕnt sif′i-lis) Infection with Treponema pallidum, after manifestations of primary and secondary syphilis have subsided (or were never noticed), and before any manifestations of tertiary syphilis have appeared.

**la·tent zone** (lā′tĕnt zōn) Portion of cerebral cortex, the stimulation of which produces no movement and a lesion of which produces no symptoms.

**lat·er·al** (lat′ĕr-ăl) [TA] **1.** In dentistry, a position either right or left of midsagittal plane. **2.** A radiographic projection made with the film in the sagittal plane. **3.** On the side. **4.** Farther from the median or midsagittal plane. [L. *lateralis,* lateral, fr. *latus,* side]

**lat·er·al al·ve·o·lar ab·scess** (lat′ĕr-ăl al-vē′ŏ-lăr ab′ses) Lesion located along lateral root surface of a tooth. SYN pericemental abscess.

**lat·er·al ca·nal** (lat′ĕr-ăl kă-nal′) SYN accessory canal.

**lat·er·al cyst** (lat′ĕr-ăl sist) Periodontal lesion located at the lateral of the root, often at the opening of the lateral canal.

**lat·er·al de·vi·a·tion** (lat′ĕr-ăl dē′vē-ā′shŭn) Movement of the mandible as it shifts from side-to-side, especially during opening or closing.

**lat·er·al ex·cur·sion** (lat′ĕr-ăl eks-kŭr′zhŭn) Movement of the mandible to the right or left side excursion.

**lat·er·al in·ci·sor** (lat′ĕr-ăl in-sī′zŏr) See this page. SYN second incisor.

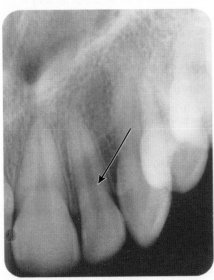

**maxilla:** lateral incisor (radiograph)

**lat·er·al·i·ty** (lat′ĕr-al′i-tē) Referring to a side of body or structure; specifically, dominance of one side of brain or body.

**lat·er·al lig·a·ment of tem·po·ro·man·dib·u·lar joint** (lat′ĕr-ăl lig′ă-mĕnt tem′pŏr-ō-man-dib′yū-lăr joynt) [TA] Capsular ligament that passes obliquely down and backward across the lateral surface of the temporomandibular joint. SYN temporomandibular ligament.

**lat·er·al lin·gual bud** (lat′ĕr-ăl ling′gwăl bŭd) SYN lateral lingual swelling.

**lat·er·al lin·gual swell·ing** (lat′ĕr-ăl lin′gwăl swel′ing) One of two oval swellings in the floor of the primordial mouth, one on each side of the median lingual swelling; they converge to form the anterior two thirds of the tongue. SYN distal tongue bud, lateral lingual bud.

**lat·er·al move·ment** (lat′ĕr-ăl mūv′mĕnt) In dentistry, motion of mandible to the side.

**lat·er·al ob·lique ra·di·o·graph** (lat′ĕr-ăl ō-blēk′ rā′dē-ō-graf) Radiographic view of mandible, revealing one side of it from symphysis to condyle by displacing other side upwards.

**lat·er·al oc·clu·sion** (lat′ĕr-ăl ŏ-klū′zhŭn) Malposition of tooth or entire dental arch in a direction away from midline.

**lat·er·al pal·a·tine pro·ces·ses** (lat′ĕr-ăl pal′ă-tīn pro′ses) Medially directed out growth of embryonic maxilla; when fused with its opposite number forms the secondary palate. SYN palatal shelves.

**lat·er·al path** (lat′ĕr-ăl path) Path of mandibular condyle during lateral mandibular movement.

**lat·er·al per·i·o·don·tal ab·scess** (lat′ĕr-ăl per′ē-ō-don′tăl ab′ses) Lesion that forms at depth of periodontal pocket due to multiplication of pyogenic microorganisms.

**lat·er·al per·i·o·don·tal cyst** (lat′ĕr-ăl per′ē-ō-don′tăl sist) Intraosseous lesion, usually encountered in the madibular cuspid-premolar region derived from remnants of dental lamina. See this page.

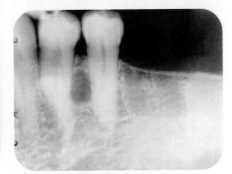

**lateral periodontal cyst:** common location and size

**lat·er·al pinch** (lat′ĕr-ăl pinch) A grasp pattern in which the object is held between the thumb pads and the radial side of the index finger. (Also referred to as a key grasp).

**lat·er·al pres·sure** (lat′ĕr-ăl presh′ŭr) Applying equal (and minimal) pressure with the index finger and thumb inward against the instrument handle to press the working-end against a calculus deposit or tooth surface (or area of soft tissue) before and during an instrumentation stroke.

kl

**lat·er·al pter·y·goid mus·cle** (lat′ĕr-ăl ter′ĭ-goyd mŭs′ĕl) [TA] Masticatory muscle of infratemporal fossa; *origin*, inferior head from lateral lamina of pterygoid process; superior head from infratemporal crest and adjacent greater wing of the sphenoid; *insertion*, into pterygoid fovea of mandible and articular disc and capsule of temporomandibular joint; *action*, protrudes lower jaw to enable opening of mouth; unilateral contraction deviates chin laterally, enabling grinding motion for chewing; *nerve supply*, nerve to lateral pterygoid from mandibular division of trigeminal. SYN external pterygoid muscle, musculus pterygoideus externus, musculus pterygoideus lateralis.

**lat·er·al ra·mus ra·di·o·graph** (lat′ĕr-ăl rā′mŭs rā′dē-ō-graf) Radiographic view of mandibular ramus and condyle.

**lat·er·o·tru·sion** (lat′ĕr-ō-trū′zhŭn) Outward thrust given by muscles of mastication to rotating mandibular condyle during movement of mandible. [L. *lateralis*, to the side, + L. *trudo*, pp. *trusus*, to thrust]

**la·tex** (lā′teks) 1. Emulsion or suspension produced by some seed plants. 2. Similar synthetic materials (e.g., polystyrene, polyvinyl chloride). [L. liquid]

**la·tex al·ler·gy** (lā′teks al′ĕr-jē) Hypersensitivity to latex-based products, those derived from similar plants, and those containing such synthetic materials. See this page.

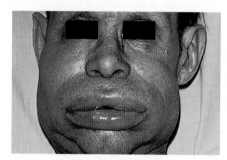

**angioedema:** latex allergy

**lathe** (lādh) Motor-driven machine with a rotating shaft that can be fitted with various types of implements; used to finish and polish dental appliances.

**lat·i·tude** (lat′i-tūd) The range of light or x-ray exposure acceptable with a given photographic emulsion. [L. *latitudo*, width, fr. *latus*, wide]

**laud·able** (law′dă-bĕl) Historic term to describe a quality of pus (thick and creamy) suggesting a wound that ultimately would heal and not be associated with sepsis and death. [L. *laudabilis*, praiseworthy]

**lau·da·num** (law′dă-nŭm) A tincture containing opium. [G. *lēdanon*, a resinous gum]

**laugh·ing gas** (laf′ing gas) Term for nitrous oxide because its inhalation could excite hilarious delirium before insensibility.

**la·vage** (lă-vahzh′) The washing out of a hollow cavity or organ by copious injections and rejections of fluid. [Fr. from L. *lavo*, to wash]

**law** (law) 1. A principle or rule. 2. A statement of fact detailing a sequence or relation of phenomena that is invariable under given conditions. [A.S. *lagu*]

**law of de·ner·va·tion** (law dē′nĕr-vā′shŭn) When a structure is denervated, its irritability to certain chemical agents is increased.

**law of in·de·pen·dent as·sort·ment** (law in′dĕ-pen′dĕnt ă-sōrt′mĕnt) Different hereditary factors assort independently when the gametes are formed. SYN Mendel second law.

**law of par·tial pres·sures** (law pahr′shăl presh′shŭrz) SYN Dalton law.

**law of re·fer·red pain** (law rĕ-fĕrd′ pān) Pain arises only from irritation of nerves that are sensitive to those stimuli that produce pain when applied to the surface of the body.

**law of seg·re·ga·tion** (law seg′rĕ-gā′shŭn) Factors that affect development retain their individuality from generation to generation, do not become contaminated when mixed in a hybrid, and become sorted out from one another when the next generation of gametes is formed. SYN Mendel first law.

**lax·a·tive** (lak′să-tiv) Mild cathartic; remedy that moves bowels gently. [L. *laxativus*, fr. *laxo*, pp. *-atus*, to slacken, relax]

**lay·er** (lā′ĕr) [TA] A sheet of one substance's lying on another and distinguishable from it by a difference in texture or color or by not being continuous with it. SEE ALSO stratum, lamina.

**LD** Abbreviation for lethal dose.

**LD₅₀** Dosage of drug or numbers of microorganisms or other pathogens that kills 50% of a test population.

**LDH** Abbreviation for lactate dehydrogenase.

**L dos·es** (dōs′ĕz) A group of terms that indicate the relative activity or potency of diphtheria toxin; the L doses are different from the minimal lethal dose and minimal reacting dose.

**LE** Abbreviation for lupus erythematosus.

**leach·ing** (lēch′ing) Removal of the soluble constituents of a substance by running water through it. [A.S. *leccan*, to wet]

**lead** (lēd) An electrocardiographic cable with connections within the electronics of the machine designated for an electrode placed at a particular point on the body surface.

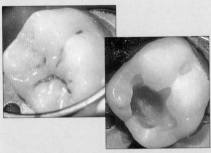

**class I caries:** before and after preparation

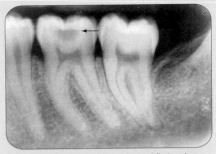

**class I caries:** below occlusal enamel first molar

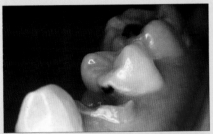

**class II caries:** mesial surface of mandibular second premolar; clearly visible because adjacent first premolar broken off at cervical line

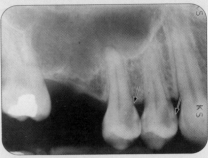

**radiographic evidence of class II caries** (arrows)

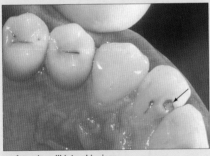

**caries:** class III lateral incisor

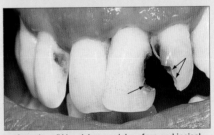

**caries:** class IV involving mesial surface and incisal angle of lateral incisor (double arrows); class III involving distal surface of central incisor

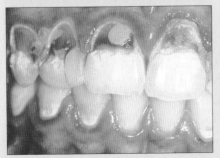

**class V caries:** maxillary anteriors

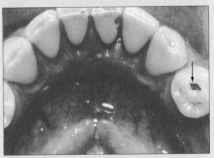

**class VI caries:** premolar cusp tip

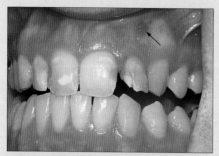

**periapical inflammation:** draining at periapical parulis

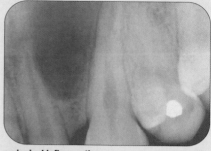

**periapical inflammation**

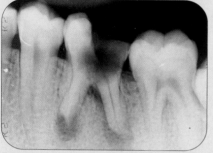

**caries and chronic periapical inflammation:** first molar

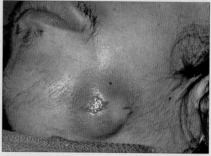

**abscess:** draining through mandible

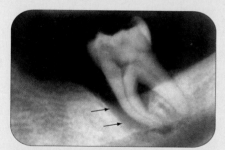

**circumferential (moat) defect** and nonvital tooth

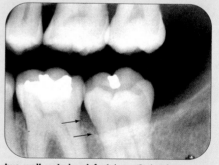

**two-wall cratering defect:** lower 2nd molar

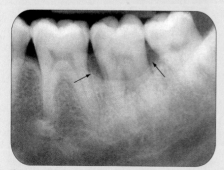

**three-wall bone defect:** second molar area

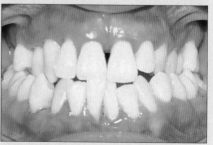

**mild periodontitis:** loss of attachment evident

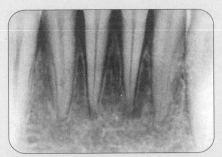

**mild periodontitis:** loss of crestal alveolar bone

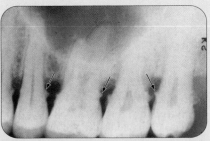

**moderate periodontitis:** horizontal bone loss and calculus (arrows point to calculus)

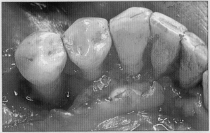

**moderate to severe periodontitis:** 4-mm moat defect

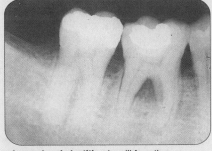

**advanced periodontitis:** class III furcation

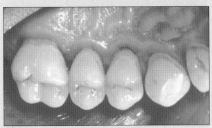

**palatal gingiva of patient with chronic periodontitis:** note calculus deposits on tooth surfaces and rolled gingival margins

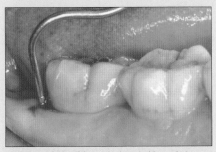

**chronic periodontitis:** probe inserted in pocket showing attachment loss

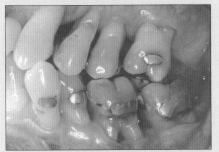

**aggressive periodontitis:** in patient with good plaque control, disease severity seems exaggerated given amount of bacterial plaque

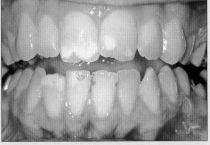

**amelogenesis imperfecta type II-C:** snow capped

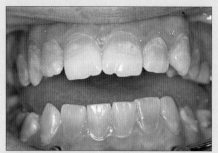

**dentinogenesis imperfecta:** Shields type I

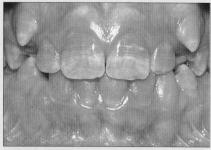

**intrinsic staining:** tetracycline staining

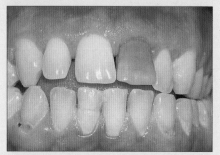

**intrinsic staining:** pink tooth of Mummery

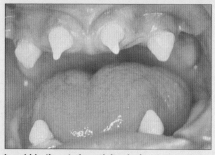

**hypohidrotic ectodermal dysplasia**

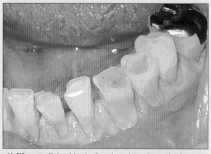

**attrition:** polished incisals; abrasion at cervical

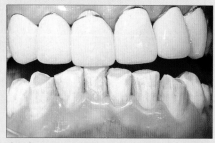

**abrasion:** worn by friction against porcelain crowns on maxillary teeth

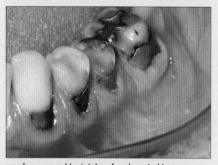

**erosion:** caused by intake of carbonated beverages

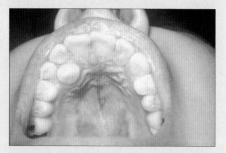

**systemic lupus erythematosus:** ulceration present on hard palate

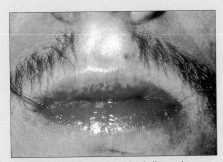

**erythema multiforme:** hemorrhagic lip crusts

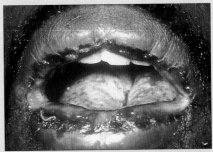

**Stevens-Johnson syndrome:** hemorrhagic, crusted lips

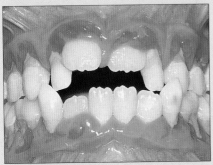

**cyclic neutropenia:** gingival erythema

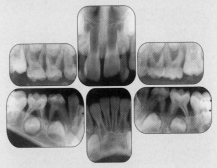

**cyclic neutropenia:** floating teeth

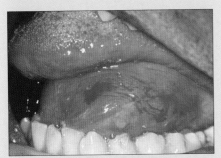

**ranula:** rare large lesion; impairs eating

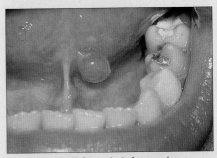

**cyst of Blandin-Nuhn:** variant of mucocele

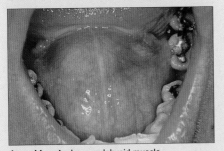

**dermoid cyst:** above mylohyoid muscle

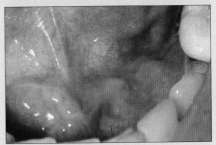

**oral lymphoepithelial cyst:** floor of mouth

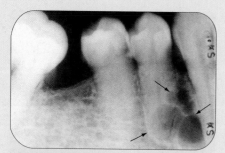

**botryoid lateral periodontal cyst:** arrows show multilobular nature of botryoid cyst

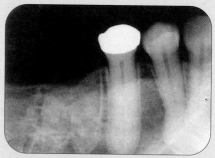

**socket sclerosis:** molar area

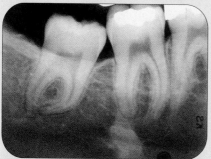

**idopathic osteosclerosis:** vital second molar

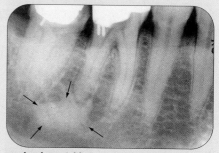

**condensing osteitis** (seen as more dense area indicated by arrows): nonvital first molar

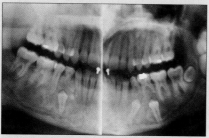

**Gardner syndrome:** osteomas, supernumerary teeth

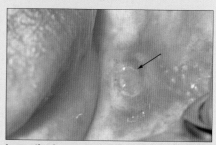

**traumatic ulcer:** molar region

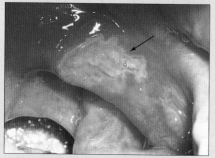

**major aphthous ulcer:** large irregular ulcer, soft palate

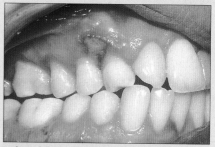

**major aphthous ulceration:** deep, painful gingival ulcers

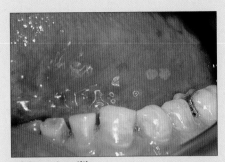

**aphthous stomatitis**

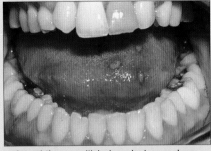

**major aphthous:** multiple, irregular tongue ulcers

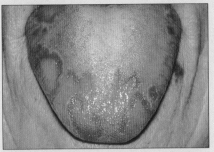

**geographic tongue**

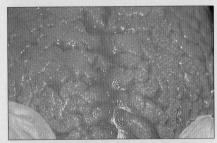

**orofacial granulomatosis:** fissured tongue due to Melkersson-Rosenthal syndrome

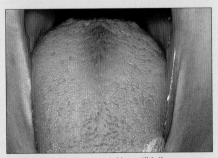

**brown hairy tongue:** caused by antibiotics

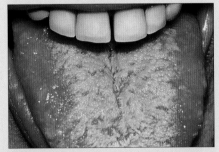

**white hairy tongue:** stomatitis medicamentosa

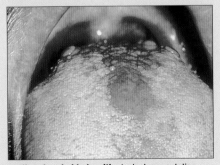

**median rhomboid glossitis:** typical presentation

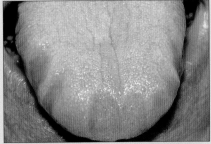

**scalloped tongue showing impressions of teeth:** associated with clenching

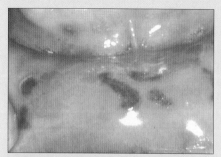

**geographic stomatitis:** symptomatic labial mucosa

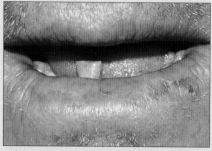

**actinic cheilosis:** vermilion border lost and scaly

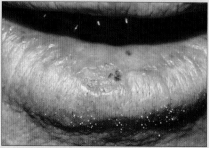

**actinic cheilosis:** everted, thickened with crusts

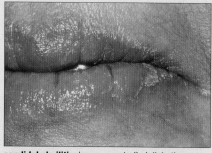

**candidal cheilitis:** in an uncontrolled diabetic

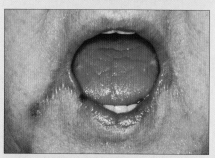

**angular cheilitis:** in older adult

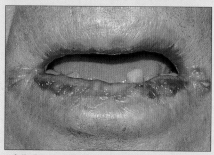

**exfoliative cheilitis:** hemorrhagic crusts

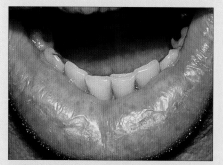

**cheilitis glandularis:** everted lip; red spots

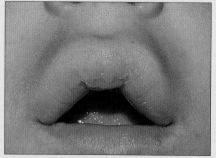

**cheilitis granulomatosa**

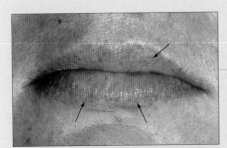

**hereditary hemorrhagic telangiectasia:** multiple lesions evident on lips

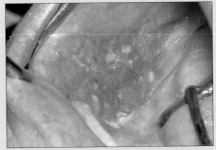

**erythroleukoplakia:** squamous cell carcinoma

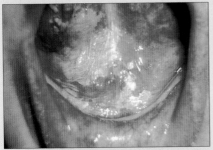

**squamous cell carcinoma:** floor of mouth

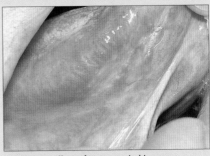

**squamous cell carcinoma:** ventral tongue

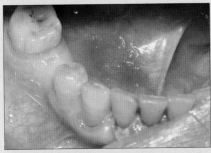

**carcinoma appearing as erythroplakia**

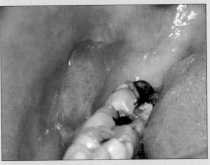

**erosive lichen planus:** buccal mucosa

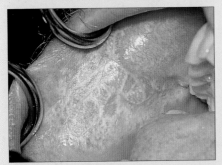

**lichen planus:** plaque form

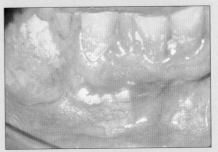

**proliferative verrucous leukoplakia**

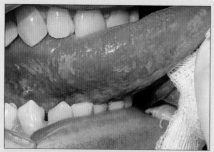

**HIV-associated hairy leukoplakia:** lateral tongue

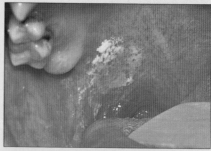

**leukoplakia:** hyperkeratosis of soft palate

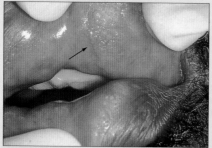

**cigarette keratosis:** labial mucosa

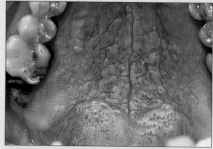

**nicotine stomatitis:** in reverse smoker

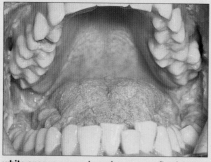

**white sponge nevus:** buccal mucosa, soft palate

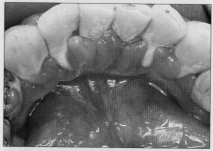

**nifedipine-induced gingival overgrowth**

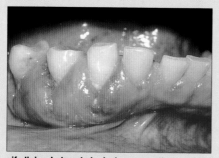

**nifedipine-induced gingival overgrowth**

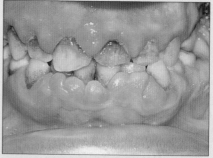

**phenytoin-induced gingival overgrowth**

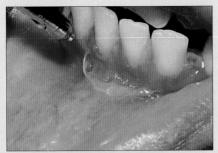

**cicatricial pemphigoid:** positive Nikolsky sign

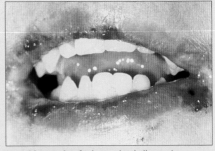

**pemphigus vulgaris:** hemorrhagic lip crusts

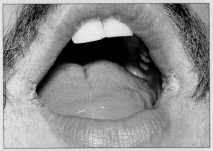

**chronic hyperplastic candidiasis:** at commissures

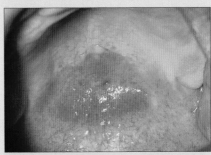

**acute atrophic candidiasis:** due to inhaled steroid use

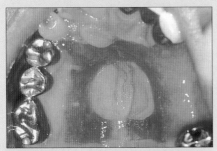

**chronic atrophic candidiasis:** denture-bearing area (denture stomatitis)

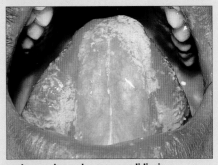

**acute pseudomembranous candidiasis**

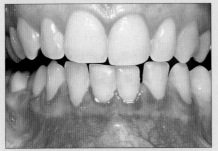

**actinomycotic gingivitis** (confirmed by biopsy)

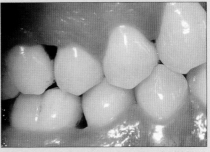

**HIV-associated necrotizing ulcerative gingivitis**

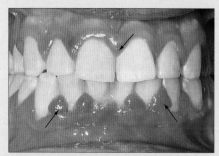

**primary herpetic gingivostomatitis:** multiple areas of gingivitis around teeth with inflammation extending to attached gingiva and mucosa

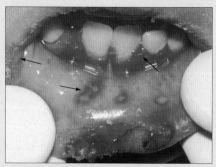

**primary herpetic gingivostomatitis:** lesions around teeth, on lip, and at corner of mouth

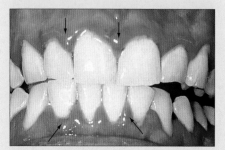

**primary herpetic gingivitis**

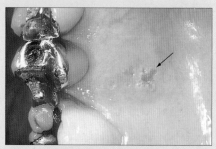

**recurrent herpes simplex:** on hard palate

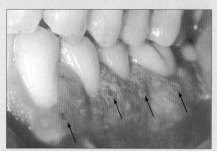

**recurrent herpes simplex:** multiple gingival ulcers

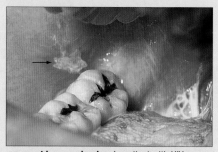

**recurrent herpes simplex:** in patient with HIV

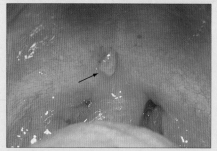

**varicella:** vesicle on palate, a common location

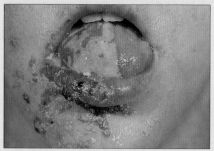

**herpes zoster:** painful oral lesions

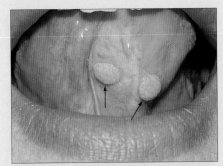

**condyloma acuminata:** ventral tongue

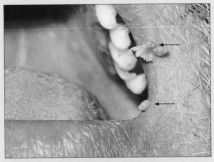

**HIV-associated condyloma acuminata**

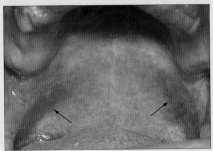

**smoker's melanosis:** lateral soft palate

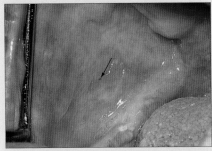

**smoker's melanosis:** buccal mucosa

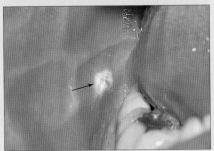

**lichenoid mucositis:** adjacent to facial alloy restoration

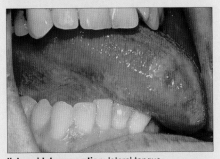

**lichenoid drug eruption:** lateral tongue

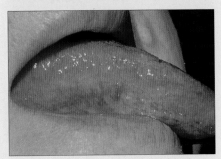

**lichenoid drug eruption:** after drug withdrawal

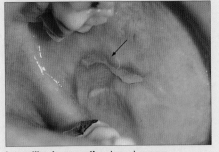

**lupus-like drug eruption:** buccal mucosa

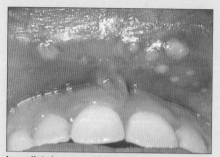

**immediate hypersensitivity:** penicillin

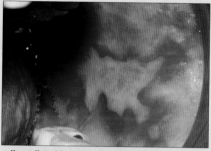

**cell-mediated hypersensitivity:** thiazide

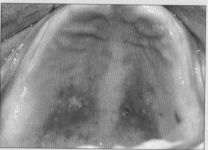

**cell-mediated hypersensitivity:** benzocaine

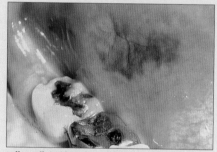

**cell-mediated hypersensitivity:** alloy contact

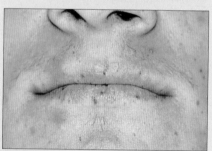

**Peutz-Jeghers syndrome:** macules on lips and perioral skin

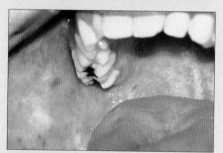

**Peutz-Jeghers syndrome:** macules on buccal mucosa

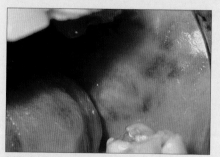

**Addison disease:** hypermelanosis on buccal mucosa

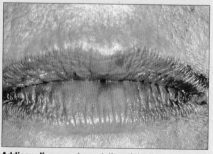

**Addison disease:** pigmentation of the lips

A14

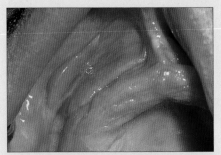

**epulis fissuratum:** in maxillary labial fornix

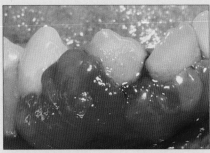

**pyogenic granuloma**

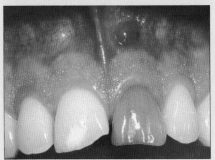

**parulis:** reddish papule above nonvital central

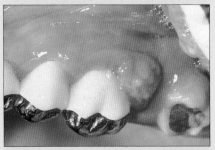

**peripheral odontogenic fibroma:** from periodontal ligament

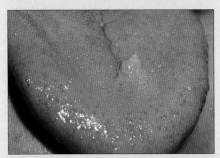

**giant cell fibroma:** dorsum of tongue

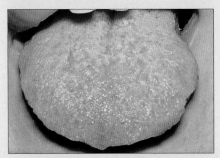

**lymphangiomas causing macroglossia**

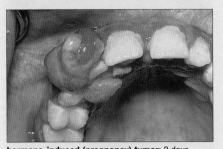

**hormone-induced (pregnancy) tumor:** 3 days after parturition

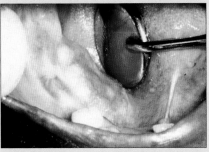

**desmoplastic fibroma:** aggressive, firm lesion

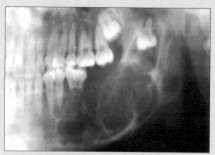

**ameloblastoma:** soap-bubble locules

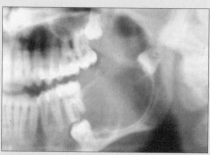

**unicystic ameloblastoma:** cystlike with locules

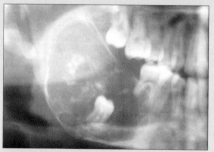

**ameloblastic fibro-odontoma**

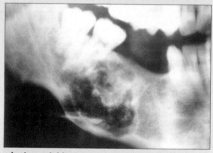

**odontoameloblastoma:** some locules with flecks

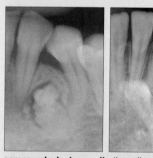

**compound odontoma:** affecting adjacent teeth

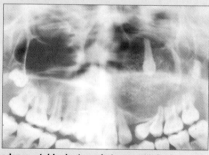

**adenomatoid odontogenic tumor** with flecks

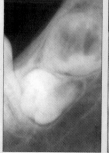

**complex odontoma:** related to impacted teeth

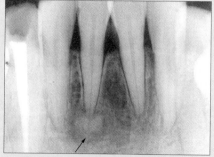

**periapical cemento-osseous dysplasia:** vital incisor

**lead** (lĕd) A metallic element, atomic no. 82, atomic wt. 207.2. [L. *plumbum*]

**lead a·ne·mi·a** (led ă-nē´mē-ă) Anemia associated with poisoning from lead.

**lead en·ceph·a·lop·a·thy, lead en·ceph·a·li·tis** (led en-sef´a-lop´ă-thē, en-sef´ ă-lī´tis) Metabolic encephalopathy, caused by the ingestion of lead compounds; seen particularly in early childhood; characterized pathologically by extensive cerebral edema, status spongiosus, and neurocytolysis; clinical manifestations include convulsions, delirium, and hallucinations.

**lead·ing-third of work·ing-end** (lēd´ing thǐrd wǒrk´ing end) Portion of the working-end of an instrument that is kept in contact with the tooth surface during instrumentation.

**lead line** (led līn) Deposits of lead sulfide in gingiva in areas of chronic inflammation. See this page.

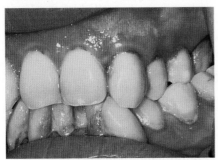

**lead line:** marginal gingiva

**lead neu·rop·a·thy** (led nūr-op´ă-thē) Polyneuropathy reportedly seen in chronic lead intoxication.

**lead-pipe ri·gid·i·ty** (led´pīp´ ri-jid´ĭ-tē) Symptom comprising increased muscle tone due to an extrapyramidal lesion in which pathologic resistance to passive extension of a joint is constant throughout the range of motion.

**lead poi·son·ing** (led poy´zŏn-ing) Acute or chronic intoxication by lead or any of its salts; symptoms of **acute lead poisoning** usually are those of acute gastroenteritis in adults or encephalopathy in children; **chronic lead poisoning** is manifested chiefly by anemia, constipation, colicky abdominal pain, finding of a bluish lead line of the gums, and interstitial nephritis; gout, convulsions, and coma may occur.

**lead sto·ma·ti·tis** (led stō´mă-tī´tis) Oral manifestation of lead poisoning consisting of a bluish-black line along contours of marginal gingiva where lead sulfide has precipitated.

**learn·ing** (lĕrn´ing) Generic term for the relatively permanent change in behavior that occurs as a result of practice.

**learn·ing dis·a·bil·i·ty** (lĕrn´ing dis´ă-bil´i-tē) Disorder in one or more basic cognitive and psychological processes involved in understanding or using written or spoken language; may be manifested in age-related impairment in ability to read, write, spell, speak, or perform mathematical calculations.

**lec·i·thin** (les´i-thin) Lecithin is a yellowish or brown waxy substance, readily miscible in water, in which it appears under the microscope as irregular elongated particles known as "myelin forms"; found in nervous tissue, especially in the myelin sheaths, in egg yolk, and as essential constituents of animal and vegetable cells. [G. *lekithos*, egg yolk]

**lec·i·thi·nase** (les´i-thi-nās) SYN phospholipase.

**ledge** (lej) In dentistry, substance (e.g., oil, water) applied to surface of sharpening stone to reduce friction between stone and implement.

**leech** (lēch) A bloodsucking aquatic annelid worm sometimes used in medicine for local withdrawal of blood.

**lee·way space** (lē´wā spās) Difference between combined mesiodistal widths of deciduous cuspids and molars and their successors.

**Le Fort I frac·ture** (lĕ fōrt´ frak´shŭr) See this page. SYN Guérin fracture.

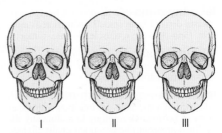

I      II      III

**Le Fort classification of facial fractures:** Guérin fracture (I), pyramidal fracture (II), craniofacial dysjunction fracture (III)

**Le Fort os·te·o·to·my** (lĕ fōrt´ os-tē-ot´ŏ-mē) Osteotomy performed along classic lines of fracture as described by Le Fort to correct a maxillary skeletal deformity; classified as Le Fort osteotomy I, lower maxillary; II, pyramidal nasoorbitomaxillary; or III, high maxillary, depending on the location.

**left ven·tric·u·lar fail·ure** (left ven-trik´yŭ-lăr fāl´yŭr) Congestive heart failure manifested by signs of pulmonary congestion and edema.

**leg** (leg) **1.** [TA] Segment of inferior limb between knee and ankle. **2.** A structure resembling a leg. **3.** Colloquially, the entire inferior limb.

**le·gal blind·ness** (lē´găl blīnd´nĕs) Generally, visual acuity of less than 6/60 or 20/200

**kl**

using Snellen test types, or visual field restriction to 20 degrees or less in the better eye; the criteria used to define legal blindness vary.

**le·gal den·tis·try** (lē′gal den′tis-trē) SYN forensic dentistry.

**Le·gen·dre sign** (lĕ-zhahn′drĕ sīn) In facial hemiplegia of central origin, when the examiner raises the lids of the actively closed eyes, the resistance on the affected side is less.

**Le·gion·el·la** (lē′jŏ-nel′ă) A genus of aerobic, motile, non-acid-fast, nonencapsulated, gram-negative bacilli; they dwell in water and are borne by air; pathogenic for humans. The type species is *L. pneumophila.*

**Le·gion·naires′ dis·ease** (lē′jŏ-nārz′ di-zēz′) Acute infectious disease, caused by *Legionella pneumophila,* with prodromal influenzalike symptoms and a rapidly rising high fever, followed by severe pneumonia and production of usually nonpurulent sputum, and sometimes mental confusion, hepatic fatty changes, and renal tubular degeneration. It has a high case-fatality rate; acquired from contaminated water, usually by aerosolization rather than being transmitted from person-to-person. [American *Legion* convention, in Philadelphia in 1976, at which many delegates took sick]

**leg·ume** (lā-gyūm′) Pod or fruit from family of plants that includes peas, lentils, and beans.

**lei·o·my·o·ma** (lī′ō-mī-ō′mă) A benign neoplasm derived from smooth (nonstriated) muscle. [*leio-* + G. *mys,* muscle, + *-oma,* tumor]

**lei·o·my·o·sar·co·ma** (lī′ō-mī′ō-sahr-kō′mă) A malignant neoplasm derived from smooth (nonstriated) muscle.

**leish·man·i·a·sis, leish·man·i·o·sis** (lēsh′mă-nī′ă-sis, -nē-ō′sis) Infection with a species of *Leishmania* resulting in a clinically ill-defined group of diseases traditionally divided into four major types: visceral leishmaniasis (kala azar); Old World cutaneous leishmaniasis; New World cutaneous leishmaniasis; and mucocutaneous leishmaniasis.

**length** (length) *Avoid the mispronunciation lenth.* Linear distance between two points.

**len·i·tive** (len′i-tiv) Soothing; relieving discomfort or pain. [L. *lenio,* pp. *lenitus,* to soften, fr. *lenis,* mild]

**len·tig·i·no·sis** (len-tij′i-nō′sis) Presence of lentigines in very large numbers or in a distinctive configuration.

**len·ti·go,** pl. **len·ti·gi·nes** (len-tī′gō, len-tij′i-nēz) A brown macule resembling a freckle except that the border is usually regular, and microscopic proliferation of rete ridges is present; scattered melanocytes are seen in the basal cell layer. It is usually caused by sun exposure in someone of middle age or older. SYN lentigo simplex. [L. fr. *lens (lent-),* a lentil]

**len·ti·go sim·plex** (len-tī′gō sĭm′pleks) SYN lentigo.

**len·tu·lo** (len′tyū-lō) Motorized, flexible, spiral wire instrument used in dentistry to apply paste filling material into the root canal(s) of a tooth.

**LEOPARD syn·drome** (lep′ărd sin′drōm) Syndrome consisting of *l*entigines (multiple), *e*lectrocardiographic abnormalities, *o*cular hypertelorism, *p*ulmonary stenosis, *a*bnormalities of genitalia, *r*etardation of growth, and *d*eafness (sensorineural).

**le·pro·ma** (lĕ-prō′mă) A discrete focus of granulomatous inflammation, caused by *Mycobacterium leprae.* [G. *lepros,* scaly, + *-oma,* tumor]

**lep·ro·sy** (lep′rŏ-sē) Chronic granulomatous infection caused by *Mycobacterium leprae* affecting the cooler body parts, especially the skin, peripheral nerves, and testes; classified into two main types, lepromatous and tuberculoid. SYN Hansen disease. [G. *lepra,* from *lepros,* scaly]

♻ **lepto-** Light, thin, frail. [G. *leptos,* slender, delicate, weak]

**lep·to·cyte** (lep′tō-sīt) SYN target cell.

**lep·to·pro·so·pi·a** (lep′tō-prō-sō′pē-ă) Narrowness of the face.

**lep·to·spi·ral jaun·dice** (lep′tō-spī′răl jawn′dis) Jaundice associated with infection by various species of *Leptospira.*

**Lep·to·trich·i·a** (lep′tō-trik′ē-ă) Genus of anaerobic, nonmotile bacteria containing gram-negative, straight or slightly curved rods, with one or both ends rounded or pointed; found in human oral cavity.

**Lesch-Ny·han syn·drome** (lesh nī′ăn sin′drōm) Disorder of purine metabolism characterized by hyperuricemia, uric acid renal stones, mental retardation, spasticity, choreoathetosis, and self-mutilation of fingers and lips by biting.

**le·sion** (lē′zhŭn) **1.** Wound or injury. **2.** Pathologic change in tissues. **3.** One of the individual points or patches of a multifocal disease. [L. *laedo,* pp. *laesus,* to injure]

**less·er pal·a·tine nerves** (les′ĕr pal′ă-tīn nĕrvz) [TA] Usually two, emerge through lesser palatine foramina and supply the mucosa and glands of the soft palate and uvula.

**less·er wing of sphe·noid (bone)** (les′ĕr wing sfē′noyd bōn) [TA] One of a bilateral pair of triangular, pointed plates extending laterally from the anterolateral body of the sphenoid bone. SYN ala minor ossis sphenoidalis.

**LET** Abbreviation for linear energy transfer.

**le·thal** (lē′thăl) Pertaining to or causing death;

especially denoting the causal agent. [L. *letalis,* deadly, fr. *letum,* death]

**le·thal dose (LD)** (lē′thăl dōs) Amount of chemical or biologic preparation (e.g., a bacterial exotoxin or a suspension of bacteria) likely to cause death; varies in relation to type of animal and route of administration; when followed by a subscript (generally "$LD_{50}$" or median lethal dose), denotes amount likely to cause death in a certain percentage (e.g., 50%) of the test animals; median lethal dose is $LD_{50}$, absolute lethal dose is $LD_{100}$, and minimal lethal dose is $LD_{05}$. [L. *dosis letalis*]

**le·thal mid·line gran·u·lo·ma** (lē′thăl mid′līn gran′yū-lō′mă) Destruction of nasal septum, hard palate, lateral nasal walls, paranasal sinuses, skin of face, orbit, and nasopharynx by an inflammatory infiltrate with atypical lymphocytic and histiocytic cells.

**le·thal mu·ta·tion** (lē′thăl myū-tā′shŭn) A mutant trait that leads to a phenotype incompatible with effective reproduction.

**leth·ar·gy** (leth′ăr-jē) Relatively mild impairment of consciousness resulting in reduced alertness and awareness. [G. *lēthargia,* drowsiness]

**Let·te·rer-Si·we dis·ease** (let′er-er-sē′vē di-zēz′) The acute disseminated form of Langerhans cell histiocytosis. SYN nonlipid histiocytosis.

**leucaemia** [Br.] SYN leukemia.

**leu·cine** (lū′sīn) The L-isomer is one of the amino acids of proteins; a nutritionally essential amino acid.

**leu·cine hy·po·gly·ce·mi·a** (lū′sīn hī′pō-glī-sē′mē-ă) Reduction in blood glucose concentration produced by administration of leucine; believed to reflect ability of this amino acid to stimulate insulin secretion.

**leucocyte** [Br.] SYN leukocyte.

**leucocytopenia** [Br.] SYN leukopenia.

**leucocytosis** [Br.] SYN leukocytosis.

**leucoderma** [Br.] SYN leukoderma.

**leuco-oedema** [Br.] SYN leukoedema.

**leucopenia** [Br.] SYN leukopenia.

**leucoplakia** [Br.] SYN leukoplakia.

**leukaemia** [Br.] SYN leukemia.

**leukaemic** [Br.] SYN leukemic.

**leukaemogen** [Br.] SYN leukemogen.

**leukaemoid reaction** [Br.] SYN leukemoid reaction.

**leu·ke·mi·a** (lū-kē′mē-ă) Progressive proliferation of abnormal leukocytes found in hemo-

poietic tissues, other organs, and usually in the blood in increased numbers; classified by dominant cell type, and by duration from onset to death. This occurs in *acute leukemia* within a few months in most cases, and is associated with acute symptoms including severe anemia, hemorrhages, and slight enlargement of lymph nodes or the spleen. *Chronic leukemia* lasts over 1 year, with a gradual onset of symptoms of anemia or marked enlargement of spleen, liver, or lymph nodes. SYN leucaemia, leukaemia. [*leuko-* + G. *haima,* blood]

**leu·ke·mic** (lū-kē′mik) Pertaining to, or having the characteristics of, any form of leukemia. SYN leukaemic.

**leu·ke·mic hy·per·plas·tic gin·gi·vi·tis** (lū-kē′mik hī′pěr-plas′tik jin′ji-vī′tis) Enlarged gingiva due to infiltration of leukemic cells and infection from local factors in the face of diminished host response.

**leu·ke·mo·gen** (lū-kē′mō-jen) Any substance or entity (e.g., benzene, ionizing radiation) considered to be a causal factor in the occurrence of leukemia. SYN leukaemogen.

**leu·ke·moid re·ac·tion** (lū-kē′moyd rē-ak′shŭn) Leukocytosis similar to that occurring in leukemia, but not the result of leukemic disease. Sometimes observed as a feature of infectious disease (tuberculosis, diphtheria), intoxication (eclampsia, mustard gas poisoning), malignant neoplasms, and acute hemorrhage or hemolysis. SYN leukaemoid reaction.

♻ **leuko-** Combining form meaning white; white blood cells. [G. *leukos,* white]

**leu·ko·cyte** (lū′kō-sīt) Cell formed in myelopoietic, lymphoid, and reticular portions of the reticuloendothelial system in various parts of the body, and normally present in those sites and in the circulating blood. SYN white blood cell, leucocyte. [*leuko-* + G. *kytos,* cell]

**leu·ko·cy·to·sis** (lū′kō-sī-tō′sis) An abnormally large number of leukocytes, as observed in acute infections, inflammation, hemorrhage, and other conditions. SYN leucocytosis. [*leukocyte* + G. *-osis,* condition]

**leu·ko·der·ma** (lū′kō-děr′mă) An absence of pigment, partial or total, in the skin. [*leuko-* + G. *derma,* skin]

**leu·ko·don·ti·a** (lū′kō-don′shē-ă) Condition of having white teeth. [*leuko-* + G. *odous,* tooth]

🔲 **leu·ko·e·de·ma** (lū′kō-ĕ-dē′mă) Bluish-white opalescence of buccal mucosa that assumes normal mucosal color on stretching affected tissue. See page 340. SYN leucoderma, leuco-oedema.

**leu·ko·pe·ni·a** (lū′kō-pē′nē-ă) Antithesis of leukocytosis; any situation in which total number of leukocytes in circulating blood is less than normal. SYN leucocytopenia, leucopenia. [*leuko-*(cyte) + G. *penia,* poverty]

kl

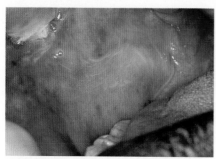

**leukoedema:** buccal mucosa, prominent in a smoker

□**leu·ko·pla·ki·a** (lū′kō-plā′kē-ă) White patch of oral or female genital mucous membrane that cannot be wiped off and cannot be diagnosed clinically as any specific disease entity; in current usage, no histologic connotation. See this page and pages A9–A10. SYN leucoplakia. [*leuko-* + G. *plax,* plate]

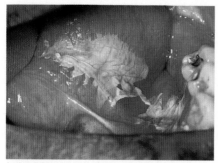

**leukoplakia:** floor of mouth and ventral tongue

**leu·ko·tax·ine** (lū′kō-tak′sēn) A cell-free nitrogenous material prepared from injured degenerating tissue and inflammatory exudates.

**le·va·tor** (lĕ-vā′tŏr) [TA] **1.** A surgical instrument for prying up the depressed part in a fracture of the skull. **2.** One of several muscles with an action to raise the part to which it inserts. [L. a lifter, fr. *levo,* pp. -*atus,* to lift, fr. *levis,* light]

**le·va·tor an·gu·li o·ris (mus·cle)** (lĕ-vā′tŏr an′yū-lī ōr′is mŭs′ĕl) [TA] Facial muscle of upper lip; *origin,* canine fossa of maxilla; *insertion,* orbicularis oris and skin at angle of mouth; *action,* raises angle of mouth; *nerve supply,* facial.

**lev·el** (lev′ĕl) Any rank, position, or status in a graded scale of values.

**lev·el of con·scious·ness (LOC)** (lev′ĕl kon′shŭs-nĕs) The degree of a patient's alertness and awareness of self and environment, varying from wakefulness to coma. Decreases often measured with the Glasgow Coma Scale (q.v.), a tool for standardizing uniformity in assessment by more than one observer as a way of standardizing subjective assessment data.

**lev·er** (lev′ĕr) An instrument used to lift or pry. [Fr. *lever,* to lift]

**lev·er·age** (lev′ĕr-ăj) Actual lift or elevating direction of a lever or elevator.

⟳**levo-** Combining form meaning left, toward or on the left side. SYN laev-, laevo-. [L. *laevus*]

**le·vo·do·pa** (lē′vō-dō′pă) Biologically active form of dopa; an antiparkinsonian agent that is converted to dopamine. SYN L-dopa, laevodopa.

**Ley·dig cells** (lī′dig selz) SYN interstitial cells (1).

**LGE** Abbreviation for linear gingival erythema.

**li·brar·y** (lī′brār-ē) A collection of cloned fragments that represent the entire genome.

**li·cense, li·cence** (lī′sĕns) Legal permission given to professional to practice in specific fields according to rules and regulations of a jurisdiction. [L. *licentia,* fr. *licet,* it is permitted]

**li·cen·sure** (lī′sĕn-shŭr) Permission granted to a professional to practice within a jurisdiction. [L. *licentia,* fr. *licet,* it is permitted, + -*ure,* noun suffix]

**li·cen·sure by cre·den·tial** (lī′sĕn-shŭr krĕ-den′shăl) Legal permission granted to a professional to practice that profession in a given jurisdiction based on holding a like license in another jurisdiction.

□**li·chen pla·nus, li·chen ru·ber pla·nus** (lī′ken plā′nŭs, rū′bĕr) Eruption of flat-topped violaceous papules on flexor surfaces and buccal mucosa of unknown cause. See this page and page A9.

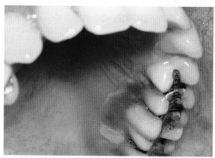

**erosion:** lichen planus on palatal gingiva

**li·do·caine hy·dro·chlor·ide (top·i·cal)** (lī′dō-kān hī′drŏ-klōr′īd top′i-kăl) Anesthetic preparation in various forms applied to skin and mucous membranes.

**li·en** (lī′en) [TA] SYN spleen. [L.]

**li·en·ter·y** (lī′en-ter-ē) Passage of undigested food in stools. [G. *leienteria,* fr. *leios,* smooth, + *enteron,* intestine]

**life stress** (līf stres) Events or experiences that produce severe strain, e.g., job loss.

**life·style** (līf′stīl) Set of habits and customs influenced by life-long process of socialization, including social use of substances such as alcohol and tobacco, and exercise.

**lig·a·ment** (lig′ă-mĕnt) [TA] **1.** Band or sheet of fibrous tissue connecting two or more bones, cartilages, or other structures, or serving as support for fasciae or muscles. **2.** Fold of peritoneum supporting any of the abdominal viscera. **3.** Any structure resembling a ligament without such function. SYN ligamentum. [L. *ligamentum,* a band, bandage]

**lig·a·ments of au·ri·cle** (lig′ă-mĕnts awr′ĭ-kĕl) [TA] Three ligaments that attach auricle to side of the head. SYN auricular ligaments.

**lig·a·men·tum** (lig-ă-men′tŭm) [TA] SYN ligament. [L. a band, tie, fr. *ligo,* to bind]

**li·gand** (lī′gand) **1.** Any individual atom, group, or molecule attached to a central metal ion by multiple coordinate bonds. **2.** An organic molecule attached to a tracer element. **3.** A molecule that binds to a macromolecule. [L. *ligo,* to bind]

**li·gate** (lī′gāt) To apply a ligature. [L. *ligo,* pp. *-atus,* to bind]

**li·ga·tion** (lī-gā′shŭn) **1.** Application of a ligature. **2.** The act of binding or annealing. [L. *ligatio,* fr. *ligo,* to bind]

**lig·a·ture** (lig′ă-chŭr) **1.** In orthodontics, a wire or other material used to secure an orthodontic attachment or tooth to an archwire. **2.** A thread, wire, fillet, or the like, tied tightly around a blood vessel or other structure to constrict it.

**lig·a·ture wire** (lig′ă-chŭr wīr) Soft thin stainless steel wire used in dentistry to tie an archwire to band attachments or brackets.

**light** (līt) That portion of electromagnetic radiation to which the retina is sensitive. SEE ALSO lamp. [A.S. *leōht*]

🔲**light-cured res·in** (līt′kyūrd rez′in) Resin that uses visible or ultraviolet light to excite a photoinitiator, used mainly in restorative dentistry. See this page.

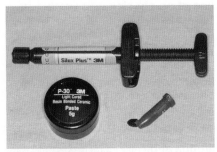

light-cure dental resin kit

🔲**light cur·ing** (līt kyūr′ing) See this page. SYN light polymerization.

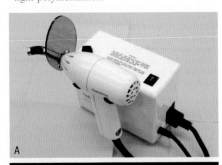

A

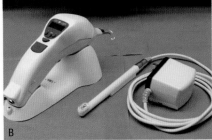

B

**dental curing lights:** (A) conventional halogen curing light with shield to protect operator's eyes from the intense light; (B) light-emitting diode curing lights

**light fog** (līt fawg) Black areas seen on a radiograph when a film is exposed to white light before processing. SYN fog.

**light leak** (līt lēk) Any white luminescence visible when lights are off in an x-ray darkroom; may be due to unsealed door frames or air vents.

**light·ning strip** (līt′ning strip) Band or ribbon of metal with abrasive on one side, used to open rough or improper contacts of proximal restorations.

**light pol·y·mer·i·za·tion** (līt pol′i-mĕr-ī-zā′shŭn) Use of visible or ultraviolet illumination to excite a photoinitiator; which can initiate polymerization, usually of a resin. SYN light curing.

**light tight** (līt tīt) Referring to a darkroom with no visible white light leaks that would interfere with the diagnostic quality of radiographs.

**light wire ap·pli·ance** (līt wīr ă-plī′ăns) Orthodontic fixture using small gauge labial wires with expansion and contraction loops formed into it and attached to bands fitted to individual teeth; sometimes called Begg light wire differential force technique.

**lig·nin** (lig′nin) A water-insoluble fiber found in wheat bran, whole grains, and vegetables. [L. *lignum,* wood]

kl

**limb** (lim) [TA] **1.** An extremity; a member; an arm (upper extremity) or leg (lower extremity). **2.** A segment of any jointed structure. [A.S. *lim*]

**lim·bic sys·tem** (lim'bik sis'tĕm) Collective term denoting a heterogeneous array of brain structures at or near the edge (limbus) of the medial wall of the cerebral hemisphere, in particular the hippocampus, amygdala, and fornicate gyrus.

**lime** (līm) **1.** An alkaline earth oxide occurring in grayish white masses (quicklime); on exposure to the atmosphere it converts into calcium hydrate and calcium carbonate (air-slaked lime); direct addition of water to calcium oxide produces calcium hydrate (slaked lime). SYN calx (1). **2.** Fruit of the lime tree, *Citrus medica* (family Rutaceae), which is a source of ascorbic acid and acts as a therapeutic antiscorbutic agent in treating scurvy. [A.S. *līm*, birdlime]

**li·mes (L)** (lī'mēz) A boundary or threshold. [L.]

**lime wa·ter** (līm waw'tĕr) Calcium hydroxide solution; prepared by mixing 3 g of calcium hydroxide in 1 L of purified cool water. Undissolved calcium hydroxide is allowed to precipitate and the solution is dispensed without agitating it; common ingredient in lotions.

**lim·i·nal** (lim'i-năl) Pertaining to a threshold.

**lim·i·nom·e·ter** (lim'i-nom'ĕ-tĕr) An instrument for measuring the strength of a stimulus that is barely sufficient to produce a reflex response.

**lim·it** (lim'it) A boundary or end. [L. *limes,* boundary]

**lim·i·ta·tions** (lim'i-tā'shŭnz) Conditions or restrictions on activity or motion of something.

**lim·i·ted treat·ment** (lim'i-tĕd trēt'mĕnt) Therapy that focuses on diagnosing and treating only the immediate concerns (i.e., complaints) or needs of the presenting patient.

**lim·i·ted use life** (lim'i-tĕd yūs līf) Denotes an item intended to be discarded because of wear or deterioration after a given period.

**lin·co·my·cin** (lin'kō-mī'sin) An antibacterial substance active against gram-positive organisms.

**line** (līn) [TA] ANATOMY long, narrow mark, strip, or streak distinguished from the adjacent tissues by color, texture, or elevation. SYN linea [TA]. [L. *linea,* a linen thread, a string, line, fr. *linum,* flax]

**lin·e·a,** pl. **lin·e·ae** (lin'ē-ă, -ē) [TA] SYN line. [L.]

**lin·e·a al·ba** (lin'ē-ă al'bă) [TA] A fibrous band running vertically the entire length of the center of the anterior abdominal wall, receiving the attachments of the oblique and transverse abdominal muscles. SYN white line (1).

**line an·gle** (līn ang'gĕl) In dentistry, the junction of two surfaces of tooth crowns, or of tooth cavities (cavity line angle). See this page.

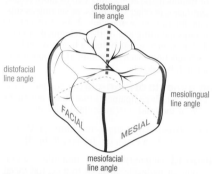

**line angle:** boundary or imaginary line formed where two tooth surfaces meet. Each tooth has four line angles: (1) mesiofacial, (2) distofacial, (3) mesiolingual, and (4) distolingual line angle. Instrumentation of a posterior tooth is usually initiated at tooth's distofacial or distolingual line angle

**lin·e·ar en·er·gy trans·fer (LET)** (lin'ē-ăr en'ĕr-jē trans'fĕr) Rate at which a charged particle deposits energy as it advances.

**lin·e·ar frac·ture** (lin'ē-ăr frak'shŭr) Breakage running parallel with the long axis of the bone. SYN fissured fracture.

**lin·e·ar gin·gi·val er·yth·e·ma (LGE)** (lin'ē-ăr jin'ji-văl er'i-thē'mă) Gingivitis in the HIV-positive patient; characterized by a well-demarcated band of intense erythema at the gingival margin, not associated with bacterial plaque; does not respond to conventional plaque-removal procedures.

**lin·en strip** (lin'ĕn strip) A piece of linen, with or without abrasive, used to polish proximal surfaces of dental restorations. SEE ALSO polishing strip.

**line of oc·clu·sion** (līn ŏ-klū'zhŭn) Alignment of occluding surfaces of teeth in horizontal plane. SEE ALSO occlusal plane.

**line of Ret·zi·us** (līn ret'zē-ŭs) SYN striae of Retzius.

**lin·er** (lī'nĕr) A layer of protective material. SYN insulating base, protective base.

**lin·gua,** pl. **lin·guae** (ling'gwă, -gwē) [TA] SYN tongue. [L. tongue]

**lin·gua al·ba** (ling'gwă al'bă) SYN white hairy tongue.

**lin·gua fis·su·ra·ta** (ling′gwă fis′ū-rā′tă) SYN fissured tongue.

**lin·gua ge·o·graphi·ca** (ling′gwă jē-ō-graf′i-kă) SYN geographic tongue.

**lin·gual** (ling′gwăl) **1.** Relating to the tongue or any tonguelike part. **2.** Next to or toward the tongue.

**lin·gual ap·o·neu·ro·sis** (ling′gwăl ap′ō-nūr-ō′sis) [TA] Thickened lamina propria of tongue to which lingual muscles attach.

**lin·gual ap·pli·ance** (ling′gwăl ă-plī′ăns) SYN lingual arch attachment.

**lin·gual a·pron** (ling′gwăl ā′prŏn) SYN lingual plate.

**lin·gual arch** (ling′gwăl ahrch) Orthodontic arch wire that approximates lingual surfaces of teeth.

**lin·gual arch at·tach·ment** (ling′gwăl ahrch ă-tach′mĕnt) Bracket on the lingual side of an orthodontic band that stabilizes the arch or aids in tooth movement. SYN lingual appliance.

**lin·gual ar·te·ry** (ling′gwăl ahr′tĕr-ē) [TA] *Origin*, external carotid; *distribution*, runs along undersurface of tongue, terminates as deep lingual artery; *branches*, suprahyoid and dorsal lingual branches and sublingual artery.

**lin·gual bar** (ling′gwăl bahr) Major connector located lingually to dental arch joining two or more bilateral parts of a mandibular removable partial denture.

**lin·gual bar ma·jor con·nec·tor** (ling′gwăl bahr mā′jŏr kŏ-nek′tŏr) A connector located lingually to the alveolar ridge that unites the right and left portions of a mandibular partial denture.

**lin·gual bone** (ling′gwăl bōn) SYN hyoid bone.

**lin·gual branch·es** (ling′gwăl branch′ĕz) [TA] Branches to tongue. *Terminologia Anatomica* lists lingual branches of 1) accessory nerve; 2) facial nerve (a finding in some patients); 3) lingual nerve; 4) and glossopharyngeal nerve.

**lin·gual crib** (ling′gwăl krib) Wire orthodontic appliance placed in a position lingual to the maxillary incisors to help a child overcome the habits of thumb sucking and tongue thrusting.

**lin·gual cross·bite** (ling′gwăl kraws′bīt) Lingual displacement of a mandibular tooth or teeth as related to the opposing (i.e., antagonistic) tooth or teeth.

**lin·gual crypt** (ling′gwăl kript) Pit lined with epithelium in lingual tonsil.

**lin·gual cusp** (ling′gwăl kŭsp) Elevation of the crown of a tooth located toward the tongue.

May be single, as on a premolar, or multiple, as on a molar. If multiple, designated as to mesial or distal sides (e.g., mesiolingual or distolingual).

**lin·gual em·bra·sure** (ling′gwăl em-brā′shŭr) Space on lingual aspect of interproximal contact area between adjacent teeth.

**lin·gual er·up·tion** (ling′gwăl ĕ-rŭp′shŭn) Eruption of a tooth in a position closer to the tongue than its normal or final position.

**lin·gual flange** (ling′gwăl flanj) Portion of flange of a mandibular denture that occupies space adjacent to tongue.

**lin·gual for·a·men** (ling′gwăl fōr-ā′mĕn) Small opening in the bone of mandible located at the midline on inside surface of mandible that permits passage of mandibular nerve. Radiographically, it appears as a round, radiolucent spot below the apices of the mandibular incisors.

**lin·gual fos·sa** (ling′gwăl fos′ă) Shallow rounded depression on the lingual surface of the maxillary incisors.

**lin·gual fren·u·lum** (ling′gwăl fren′yū-lŭm) SYN frenulum of tongue.

**lin·gual fre·num** (ling′gwăl frē′nŭm) SYN frenulum of tongue.

**lin·gual gin·gi·va** (ling′gwăl jin′ji-vă) Portion of gingiva that covers lingual surfaces of teeth and alveolar process.

**lin·gual gin·gi·val pa·pil·la** (ling′gwăl jin′ji-văl pă-pil′ă) Lingual portions of gingiva filling interproximal space between adjacent teeth; in molar and premolar areas, lingual and buccal interdental papillae may be separate. SYN lingual papillae.

**lin·gual glands** (ling′gwăl glandz) [TA] Minor salivary glands of tongue.

**lin·gual groove** (ling′gwăl grūv) A linear area or depression found on the lingual surface of maxillary molars, extending from the occlusal third to the middle third of the tooth.

**lin·gual hem·i·at·ro·phy** (ling′gwăl hem′ē-at′rŏ-fē) Atrophy of one lateral half of tongue.

**lin·gual lobe** (ling′gwăl lōb) SYN cingulum of tooth.

**lin·gual lymph nodes** (ling′gwăl limf nōdz) [TA] Those along lingual vein receiving drainage from the tongue (except tip); drain to submandibular lymph nodes.

**lin·gual mu·co·sa** (ling′gwăl myū-kō′să) SYN mucosa of tongue.

**lin·gual mus·cles** (ling′gwăl mŭs′ĕlz) SYN muscles of tongue.

**lin·gual nerve** (ling′gwăl nĕrv) [TA] Branch

kl

of mandibular nerve [CN V3], passing medial to the lateral pterygoid muscle, between medial pterygoid and mandible, and beneath mucous membrane of floor of mouth to side of the tongue over anterior two thirds of which it is distributed: also supplies mucous membrane of floor of mouth and passes close to lingual side of roots of second and third mandibular molar teeth; is endangered during tooth extractions.

**lin·gual oc·clu·sion** (ling´gwăl ŏ-klū´zhŭn) **1.** SYN linguoclusion. **2.** Interdigitation of teeth as seen from internal or lingual aspect.

**lin·gual pa·pil·la** (ling´gwăl pă-pil´ă) **1.** One of numerous variously shaped projections of mucous membrane of dorsum of tongue. **2.** Lingual portion of gingiva filling interproximal space between adjacent teeth; in molar and premolar areas, there may be separate lingual and buccal interdental papillae. SEE ALSO interdental papilla.

**lin·gual pa·pil·lae** (ling´gwăl pă-pil´ē) SYN lingual gingival papilla.

**lin·gual plate** (ling´gwăl plāt) Major connector portion of a mandibular removable partial denture (i.e., prosthesis) that connects the posterior segments and contacts the lingual surfaces of the natural anterior teeth. SYN lingual apron, lingual strap, linguoplate.

**lin·gual plex·us** (ling´gwăl pleks´ŭs) SYN periarterial plexus of lingual artery.

**lin·gual rest** (ling´gwăl rest) Metallic extension onto lingual surface of a tooth to provide support or indirect retention for a removable partial denture.

**lin·gual sal·i·var·y gland de·pres·sion** (ling´gwăl sal´i-var-ē gland dĕ-presh´ŭn) Indentation on lingual surface of mandible within which part of submandibular gland lies; appears radiographically as a sharply circumscribed ovoid radiolucency.

**lin·gual splint** (ling´gwăl splint) Appliance similar to the splint, but conforming to inner aspect of dental arch.

**lin·gual strap** (ling´gwăl strap) SYN lingual plate.

**lin·gual sur·face of tooth** (ling´gwăl sŭr´făs tūth) [TA] Oral surface of mandibular tooth that faces the tongue, opposite to its vestibular surface. SYN facies lingualis dentis.

**lin·gual thy·roid** (ling´gwăl thī´royd) Ectopic thyroid tissue found at base of tongue.

🄴**lin·gual ton·sil** (ling´gwăl ton´sil) [TA] Collection of lymphoid follicles on posterior or pharyngeal portion of dorsum of the tongue. See this page. SYN tonsilla lingualis.

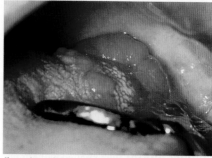

lingual tonsil at dorsolateral aspect of tongue

**lin·gual vein** (ling´gwăl vān) [TA] Vein that receives blood from tongue, sublingual and submandibular glands, and muscles of floor of mouth; empties into internal jugular or the facial vein.

**lin·gua ni·gra** (ling´gwă nī´gră) SYN black tongue.

**lin·gua pli·ca·ta** (ling´gwă plī-kā´tă) SYN fissured tongue.

**lin·gua vil·lo·sa al·ba** (ling´gwăl vil-ō´să al´bă) SYN white hairy tongue.

**lin·gui·form** (ling´gwi-fōrm) Tongue-shaped.

**lin·gu·la,** pl. **lin·gu·lae** (ling´gyū-lă, -lē) [TA] A tongue-shaped process. [L. dim. of *lingua,* tongue]

**lin·gu·la of man·di·ble** (ling´gyū-lă man´di-bĕl) [TA] Pointed tongue of bone overlapping mandibular foramen, giving attachment to sphenomandibular ligament. SYN mandibular tongue.

**lin·gu·lec·to·my** (ling´gyū-lek´tŏ-mē) **1.** SYN glossectomy. **2.** Excision of the lingular portion of the upper lobe of the left lung.

♻ **linguo-** Combining form denoting the tongue. [L. *lingua*]

**lin·guo·cer·vi·cal ridge** (ling´gwō-sĕr´vi-kăl rij) SYN linguogingival ridge.

**lin·guo·cli·na·tion** (ling´gwō-kli-nā´shŭn) Axial inclination of a tooth when crown is inclined more toward tongue than normal.

**lin·guo·clu·sion** (ling´gwō-klū´zhŭn) Displacement of tooth toward interior of dental arch, or toward tongue. SEE ALSO lingual occlusion (2). SYN lingual occlusion (1).

**lin·guo·dis·tal** (ling´gwō-dis´tăl) Relating to lingual and distal parts of the tooth.

**lin·guo·gin·gi·val** (ling´gwō-jin´ji-văl) **1.** Relating to gingival third of lingual surface of a tooth. **2.** Relating to angle or point of junction of lingual border and gingival line on distal or mesial surface of an incisor tooth.

**lin·guo·gin·gi·val fis·sure** (ling´gwō-jin´ji-văl fish´ŭr) Fissure of lingual surface of upper incisors extending into cementum.

**lin·guo·gin·gi·val groove** (ling´gwō-jin´ji-văl grūv) Groove separating embryonic mandibular portion of tongue from remainder of mandibular process.

**lin·guo·gin·gi·val ridge** (ling´gwō-jin´ji-văl rij) Ridge on lingual surface, near cervix, of incisor and cuspid teeth. SYN linguocervical ridge.

**lin·guo·gin·gi·val shoul·der** (ling´gwō-jin´ji-văl shōl´dĕr) In tooth preparation, the ledge or step formed by the gingival and lingual axial line angles.

**lin·guo·oc·clu·sal** (ling´gwō-ŏ-klū´săl) Relating to the line of junction of the lingual and occlusal surfaces of a tooth.

**lin·guo·pap·il·li·tis** (ling´gwō-pap´i-lī´tis) Small painful ulcers involving papillae on tongue margins.

**lin·guo·plate** (ling´gwō-plāt) SYN lingual plate.

**lin·guo·plate ma·jor con·nec·tor** (ling´gwō-plāt mā´jŏr kŏ-nek´tŏr) Attachment that extends a plate across the gingiva to the cingulum of the anterior teeth.

**lin·guo·ver·sion** (ling´gwō-vĕr´zhŭn) Malposition of tooth lingual to the normal position.

**lin·i·ment** (lin´i-mĕnt) Liquid preparation for external application or application to gingiva; frequently applied by friction to skin; used as counterirritants, rubefacients, or cleansing agents.

**lin·ing** (līn´ing) Coating applied to pulpal wall(s) of restorative dental preparation to protect pulp from thermal or chemical irritation; usually a vehicle containing a varnish, resin, and/or calcium hydroxide.

**lin·ing mu·co·sa** (līn´ing myū-kō´să) Mucosa that lines a cavity (e.g., oral cavity).

**link·age** (lingk´ăj) **1.** A chemical covalent bond. **2.** Form of connection between and among things.

**li·no·le·ate** (li-nō´lē-āt) Salt of linoleic acid.

**lip** (lip) [TA] **1.** One of two muscular folds with outer membrane having a stratified squamous cell epithelial surface layer around mouth. **2.** Any liplike structure bounding a cavity or groove. [A.S. *lippa*]

**lipaemia** [Br.] SYN lipemia.

**li·pase** (lip´ās) Any fat-splitting or lipolytic enzyme; a carboxylesterase.

**li·pe·mi·a** (li-pē´mē-ă) Presence of abnormally high concentration of lipids in circulating blood. SYN lipaemia. [*lipid* + G. *haima,* blood]

**lip·id** (lip´id) "Fat-soluble," operational term describing a solubility characteristic, not a chemical substance, i.e., denoting substances extracted from animal or vegetable cells by nonpolar solvents.

**lip·i·do·ly·tic** (lip´i-dō-lit´ik) Causing breakdown of lipids. [*lipid* + G. *lysis,* loosening]

**lip·i·do·sis,** pl. **lip·i·do·ses** (lip´i-dō´sis, -sēz) Hereditary abnormality of lipid metabolism that results in abnormal amounts of lipid deposition. [*lipid* + G. *-ōsis,* condition]

**lip·o·at·ro·phy** (lip´ō-at´rŏ-fē) Loss of subcutaneous fat, which may be total, congenital, and associated with various disorders.

**lip·o·dys·tro·phy** (lip´ō-dis´trŏ-fē) **1.** Defective metabolism of fat. **2.** Abnormal depositions or wastings of adipose tissue, or combinations of these changes. [*lipo-* + G. *dys-,* bad, difficult, + *trophē,* nourishment]

**lip·o·fus·ci·no·sis** (lip´ō-fyūs´i-nō´sis) Abnormal storage of any one of a group of fatty pigments.

**lip·o·gen·e·sis** (lip´ō-jen´ĕ-sis) Production of fat as either fatty degeneration or fatty infiltration. [*lipo-* + G. *genesis,* production]

**lip·o·gen·ic** (lip´ō-jen´ik) Relating to lipogenesis.

**lip·o·gran·u·lo·ma·to·sis** (lip´ō-gran´yŭ-lō´mă-tō´sis) **1.** Presence of lipogranulomas. **2.** Local inflammatory reaction to necrosis of adipose tissue.

**lip·oid** (lip´oyd) **1.** Resembling fat. **2.** Former term for lipid. SYN adipoid.

**lip·oi·do·sis** (lip´oy-dō´sis) Presence of anisotropic lipoids in cells.

**lip·oid pro·tein·o·sis** (lip´oyd prō´tēn-ō´sis) Disturbance of lipid metabolism with deposits of a protein-lipid complex on tongue and sublingual and faucial areas leading to hoarseness and translucent keratotic papillomatous eyelid lesions.

**li·pol·y·sis** (li-pol´i-sis) The splitting up (hydrolysis), or chemical decomposition, of fat. [*lipo-* + G. *lysis,* dissolution]

**li·po·ma,** pl. **li·po·mas** (li-pō´mă, -măz) A benign neoplasm of adipose tissue, composed of mature fat cells. See page 346. [*lipo-* + G. *-oma,* tumor]

**lip·o·ox·y·gen·ase, lip·ox·y·gen·ase** (lip´ō-oks´i-jĕ-nās, li-poks´) An enzyme that converts unsaturated fatty acids to peroxides acid. [*lipo-* + oxygen + -ase]

**lip·o·pe·nic** (lip´ō-pē´nik) An agent or drug that reduces concentration of lipids in the blood.

kl

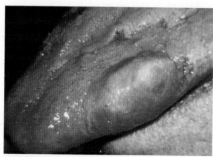

lipoma: lateral margin of tongue

**lip·o·phil·ic** (lip'ō-fil'ik) Capable of dissolving, of being dissolved in, or of absorbing lipids.

**li·po·sis** (li-pō'sis) Fatty infiltration.

**lip·o·troph·ic** (lip'ō-trō'fik) Relating to lipotrophy.

**li·pot·ro·phy** (li-pot'rŏ-fē) An increase of fat in the body. [lipo- + G. trophē, nourishment]

**lip·o·trop·ic** (lip'ō-trō'pik) 1. Pertaining to substances preventing or correcting excessive fat deposits in liver. 2. Relating to lipotropy.

**lip·o·tro·pin** (lip'ō-trō'pin) Pituitary hormone mobilizing fat from adipose tissue.

**lipoxidase** SYN lipoxygenase.

**li·pox·y·ge·nase** (li-poks'ē-jĕ-nās) An enzyme that catalyzes the oxidation of unsaturated fatty acids with $O_2$ to yield lipoperoxides of the fatty acids. SYN lipoxidase.

**lip pits** (lip pits) Malformations of lip seen in unilateral or bilateral depressions or fistulae. May be hereditary or associated with cleft lip and/or palate. See this page.

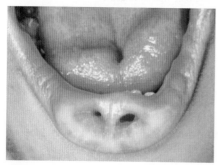

lip pits

**lip read·ing** (lip rēd'ing) SYN speech reading.

**lip re·flex** (lip rē'fleks) Pouting movement of lips provoked in young infants by tapping near the angle of the mouth.

**lip re·trac·tors** (lip rĕ-trak'tŏrz) Instruments used during dental procedures to hold back lips for improved access to oral areas.

**lips of mouth** (lips mowth) [TA] Fleshy folds with skin externally and oral mucosa internally that surround oval fissure and form anterior walls of oral vestibule; with the enclosed orbicularis oris and various dilator muscles, constitute cranial sphincter of the alimentary tract.

**lip sul·cus** (lip sŭl'kŭs) SYN labial sulcus.

**liq·ue·fa·cient** (lik'wĕ-fā'shĕnt) 1. Making liquid. 2. Denoting a resolvant supposed to cause resolution of a solid tumor by liquefying its contents.

**liq·ue·fied phe·nol** (lik'wi-fīd fē'nol) Liquefied carbolic acid.

**li·queur** (li-kur') A cordial; a spirit containing sugar and aromatics. [Fr.]

**liq·uid glu·cose** (lik'wid glū'kōs) Pharmaceutic aid consisting of dextrose, dextrins, maltose, and water, obtained by incomplete hydrolysis of starch.

**liq·uid hu·man se·rum** (lik'wid hyū'măn sēr'ŭm) Pool of fluids separated from blood withdrawn from human subjects and allowed to clot in the absence of any anticoagulant.

**liq·uid par·af·fin** (lik'wid par'ă-fin) SYN mineral oil.

**liq·uid pe·tro·le·um** (lik'wid pĕ-trō'lē-ŭm) SYN mineral oil.

**li·quor,** pl. **li·quo·res** (lī'kwōr, lī-kwōr'ēz) [TA] As a Latin word, liquor is pronounced lī'kwōr. As an English word it is pronounced lik'ĕr. 1. Any liquid or fluid. 2. A term used for certain body fluids. 3. Pharmacopoeial term for any aqueous solution of a nonvolatile substance.

**li·quo·rice** (li-kŏ-ris) SYN glycyrrhiza.

**li·quor pu·ris** (lī'kwōr pū'ris) Fluid portion of pus.

**lis·pro in·su·lin** (lis'prō in'sŭ-lin) A modified version of natural human insulin, with a much faster onset of action, which reaches its peak effect earlier than regular insulin; available only by prescription.

**Lis·ter·i·a** (lis-tēr'ē-ă) Genus of aerobic to microaerophilic, motile, peritrichous bacteria containing small, coccoid, gram-positive rods; found in the feces of humans and other animals, on vegetation, and in silage. The type species is L. monocytogenes.

**li·ter (L)** (lē'tĕr) A measure of capacity of 1000 cubic centimeters or 1 cubic decimeter; equivalent to 1.056688 quarts (U.S., liquid). SYN litre. [Fr., fr. G. litra, a pound]

**lith·a·gogue** (lith′ă-gog) A substance or agent that causes dislodgment or expulsion of calculi, especially urinary. [*litho-* + G. *agōgos,* drawing forth]

**lith·i·um car·bon·ate** (lith′ē-ŭm kahr′bŏ-nāt) Agent used to treat depressive, hypomanic, and manic phases of bipolar affective disorders.

✪ **litho-** Combining form denoting a stone, calculus, calcification. [G. *lithos*]

**lith·o·lyt·ic** (lith′ō-lit′ik) Agent tending to dissolve calculi. [*litho-* + G. *lysis,* dissolution]

**litre** [Br.] SYN liter.

**live·birth, live birth** (līv-bĭrth) The birth of an infant who shows postnatal evidence of life.

**liv·er** (liv′ĕr) [TA] The largest gland of the body, lying beneath the diaphragm in the right hypochondrium and upper part of the epigastric region; it is of irregular shape and weighs from 1–2 kg, or about one fortieth weight of body. Detoxifies drugs and many exogeneous substances and is also of great importance in fat, carbohydrate, and protein metabolism.

**liv·er breath** (liv′ĕr breth) SYN fetor hepaticus.

**live vac·cine** (līv vak-sēn′) Vaccine prepared from living attenuated organisms.

**liv·ing will** (liv′ing wil) Advance directive that specifies the types of care a person does or does not want to receive in the event of becoming mentally incompetent during the course of a terminal illness, or becoming permanently comatose. A document that may also name another person to make such decisions is known as a durable power-of-attorney for health care decisions. An advance directive can contain both types of instruction.

**LJP** Abbreviation for localized juvenile periodontitis.

**LLQ** Abbreviation for lower left quadrant (of mouth).

**LN** Abbreviation for laminin.

**LOA** Abbreviation for loss of attachment.

**load** (lōd) Departure from normal body content; positive loads are quantities in excess of normal; negative loads are quantities in deficit.

**load·ing** (lōd′ing) 1. Process in which dental prosthesis is placed into functional occlusion. 2. Administration of a substance for the purpose of testing metabolic function.

**load·ing dose** (lōd-ing′ dōs) Comparatively large dose given at beginning of treatment to start getting the effect of a drug. SYN initial dose.

**lobe** (lōb) [TA] 1. One of the larger divisions of tooth crown, formed from a distinct point of calcification. 2. One of the subdivisions of an organ or other part, bounded by fissures, sulci, connective tissue septa, or other structural demarcations. [G. *lobos,* lobe]

**lo·bec·to·my** (lō-bek′tŏ-mē) Excision of a lobe of any organ or gland. [G. *lobos,* lobe, + *ektomē,* excision]

**lob·ule of au·ri·cle** (lob′yūl awr′i-kĕl) [TA] The lowest part of the auricle; it consists of fat and fibrous tissue not reinforced by the auricular cartilage; it is often used as a site to obtain a small sample of blood with a lancet.

**LOC** Abbreviation for level of consciousness.

**lo·cal** (lō′kăl) Having reference or confined to a limited part; not general or systemic. [L. *localis,* fr. *locus,* place]

**lo·cal an·al·ge·si·a** (lō′kăl an′al-jē′zē-ă) Localized palliation of pain. SEE ALSO analgesia.

**lo·cal an·es·the·si·a** (lō′kăl an′es-thē′zē-ă) General term referring to topical, infiltration, field block, or nerve block anesthesia but usually not to spinal or epidural anesthesia; may mean pharmacologic agents used to achieve local anesthesia. SEE ALSO local anesthetics.

**lo·cal an·es·thet·ic re·ac·tion** (lō′kăl an′ĕs-thet′ik rē′ak′shŭn) Toxic reaction due to absorption of local anesthetic drug during regional anesthesia, ranging from drowsiness to convulsions and cardiovascular collapse.

**lo·cal an·es·thet·ics** (lō′kăl an′ĕs-thet′iks) Drugs used for the interruption of the nerve transmission of pain sensations; act at site of application to prevent perception of pain.

**lo·cal hor·mone** (lō′kăl hōr′mōn) Metabolic product secreted by one set of cells that affects function of nearby cells; an autacoid.

**lo·cal·i·za·tion** (lō′kăl-i-zā′shŭn) 1. Limitation to a definite area. 2. Reference of sensation to its point of origin. 3. Determination of location of a morbid process.

**lo·cal·ized juv·e·nile per·i·o·don·ti·tis (LJP)** (lō′kăl-īzd jū′vĕ-nil per′ē-ō-don-tī′tis) SYN juvenile periodontitis.

**lo·cal syn·cope** (lō′kăl sing′kŏ-pē) Limited numbness in a body part, especially fingers; usually associated with local asphyxia or Raynaud disease.

**lo·ca·tor** (lō′kā-tŏr) An instrument or apparatus for finding the position of a foreign object in tissue.

**lock·ed bite** (lokt bīt) Occlusion in which lateral mandibular movements (excursions) are restricted by the cusp arrangement of the teeth.

**lock·jaw** (lok′jaw) SYN trismus.

**lo·co·mo·tor a·tax·i·a** (lō′kō-mō′tŏr ă-

kl

tak´sē-ă) Severe gait ataxia seen with tabetic neurosyphilis.

**lo·cus**, pl. **lo·ci** (lō´kŭs, -sī) **1.** A place or site. **2.** The position that a gene occupies on a chromosome. **3.** The position of a point, as defined by graph coordinates.

**lo·cus of con·trol** (lō´kŭs kŏn-trōl´) A theoretic construct designed to assess a person's perceived control over personal behavior; classified as internal if the person feels in control of events, external if others are perceived to have that control.

**lod score** (lod skōr) A number used in genetic linkage studies; logarithm (base 10) of the odds in favor of genetic linkage. [*logarithm + od*ds]

**log·o·pe·dics, log·o·pe·di·a** (log´ō-pē´diks, -pē´dē-ă) A branch of science concerned with the physiology and pathology of the organs of speech and with the correction of speech defects.

**lo·mus·tine** (lō-mŭs´tēn) An antineoplastic agent.

**long-act·ing thy·roid stim·u·la·tor** (lawng´ak´ting thī´royd stim´yū-lā-tŏr) A hematologic substance that exerts a prolonged stimulatory effect on the thyroid gland.

**long ax·is** (lawng aks´is) **1.** In dentistry, line extending incisocervically (occlusocervically) parallel to axial tooth surfaces. **2.** Line extending through the center of an object lengthwise.

**long buc·cal nerve** (lawng bŭk´ăl nĕrv) SYN buccal nerve.

**long-cone tech·nique** (lawng-kōn´ tek-nēk´) A radiographic method for oral x-rays used in dentistry wherein the cone used for alignment of the head of the radiographic machine with the film is about 35 cm (14 in) long.

**lon·gev·i·ty** (lawn-jev´i-tē) Duration of a given life beyond the norm for the species.

**lon·gi·tu·di·nal sec·tion** (lon´ji-tū´di-nǎl sek´shŭn) A cross-section attained by slicing in any plane parallel to the long or vertical axis, actually or through imaging techniques, the body or any part of the body or anatomic structure.

**lon·gi·tu·di·nal stud·y** (lon´ji-tū´di-nǎl stŭd´ē) A study of the natural course of life or disorder in which a cohort of subjects is serially observed over a period of time and no assumptions need be made about the stability of the system.

**long junc·tion·al ep·i·the·li·um** (lawng jŭngk´shŭn-ăl ep´i-thē´lē-ŭm) Primary pattern of healing that occurs after periodontal débridement; no new periodontal ligament or bone forms.

**long-scale con·trast** (lawng-skāl´ kon´

trast) A radiographic image that shows many shades of gray and thus has low contrast.

**long-term mem·o·ry (LTM)** (lawng´tĕrm mem´ŏ-rē) Phase of memory process considered as the permanent storehouse of information that has been registered, encoded, passed into the short-term memory, then coded, rehearsed, and finally transferred and stored for future retrieval.

**loop** (lūp) **1.** A sharp curve or complete bend in a vessel, cord, or other cylindric body, forming an oval or circular ring. **2.** A wire (usually of platinum or nichrome) fixed into a handle at one end and bent into a circle at the other, rendered sterile by flaming, and used to transfer microorganisms. [M.E. *loupe*]

**loop di·u·ret·ic** (lūp dī´yūr-et´ik) Class of diuretic agents that acts by inhibiting reabsorption of sodium and chloride.

**loph·o·dont** (lof´ŏ-dont) Having crowns of molar teeth formed in transverse or longitudinal crests or ridges.

**lor·do·sis** (lōr-dō´sis) [TA] A normal anteriorly convex curvature of the vertebral column. [G. *lordōsis*, a bending backward]

**loss of at·tach·ment (LOA)** (laws ă-tach´mĕnt) Damage to the structures that support the tooth; results from periodontitis and is characterized by relocation of the junctional epithelium to the tooth root, destruction of the fibers of the gingiva, destruction of the periodontal ligament fibers, and loss of alveolar bone support from around the tooth.

**lo·tion** (lō´shŭn) A class of pharmacopeial preparations that are liquid suspensions or dispersions intended for external application. [L. *lotio*, a washing, fr. *lavo*, to wash]

**loupe** (lūp) A magnifying lens. [Fr.]

**low-cal·o·rie di·et** (lō-kal´ŏr-ē dī´ĕt) Dietary regimen of 1,200 or fewer calories per day.

**low·er cut·ting edge** (lō´wĕr kŭt´ing ej) Cutting edge of an area-specific curette used for periodontal débridement.

**low·er den·tal ar·cade** (lō´wĕr den´tăl ahr-kād´) SYN mandibular dental arcade.

**low·er jaw** (lō´wĕr jaw) SYN mandible.

**low·er left quad·rant (of mouth) (LLQ)** (lō´ĕr left kwah´drănt mowth) One of four areas in the oral cavity comprising (according to the numeration system of the American Dental Association) lower mandibular teeth 17 to 24.

**low·er mo·tor neu·ron le·sion** (lō´wĕr mō´tŏr nūr´on le´zhŭn) Injury to motor cells in the brainstem or spinal cord.

**low·er ridge slope** (lō´wĕr rij slōp) Slope

of mandibular residual ridge in second and third molars as seen from the buccal side.

**low·er right quad·rant (of mouth) (LRQ)** (lō′ĕr rīt kwah′drănt mowth) One of four areas in the oral cavity comprising (according to the numeration system of the American Dental Association) lower mandibular teeth 17 to 24.

**low·er shank** (lō′ĕr shangk) Portion of the functional shank nearest to the working-end; provides an important visual clue when selecting the correct working-end of an instrument. SYN terminal shank.

**low-fat di·et** (lō-fat dī′ĕt) Diet containing a minimal proportion of fat designed to reduce the risk of cardiovascular disease, specifically atherosclerosis.

**low lip line** (lō lip līn) 1. Lowest position of lower lip during the act of smiling or voluntary retraction. 2. Lowest position of upper lip at rest.

**low res·i·due di·et** (lō rez′i-dū dī′ĕt ) Diet that leaves few unabsorbed components in the intestine to minimize functional colonic stress.

**low salt di·et** (lō sawlt dī′ĕt) Diet with restricted amounts of sodium chloride; useful in the treatment of some cases of hypertension, heart failure, and other syndromes.

**low-tem·per·a·ture ster·i·li·za·tion** (lō tem′pĕr-ă-chŭr ster′i-lī-zā′shŭn) Disinfection of items customarily with ethylene oxide gas; usually accomplished at ambient temperatures or temperatures below those used for autoclave, chemical vapor, or dry-heat oven sterilization. SYN gas sterilization.

**loz·enge** (loz′ĕnj) SYN troche. [Fr. *losange,* fr. *lozangé,* rhombic]

**LRQ** Abbreviation for lower right quadrant (of mouth).

**LSD** Abbreviation for lysergic acid diethylamide.

**LTM** Abbreviation for long-term memory.

**lu·cid** (lū′sid) Clear, not obscured or confused. [L. *lucidus,* clear]

**lu·cid·i·ty** (lū-sid′i-tē) The quality or state of being lucid.

**Lud·wig an·gi·na** (lud′vig an′ji-nă) Cellulitis, usually of odontogenic origin, bilaterally involving submaxillary, sublingual, and submental spaces, resulting in painful swelling of floor of mouth, elevation of tongue, dysphagia, and dysphonia. See this page. [W.F. *Ludwig*]

**lu·es** (lū′ēz) A plague or pestilence; specifically, syphilis. [L. pestilence]

**lu·et·ic** (lū-et′ik) SYN syphilitic.

**lu·men,** pl. **lu·mi·na** (lū′mĕn, -mi-nă) 1.

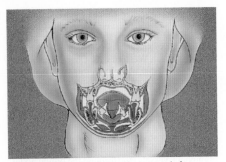

**Ludwig angina:** pink arrows show spread of infection

Space in interior of a hollow tubular structure (e.g., artery or intestine). 2. The bore of a catheter or hollow needle. [L. light, window]

**lu·mi·nes·cence** (lū′mi-nes′ĕns) Emission of light from a body as a result of a chemical reaction. [L. *lumen,* light]

**lung** (lŭng) [TA] One of a pair of viscera occupying thoracic pulmonary cavities; organs of respiration in which blood is aerated. [A.S. *lungen*]

**lu·pus** (lū′pŭs) A term originally used to depict erosion (as if gnawed) of the skin, now used with modifying terms designating various diseases. [L. wolf]

**lu·pus er·y·the·ma·to·sus (LE)** (lū′pŭs ĕr-i′thĕ-mă-tō′sŭs) An illness that may be characterized by skin lesions alone or systemic (disseminated) with antinuclear antibodies present and usually involvement of vital structures. See page A4.

**lu·pus·like syn·drome** (lū′pŭs-līk sin′drōm) Clinical syndrome resembling systemic lupus erythematosus, but due to another cause.

**lu·pus vul·ga·ris** (lū′pŭs vŭl-gā′ris) Cutaneous tuberculosis with characteristic nodular lesions on the face.

**lute** (lūt) To seal or fasten with wax or cement. [L. *lutum,* mud]

**lu·te·in** (lū′tē-in) Yellow pigment in corpus luteum, in egg yolk, or any lipochrome. [L. *luteus,* saffron-yellow]

**lut·ing a·gent** (lūt′ing ā′jĕnt) In dentistry, fastening material or cement (e.g., plaster or wax to hold casts to an articulator, or material to hold crowns to teeth).

**lux·a·tion** (lŭk-sā′shŭn) 1. In dentistry, dislocation or displacement of condyle in temporomandibular fossa, or of a tooth from the alveolus. 2. SYN dislocation. [L. *luxatio*]

**lye** (lī) Liquid obtained by leaching wood ashes. [A.S. *leáh*]

**Lyme dis·ease** (līm di-zēz′) Subacute inflammatory disorder caused by infection with Borrelia burgdorferi, a nonpyogenic spirochete transmitted by Ixodes scapularis, deer tick, in eastern U.S. and I. pacificus, western black-legged tick, in Western U.S. Characteristic skin lesion, erythema chronicum migrans, is usually preceded or accompanied by fever, malaise, fatigue, headache, and stiff neck. [Old Lyme, CT, where first observed]

**lymph** (limf) [TA] A clear, sometimes faintly yellow, and slightly opalescent fluid collected from tissues throughout the body, flows in the lymphatic vessels, and through the lymph nodes, and is eventually added to the venous blood circulation.

**lym·phad·e·ni·tis** (lim-fad′ĕ-nī′tis) Inflammation of one or more lymph nodes. [lymphadeno- + G. -itis, inflammation]

**lym·phad·e·nop·a·thy** (lim-fad′ĕ-nop′ă-thē) 1. Any disease process affecting lymph nodes. 2. The appearance of enlarged lymph nodes found on x-rays. [G. lympha spring water + aden gland + G. pathos, suffering]

**lym·phan·gi·o·ma** (lim-fan′jē-ō′mă) General term for tumors formed by a mass of anomalous lymphatic vessels or channels that vary in size, are usually greatly dilated, and are lined with normal endothelial cells. They occur most frequently in the neck and axilla, but may also develop in the arm, mesentery, and other sites. See this page and page A15. [G. lympha spring water + angeion vessel + G. -oma, tumor]

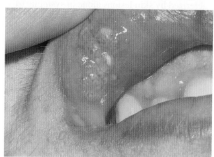
labial lymphangioma

**lym·phat·ic** (lim-fat′ik) 1. Pertaining to lymph. 2. A vascular channel that transports lymph. [L. lymphaticus, frenzied]

**lymph cir·cu·la·tion** (limf sir′kyū-lā′shŭn) Slow passage of lymph through lymphatic vessels and glands.

**lymph·e·de·ma** (lim′fĕ-dē′mă) Swelling (especially in subcutaneous tissues) due to obstruction of lymphatic vessels or lymph nodes and accumulation of large amounts of lymph in affected region. SYN lymphoedema. [lymph + G. oidēma, a swelling]

**lymph node** (limf nōd) [TA] One of numerous round, oval, or bean-shaped bodies located along the course of lymphatic vessels, varying greatly in size and usually presenting a depressed area, the hilum. See this page.

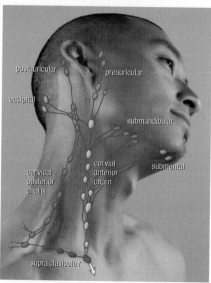
location of lymph nodes of head and neck

**lympho-** Combining form denoting lymph. [L. lympha, spring water]

**lym·pho·cyte** (lim′fŏ-sīt) A white blood cell formed in bone marrow and distributed throughout the body in lymphatic tissue (e.g., lymph nodes, spleen, thymus, tonsils, Peyer patches), where it undergoes proliferation. [lympho- + G. kytos, call]

**lymphocythaemia** [Br.] SYN lymphocytosis.

**lymphocythemia** SYN lymphocytosis.

**lymphocytic leukemia** SYN lymphatic leukemia.

**lym·pho·cy·to·sis** (lim′fŏ-sī-tō′sis) A form of leukocytosis in which there is an actual or relative increase in the number of lymphocytes. SYN lymphocytheto prevent mia, lymphocythaemia.

**lymphoedema** [Br.] SYN lymphedema.

**lym·pho·ep·i·the·li·al cyst** (lim′fŏ-ep′i-thē′lē-ăl sist) Cervical cyst arising from salivary gland epithelium entrapped in lymph nodes during embryogenesis, also seen within the oral cavity. See page 351 and page A5.

**lym·pho·ep·i·the·li·o·ma** (lim′fŏ-ep′i-thē′lē-ō′mă) A poorly differentiated radiosensitive

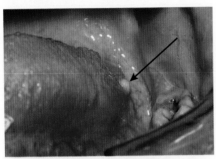

**oral lymphoepithelial cyst:** lateral tongue

squamous cell carcinoma involving lymphoid tissue in the region of the tonsils and nasopharynx; metastasizes early to cervical lymph nodes. [*lympho-* + epithelium + *-oma,* tumor]

**lym·pho·gran·u·lo·ma** (lim′fō-gran-yū-lō′ mă) Older nonspecific term used with reference to a few basically dissimilar diseases in which the pathologic processes result in granulomas or granulomalike lesions.

**lym·pho·ma** (lim-fō′mă) Any neoplasm of lymphoid or reticuloendothelial tissues; in general use, synonymous with malignant lymphoma; presents as apparently solid tumors composed of cells that appear primitive or resemble lymphocytes, plasma cells, or histiocytes; appear most frequently in the lymph nodes, spleen, or other normal sites of lymphoreticular cells. [*lympho-* + G. *-oma,* tumor]

**lym·phop·a·thy** (lim-fop′ă-thē) Any disease of the lymphatic vessels or lymph nodes. [*lympho-* + G. *pathos,* suffering]

**lym·pho·pe·ni·a** (lim′fō-pē′nē-ă) Reduction, relative or absolute, in the number of lymphocytes in circulating blood. [*lympho-* + G. *penia,* poverty]

**ly·pres·sin** (lī-pres′in) An antidiuretic and vasopressor hormone.

**Lys** Abbreviation for lysine.

**ly·ser·gic ac·id** (lī-ser′jik as′id) The D-isomer is a cleavage product of alkaline hydrolysis of ergot alkaloids; a psychotomimetic.

**ly·ser·gic ac·id am·ide** (lī-sĕr′jik as′id am′īd) Psychotomimetic agent present in *Rivea corymbosa* and *Ipomoea tricolor;* possesses less hallucinogenic potency than lysergic acid diethylamide (LSD) (q.v.).

**ly·ser·gic ac·id di·eth·yl·am·ide (LSD)** (lī-sĕr′jik as′id dī-eth′il-am′īd) Peripherally, a serotonin antagonist; 1–2 mcg or less per kg induces hallucinatory states; its use may precipitate psychoses.

**ly·sin** (lī′sin) **1.** A complement-fixing antibody that acts destructively on cells and tissues; the various types are designated in accordance with the form of antigen that stimulates the production of the lysin, e.g., hemolysin, bacteriolysin. **2.** Any substance that causes lysis.

**ly·sine (Lys)** (lī′sēn) A nutritionally essential α-amino acid found in many proteins.

**ly·sis** (lī′sis) **1.** Destruction of red blood cells, bacteria, and other structures by a specific lysin, usually referred to by structure destroyed (e.g., hemolysis, bacteriolysis, nephrolysis). **2.** Gradual subsidence of symptoms of an acute disease, a form of recovery. [G. dissolution or loosening]

**ly·so·so·mal dis·ease** (lī′sō-sō′măl di-zēz′) Disorder due to inadequate functioning of a lysosomal enzyme.

**ly·so·some** (lī′sō-sōm) A cytoplasmic membrane-bound vesicle (primary lysosome) and containing a wide variety of glycoprotein hydrolytic enzymes active at an acid pH; serves to digest exogenous material, such as bacteria. [*lyso-* + G. *soma,* body]

**ly·so·zyme** (lī′sō-zīm) An enzyme destructive to cell walls of certain bacteria; present in tears, egg white, and some plant tissues; used in caries to prevent. SYN muramidase.

**lyt·ic** (lit′ik) Pertaining to lysis; used colloquially as an abbreviation for osteolytic.

kl

# M

**M** Abbreviation for methionine.

**m** Abbreviation for meter.

**mac·er·ate** (mas′ĕr-āt) To soften by steeping or soaking.

**mac·er·a·tion** (mas′ĕr-ā′shŭn) Softening by the action of a liquid. [L. *macero*, pp. *-atus*, to soften by soaking]

**Mac·ew·en sign** (măk-yū′ĕn sīn) Percussion of cranium gives a cracked-pot sound in cases of hydrocephalus.

**Ma·cha·do-Jo·seph dis·ease** (mă-shah′dū-jō′sef di-zēz′) Rare form of hereditary ataxia, found predominantly in people of Azorean ancestry.

**macro-, macr-** Combining forms meaning large, long. [G. *makros*]

**mac·ro·bi·ot·ics** (mak′rō-bī-ot′iks) The study of the prolongation of life.

**mac·ro·chei·li·a, mac·ro·chi·li·a** (mak′rō-kī′lē-ă) **1.** Abnormally enlarged lips. **2.** Cavernous lymphangioma of the lip, a condition of permanent swelling due to greatly distended lymphatic spaces.

**mac·ro·cyte** (mak′rō-sīt) A large erythrocyte, such as those observed in pernicious anemia. [*macro-* + G. *kytos*, a hollow (cell)]

**mac·ro·cyt·ic a·ne·mi·a** (mak′rō-sit′ik ă-nē′mē-ă) Any anemia in which average size of circulating erythrocytes is greater than normal; i.e., comprises syndromes such as pernicious anemia, sprue, celiac disease, and others.

**mac·ro·cyt·ic a·ne·mi·a of preg·nan·cy** (mak′rō-sit′ik ă-nē′mē-ă preg′năn-sē) Anemia related to folate deficiency characterized by a low level of hemoglobin and a reduced number of enlarged erythrocytes.

**mac·ro·dont** (mak′rō-dont) **1.** Tooth of proportions; may be localized or generalized. **2.** Denoting a cranium with a dental index exceeding 44. SYN megadont enlarged. [*macro-* + G. *odous* (*odont-*), tooth]

**mac·ro·don·ti·a, mac·ro·don·tism** (mak′rō-don′shē-ă, -tizm) Having abnormally large teeth. See this page. SYN megadontism, megalodontia.

**ma·cro·fill·ed com·pos·ite** (mak′rō-fild kŏm-poz′īt) Resin compound with a high proportion of filler particles to make it more resistant to wear.

**mac·ro·glos·si·a** (mak′rō-glos′ē-ă) Enlargement of tongue, either developmentally or due to a neoplasm or vascular hamartoma. See this page. SYN megaloglossia. [*macro-* + G. *glōssa*, tongue]

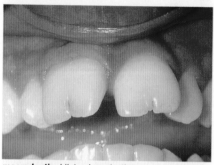
**macrodontia:** bilateral gemination

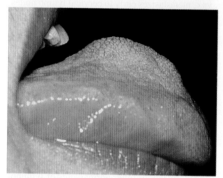
**macroglossia:** caused by hemangioma

**mac·ro·gna·thi·a** (mak′rog-nā′thē-ă) Enlargement or elongation of the jaw. SYN megagnathia. [*macro-* + G. *gnathos*, jaw]

**mac·ro·lides** (mak′rō-līdz) Class of antibiotics discovered in streptomycetes, e.g., erythromycin; many inhibit protein biosynthesis.

**mac·ro·mol·e·cule** (mak′rō-mol′ĕ-kyūl) A molecule of colloidal size (e.g., proteins, polynucleic acids, polysaccharides).

**mac·ro·nu·tri·ents** (mak′rō-nū′trē-ĕnts) Nutrients required in the greatest amount; e.g., carbohydrates, protein, fats.

**mac·ro·phage** (mak′rō-fāj) Any mononuclear, actively phagocytic cell arising from monocytic stem cells in bone marrow; widely distributed in body and vary in morphology and motility. [*macro-* + G. *phagō*, to eat]

**mac·ro·scop·ic** (mak′rō-skop′ik) **1.** Of a size visible with the naked eye or without the use of a microscope. **2.** Relating to macroscopy.

**macroscopy** SYN macroscopic.

**mac·ro·so·mi·a** (mak′rō-sō′mē-ă) Abnormally large body size. [*macro-* + G. *sōma*, body]

**mac·ro·sto·mi·a** (mak′rō-stō′mē-ă) Abnormally large mouth resulting from embryonic failure of fusion between maxillary and mandibular prominences. [*macro-* + G. *stoma*, mouth]

**mac·ro·ti·a** (mak-rō′shē-ă) Congenital excessive enlargement of the auricle. [G. *makros*, large, + *ous, gen. otos*, ear, + *-ia*, noun suffix]

**mac·u·la**, pl. **mac·u·lae** (mak′yū-lă, -lē) **1.** [TA] Circumscribed flat area, differing perceptibly in color from surrounding tissue. **2.** Small discolored patch on skin, neither elevated above nor depressed below skin's surface. **3.** Neuroepithelial sensory receptors of utricle and saccule of vestibular labyrinth collectively. See this page. SYN spot (1). [L. a spot]

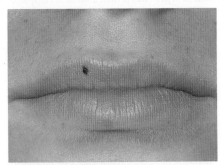

oral (labial) melanotic macula

**mag·al·drate** (mag′al-drāt) A chemical combination used as an antacid.

**ma·gen·ta tongue** (mă-jen′tă tŭng) Purplish red coloration of tongue, with edema and flattening of the filiform papillae, occurring in riboflavin deficiency. Cf. cyanosis.

**mag·ic·al think·ing** (maj′i-kăl thingk′ing) Irrational belief that one can bring about a circumstance or event by thinking about it or wishing for it.

**Ma·gill for·ceps** (mă-gil′ fōr′seps) A bent blunt instrument used to facilitate nasotracheal intubation.

**mag·is·tral** (maj′is-trăl) Denoting a preparation compounded according to a physician's prescription, in contrast to officinal (derived from a pharmacist's stock). [L. *magister*, master]

**Mag·nan trom·bone move·ment** (mahnyahn′ trom-bōn′ mūv′měnt) Involuntary back-and-forth tongue motion when it is drawn out of the mouth; seen in basal ganglia disorders.

**mag·ne·si·um** (mag-nē′zē-ŭm) An alkaline earth element, which oxidizes to magnesia; a bioelement, many salts have clinical applications. [Mod. L. fr. G. *Magnēsia*, a region in Thessaly in Greece]

**mag·ne·si·um sul·fate (MS)** (mag-nē′zē-ŭm sŭl′fāt) Active ingredient of most natural laxative waters; used as a promptly acting cathartic in certain poisonings, in treatment of increased intracranial pressure and edema, as an anticonvulsant in eclampsia (when administered intravenously), and as an antiinflammatory. SYN Epsom salts.

**mag·net·ic im·plant** (mag-net′ik im′plant) Tissue-tolerated, magnetized metal placed within the bone to aid in denture retention; a similar magnet is placed in overlying denture to complete the field.

**mag·net·ic res·o·nance im·a·ging** (mag-net′ik rez′ŏ-năns im′ăj-ing) Diagnostic radiologic modality, using nuclear magnetic resonance technology, in which magnetic nuclei (especially protons) of a patient are aligned in a strong, uniform magnetic field, absorb energy from tuned radiofrequency pulses, and emit radiofrequency signals as their excitation decays. These signals, which vary in intensity according to nuclear abundance and molecular chemical environment, are converted into sets of tomographic images.

**mag·ne·to·en·ceph·a·lo·gram (MEG)** (mag-nē′tō-en-sef′ă-lō-gram) A Gauss-time record of the magnetic field of the brain.

**mag·ne·tom·e·ter** (mag′ně-tom′ě-těr) An instrument for detecting and measuring the magnetic field.

**mag·ne·to·stric·tive ul·tra·son·ic de·vice** (mag-nē′tō-strik′tiv ŭl′tră-son′ik dě-vīs′) Electronically powered tool that used rapid energy vibrations of a powered instrument tip to fracture calculus from tooth surfaces and cleanse environment of a periodontal pocket; consists of a portable unit that contains an electronic generator, a handpiece, and interchangeable instrument inserts. See this page. SYN ultrasonic scaler.

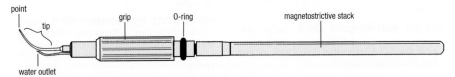

**magnetostrictive ultrasonic device:** handpiece insert, design with external water delivery tube

mn

**mag·ni·fi·ca·tion loupes** (mag′ni-fi-kā′ shŭn lūps) Visual enlargement of the treatment area through surgical telescopes during dental or periodontal procedures.

**ma-huang** (mah-hwahng) Chinese name for *Ephedra equisetina*. [Chinese]

**main·stream smoke** (mān′strēm smōk) Smoke that is inhaled directly into the smoker's lungs.

**main·tain·er** (mān-tān′ĕr) Device used to hold or keep teeth in a given position.

**main·te·nance** (mān′tĕ-nǎns) **1.** Therapeutic regimen intended to preserve health benefit. **2.** Extent to which patient continues good health practices without supervision, incorporating them into a general lifestyle.

**main·te·nance drug ther·a·py** (mān′tĕ-nǎns drŭg thār′ǎ-pē) In pharmacotherapy, systematic dosage at a level that maintains protection against exacerbation of disease.

**main·te·nance phase per·i·o·don·tal dis·ease** (mān′tĕ-nǎns fāz per′ē-ō-don′tǎl di-zēz′) Reexamination, assessment, and patient self-care as well as oral prophylaxis.

**ma·jor con·nec·tor** (mā′jŏr kŏ-nek′tŏr) Plate or bar (e.g., lingual bar, palatal bar or plate) used to unite partial denture bases.

**ma·jor de·pres·sion, ma·jor de·pres·sive dis·or·der** (mā′jŏr dĕ-presh′ŭn, dĕ-pres′iv dis-ōr′dĕr) Mental disorder characterized by sustained depression of mood, anhedonia, sleep and appetite disturbances, and feelings of worthlessness, guilt, and hopelessness.

**ma·jor his·to·com·pat·i·bil·i·ty com·plex (MHC)** (mā′jŏr his′tō-kŏm-pat′i-bil′i-tē kom′pleks) A group of linked loci, collectively termed HLA complex in humans, which codes for cell-surface histocompatibility antigens and is the principal determinant of tissue type and transplant compatibility.

**ma·jor hyp·no·sis** (mā′jŏr hip-nō′sis) State of extreme suggestibility in hypnosis in which the subject is insensible to all outside impressions except the commands of the hypnotist.

**ma·jor sal·i·var·y glands** (mā′jŏr sal′i-var-ē glandz) [TA] Category of salivary glands that secrete intermittently; includes three largest glands of oral cavity, which also secrete most saliva: parotid, submandibular, and sublingual glands.

**ma·jor sub·lin·gual duct** (mā′jŏr sŭb-ling′ gwǎl dŭkt) [TA] Duct that drains anterior portion of sublingual gland.

**ma·la** (mā′lǎ) **1.** SYN cheek. **2.** SYN zygomatic bone. [L. cheek bone]

**mal·ab·sorp·tion** (mal′ab-sōrp′shŭn) Imperfect or disordered gastrointestinal absorption.

**mal·ab·sorp·tion syn·drome** (mal′ab-sōrp′shŭn sin′drōm) State characterized by diverse features; caused by conditions in which there is ineffective absorption of nutrients.

**mal·a·chite green** (mal′ǎ-kīt grēn) [C.I. 42000] Dye used as a wound antiseptic, treatment for mycotic skin infections, and in stains. [G. *malachē*, a mallow]

**ma·laise** (mǎ-lāz′) A feeling of general discomfort or uneasiness, may be first indication of disease.

**mal·a·lign·ment** (mal′ǎ-līn′mĕnt) Displacement of one or more teeth from a normal position in dental arch.

**ma·lar** (mā′lǎr) Relating to mala, the cheek or cheek bones.

**ma·lar arch** (mā′lǎr ahrch) SYN zygomatic arch.

**ma·lar bone** (mā′lǎr bōn) SYN zygomatic bone.

**ma·lar·i·a** (mǎ-lar′ē-ǎ) Disease caused by the sporozoan *Plasmodium*, usually transmitted to humans by the bite of an infected female mosquito of the genus *Anopheles* that previously sucked blood from a person with malaria.

**ma·lar pro·cess** (mā′lǎr pros′es) SYN zygomatic process of maxilla.

**Ma·las·sez ep·i·the·li·al rests** (mal′ah-sā ep′i-thē′lē-ǎl rests) Epithelial remains of Hertwig root sheath in periodontal ligament.

**mal·e·rup·tion** (mal′ē-rŭp′shŭn) Faulty eruption of teeth.

**mal·for·ma·tion** (mal′fōr-mā′shŭn) Failure of normal development; more specifically, a primary structural defect that results from a localized error of morphogenesis; e.g., cleft lip.

**mal·func·tion** (mal-fŭngk′shŭn) Disordered, inadequate, or abnormal function.

**ma·lig·nant** (mǎ-lig′nǎnt) **1.** Resistant to treatment; occurring in severe form and frequently fatal; tending to become worse. **2.** In reference to a neoplasm, having the properties of locally invasive and destructive growth.

**ma·lig·nant hy·per·ten·sion** (mǎ-lig′ nǎnt hī′pĕr-ten′shŭn) Severe hypertension that runs a rapid course, causing necrosis of arteriolar walls.

**ma·lig·nant hy·per·ther·mi·a** (mǎ-lig′ nǎnt hī′pĕr-thĕr′mē-ǎ) Rapid onset of extremely high fever with muscle rigidity, precipitated by exogenous agents in genetically susceptible people.

**ma·lin·ger·ing** (mǎ-ling′gĕr-ing) Feigning illness or disability to escape work, excite sympathy, or gain compensation. [Fr. *malingre*, poor, weakly]

**mal·in·ter·dig·i·ta·tion** (mal'in-tĕr-dij'i-tā'shŭn) Faulty intercuspation of teeth.

**mal·nu·tri·tion** (mal'nū-trish'ŭn) Faulty nutrition resulting from malabsorption, poor diet, or overeating.

**mal·oc·clu·sion** (mal'ŏ-klū'zhŭn) **1.** Any deviation from a physiologically acceptable contact of opposing dentitions. **2.** Any deviation from a normal occlusion.

**mal·po·si·tion** (mal'pŏ-zish'ŭn) SYN dystopia.

**mal·prac·tice** (mal-prak'tis) Mistreatment of a patient through ignorance, carelessness, neglect, or criminal intent.

**mal·tose** (mawl'tōs) A disaccharide formed in the hydrolysis of starch and consisting of two D-glucose residues.

**mam·e·lon** (mam'ĕ-lon) One of three rounded prominences on cutting edge of an incisor tooth when it first pierces the gum. [Fr. nipple]

**man·aged care** (man'ăjd kār) Contractual arrangement whereby a third-party payer (e.g., insurance company) mediates between physicians and patients, negotiating fees for service and overseeing treatment.

**man·age·ment** (man'ăj-mĕnt) The process of supervising or controlling the affairs or activities of a group. [It. *maneggiare*, to control, fr. L. *manus*, hand]

**man·di·ble** (man'di-bĕl) [TA] U-shaped bone (in superior view), forming lower jaw, articulating by its upturned extremities with temporal bone on either side. See this page. SYN jaw bone, lower jaw, mandibulum, submaxilla.

**man·dib·u·lar** (man-dib'yū-lăr) Relating to the lower jaw. SYN inframaxillary, submaxillary (1).

**man·dib·u·lar an·gle** (man-dib'yū-lăr ang'gĕl) SYN angle of mandible.

**man·dib·u·lar arch** (man-dib'yū-lăr ahrch) SYN first pharyngeal arch.

**man·dib·u·lar ax·is** (man-dib'yū-lăr ak'sis) **1.** SYN transverse horizontal axis. **2.** SYN condylar axis.

**man·dib·u·lar bor·der** (man-dib'yū-lăr bōr'dĕr) SYN inferior border of the mandible.

**man·dib·u·lar ca·nal** (man-dib'yū-lăr kă-nal') [TA] Canal within mandible that transmits inferior alveolar nerve and vessels. Its posterior opening is the mandibular foramen. See this page. SYN inferior dental canal.

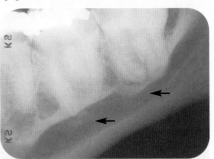

**mandibular molar area (radiograph):** mandibular canal containing nerves and blood vessels, running from lower left to upper right of figure, is prominent within bone (arrows)

**man·dib·u·lar car·ti·lage** (man-dib'yū-lăr kahr'ti-lăj) SYN pharyngeal arch cartilage.

**mn**

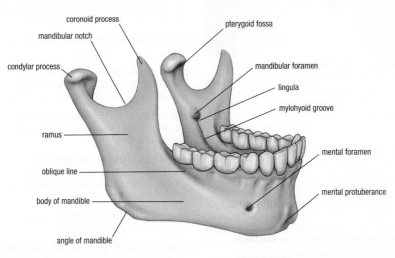

coronoid process
mandibular notch
condylar process
pterygoid fossa
mandibular foramen
lingula
mylohyoid groove
ramus
oblique line
mental foramen
body of mandible
mental protuberance
angle of mandible

**mandible**

**man·dib·u·lar den·tal ar·cade** (man-dib´yū-lăr den´tăl ahr-kād´) [TA] Teeth supported by alveolar part of mandible. SYN arcus dentalis inferior, inferior dental arch, lower dental arcade.

**man·dib·u·lar disc** (man-dib´yū-lăr disk) SYN articular disc of temporomandibular joint.

**man·dib·u·lar for·a·men** (man-dib´yū-lăr fōr-ā´měn) [TA] Opening on medial surface of ramus of mandible through which inferior alveolar artery, vein, and nerve pass to supply lower teeth. SYN inferior dental foramen.

**man·dib·u·lar fos·sa** (man-dib´yū-lăr fos´ă) [TA] Deep hollow in squamous portion of temporal bone at root of zygoma, in which condyle of mandible rests.

**man·dib·u·lar frac·ture** (man-dib´yū-lăr frak´shŭr) Breakage or other forms of osseous trauma involving the mandible. See this page.

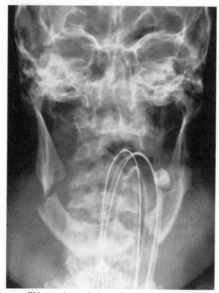

**mandible:** posteroanterior radiograph shows displaced fractures near right angle, with the body, and another to left of symphysis. Maxillary fractures are evident. Radiopaque loops are part of an endotracheal tube

**man·dib·u·lar glide** (man-dib´yū-lăr glīd) Side-to-side, protrusive, and intermediate movement of mandible occurring when teeth or other occluding surfaces are in contact.

**man·dib·u·lar guide pros·the·sis** (man-dib´yū-lăr gīd pros-thē´sis) Appliance with an extension designed to direct a resected mandible into functional relation to the maxilla.

**man·dib·u·lar hinge po·si·tion** (man-dib´yū-lăr hinj pŏ-zish´ŭn) Position of the man-dible with respect to the maxilla at which opening and closing movements can be made about the hinge axis.

**man·dib·u·lar joint** (man-dib´yū-lăr joynt) SYN temporomandibular joint.

**man·dib·u·lar la·bi·al fren·u·lum** (man-dib´yū-lăr lā´bē-ăl fren´yū-lŭm) SYN frenulum of lower lip.

**man·dib·u·lar lymph node** (man-dib´yū-lăr limf nōd) [TA] Facial lymph nodes located by the facial artery near point where it crosses mandible. SYN mandibular nodes.

**man·dib·u·lar move·ment** (man-dib´yū-lăr mūv´měnt) Motion or changes in position of which lower jaw is capable.

**man·dib·u·lar nerve [CN V3]** (man-dib´yū-lăr něrv) [TA] Third division of trigeminal nerve formed by union of sensory fibers from trigeminal ganglion and motor root of trigeminal nerve in the foramen ovale, through which nerve emerges. SYN inferior maxillary nerve, nervus mandibularis [CN V3].

**man·dib·u·lar nodes** (man-dib´yū-lăr nōdz) SYN mandibular lymph node.

**man·dib·u·lar notch** (man-dib´yū-lăr noch) [TA] Deep notch between condylar and coronoid processes of mandible. SYN sigmoid notch.

**man·dib·u·lar pro·cess** (man-dib´yū-lăr pro´ses) SEE pharyngeal arch.

**man·dib·u·lar pro·trac·tion** (man-dib´yū-lăr prō-trak´shŭn) Facial anomaly in which the gnathion lies anterior to orbital plane.

**man·dib·u·lar ra·mus** (man-dib´yū-lăr rā´mŭs) The upturned perpendicular extremity of the mandible on either side; it gives attachment on its lateral surface to the masseter muscle.

**man·dib·u·lar re·flex** (man-dib´yū-lăr rē´fleks) SYN jaw reflex.

**man·dib·u·lar re·trac·tion** (man-dib´yū-lăr rě-trak´shŭn) Facial anomaly in which the gnathion lies posterior to the orbital plane.

**man·dib·u·lar re·tru·sion** (man-dib´yū-lăr rě-trū´zhŭn) Movement of the mandible in a dorsal direction.

**man·dib·u·lar sym·phy·sis** (man-dib´yū-lăr sim´fi-sis) [TA] Fibrocartilaginous union of two halves of mandible in fetus. SYN mental symphysis.

**man·dib·u·lar tongue** (man-dib´yū-lăr tŭng) SYN lingula of mandible.

**man·dib·u·lar to·rus, to·rus man·di·bu·la·ris** (man-dib´yū-lăr tōr´ŭs, man-dib´yū-lā´ris) Exostosis protruding from lingual aspect of mandible, usually opposite premolar teeth. See this page.

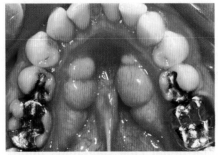

**mandibular tori:** lobulated, bilaterally symmetric

**man·dib·u·lec·to·my** (man-dib′yū-lek′tŏ-mē) Resection of the lower jaw. [L. *mandibula*, jaw + G. *ektomē*, excision]

**man·dib·u·lo·ac·ral dys·os·to·sis** (man-dib′yū-lō-ak′răl dis′os-tō′sis) Disorder characterized by hypoplastic mandible, dental crowding, acroosteolysis, stiff joints, and atrophy of skin of hands and feet.

**man·dib·u·lo·ac·ral dys·pla·si·a** (man-dib′yū-lō-ak′răl dis-plā′zē-ă) Disorder characterized by dental crowding, acroosteolysis, stiff joints, and atrophy of skin of hands and feet.

**man·dib·u·lo·fa·cial** (man-dib′yū-lō-fā′shăl) Relating to mandible and face.

**man·dib·u·lo·fa·cial dys·os·to·sis** (man-dib′yū-lō-fā′shăl dis′os-tō′sis) Variable syndrome of malformations primarily of derivatives of pharyngeal arch; characterized by bony defects or hypoplasia of malar and zygomatic bones, hypoplasia of mandible, macrostomia with high or cleft palate, malposition and malocclusion of teeth. SYN mandibulofacial dysplasia.

**man·dib·u·lo·fa·cial dys·pla·si·a** (man-dib′yū-lō-fā′shăl dis-plā′zē-ă) SYN mandibulofacial dysostosis.

**man·dib·u·lo·max·il·lar·y fix·a·tion** (man-dib′yū-lō-mak′si-lar-ē fik-sā′shŭn) SYN intermaxillary fixation.

**man·dib·u·lo·oc·u·lo·fa·cial** (man-dib′yū-lō-ok′yū-lō-fā′shăl) Relating to mandible and orbital part of face.

**man·dib·u·lo·pha·ryn·ge·al** (man-dib′yū-lō-fă-rin′jē-ăl) Relating to mandible and pharynx; denoting region between pharynx and ramus of mandible, in which are found internal carotid artery, internal jugular vein, and the vagus, glossopharyngeal, accessory, and hypoglossal nerves.

**man·dib·u·lum** (man-dib′yū-lŭm) SYN mandible.

**man·drel, man·dril** (man′drĕl, -dril) In dentistry, an instrument fitted in a handpiece to hold a disc, stone, or cup used for grinding, smoothing, or finishing.

**ma·neu·ver** (mă-nū′vĕr) A planned movement or procedure. SYN manoeuvre. [Fr. *manoeuvre,* fr. L. *manu operari,* to work by hand]

**man·ga·nese** (mang′gă-nēz) A metallic element resembling iron; salts are often used in medicine. [Mod. L. *manganesium, manganum,* an altered form of *magnesium*]

♻ **-mania** Suffix denoting an abnormal love for, or morbid impulse toward, some specific object, place, or action. [G. frenzy]

**ma·ni·a** (mā′nē-ă) SEE bipolar disorder. [G. frenzy]

**man·ic-de·pres·sive** (man′ik dĕ-pres′siv) SEE bipolar disorder.

**man·ic-de·pres·sive ill·ness** (man′ik dĕ-pres′iv il′nĕs) SEE bipolar disorder.

**man·ic-de·pres·sive psy·cho·sis** (man′ik dĕ-pres′iv sī-kō′sis) SYN bipolar disorder.

**man·i·fes·ta·tion** (man′i-fes-tā′shŭn) Display or disclosure of characteristic signs or symptoms of an illness. [L. *manifestus,* caught in the act]

**man·ne·quin, man·ni·kin** (man′i-kin) A model, especially one with removable pieces, of the human body or any of its parts.

**D-man·ni·tol** (man′i-tol) The hexahydric alcohol, widespread in plants, used in renal function testing and intravenously as an osmotic diuretic.

**man·no·si·do·sis** (man′ō-si-dō′sis) Congenital deficiency of α-mannosidase; associated with coarse facial features, enlarged tongue and other findings.

**manoeuvre** [Br.] SYN maneuver.

**ma·nom·e·ter** (mă-nom′ĕ-tĕr) An instrument for measuring the pressure of fluids.

**man. pr.** Abbreviation for L. *mane primo,* early morning, first thing in the morning.

**man·u·al film pro·ces·sing** (man′yū-ăl film pros′es-ing) Processing of exposed radiographic film by hand through timed steps of developing, rinsing, fixing, and washing.

**man·u·al·ly tuned** (man′yū-ăl-lē tūnd) Denotes ultrasonic device with a tuning control knob or button that can be used to set the vibration frequency of the tip at a level above or below resonant frequency.

**man·u·al scal·ing** (man′yū-ăl skāl′ing) Use of a hand-held scaling instrument as opposed to a mechanical or ultrasonic device.

**man·u·al ven·ti·la·tion** (man′yū-ăl ven′ti-lā′shŭn) Intermittent manual compression of a gas-filled reservoir bag to force gases into a patient's lungs and thus maintain oxygenation and carbon dioxide elimination.

**man·u·dy·na·mom·e·ter** (man′yū-dī′nă-

mn

mom′ĕ-tĕr) In dentistry, device for measuring force exerted by thrust of an instrument. [L. *manus,* hand, + G. *dynamis,* force, + *metron,* measure]

**MAOI** Abbreviation for monoamine oxidase inhibitor.

**map** (map) A representation of a region or structure, e.g., of a stretch of DNA.

**ma·ras·mus** (mă-raz′mŭs) Cachexia primarily due to prolonged dietary deficiency of protein and calories.

**Mar·chi·a·fa·va-Big·na·mi dis·ease** (mahr-kē-ă-fah′vah-bēn-yah′mē di-zēz′) Disorder recognized primarily by its pathologic features, consisting of demyelination of corpus callosum and cortical laminar necrosis involving frontal and temporal lobes.

**mar·cid** (mahr′sid) Emaciating; wasting away. [L. *marcidus;* fr. *marceo,* to wither]

**Mar·cus Gunn phe·nom·e·non, Mar·cus Gunn syn·drome** (mahr′kŭs gŭn fĕ-nom′ĕ-non, sin′drōm) SYN jaw-winking syndrome.

**mar·fan·oid** (mahr′fă-noyd) A term used to describe those whose phenotype bears a superficial resemblance to that of Marfan syndrome.

**Mar·fan syn·drome** (mahr-fahn′ sin′drōm) Connective tissue multisystemic disorder characterized by skeletal changes (arachnodactyly, long limbs, joint laxity, pectus), cardiovascular defects (aortic aneurysm that may dissect, mitral valve prolapse), and ectopia lentis.

**mar·gin** (mahr′jin) [TA] A boundary, edge, or border, as of a surface or structure.

**mar·gi·nal crest of tooth** (mahr′ji-năl krest tūth) [TA] SYN marginal ridge.

**mar·gi·nal gin·gi·va** (mahr′ji-năl jin′ji-vă) SYN free gingiva.

**mar·gi·nal gin·gi·vi·tis** (mahr′ji-năl jin′ji-vī′tis) Gingivitis in which the clinical alterations are confined to the marginal gingiva and do not involve the attached gingiva. See this page.

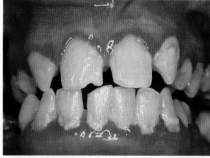

marginal gingivitis

**mar·gi·nal groove** (mahr′ji-năl grūv) Free gingival groove/shallow depression on outer surface of gingiva; separates free gingiva from attached gingiva.

**mar·gi·nal in·teg·ri·ty of a·mal·gam** (mahr′ji-năl in-teg′ri-tē ă-mal′găm) Ability of dental amalgam restoration to maintain its original marginal form at cavosurface margins.

**mar·gi·nal ir·ri·ga·tion** (mahr′ji-năl ir′i-gā′shŭn) Point of delivery of the irrigation angled at, or placed apically to, the gingival margin.

**Mar·gi·nal Line Cal·cu·lus In·dex (MLC)** (mahr′ji-năl līn kal′kyū-lŭs in′deks) Measure that assesses supragingival calculus found in cervical areas paralleling marginal gingiva.

**mar·gi·nal per·i·o·don·ti·tis** (mahr′ji-năl per′ē-ō-don-tī′tis) Formerly used term more accurately replaced in current dental terminology by chronic periodontitis, necrotizing periodontal diseases, and pericoronal abscesses of the periodontium.

**mar·gi·nal ridge** (mahr′ji-năl rij) [TA] Rounded edges of a tooth where the occlusal surface meets the mesial or distal surfaces and forms a ridge or crest. SYN marginal crest of tooth [TA], crista marginalis dentis.

**mar·gin·a·tion** (mahr′ji-nā′shŭn) A hematologic phenomenon that occurs during the relatively early phases of inflammation.

**mar·gin of safe·ty** (mahr′jin sāf′tē) The gap (i.e., range) between the minimal therapeutic dose of a drug and its minimal toxic dose.

**mar·gin trim·mer** (mahr′jin trim′ĕr) SYN gingival margin trimmer.

**mar·go in·ci·sa·lis** (mahr′gō in′si-sā′lis) [TA] SYN incisal margin.

**mark·er** (mahrk′ĕr) **1.** A device used to make a mark or to indicate measurement. **2.** A locus containing two or more alleles that, being harmless, are common and therefore yield high frequencies of heterozygotes, which facilitate linkage analysis.

**mark·ing** (mahrk′ing) The act of indicating or distinguishing a thing by placing on it a sign, symbol, or other perceptible trace.

**mar·row ca·nal** (mar′ō kă-nal′) SYN root canal of tooth.

**mar·su·pi·al·i·za·tion** (mahr-sū′pē-ăl-ī-zā′shŭn) Exteriorization of a cyst or other such enclosed cavity by resecting the anterior wall and suturing the cut edges of the remaining wall to adjacent edges of the skin, thereby creating a pouch. [L. *marsupium,* pouch]

**mask** (mask) **1.** Any of a variety of disease states or disorders that cause alteration or discoloration of facial skin. **2.** Expressionless appearance seen in association with some diseases, e.g., Parkinson facies. **3.** Facial bandage. **4.** Shield designed to cover mouth and nose for maintenance of antiseptic conditions. **5.** Device designed to cover mouth and nose for administration of inhalation anesthetics, oxygen, or other gases. See this page.

**mask·ing** (mask′ing) **1.** In dentistry, an opaque covering used to camouflage the metal parts of a prosthesis. **2.** In radiography, superimposition of an altered positive image on the original negative to produce an enhanced copy photographically.

**Mas·low hi·er·ar·chy** (maz′lō hī′ĕr-ahr-kē) Ranking of needs that humans presumably fill successively from lowest to highest: physiologic needs, love and belonging, self-esteem, and self-actualization.

mn

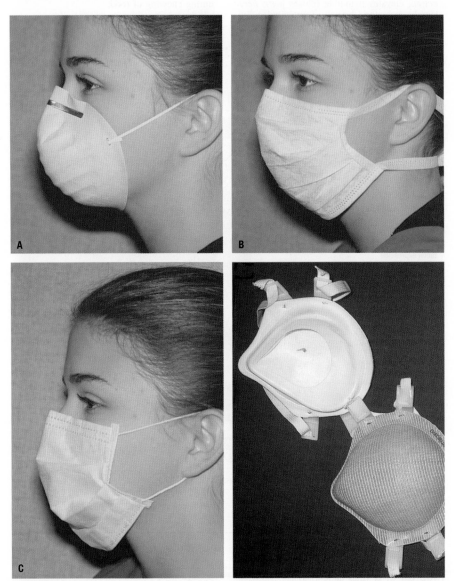

**face masks:** (A) preformed cone; (B) soft, with ties for head and neck; (C) soft, with elasticized over-the-ear loops; (D) EPA filtration mask

**mas·se·ter·ic ar·te·ry** (mas′ĕ-ter′ik ahr′ tĕr-ē) [TA] *Origin*, second (infratemporal) part of maxillary; *distribution*, masseter muscle via mandibular notch, temporomandibular joint; *anastomoses*, branches of transverse facial and masseteric branches of facial.

**mas·se·ter mus·cle** (mas′ĕ-tĕr mŭs′ĕl) *Origin*, superficial part: inferior border of the anterior two thirds of the zygomatic arch; deep part: inferior border and medial surface of the zygomatic arch; *insertion*, lateral surface of ramus and coronoid process of the mandible; *action*, elevates mandible (closes jaw); *nerve supply*, masseteric branch of mandibular division of trigeminal. SYN musculus masseter [TA].

**mas·se·ter re·flex** (mas′ĕ-tĕr rē′fleks) SYN jaw reflex.

**mass screen·ing** (mas skrēn′ing) Examination of a large population to detect manifesta-

that contains coarse, basophilic, metachromatic secretory granules that contain, among other pharmacologic agents, heparin, histamine, and eosinophilic chemotactic factor.

**mas·ter cast** (mas′tĕr kast) Replica of prepared tooth surfaces, residual ridge areas, and/ or other parts of dental arch as reproduced from an impression.

**mas·ti·cate** (mas′ti-kāt) To chew.

**mas·ti·cat·ing cy·cles** (mas′ti-kāt-ing sī′ kĕlz) Patterns of mandibular movements formed during chewing of food.

**mas·ti·cat·ing sur·face** (mas′ti-kāt-ing sŭr′făs) SYN denture occlusal surface.

**▣mas·ti·ca·tion** (mas′ti-kā′shŭn) Process of chewing food in preparation for deglutition and digestion. See this page. [L. *mastico*, pp. *-atus*, to chew]

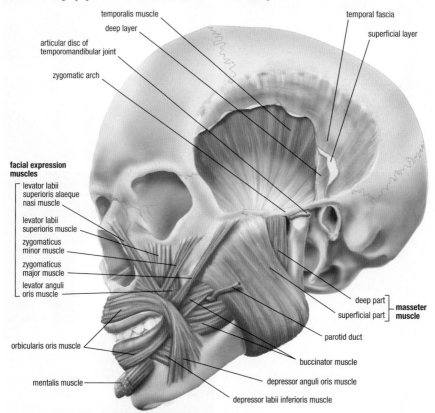

temporalis muscle
deep layer
articular disc of temporomandibular joint
zygomatic arch
temporal fascia
superficial layer

**facial expression muscles**
levator labii superioris alaeque nasi muscle
levator labii superioris muscle
zygomaticus minor muscle
zygomaticus major muscle
levator anguli oris muscle

orbicularis oris muscle
mentalis muscle

deep part ⎤
superficial part ⎦ **masseter muscle**
parotid duct
buccinator muscle
depressor anguli oris muscle
depressor labii inferioris muscle

**muscles of mastication** (oblique view)

tion of disease to initiate treatment or prevent its spread.

**mas·tal·gi·a** (mas-tal′jē-ă) SYN mastodynia. [*masto-* + G. *algos*, pain]

**mast cell** (mast sel) Connective tissue cell

**mas·ti·ca·tor nerve** (mas′ti-kā-tŏr nĕrv) SYN motor root of trigeminal nerve.

**mas·ti·ca·tor space** (mas′ti-kā-tŏr spās) Area subtended by superficial layer of deep cervical fascia that splits into lateral and medial slings at inferior border of mandible to enclose the masseter muscle, part of the temporalis muscle, and medial and lateral pterygoid muscles.

**mas·ti·ca·to·ry** (mas′ti-kă-tōr-ē) Relating to mastication.

**mas·ti·ca·to·ry ap·pa·ra·tus** (mas′ti-kă-tōr-ē ap″ă-rat′ŭs) SYN stomatognathic system.

**mas·ti·ca·to·ry di·ple·gi·a** (mas′ti-kā-tōr-ē dī-plē′jē-ă) Paralysis of all the muscles of mastication.

**mas·ti·ca·to·ry force** (mas′ti-kă-tōr-ē fōrs) SYN force of mastication.

**mas·ti·ca·to·ry mu·co·sa** (mas′ti-kă-tōr-ē myū-kō′să) Oral mucosa covered by stratified squamous epithelium that can withstand forces of mastication.

**mas·ti·ca·to·ry mus·cles** (mas′ti-kă-tōr-ē mŭs′ĕlz) [TA] Muscles derived from first (mandibular) arch used in chewing; all receive innervation from motor root of trigeminal nerve via its mandibular division; includes masseter muscle, temporalis muscle, lateral pterygoid muscle, and medial pterygoid muscle.

**mas·ti·ca·to·ry si·lent pe·ri·od** (mas′ti-kā-tōr-ē sī′lĕnt pēr′ē-ŏd) Pause in electromyographic patterns associated with tooth contacts during chewing and biting.

**mas·ti·ca·to·ry spasm** (mas′ti-kā-tōr-ē spazm) Involuntary convulsive muscular contraction affecting muscles of mastication.

**mas·ti·ca·to·ry sur·face** (mas′ti-kā-tōr-ē sŭr′făs) SYN denture occlusal surface.

**mas·ti·ca·to·ry sys·tem** (mas′ti-kă-tōr-ē sis′tĕm) Organs and structures primarily functioning in mastication: jaws, teeth with their supporting structures, temporomandibular joint, muscles of mastication, tongue, lips, cheeks, and oral mucosa. SYN dental apparatus.

**mas·to·dy·ni·a** (mas′tō-din′ē-ă) SYN mastalgia.

**mas·toid** (mas′toyd) Relating to the mastoid process, antrum, and cells. [masto- + G. eidos, resemblance]

**mas·toi·da·le** (mas-toy-dā′lē) The lowest point on the contour of the mastoid process.

**mas·toid an·gle of pa·ri·e·tal bone** (mas′toyd ang′gĕl păr-ī′ĕ-tăl bōn) [TA] The posteroinferior point of the parietal bone. SYN angulus mastoideus ossis parietalis.

**mas·toid an·trum** (mas′toyd an′trŭm) [TA] A cavity in the petrous portion of the temporal bone, communicating posteriorly with the mastoid cells and anteriorly with the epitympanic recess of the middle ear via the aditus to the mastoid antrum. SYN antrum mastoideum.

**mas·toid fon·ta·nelle** (mas′toyd fon′tă-nel′) [TA] Membranous interval on either side between mastoid angle of parietal bone, petrous portion of temporal bone, and occipital bone.

**mas·to·oc·cip·i·tal** (mas′tō-ok-sip′i-tăl) Relating to mastoid portion of temporal bone and occipital bone.

**mas·to·pa·ri·e·tal** (mas′tō-pă-rī′ĕ-tăl) Relating to mastoid portion of temporal bone and parietal bone, denoting suture uniting them.

**match·ed groups** (macht grŭps) A method of experimental control in which subjects in one group are matched on a one-to-one basis with subjects in other groups concerning all organism variables, which the experimenter believes could influence findings.

**match·ing** (mach′ing) Process of making a study group and a comparison group in an epidemiologic study comparable with respect to extraneous or confounding factors.

**ma·te·ri·a al·ba** (mă-tē′rē-ă al′bă) Accumulation or aggregation of microorganisms, desquamated epithelial cells, blood cells, and food debris loosely adherent to surfaces of plaques, teeth, gingiva or dental appliances. [L. white matter]

**ma·te·ri·al** (mă-tēr′ē-ăl) That of which something is made or composed. [L. materialis, fr. materia, substance]

**ma·te·ri·a med·i·ca** (mă-tē′rē-ă med′i-kă) Aspect of medical science concerned with origin and preparation of drugs, their doses, and mode of administration. [L. medical matter]

**ma·te·ri·es mor·bi** (mă-tē′rē-ēz mōr′bī) Substance acting as immediate cause of a disease. [L. the matter of disease]

**mat gold** (mat gōld) Powdered gold formed by electrolytic precipitation, compressed into strips, and sintered.

**ma·trix,** pl. **ma·tri·ces** (mā′triks, -tri-sēz) **1.** [TA] A mold in which anything is cast or swaged; material shaped for holding and shaping the material used to fill a tooth cavity. **2.** [TA] The formative portion of a nail. **3.** The intercellular substance of a tissue. [L. womb; female breeding animal]

**ma·trix band** (mā′triks band) Metal or plastic band secured around tooth crown to confine restorative material to be adapted into a prepared cavity.

**ma·trix re·tain·er** (mā′triks rĕ-tā′nĕr) Mechanical device designed to hold a matrix around a tooth during restorative procedures.

**mat·tress su·ture** (mat′trĕs sū′chŭr) A suture using a double stitch that forms a loop about the tissue on both sides of a wound, producing eversion of the edges when tied.

mn

**mat·u·ra·tion** (mach'ūr-ā'shŭn) Achievement of full development or growth.

**ma·ture** (mă-chūr') Ripe; fully developed. [L. *maturus,* ripe]

**ma·tu·ri·ty** (mă-chūr'i-tē) A state of full development or completed growth.

**ma·tu·ri·ty-on·set di·a·be·tes of youth** (mă-chūr'i-tē on'set dī'ă-bē'tēz yūth) SEE Type 2 diabetes.

**max·il·la,** pl. **max·il·lae** (mak-sil'ă, -ē) [TA] Irregularly shaped pneumatized bone, supporting superior teeth and taking part in formation of orbit, hard palate, and nasal cavity. See this page. [L. jawbone]

**max·il·lar·y den·tal ar·cade** (mak'si-lar-ē den'tăl ahr-kād') [TA] Teeth supported by alveolar process of two maxillae, whether 10 deciduous or 16 permanent teeth. SYN arcus dentalis superior, superior dental arch.

**max·il·lar·y em·i·nence** (mak'si-lar-ē em'i-nĕns) SYN maxillary tuberosity.

**max·il·lar·y gland** (mak'si-lar-ē gland) SYN submandibular gland.

**max·il·lar·y hi·a·tus** (mak'si-lar-ē hī-ā'tŭs) [TA] Large opening into maxillary sinus on nasal surface of maxilla.

**max·il·lar·y la·bi·al fre·num** (mak'si-

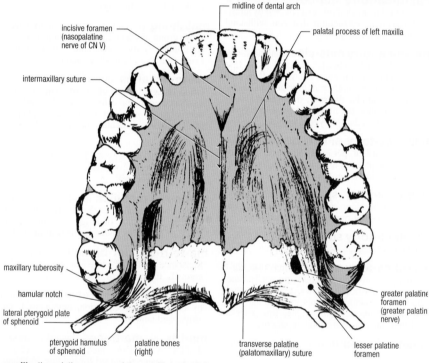

maxilla: the palatine process of the maxilla is shaded

Labels: midline of dental arch — incisive foramen (nasopalatine nerve of CN V) — palatal process of left maxilla — intermaxillary suture — maxillary tuberosity — hamular notch — lateral pterygoid plate of sphenoid — pterygoid hamulus of sphenoid — palatine bones (right) — transverse palatine (palatomaxillary) suture — greater palatine foramen (greater palatine nerve) — lesser palatine foramen

**max·il·lar·y** (mak'si-lar-ē) Relating to the maxilla, or upper jaw.

**max·il·lar·y an·gle** (mak'si-lar-ē ang'gĕl) Area formed by line drawn from ophryon and another from point of mandible and meeting at contact between maxillary and mandibular incisor teeth.

**max·il·lar·y arch** (mak'si-lar-ē ahrch) Curved composite structure of the natural dentition or residual ridge of the upper jaw or maxilla. SEE arch, dental arch.

**max·il·lar·y ar·te·ry** (mak'si-lar-ē ahr'tĕr-ē) [TA] Primary artery of the infratemporal fossa. See page 363.

lar-ē lā'bē-ăl frē'nŭm) SYN frenulum of upper lip.

**max·il·lar·y nerve [CN V2]** (mak'si-lar-ē nĕrv) Second division of the trigeminal nerve, passing from trigeminal ganglion in middle cranial fossa through foramen rotundum into pterygopalatine fossa, where it gives off ganglionic branches to the pterygopalatine ganglion and continues forward to give off the zygomatic nerve and enter the orbit, where it continues as the infraorbital nerve. Its sensory fibers are distributed to skin and conjunctiva of lower eyelid, skin and mucosa of upper lip and cheek, palate, upper teeth and gingiva, maxillary sinus, wings of the nose, and posterior/interior nasal cavity. SYN nervus maxillaris [CN V2].

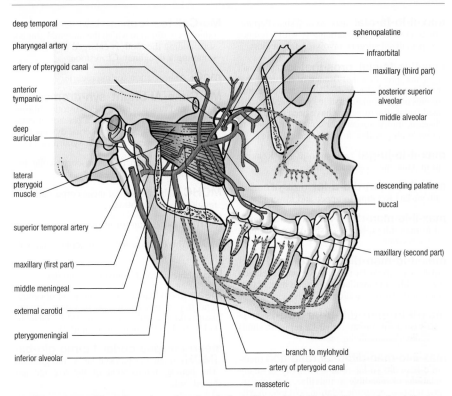

deep temporal

pharyngeal artery

artery of pterygoid canal

anterior tympanic

deep auricular

lateral pterygoid muscle

superior temporal artery

maxillary (first part)

middle meningeal

external carotid

pterygomeningial

inferior alveolar

sphenopalatine

infraorbital

maxillary (third part)

posterior superior alveolar

middle alveolar

descending palatine

buccal

maxillary (second part)

branch to mylohyoid

artery of pterygoid canal

masseteric

**maxillary artery and branches:** artery arises at neck of mandible and is divided into three parts in relation to lateral pterygoid muscle; may pass medially or laterally to this muscle. Examine branches of first (mandibular) part that pass through the foramina or canals

**max·il·lar·y ple·xus** (mak´si-lar-ē pleks´ ŭs) SYN periarterial plexus of maxillary artery.

**max·il·lary pro·cess** (mak´si-lar-ē pro´ses) A thin plate of irregular form projecting from the middle of the upper border of the inferior concha, articulating with the maxilla bone and partly closing the orifice of the maxillary sinus.

**max·il·lar·y pro·cess of in·fe·ri·or na·sal con·cha** (mak´si-lar-ē pro´ses in-fēr´ē-ŏr nā´zăl kong´kă) [TA] Thin plate of irregular form projecting from middle of upper border of inferior concha, articulating with maxilla and partly closing orifice of the maxillary sinus.

**max·il·lar·y pro·trac·tion** (mak´si-lar-ē prō-trak´shŭn) Facial anomaly in which subnasion lies anterior to the orbital plane.

**max·il·lar·y si·nus** (mak´si-lar-ē sī´nŭs) [TA] Largest of the paranasal sinuses occupying body of maxilla, communicating with middle meatus of nose. SYN antrum of Highmore, genyantrum.

**max·il·lar·y si·nus ra·di·o·graph** (mak´ si-lar-ē sī´nŭs rā´dē-ō-graf) Radiographic frontal view of maxillary sinuses, orbits, nasal structures and zygomas.

**max·il·lar·y sur·face of great·er wing of sphe·noid bone** (mak´si-lar-ē sŭr´făs grā´tĕr wing sfē´noyd bōn) [TA] Part of anterior surface of greater wing of sphenoid bone perforated by foramen rotundum.

**max·il·lar·y sur·face of pal·a·tine bone** (mak´si-lar-ē sŭr´făs pal´ă-tīn bōn) Lateral surface of perpendicular plate of palatine bone. SYN facies maxillaris ossis palatini.

**max·il·lar·y torus** (mak´si-lar-ē tōr´ŭs) SYN torus palatinus.

**max·il·lar·y tu·ber·os·i·ty** (mak´si-lar-ē tū´bĕr-os´i-tē) [TA] Bulging lower extremity of posterior surface of body of the maxilla, behind root of last molar tooth. SYN maxillary eminence.

**max·il·lar·y vein** (mak´si-lar-ē vān) [TA] Posterior continuation of pterygoid plexus; joins superficial temporal vein to form the retromandibular vein.

**max·il·li·tis** (mak´si-lī´tis) Inflammation of maxilla.

**max·il·lo·den·tal** (mak-sil´ō-den´tăl) Relating to upper jaw and its associated teeth.

mn

**max·il·lo·fa·cial** (mak-sil′ō-fā′shăl) Pertaining to jaws and face, particularly with reference to specialized surgery involving this region.

**max·il·lo·fa·cial pros·thet·ics** (mak-sil′ō-fā′shăl pros′thet′iks) Branch of dentistry that provides prostheses or devices to treat or restore tissues of the stomatognathic system and associated facial structures that have been affected by disease, injury, surgery, or congenital defect to provide all possible function and esthetics.

**max·il·lo·ju·gal** (mak-sil′ō-jū′găl) Relating to maxilla and zygomatic bone.

**max·il·lo·man·dib·u·lar** (mak-sil′ō-man-dib′yū-lăr) Relating to upper and lower jaws.

**max·il·lo·man·dib·u·lar fix·a·tion** (mak′si-lō-man-dib′yū-lăr fik-sā′shŭn) SYN intermaxillary fixation.

**max·il·lo·man·dib·u·lar re·cord** (mak-sil′ō-man-dib′yū-lăr rek′ŏrd) Record of relation of mandible to maxillae. SYN biscuit bite, maxillomandibular registration.

**max·il·lo·man·dib·u·lar reg·is·tra·tion** (mak-sil′ō-man-dib′yū-lăr rej′is-trā′shŭn) SYN maxillomandibular record.

**max·il·lo·man·dib·u·lar re·la·tion** (mak-sil′ō-man-dib′yū-lăr rĕ-lā′shŭn) Any of many relations of mandible to maxillae, e.g., centric jaw relation, eccentric relation. SYN intermaxillary relation.

**max·il·lo·man·dib·u·lar trac·tion** (mak-sil′ō-man-dib′yū-lăr trak′shŭn) Pulling force developed by using elastic or wire ligatures and interdental wiring or splints, or both. SYN intermaxillary traction.

**max·il·lo·pal·a·tine** (mak-sil′ō-pal′ă-tīn) Relating to maxilla and palatine bone.

**max·il·lot·o·my** (mak′si-lot′ŏ-mē) Surgical sectioning of maxilla to allow movement of all or a part of the maxilla into desired portion. [*maxilla* + G. *tomē*, incision]

**max·il·lo·tur·bi·nal** (mak-sil′lō-tŭr′bi-năl) Relating to the inferior nasal concha.

**max·i·mal dose** (mak′si-măl dōs) Largest amount of a drug or physical procedure an adult can take safely.

**max·i·mal stim·u·lus** (mak′si-măl stim′yū-lŭs) A stimulus strong enough to evoke a maximal response.

**max·i·mum per·mis·si·ble dose (MPD)** (mak′si-mŭm per-mis′i-bĕl dōs) Greatest dose of radiation which, in the light of present knowledge, is not expected to cause detectable bodily injury to people at any time during their lifetime.

**mc** Abbreviation for millicurie.

**Mc·Call fes·toon** (mĕ-kawl′ fes-tūn′) Periodontal condition in which the marginal gingiva surrounding the tooth is enlarged in a form resembling a doughnut. Cf. festoon.

**mcCi** Abbreviation for microcurie.

**Mc·Cune-Al·bright syn·drome** (mik-kyūn′ awl′brīt sin′drōm) Polyostotic fibrous dysplasia with irregular brown patches of cutaneous pigmentation and endocrine dysfunction. SYN Albright disease, Albright syndrome (1).

**MCH** Abbreviation for mean corpuscular hemoglobin.

**MCHC** Abbreviation for mean corpuscular hemoglobin concentration.

**mcm** Abbreviation for micrometer.

**MCV** Abbreviation for mean corpuscular volume.

**ME** Abbreviation for medical examiner.

**mean** (mēn) Statistical measurement of central tendency or average of a set of values, usually assumed to be arithmetic mean. [M.E., *mene* fr. O.Fr., fr. L. *medianus*, in the middle]

**mean cor·pus·cu·lar he·mo·glo·bin (MCH)** (mēn kōr-pŭs′kyū-lăr hē′mŏ-glō-bin) The hemoglobin content of the average red blood cell.

**mean cor·pus·cu·lar he·mo·glo·bin con·cen·tra·tion (MCHC)** (mēn kōr-pŭs′kyū-lăr hē′mŏ-glō-bin kon′sĕn-trā′shŭn) The average hemoglobin concentration in a given volume of packed red blood cells.

**mean cor·pus·cu·lar vol·ume (MCV)** (mēn kōr-pŭs′kū-lăr vol′yūm) The average volume of red blood cells.

**mean foun·da·tion plane** (mēn fown-dā′shŭn plān) Mean of various irregularities in form and inclination of basal seat; condition for denture stability is ideal when mean foundation plane is most nearly at right angles to direction of force.

**mean life** (mēn līf) The average lifetime of decay of a radioactive atom. SYN average life.

**mea·sles** (mē′zĕlz) An acute exanthematous disease, caused by measles virus, marked by fever and other constitutional disturbances, catarrhal inflammation of respiratory mucous membranes, and a generalized dusky red maculopapular eruption. Eruption occurs early on buccal mucous membrane in the form of Koplik spots, a manifestation useful in early diagnosis. SYN morbilli. [D. *maselen*]

**me·a·tus,** pl. **me·a·tus** (mē-ā′tŭs) [TA] Passage, especially external opening of a canal.

**me·chan·ic·al con·den·ser** (mĕ-kan′i-kăl kŏn-den′sĕr) Device that compacts restorative material into a dental cavity using force generated by a spring-loaded device, either pneumatically or electrically.

**me·chan·i·cal ir·ri·tant** (mĕ-kan′i-kăl ir′i-tănt) In dentistry, irritation of dental pulp due to trauma from use of dental handpieces or instruments.

**me·chan·i·cal·ly bal·anced oc·clu·sion** (mĕ-kan′i-kă-lē bal″ănst ŏ-klū″zhŭn) Balanced occlusion without reference to physiologic considerations, as on an articulator.

**me·chan·i·cal plaque con·trol** (mĕ-kan′i-kăl plak kon-trōl′) Oral hygiene procedures to remove dental biofilm from tooth surfaces using a toothbrush and selected devices for interdental cleaning.

**mech·a·nism** (mek′ă-nizm) **1.** Arrangement or grouping of parts of anything that has a definite action. **2.** Means by which an effect is obtained. **3.** Chain of events in a particular process. [G. *mēchanē,* a contrivance]

**mech·a·no·re·cep·tor** (mek″ă-nō-rĕ-sep′tŏr) Receptor that responds to mechanical pressure, e.g., receptors in the carotid sinuses.

**mech·a·no·re·flex** (mek′ă-nō-rē′fleks) A reflex triggered by stimulation of a mechanoreceptor.

**mech·a·no·ther·a·py** (mek′ă-nō-thār′ă-pē) Treatment of disease with any apparatus or mechanical appliances.

**Mec·kel car·ti·lage** (mek′el kahr′ti-lăj) SYN mandibular cartilage.

**me·di·a** (mē′dē-ă) **1.** SYN tunica media. **2.** Plural of medium. [L. fem. of *medius,* middle]

**me·di·al** (mē′dē-ăl) [TA] Relating to the middle or center; nearer to the median or midsagittal plane or center of dental arch. [L. *medialis,* middle]

**me·di·al lig·a·ment of tem·po·ro·man·dib·u·lar joint** (mē′dē-ăl lig″ă-mĕnt tem′pŏr-ō-man-dib′yū-lăr joynt) [TA] Intracapsular bundle of fibers strengthening medial part of the articular capsule of temporomandibular joint; not as apparent as lateral ligament.

**me·di·al na·sal prom·i·nence, me·di·al na·sal pro·cess** (mē′dē-ăl nā′zăl prom′i-nĕns, pro′ses) Ectodermally covered mesenchymal swelling lying medial to the olfactory placode or pit in embryos.

**me·di·an** (mē′dē-ăn) **1.** Central; middle; lying in the midline. **2.** The middle value in a set of measurements.

**me·di·an an·te·ri·or max·il·lar·y cyst** (mē′dē-ăn an-tēr′ē-ŏr mak′si-lar-ē sist) SYN incisive canal cyst.

**me·di·an ef·fec·tive dose (ED₅₀)** (mē′dē-ăn e-fekt′iv dōs) SEE effective dose.

**me·di·an lin·gual swell·ing** (mē′dē-ăn ling′gwăl swel′ing) In embryo, small elevation in floor of mouth between first and second pharyngeal arches; overgrown by lateral lingual swellings; forms a small part of posterior region of anterior two thirds of tongue.

**me·di·an lon·gi·tu·di·nal ra·phe of tongue** (mē′dē-ăn lon′ji-tū′di-năl rā′fē tŭng) SYN median sulcus of tongue.

**me·di·an man·dib·u·lar point** (mē′dē-ăn man-dib′yū-lăr poynt) Position on anteroposterior center of mandibular ridge in median sagittal plane.

**me·di·an max·il·lar·y an·te·ri·or al·ve·o·lar cleft** (mē′dē-ăn mak′si-lar-ē an-tēr′ē-ŏr al-vē′ō-lăr kleft) Asymptomatic midline defect of maxillary anterior ridge; result of failure of fusion or development of lateral halves of palate.

**me·di·an nerve** (mē′dē-ăn nĕrv) [TA] Formed by the union of medial and lateral roots from the medial and lateral cords of the brachial plexus, respectively; it supplies all the muscles in the anterior compartment of the forearm with the exception of the flexor carpi ulnaris and ulnar half of the flexor digitorum profundus.

**me·di·an pal·a·tal cyst** (mē′dē-ăn pal′ă-tăl sist) Developmental lesion located in midline of hard palate.

**me·di·an pal·a·tine su·ture** (mē′dē-ăn pal′ă-tīn sū′chŭr) [TA] Juncture of right and left palatine bones.

**me·di·an plane** (mē′dē-ăn plān) [TA] A plane vertical in the anatomic position, through the midline of the body that divides the body into right and left halves.

**me·di·an re·trud·ed re·la·tion, me·di·an re·la·tion** (mē′dē-ăn rĕ-trū′dĕd rĕ-lā′shŭn) SYN centric jaw relation.

🔲**me·di·an rhom·boid glos·si·tis** (mē′dē-ăn rom′boyd glos-ī′tis) Asymptomatic, ovoid or rhomboid, macular, erythematous area with absence of papillae on the median portion of the dorsum of the tongue just anterior to circumvallate papillae. See page A7.

**me·di·an sul·cus of tongue** (mē′dē-ăn sŭl′kŭs tŭng) [TA] Slight longitudinal depression on dorsal surface of tongue extending from foramen cecum and dividing dorsum into right and left halves. SYN median longitudinal raphe of tongue.

**me·di·as·ti·nal space** (mē′dē-ă-stī′năl spās) SYN mediastinum (2).

**me·di·as·ti·ni·tis** (mē′dē-as′ti-nī′tis) Inflammation of the cellular tissue of the mediastinum.

mn

**me·di·as·ti·num** (me′dē-ă-stī′nŭm) [TA] **1.** A septum between two parts of an organ or a cavity. **2.** The median partition of the thoracic cavity, covered by the mediastinal part of the parietal pleura and containing all the thoracic viscera and structures except the lungs.

**me·di·ate per·cus·sion** (mē′dē-ăt pĕr-kŭsh′ŭn) Percussion effected by intervention of a finger or a plessimeter between striking finger or plessor and part percussed.

**Med·i·caid** (medi-kād) A nationwide health insurance program in the U.S. that provides coverage to qualified low-income citizens and qualified legal residents; funded jointly by the state and federal governments, the program has federal guidelines that give the individual states wide discretion to determine eligibility and to set benefits. Cf. Medicare (1).

**med·i·cal** (med′i-kăl) Relating to medicine or the practice of medicine. SYN medicinal (2). [L. *medicalis,* fr *medicus,* physician]

**med·i·cal a·nat·o·my** (med′i-kăl ă-nat′ŏ-mē) Anatomy in its bearing on diagnosis and treatment of diseases.

**med·i·cal corps** (med′i-kăl kōr) Subdivision of a military organization, such as the U.S. Army, devoted to medical care of its troops.

**med·i·cal eth·ics** (med′i-kăl eth′iks) Principles of proper professional conduct concerning the rights and duties of the physician, patients, and fellow practitioners, as well as the physician's actions in the care of patients and in relations with their families.

**med·i·cal ex·am·i·ner (ME)** (med′i-kăl eg-zam′in-ĕr) **1.** Physician who examines a person and reports on that person's physical condition to the company or individual at whose request the examination was made. **2.** In jurisdictions where coroner's office has been abolished, physician appointed to investigate all cases of sudden, violent, or suspicious death.

**med·i·cal ju·ris·pru·dence** (med′i-kăl jŭr′is-prū′dĕns) SYN forensic medicine.

**Med·i·cal Lit·er·a·ture A·nal·y·sis and Re·trie·val Sys·tem (MEDLARS)** (med′ i-kăl lit′ĕr-ă-chŭr ă-nal′i-sis rē-trē′văl sis′tĕm) A computerized system of databases and databanks maintained by the U.S. National Library of Medicine.

**med·i·cal mod·el** (med′i-kăl mod′ĕl) A set of assumptions that views behavioral abnormalities in the same framework as physical disease or abnormalities.

**med·i·cal re·cord** (med′i-kăl rek′ŏrd) SYN record (1).

**med·i·cal tran·scrip·tion·ist (MT)** (med′i-kăl tran-skrip′shŭn-ist) One who performs machine transcription of physician-dictated medi-

cal reports concerning a patient's health care, which become part of the patient's permanent medical record; a certified medical transcriptionist (CMT) has satisfied the requirements for certification by the American Association for Medical Transcription.

**med·i·cal treat·ment** (med′i-kăl trēt′mĕnt) Treatment of disease by hygienic and pharmacologic remedies rather than invasive surgical procedures.

**me·di·ca·ment** (med′i-kă-ment, me-dik′ă-ment) Medicine, medicinal application, or remedy. [L. *medicamentum,* medicine]

**med·i·ca·men·to·sus** (med′i-kă-men-tō′sŭs) Relating to a drug. [L.]

**Med·i·care** (med′i-kār) **1.** A national health insurance plan managed by the U.S. government that covers Social Security and Railroad Retirement beneficiaries age 65 years and older, people who have been entitled for at least 24 months to receive Social Security or Railroad Retirement disability benefits, and some people with end-stage renal disease; established in 1965 by an amendment to the Social Security Act. Cf. Medicaid. **2.** The universal public health insurance system of Canada, administered by the provincial governments under guidelines set by the Canadian federal government; initiated under the Canada Health Act in 1984. **3.** A national public health insurance system in Australia; provides for free care in public hospitals, and free or subsidized care in clinical settings for certain conditions; established in 1984.

**med·i·cate** (med′i-kāt) **1.** To treat disease by dispensing (i.e., prescribing) drugs. **2.** To impregnate with medicinal substance. [L. *medico,* pp. *-atus,* to heal]

**med·i·cat·ed** (med′i-kāt′ĕd) **1.** Impregnated with a medicinal substance. **2.** Treated, as a patient.

**med·i·ca·tion** (med′i-kā′shŭn) **1.** Act of medicating. **2.** Medicinal substance or medicament.

**med·i·ca·tor** (med′i-kā′tŏr) Instrument used to make therapeutic applications to deeper body parts.

**me·dic·i·nal** (mĕ-dis′i-năl) **1.** Relating to medicine having curative properties. **2.** SYN medical.

**med·i·cine** (med′i-sin) **1.** A drug. **2.** Art of preventing or curing disease. **3.** Study and treatment of general diseases or those affecting the internal parts of the body.

⚙ **medico-** Combining form meaning medical. [L. *medicus,* physician]

**med·i·co·bi·o·log·ic, med·i·co·bi·o·log·i·cal** (med′i-kō-bī′ŏ-loj′ik, -i-kăl) Pertaining to the biologic aspects of medicine.

**med·i·co·chi·rur·gi·cal** (med′i-kō-kī-rŭr′

ji-kăl) Relating to both medicine and surgery, or to both physicians and surgeons. [*medico-* + G. *cheirourgia,* surgery]

**med·i·co·le·gal** (med'i-kō-lē'găl) Relating to both medicine and the law. SEE ALSO forensic medicine. [*medico-* + L. *legalis,* legal]

**med·i·co·me·chan·i·cal** (med'i-kō-mĕ-kan'i-kăl) Relating to both medicinal and mechanical measures in therapeutics.

**med·i·co·phys·i·cal** (med'i-kō-fiz'i-kăl) Relating to disease and body's general condition considered as an entity.

**med·i·co·psy·chol·o·gy** (med'i-kō-sī-kol'ŏ-jē) Psychology in its relation to medicine.

♻ **medio-** Middle, median. [L. *medius*]

**me·di·o·dens** (mē'dē-ō-dens) SYN mesiodens. [L. *medio-* middle + L. *dens,* tooth]

**me·di·o·tru·sion** (mē'dē-ō-trū'zhŭn) Thrusting of mandibular condyle toward midline during movement of mandible.

**me·di·um,** pl. **me·di·a** (mē'dē-ŭm, -ă) **1.** A means; that through or by which an action is performed. **2.** Liquid holding another substance in solution or suspension.

**MEDLARS** (med'lahrz) Acronym for Medical Literature Analysis and Retrieval System.

**MEDLINE** (med'līn) Internet-based linkage to MEDLARS for rapid provision of medical bibliographies. [fr. MEDLARS online]

**me·dul·la,** pl. **me·dul·lae** (me-dŭl'ă, -ē) [TA] Any soft marrowlike structure, especially in the center of a part. SYN substantia medullaris (1).

**me·dul·la ob·lon·ga·ta** (mĕ-dŭl'ă ob-long-gă'tă) [TA] The most caudal subdivision of the brainstem, continuous with the spinal cord, extending from the lower border of the decussation of the pyramid to the pons. SYN myelencephalon, oblongata.

**med·ul·lar·y mem·brane** (med'ŭ-lar'ē mem'brăn) SYN endosteum.

**me·dul·la spi·na·lis** (mĕ-dŭl'ă spī-nā'lis) [TA] SYN spinal cord.

**MEG** Abbreviation for magnetoencephalogram.

♻ **mega-** Combining form meaning large, oversize; opposite of micro-. [G. *megas,* big]

**meg·a·co·lon** (meg'ă-kō-lŏn) Condition involving extreme dilation of the colon.

**meg·a·dont** (meg'ă-dont) SYN macrodont. [*mega-* + G. *odous* (*odont-*), tooth]

**meg·a·don·tism** (meg'ă-don'tizm) SYN macrodontia.

**meg·a·gna·thi·a** (meg'ăg-nā'thē-ă) SYN macrognathia.

**meg·al·gi·a** (meg-al'jē-ă) Very severe pain. [*mega-* + G. *algos,* pain]

**meg·a·lo·blas·tic a·ne·mi·a** (meg'ă-lō-blast'ik ă-nē'mē-ă) Anemia with a predominant number of megaloblastic erythroblasts and relatively few normoblasts, among hyperplastic erythroid cells in bone marrow.

**meg·a·lo·don·ti·a** (meg'ă-lō-don'shē-ă) SYN macrodontia.

**meg·a·lo·glos·si·a** (meg'ă-lō-glos'sē-ă) SYN macroglossia. [*megalo-* + G. *glōssa,* tongue]

**mei·o·sis** (mī-ō'sis) Special process of cell division comprising two nuclear divisions in rapid succession that result in four gametocytes, each containing half the number of chromosomes found in somatic cells.

**Meiss·ner cor·pus·cle** (mīs'ner kōr'pŭs-ĕl) SYN tactile corpuscle.

**melaena** [Br.] SYN melena.

**mel·a·nin** (mel'ă-nin) Any of the dark brown to black pigments that occur in the skin, hair, pigmented coat of the retina, and medulla and zona reticularis of the suprarenal gland. [G. *melas* (*melan-*), black]

**mel·a·nin pig·men·ta·tion** (mel'ă-nin pig'mĕn-tā'shŭn) Coloration due to melanin within soft tissue; may be normal or connected with disease or disorder.

♻ **melano-** Combining form meaning black, extreme darkness of hue. [G. *melas*]

**mel·a·no·cyte-stim·u·lat·ing hor·mone (MSH)** (mel'ă-nō-sīt-stim'yū-lā-ting hōr'mōn) SYN melanotropin, bioregulator.

▪ **mel·a·no·ma** (mel'ă-nō'mă) Malignant neoplasm, derived from cells capable of forming melanin, arising in skin of any part of the body, or in the eye, and, rarely, in mucous membranes of the genitalia, anus, oral cavity, or other sites. See this page.

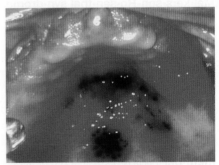

**melanoma:** satellite lesions of palate

**mn**

⊞**mel·a·no·pla·ki·a** (mel′ă-nō-plă′kē-ă) The occurrence of pigmented patches on the tongue and buccal mucous membrane. See this page. [*melano-* + G. *plax,* plate, plaque]

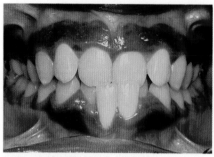

**melanoplakia with attached gingiva**

⊞**mel·a·no·sis** (mel′ă-nō′sis) Abnormal dark brown or brown-black pigmentation of various tissues or organs, as the result of melanin or, in some situations, other substances that resemble melanin to varying degrees. See page A13. [*melano-* + G. *-osis,* condition]

**mel·a·not·ic neu·ro·ec·to·der·mal tu·mor of in·fan·cy** (mel′ă-not′ĭk nū′rō-ek′tō-dĕr-măl tū′mŏr in′făn-sē) Benign neoplasm of neuroectodermal origin that most often involves the anterior maxilla of infants in the first year of life.

**mel·a·no·tro·pin** (mel′ă-nō-trō′pin) A polypeptide hormone secreted by the intermediate lobe of the hypophysis in humans. SYN melanocyte-stimulating hormone.

**mel·a·to·nin** (mel′ă-tōn′in) Substance formed by mammalian pineal body, which appears to depress gonadal function in mammals; a precursor is serotonin. [*melanophore* + G. *tonos,* contraction, + *-in*]

**me·le·na** (mĕ-lē′nă) Passage of dark-colored, tarry stools, due to presence of blood altered by intestinal juices. Cf. hematochezia. [G. *melaina,* fem. of *melas,* black]

⊞**Mel·kers·son-Ro·sen·thal syn·drome** (mel′kĕr-sŏn rō′zen-thahl sin′drŏm) Cheilitis granulomatosa, fissured tongue, and recurrent facial nerve paralysis. See page A7.

**Mel·nick-Nee·dles os·te·o·dys·plas·ty** (mel′nik nē′dĕlz os′tē-ō-dis-plas′tē) A generalized skeletal dysplasia with prominent forehead and small mandible. SYN osteodysplasty.

**me·los·chi·sis** (me-los′ki-sis) Congenital cleft in the face. [G. *mēlon,* cheek, + *schisis,* a cleaving]

**mem·ber** (mem′bĕr) SYN limb (1). [L. *membrum*]

**mem·bra·na ad·a·man·ti·na** (mem-brā′nă ad′ă-man-tī′nă) SYN enamel cuticle.

**mem·bra·na e·bor·is** (mem-brā′nă ē-bō′ris) Lining membrane of pulp cavity of a tooth, consisting of the odontoblastic layer.

**mem·brane** (mem′brān) A thin sheet or layer of pliable tissue, serving as a covering or envelope of a part, as the lining of a cavity, as a partition or septum, or as a connector.

**mem·brane bone** (mem′brān bōn) Bone that develops embryologically within a membrane of vascularized primordial mesenchymal tissue without prior formation of cartilage.

**mem·bra·nous am·pul·lae of the sem·i·cir·cu·lar ducts** (mem′bră-nŭs am-pul′ē sem′ē-sĭr′kyū-lăr dŭkts) [TA] A nearly spheric enlargement of one end of each of the three semicircular ducts, anterior, posterior, and lateral, where they connect with the utricle. SYN ampulla membranacea.

**mem·bra·nous lab·y·rinth** (mem′bră-nŭs lab′i-rinth) [TA] Complex arrangement of communicating membranous canaliculi and sacs, filled with endolymph and surrounded by perilymph, suspended within cavity of the bony labyrinth.

**mem·o·ry** (mem′ŏ-rē) **1.** General term for recollection of that which was earlier experienced or learned. **2.** Mental information processing system that receives (registers), modifies, stores, and retrieves informational stimuli.

**MEN** Abbreviation for multiple endocrine neoplasia.

**men·a·di·ol di·ac·e·tate** (men′ă-dī′ol dī-as′ĕ-tāt) Menadiol acetylated at both hydroxyl groups; a prothrombogenic vitamin. SYN vitamin K4.

**men·a·di·one** (men′ă-dī′ōn) Root of compounds that are 3-multiprenyl derivatives of menadione and known as the menaquinones or vitamins K2. SYN vitamin K3.

**me·nar·che** (men-ahr′kē) Establishment of the menstrual function; the time of the first menstrual period. [G. *mēn,* month, + *archē,* beginning]

**Men·del first law** (men′dĕl fĭrst law) SYN law of segregation.

**men·de·li·an in·her·i·tance** (men-dē′lē-ăn in-her′i-tăns) Inheritance in which stable and undecomposable characters controlled entirely or overwhelmingly by a single genetic locus are transmitted over many generations.

**Men·del sec·ond law** (men′dĕl sek′ŏnd law) SYN law of independent assortment.

**Mé·ni·ère dis·ease, Mé·ni·ère syn·drome** (men-yār′ di-zēz′, sin′drŏm) An affliction characterized clinically by vertigo, nausea, vomiting, tinnitus, and progressive hearing loss.

♻ **mening-** *Avoid mispronouncing this combining form men-in´jō.* The meninges. [G. *mēninx,* membrane]

**me·nin·gi·o·ma** (mĕ-nin´jē-ō´mă) A benign, encapsulated neoplasm of arachnoidal origin, occurring most frequently in adults; tends to occur along the superior sagittal sinus, along the sphenoid ridge, or in the vicinity of the optic chiasm. [*mening-* + G. *-oma,* tumor]

**me·nin·gism** (men´in-jizm) Condition in which symptoms simulate meningitis, without actual inflammation of these membranes.

**men·in·gi·tis,** pl. **men·in·git·i·des** (men´ in-jī´tis, -jit´ti-dēz) Inflammation of membranes of brain or spinal cord. SYN cerebrospinal meningitis. [*mening-* + G. *itis,* inflammation]

**me·nin·go·cele** (mĕ-ning´gō-sēl) Protrusion of membranes of the brain or spinal cord through defect in cranium or spinal column. [*meningo-* + G. *kēlē,* tumor]

**me·nin·go·en·ceph·a·li·tis** (mĕ-ning´gō-en-sef´ăl-ī´tis) Inflammation of brain and its membranes. SYN cerebromeningitis. [*meningo-* + G. *enkephalos,* brain, + *-itis,* inflammation]

**me·nin·go·hy·dro·en·ceph·a·lo·cele** (mĕ-ning´gō-hī´drō-en-sef´ă-lō-sēl) Large ossification defect of cranial bones, usually squamous part of occipital bone, through which part of brain and ventricle pass into an external meningeal sac.

**me·nin·go·my·e·lo·cele** (mĕ-ning´gō-mī´ĕ-lō-sēl) Protrusion of meninges and spinal cord through a defect in the vertebral column. [*meningo-* + G. *myelos,* marrow, + *kēlē,* tumor]

**me·ninx,** pl. **me·nin·ges** (mē´ningks, me-nin´jēz) [TA] Any membrane; specifically, membranous covering of brain and spinal cord. [Mod. L. fr. G. *mēninx,* membrane]

**men·is·cec·to·my** (men´i-sek´tŏ-mē) Excision of a meniscus. [G. *mēniskos,* crescent (meniscus) + *ektomē,* excision]

**me·nis·cus,** pl. **me·nis·ci** (mĕ-nis´kŭs, -kī) [TA] **1.** [TA] Any crescent-shaped structure. **2.** A crescent-shaped fibrocartilaginous structure of the knee, the acromio- and sternoclavicular and the temporomandibular joints. **3.** The crescentic curvature of the surface of a liquid standing in a narrow vessel. SYN meniscus lens. [G. *mēniskos,* crescent]

**me·nis·cus lens** (mĕ-nis´kŭs lenz) SYN meniscus.

♻ **meno-** The menses, menstruation. [G. *mēn,* month]

**men·o·pause** (men´ŏ-pawz) Permanent cessation of the menses. [*meno-* + G. *pausis,* cessation]

**men·or·rha·gi·a** (men´ŏ-rā´jē-ă) SYN hypermenorrhea. [*meno-* + G. *rhēgnymi,* to burst forth]

**men·ses** (men´sēz) A periodic physiologic hemorrhage, which occurs at approximately 4-week intervals; its source is the uterine mucous membrane; usually the bleeding is preceded by ovulation and predecidual changes in the endometrium. SYN emmenia. [L. pl. of *mensis,* month]

**men·stru·al cy·cle** (men´strū-ăl sī´kĕl) The period in which an oocyte matures, is ovulated, and enters the uterine lumen through the uterine tube; ovarian hormonal secretions effect endometrial changes such that, if fertilization occurs, nidation will be possible; in the absence of fertilization, ovarian secretions wane, the endometrium sloughs, and menstruation begins; this cycle lasts an average of 28 days, with day 1 of the cycle designated as that day on which menstrual flow begins.

**men·stru·al mo·li·mi·na** (men´strū-ăl mŏ-lim´i-nă) SYN premenstrual syndrome.

**men·stru·al phase** (men´strū-ăl fāz) First day of menstruation; indicates beginning of endometrial menstrual cycle; lasts 4–5 days and coincides with bleeding and shedding of degenerated endometrium from previous menstrual cycle.

**men·tal** (men´tăl) **1.** Relating to the mind. **2.** Relating to the chin. [L. *mens (ment-),* mind]

**men·tal ab·er·ra·tion** (men´tăl ab´ĕr-ā´shŭn) Disturbed loosening of association, ambivalence, hallucination, or behavior.

**men·tal ar·te·ry** (men´tăl ahr´tĕr-ē) *Distribution,* chin; the terminal branch of the inferior alveolar; *anastomoses,* inferior labial artery. SYN arteria mentalis [TA].

**men·tal dis·or·der** (men´tăl dis-ōr´dĕr) Psychological syndrome or behavioral pattern associated with subjective distress and/or objective impairment.

**men·tal for·a·men** (men´tăl fōr-ā´mĕn) [TA] The anterior opening of the mandibular canal on the body of the mandible lateral to and above the mental tubercle giving passage to the mental artery and nerve.

**men·tal health** (men´tăl helth) Emotional, behavioral, and social maturity or normality; absence of a mental or behavioral disorder; state of psychological well-being in which one has achieved a satisfactory integration of one's instinctual drives acceptable to both oneself and one's social milieu.

**men·tal ill·ness** (men´tăl il´nĕs) Broadly inclusive term, generally denoting one or all of the following: 1) a disease of the brain, with predominant behavioral symptoms; as in paresis 2) a disease of the "mind" or personality, evi-

**mn**

denced by abnormal behavior, as in hysteria or schizophrenia.

**men·ta·lis mus·cle** (men-tā′lis mŭs′ĕl) *Origin,* incisor fossa of mandible; *insertion,* skin of chin; *action,* raises and wrinkles skin of chin, thus elevating the lower lip; *nerve supply,* facial. SYN musculus mentalis [TA].

**men·tal nerve** (men′tăl nĕrv) [TA] Branch of inferior alveolar nerve, arising in mandibular canal and passing through mental foramen to chin and lower lip.

**men·tal pro·cess** (men′tăl prŏ′ses) SYN mental protuberance.

**men·tal pro·tu·ber·ance** (men′tăl prŏ-tū′bĕr-ăns) [TA] Chin prominence at anterior part of mandible. SYN mental process.

**men·tal re·tar·da·tion** (men′tăl rē′tahr-dā′shŭn) Subaverage general intellectual functioning starting with developmental period, associated with impairment in adaptive behavior.

**men·tal ridge** (men′tăl rij) Radiographic radiopaque image of ridge of bone on labial aspect of mandible below the apices of canines and incisors toward the mandibular symphysis.

**men·tal spine** (men′tăl spīn) [TA] SYN genial tubercle.

**men·tal sym·phy·sis** (men′tăl sim′fi-sis) SYN mandibular symphysis.

**men·tal tu·ber·cle (of man·di·ble)** (men′tăl tū′bĕr-kĕl man′di-bĕl) [TA] Paired eminence on mandibular mental protuberance.

**men·ta·tion** (men-tā′shŭn) Process of reasoning and thinking.

**men·thol** (men′thol) An alcohol obtained from peppermint or other mint oils, or prepared synthetically; used as an antipruritic and topical anesthetic; in nasal sprays, cough drops, and inhalers; and as a flavoring agent. [L. *menta,* mint]

**men·to·la·bi·a·lis** (men′tō-lā′bē-ā′lis) Mentalis and depressor labii inferioris muscles considered as one entity. [L.]

**men·to·la·bi·al sul·cus** (men′tō-lā′bē-ăl sŭl′kŭs) [TA] Indistinct line separating lower lip from chin.

**men·ton** (men′tŏn) In cephalometrics, the lowermost point in the symphysial shadow as seen on a lateral jaw projection. [L. *mentum,* chin]

**me·per·i·dine hy·dro·chlor·ide** (mĕ-per′i-dēn hī′drŏ-klōr′īd) A widely used narcotic analgesic.

**me·phit·ic** (mĕ-fit′ik) Foul, poisonous, or noxious. [L. *mephitis,* a noxious exhalation]

**me·pro·ba·mate** (mĕ-prō′bă-māt) Oral anxiolytic with potential for dependency and addiction.

**mer·bro·min** (mer-brō′min) Organic mercurial antiseptic compound that also has staining properties similar to those of eosin and phloxine. SYN mercurochrome.

**mer·cap·tan** (mĕr-kap′tan) In dentistry, class of elastic impression compounds sometimes called rubber base materials.

**mer·cu·ri·al** (mĕr-kyūr′ē-ăl) **1.** Any salt of mercury used medicinally. **2.** Relating to mercury.

**mer·cu·ri·al line** (mĕr-kyūr′ē-ăl līn) Bluish brown pigmentation seen at gingival margin and associated with mercury poisoning.

**mer·cu·ri·al sto·ma·ti·tis** (mĕr-kyūr′ē-ăl stō′mă-tī′tis) Alterations of oral mucosa arising from chronic mercury poisoning; may consist of mucosal erythema and edema, ulceration, and deposition of mercurial sulfide in inflamed tissues, resulting in oral pigmentation resembling that of lead stomatitis.

**mer·cu·ric** (mĕr-kyūr′ik) Denoting mercury salt in which ion of the metal is bivalent, as in corrosive sublimate, mercuric chloride: the mercurous chloride is termed calomel.

**mer·cu·ro·chrome** (mĕr-kyūr′ŏ-krōm) SYN merbromin.

**mer·cu·rous** (mĕr-kyūr′ŭs) Denoting a salt of mercury in which the ion of the metal is univalent.

**mer·cu·ry** (mĕr′kyūr-ē) A dense liquid metallic element; used in thermometers, barometers, manometers, and other scientific instruments; some salts and organic mercurials are used medicinally; must be handled with care.

**mer·cu·ry poi·son·ing** (mĕr′kyūr-ē poy′zŏn-ing) Disease usually caused by ingestion or inhalation of mercury or mercury compounds, which are toxic in relation to their ability to produce mercuric ions; **acute mercury poisoning** is associated with ulcerations of mouth (including loosening of teeth), stomach, and intestine in addition to toxic changes in the renal tubules; anuria and anemia may occur; respiratory distress and pneumonia can follow inhalation; **chronic mercury poisoning** is due to industrial pollution; causes gastrointestinal or central nervous system manifestations including stomatitis, diarrhea, headaches, ataxia, tremor, hyperreflexia, sensorineural impairment, and emotional instability and sometimes delirium.

**me·rid·i·an** (mĕr-id′ē-an) Line encircling a globular body at right angles to its equator and touching both poles, or the half of such a circle extending from pole to pole.

**Mer·kel cor·pus·cle** (mer′kel kōr′pŭs-ĕl) SYN tactile meniscus.

**mer·o·crine gland** (mer′ŏ-krin gland)

Gland that releases only an acellular secretory product, in contrast to a holocrine gland.

**Mer·ri·field knife** (mer'i-fēld nīf) A long, narrow, triangularly or spear-shaped bladed instrument used for dental periodontal surgery, specifically to cut interdental tissues.

**mes·ca·line** (mes'kă-lin) The most active alkaloid present in the buttons of the mescal cactus, *Lophophora williamsii*. Has psychotomimetic effects similar to those produced by lysergic acid diethylamide (LSD). [Sp. *mezcal*]

**me·sec·to·derm** (mes-ek'tō-dĕrm) 1. Cells in the area around the dorsal lip of the blastopore where mesoderm and ectoderm undergo a process of separation. 2. That part of the mesenchyme derived from ectoderm. [*mes- + ectoderm*]

**mes·en·ceph·a·lon** (mes'en-sef'ă-lon) [TA] That part of the brainstem developing from the middle of the three primary cerebral vesicles of the embryo. In an adult, the mesencephalon is characterized by the unique conformation of its roof plate, the lamina of the mesencephalic tectum, composed of the bilaterally paired superior and inferior colliculi, and by the massive paired prominence of the crus cerebri at its ventral surface. SYN midbrain. [G. *mes-* middle + G. *enkephalos,* brain]

**me·sen·chy·mal cells** (mez'ĕn-kī'măl selz) Fusiform or stellate cells located between ectoderm and endoderm of young embryos.

**mes·en·chyme** (mez'ĕn-kīm) An aggregation of mesenchymal or fibroblastlike cells. [G. *mes-* middle + G. *enkyma,* infusion]

**me·si·al** (mē'zē-ăl) Nearer to midline or most anterior part of dental arch. SEE ALSO proximal. [G. *mesos,* middle]

**me·si·al an·gle** (mē'zē-ăl ang'gĕl) Area formed by meeting of mesial with labial (or buccal) or lingual tooth surface.

**me·si·al ca·ries** (mē'zē-ăl kar'ēz) Caries on tooth surface directed toward median plane of dental arch.

**me·si·al dis·place·ment** (mē'zē-ăl dis-plās'mĕnt) SYN mesioversion.

**me·si·al drift** (mē'zē-ăl drift) SYN drift.

**me·si·al fo·ve·a of tooth** (mē'zē-ăl fō'vē-ă tūth) [TA] Shallow depression related to cusps on anterior aspect of a molar.

**me·si·al oc·clu·sion** (mē'zē-ăl ŏ-klū'zhŭn) Occlusion in which the mandibular articulate with maxillary teeth in a position more anterior than normal. SYN anterior occlusion (2), mesiooocclusion.

**me·si·al root of tooth** (mē'zē-ăl rūt tūth) [TA] Root of multirooted tooth that is located toward the mesial side of the tooth.

**me·si·al step** (mē'zē-ăl step) Projection of a cavity prepared in a tooth into the mesial surface perpendicular to the main part of the cavity to prevent displacement of the restoration (filling) by forces of mastication.

**me·si·al sur·face of tooth** (mē'zē-ăl sŭr'făs tūth) [TA] Contact tooth surface directed toward median plane of dental arch; opposite facies distalis dentis. SYN facies mesialis dentis.

🔧 **mesio-** Combining form meaning mesial (especially in dentistry). [G. *mesos,* middle]

**me·si·o·buc·cal** (mē'zē-ō-bŭk'ăl) Relating to mesial and buccal tooth surfaces; denoting especially angle formed by junction of these two surfaces.

**me·si·o·buc·cal root of tooth** (mē'zē-ō-bŭk'ăl rūt tūth) [TA] Root of a multirooted tooth located toward mesial aspect of tooth and buccal side of alveolar ridge.

**me·si·o·buc·co·oc·clu·sal** (mē'zē-ō-bŭk'ō-ŏ-klū'zăl) Relating to angle formed by junction of mesial, buccal, and occlusal surfaces of a premolar or molar tooth.

**me·si·o·buc·co·pul·pal** (mē'zē-ō-bŭk'ō-pŭl'păl) Relating to angle denoting junction of mesial, buccal, and pulpal surfaces in a tooth cavity preparation.

**me·si·oc·clu·sion** (mē'zē-ō-klū'zhŭn) A malocclusion in which the mandibular arch articulates with the maxillary arch in a position mesial to normal; in Angle classification, a Class III malocclusion. SYN mesial occlusion (2).

**me·si·o·cer·vi·cal** (mē'zē-ō-sĕr'vi-kăl) 1. Relating to line angle of cavity preparation at junction of mesial and cervical walls. 2. Pertaining to tooth area at junction of mesial surface and cervical region.

**me·si·o·clu·sion** (mē'zē-ō-klū'zhŭn) Malocclusion in which mandibular arch articulates with maxillary arch more mesially than normal; in Angle classification, a Class III malocclusion.

**me·si·o·dens** (mē'zē-ō-denz) Supernumerary tooth in midline of anterior maxillae, between maxillary central incisor teeth. SYN mediodens. [*mesio- + L. dens,* tooth]

**me·si·o·dis·tal** (mē'zē-ō-dis'tăl) Denoting plane or diameter of a tooth cutting its mesial and distal surfaces.

**me·si·o·dis·tal clasp** (mē'zē-ō-dis'tăl klasp) Type of fitting on removable partial dentures that embraces distolingual and mesial surfaces of a tooth and establishes retention in either mesial or distal undercuts (or both). [*mesio-,* toward the midline, fr. G. *mesos,* middle, + *distal*]

**me·si·o·dis·toc·clu·sal (MOD)** (mē'zē-ō-dis'tō-klū'zăl) Denoting three-surface cavity

mn

or cavity preparation or restoration (class 2, Black classification) in the premolars (bicuspids) and molars.

**me·si·o·gin·gi·val** (mē′zē-ō-jin′ji-văl) Relating to angle formed by junction of mesial surface with gingival line of a tooth.

**me·si·o·gnath·ic** (mē′zē-ōg-nath′ik) Denoting malposition of one or both jaws in a more forward position than normal.

**me·si·o·in·ci·sal** (mē′zē-ō-in-sī′zăl) Relating to mesial and tooth incisal surfaces; denoting angle formed by their junction.

**me·si·o·la·bi·al** (mē′zē-ō-lā′bē-ăl) Relating to mesial and labial tooth surfaces; denoting especially angle formed by their junction.

**me·si·o·lin·gual** (mē′zē-ō-ling′gwăl) Relating to mesial and lingual tooth surfaces; denoting especially angle formed by their junction.

**me·si·o·lin·gual root of tooth** (mē′zē-ō-ling′gwăl rūt tūth) [TA] Root of a multirooted tooth located toward mesial aspect of tooth and lingual side of alveolar ridge.

**me·si·o·lin·guo·oc·clu·sal** (mē′zē-ō-ling′ gwō-ŏ-klū′zăl) Denoting angle formed by junction of the mesial, lingual, and occlusal surfaces of a premolar or molar tooth.

**me·si·o·lin·guo·pul·pal** (mē′zē-ō-ling′ gwō-pŭl′păl) Relating to angle denoting junction of mesial, lingual, and pulpal surfaces in a tooth cavity preparation.

**me·si·o·oc·clu·sal** (mē′zē-ō-ŏ-klū′zăl) Denoting angle formed by junction of mesial and occlusal surfaces of a premolar or molar tooth.

**me·si·o·oc·clu·sion** (mē′zē-ō-ŏ-klū′zhŭn) SYN mesial occlusion.

**me·si·o·place·ment** (mē′zē-ō-plās′měnt) SYN mesioversion.

**me·si·o·pul·pal** (mē′zē-ō-pŭl′păl) Pertaining to inner wall or floor of a cavity preparation on mesial tooth side.

**me·si·o·ver·sion** (mē′zē-ō-věr′zhŭn) Malposition of a tooth mesial to normal, in an anterior direction following curvature of dental arch. SYN mesial displacement, mesioplacement.

**mes·mer·ism** (mes′měr-izm) A system of therapeutics from which hypnotism and therapeutic suggestion developed.

♻ **meso-, mes-** Combining forms denoting **1.** Middle, mean, intermediacy. **2.** A mesentery or mesentery like structure. **3.** A compound, containing more than one chiral center, having an internal plane of symmetry.

**mes·o·ce·phal·ic** (mez′ō-se-fal′ik) Having a head of medium length. SYN mesaticephalic, normocephalic.

**mesocephalous** SYN mesocephalic.

**mes·o·derm** (mez′ō-děrm) Middle of three primary germ layers of embryo (the others being ectoderm and endoderm). [G. *meso-* middle + G. *derma,* skin]

**mes·o·dont** (mez′ō-dont) Having teeth of medium size. [G. *meso-* middle + G. *odous,* tooth]

**mes·og·nath·ic** (mez′og-nath′ik) **1.** Relating to the mesognathion. **2.** SYN mesognathous.

**mes·og·nath·i·on** (mez′og-nā′thē-on) Lateral segment of premaxillary or incisive bone external to the endognathion. [G. *meso-* middle + G. *gnathos,* jaw]

**me·sog·na·thous** (měz-og′nă-thŭs) Having a face with slightly projecting jaw. SYN mesognathic.

**mes·o·neph·ros,** pl. **mes·o·neph·roi** (mez′ō-nef′ros, -roy) One of three excretory organs appearing in the evolution of vertebrates. SYN wolffian body. [G. *meso-* middle + G. *nephros,* kidney]

**mes·oph·ry·on** (mez-of′rē-on) SYN glabella (2). [G. *meso-* middle + Gr. *ophrys,* eyebrow]

♻ **meta-** In medicine and biology, a prefix denoting the concept of after, subsequent to, behind, or hindmost. [G. after, between, over]

**met·a·anal·y·sis** (met′ă-nal′i-sis) The systematic process of using statistical methods to combine the results of different studies.

**met·a·bol·ic ac·id·o·sis** (met′ă-bol′ik as′i-dō′sis) Decreased pH and bicarbonate concentration in body fluids caused either by accumulation of acids or abnormal losses of fixed base from the body.

**met·a·bol·ic cal·cu·lus** (met′ă-bol′ik kal′ kyū-lŭs) Stone, usually renal, caused by metabolic abnormality resulting in increased excretion of a substance of low solubility in urine.

**met·a·bol·ic syn·drome** (met′ă-bol′ik sin′ drōm) Group of metabolic risk factors linked to insulin resistance and associated with increased risk of cardiovascular disease.

**me·tab·o·lism** (mě-tab′ŏ-lizm) Sum of chemical and physical changes occurring in tissue, consisting of anabolism (those reactions that convert small molecules into large), and catabolism (those reactions that convert large molecules into small), including both endogenous large molecules and biodegradation of xenobiotics. [G. *metabolē,* change]

**met·a·car·pal** (met′ă-kahr′păl) **1.** Relating to the metacarpus. **2.** Any one of the metacarpal bones.

**met·a·car·pus,** pl. **met·a·car·pi** (met′ă-kahr′pŭs, -pī) [TA] The five bones of the hand between the carpus and the phalanges. [*meta-* + G. *karpos,* wrist]

**met·a·in·fec·tive** (met′ă-in-fek′tiv) Occurring subsequent to an infection.

**met·al** (met′ăl) One of the electropositive elements, either amphoteric or basic, characterized by luster, malleability, ductility, the ability to conduct electricity and heat, and the tendency to lose rather than gain electrons in chemical reactions. [L. *metallum,* a mine, a mineral, fr. G. *metallon,* a mine, pit]

**met·al base** (met′ăl bās) Metallic portion of a denture base forming part of wall of basal surface of denture; serves as base for attachment of plastic (resin) part of denture and teeth.

**met·al burs** (met′ăl bŭrz) Minute metallic shards that project from cutting edge of the working-end of an improperly sharpened instrument.

**met·al in·sert teeth** (met′ăl in′sĕrt tēth) Prosthetic teeth containing metal cutting surfaces in occlusal surfaces.

**met·al in·ter·face** (met′ăl in′tĕr-fās) In dentistry, boundary between metal and nonsolvent solder, or between metal and surface oxide.

**me·tal·lic stain** (mĕ-tal′ik stān) Dental discolorations generally caused by orally inhaling metal-containing dust or by ingestion of some orally administered medications.

**met·al·loid** (met′ă-loyd) Resembling a metal in at least one amphoteric form. [*metal* + G. *eidos,* resemblance]

**me·tal·lo·pho·bi·a** (mĕ-tal′ō-fō′bē-ă) Morbid fear of metal objects. [G. *metallon,* metal, + *phobos,* fear]

**me·tal·lo·pro·tein** (mĕ-tal′ō-prō′tēn) A protein with a tightly bound metal ion or ions.

**met·a·neph·rine** (met′ă-nef′rin) A catabolite of epinephrine found in the serum, urine, and some tissue types, due to action of catechol-*O*-methyltransferase on epinephrine.

**me·taph·y·sis,** pl. **me·taph·y·ses** (mĕ-taf′i-sis, -sēz) [TA] A conic segment between the epiphysis and diaphysis of a long bone. [*meta-* + G. *physis,* growth]

**met·a·pla·si·a** (met′ă-plā′zē-ă) Abnormal transformation of an adult, fully differentiated tissue of one kind into a differentiated tissue of another kind; an acquired condition, in contrast to heteroplasia. [G. *metaplasis,* transformation]

**met·a·py·ret·ic** (met′ă-pī-ret′ik) SYN postfebrile. [*meta-* + G. *pyretos,* fever]

**me·tas·ta·sis,** pl. **me·tas·ta·ses** (mĕ-tas′tă-sis, -sēz) **1.** Spread of a disease process from one part of the body to another, as in the appearance of neoplasms in parts of the body

remote from the site of the primary tumor; results from dissemination of tumor cells by the lymphatics or blood vessels or by direct extension through serous cavities or subarachnoid or other spaces. **2.** Transportation of bacteria from one part of the body to another, through the bloodstream or through lymph channels.

**me·tas·ta·siz·ing sep·ti·ce·mi·a** (mĕ-tas′tă-sīz-ing sep′ti-sē′mē-ă) Sepsis, with entry of microorganisms into bloodstream leading to abscess formation distant from original infection site.

**met·a·stat·ic cal·ci·fi·ca·tion** (met′ă-stat′ik kal′si-fi-kā′shŭn) Calcification occurring in nonosseous viable tissue in hypercalcemia.

**me·te·or·o·trop·ic** (mē′tē-ŏr-ō-trō′pik) Denoting diseases affected by the weather.

**me·ter (m)** (mē′tĕr) **1.** Fundamental unit of length in the SI and metric system, equivalent to 39.37007874 inches. **2.** A device for measuring the quantity of that which passes through it. SYN metre. [Fr. *metre;* G. *metron,* measure]

**me·ter·ed spray** (mē′tĕrd sprā) Method for dispensing topical anesthetic that administers a fixed volume of drug and then stops automatically.

**meth·ac·ry·late res·in** (meth′ă-kril′āt rez′in) Translucent plastic material, used to manufacture various medical appliances, surgical instruments, and seating components used in total joint replacement.

**meth·a·cryl·ic ac·id** (meth′ă-kril′ik as′id) A chemical in oil made from Roman camomile; used to manufacture resins and plastics.

**meth·a·done hy·dro·chlor·ide** (meth′ă-dōn hī′drŏ-klōr′īd) Synthetic narcotic drug; orally effective analgesic similar in action to morphine but with slightly greater potency and longer duration; produces psychic and physical dependence, as does morphine, but withdrawal symptoms are somewhat milder; used as a replacement (by oral route) for morphine and heroin; also used during withdrawal treatment in morphine and heroin addiction.

**methaemoglobinaemia** [Br.] SYN methemoglobinemia.

**meth·am·phet·a·mine hy·dro·chlor·ide** (meth′am-fet′ă-mēn hī′drŏ-klōr′īd) Sympathomimetic agent that exerts greater stimulating effects on the central nervous system than amphetamine (hence street name, ''speed''); widely used by drug abusers through oral and intravenous (''mainlining'') routes; strong psychic dependence may develop. When converted to the freebase (methamphetamine), it can be smoked like crack cocaine and is commonly referred to by various street names.

**meth·a·nol** (meth′ă-nol) SYN methyl alcohol.

mn

**met·he·mo·glo·bi·ne·mi·a** (met-hē'mŏ-glō-bi-nē'mē-ă) The presence of methemoglobin in the circulating blood. SYN methaemoglobinaemia. [methemoglobin + G. *haima*, blood]

**meth·i·cil·lin so·di·um** (meth'i-sil'in sō'dē-ŭm) A semisynthetic penicillin salt for parenteral administration; restriction of its use to infections caused by penicillin G-resistant staphylococci is recommended; less effective than penicillin G in infections caused by hemolytic streptococci, pneumococci, gonococci, and penicillin G–sensitive staphylococci.

**me·thi·o·nine (M)** (me-thī'ō-nēn) The L-isomer is a nutritionally essential amino acid and the most important natural source of ''active methyl'' groups in the body.

**meth·od** (meth'ŏd) The mode or manner or orderly sequence of events of a process or procedure. [G. *methodos;* fr. *meta,* after, + *hodos,* way]

**meth·o·trex·ate** (meth'ō-trek'sāt) Folic acid antagonist used as an antineoplastic agent and to treat psoriasis and rheumatoid arthritis.

**meth·yl al·co·hol** (meth'il al'kŏ-hol) Flammable toxic liquid, used as an industrial solvent, antifreeze, and in chemical manufacture; ingestion may result in severe acidosis and other effects on the central nervous system. SYN methanol.

**meth·yl·a·tion** (meth'i-lā'shŭn) Addition of methyl groups; in histochemistry, used to esterify carboxyl groups and remove sulfate groups by treating tissue sections with hot methanol in the presence of hydrochloric acid.

**meth·y·lene blue** (meth'i-lēn blū) A basic dye easily oxidized to azure, with dye mixtures; used in histology and microbiology.

**meth·yl·ma·lon·ic ac·i·de·mi·a** (meth'il-mă-lon'ik as'i-dē'mē-ă) SYN ketotic hyperglycinemia.

**meth·yl meth·ac·ry·late** (meth'il meth'ă-kril'āt) Thermoplastic material used for denture bases and as an embedding material for electron microscopy.

**meth·yl·par·a·ben** (meth'il-par'ă-ben) An antifungal preservative.

**metre** [Br.] SYN meter.

**met·ric sys·tem** (met'rik sis'tĕm) A system of weights and measures, universal for scientific use, based on the meter, the gram, and the liter.

**Mex·i·can hat cell** (mek'si-kăn hat sel) SYN target cell.

**MHC** Abbreviation for major histocompatibility complex.

**MI** Abbreviation for myocardial infarction.

**mi·celle** (mi-sel') 1. Elongated sub(light)microscopic particles, detected in hydrogels, of supramolecular character and crystalline structure. 2. Any water-soluble aggregate, spontaneously and reversibly, formed from amphiphile molecules. 3. A hypothetical ordered region in a natural fiber such as cellulose. [L. *micella,* small morsel, dim. of *mica,* morsel, grain]

○ **micro-** 1. Prefixes denoting smallness. 2. μ *It is recommended that, in handwritten material and in computer work, names of units formed with this prefix be written in full, because both human beings and computers may misread the Greek letter μ as the Roman letter m. Alternatively the abbreviation mc may be substituted for μ thus, mcg, mcL, mcm, mcmol instead of μg, μL, μm, μmol. The Roman letter u is not in any circumstances a suitable substitute for* μ. Prefix used in the SI and the metric system to signify submultiples of one-millionth ($10^{-6}$) of such unit. 3. CHEMISTRY prefix to terms denoting procedures that utilize minimal quantities of the substance to be examined; e.g., a drop or two in place of 1 or more mL. 4. Combining forms meaning microscopic. [G. *mikros,* small]

**mi·cro·aer·o·sol** (mī'krō-ăr'ŏ-sol) A suspension in air of particles that are submicronic or from 1–10 mcm in diameter.

**mi·cro·al·bu·mi·nu·ria** (mī'krō-al-bū'min-yūr'ē-ă) A slight increase in urinary albumin excretion that can be detected using immunoassays but not by means of conventional urine protein measurements; an early marker for renal disease in patients with diabetes. [*micro-* + *albuminuria*]

**mi·cro·a·nal·y·sis** (mī'krō-ă-nal'i-sis) Analytic techniques involving unusually small samples.

**mi·cro·an·gi·op·a·thy** (mī'krō-an-jē-op'ă-thē) SYN capillaropathy.

**mi·cro·bi·al aer·o·sol** (mī-krō'bē-ăl ār'ŏ-sol) Airborne suspension of particles smaller than 10 mcm in diameter that consists partially or wholly of microorganisms.

**mi·cro·bi·cide** (mī-krō'bi-sīd) Agent destructive to microbes; germicide; antiseptic. [*microbe* + L. *caedo,* to kill]

**mi·cro·bi·ol·o·gy** (mī'krō-bī-ol'ŏ-jē) The science concerned with microorganisms, including fungi, protozoa, bacteria, and viruses.

**mi·cro·bi·o·ta** (mī'krō-bī-ō'tă) Collective term for microflora (i.e., any type of minute organism) that may be found within a given environment.

**mi·cro·ceph·a·ly, mi·cro·ceph·a·li·a** (mī'krō-sef'ă-lē, -sĕ-fā'lē-ă) Abnormal smallness of the head; often associated with mental retardation. [*micro-* + G. *kephalē,* head]

**mi·cro·chei·li·a, mi·cro·chi·li·a** (mī-krō-kī'lē-ă) Abnormal smallness of the lips. [*micro-* + G. *cheilos,* lip]

**mi·cro·chem·is·try** (mī′krō-kem′is-trē) Use of chemical procedures involving minute quantities or reactions invisible to an unaided eye.

**mi·cro·cir·cu·la·tion** (mī′krō-sĭr-kyū-lā′shŭn) Passage of blood in the smallest vessels, namely arterioles, capillaries, and venules.

**mi·cro·cu·rie (mcCi)** (mī′krō-kyūr′ē) One millionth of a curie; a quantity of any radionuclide with $3.7 \times 10^4$ disintegrations per second.

**mi·cro·cyte** (mī′krō-sīt) A small (i.e., 5 mcm or less) nonnucleated red blood cell; with decreased mean corpuscular volume. SYN microerythrocyte. [*micro-* + G. *kytos*, cell]

**mi·cro·cyt·ic hy·po·chrom·ic a·ne·mi·a** (mī′krō-sit′ik hī′pō-krō′mik ă-nē′mē-ă) Any anemia with microcytes that are reduced in size and in hemoglobin content.

**mi·cro·di·al·y·sis** (mī′krō-dī-al′i-sis) Method of studying extracellular fluid composition and response to exogenous agents.

**mi·cro·dont** (mī′krō-dont) Having a very small tooth or teeth. [*micro-* + G. *odous* (*odont-*), tooth]

**⬛mi·cro·don·ti·a, mi·cro·don·tism** (mī′krō-don′shē-ă, -tizm) Condition in which a single tooth, pairs of teeth, or whole dentition, may be disproportionately small. See this page. [*micro-* + G. *odous,* tooth]

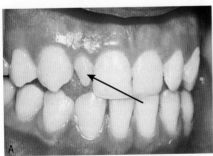

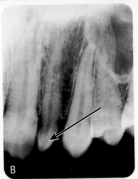

**microdontia:** (A) photo of peg lateral incisor; (B) radiograph of peg lateral incisor

**mi·cro·dose** (mī′krō-dōs) A very small dose.

**mi·cro·e·lec·trode** (mī′krō-ĕ-lek′trōd) An electrode of very fine caliber consisting usually of a fine wire or a glass tube of capillary diameter (10 mcm–1 mm) drawn to a fine point and filled with saline or a metal such as gallium or indium (while melted); used in physiologic experiments to stimulate or to record action currents of extracellular or intracellular origin.

**mi·cro·e·ryth·ro·cyte** (mī′krō-ĕ-rith′rō-sīt) SYN microcyte.

**mi·cro·etch·ing tech·nique** (mī′krō-ech′ing tek-nēk′) Method of roughening natural tooth surface or a dental restoration using a gas-impelled jet of fine abrasive; enhances attachment of resin cements or restorative materials to surface.

**mi·cro·fil res·in** (mī′krō-fil rez′in) Colloq. for microfine composite resin (q.v.).

**mi·cro·fine com·pos·ite res·in** (mī′krō-fīn kŏm-poz′it rez′in) Restorative compound that contains high surface area silicate particles (0.04–0.2 mcm) at about 25% volume; may be prepared in polymerized oligopolymers and ground into small particles so that inorganic content may be increased.

**mi·cro·flo·ra** (mī′krō-flōr′ă) Bacteria and fungi that inhabit an environment.

**mi·cro·gen·i·a** (mī′krō-jē′nē-ă) Abnormal chin smallness resulting from underdevelopment of mental symphysis.

**mi·cro·glos·si·a** (mī′krō-glos′ē-ă) Abnormal smallness of tongue.

**mi·cro·gna·thi·a** (mī′krog-nā′thē-ă) Abnormal smallness of the jaws, especially of mandible.

**mi·cro·gna·thi·a with pe·ro·me·li·a** (mī′krog-nath′ē-ă per-o′-mē-lē-ă) Hypoplasia of mandible with malformed and missing teeth, birdlike face, and severe deformities of the hands, forearms, feet, legs.

**mi·cro·gram** (mī′krō-gram) One millionth of a gram.

**⬛mi·cro·leak·age** (mī′krō-lē′kăj) Passage of microorganisms and saliva-borne constituents through the interstices between the sides of a cavity preparation and a restoration, due to incomplete sealing of the interface. See page 376.

**mi·cro·me·ter (mcm)** (mī′krō-mē′tĕr, mī-krom′ĕ-tĕr) **1.** One millionth of a meter; formerly called a micron. **2.** A device for measuring various objects in an accurate and precise manner. **3.** In medicine and biology, the term is usually used with reference to a glass slide or lens that is accurately marked for measuring microscopic forms. SYN micrometre. [*micro-* + G. *metron,* measure]

mn

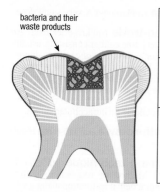

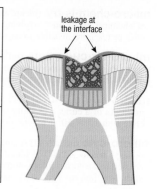

bacteria and their waste products

with colder temperatures, uneven shrinkage occurs →

with warmer temperatures, uneven expansion occurs ←

with cyclic temperatures, repeated shrinkage and expansion occurs, resulting in percolation

leakage at the interface

**microleakage and effects of alteration of temperature**

**micrometre** [Br.] SYN micrometer.

**mi·cron** (mī′kron) SEE micrometer.

**mi·cro·nu·tri·ents** (mī′krō-nū′trē-ĕnts) Essential food factors required in only small quantities by the body; e.g., vitamins, trace minerals.

**mi·cro·or·gan·ism** (mī′krō-ōr′găn-izm) A microscopic organism (plant or animal).

**mi·croph·thal·mos, mi·croph·thal·mi·a** (mī′krof-thal′mŏs, -mē-ă) Abnormal smallness of the eye. [micro- + G. ophthalmos, eye]

**mi·cro·pore** (mī′krō-pōr) An organelle formed by the pellicle of all stages of sporozoan protozoa of the subphylum Apicomplexa and also found in developmental stages that may lack the inner pellicle layer. [micro- + G. poros, pore]

**mi·cro·pro·so·pi·a** (mī′krō-prō-sō′pē-ă) A condition characterized by an abnormally small or imperfectly developed face. [micro- + G. prosōpon, face]

**mi·cro·ra·di·og·ra·phy** (mī′krō-rā′dē-og′ră-fē) Making radiographs of histologic sections of tissue for enlargement.

**mi·cro·scope** (mī′krŏ-skōp) An instrument that gives an enlarged image of an object or substance that is minute or not visible with the unaided eye; usually denotes a compound microscope; for low magnifications, the term simple microscope, or magnifying glass, is used. [micro- + G. skopeō, to view]

**mi·cros·co·py** (mī-kros′kŏ-pē) Investigation of minute objects with a microscope.

**Mi·cros·po·rum** (mī′krō-spō′rŭm) A genus of pathogenic fungi causing dermatophytosis. [micro- + G. sporos, seed]

**mi·cro·steth·o·scope** (mī′krō-steth′ŏ-skōp) Very small stethoscope that amplifies sounds heard.

**mi·cro·sto·mi·a** (mī′krō-stō′mē-ă) Abnormal smallness of oral fissure or opening.

**mi·cro·strain** (mī′krō-strān) This technique of digital stereoimaging is used to measure the microstructural strain (also known as microstrain) fields in cortical bone. The measurement of microstrains is made by comparing images acquired from a specimen at two distinct stress states.

**mi·cro·sur·ger·y** (mī′krō-sŭr′jĕr-ē) Surgical procedures performed under the magnification of a surgical microscope.

**mi·cro·sy·ringe** (mī′krō-si-rinj′) Hypodermic syringe with a micrometer screw attached to the piston, so accurately measured minute quantities of fluid may be injected.

**mi·cro·ti·a** (mī-krō′shē-ă) Abnormal smallness of the auricle of the acoustic external ear with a blind or absent external auditory meatus. [micro- + G. ous, ear]

**mi·cro·trau·ma** (mī′krō-traw′mă) SYN cumulative trauma disorder.

**mi·cro·tu·bule** (mī′krō-tū′byūl) A cylindric cytoplasmic element that occurs widely in the cytoskeleton of plant and animal cells; microtubules increase in number during mitosis and meiosis.

**mid·brain** (mid′brān) SYN mesencephalon.

**mid·dle ear** (mid′ĕl ēr) SEE ear.

**mid·dle me·nin·ge·al ar·te·ry** (mid′ĕl mĕ-nin′jē-ăl ahr′tĕr-ē) [TA] Origin, maxillary; branches, petrosal, superior tympanic, frontal and parietal; distribution, to parts mentioned and through terminal branches to anterior and middle cranial fossae; anastomoses, meningeal branches of occipital, ascending pharyngeal, ophthalmic and lacrimal, stylomastoid, accessory meningeal branch of maxillary, and deep temporal.

**mid·dle me·nin·ge·al veins** (mid′dĕl mĕ-nin′jē-ăl vānz) [TA] Venae comitantes of the middle meningeal artery that empty into the pterygoid plexus.

**mid·dle na·sal con·cha** (mid′ĕl nā′zăl kong′kă) [TA] Middle thin, spongy, bony plate with curved margins, part of ethmoidal labyrinth.

**mid·line le·thal gran·u·lo·ma** (mid′līn lē′thăl gran′yū-lō′mă) Destruction of nasal septum, hard palate, lateral nasal walls, paranasal sinuses, facial skin, orbit, and nasopharynx by an inflammatory infiltrate with atypical lymphocytic and histiocytic cells.

**mid·sag·it·tal plane** (mid-saj′i-tăl plān) SYN median plane.

**mid·wife** (mid′wīf) A person qualified to practice midwifery, having received specialized training in obstetrics and child care.

**mi·graine** (mī′grān) A familial, recurrent syndrome usually characterized by unilateral head pain, accompanied by various focal disturbances of the nervous system, particularly in regard to visual phenomenon, e.g., scintillating scotomas.

**mi·grat·ing teeth** (mī′grāt-ing tēth) SYN drift.

**mi·gra·tion** (mī-grā′shŭn) **1.** Movement of a tooth or teeth out of normal position. **2.** Passing from one part to another, said of certain morbid processes or symptoms. See this page. [L. migro, pp.-atus, to move from place to place]

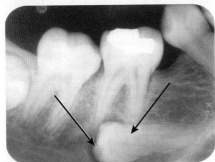

migration of second premolar and partial eruption buccal to first molar

**Mi·ku·licz aph·thae** (mē′kū-lich af′thē) SYN periadenitis mucosa necrotica recurrens.

**Mi·ku·licz dis·ease** (mē′kū-lich di-zēz′) Benign swelling of lacrimal and, usually, also of the salivary glands, due to infiltration and replacement of the normal gland structure by lymphoid tissue.

**Mi·ku·licz syn·drome** (mē′kū-lich sin′drōm) The symptoms characteristic of Mikulicz disease occurring as a complication of some other disease.

**milk** (milk) **1.** White liquid, containing proteins, sugar, and lipids, secreted by mammary glands, designed to nourish young. **2.** Any whitish milky fluid, e.g., juice of coconut or a suspension of various metallic oxides. **3.** A pharmaco-

peial preparation that is a suspension of insoluble drugs in a water medium; distinguished from gels mainly in that the suspended particles of milk are larger. **4.** SYN strip (1). [A.S. meolc]

**milk den·ti·tion** (milk den-tish′ŭn) SYN deciduous tooth.

**milk of mag·ne·si·a (MOM)** (milk mag-nē′zē-ă) Mixture of magnesium hydroxide; aqueous solution of magnesium hydroxide, used as an antacid and laxative.

**milk sug·ar** (milk shug′ăr) SYN lactose.

**milk tooth** (milk tūth) SYN deciduous tooth.

**mill·ed-in curves** (mild-in′ kŭrvz) SYN milled-in paths.

**mill·ed-in paths** (mild-in′ padhz) **1.** Contours carved by various mandibular movements into occluding surface of occlusion rim, by teeth or studs placed in opposing occlusion rim; curves or contours may be carved into wax, modeling plastic, or plaster of Paris. **2.** Occlusal curves developed by masticatory or gliding movements of occlusion rims that are composed of materials including abrasives. SYN milled-in curves.

**Mil·ler chem·i·co·par·a·sit·ic the·o·ry** (mil′ĕr kem′i-kō-par-ă-sit′ik thē′ŏr-ē) Tenet that dental caries are due to oral microorganisms fermenting dietary carbohydrates and thus producing acids that demineralize teeth.

**mil·li·am·pere** (mil′ē-am′pēr) One thousandth of an ampere.

**mil·li·cu·rie (mc)** (mil′i-kyūr′ē) A unit of radioactivity equivalent to $3.7 \times 10^7$ disintegrations per second.

**mil·li·li·ter (mL, ml)** (mil′i-lē′tĕr) One thousandth of a liter. SYN millilitre.

**millilitre** [Br.] SYN milliliter.

**mill·ing-in** (mil′ing-in′) Refining occlusion of teeth with abrasives between their occluding surfaces while the dentures are rubbed together in the mouth or on an articulator.

**mil·li·volt** (mil′i-vōlt) One thousandth of a volt.

**min·er·al·i·za·tion** (min′ĕr-ăl-ī-zā′shŭn) The introduction of minerals into a structure, as in the normal mineralization of bones and teeth or the pathologic mineralization of tissues.

**min·er·al·o·cor·ti·coid** (min′ĕr-ăl-ō-kōr′ti-koyd) One of the steroids of the cortex of the suprarenal gland that influences water and electrolyte metabolism and balance.

**min·er·al oil (MO)** (min′ĕr-ăl oyl) Mixture of liquid hydrocarbons obtained from petroleum, used as a vehicle in pharmaceutical preparations; occasionally used as an intestinal lubricant. SYN heavy liquid petrolatum, liquid paraffin, liquid petroleum.

**mn**

**min·er·al wa·ter** (min'ĕr-ăl waw'tĕr) Water that contains appreciable amounts of particular salts, which give it therapeutic properties.

**min·er·al wax** (min'ĕr-ăl waks) **1.** SYN ceresin. **2.** Mineral substance with physical properties similar to those of wax.

**min·i·a·ture work·ing-end** (min'ē-ă-chŭr wŏrk'ing end) Curette with a shorter thinner working-end and a longer lower shank than that of a standard Gracey curette.

**min·im** (min'im) A fluid measure, 1/60 of a fluidrachm. Smallest; least; the smallest of several similar structures. [L. *minimus,* least]

**min·i·mal dose** (min'i-măl dōs) Smallest amount of drug or physical procedure that will produce a desired physiologic effect in an adult.

**min·i·mal le·thal dose (MLD)** (min'i-măl lē'thăl dōs) Lowest dose of a toxic substance or infectious agent that will cause death, as assayed in various experimental animals.

**min·i·plate os·te·o·syn·the·sis** (min'ē-plāt os'tē-ō-sin'thĕ-sis) Method of internal fixation of mandibular fractures using miniaturized metal plates and screws made of titanium, stainless steel, or biodegradable or resorbable synthetic materials.

**mi·nor** (mī'nŏr ) Smaller; lesser; denoting the smaller of two similar structures. [L.]

**mi·nor a·lar ca·rti·lage of nose** (mī'nŏr ā'lăr kahr'ti-lăj nōz) [TA] The 2–4 cartilaginous plates of the wing of the nose posterior to the greater alar cartilage. SYN accessory quadrate cartilage.

**mi·nor con·nec·tor** (mī'nŏr kŏ-nek'tŏr) Connecting link between major connector or base of partial denture and other units of prosthesis (e.g., clasps, indirect retainers, and occlusal rests).

**mi·nor sal·i·var·y glands** (mī'nŏr sal'i-var-ē glandz) [TA] Mucus-secreting exocrine glands of the oral cavity, consisting of the labial, buccal, molar, lingual, and palatine; unlike major salivary glands, these secrete continuously.

**mi·nor sub·lin·gual ducts** (mī'nŏr sŭb-ling'gwăl dŭkts) [TA] About 8–20 small ducts of the sublingual salivary gland that open into the mouth on surface of sublingual fold; a few join submandibular ducts.

**mi·nor tran·quil·iz·er** (mī'nŏr trangk'wi-lī-zĕr) SYN antianxiety agent.

**mi·o·sis** (mī-ō'sis) Contraction of the pupil. [G. *meiōsis,* a lessening]

**mi·ot·ic** (mī-ot'ik) An agent that causes the pupil to constrict so that the pupils are smaller.

**mir·ror** (mir'ŏr) A polished surface reflecting the rays of light reflected from objects in front of it; particularly useful in visualizing structures in the oral cavity.

**mis·ci·ble** (mis'i-bĕl) Capable of being mixed and remaining so after the mixing process ceases. [L. *misceo,* to mix]

**mis·di·ag·no·sis** (mis'dī-ag-nō'sis) A wrong or mistaken diagnosis.

**mi·so·pros·tol** (mī'sō-prost'ol) A prostaglandin analogue used to prevent gastric and duodenal ulcers; particularly useful in patients taking nonsteroidal antiinflammatory drugs.

**mith·ra·my·cin** (mith'ră-mī'sin) An antibiotic produced by *Streptomyces argillaceus* and *S. tanashiensis;* possesses antineoplastic activity.

**mit·i·gate** (mit'i-gāt) SYN palliate.

**mi·to·chon·dri·al dis·or·ders** (mī'-tō-kon'drē-ăl dis-ōr'dĕrz) Diverse hereditary disorders caused by genetic mutation of mitochondrial DNA.

**mi·to·gen** (mī'tō-jen) A substance that stimulates mitosis and lymphocyte transformation; includes not only lectins such as phytohemagglutinins and concanavalin A, but also substances from streptococci and from strains of α-toxin-producing staphylococci.

**mi·to·my·cin** (mī'tō-mī'sin) Antibiotic produced by *Streptomyces caespitosus,* variants of which are designated mitomycin A, mitomycin B, C, which is an antineoplastic agent and a bacteriocide; inhibits DNA synthesis.

**mi·to·sis,** pl. **mi·to·ses** (mī-tō'sis, -sēz) Usual process of somatic reproduction of cells consisting of a sequence of modifications of the nucleus that result in the formation of two daughter cells with exactly the same chromosome and nuclear DNA content as that of the original cell. [G. *mitos,* thread]

**mi·tral mur·mur** (mī'trăl mŭr'mŭr) Sound produced at the mitral valve.

**mi·tral valve** (mī'trăl valv) [TA] Valve closing orifice between left atrium and left ventricle of heart; its two cusps are called anterior and posterior.

**mi·tral valve pro·lapse** (mī'trăl valv prō'laps) Excessive retrograde movement of one or both mitral valve leaflets into the left atrium during left ventricular systole.

**mixed den·ti·tion** (mikst den-tish'ŭn) Combination of primary and permanent teeth, usually present between ages 6 and 12 years when primary teeth are being replaced; starts with the eruption of the first permanent tooth. SYN transitional dentition.

**mixed ep·i·sode** (mikst ep'i-sōd) Manifestation of major mood disorder involving simultaneous symptoms of a manic episode and a major depressive episode.

**mixed hear·ing loss** (mikst hēr'ing laws) Combination of conductive and sensorineural hearing loss.

**mix·ed tu·mor** (mikst tū′mŏr) A tumor composed of two or more varieties of tissue.

**mix·ture** (miks′chŭr) A mutual incorporation of two or more substances, without chemical union, the physical characteristics of each component is retained. A **mechanical mixture** has particles or masses distinguishable as such under the microscope or in other ways; a **physical mixture** is a more intimate blending of molecules. [L. *mixtura* or *mistura* ]

**mL** Abbreviation for milliliter.

**ml** Abbreviation for milliliter.

**MLC** Abbreviation for Marginal Line Calculus Index.

**MLD** Abbreviation for minimal lethal dose.

**MND** Abbreviation for motor neuron disease.

**MO** Abbreviation for mineral oil.

**Mo** Symbol for molybdenum.

**mo·bil·i·ty** (mō-bil′i-tē) Loosening of a tooth in its socket; may result from loss of bone support to tooth. Horizontal tooth mobility is ability to move tooth in a facial-lingual direction in its socket. Vertical tooth mobility is the ability to depress the tooth in its socket.

**MO cav·i·ty** (kav′i-tē) The presence of a carious lesion involving the mesial (M) and occlusal (O) surfaces of a tooth.

**MOD** Abbreviation for mesiodistocclusal.

**mo·dal·i·ty** (mō-dal′i-tē) **1.** A form of application or employment of a therapeutic agent or regimen. **2.** Various forms of sensation. [Mediev. L. *modalitas,* fr. L. *modus,* a mode]

**mode** (mōd) In a set of measurements, most frequent value. [L. *modus,* a measure, quantity]

**mod·el** (mod′ĕl) **1.** In dentistry, a cast. **2.** A representation of something. [It. *midello,* fr. L. *modus,* measure, standard]

**mod·el·ing** (mod′ĕl-ing) **1.** A continuous process by which a bone is altered in size and shape during its growth by resorption and formation of bone at different sites and rates. **2.** A process by which a representation of an entity is formed. SYN modelling.

**mod·el·ing plas·tic** (mod′ĕl-ing plas′tik) Thermoplastic material usually composed of gum damar and prepared chalk, used especially for making dental impressions. SYN impression compound.

**modelling** [Br.] SYN modeling.

**mod·el trim·mer** (mod′ĕl trim′ĕr) A grinding instrument used to shape and remove excess plaster or dental stone from a model or cast of the dentition.

**mod·i·fied in·tra·o·ral ful·crum** (mod′i-fīd in′tră-ōr′ăl ful′krŭm) Advanced intraoral stabilizing point that involves and alters the point of contact between the middle and ring fingers in the grasp.

**mod·i·fied pen grasp** (mod′i-fīd pen grasp) Common posture for holding a dental instrument between thumb pads and index finger, with side of middle finger either supporting shank or placed lower on the handle. The fourth finger is used as a fulcrum (finger rest). See this page.

**mn**

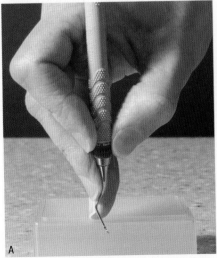
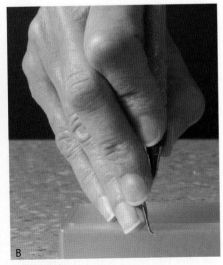

**modified pen grasp, right-handed clinician:** (A) side view; (B) front view

**mod·i·fied Still·man meth·od** (mod´i-fīd stil´măn meth´ŏd) Toothbrushing technique that places toothbrush bristles on gingiva and cervical areas to massage and stimulate them.

**mod·i·fied zinc ox·ide-eu·ge·nol ce·ment** (mod´i-fīd zingk ok´sīd yū´jĕ-nol sĕ-ment´) Dental cement obtained by mixing zinc oxide and eugenol with one or more additives.

**mo·di·o·lus,** pl. **mo·di·o·li** (mō-dī´ō-lŭs, -lī) The central cone-shaped core of spongy bone about which the spiral canal of the cochlea turns. [L., the nave of a wheel]

**mo·di·o·lus la·bi·i** (mō-dī´ō-lŭs lā´bē-ī) A point near the corner of the mouth where several muscles of facial expression converge.

**mo·di·o·lus of an·gle of mouth** (mō-dī´ō-lŭs ang´gĕl mowth) [TA] Point near corner of mouth where several muscles of facial expression converge. SYN columella cochleae.

**mo·du·lus** (mod´yū-lŭs) A coefficient expressing the magnitude of a physical property by a numerical value.

**Moe·bi·us syn·drome** (mĕr´bē-ŭs sin´drōm) Congenital paralysis, usually bilateral, of facial and ocular muscles due to failure of development of nerve cells. SYN congenital facial diplegia, nuclear agenesis, oculofacial paralysis, von Graefe syndrome II.

**Moel·ler glos·si·tis** (mĕr´ler glos-ī´tis) SYN smooth tongue.

**moist gan·grene** (moyst gang-grēn´) SYN wet gangrene.

**mol** Abbreviation for mole.

▪**mo·lar** (mō´lăr) 1. SYN molar tooth. 2. Denoting a grinding or wearing away. 3. Massive; relating to a mass; not molecular. 4. Denoting a concentration of 1 g.-molecular weight (1 mol) of solute per liter of solution, the common unit of concentration in chemistry. See this page. [L. molaris, relating to a mill, millstone]

**mo·lar glands** (mō´lăr glandz) [TA] The 4–5 large buccal glands around the last molar tooth.

**mo·lar·i·form** (mō-lar´i-fōrm) Having the form of a molar tooth. [molar (tooth) + L. forma, form]

**mo·lar tooth** (mō´lăr tūth) [TA] Tooth with a somewhat quadrangular crown with four or five cusps on grinding surface; root is bifid in lower jaw, but there are three conic roots in the upper jaw; there are six molars in each jaw, three on either side behind premolars in permanent dentition; deciduous dentition has only four mo-

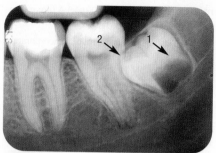

**mandibular first, second, and third molars (radiograph):** incompletely formed third molar (1) has not erupted. Its crown appears trapped below distal contour of adjacent second molar so that tooth may be blocked from full eruption (2)

lars in each jaw, two on either side behind the canines. SYN dens molaris [TA], cheek tooth, molar (1).

**mold** (mōld) 1. A shaped receptacle into which wax is pressed or fluid plaster is poured in making a cast. 2. To shape a mass of plastic material according to a definite pattern. 3. The term used to specify the shape of an artificial tooth (or teeth). SYN mould.

**mold guide** (mōld gīd) Guide used to specify shape of artificial tooth (or teeth).

**mold·ing** (mōld´ing) Shaping with a mold.

**mole (mol)** (mōl) 1. SYN nevus (2). 2. SYN nevus pigmentosus. 3. An intrauterine mass formed by the degeneration of the partly developed products of conception. [A.S. mǣl (L. macula), a spot]

**mo·lec·u·lar bi·ol·o·gy** (mŏ-lek´yū-lăr bī-ol´ō-jē) Study of phenomena in terms of molecular interactions.

**mo·lec·u·lar dis·ease** (mŏ-lek´yū-lăr di-zēz´) Disease with manifestations due to alterations in molecular structure and function.

**mo·lec·u·lar weight (mol wt, MW)** (mŏ-lek´yū-lăr wāt) The sum of the atomic weights of all the atoms constituting a molecule. SYN molecular weight ratio, relative molecular mass.

**mol·e·cule** (mol´ĕ-kyūl) The smallest possible quantity of a di-, tri-, or polyatomic substance that retains the chemical properties of the substance.

**mol·lus·cum con·ta·gi·o·sum** (mo-lŭs´kŭm kon-tā´jē-ō´sŭm) A contagious disease of the skin caused by intranuclear proliferation of a virus of the family Poxviridae characterized by the appearance of small, pearly, umbilicated papular epidermal growths.

**mol wt** Abbreviation for molecular weight.

**mo·lyb·de·num (Mo)** (mō-lib′dĕ-nŭm) A silvery white metallic element; bioelement found in proteins. [G. *molybdaina,* a piece of lead; a metal, prob. galena, fr. *molybdos,* lead]

**mo·lyb·de·num tar·get tube** (mō-lib′ dĕ-nŭm tahr′get tyūb) SYN molybdenum (Mo).

**MOM** Abbreviation for milk of magnesia.

**mo·men·tum** (mō-men′tŭm) The tendency of an object in motion to continue in motion. [L., abridgment of *movimentum,* movement]

**mon·an·gle** (mon′ang-gĕl) Having only one angle, e.g., dental instrument that has only one angle between handle or shaft and working portion (blade or nib).

**mon·i·li·a·sis** (mō′ni-lī′ă-sis) SYN candidiasis.

**mo·nism** (mō′nizm) A metaphysical system in which all of reality is conceived as a unified whole. [G. *monos,* single]

**mon·i·tor** (mon′i-tŏr) **1.** A device that displays and/or records specified data for a given series of events, operations, or circumstances. **2.** To observe over time. [L., one who warns, fr. *moneo,* pp. *monitum,* to warn]

**mon·i·tor·ing** (mon′i-tŏr′ing) **1.** Performance and analysis of routine measurements aimed at detecting a change in the environment or health status of a population. **2.** Ongoing measurement of performance of a health service.

✿ **mono-** The participation or involvement of a single element or part. [G. *monos,* single]

**mon·o·a·mine ox·i·dase in·hib·it·or (MAOI)** (mon′ō-ă-mēn′ ok′si-dās in-hib′i-tŏr) An older antidepressant.

**mon·o·bac·tam** (mon′ō-bak′tam) Class of antibiotic with a monocyclic β-lactam nucleus: structurally different from other β-lactams.

**mon·o·chro·mat·ic ra·di·a·tion** (mon′ ō-krō-mat′ik rā′dē-ā′shŭn) Light rays or ionizing radiation of a very narrow band of wavelengths.

**mon·o·chro·ma·tism** (mon′ō-krō′mă-tizm) **1.** The state of having or exhibiting only one color. **2.** SYN achromatopsia. [*mono-* + G. *chrōma,* color]

**mon·o·clo·nal an·ti·bod·y** (mon′ō-klō′ năl an′ti-bod-ē) An antibody produced by a clone or genetically homogeneous population of hybrid cells.

**mon·o·cyte** (mon′ō-sīt) A relatively large mononuclear leukocyte that normally constitutes 3–7% of the leukocytes in circulating blood. [*mono-* + G. *kytos,* cell]

**mon·o·cyt·ic leu·ke·mi·a** (mon′ō-sit′ik lū-kē′mē-ă) A form of leukemia characterized by large numbers of cells that can be definitely identified as monocytes, in addition to larger, apparently related cells formed from the uncontrolled proliferation of the reticuloendothelial tissue.

**mon·o·cy·to·sis** (mon′ō-sī-tō′sis) An abnormal increase in the number of monocytes in the circulating blood.

**mon·o·gen·ic** (mon′ō-jen′ik) Relating to a hereditary disease or syndrome, or to an inherited characteristic.

**mon·o·mer** (mon′ō-mĕr) **1.** The molecular unit that, by repetition, constitutes a large structure or polymer. **2.** The protein structural unit of a virion capsid.

**mo·nop·a·thy** (mon-op′ă-thē) **1.** Single uncomplicated disease. **2.** Local disease affecting only one organ or part. [*mono-* + G. *pathos,* suffering]

**mon·o·phy·o·dont** (mon′ō-fī′ō-dont) Having only one set of teeth. [*mono-* + G. *phyō,* to grow, + *odous* (*odont-*), tooth]

**mon·o·ple·gi·a mas·ti·ca·to·ri·a** (mon′ ō-plē′jē-ă mas′ti-kă-tō′rē-ă) Unilateral paralysis of the muscles of mastication (masseter, temporal, pterygoid).

**mon·o·so·di·um glu·ta·mate (MSG)** (mon′ō-sō′dē-ŭm glū′tă-māt) Monosodium salt of naturally occurring levorotatory form of glutamic acid; used as a flavor enhancer that is a cause or contributing factor to the colloquially named ''Chinese restaurant'' syndrome.

**mon·os·tot·ic** (mon′os-tot′ik) Involving only one bone. [*mono-* + G. *osteon,* bone]

**mon·o·symp·to·mat·ic** (mon′ō-simp-tŏ-mat′ik) Denoting a disease or morbid condition manifested by only one marked symptom.

**mon·o·ther·mi·a** (mon′ō-thĕr′mē-ă) Evenness of bodily temperature. [*mono-* + G. *thermē,* heat]

**Mon·son curve** (mon′sŏn kŭrv) Curve of occlusion in which each cusp and incisal edge touches or conforms to a segment of the surface of a sphere 8 inches in diameter with its center in region of the glabella.

**mood sta·bil·iz·ing a·gent** (mūd stā′bil-īz-ing ā′jĕnt) Functional category of drugs used to dampen mood swings.

**moon fa·ci·es** (mūn fash′ē-ēz) Roundness of face (often with attendant redness) due to increased fat deposition laterally seen in patients with hyperadrenocorticalism.

**Moon mo·lars** (mūn mō′lărz) Small dome-shaped first molar teeth in congenital syphilis.

**mor·al** (mōr′ăl) **1.** Pertaining to the rightness

**mn**

or wrongness of an act. **2.** Ethical; in accord with accepted rules of what is right.

**mor·bid·i·ty** (mōr-bid′ĭ-tē) **1.** A diseased state. **2.** Ratio of sick:well people. SEE ALSO morbidity rate. **3.** Frequency of appearance of complications after surgery or other treatment.

**mor·bid·i·ty rate** (mōr-bid′ĭ-tē rāt) Proportion of patients with a particular disease during a given year per given unit of population.

**mor·bid o·be·si·ty** (mōr′bid ō-bē′si-tē) Obesity sufficient to prevent normal activity or physiologic function or to cause the onset of a pathologic condition.

**mor·bil·li** (mōr-bil′ī) SYN measles. [Mediev. L. *morbillus,* dim. of L. *morbus,* disease]

**mor·cel** (mor′sĕl) To remove piecemeal; to morcelize. [Fr. *morceler,* to subdivide]

**Mor·ga·gni dis·ease** (mōr-gahn′yē di-zēz′) SYN Adams-Stokes syndrome.

**Mor·ga·gni syn·drome** (mōr-gahn′yē sin′drōm) Hyperostosis frontalis interna in elderly women, with obesity and neuropsychiatric disorders of uncertain cause.

**mor·phine** (mōr′fēn) The major phenanthrene alkaloid of opium. Used as an analgesic, sedative, and anxiolytic. [L. *Morpheus,* god of dreams and sleep]

**mor·phine sul·fate (MS)** (mōr′fēn sŭl′fāt) Morphine used for parenteral, epidural, or intrathecal injection to relieve pain.

**morpho-** Combining form meaning form, shape, structure. [G. *morphē*]

**mor·pho·gen·e·sis** (mōr′fō-jen′ĕ-sis) **1.** Differentiation of cells and tissues in early embryo that establishes form and structure of various organs and parts of the body. **2.** Ability of a molecule or group of molecules to assume a shape.

**mor·phol·o·gy** (mōr-fol′ŏ-jē) The science concerned with the configuration or the structure of animals and plants. [*morpho-* + G. *logos,* study]

**mors** (mōrz) SYN death. [L.]

**mor·si·ca·ti·o** (mor-sik′că-shē-ō) Habitual nibbling of the lips (morsicatio labiorum), tongue (morsicatio linguae), or buccal mucosa (morsicatio buccarum); often produces a shaggy white lesion. See this page. [L. biting, fr. *mordeo,* to bite]

**mor. sol.** Abbreviation for L. *more solito,* as usual, as customary.

**mor·su·lus** (mōr′sū-lŭs) SYN troche. [Mod. L. dim. of L. *morsus,* a bite]

**mor·tal·i·ty** (mōr-tal′ĭ-tē) **1.** State of being mortal. **2.** A fatal outcome.

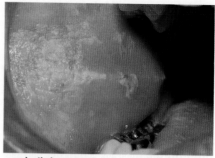

**morsicatio buccarum**

**mor·tar** (mōr′tăr) Vessel with rounded interior in which substances may be crushed with a pestle. [L. *mortarium*]

**mo·tile** (mō′til) Having the power of spontaneous movement.

**mo·tion** (mō′shŭn) **1.** A change of place or position. Cf. movement (1). **2.** SYN defecation. **3.** SYN stool. [L. *motio,* movement, fr. *moveo,* pp. *motus,* to move]

**mo·tion ac·ti·va·tion** (mō′shŭn ak′ti-vā′shŭn) Moving the dental instrument to produce an instrumentation stroke on the tooth surface. SEE ALSO wrist motion activation, digital motion activation.

**mo·ti·va·tion** (mō′ti-vā′shŭn) Aggregate of all individual motives, needs, and drives operative in a person at any given moment that influence the will and cause a given behavior. [ML. *motivus,* moving]

**motoneuron** SYN motor neuron.

**motoneurone** [Br.] SYN motor neuron.

**mo·tor** (mō′tŏr) In anatomy and physiology, denoting those neural structures that, because of the impulses generated and transmitted by them, cause muscle fibers or pigment cells to contract or glands to secrete. [L. a mover, fr. *moveo,* to move]

**mo·tor end·plate** (mō′tŏr end′plāt) The large and complex end-formation by which the axon of a motor neuron establishes synaptic contact with a striated muscle fiber (cell).

**mo·tor nerve** (mō′tŏr nĕrv) [TA] Nerve composed mostly or entirely of efferent (motor) nerve fibers conveying impulses that excite muscular contraction; those in autonomic nervous system also elicit secretions from glandular epithelia.

**mo·tor nerve of face** (mō′tŏr nĕrv fās) SYN facial nerve [CN VII].

**mo·tor neu·ron** (mō′tŏr nūr′on) A nerve cell in the spinal cord, rhombencephalon, or mesencephalon characterized by an axon that leaves the central nervous system to establish a functional connection with an effector (muscle or glandular) tissue. SYN motoneuron, motoneurone.

**mo·tor neu·ron dis·ease (MND)** (mō′tŏr nūr′on di-zēz′) **1.** SYN amyotrophic lateral sclerosis. **2.** In the plural (i.e., diseases) generic term for heterogenous group of disorders, all affecting motor neurons in the brain, spinal cord, or both.

**mo·tor pa·ral·y·sis** (mō′tŏr păr-al′i-sis) Loss of the power of muscular contraction.

**mo·tor root of tri·gem·i·nal nerve** (mō′tŏr rūt trī-jem′i-năl nĕrv) [TA] The smaller root of the trigeminal nerve, composed of fibers originating from the trigeminal motor nucleus and emerging from the pons medial to the much larger sensory root, to join the mandibular nerve; it carries motor and proprioceptive fibers to the muscles derived from the first branchial (mandibular) arch (pharyngeal is preferred for humans), including the four muscles of mastication, plus the mylohyoid, anterior belly of the digastric, and the tensores tympani and veli palati. SYN masticator nerve.

**mo·tor u·nit** (mō′tŏr yū′nit) A single somatic motor neuron and the group of muscle fibers innervated by it.

**mot·tled e·nam·el** (mŏt′ĕld ĕ-nam′ĕl) Alterations in enamel structure often due to excessive fluoride ingestion during tooth formation.

**mou·lage** (mū-lahzh′) A reproduction in wax of a skin lesion, tumor, or other pathologic state. [F. a molding]

**mould** (mōld) SYN mold.

**mount·ing** (mownt′ing) In dentistry, laboratory procedure of attaching maxillary and/or mandibular cast to an articulator.

◨ **mouth** (mowth) **1.** SYN oral cavity. **2.** Opening, usually external, of a cavity or canal. SEE ostium, orifice, stoma (2). See this page. [A.S. *mūth*]

◨ **mouth breath·ing** (mowth brēdh′ing) Habitual respiration through the mouth instead of the nose, usually due to obstruction of the nasal airways. See this page.

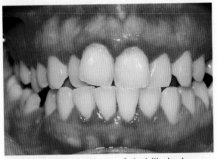

**mouth breathing:** mild case of gingivitis due to mouth breathing

◨ **mouth guard** (mowth gahrd) Pliable plastic device, adapted to cover maxillary teeth, which is worn to reduce potential injury to oral structures during participation in contact sports. See page 384.

◨ **mouth mir·ror** (mowth mir′ŏr) Small reflector on a handle used to facilitate clinicians' visualization in examination of teeth. See page 384.

**mouth re·ha·bil·i·ta·tion** (mowth rē′hă-bil′i-tā′shŭn) Restoration of form and function of masticatory apparatus as close to normal as possible.

**mouth stick** (mowth stik) Prosthesis held by teeth and used by handicapped people to perform such actions as computer keyboarding, painting, and lifting small objects.

**mouth-to-mouth res·pi·ra·tion** (mowth-mowth res′pir-ā′shŭn) Method of artificial ven-

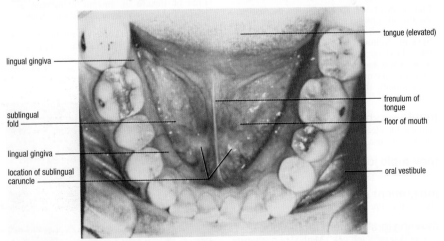

tongue (elevated)

lingual gingiva

frenulum of tongue

sublingual fold

floor of mouth

lingual gingiva

location of sublingual caruncle

oral vestibule

**floor of mouth and vestibule of oral cavity (superior view):** tongue is elevated and retracted superiorly; observe mucous membrane, lingual gingiva, and frenulum of tongue

**mn**

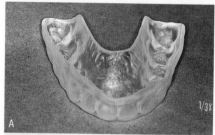

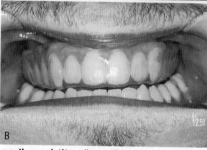

**mouth guard:** (A) appliance; (B) appliance in place

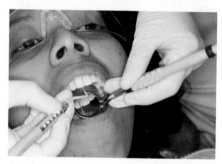

**dental or mouth mirror**

tilation involving an overlap of the patient's mouth (and nose in small children) with the operator's mouth to inflate the patient's lungs by blowing, followed by an unassisted expiratory phase brought about by elastic recoil of the patient's chest and lungs; repeated 12–16 times a minute; if the nose is not covered by the operator's mouth, the nostrils must be closed by pinching.

**mouth·wash** (mowth'wawsh) Medicated liquid used to clean oral cavity and treat disorders of oral mucosa. Also called mouth rinse.

**mov·a·ble joint** (mūv'ă-běl joynt) SYN synovial joint, moveable joint.

**move·ment** (mūv'měnt) The act of motion. [L. *moveo*, pp. *motus*, to move]

**mov·ing in·stru·ment tech·nique** (mūv' ing in'strŭ-měnt tek-nēk') Method of instrument sharpening done by moving the working-end over a stabilized sharpening stone.

**mov·ing stone tech·nique** (mūv'ing stōn tek-nēk') Method of instrument sharpening accomplished by moving a sharpening stone over the working-end of a stabilized instrument.

**mox·a** (mok'să) A cone or cylinder of cotton wool or other combustible material, placed on the skin and ignited to produce counterirritation. [Jap. *moe kusa*, burning herb]

**mox·a·lac·tam** (moks'ă-lak'tam) Third-generation cephalosporin with a broad spectrum of antibacterial action.

**mox·i·bus·tion** (mok'sē-bŭs'chŭn) Burning of herbal agents, such as moxa, on the skin as a counterirritant in the treatment of disease.

**MPD** Abbreviation for maximum permissible dose.

**MS** Abbreviation for morphine sulfate; multiple sclerosis; magnesium sulfate.

**MSA** Abbreviation for multiple-system atrophy.

**MSG** Abbreviation for monosodium glutamate.

**MSH** Abbreviation for melanocyte-stimulating hormone.

**MSM** Abbreviation for men who have sex with men.

**MT** Abbreviation for medical transcriptionist.

**mu·ci·lage** (myū'si-lăj) Pharmacopeial preparation consisting of a solution with mucilaginous principles of vegetable substances.

**mu·cin** (myū'sin) The hydrated form of mucinogen that lubricates and protects body cavity linings.

**mu·cip·a·rous gland** (myū-sip'ăr-ŭs gland) SYN mucous gland.

**mu·co·buc·cal fold** (myū'kō-bŭk'ăl fōld) Line of flexure of mucous membrane as it passes from mandible or maxilla to cheek.

**mu·co·cele** (myū'kō-sēl) A retention cyst of the salivary gland, lacrimal sac, paranasal sinuses, appendix, gallbladder, and other sites. See this page and page A5. [*muco-* + G. *kēlē*, tumor, hernia]

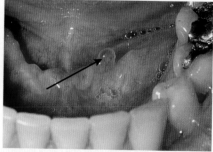

**mucocele:** superficial translucent lesion

**mu·co·cu·ta·ne·ous** (myū′kō-kyū-tā′nē-ŭs) Relating to mucous membrane and skin; denoting line of junction of two at nasal, oral, vaginal, and anal orifices.

**mu·co·cu·ta·ne·ous lymph node syn·drome** (myū′kō-kyū-tā′nē-ŭs limf nōd sin′drōm) Systemic vasculitis of unknown origin that occurs primarily in children younger than 8 years of age. SYN Kawasaki disease.

**mu·co·en·ter·i·tis** (myū′kō-en-tĕr-ī′tis) Inflammation of the intestinal mucous membrane.

**mu·co·ep·i·the·li·al dys·pla·si·a** (myū′kō-ep′i-thē′lē-ăl dis-plā′zē-ă) Epithelial cell periorofacial disease characterized by red, periorificial mucosal lesions of oral, nasal, vaginal, urethral, anal, bladder, and conjunctival mucosa.

ℹ **mu·co·gin·gi·val junc·tion** (myū′kō-jin′ji-văl jungk′shŭn) Area visible in the oral cavity where the tissues forming gingiva and oral mucosa join. There is a distinct contrast in color of the two tissues; gingiva more coral pink; compared with the redder shiny alveolar mucosa. See this page. SYN mucogingival line.

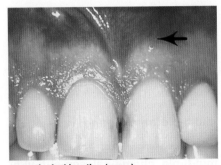

**mucogingival junction (arrow)**

**mu·co·gin·gi·val line** (myū′kō-jin′ji-văl līn) SYN mucogingival junction.

**mu·co·gin·gi·val sur·ger·y** (myū′kō-jin′ji-văl sŭr′jĕr-ē) Clinical operation involving oral mucosa and gingival tissues.

**mu·coid im·pac·tion of bron·chus** (myū′koyd im-pak′shŭn brongk′ŭs) Plugging of lumen of bronchi due to thickened mucus.

**mu·co·lip·i·do·sis,** pl. **mu·co·lip·i·do·ses** (myū′kō-lip-i-dō′sis, -sēz) A lysosomal storage disease in which symptoms of visceral and mesenchymal mucopolysaccharide, glycoprotein, oligosaccharide, or glycolipid storage are present. [*muco-* + *lipid* + *-osis*, condition]

**mu·co·lip·i·do·sis I** (myū′kō-lip-i-dō′sis) Lysosomal storage disease resembling mild form of Hurler syndrome with coarse facial features, macular cherry red spots, and other findings.

**mu·co·lip·i·do·sis II** (myū′kō-lip-i-dō′sis) Metabolic disorder with onset in early childhood characterized by clinical and radiographic findings similar to those in Hurler syndrome including gum hypertrophy and thoracic dysplasia. SYN I-cell disease.

**mu·co·lip·i·do·sis III** (myū′kō-lip-i-dō′sis) Mucolipidosis with mild Hurler-like symptoms, restricted joint mobility and short stature.

**mu·co·lip·i·do·sis IV** (myū′kō-lip-i-dō′sis) Psychomotor retardation with cloudy corneas and retinal degeneration, with inclusion cells in cultured fibroblasts; pathogenesis uncertain.

**mu·co·mem·bra·nous** (myū′kō-mem′bră-nŭs) Relating to a mucous membrane.

**mu·co·per·i·chon·dri·al flap** (myū′kō-per′i-kon′drē-ăl flap) Flap composed of mucous membrane and perichondrium, e.g., nasal septum.

**mu·co·per·i·os·te·al flap** (myū′kō-per′ē-os′tē-ăl flap) Flap composed of mucous membrane and periosteum, e.g., hard palate.

**mu·co·per·i·os·te·um** (myū′kō-per′ē-os′tē-ŭm) Mucous membrane and periosteum so intimately united as to form practically a single membrane.

**mu·co·pol·y·sac·cha·ride** (myū′kō-pol′ē-sak′ă-rīd) General term for a protein-polysaccharide complex obtained from proteoglycans and containing as much as 95% polysaccharide.

**mu·co·pol·y·sac·cha·ride ker·a·tin dys·tro·phy** (myū′kō-pol′ē-sak′ăr-īd ker′ă-tin dis′trŏ-fē) Histologic finding seen on surface epithelium of oral inflammatory fibrous hyperplasia.

**mu·co·pol·y·sac·cha·ri·do·sis,** pl. **mu·co·pol·y·sac·cha·ri·do·ses** (myū′kō-pol′ē-sak′ă-ri-dō′sis, -sēz) Any of a group of lysosomal storage diseases that share a disorder in metabolism of mucopolysaccharides.

**mu·co·pu·ru·lent** (myū′kō-pyūr′ŭ-lĕnt) Pertaining to an exudate that is chiefly purulent (pus), but containing significant mucous material.

**mu·co·pus** (myū′kō-pŭs) A mucopurulent discharge; mixture of mucous material and pus.

**mu·co·sa,** pl. **mu·co·sae** (myū-kō′să, -sē) [TA] Mucous tissue lining various tubular structures consisting of epithelium, lamina propria, and, in the digestive tract, a layer of smooth muscle (muscularis mucosae). SYN mucous membrane. [L. fem. form of *mucosus,* mucous]

**mu·co·san·guin·e·ous, mu·co·san·guin·o·lent** (myū′kō-sang-gwin′ē-ŭs, -ŏ-lĕnt) Pertaining to exudate or other fluid material with a relatively high content of blood and mucus. [*muco-* + L. *sanguis,* blood]

**mn**

**mu·co·sa of mouth** (myū-kō´să mowth) [TA] Mucous membrane of oral cavity, including gingiva. SYN oral mucosa [TA].

**mu·co·sa of nose** (myū-kō´să nōz) [TA] Lining of the nasal cavity, continuous with skin in vestibule of nose and with mucosa of nasopharynx, paranasal sinuses, and nasolacrimal duct.

**mu·co·sa of pha·ryng·o·tym·pan·ic (au·di·to·ry) tube** (myū-kō´să fă-ring´gō-tim-pan´ik aw´di-tōr-ē tūb) [TA] Lining coat of auditory tube.

**mu·co·sa of phar·ynx** (myū-kō´să far´ingks) [TA] Mucous coat of pharynx.

**mu·co·sa of tongue** (myū-kō´să tŭng) [TA] Mucosa forming lingual surface; that of the dorsum of the tongue appears velvety due to the presence of vast numbers of papillae; that of the inferior surface is smooth and thinner. SYN lingual mucosa.

**mu·co·se·rous** (myū´kō-sēr´ŭs) Pertaining to an exudate or secretion that consists of both mucus and serum or a watery component.

**mu·co·si·tis** (myū´kō-sī´tis) Inflammation of a mucous membrane. See page A13. [*mucosa* + *-itis*]

**mu·co·stat·ic** (myū´kō-stat´ik) 1. Denoting normal relaxed condition of mucosal tissues covering the jaws. 2. Arresting secretion of mucus. [*muco-* + G. *stasis,* a standing]

**mu·cous cell** (myū´kŭs sel) A cell that secretes mucus (e.g., a goblet cell).

**mu·cous cyst** (myū´kŭs sist) SEE mucocele (1).

**mu·cous gland** (myū´kŭs gland) Gland that secretes mucus. SYN muciparous gland.

**mu·cous mem·brane** (myū´kŭs mem´brān) SYN mucosa.

**mu·cous rale** (myū´kŭs rahl) Bubbling rale heard on auscultation over bronchial tubes containing mucus.

**mu·co·vis·ci·do·sis** (myū´kō-vis´i-dō´sis) SYN cystic fibrosis. [*muco-* + G. *toxikon,* poison, + *-osis,* condition]

**mu·cus** (myū´kŭs) *Do not confuse this noun with the adjective mucous.* Clear viscid secretion of the mucous membranes, consisting of mucin, epithelial cells, leukocytes, and various inorganic salts dissolved in water. [L.]

**mu·cus im·pac·tion** (myū´kŭs im-pak´shŭn) Filling of the proximal bronchi and bronchioles with mucus.

**muf·fle fur·nace** (mŭf´ĕl fŭr´năs) Dental furnace heated by resistant muffle.

**mul·ber·ry mo·lar** (mŭl´ber-ē mō´lăr) Molar tooth with alternating nonanatomic depressions and rounded enamel nodules on its crown surface.

**mull·ing** (mŭl´ing) In dentistry, final step of mixing dental amalgam, when the triturated mass is kneaded to complete amalgamation.

**mul·ti·core dis·ease** (mŭl´tē-kōr di-zēz´) Nonprogressive congenital myopathy characterized by weakness of proximal muscles, multifocal degeneration of the muscle fibers, and eccentric areas of decreased or absent oxidative enzyme activity in muscles.

**mul·ti·cus·pi·date** (mŭl´tē-kŭs´pi-dāt) 1. Having more than two cusps. 2. A molar tooth with three or more cusps on the crown.

**mul·ti·di·rec·tion·al strokes** (mŭl´tē-di-rek´shŭn-ăl strōks) Instrumentation strokes made using a combination of vertical, oblique, and horizontal actions; used to assess or débride a subgingival tooth surface.

**mul·ti·fac·to·ri·al in·her·i·tance** (mŭl´tē-fak-tōr´ē-ăl in-her´i-tăns) Inheritance involving many factors, of which at least one is genetic but none is of overwhelming importance.

**mul·ti·loc·u·lar** (mŭl´tē-lok´yū-lăr) Many-celled; having many compartments or loculi.

**mul·ti·loc·u·lar cyst** (mŭl´tē-lok´yū-lăr sist) Lesion containing several compartments formed by membranous septa.

**mul·ti·ple** (mŭl´ti-pĕl) Manifold; repeated several times. [L. *multiplex,* fr. *multus,* many, + *plico,* pp. *-atus,* to fold]

**mul·ti·ple an·chor·age** (mŭl´ti-pĕl ang´kŏr-ăj) Anchorage in which more than one type of resistance unit is used.

**mul·ti·ple chem·i·cal sen·si·ti·vi·ty** (mŭl´ti-pĕl kem´i-kăl sen´si-tiv´i-tē) Symptom array of variable presentation attributed to recurrent exposure to known environmental chemicals at dosages generally below levels established as harmful.

**mul·ti·ple en·do·crine de·fi·cien·cy syn·drome** (mŭl´ti-pĕl en´dō-krin dĕ-fish´ĕn-sē sin´drōm) Acquired deficiency of function of several endocrine glands.

**mul·ti·ple en·do·crine ne·o·pla·si·a (MEN)** (mŭl´ti-pĕl en´dō-krin nē´ō-plā´zē-ă) Group of disorders characterized by functioning tumors in more than one endocrine gland.

**mul·ti·ple en·do·crine ne·o·pla·si·a I** (mŭl´ti-pĕl en´dō-krin nē´ō-plā´zē-ă) Syndrome characterized by tumors of the pituitary gland, pancreatic islet cells, and parathyroid glands and may be associated with Zollinger-Ellison syndrome; also called MEN1.

**mul·ti·ple en·do·crine ne·o·pla·si·a II** (mŭl´ti-pĕl en´dō-krin nē´ō-plā´zē-ă) Syndrome associated with pheochromocytoma, parathyroid adenoma, and medullary thyroid carcinoma; also called MEN2.

**mul·ti·ple en·do·crine ne·o·pla·sia IIB** (mŭl′ti-pĕl en′dō-krin nē′ō-plā′zē-ă) SYN multiple endocrine neoplasia III.

**mul·ti·ple en·do·crine ne·o·pla·si·a III** (mŭl′ti-pĕl en′dō-krin nē′ō-plā′zē-ă) Syndrome characterized by tumors found in MEN2, tall, thin habitus, prominent lips, and neuromas of the tongue and eyelids; also called MEN3. SYN multiple endocrine neoplasia IIB.

**mul·ti·ple mu·co·sal neu·ro·mas syn·drome** (mŭl′ti-pĕl myū-kō′săl nūr-ō′mă sin′ drōm) Multiple submucosal neuromas or neurofibromas of the tongue, lips, and eyelids in young people.

**mul·ti·ple my·e·lo·ma, my·e·lo·ma mul·ti·plex** (mŭl′ti-pĕl mī′ĕ-lō′mă, mī-ĕ-lō′mă mŭl′tē-pleks) An uncommon disease that occurs more frequently in men associated with anemia, hemorrhage, recurrent infections, and weakness. SYN plasma cell myeloma (1).

**mul·ti·ple scle·ro·sis (MS)** (mŭl′ti-pĕl skler-ō′sis) Common demyelinating disorder of central nervous system, causing patches of sclerosis (plaques) in brain and spinal cord; occurs primarily in young adults, and has protean clinical manifestations. [F. *sclerose en plaques*]

**mul·ti·ple self-heal·ing squa·mous ep·i·the·li·o·ma** (mŭl′ti-pĕl self-hēl′ing skwā′mŭs ep′i-thē′lē-ō′mă) Skin tumors, most frequently on the head, each resembling a well-differentiated squamous carcinoma or keratoacanthoma; individual tumors resolve spontaneously after several months, leaving deep-pitted scars with irregular crenellated borders.

**mul·ti·ple-sys·tem at·ro·phy (MSA)** (mŭl′ti-pĕl sis′tĕm at′rŏ-fē) Nonhereditary, neurodegenerative disease of unknown cause, characterized clinically by the development of parkinsonism, ataxia, autonomic failure, or pyramidal track signs, in various combinations.

**mul·ti·root·ed** (mŭl′tē-rū′tĕd) Having two or more tooth roots.

**mum·mi·fi·ca·tion** (mŭm′i-fi-kā′shŭn) In dentistry, treatment of inflamed dental pulp with fixative drugs (usually formaldehyde derivatives) to retain teeth so treated for relatively short periods; generally acceptable only for primary (deciduous) teeth.

**mum·mi·fied pulp** (mŭm′i-fīd pŭlp) Misnomer for pulp treated with a formaldehyde derivative.

**mumps** (mŭmps) An acute infectious and contagious disease caused by a mumps virus of the genus *Rubulavirus* and characterized by fever, inflammation, and swelling of the parotid gland, and sometimes of other salivary glands, and oc-casionally by inflammation of the testis, ovary, pancreas, or meninges. SYN epidemic parotitis.

**Mun·chau·sen by prox·y syn·drome** (mūn′chow-zĕn prok′sē sin′drōm) Form of child maltreatment or abuse inflicted by a caretaker (usually the mother) with fabrications of symptoms and/or induction of signs of disease, leading to unnecessary investigations and interventions, with occasional serious health consequences, including death of the child. SYN factitious illness by proxy.

**Mun·chau·sen syn·drome** (mūn′chow-zĕn sin′drōm) Repeated fabrication of clinically convincing simulations of disease to gain medical attention.

**mu·ram·i·dase** (myū-ram′i-dās) SYN lysozyme.

**mu·ri·at·ic** (myū′rē-at′ik) Relating to brine. [L. *muriaticus*, pickled in brine, fr. *muria*, brine]

**mu·ri·at·ic ac·id** (myūr′ē-at′ik as′id) SYN hydrochloric acid.

**mur·mur** (mŭr′mŭr) **1.** A soft sound, like that made by a somewhat forcible expiration with the mouth open, heard on auscultation of the heart, lungs, or blood vessels. **2.** An other-than-soft sound, which may be loud, harsh, or frictional. [L.]

**mus·cle** (mŭs′ĕl) [TA] Primary tissue, consisting predominantly of highly specialized contractile cells, which may be classified as skeletal muscle, cardiac muscle, or smooth muscle. SYN musculus [TA]. [L. *musculus*]

**mus·cle fa·tigue** (mus′ĕl fă-tēg′) A state of exhaustion or loss of strength and/or muscle endurance following strenuous activity associated with the accumulation of lactic acid in muscles.

**mus·cle re·lax·ant** (mŭs′ĕl rĕ-lak′sănt) Drug with capacity to reduce muscle tone; may be either a peripherally acting muscle relaxant such as curare and act to produce blockade at the neuromuscular junction (and thus useful in surgery), or act as a centrally acting muscle relaxant exerting its effects within the brain and spinal cord to diminish muscle tone (and thus useful in muscle spasm or spasticity).

**mus·cles of tongue** (mŭs′ĕlz tŭng) [TA] Extrinsic muscles include the genioglossus, hyoglossus, chondroglossus, and styloglossus muscles; intrinsic muscles comprise the vertical, transverse, and the superior and inferior longitudinal; all are innervated by the hypoglossal nerve. SYN lingual muscles.

**mus·cle spasm** (mŭs′ĕl spazm) SYN spasm.

**mus·cu·lar at·ro·phy** (mŭs′kyū-lăr at′rŏ-fē) Wasting of muscular tissue.

**mus·cu·lar dys·tro·phy** (mŭs′kyū-lăr dis′ trŏ-fē) General term for hereditary progressive

**mn**

degenerative disorders affecting skeletal muscles and other organ systems.

**mus·cu·lar in·suf·fi·cien·cy** (mŭs´kyū-lăr in´sŭ-fish´ĕn-sē) Failure of any muscle to contract with its normal force.

**mus·cu·la·ture** (mŭs´kyū-lă-chŭr) The arrangement of the muscles in the body.

**mus·cu·lo·skel·e·tal dis·or·der** (mŭs´kyū-lō-skel´ĕ-tăl dis-ōr´dĕr) Condition affecting the musculoskeletal, peripheral nervous, and neurovascular systems, which is caused or aggravated by prolonged repetitive forceful or awkward movements, poor posture, badly fitted chairs and equipment, or a fast-paced workload.

**mus·cu·lus,** pl. **mus·cu·li** (mŭs´kyū-lŭs, -lī) [TA] SYN muscle. [L. a little mouse, a muscle, fr. *mus* (*mur*-), a mouse]

**mus·cu·lus buc·ci·na·tor** (mŭs´kyū-lŭs buk-sin-ā´tōr) [TA] SYN buccinator muscle.

**mus·cu·lus cil·i·ar·is** (mŭs´kyū-lŭs sil´ē-ā´ris) [TA] SYN ciliary muscle.

**mus·cu·lus ge·ni·o·hy·oi·de·us** (mŭs´kyū-lŭs jē´nē-ō-hī-oyd´ē-ŭs) [TA] SYN geniohyoid muscle.

**mus·cu·lus men·ta·lis** (mŭs´kyū-lŭs men-tā´lis) [TA] SYN mentalis muscle.

**mus·cu·lus o·mo·hy·oi·de·us** (mŭs´kyū-ŭs ō´mō-hī-oy´dē-ŭs) [TA] SYN omohyoid muscle.

**mus·cu·lus or·bic·u·la·ris o·ris** (mŭs´kyū-lŭs ōr-bik´yū-lā´ris ō´ris) [TA] SYN orbicularis oris muscle.

**mus·cu·lus ster·no·thy·roid·e·us** (mŭs´kyū-lŭs stĕr´nō-thī-roy´dē-ŭs) [TA] SYN sternothyroid muscle.

**mus·cu·lus sty·lo·glos·sus** (mŭs´kyū-lŭs stī´lō-glos´ŭs) [TA] SYN styloglossus muscle.

**mus·cu·lus thy·ro·hy·oi·de·us** (mŭs´kyū-lŭs thī-rō-hī-oy´dē-ŭs) [TA] SYN thyrohyoid (muscle).

**mush·bite** (mŭsh´bīt) Maxillomandibular record made by introducing a mass of soft wax into patient's mouth and telling patient to bite into it as necessary; procedure not generally accepted.

**mus·si·ta·tion** (mŭs´i-tā´shŭn) Lip movements as if speaking, but without sound; observed in delirium and other disease.

**mu·ta·gen** (myū´tă-jen) Any agent that promotes a mutation or increases rate of mutational events. [L. *muto*, to change, + G. *-gen*, producing]

**mu·ta·gen·e·sis** (myū´tă-jen´ē-sis) **1.** Production of a mutation. **2.** Production of genetic alteration through use of chemicals or radiation.

**mu·tant** (myū´tănt) A phenotype in which a mutation is manifested.

**mu·ta·tion** (myū-tā´shŭn) Change in gene chemistry perpetuated in subsequent divisions of cell in which it occurs. [L. *muto*, pp. *-atus*, to change]

**mut·ism** (myū´tizm) **1.** State of being silent. **2.** Organic or functional absence of faculty of speech. [L. *mutus*, mute]

**MW** Abbreviation for molecular weight.

**my·al·gi·a** (mī-al´jē-ă) Muscular pain. [G. *mys*, muscle, + *algos*, pain]

**my·as·the·ni·a** (mī´as-thē´nē-ă) Muscular weakness. [G. *mys*, muscle, + *astheneia*, weakness]

**my·as·the·ni·a gra·vis** (mī´as-thē´nē-ă grā´vis) Disorder of neuromuscular transmission marked by fluctuating weakness and fatigue of some voluntary muscles.

**my·as·then·ic cri·sis** (mī´as-then´ik krī´sis) Severe, life-threatening exacerbation of the manifestations of myasthenia gravis requiring intensive treatment.

**my·as·then·ic fa·ci·es** (mī´as-then´ik fash´ē-ēz) Facial expression in myasthenia gravis, caused by drooping eyelids and corners of mouth, and of facial muscle weakness.

**my·a·to·ni·a, my·at·o·ny** (mī´ă-tō´nē-ă, mī-at´ŏ-nē) Abnormal extensibility of a muscle. [G. *mys*, muscle, + *a* priv. + *tonos*, tone]

**my·ce·li·um,** pl. **my·ce·li·a** (mī-sē´lē-ŭm, -ă) The mass of hyphae making up a colony of fungi. [G. *mykēs*, fungus, + *hēlos*, nail, wart, excrescence on animal or plant]

**my·ce·tism, my·ce·tis·mus** (mī´sĕ-tizm, -tiz´mŭs) Poisoning by some species of mushrooms. [G. *mykēs*, fungus]

✿ **myco-** Fungus. [G. *mykēs*, fungus]

**my·co·bac·te·ri·a** (mī´kō-bak-tēr´ē-ă) Organisms belonging to the genus *Mycobacterium*.

**My·co·bac·te·ri·um** (mī´kō-bak-tēr´ē-ŭm) A genus of aerobic, nonmotile bacteria. Some species are associated with infections in immunocompromised people, especially those with AIDS. The type species is *M. tuberculosis*. [*myco-* + *bacterium*]

**my·co·gas·tri·tis** (mī´kō-gas-trī´tis) Inflammation of stomach due to presence of a fungus. [*myco-* + G. *gastēr*, stomach, + *-itis*, inflammation]

**my·col·o·gy** (mī-kol´ŏ-jē) The study of fungi: their identification, classification, edibility, cultivation, and biology, including pathogenicity. [*myco-* + G. *logos,* study]

**My·co·plas·ma** (mī′kō-plaz′mă) A genus of aerobic to facultatively anaerobic bacteria found in humans and other animals; range from parasitic to pathogenic. [*myco-* + G. *plasma,* something formed (plasm)]

**my·co·sis** (mī-kō′sis) Any disease caused by a fungus (filamentous or yeast). [*myco-* + G. *-osis,* condition]

**my·co·sis fun·goi·des** (mī-kō′sis fung-goyd′ēz) A chronic progressive lymphoma arising in the skin that initially simulates eczema or other inflammatory dermatoses; in advanced cases, ulcerated tumors and infiltrations of lymph nodes may occur.

**my·co·tox·i·co·sis** (mī′kō-tok-si-kō′sis) Poisoning due to ingestion of preformed substances produced by action of some fungi on particular foodstuffs or ingestion of fungi themselves; e.g., ergotism. [*myco-* + G. *toxikon,* poison, + *-osis,* condition]

**my·co·tox·in** (mī′kō-tok′sin) Toxic compound produced by certain fungi; some are used for medicinal purposes; e.g., muscarine, psilocybin.

**my·dri·a·sis** (mi-drī′ă-sis) Dilation of the pupil. [G.]

**myd·ri·at·ic** (mid′rē-at′ik) **1.** Causing mydriasis or dilation of the pupil. **2.** An agent that dilates the pupil.

**my·e·lin** (mī′ĕ-lin) Lipoproteinaceous material, composed of regularly alternating membranes of lipid lamellae (e.g., cholesterol, phospholipids, sphingolipids, and phosphatidates) and protein, of the myelin sheath.

♻ **myelo-** *Do not confuse this combining form with mylo- or myo-.* **1.** The bone marrow. **2.** The spinal cord and medulla oblongata. **3.** The myelin sheath of nerve fibers. [G. *myelos,* medulla, marrow]

**my·e·lo·cyte** (mī′ĕ-lō-sīt) **1.** A young cell of the granulocytic series, occurring normally in bone marrow, but not in circulating blood. **2.** A nerve cell of the gray matter of the brain or spinal cord. [*myelo-* + G. *kytos,* cell]

**my·e·lo·ma** (mī′ĕ-lō′mă) **1.** A tumor composed of cells derived from hemopoietic tissues of bone marrow. **2.** A plasma cell tumor. [*myelo-* + G. *-oma,* tumor]

**my·e·lop·a·thy** (mī′ĕ-lop′ă-thē) **1.** Disorder of the spinal cord. **2.** A disease of the myelopoietic tissues. [*myelo-* + G. *pathos,* suffering]

**my·e·loph·this·ic a·ne·mi·a, my·e·lo·path·ic a·ne·mi·a** (mī′ĕ-lof-thiz′ik ă-nē′mē-ă, mī′ĕ-lō-path′ik) SYN leukoerythroblastosis.

**my·e·loph·thi·sis** (mī′ĕ-lof′thi-sis) Wasting or atrophy of the spinal cord. Replacement of hemopoietic tissue in the bone marrow by abnormal tissue. SYN panmyelophthisis. [*myelo-* + G. *phthisis,* a wasting away]

**my·e·lo·pro·lif·er·a·tive syn·dromes** (mī′ĕ-lō-prō-lif′ĕr-ă-tiv sin′drōmz) Group of conditions due to disorder in the rate of cell formation.

**my·e·lo·ra·dic·u·li·tis** (mī′ĕ-lō-ră-dik′yū-lī′tis) Inflammation of spinal cord and nerve roots. [*myelo-* + L. *radicula,* root, + G. *-itis,* inflammation]

**my·e·lo·ra·dic·u·lop·a·thy** (mī′ĕ-lō-ră-dik′yū-lop′ă-thē) Disease involving spinal cord and nerve roots. [*myelo-* + L. *radicula,* root, + G. *pathos,* disease]

**my·e·lo·sup·pres·sion** (mī′ĕ-lō-sŭ-pre-sh′ŭn) A reduction in the ability of the bone marrow to produce blood cells: platelets, red blood cells, and white blood cells. [G. *myelos,* marrow, + L. *suppressio,* pressing under]

**my·i·a·sis** (mī-ī′ă-sis) Any infection due to invasion of tissues or cavities of the body by larvae of dipterous insects. [G. *myia,* a fly]

**my·lo·hy·oid** (mī′lō-hī′oyd) Relating to molar teeth, posterior portion of lower jaw, and hyoid bone; denoting various structures. [G. *mylē,* a mill, in pl. *mylai,* molar teeth]

**my·lo·hy·oid groove** (mī′lō-hī′oyd grūv) [TA] Groove on medial surface of ramus of mandible beginning at lingula; lodges the mylohyoid artery and nerve.

**my·lo·hy·oid line** (mī′lō-hī′oyd līn) [TA] Ridge on inner surface of mandible running from a point inferior to the mental spine upward and backward to ramus behind last molar tooth; gives attachment to muscle and the lowermost part of the superior constrictor of the pharynx.

**my·lo·hy·oid (mus·cle)** (mī′lō-hī′oyd mŭs′ĕl) [TA] Muscle of floor of mouth; *origin,* mylohyoid line of mandible; *insertion,* upper border of hyoid bone and raphe separating muscle from its fellow; *action,* elevates floor of mouth and the tongue, depresses jaw when hyoid is fixed; *nerve supply,* nerve to mylohyoid from mandibular division of trigeminal. SYN diaphragm of mouth, musculus hyoideus [TA].

**my·lo·hy·oid nerve** (mī′lō-hī′oyd nĕrv) SYN nerve to mylohyoid.

**my·lo·hy·oid ridge** (mī′lō-hī′oyd rij) SYN internal oblique ridge.

♻ **myo-** *Do not confuse this combining form with myelo- or mylo-.* Muscle. [G. *mys,* muscle]

**my·o·blast** (mī′ō-blast) A primordial muscle cell with the potentiality of developing into a muscle fiber. [*myo-* + G. *blastos,* germ]

**mn**

**my·o·blas·to·ma** (mī′ō-blas-tō′mă) A tumor of immature muscle cells. [*myo-* + G. *blastos,* germ, + *-oma,* tumor]

**my·o·bra·di·a** (mī′ō-brā′dē-ă) Sluggish reaction of muscle to stimulation. [*myo-* + G. *bradys,* slow]

**my·o·car·di·al in·farc·tion (MI)** (mī′ō-kahr′dē-ăl in-fahrk′shŭn) Infarction of an area of the heart muscle, usually as a result of occlusion of a coronary artery. SYN heart attack.

**my·o·car·di·al in·suf·fi·cien·cy** (mī′ō-kahr′dē-ăl in′sŭ-fish′ĕn-sē) SYN heart failure (1).

**my·o·car·di·tis** (mī′ō-kahr-dī′tis) Inflammation of the muscular walls of heart.

**my·o·car·di·um,** pl. **my·o·car·di·a** (mī′ō-kahr′dē-ŭm, -ă) [TA] The middle layer of the heart, consisting of cardiac muscle. [*myo-* + G. *kardia,* heart]

**my·o·clon·ic sei·zure** (mī′ō-klon′ik sē′zhŭr) Seizure characterized by sudden, brief (200-msec) contractions of muscle fibers, muscles, or groups of muscles.

**my·oc·lo·nus** (mī′ok′lŏ-nŭs) One or a series of shocklike contractions of a group of muscles, of variable regularity, synchrony, and symmetry. [*myo-* + G. *klonos,* tumult]

**my·o·fas·ci·al pain-dys·func·tion syn·drome** (mī′ō-fash′ē-ăl pān-dis-fŭngk′shŭn sin′drōm) Dysfunction of masticatory apparatus related to spasm of muscles of mastication precipitated by lack of occlusal harmony or alteration in vertical dimension of jaws, and exacerbated by emotional stress; characterized by pain in the preauricular region, muscle tenderness, popping noise in temporomandibular joint, and limitation of jaw motion. SYN temporomandibular joint pain-dysfunction syndrome, TMJ syndrome.

**my·o·fi·bro·ma·to·sis** (mī′ō-fī′brō-mă-tō′sis) Solitary or multiple tumors of muscle and fibrous tissue, or tumors composed by myofibroblasts. [*myo-* + L. *fibra,* fiber, + G. suffix, *-ōma,* tumor, + suffix *-osis,* condition]

**my·o·func·tion·al** (mī′ō-fŭngk′shŭn-ăl) **1.** In dentistry, relating to the role of muscle function in etiology or correction of orthodontic problems. **2.** Relating to function of muscles.

**my·o·func·tion·al ther·a·py** (mī′ō-fŭngk′shŭn-ăl thār′ă-pē) Treatment of malocclusion and other dental and speech disorders using muscular exercises of tongue and lips; most often intended to alter a tongue thrust swallowing pattern.

**my·o·li·po·ma** (mī′ō-li-pō′mă) A benign neoplasm that consists chiefly of fat cells (adipose tissue).

**my·o·ma** (mī-ō′mă) A benign neoplasm of muscular tissue. [*myo-* + G. *-oma,* tumor]

**my·o·path·ic fa·cies** (mī′ō-path′ik fash′ē-ēz) Facial appearance of some patients with myopathies and with myasthenia gravis, consisting of bilateral ptosis and inability to elevate corners of mouth due to muscle weakness.

**my·op·a·thy** (mī-op′ă-thē) Any abnormal condition or disease of the muscular tissues; commonly designates a disorder involving skeletal muscle. [*myo-* + G. *pathos,* suffering]

**my·o·pi·a** (mī-ō′pē-ă) The optic condition in which parallel light rays are brought by the ocular media to focus in front of the retina. SYN nearsightedness, shortsightedness. [G. fr. *myo,* to shut, + *ōps,* eye]

**my·o·sin** (mī′ō-sin) A globulin present in muscle; in combination with actin, it forms actomyosin.

**my·o·si·tis** (mī′ō-sī′tis) Inflammation of a muscle. [*myo-* + G. *-itis,* inflammation]

**my·o·spasm, my·o·spas·mus** (mī′ō-spazm, -spaz′mŭs) Spasmodic muscular contraction.

**my·o·tat·ic re·flex** (mī′ō-tat′ik rē′fleks) Tonic contraction of the muscles in response to a stretching force, due to stimulation of muscle proprioceptors.

**my·ot·o·my** (mī-ot′ŏ-mē) **1.** Anatomy or dissection of the muscles. **2.** Surgical division of a muscle. [*myo-* + G. *tomē,* excision]

**my·o·to·ni·a** (mī′ō-tō′nē-ă) Delayed relaxation of a muscle after a strong contraction, or prolonged contraction after mechanical stimulation (as by percussion) or brief electrical stimulation; due to abnormality of muscle membrane, specifically ion channels. [*myo-* + G. *tonos,* tension, stretching]

**my·o·ton·ic dys·tro·phy** (mī′ō-ton′ik dis′trŏ-fē) Most common adult muscular dystrophy, characterized by progressive muscle weakness and wasting of some of cranial innervated muscles, as well as the distal limb muscles.

**my·ot·o·noid** (mī-ot′ŏ-noyd) Denoting a muscular reaction, naturally or electrically excited, characterized by slow contraction and slow relaxation.

**my·ot·o·nus** (mī-ot′ŏ-nŭs) Tonic spasm or temporary rigidity of a muscle or group of muscles. [*myo-* + G. *tonos,* tension, stretching]

**My·Pyr·a·mid** (mī′pir′ă-mid) SYN Food Guide Pyramid.

**myrrh** (mĕr) Gum resin used as an astringent, tonic, and stimulant, and locally for diseases of oral cavity and in mouthwashes. [G. *myrrha*]

**myx·e·de·ma** (miks′ĕ-dē′mă) Hypothyroidism with a relatively hard edema of subcutaneous tissue, with increased content of mucins (proteoglycans) in the interstitial fluid; characterized by somnolence, slow mentation, dryness and loss of hair, increased fluid in body cavities such as the pericardial sac, subnormal temperature, hoarseness, muscle weakness, and slow return of a muscle to the neutral position after a tendon jerk. SYN myxoedema. [*myx-* + G. *oidēma,* swelling]

♻ **myxo-** Combining form meaning mucus. [G. *myxa,* mucus]

**myxoedema** [Br.] SYN myxedema.

**myx·o·fi·bro·ma** (mik′sō-fī-brō′mă) A be-

nign neoplasm of fibrous connective tissue that resembles primitive mesenchymal tissue. [*myxo-* + L. *fibra,* fiber, + G. *-ōma,* tumor]

**myx·o·ma** (mik-sō′mă) Benign neoplasm derived from connective tissue, found intramuscularly and in jaw bones. [*myxo-* + G. *-ōma,* tumor]

**myx·o·sar·co·ma** (mik′sō-sahr-kō′mă) A sarcoma, usually a liposarcoma or malignant fibrous histiocytoma, with an abundant component of myxoid tissue resembling primitive mesenchyme containing connective tissue mucin. [*myxo-* + G. *sarx,* flesh, + *-ōma,* tumor]

mn

# N

**N** Abbreviation for nitrogen; normal.

**Na** Symbol for sodium; natrium.

**Na·bers probe** (nă′bĕrz prōb) Calibrated curved probe used to measure bone loss.

**naevus** [Br.] SYN nevus.

**naevus pigmentosus** [Br.] SYN nevus pigmentosus.

**nail** (nāl) **1.** One of the thin, horny, translucent plates covering dorsal surface of distal end of each terminal phalanx of fingers and toes. **2.** Generally, a metal rod, used in operations to attach fragments of a broken bone.

**nal·i·dix·ic ac·id** (nal′i-dik′sik as′id) Orally effective antibacterial agent used to treat genitourinary tract infections.

**nal·ox·one hy·dro·chlor·ide** (nal-ok′sōn hī′drŏ-klōr′īd) Synthetic congener of oxymorphone, a potent antagonist of both endorphins and narcotics. Used to treat opiate overdose and to reverse coma and respiratory depression.

**nal·trex·one** (nal-treks′ōn) Orally active narcotic antagonist; devoid of pharmacologic action when administered in absence of narcotics.

**NANB** Abbreviation for hepatitis, viral, non-A, non-B.

**nan·oid e·nam·el** (nan′oyd ĕ-nam′ĕl) Condition involving abnormal thinness of enamel. SYN dwarfed enamel.

**na·nom·e·ter (nm)** (nan′ŏ-mē-tĕr) One billionth of a meter ($10^{-9}$ m). SYN nanometre.

**nanometre** [Br.] SYN nanometer.

**nar·cis·sism** (nahr′si-sizm) **1.** State in which one interprets everything in relation to oneself and not to other people or things. **2.** Self-love, which may include sexual attraction to oneself. [*Narkissos,* G. myth. char.]

**nar·co·lep·sy** (nahr′kō-lep-sē) Sleep disorder, mostly in young adults, with recurring diurnal episodes of sleep and often disrupted nocturnal sleep.

**nar·co·sis** (nahr-kō′sis) General and nonspecific reversible depression of neuronal excitability, produced by physical and chemical agents, usually resulting in stupor rather than in anesthesia. [G. *narkōtikos,* a benumbing]

**nar·cot·ic** (nahr-kot′ik) **1.** Any drug, synthetic or naturally occurring, with effects similar to those of opium and opium derivatives, including meperidine, fentanyl, and their derivatives. **2.** Capable of inducing stuporous analgesia. [G. *narkōtikos,* a benumbing]

**nar·cot·ic an·tag·o·nist** (nahr-kot′ik an-tag′ŏ-nist) SEE opioid antagonist.

**nar·cot·ic block·ade** (nahr-kot′ik blok-ād′) Use of drugs to inhibit effects of narcotic substances, as with naloxone.

**nar·cot·ic re·ver·sal** (nahr-kot′ik rĕ-vĕr′săl) Use of narcotic antagonists, such as naloxone, to terminate the action of narcotics.

**nar·co·tism** (nar′kō-tizm) Stuporous analgesia induced by a narcotic.

**na·ris,** pl. **na·res** (nā′ris, -rēz) [TA] Anterior opening to nasal cavity. SYN anterior naris. [L.]

**na·sal arch** (nā′zăl ahrch) Bridge of nose.

**na·sal a·tri·um** (nā′zăl ā′trē-ŭm) SYN atrium of middle nasal meatus.

**na·sal can·nu·la** (nā′zăl kan′yū-lă) Structure to deliver oxygen to the nostrils. Also called nasal prongs.

**na·sal cap·sule** (nā′zăl kap′sŭl) Cartilage around developing nasal cavity of embryo.

**na·sal cav·i·ty** (nā′zăl kav′i-tē) [TA] Space around nasal septum, lined with ciliated respiratory mucosa, extending from naris anteriorly to choana posteriorly, and communicating with paranasal sinuses through their orifices in lateral wall, from which three conchae also project.

**na·sal feed·ing** (nā′zăl fēd′ing) Giving of nourishment through a flexible tube passed through nasal passages into stomach.

**na·sal height** (nā′zăl hīt) Distance between nasion and lower border of the nasal aperture.

**na·sa·lis (mus·cle)** (nā-sā′lis mŭs′ĕl) [TA] Facial muscle of nose; compound muscle consisting of: a transverse part [TA] (pars transversa [TA], musculus compressor naris) arising from the maxilla above the root of the canine tooth on each side and forming an aponeurosis across the bridge of the nose; and an alar part [TA] (pars alaris [TA], musculus dilator naris) arising from the maxilla above the lateral incisor and attaching to the wing of the nose; the alar part dilates the nostril; *nerve supply,* facial.

**na·sal pits** (nā′zăl pits) Paired depressions formed when nasal placodes come to lie below general external contour of developing face as a result of the rapid growth of the adjacent nasal elevations.

**na·sal plac·odes** (nā′zăl plak′ōdz) Paired ectodermal plates that come to lie in bottom of olfactory pits as they deepen by growth of surrounding medial and lateral nasal processes.

**na·sal sacs** (nā′zăl saks) Deepened nasal pits that develop into definitive nasal cavities.

**na·sal sep·tum** (nā′zăl sep′tŭm) [TA] The wall dividing the nasal cavity into halves; it is composed of a central supporting skeleton covered on each side by a mucous membrane.

**na·sal sur·face of bod·y of max·il·la** (nā′zăl sŭr′făs bod′ē mak-sil′ă) [TA] The surface of the maxilla that forms part of the lateral nasal wall with a large defect (maxillary hiatus) posteriorly and the lacrimal sulcus in its midportion. SYN facies nasalis corporis maxillae.

**na·sal sur·face of hor·i·zon·tal plate of pal·a·tine bone** (nā′zăl sŭr′făs hōr′i-zon′tăl plāt pal′ă-tīn bōn) Superiorly (nasally) directed bony crest, formed at the meeting of the horizontal processes of the right and left palatine bones, for attachment of the nasal septum. SYN facies nasalis laminae horizontalis ossis palatini.

**na·sal surface of pal·a·tine bone** (nā′zăl sŭr′făs pal′ă-tīn bōn) [TA] **1.** Nasal surface of the perpendicular lamina of the palatine bone that forms part of the lateral wall of the nasal cavity (facies nasalis lamina perpendicularis ossis palatini [TA]). **2.** Nasal surface of the horizontal lamina of the palatine bone that forms part of the floor of the nasal cavity (facies nasalis lamina horizontalis ossis palatini [TA]). SYN facies nasalis ossis palatini.

**nas·cent** (nā′sĕnt) **1.** Beginning; being born or produced. **2.** Denoting the state of a chemical element at the moment it is set free from one of its compounds. [L. *nascor*, pres. p. *nascens*, to be born]

**na·si·o·in·i·ac** (nā′zē-ō-in′ē-ak) Relating to nasion and inion.

**na·si·on** (nā′zē-on) [TA] Point on cranium corresponding to middle of nasofrontal suture.

**na·si·on-po·go·ni·on mea·sure·ment** (nā′zē-on-pŏ-gō′nē-on mezh′ŭr-mĕnt) SYN facial plane.

**na·si·on soft tis·sue** (nā′zē-on sawft tish′ū) Outer point of intersection between the nasion-sella line and the soft tissue profile.

🔲**na·so·al·ve·o·lar cyst** (nā′zō-al-vē′ŏ-lăr sist) Soft tissue lesion located near attachment of ala over maxilla. See this page. SYN nasolabial cyst.

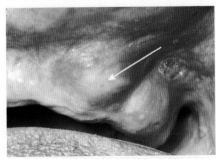
**nasoalveolar cyst:** nodule fluctuant on palpation

**na·so·an·tral** (nā′zō-an′trăl) Relating to nose and maxillary sinus.

**na·so·cil·i·ar·y nerve** (nā′zō-sil′ē-ar-ē nĕrv) [TA] A branch of the ophthalmic nerve in the superior orbital fissure, passing through the orbit, giving rise to the communicating branch to the ciliary ganglion, the long ciliary nerves, and the posterior and anterior ethmoidal nerves. SYN nervus nasociliaris [TA].

**na·so·fron·tal** (nā′zō-frŭn′tăl) Relating to nose and forehead, or to nasal cavity and frontal sinuses.

**na·so·gas·tric** (nā′zō-gas′trik) Pertaining to or involving both nasal passages and stomach, as in nasogastric intubation.

**na·so·gas·tric tube** (nā′zō-gas′trik tūb) A tube used for feeding or suctioning stomach contents; inserted through the nose and down the esophagus into the stomach.

**na·so·la·bi·al** (nā′zō-lā′bē-ăl) Relating to nose and upper lip. [*naso-* + L. *labium*, lip]

**na·so·la·bi·al cyst** (nā′zō-lā′bē-ăl sist) SYN nasoalveolar cyst.

**na·so·lac·ri·mal** (nā′zō-lak′ri-măl) Relating to nasal and lacrimal bones, or to nasal cavity and lacrimal ducts.

**na·so·lac·ri·mal duct** (nā′zō-lak′ri-măl dŭkt) [TA] The passage leading downward from the lacrimal sac on each side to the anterior portion of the inferior meatus of the nose, through which tears are conducted into the nasal cavity.

**na·so·man·dib·u·lar fix·a·tion** (nā′zō-man-dib′yū-lăr fik-sā′shŭn) Mandibular immobilization, especially for edentulous jaws, with maxillomandibular splints, attached by connecting a circummandibular wire with an intraoral interosseous wire passed through a hole drilled into anterior nasal spine of maxillae.

**na·so·max·il·lar·y su·ture** (nā′zō-mak′si-lar-ē sū′chŭr) [TA] Line of union of lateral margin of nasal bone with frontal process of maxilla.

**na·so·men·tal re·flex** (nā′zō-men′tăl rē′fleks) Contraction of mentalis muscle after a tap on side of nose.

**na·so·o·ral** (nā′zō-ōr′ăl) Relating to the nose and mouth.

**na·so·pal·a·tine** (nā′zō-pal′ă-tīn) Relating to nose and palate.

**na·so·pal·a·tine groove** (nā′zō-pal′ă-tīn grūv) Notch on vomer lodging nasopalatine nerve.

**na·so·pal·a·tine nerve** (nā′zō-pal′ă-tīn nĕrv) [TA] Branch from pterygopalatine ganglion, passing through sphenopalatine foramen,

mn

crossing to and then down nasal septum to supply mucous membrane of hard palate.

**na·so·pha·ryn·ge·al** (nā′zō-fă-rin′jē-ăl) Relating to the nasopharynx. SYN rhinopharyngeal (1).

**na·so·phar·ynx** (nā′zō-far′ingks) [TA] Part of pharynx that lies above soft palate; anteriorly opens into nasal cavities through choanae; inferiorly, communicates with oropharynx through isthmus of pharynx. SYN rhinopharynx.

◼**na·tal tooth** (nā′tăl tūth) Predeciduous supernumerary tooth present at birth. See this page.

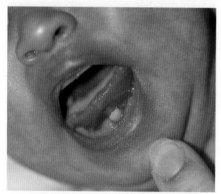

**natal tooth:** this 16-day-old neonate presented for medical care due to difficulty feeding

**Na·tion·al Board Den·tal Hy·giene Ex·am·i·na·tion** (nash′ŏ-năl bōrd den′tăl hī′jēn eg-zam′i-nā′shŭn) Standardized written examination sponsored by the American Dental Association; normally part of the dental hygiene licensure process.

**Na·tion·al Den·tal Hy·gien·ists As·so·ci·a·tion (NDHA)** (nash′ŏ-năl den′tăl hī-jēn′ists ă-sō′sē-ā′shŭn) A professional association whose efforts are directed toward enhancing access to oral health care and providing an organization for minority dental hygienists and dental hygiene students.

**Na·tion·al For·mu·la·ry (NF)** (nash′ŏ-năl fōr′myū-lar-ē) An official compendium issued by the United States Pharmacopeial Convention to provide standards and specifications used to evaluate quality of pharmaceuticals and therapeutic agents.

**Na·tion·al In·sti·tute for Oc·cu·pa·tion·al Safe·ty and Health (NIOSH)** (nash′ŏ-năl in′sti-tūt ok′yū-pā′shŭn-ăl sāf′tē helth) U.S. federal agency established to perform epidemiologic and laboratory research into the causes of occupational diseases and injuries and methods to prevent them.

**Na·tion·al In·sti·tutes of Health (NIH)** (nash′ŏ-năl in′sti-tūts helth) A nonregulatory

U.S. federal agency that oversees research activities funded by the Institute.

**nat·u·ral im·mu·ni·ty, non·spe·cif·ic im·mu·ni·ty** (nach′ŭr-ăl i-myū′ni-tē, non′ spĕ-sif′ik) SYN innate immunity.

**nau·se·a** (naw′zē-ă) An inclination to vomit. [L. fr. G. *nausia,* seasickness, fr. *naus,* ship]

**nau·seous** (naw′shŭs) Nauseated; causing nausea.

**Nb** Symbol for niobium.

**NDHA** Abbreviation for National Dental Hygienists Association.

**near·sight·ed·ness** (nēr-sīt′ĕd-nĕs) SYN myopia.

**neb·u·lize** (neb′yū-līz) To break up a liquid into a fine spray or vapor; to vaporize.

**neb·u·liz·er** (neb′yū-lī-zĕr) A device used to reduce a liquid medication to extremely fine cloudlike particles.

**ne·ca·to·ri·a·sis** (nĕ-kā′tōr-ī′ă-sis) Hookworm disease caused by *Necator.*

**neck** (nek) **1.** [TA] Part of body by which head is connected to trunk; extends from cranial base to top of the shoulders. **2.** In anatomy, any constricted portion having a fancied resemblance to the neck of an animal. SYN cervix (1) [TA].

**neck of tooth** (nek tūth) [TA] Slightly constricted tooth part, between crown and root. SYN cervix dentis [TA], cervical margin of tooth, cervical zone of tooth, cervix of tooth, dental neck.

**neck re·flex·es** (nek rē′fleks′ĕz) Changes in head position alter tone of neck muscles through stimulation of proprioceptors in labyrinth that bring head into its correct position.

**nec·ro·phil·i·a, ne·croph·i·lism** (nek′ rō-fil′ē-ă, nĕ-krof′i-lizm) Impulse to have sexual contact, or the act of such contact, with a dead body, usually involving men with female corpses.

**ne·cro·sis,** pl. **ne·cro·ses** (nĕ-krō′sis, -sēz) Pathologic death of one or more cells, or of a portion of tissue or organ, resulting from irreversible damage. [G. *nekrōsis,* death, fr. *nekroō,* to make dead]

**ne·crot·ic pulp** (nĕ-krot′ik pŭlp) Necrosis of dental pulp that clinically does not respond to thermal stimulation; tooth may be asymptomatic or sensitive to percussion and palpation. SYN dead pulp, nonvital pulp.

**nec·ro·tiz·ing si·a·lo·met·a·pla·si·a** (nek′rō-tīz-ing sī′ă-lō-met-ă-plā′zē-ă) Squamous cell metaplasia of the salivary gland ducts and lobules; seen most frequently in the hard palate. [G. *sialon,* saliva, + *metaplasia*]

**nec·ro·tiz·ing ul·cer·a·tive gin·gi·vi·tis (NUG)** (nek′rō-tīz-ing ŭl′sĕr-ă-tiv jin′ji-vī′tis) Gingivitis of young and middle-aged adults characterized clinically by gingival erythema and pain, fetid odor, necrosis, and sloughing of interdental papillae and marginal gingiva that gives rise to a gray pseudomembrane. See this page and page A11. SYN fusospirochetal gingivitis, trench mouth, ulceromembranous gingivitis, Vincent gingivitis.

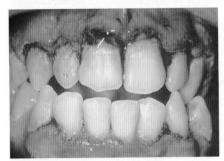

**acute necrotizing ulcerative gingivitis**

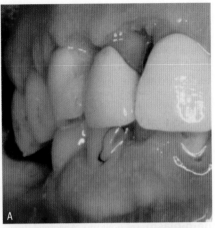

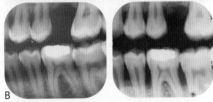

**necrotizing ulcerative periodontitis:** (A) anterior and (B) posterior bone loss (films taken 6 months apart)

**nec·ro·tiz·ing ul·cer·a·tive per·i·o·don·ti·tis** (nek′rŏ-tīz-ing ŭl′sĕr-ă-tiv per′ē-ō-don-tī′tis) Severe and rapidly progressive disease with distinctive erythema of the free gingiva, attached gingiva, and the alveolar mucosa; extensive soft tissue necrosis that usually starts with the interdental papillae and marked loss of periodontal attachment. See this page.

**nee·dle** (nē′dĕl) **1.** Slender, usually sharp-pointed instrument used to puncture tissues, suture, or pass a ligature around or through a vessel. **2.** Hollow device used for injection, aspiration, biopsy, or to guide introduction of a catheter into a space. [M.E. *nedle*, fr. A.S. *nāedl*]

**nee·dle bi·op·sy** (nē′dĕl bī′op-sē) Method in which the specimen for biopsy is removed by aspirating it through an appropriate needle or trocar that pierces the skin. SYN aspiration biopsy.

**nee·dle·point trac·ing** (nēd′ĕl-poynt trās′ing) SYN intraoral tracing.

**nee·dle·stick** (nē′dĕl-stik) Accidental puncture of a health care worker's skin with a contaminated needle.

**neg·a·tive** (neg′ă-tiv) Not affirmative; refutative; not positive. [L. *negativus*, fr. *nego*, to deny]

**neg·a·tive ni·tro·gen bal·ance** (neg′ă-tiv nī′trŏ-jĕn bal′ăns) Nonphysiologic state wherein nitrogenous output exceeds intake.

**ne·glect** (nĕg-lekt′) To fail to perform a duty or give proper care.

**neg·li·gence** (neg′li-jĕns) Failure to perform duties or activities with due diligence and attention or to meet the standards of regular care.

**Ne·gri bod·ies** (nā′grē bod′ēz) Eosinophilic, sharply outlined, pathognomonic inclusion bodies found in the cytoplasm of some nerve cells containing the rabies virus.

**Neis·se·ri·a** (nī-sē′rē-ă) A genus of aerobic to facultatively anaerobic bacteria containing gram-negative cocci that occur in pairs with the adjacent sides flattened. [A. *Neisser*]

**Nel·son syn·drome** (nel′sŏn sin′drŏm) Disorder of hyperpigmentation, third cranial nerve damage, and enlarging sella turcica caused by pituitary adenomas presumably present before adrenalectomy for Cushing syndrome.

**nem·a·tode** (nem′ă-tōd) A common name for any roundworm of the phylum Nematoda.

**ne·o·blas·tic** (nē′ō-blas′tik) Developing in or characteristic of new tissue. [*neo-* + G. *blastos*, germ, offspring]

**ne·o·my·cin sul·fate** (nē′ō-mī′sin sŭl′fāt) Antibacterial antibiotic substance produced by the growth of *Streptomyces fradiae*, active against gram-positive and gram-negative bacteria.

**ne·o·na·tal** (nē′ō-nā′tăl) Relating to period immediately after birth through first 28 days of

mn

extrauterine life. [*neo-* + L. *natalis,* relating to birth]

**ne·o·na·tal hep·a·ti·tis** (nē′ō-nā′tăl hep′ă-tī′tis) Neonatal disorder due to chiefly viral pathogens.

**ne·o·na·tal line** (nē′ō-nā′tăl līn) In deciduous teeth, line of demarcation between prenatal and postnatal enamel.

**ne·o·na·tal tooth** (nē′ō-nā′tăl tūth) Tooth erupting within 28 days after birth.

**ne·o·nate** (nē′ō-nāt) Infant aged up to 1 month.

**ne·o·pla·si·a** (nē′ō-plā′zē-ă) The pathologic process that results in formation and growth of a neoplasm. [*neo-* + G. *plasis,* a molding]

**ne·o·plasm** (nē′ō-plazm) Abnormal tissue that grows by cellular proliferation more rapidly than normal and continues to grow after the stimuli that initiated the new growth cease; may be either benign or malignant. [G. *neo-* new + G. *plasma,* thing formed]

**neph·ric** (nef′rik) Relating to the kidney. SYN renal.

**neph·ro·cal·ci·no·sis** (nef′rō-kal-si-nō′sis) Renal lithiasis characterized by diffusely scattered foci of calcification in the renal parenchyma.

**ne·phrol·o·gy** (nĕ-frol′ŏ-jē) Medical branch concerned with kidney diseases. [*nephro-* + G. *logos,* study]

**ne·phrop·a·thy** (nĕ-frop′ă-thē) Any disease of the kidney. [*nephro-* + G. *pathos,* suffering]

**neph·rot·ic syn·drome** (nef-rot′ik sin′ drōm) Clinical state characterized by edema, albuminuria, decreased plasma albumin, doubly refractile bodies in the urine, and usually increased blood cholesterol.

**nerve** (nĕrv) [TA] A whitish cordlike structure composed of one or more bundles (fascicles) of myelinated or unmyelinated nerve fibers, or more often mixtures of both, coursing outside the central nervous system, together with connective tissue within the fascicle and around the neurolemma of individual nerve fibers (endoneurium), around each fascicle (perineurium), and around the entire nerve and its nourishing blood vessels (epineurium). See this page. [L. *nervus*]

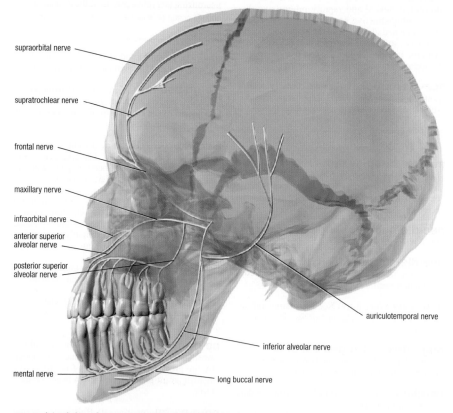

supraorbital nerve

supratrochlear nerve

frontal nerve

maxillary nerve

infraorbital nerve

anterior superior alveolar nerve

posterior superior alveolar nerve

auriculotemporal nerve

inferior alveolar nerve

mental nerve

long buccal nerve

**nerves:** lateral view of nerve supply to teeth; image of head and jaw is transparent

**nerve a·vul·sion** (nĕrv ă-vŭl´shŭn) Tearing away of a peripheral nerve at its point of origin from its parent nerve as a result of traction.

**nerve block** (nĕrv blok) Interruption of conduction of impulses in peripheral nerves or nerve trunks by injection of local anesthetic solution.

**nerve block an·es·the·si·a** (nĕrv blok an´es-thē´zē-ă) Conduction anesthesia in which local anesthetic solution is injected about nerves, nerve trunks, or nerve plexuses.

**nerve con·duc·tion** (nĕrv kŏn-dŭk´shŭn) Transmission of an impulse along a nerve fiber.

**nerve de·com·pres·sion** (nĕrv dē-kŏm-presh´ŭn) Release of pressure on a nerve trunk by the surgical excision of constricting bands or widening of a bony canal.

**nerve end·ing** (nĕrv end´ing) A specialized termination of peripheral sensory nerve fibers. See this page.

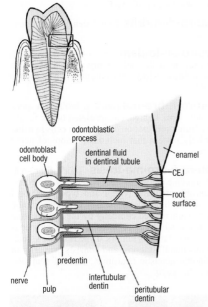

odontoblastic process

odontoblast cell body

dentinal fluid in dentinal tubule

enamel

CEJ

root surface

predentin

intertubular dentin

nerve

pulp

peritubular dentin

**relationship of dentin tubules and pulpal nerve endings:** nerve endings from pulp wrap themselves around odontoblasts that extend only a short distance into tubule; fluid-filled dentin tubules transmit fluid disturbances through mechanism known as hydraulic conductance

**nerve fi·ber** (nĕrv fī´bĕr) Nerve cell axon, ensheathed by oligodendroglial cells in brain and spinal cord.

**nerve root** (nĕrv rūt) One of two bundles of nerve fibers emerging from the spinal cord that

join to form a single segmental (mixed) spinal nerve.

**nerve stro·ma** (nĕrv strō´mă) Connective tissue supporting structures of peripheral nerve fibers, consisting of endoneurium, perineurium, and epineurium.

**nerve to my·lo·hy·oid** (nĕrv mī´lō-hī´oyd) [TA] Small branch of inferior alveolar nerve given off posteriorly just before it enters mandibular foramen, distributed to anterior belly of digastric muscle and mylohyoid muscle. SYN mylohyoid nerve, nervus mylohyoideus.

**nerve trunk** (nĕrv trŭngk) Collection of funiculi or bundles of nerve fibers enclosed in a connective tissue sheath, the epineurium.

**ner·vi spi·na·les** (nĕr´vī spī-nā´lēz) [TA] SYN spinal nerves.

**ner·vous sys·tem** (nĕr´vŭs sis´tĕm) [TA] The entire neural apparatus, composed of a central part, the brain and spinal cord, and a peripheral part, the cranial and spinal nerves, autonomic ganglia, and plexuses.

**ner·vus ab·du·cens [CN VI]** (nĕr´vŭs ab-dū´senz) [TA] SYN abducent nerve [CN VI].

**ner·vus ac·ces·so·ri·us [CN XI]** (nĕr´vŭs ak-ses-sō´rē-ŭs) [TA] SYN accessory nerve [CN XI].

**ner·vus a·cus·ti·cus [CN VIII]** (nĕr´vŭs ă-kū´sti-kŭs) SYN vestibulocochlear nerve [CN VIII].

**ner·vus al·ve·o·la·ris in·fe·ri·or** (nĕr´vŭs al-vē-ō-lā´ris in-fēr´ē-ŏr) [TA] SYN inferior alveolar nerve.

**ner·vus au·ric·u·lo·tem·po·ra·lis** (nĕr´vŭs aw-rik´yū-lō-tem-pō-rā´lis) [TA] SYN auriculotemporal nerve.

**ner·vus fa·ci·a·lis [CN VII]** (nĕr´vŭs fā-shē-ā´lis) [TA] SYN facial nerve [CN VII].

**ner·vus glos·so·pha·ryn·ge·us [CN IX]** (nĕr´vŭs glos-ō-fă-rin´jē-ŭs) [TA] SYN glossopharyngeal nerve [CN IX].

**ner·vus hy·po·glos·sus [CN XII]** (nĕr´vŭs hī-pō-glos´ŭs) [TA] SYN hypoglossal nerve [CN XII].

**ner·vus la·cri·ma·lis** (nĕr´vŭs lak´ri-mā´lis) [TA] SYN lacrimal nerve.

**ner·vus man·di·bu·la·ris [CN V3]** (nĕr´vŭs man-di-byū-lā´ris) [TA] SYN mandibular nerve [CN V3].

**ner·vus max·il·la·ris [CN V2]** (nĕr´vŭs maks´i-lā´ris) [TA] SYN maxillary nerve [CN V2].

**ner·vus my·lo·hy·oi·de·us** (nĕr´vŭs mī´lō-hī-oyd´ē-ŭs) SYN nerve to mylohyoid.

mn

**ner·vus na·so·cil·i·a·ris** (nĕr′vŭs nā′so-sil′ē-ā′ris) [TA] SYN nasociliary nerve.

**ner·vus oc·ta·vus [CN VIII]** (nĕr′vŭs ok-tā′vŭs) SYN vestibulocochlear nerve [CN VIII].

**ner·vus o·cu·lo·mo·to·ri·us [CN III]** (nĕr′vŭs ok-yū-lō-mō-tō′rē-ŭs) [TA] SYN oculomotor nerve [CN III].

**ner·vus ol·fac·to·ri·i [CN I]** (nĕr′vŭs olfak-tō′rē-ī) [TA] SYN olfactory nerve [CN I].

**ner·vus oph·thal·mi·cus [CN V1]** (nĕr′vŭs of-thal′mi-kŭs) [TA] SYN ophthalmic nerve [CN V1].

**ner·vus op·ti·cus [CN II]** (nĕr′vŭs op′ti-kŭs) [TA] SYN optic nerve [CN II].

**ner·vus pe·tro·sus ma·jor** (nĕr′vŭs petrō′sŭs mā′jor) [TA] SYN greater petrosal nerve.

**ner·vus stat·o·a·cus·ti·cus [CN VIII]** (nĕr′vŭs stat′ō-ă-kū′sti-kŭs) SYN vestibulocochlear nerve [CN VIII].

**ner·vus tri·gem·i·nus [CN V]** (nĕr′vŭs trī-jem′i-nŭs) [TA] SYN trigeminal nerve [CN V].

**ner·vus troch·le·a·ris [CN IV]** (nĕr′vŭs trō-klē-ā′ris) [TA] SYN trochlear nerve [CN IV].

**ner·vus va·gus [CN X]** (nĕr′vŭs vā′gŭs) [TA] SYN vagus nerve [CN X].

**ner·vus ves·ti·bu·lo·co·chle·a·ris [CN VIII]** (nĕr′vŭs ves-tib′yū-lō-kok-lē-ā′ris) [TA] SYN vestibulocochlear nerve [CN VIII].

**neur-** Combining form meaning nerve, nerve tissue, the nervous system. [G. neuron]

**neu·ral crest syn·drome** (nūr′ăl krest sin′drōm) Disorder involving loss of pain sensibility and other symptoms.

**neu·ral de·pol·a·ri·za·tion mech·a·nism** (nūr′ăl dē-pō′lăr-ī-zā′shŭn mek′ă-nizm) Reduction of resting potential of nerve membrane so that a nerve impulse is fired.

**neu·ral·gi·a** (nūr-al′jē-ă) Variable pain along the course or distribution of a nerve. [neur- + G. algos, pain]

**neu·ra·prax·i·a** (nūr′ă-prak′sē-ă) Mildest type of focal nerve lesion that produces clinical deficits. [neur- + G. a- priv. + praxis, action]

**neur·as·the·ni·a** (nūr′as-thē′nē-ă) An ill-defined condition, commonly accompanying or following depression, characterized by vague fatigue believed to be brought on by psychological factors. [neur- + G. astheneia, weakness]

**neu·rec·to·my** (nūr-ek′tŏ-mē) Excision of a segment.

**neu·rec·to·pi·a, neur·ec·to·py** (nūr′ek-tō′pē-ă, nūr-ek′tō-pē) Condition in which a nerve follows an anomalous course. [neur- + G. ektopos, fr. ek, out of, + topos, place]

**neu·ri·lem·ma** (nūr′i-lem′ă) A cell that enfolds axons of the peripheral nervous system. SYN sheath of Schwann. [neuri- + G. lemma, husk]

**neu·ri·lem·mo·ma** (nūr′i-lĕ-mō′mă) SYN schwannoma. [neurilemma + G. -oma, tumor]

**neu·ri·no·ma** (nūr′i-nō′mă) Obsolete term for schwannoma.

**neu·ri·tis,** pl. **neu·ri·ti·des** (nūr-ī′tis, -it′i-dēz) 1. Inflammation of a nerve. 2. SYN neuropathy. [neuri- + G. -itis, inflammation]

**neu·ro·a·nat·o·my** (nūr′ō-ă-nat′ŏ-mē) The anatomy of the nervous system, usually specific to the central nervous system.

**neu·ro·blas·to·ma** (nūr′ō-blas-tō′mă) Malignant neoplasm characterized by immature, only slightly differentiated nerve cells of embryonic type, i.e., neuroblasts.

**neu·ro·cu·ta·ne·ous syn·drome** (nūr′ō-kyū-tā′nē-ŭs sin′drōm) Heterogenous disorders with finding that central nervous system and skin lesions coexist.

**neu·ro·den·drite** (nūr′ō-den′drīt) SYN dendrite (1).

**neu·ro·ec·to·derm** (nūr′ō-ek′tō-dĕrm) Central region of the early embryonic ectoderm that on further development forms the brain and spinal cord.

**neu·ro·fi·bro·ma** (nūr′ō-fī-brō′mă) A moderately firm, benign, encapsulated tumor resulting from proliferation of Schwann cells in a disorderly pattern that includes portions of nerve fibers.

**neu·ro·fi·bro·ma·to·sis** (nūr′ō-fī-brō-mă-tō′sis) One of two distinct hereditary disorders: neurofibromatosis type I and type II. Type I (von Recklinghausen disease), is more common and characterized clinically by the combination of patches of hyperpigmentation and cutaneous and subcutaneous tumors. Type II has few cutaneous manifestations, and consists primarily of bilateral acoustic neuromas, causing deafness. See this page.

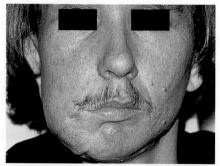

**neurofibromatosis:** asymmetric enlargement

**neu·rog·li·a** (nūr-og′lē-ă) [TA] Nonneuronal cellular elements in the central and peripheral nervous systems that are supporting cells; thought have important metabolic functions. [G. *neuron*, tendon, nerve, + *glia*, glue]

**neu·ro·ki·nins** (nūr′ō-kī′ninz) Neuropeptides with vasoactive and bronchospastic properties.

**neu·ro·lab·y·rin·thi·tis** (nūr′ō-lab′i-rin-thī′tis) Idiopathic inflammation of the vestibular nerve; presents with vertigo, nausea, and imbalance; usually no involvement of cochlear nerve, and thus neither tinnitus nor hearing loss.

**neu·ro·lept·an·al·ge·si·a** (nūr′ō-lept-an-ăl-jē′zē-ă) An intense analgesic and amnesic state produced by narcotic analgesics and neuroleptic drugs; unconsciousness may occur; cardiorespiratory function may be altered.

**neu·rol·o·gy** (nūr-ol′ŏ-jē) Branch of medical science concerned with various nervous systems (central, peripheral, and autonomic), plus the neuromuscular junction and muscle, and related disorders. [*neuro-* + G. *logos*, study]

**neu·rol·y·sis** (nūr-ol′i-sis) **1.** Destruction of nerve tissue. **2.** Procedure to free a nerve from inflammatory adhesions or incising its epineurium for decompression. [*neuro-* + G. *lysis*, dissolution]

**neu·ro·lyt·ic** (nūr′ō-lit′ik) Relating to neurolysis.

**neu·ro·ma,** pl. **neu·ro·ma·ta,** pl. **neu·ro·mas** (nūr-ō′mă, -mă-tă, -măz) General term for any neoplasm derived from cells of the nervous system. [*neuro-* + G. *-oma*, tumor]

**neu·ro·mus·cu·lar** (nūr′ō-mŭs′kyū-lăr) Referring to relationship between nerve and muscle.

**neu·ro·mus·cu·lar block·ing a·gents** (nūr′ō-mŭs′kyū-lăr blok′ing ā′jĕnts) Drugs that prevent motor nerve endings from exciting skeletal muscle.

**neu·ron** (nūr′on) [TA] Morphologic and functional unit of nervous system, consisting of nerve cell body, dendrites, and the axons. SYN neurone. [G. *neuron*, a nerve]

**neurone** [Br.] SYN neuron.

**neu·ro·o·tol·o·gy** (nūr′ō-ō-tol′ŏ-jē) Branch of medicine concerned with the auditory and vestibular systems and with related structures.

**neu·ro·pa·ral·y·sis** (nūr′ō-pă-ral′i-sis) Paralysis resulting from disease of the nerve supplying affected part.

**neu·ro·path·ic ar·throp·a·thy** (nūr′ō-path′ik ahr-throp′ă-thē) SYN neuropathic joint.

**neu·ro·path·ic joint** (nūr′ō-path′ik joynt) Joint disease caused by diminished propriocep-

tive sensation, with gradual destruction of the joint by repeated subliminal injury. SYN Charcot joint.

**neu·ro·path·o·gen·e·sis** (nūr′ō-path-ŏ-jen′ě-sis) Origin or causation of disease of nervous system. [*neuro-* + G. *pathos*, suffering, + *genesis*, origin]

**neu·rop·a·thy** (nūr-op′ă-thē) **1.** Classic term for any disorder affecting any segment of nervous system. **2.** In contemporary usage, disease involving the cranial nerves or the peripheral or autonomic nervous system. SYN neuritis (2). [*neuro-* + G. *pathos*, suffering]

**neu·ro·pep·tide** (nūr′ō-pep′tīd) Any of a variety of peptides found in neural tissue.

**neu·ro·psy·cho·log·i·cal dis·or·der** (nū′rō-sī-kŏ-loj′ik-ăl dis-ōr′dĕr) Cerebral dysfunction from any physical cause manifested by changes in mood, behavior, perception, memory, cognition, or judgment and/or psychophysiology.

**neu·ro·reg·u·la·tor** (nūr′ō-reg′yū-lā-tŏr) Chemical factor with a modulatory effect on neurons.

**neu·ro·sis,** pl. **neu·ro·ses** (nūr-ō′sis, -sēz) **1.** Psychological or behavioral disorder with anxiety as primary characteristic; affected patients may be as disabled as those with a psychosis. **2.** A functional nervous disease, or one in which there is no evident lesion. **3.** A peculiar state of tension or irritability of the nervous system.

**neu·ro·sur·ger·y** (nūr′ō-sŭr′jĕr-ē) Surgery of the nervous system.

**neu·ro·ten·sin** (nū′rō-ten′sin) A 13-amino acid peptide neurotransmitter in synapsomes in the hypothalamus, amygdala, basal ganglia, and dorsal gray matter of the spinal cord.

**neu·rot·o·my** (nūr-ot′ŏ-mē) Operative division of a nerve. [*neuro-* + G. *tomē*, a cutting]

**neu·ro·trans·mit·ter** (nūr′ō-trans′mit-ĕr) Any specific chemical agent released by a presynaptic cell that, on excitation, crosses synapse to stimulate or inhibit the postsynaptic cell. [*neuro-* + L. *transmitto*, to send across]

**neu·ro·tro·phins** (nū′rō-trō′finz) Growth factors of nervous system (e.g., brain-derived neurotrophic factor). [*neuro-* + G. *trophē*, nourishment, + *-in*]

**neu·tral** (nū′trăl) **1.** Exhibiting no positive properties. **2.** CHEMISTRY neither acid nor alkaline. [L. *neutralis*, fr. *neuter*, neither]

**neutralisation** [Br.] SYN neutralization.

**neu·tral·i·za·tion** (nū′trăl-ī-zā′shŭn) **1.** The change in reaction of a solution from acid or alkaline to neutral by the addition of a sufficient amount of an alkaline or an acid substance, respectively. **2.** The rendering ineffective of any action, process, or potential. SYN neutralisation.

**neu·tral oc·clu·sion** (nū′trăl ŏ-klū′zhŭn) Arrangement of teeth with maxillary and mandibular first permanent molars in normal anteroposterior relation. SYN normal occlusion (2).

**neu·tral po·si·tion** (nū′trăl pŏ-zish′ŭn) Ideal positioning of the body while performing work activities associated with decreased risk of musculoskeletal injury.

**neu·tral wrist po·si·tion** (nū′trăl rist pŏ-zish′ŭn) Ideal position of the wrist while performing work activities that is associated with decreased risk of musculoskeletal injury.

**neu·tral zone** (nū′trăl zōn) In dentistry, potential space between the lips and cheeks on one side and tongue on the other; natural or artificial teeth in this area are subject to equal and opposite forces from the surrounding musculature.

**neu·tro·clu·sion** (nū′trō-klū′zhŭn) Malocclusion with a normal anteroposterior relationship between the maxilla and mandible; in Angle classification, a Class I malocclusion.

**neu·tron** (nū′tron) An electrically neutral particle in the nuclei of all atoms (except hydrogen-1) with a mass slightly larger than that of a proton; in isolation, it breaks down to a proton and an electron with a half-life of about 10.3 minutes. [L. *neuter,* neither]

**neu·tro·pe·ni·a** (nū′trō-pē′nē-ă) The presence of abnormally small numbers of neutrophils in the circulating blood. [*neutrophil* + G. *penia,* poverty]

**neu·tro·phil, neu·tro·phile** (nū′trō-fil, -fīl) A mature white blood cell in granulocytic series, formed by myelopoietic tissue of bone marrow and released into circulating blood. [*neutro-* + G. *philos,* fond]

**neu·tro·phil·i·a** (nū′trō-fil′ē-ă) An increase of neutrophils in blood or tissues.

**ne·vus,** pl. **ne·vi** (nē′vŭs, -vī) Circumscribed dermal malformation, especially if hyperpigmented or with increased vascularity; may be predominantly epidermal, adnexal, melanocytic, vascular, or mesodermal, or a composite. SYN naevus. [L. *naevus,* mole, birthmark]

**ne·vus pig·men·to·sus** (nē′vŭs pig-men-tō′sŭs) A benign pigmented melanocytic proliferation; raised or level with the skin, present at birth or arising early in life. SYN mole (2), naevus pigmentosus.

**new at·tach·ment** (nū ă-tach′mĕnt) Union of connective tissue or epithelium with a root surface that has been deprived of its original attachment apparatus; the new attachment may be epithelial adhesion and/or connective tissue adaptation or attachment and may include new cementum.

**NF** Abbreviation for National Formulary.

**Ni** Symbol for nickel.

**ni·a·cin** (nī′ă-sin) SYN nicotinic acid.

**nib** (nib) In dentistry, the portion of a condensing instrument that comes into contact with the restorative material being condensed; its end, the face, is smooth or serrated.

**NIC** Abbreviation for Nursing Interventions Classification.

**nick·el (Ni)** (nik′ĕl) A metallic bioelement; closely resembles cobalt and often associated with it. A deficiency of nickel causes changes in the ultrastructure of the liver.

**nick·el-chro·mi·um al·loy** (nik′ĕl-krō′mē-ŭm al′oy) An alloy used in the construction of crowns, bridges, and removable partial dental frameworks. It is usually given a porcelain veneer when used in crowns and bridges, but at present, its use is declining as the number of patients sensitive to nickel increases.

**nic·o·tine** (nik′ŏ-tēn) A poisonous volatile alkaloid derived from tobacco (*Nicotiana* spp.) and responsible for many of its effects; it first stimulates (small doses), then depresses (large doses) at autonomic ganglia and myoneural junctions; an important tool in physiologic and pharmacologic investigation; used as an insecticide and fumigant.

**nic·o·tine gum** (nik′ŏ-tēn gŭm) Polacrilex chewing gum that contains nicotine; developed as an aid in smoking cessation; now available as an over-the-counter product in various dosages.

**nic·o·tine loz·enge** (nik′ŏ-tēn loz′enj) A slow-dissolving troche developed as an aid in smoking cessation.

**nic·o·tine na·sal spray** (nik′ŏ-tēn nā′zăl sprā) A nicotine withdrawal product for patients' intranasal use to aid in smoking cessation.

**nic·o·tine patch** (nik′ŏ-tēn pach) A transdermal form of nicotine withdrawal therapy available in various dosages.

■**nic·o·tine sto·ma·ti·tis** (nik′ŏ-tēn stō′mă-tī′tis) Heat-stimulated lesions, usually on palate, which begin with erythema and progress to multiple white papules with a red dot in the center. The red dot represents a dilated, inflamed salivary duct orifice. See page A10.

**nic·o·tin·ic ac·id** (nik′ō-tin′ik as′id) A part of the vitamin B3 complex; used in the prevention and treatment of pellagra, as a vasodilator, and as an agent to increase levels of high-density lipoproteins. SYN niacin.

**nic·o·tin·ic cho·lin·er·gic re·cep·tor** (nik′ŏ-tin′ik kō′li-nĕr′jik rĕ-sep′tŏr) Receptors responsive to acetylcholine that also are activated by nicotine.

**nic·ti·tate** (nik'ti-tāt) To wink.

**nic·ti·tat·ing spasm** (nik'ti-tāt-ing spazm) Involuntary spasmodic winking.

**nic·ti·ta·tion** (nik'ti-tā'shŭn) Winking. [L. *nicto,* pp. *-atus,* to wink, fr. *nico,* to beckon]

**ni·dus,** pl. **ni·di** (nī'dŭs, -dī) 1. A nest. 2. Nucleus or central point of origin of a nerve. 3. Focus of infection. [L. nest]

**night guard** (nīt gahrd) Removable acrylic appliance intended to relieve temporomandibular joint pain and other effects of bruxism. SYN occlusal guard.

**Ni·kol·sky sign** (ni-kol'skē sīn) A peculiar vulnerability of the skin in pemphigus vulgaris; the apparently normal epidermis can be separated at the basal layer and rubbed off when pressed with a sliding motion.

**ninth cra·ni·al nerve [CN IX]** (nīnth krā'nē-ăl nĕrv) SYN glossopharyngeal nerve [CN IX].

**NIOSH** Abbreviation for National Institute for Occupational Safety and Health.

**ni·trite** (nī'trīt) A salt of nitrous acid.

**ni·tri·toid re·ac·tion** (nī'troyd rē-ak'shŭn) Severe reaction resembling that following the administration of nitrites, sometimes following intravenous administration of arsphenamine or other drugs; involves facial flushing, edema of tongue and lips, vomiting, profuse sweating, falling blood pressure, and sometimes death.

**ni·tro·fu·rans** (nī'trō-fyūr'anz) Antimicrobials (e.g., nitrofurazone) effective against gram-positive and gram-negative organisms.

**ni·tro·fu·ran·to·in** (nī'trō-fyūr-an'tō-in) Urinary antibacterial agent with a wide range of activity against both gram-positive and gram-negative organisms.

**ni·tro·gen (N)** (nī'trō-jĕn) A gaseous element that forms about 78.084% by volume of dry atmosphere; used as a diluent for medicinal gases, and for air replacement in pharmaceutical preparations. [L. *nitrum,* niter, + *-gen,* to produce]

**ni·tro·gen bal·ance** (nī'trŏ-jĕn bal'ăns) The difference between the total nitrogen intake by an organism and its total nitrogen loss.

**ni·tro·glyc·er·in** (nī'trō-glis'ĕr-in) Explosive, yellowish, oily fluid formed by action of sulfuric and nitric acids on glycerin; used as a vasodilator, especially in angina pectoris.

**ni·tro·sa·mines** (nī-trō'să-mēnz) Amines substituted by a nitroso (NO) group, usually on a nitrogen atom, to yield *N*-nitrosamines; some are mutagenic and/or carcinogenic.

**ni·trous ac·id (HNO₂)** (nī'trŭs as'id) A standard biologic and clinical laboratory reagent.

**ni·trous ox·ide** (nī'trŭs ok'sīd) Nonflammable, nonexplosive gas that will support combustion; widely used as a quick acting, reversible, nondepressant, and nontoxic inhalation analgesic to supplement other anesthetics and analgesics.

**NKA** Abbreviation for no known allergies.

**nm** Abbreviation for nanometer.

**NMR** Abbreviation for nuclear magnetic resonance.

**no·ble met·al** (nō'bĕl met'ăl) Any metallic element used in dental restorations and appliances that resists tarnish, corrosion, and oxidation during heating or in intraoral environments (e.g., gold, platinum).

**No·car·di·a** (nō-kahr'dē-ă) A genus of aerobic, higher bacteria, containing weakly acid-fast, slender rods or filaments, frequently swollen and occasionally branched, forming a mycelium; mainly saprophytic but may cause mycetoma or nocardiosis.

**no·car·di·o·sis** (nō-kahr'dē-ō'sis) Generalized disease caused by *Nocardia asteroides* and other species; characterized by primary pulmonary lesions that may be subclinical or chronic with hematogenous spread to deep viscera, including central nervous system; most common in immunosuppressed patients.

**noci-** Combining form meaning hurt, pain, injury. [L. *noceo*]

**no·ci·cep·tive** (nō'si-sep'tiv) Capable of appreciation or transmission of pain.

**no·ci·cep·tor** (nō'si-sep'tŏr) Peripheral nerve organ or mechanism for the reception and transmission of painful or injurious stimuli. [*noci-* + L. *capio,* to take]

**no·ci·fen·sor re·flex** (nō'si-fen'sŏr rē'fleks) Vascular dilation in a body part surrounding an injury or in its neighborhood.

**node** (nōd) [TA] 1. A knob or nodosity; a circumscribed swelling; in anatomy, a circumscribed mass of tissue. 2. A circumscribed mass of differentiated tissue. [L. *nodus,* a knot]

**nod·ule** (nod'yūl) 1. A small node; in skin, a node up to 1.0 cm in diameter, solid, with palpable depth. See page 402. 2. A pulmonary or pleural lesion seen on a radiographic image as a well-defined, discrete, roughly circular opacity. [L. *nodulus,* dim. of *nodus,* knot]

**no·ma** (nō'mă) Gangrenous stomatitis, usually beginning in mucous membrane of corner of mouth or cheek, then progressing fairly rapidly to involve entire thickness of lips or cheek (or both), with conspicuous necrosis and complete sloughing of tissue; usually observed in poorly nourished children and debilitated adults, espe-

mn

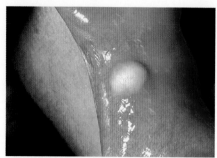

**nodule:** irritation fibroma at commissure

cially in poorer socioeconomic groups, and frequently preceded by another disease, e.g., kala azar, dysentery, or scarlet fever. SYN cancrum oris. [G. *nomē,* a spreading (sore)]

**no·men·cla·ture** (nō′měn-klā-chŭr) A set system of names used in any science, as of anatomic structures, organisms, and other classifications. [L. *nomenclatura,* a listing of names, fr. *nomen,* name, + *calo,* to proclaim]

**nom·o·gram** (nō′mō-gram) Linear chart showing scales for the variables involved in a particular formula such that corresponding values for each variable lie in a straight line intersecting all the scales. [G. *nomos,* law, + *gramma,* something written]

**non·ab·sorb·a·ble sur·gi·cal su·ture** (non′ăb-sōr′bă-ĕl sŭr′ji-kăl sū′chŭr) Type of suture material relatively unaffected by biologic activities of body tissues and therefore permanent unless removed; e.g., stainless steel, silk, cotton, and nylon and other synthetic materials.

**non·an·a·tom·ic teeth** (non′an′ă-tom′ik tēth) **1.** Teeth with occlusal surfaces not based on anatomic forms. **2.** Artificial teeth so designed that occlusal surfaces are not copied from natural forms, but rather are given forms that, in the opinion of the designer, seem more nearly to fulfill requirements of mastication, tissue tolerance, and other considerations.

**non·ar·con ar·tic·u·la·tor** (non-ahr′kon ahrtik′yū-lā-tŏr) Articulator type with equivalent condylar guides attached to lower member and hinge axis to upper.

**non·car·i·o·gen·ic** (non-kar′ē-ō-jen′ik) Not producing caries.

**non·car·i·ous den·tal le·sion** (non-kar′ē-ŭs den′tăl lē′zhŭn) A defect occurring in the enamel of the tooth not classified as decay unless (or until) it progresses. Incipient lesions are considered the initial breakdown of tooth structure. Abrasion, abfraction lesions, and erosion are other forms of noncarious lesions caused by mechanical or chemical factors.

**non·co·he·sive gold** (non′kō-hē′siv gōld) Gold that will not weld because gases adsorb to

the surface; some forms may be made cohesive by heat treatment; in dentistry, used as a direct filling material.

**non·com·pli·ance** (non′kŏm-plī′ăns) Failure by a patient to carry out a prescribed or agreed on regimen of dental or medical therapy.

**non·con·vul·sive sei·zure** (non′kŏn-vŭl′ siv sē′zhŭr) Seizure without clonic, tonic, or other convulsive motor activity.

**non·de·po·lar·iz·ing re·lax·ant** (non′dē-pō′lăr-īz-ing rĕ-laks′ănt) Agent (e.g., tubocurarine) that paralyzes skeletal muscle without depolarization of motor endplate.

**non·dis·ease** (non′di-zēz′) Absence of disease when a specific disease is suspected but not found.

**non·dom·i·nant hand** (non-dom′i-nănt hand) Hand not used for writing or other activities requiring fine motor skills.

**non·es·sen·tial a·mi·no ac·id** (non′ĕ-sen′shăl ă-mē′nō as′id) Any alpha-amino acid required for normal health and growth that can be synthesized within the body without requiring regular consumption of said amino acid.

**non-Hodg·kin lym·pho·ma** (non-hoj′kin lim-fō′mă) A lymphoma other than Hodgkin disease, classified nodular or diffuse tumor pattern and cell type.

**non·in·fec·tious** (non′in-fek′shŭs) Not infectious; not able to spread disease.

**non·in·su·lin-de·pen·dent di·a·be·tes mel·li·tus** (non-in′sŭ-lin-dĕ-pen′dĕnt dī′ă-bē′tēz mel′i-tŭs) Former designation for Type 2 diabetes (q.v.).

**non·in·va·sive** (non′in-vā′siv) Denoting procedure that does not require insertion of an instrument or device through the skin or a body orifice for diagnosis or treatment.

**non·ker·at·i·niz·ed mu·co·sa** (non-ker′ă-ti-nīzd myū-kō′să) Lining mucosa in which the stratified squamous epithelial cells retain their nuclei and cytoplasm.

**non·la·mel·lar bone** (non′lă-mel′ăr bōn) SYN woven bone.

**non·nu·tri·tive suck·ing** (non-nū′tri-tiv sŭk′ing) The sucking patterns used by infants to self-calm, regulate, organize, and explore; not associated with feeding.

**non·oc·clu·sion** (non′ŏ-klū′shŭn) Failure of a tooth to contact an opposing tooth.

**non·pit·ting e·de·ma** (non-pit′ing ĕ-dē′mă) Swelling of subcutaneous tissues that cannot be easily indented by compression.

**non-plaque-in·duc·ed gin·gi·vi·tis** (non-plak′in-dūst′ jin′ji-vī′tis) Inflammation, tenderness, and bleeding of gums associated with local irritants.

**non·pro·pri·e·tar·y name** (non'prŏ-prī'ĕ-tar-ē năm) Short name (often called a generic name) of a chemical, drug, or other substance not subject to trademark (proprietary) rights but is, in contrast to a trivial name, recognized or recommended by government agencies (e.g., U.S. Food and Drug Administration) and by quasiofficial organizations (e.g., U.S. Adopted Names Council) for general public use. Like a proprietary name, it is almost always a coined designation derived without set criteria.

**non·pro·tein ni·tro·gen (NPN)** (non-prō'tēn nī'trŏ-jĕn) The nitrogen content of other than protein bodies.

**non·re·breath·ing an·es·the·si·a** (non' rē-brēdh'ing an'es-thē'zē-ă) Technique for inhalation anesthesia in which valves exhaust all exhaled air from the circuit.

**non·re·breath·ing mask** (non'rē-brēdh'ing mask) Mask fitted with both inhalation and exhalation valves so that all exhaled gas is vented to external atmosphere and inhaled gas comes only from a reservoir connected to the mask.

**non·re·breath·ing valve** (non'rē-brēdh' ing valv) Type of valve that prevents mixture of inhaled and exhaled gases.

**non·rig·id con·nec·tor** (non-rij'id kŏ-nek' tŏr) A connector or joint in a dental appliance that is not rigid or solid.

**non·ste·roi·dal an·ti·in·flam·ma·to·ry drugs (NSAIDs)** (non'ster-oyd'ăl an'tē-in-flam'ă-tōr-ē drŭgz) Agents exerting antiinflammatory (and also usually analgesic and antipyretic) actions; examples include aspirin and ibuprofen.

**non·sur·gi·cal per·i·o·don·tal ther·a·py** (non-sŭr'ji-kăl per'ē-ō-don'tăl thār'ă-pē) Dental biofilm removal and control, supragingival and subgingival scaling, root planing, and adjunctive treatments such as use of pharmacotherapy; basic objectives are to restore periodontal health, arrest or slow progression of early periodontal disease, or, for patients with more advanced disease, to prepare tissues for further and more complex periodontal therapy.

**non·throm·bo·cy·to·pe·nic pur·pu·ra** (non-throm'bō-sī'tō-pē'nik pŭr'pyŭr-ă) SYN purpura simplex.

**non·vi·tal bleach·ing** (non-vī'tăl blēch' ing) Bleaching of a tooth or teeth, usually after endodontic treatment, to remove stains.

**non·vi·tal pulp** (non-vī'tăl pŭlp) SYN necrotic pulp.

**non·work·ing cut·ting edge** (non'wŏrk' ing kŭt'ing ej) Cutting edge on the working-end

of an area-specific curette not used for calculus removal.

**non·work·ing side con·dyle** (non'wŏrk' ng sīd kon'dīl) Condyle that moves on the side of the mandible that moves toward the midline in a lateral excursion. SYN orbiting condyle.

**nor-** Chemical prefix denoting: **1.** Elimination of one methylene group from a chain, the highest permissible locant being used. **2.** Contraction of a (steroid) ring by one $CH_2$ unit. **3.** Chemical prefix denoting "normal," i.e., unbranched chain of carbon atoms in aliphatic compounds.

**nor·ep·i·neph·rine** (nōr'ep-i-nef'rin) Catecholamine hormone with strong vasoconstrictive effects; used pharmacologically as a vasopressor, primarily as the bitartrate salt.

**norm** (nōrm) **1.** The usual value. **2.** The desirable value or behavior.

**nor·mal (N)** (nōr'măl) **1.** Typical; usual; according to the rule or standard. **2.** Referring to a straight line (or plane) at a right angle to another line (or plane). **3.** Not diseased or having been subjected to an experimental procedure. [L. *normalis,* according to pattern]

**nor·mal bite** (nōr'măl bīt) SYN normal occlusion.

**nor·mal dis·tri·bu·tion** (nōr'măl dis'tri-byū'shŭn) Specific bell-shaped frequency distribution commonly assumed by statisticians to represent the infinite population of measurements from which a sample has been drawn.

**nor·mal hu·man plas·ma** (nōr'măl hyū' măn plaz'mă) Sterile plasma obtained by pooling approximately equal amounts of the liquid portion of citrated whole blood from eight or more adult humans who have been certified as free from any disease that is transmissible by transfusion, and treating it with ultraviolet irradiation to destroy possible bacterial and viral contaminants.

**normalisation** [Br.] SYN normalization.

**nor·mal·i·za·tion** (nōr'măl-ī-zā'shŭn) Bringing something into conformance with a standard or norm. SYN normalisation.

**nor·mal·ly posed tooth** (nōr'mă-lē pōzd tūth) Tooth in correct spatial relationship with its antagonist.

**nor·mal oc·clu·sion** (nōr'măl ŏ-klū'zhŭn) **1.** Arrangement of teeth and their supporting structures that is usually found in health and approaches ideal or standard arrangement. **2.** SYN neutral occlusion.

**normo-** Combining form denoting normal, usual. [L. *normalis,* according to pattern]

**nor·mo·blast** (nōr'mō-blast) A nucleated red blood cell, the immediate precursor of a normal erythrocyte in humans. [*normo-* + G. *blastos,* sprout, germ]

**norm·os·mi·a** (nōrm-oz′mē-ă) Normal sense of smell. [*normo-* + G. *osmē,* smell, + *-ia*]

**norm·os·mic** (nōrm-oz′mik) Having normal olfactory sensation. [*normo-* + G. *osmē,* smell]

**nor·mo·ten·sive** (nōr′mō-ten′siv) Indicating a normal arterial blood pressure. SYN normotonic (2).

**nor·mo·ton·ic** (nōr′mō-ton′ik) 1. Relating to or characterized by normal muscular tone. SYN eutonic. 2. SYN normotensive.

**Nor·walk vi·rus** (nōr′wawk vī′rŭs) A virus associated with acute viral gastroenteritis.

**nose** (nōz) Specialized organ at entrance of respiratory system that conducts, warms, humidifies, and cleans inspired air and houses olfactory neuroepithelium; includes both external nose and nasal cavities. [A.S. *nosu*]

**nose·bleed** (nōz′blēd) SYN epistaxis.

**nose drops** (nōz drops) Liquid preparation intended for intranasal administration with a medicine dropper. Most frequently used for decongestion of the nasal passages but can be used for any other appropriate indication.

**nos·o·co·mi·al** (nō′zō-kō′mē-ăl) 1. Relating to a hospital. 2. Denoting a new disorder (not the patient's original condition) associated with being treated in a hospital, such as a hospital-acquired infection. [G. *nosokomeion,* hospital, fr. *nosos,* disease, + *komeō,* to take care of]

**no·so·hu·si·al** (nō′zō-hū′zē-ăl) Denotes those infections acquired by patients receiving home-based care.

**no·so·trop·ic** (nō′zō-trō′pik) Therapy directed against pathologic changes or symptoms of a disease. [G. *nosos,* disease + *tropē,* a turning]

**nos·trum** (nos′trŭm) General term for therapeutic agent, sometimes patented but usually of secret composition, offered to the general public as a specific remedy for any disease or class of diseases. Term currently carries a pejorative connotation. [L. neuter of *noster,* our, "our own remedy"]

**notch** (noch) [TA] 1. An indentation at the edge of any structure. 2. Any short, narrow, V-shaped deviation, whether positive or negative, in a linear tracing.

**notch·ed teeth** (nocht tēth) SYN Hutchinson teeth.

**no·ti·fi·a·ble dis·ease** (nō′ti-fī′ă-běl di-zēz′) Disease that, by statutory requirements, must be reported to the public health or veterinary authorities when the diagnosis is made because of its importance to human or animal health. SYN reportable disease.

**no·to·chord** (nō′tō-kōrd) In embryos, the axial fibrocellular cord about which vertebral primordia develop; vestiges persist in the adult as the nuclei pulposi of the intervertebral discs. [G. *nōtos,* back, + *chordē,* cord, string]

**nour·ish·ment** (nŭr′ish-měnt) A substance used to feed or to sustain life and growth of an organism. SYN aliment.

**nox·a** (nok′să) Anything that exerts a harmful influence (e.g., trauma, poison). [L. injury, fr. *noceo,* to injure]

**nox·ious** (nok′shŭs) Injurious; harmful. [L. *noxius,* injurious, fr. *noceo,* to injure]

**NPH in·su·lin** (in′sŭ-lin) Modified form of insulin composed of insulin, protamine, and zinc; an intermediate-acting preparation used for the treatment of diabetes mellitus. SYN isophane insulin. [*N*eutral *P*rotamine *H*agedorn]

**NPN** Abbreviation for nonprotein nitrogen.

**NPO, npo** Abbreviation for L. *non per os* or *nil per os,* nothing by mouth.

**NPU** Abbreviation for net protein utilization.

**NSAIDs** Abbreviation for nonsteroidal anti-inflammatory drugs.

**nu·chal ri·gid·i·ty** (nū′kăl ri-jid′i-tē) Impaired neck flexion due to muscle spasm (not actual rigidity) of the extensor muscles of the neck; usually attributed to meningeal irritation.

**nu·cle·ar a·gen·e·sis** (nū′klē-ăr ā-jen′ĕ-sis) SYN Moebius syndrome.

**nu·cle·ar fam·i·ly** (nū′klē-ăr fam′i-lē) In genetics, two parents and their progeny in common.

**nu·cle·ar mag·net·ic res·o·nance (NMR)** (nū′klē-ăr mag-net′ik rez′ŏ-năns) The phenomenon in which certain atomic nuclei possessing a magnetic moment will precess around the axis of a strong external magnetic field, the frequency of precession being specific for each nucleus and the strength of the magnetic field; spinning nuclei induce their own oscillating magnetic fields and therefore emit electromagnetic radiation that can produce a detectable signal. NMR is used as a method of identifying covalent bonds and is applied clinically in magnetic resonance imaging.

**nu·cle·ic ac·id** (nū-klē′ik as′id) A family of macromolecules found in chromosomes, nucleoli, mitochondria, and cytoplasm of all cells; in complexes with proteins, called nucleoproteins.

**nu·cle·i·form** (nū′klē-i-fōrm) Shaped like or having the appearance of a nucleus.

**nu·cle·oid** (nū′klē-oyd) **1.** A nuclear inclusion body. **2.** SYN nucleus (2). [*nucleo-* + G. *eidos,* resemblance]

**nu·cle·o·pro·tein** (nū′klē-ō-prō′tēn) A complex of protein and nucleic acid, the form in which essentially all nucleic acids exist in nature.

**nu·cle·o·side** (nū′klē-ō-sīd) A compound of a sugar (usually ribose or deoxyribose) with a purine or pyrimidine base.

**nu·cle·us,** pl. **nu·cle·us·es** (nū′klē-ŭs, -ĕz) **1.** [TA] In cytology, typically a rounded or oval mass of protoplasm within the cytoplasm of a plant or animal cell. **2.** By extension, because of similar function, genome of microorganisms (microbes), which is relatively simple in structure, lacks a nuclear envelope or membrane and does not undergo mitosis during replication. SYN nucleoid (3). **3.** [TA] In neuroanatomy, group of nerve cell bodies in brain or spinal cord that can be demarcated from neighboring groups on the basis of either differences in cell type or the presence of a surrounding zone of nerve fibers or cell-poor neuropil. **4.** Any substance (e.g., foreign body, mucus, crystal) around which a urinary or other calculus has formed.

**NUG** Abbreviation for necrotizing ulcerative gingivitis.

**Nuhn gland** (nūn gland) SYN anterior lingual gland.

**null hy·poth·e·sis** (nŭl hī-poth′ĕ-sis) Statistical proposition that one variable has no association with another variable or set of variables, or that two or more populations do not differ from each other; the statement that results do not differ from those that might be expected by the operation of chance alone; if rejected, it increases confidence in the hypothesis.

**numb chin syn·drome** (nŭm chin sin′ drōm) Paresthesia and sensory loss affecting one side of chin and lower lip, resulting from neoplastic infiltration of the ipsilateral mental nerve; common causes include multiple myeloma and carcinoma of breast or prostate.

**num·ber** (nŭm′bĕr) **1.** A symbol expressive of a certain value or of a specific quantity determined by count. **2.** The place of any unit in a series. [L. *numero*]

**numb·ness** (nŭm′nĕs) Imprecise term for abnormal sensation, including absent or reduced sensory perception as well as paresthesias.

**num·mu·lar** (nŭm′yū-lăr) Discoid or coin-shaped; denoting thick mucous or mucopurulent sputum in certain respiratory diseases, so called because of the disc shape assumed when it is flattened on the bottom of a sputum mug containing water or transparent disinfectant or shape of lesions in nummular eczema. [L. *nummulus,* small coin, dim. of *nummus,* coin]

**NUP** Abbreviation for necrotizing ulcerative periodontitis.

**nurse** (nŭrs) **1.** To breast-feed; suckle. **2.** To provide care for the sick. **3.** One who is educated in the scientific basis of nursing under defined standards of education and is concerned with the diagnosis and treatment of human responses to actual or potential health problems.

**nurse a·nes·the·tist** (nŭrs ă-nes′thĕ-tist) A registered nurse qualified to administer anesthesia, in both inpatient and outpatient settings; in the U.S., the title "certified registered nurse anesthetist" (CRNA) is conferred on registered nurses with at least 1 year of acute care experience who complete a graduate program recognized by the American Association of Nurse Anesthetists and pass a national certification examination; CRNAs are the sole providers of anesthesia in most rural U.S. hospitals.

**nurse mid·wife** (nŭrs mid′wīf) A registered nurse who specializes in midwifery; in some governmental jurisdictions, requires additional training and special licensure.

**nurse prac·ti·tion·er** (nŭrs prak-tish′ŭn-ĕr) Registered nurse with at least a master's degree in nursing and advanced education in primary care of particular groups of patients.

**nurs·ing** (nŭrs′ing) **1.** Feeding an infant at the breast; tending and caring for a child. **2.** The scientific application of principles of care related to prevention of illness and care during illness.

**nurs·ing bot·tle ca·ries** (nŭrs′ing bot′ĕl kar′ēz) SYN baby bottle tooth decay.

**nurs·ing home** (nŭrs′ing hōm) SYN extended-care facility.

**Nurs·ing In·ter·ven·tions Clas·si·fi·ca·tion (NIC)** (nŭrs′ing in-tĕr-ven′shŭnz klas′i-fi-kā′shŭn) Standardized classification of patient/client outcomes for evaluating effects of nursing interventions.

**nu·tra·ceu·ti·cal** (nū′tră-sū′ti-kăl) A chemical substance or group of substances that for legal purposes is defined as a nutrient but in fact is marketed and used to prevent or treat disease. [*nutr*-ient + pharm-*aceutical*]

**nu·tri·ent** (nū′trē-ĕnt) Constituent of food necessary for normal physiologic function. [L. *nutriens,* fr. *nutrio,* to nourish]

**nu·tri·ent ca·nal** (nū′trē-ĕnt kă-nal′) [TA] A canal in the shaft of a long bone or in other locations in irregular bones through which the nutrient artery enters a bone. SYN canalis nutricius [TA].

**nu·tri·ent dense** (nū′trē-ĕnt dens) Denotes foods providing a higher nutrient value in relationship to calories than other foods.

**nu·tri·tion** (nū-trish′ŭn) **1.** Function of living

plants and animals, consisting of ingestion and metabolism of food material whereby tissue is built up and energy liberated. **2.** Study of dietary requirements of human beings or animals for normal physiologic function. [L. *nutritio,* fr. *nutrio,* to nourish]

**nu·tri·tion·al de·fi·cien·cy** (nū-trish´ŭn-ăl dĕ-fish´ĕn-sē) Inadequacy of nutrients in tissues; result of inadequate dietary intake or impairment of digestion, absorption, transport, or metabolism.

**nu·tri·tive e·qui·lib·ri·um** (nū´tri-tiv ē´kwi-lib´rē-ŭm) Condition in which there is a perfect balance between intake and excretion of nutritive material, so that no weight is gained or lost.

**nu·tri·ture** (nū´tri-chŭr) State or condition of body nutrition. [L. *nutritura,* a nursing, fr. *nutrio,* to nourish]

**nyc·tal·gi·a** (nik-tal´jē-ă) Pain that characteristically occurs at night (e.g., nocturnal bone pain experienced by patients with syphilis).

**nys·tag·mus** (nis-tag´mŭs) Involuntary rhythmic oscillation of the eyeballs. [G. *nystagmos,* a nodding, fr. *nystazō,* to be sleepy, nod]

**ny·stat·in** (nī-stat´in) Antibiotic substance isolated from cultures of *Streptomyces noursei,* effective in treatment of all forms of candidiasis, particularly candidal infections of intestine, skin, and mucous membranes. [*New York State* + *-in*]

# O

**oath** (ōth) A solemn affirmation or attestation.

**OB** Abbreviation for obstetrics.

**o·be·si·ty** (ō-bē'si-tē) Excess of subcutaneous fat in proportion to lean body mass. Excess fat accumulation is associated with increase in size (hypertrophy) as well as number (hyperplasia) of adipose tissue cells. Obesity is variously defined in terms of absolute weight, weight:height ratio, distribution of subcutaneous fat, and societal and esthetic norms. Although faulty eating habits related to failure of normal satiety feedback mechanisms may be responsible for some cases, many obese people neither consume more calories nor eat different proportions of foodstuffs than nonobese people. Contrary to popular belief, obesity is not caused by disorders of pituitary, thyroid, or suprarenal gland metabolism. However, it is often associated with hyperinsulinism and relative insulin resistance. Studies of obese twins strongly suggest the presence of genetic influences on resting metabolic rate, feeding behavior, changes in energy expenditures in response to overfeeding, lipoprotein lipase activity, and basal rate of lipolysis. Environmental factors associated with obesity include socioeconomic status, race, geographic region of residence, season, urban, or rural residence, and being a member of a smaller family. Prevalence is greater when weight is measured during winter rather than summer; is much more common in the southeastern U.S., although northeastern and midwestern states also have high rates, a phenomenon independent of race, population density, and season. SYN adiposity (1). [L. *obesus*, pp. of *obedo*, to eat up, + *-ity*]

**ob·jec·tive** (ŏb-jek'tiv) Lens or lenses in object end of the body tube of a microscope by means of which rays coming from object examined are brought to a focus. [L. *ob-jicio*, pp. *-jectus*, to throw before]

**ob·lique** (ō-blēk') **1.** Slanting; deviating from perpendicular, horizontal, sagittal, or coronal plane of body. **2.** In radiography, projection that is neither frontal nor lateral. [L. *obliquus*]

**ob·lique pro·jec·tion** (ō-blēk' prŏ-jek'shŭn) Radiographic projection between frontal and lateral.

**ob·lique ridge** (ō-blēk' rij) Bony ridge on lateral aspect of anterior border of ramus of mandible that runs downward and onto body of the mandible laterally to third and second molar teeth.

**ob·lique strokes** (ō-blēk' strōks) Instrumentation strokes using a pulling action diagonal to the long axis of the tooth; used most commonly on facial and lingual surfaces.

**ob·lique tech·nique** (ō-blēk' tek-nēk') Using the working-end of an electronically powered instrument with lateral surface in an oblique—almost horizontal—orientation to long axis of tooth. The tip is positioned in a similar manner to that of the working-end of a curette.

**ob·lit·er·a·tion** (ŏb-lit'ĕr-ā'shŭn) In radiology, disappearance of organ contour when adjacent tissue has same x-ray absorption.

**ob·lit·er·a·tive bron·chi·tis, bron·chi·tis ob·lit·e·rans** (ŏb-lit'ĕr-ă'tiv brong-kī' tis, ŏb-lit'ĕr-anz) Fibrinous bronchitis in which exudate becomes organized, obliterating affected portion of bronchial tubes with consequent permanent collapse of affected portions of lung.

**ob·ses·sive-com·pul·sive dis·or·der (OCD)** (ŏb-ses'iv-kŏm-pŭl'siv dis-ōr'dĕr) Type of anxiety disorder the essential features of which include recurrent obsessions, persistent intrusive ideas, thoughts, impulses or images, or compulsions.

**ob·ste·tri·cian** (ŏb'stĕ-trish'ŭn) A physician specializing in the medical care of women during pregnancy and childbirth. SEE obstetrics.

**ob·stet·rics (OB)** (ob-stet'riks) The specialty of medicine concerned with the care of women during pregnancy, parturition, and the puerperium. [L. *obstetrix*, a midwife, fr. *ob-sto*, to stand before, denoting the position formerly taken by the midwife]

**ob·struc·tion** (ŏb-strŭk'shŭn) Blockage, clogging, or impeded flow. [L. *obstructio*]

**ob·struc·tive jaun·dice** (ŏb-strŭk'tiv jawn' dis) Hepatic disorder resulting from obstruction to the flow of bile into the duodenum, whether intra- or extrahepatic. SYN mechanical jaundice.

**ob·struc·tive pneu·mo·ni·a** (ŏb-strŭk' tiv nū-mō'nē-ă) Pulmonary infection of airway due to obstruction by narrowing resulting from disease process, persistent bronchospasm, thick secretions, or by foreign body aspiration.

**ob·tund** (ob-tŭnd') To dull or blunt, especially to blunt sensation or deaden pain. [L. *ob-tundo*, pp. *-tusus*, to beat against, blunt]

**ob·tu·ra·tion** (ob'tŭr-ā'shŭn) Obstruction or occlusion. SEE obturator.

**ob·tu·ra·tor** (ob'tŭr-ā-tŏr) **1.** A prosthesis used to close an opening in the hard palate, usually in a cleft palate. **2.** Any structure that occludes an opening. **3.** Denoting obturator foramen, obturator membrane, or any of several parts in relation to this foramen. **4.** The stylus or removable plug used during the insertion of many tubular instruments. [L. *obturo*, pp. *-atus*, to occlude or stop up]

**ob·tu·ra·tor ap·pli·ance** (ob'tŭr-ā-tŏr ă-plī'ăns) Device used to obliterate congenital or acquired defects of palate and surrounding structures, usually made of acrylic or rubber.

**ob·tu·sion** (ŏb-tū´zhŭn) A dulling or deadening of sensibility.

**oc·cip·i·tal** (ok-sip´i-tăl) Relating to occiput; referring to occipital bone or back of the head.

**oc·cip·i·tal an·chor·age** (ok-sip´i-tăl ang´kŏr-ăj) Anchorage in which top and back of head are used for resistance by means of a headgear.

**oc·cip·i·tal an·gle of pa·ri·e·tal bone** (ok-sip´i-tăl ang´gĕl păr-ī´ĕ-tăl bōn) [TA] **1.** The posterior superior angle of the parietal bone. SYN Broca angles (3). **2.** An angle formed by junction, at the opisthion, of lines coming from the basion and from the projection in the median plane of the lower border of the orbits. SYN angulus occipitalis ossis parietalis.

**oc·cip·i·tal bone** (ok-sip´i-tăl bōn) [TA] Bone at lower and posterior part of cranium, consisting of three parts (basilar, condylar, and squamous), enclosing a large oval hole, the foramen magnum.

**oc·cip·i·tal branch** (ok-sip´i-tăl branch) [TA] *Terminologia Anatomica* lists occipital branches of 1) posterior auricular artery; 2) posterior auricular nerve; and 3) occipital artery.

**oc·cip·i·tal con·dyle** (ok-sip´i-tăl kon´dīl) [TA] One of two elongated oval facets on the undersurface of the occipital bone, one on each side of the foramen magnum, which articulate with the atlas.

**oc·cip·i·tal groove** (ok-sip´i-tăl grūv) [TA] Narrow groove medial to mastoid notch of temporal bone that lodges occipital artery.

**oc·cip·i·tal lymph nodes** (ok-sip´i-tăl limf nōdz) [TA] Lymphoid tissue located ner the occipital bone.

**oc·cip·i·tal plane** (ok-sip´i-tăl plān) [TA] External surface of occipital bone above superior nuchal line.

**oc·clude** (ŏ-klūd´) **1.** To close or bring together. **2.** To enclose, as in an occluded virus.

**oc·clud·er** (ŏ-klūd´ĕr) In dentistry, specific type of articulator.

**oc·clud·ing cen·tric re·la·tion re·cord** (ŏ-klūd´ing sen´trik rĕ-lā´shŭn rek´ŏrd) Registration of centric relation made at established occlusal vertical dimension.

**oc·clud·ing frame** (ŏ-klūd´ing frām) SYN articulator.

**oc·clud·ing paper** (ŏ-klūd´ing pā´pĕr) Inked paper or ribbon interposed between natural or artificial teeth to determine tooth contacts. SYN articulating paper.

**oc·clud·ing re·la·tion** (ŏ-klūd´ing rĕ-lā´shŭn) Jaw relation at which opposing teeth occlude.

**oc·clu·sal** (ŏ-klū´zăl) **1.** Pertaining to occlusion or closure. **2.** In dentistry, pertaining to the contacting surfaces of opposing occlusal units (teeth or occlusion rims) or masticating surfaces of posterior teeth.

**oc·clu·sal ad·just·ment** (ŏ-klū´zăl ă-jŭst´mĕnt) Modification of occluding and incising surfaces of teeth to develop harmonious relationships between these surfaces.

**oc·clu·sal a·nal·y·sis** (ŏ-klū´zăl ă-nal´i-sis) Study of relations of occlusal surfaces of opposing teeth and their effect on related structures. SYN bite analysis.

**oc·clu·sal bal·ance** (ŏ-klū´zăl bal´ăns) Condition in which simultaneous contacts of occluding units of opposing dental arches in centric and eccentric positions are present within functional range.

**oc·clu·sal ca·ries** (ŏ-klū´zăl kar´ēz) Caries starting from occlusal tooth surface.

**oc·clu·sal clear·ance** (ŏ-klū´zăl klēr´ăns) Condition in which opposing occlusal surfaces may glide over one another without any interfering projection.

**oc·clu·sal con·tact** (ŏ-klū´zăl kon´takt) Touching of opposing teeth on elevation of the mandible.

**oc·clu·sal con·tour·ing** (ŏ-klū´zăl kon´tūr-ing) Shaping occlusal surface of tooth or of dental restoration to facilitate function.

**oc·clu·sal cor·rec·tion** (ŏ-klū´zăl kŏr-ek´shŭn) **1.** Correction of malocclusion by whatever means. **2.** Elimination of disharmony of occlusal contacts.

**oc·clu·sal cur·va·ture** (ŏ-klū´zăl kŭr´vă-chŭr) SYN curve of occlusion.

**oc·clu·sal dis·har·mo·ny** (ŏ-klū´zăl dis-hahr´mŏ-nē) **1.** Contacts of opposing occlusal surfaces of teeth that are not in harmony with other tooth contacts and with anatomic and physiologic control of mandible. **2.** Occlusions that do not coincide with their respective jaw relations. SEE ALSO deflective occlusal contact.

**oc·clu·sal em·bra·sure** (ŏ-klū´zăl em-brā´shŭr) Space existing on occlusal aspect of interproximal contact areas between adjacent posterior teeth.

**oc·clu·sal e·quil·i·bra·tion** (ŏ-klū´zăl ē-kwil´i-brā´shŭn) Modification of occlusal forms of teeth by grinding to equalize occlusal stress, or of producing simultaneous occlusal contacts, or of harmonizing cuspal relations.

**oc·clu·sal film** (ŏ-klū´zăl film) SYN occlusal radiograph.

**oc·clu·sal force** (ŏ-klū´zăl fōrs) Result of muscular force applied on opposing teeth.

**oc·clu·sal form** (ŏ-klū´zăl fōrm) Form of the occlusal surface of a tooth or a row of teeth.

**oc·clu·sal glide** (ŏ-klū´zăl glīd) SYN articulation.

**oc·clu·sal guard** (ŏ-klū´zăl gahrd) SYN night guard.

**oc·clu·sal har·mo·ny** (ŏ-klū´zăl hahr´mŏ-nē) Occlusion without deflective or interceptive occlusal contacts in centric jaw relation as well as eccentric movements.

**oc·clu·sal im·bal·ance** (ŏ-klū´zăl im-bal´ăns) Inharmonious relationship between the teeth of the maxilla and mandible during closing or functional movements of the jaw.

**oc·clu·sal in·ter·fer·ence** (ŏ-klū´zăl in´tĕr-fēr´ăns) Tooth cusp contacts that restrict or otherwise impede mandibular movement.

**oc·clu·sal path** (ŏ-klū´zăl path) SYN occlusal pattern.

**oc·clu·sal pat·tern** (ŏ-klū´zăl pat´ĕrn) **1.** Gliding occlusal contact of mandibular teeth against a reference surface attached to maxillary teeth. **2.** Recording of movement of occlusal surfaces. SYN occlusal path.

**oc·clu·sal per·cep·tion** (ŏ-klū´zăl pĕr-sep´shŭn) Denotes the minimal thickness of a material placed between the teeth that can be discriminated; more pronounced in incisors than in canines, premolars, and molars.

**oc·clu·sal piv·ot** (ŏ-klū´zăl piv´ŏt) Artificial elevation placed in the molar region either on the occlusal surface of a tooth or on an interocclusal appliance to cause closing rotation of the mandible and consequently distraction of the mandibular condyle whenever a patient closes on this pivot. This was proposed to reduce compression in patients with inflamed temporomandibular joints. Biomechanically, in the sagittal plane, this distraction does not occur because the combined closing forces of the masticatory muscles are always posterior to the teeth (and thus any pivot point), which will therefore cause compression of the condyle. In the frontal plane, it may be possible to cause a unilateral distraction of a condyle with such a pivot.

**oc·clu·sal plane, plane of oc·clu·sion** (ŏ-klū´zăl plān, ŏ-klū´zhŭn) **1.** Plane established by incisal and occlusal surfaces of teeth. Because occlusal surfaces of teeth do not all lie on a flat surface, the plane is an ''average'' one. SEE ALSO curve of occlusion. **2.** In complete denture fabrication, surface of wax occlusion runs contoured to position teeth in denture. SYN bite plane.

**oc·clu·sal po·si·tion** (ŏ-klū´zăl pŏ-zish´ŏn) Relationship of mandible and maxillae when jaws are closed and teeth are in contact; may or may not coincide with centric occlusion.

**oc·clu·sal pre·ma·tur·i·ty** (ŏ-klū´zăl prē´mă-chŭr´i-tē) Any contact of opposing teeth that occurs before the desirable intercuspation.

**oc·clu·sal pres·sure** (ŏ-klū´zăl presh´ŭr) Any force exerted on occlusal surfaces of teeth.

**oc·clu·sal ra·di·o·graph** (ŏ-klū´zăl rā´dē-ō-graf) Intraoral section film positioned on occlusal plane and used in visualizing entire sections of jaw; especially useful in exploring calcifications of sublingual salivary glands and in viewing eruption patterns of teeth. SYN occlusal film.

**oc·clu·sal rest** (ŏ-klū´zăl rest) Rigid extension of removable partial denture onto occlusal surface of a posterior tooth to support prosthesis. SYN occlusal stop.

**oc·clu·sal rest bar** (ŏ-klū´zăl rest bahr) Minor connector used to attach an occlusal rest to a major part of a removable partial denture.

**oc·clu·sal rim** (ŏ-klū´zăl rim) SYN occlusion rim.

**oc·clu·sal splint** (ŏ-klū´zăl splint) SYN night guard.

**oc·clu·sal stop** (ŏ-klū´zăl stop) SYN occlusal rest.

**oc·clu·sal sur·face of tooth** (ŏ-klū´zăl sŭr´făs tūth) [TA] **1.** Tooth surface that occludes with or contacts an opposing tooth surface in opposing jaw. **2.** SYN denture occlusal surface.

**oc·clu·sal sys·tem** (ŏ-klū´zăl sis´tĕm) Form or design and arrangement of occlusal and incisal units of dentition or teeth on a denture.

**oc·clu·sal ta·ble** (ŏ-klū´zăl tā´bĕl) Occlusal or grinding surfaces of premolar and molar teeth.

**oc·clu·sal trau·ma** (ŏ-klū´zăl traw´mă) Abnormal occlusal stresses that are capable of producing or have produced pathologic changes in teeth and surrounding structures.

**oc·clu·sal ver·ti·cal di·men·sion** (ŏ-klū´zăl vĕr´ti-kăl di-men´shŭn) Dimension of face when teeth or occlusion rims are in contact in centric occlusion; *decrease* may result from modification of tooth form by attrition or grinding, drifting of teeth, or, in edentulous patients, by resorption of residual ridges; *increase* may result from modifications of tooth form, tooth position, height of occlusion rims, rebasing or relining, or occlusal splints.

**oc·clu·sal wear** (ŏ-klū´zăl wār) Attritional loss of substance on opposing occlusal units or surfaces. SEE ALSO abrasion (1).

**oc·clu·sion** (ŏ-klū´zhŭn) **1.** The act of closing or the state of being closed. **2.** Any contact between the incising or masticating surfaces of upper and lower teeth. **3.** Relationship between

**op**

occlusal surfaces of maxillary and mandibular teeth when in contact.

**oc·clu·sion rim** (ŏ-klū´zhŭn rim) **1.** Occluding surfaces built on temporary or permanent denture bases to make maxillomandibular relation records and for arranging teeth. **2.** Baseplate wax fabricated to form a denture base and to support denture teeth during laboratory fabrication of a complete denture. SYN bite rim, record rim.

**oc·cult** (ŏ-kŭlt´) Hidden; concealed; not manifest.

**oc·cu·pa·tion·al der·ma·ti·tis** (ok´yū-pā´shŭn-ăl dĕr´mă-tī´tis) A form of contact dermatitis characterized by erythema, edema, and vesiculation; occupational hazard in dentistry.

**oc·cu·pa·tion·al dis·ease** (ok´yū-pā´shŭn-ăl di-zēz´) Morbid condition resulting from exposure to an agent during usual performance of one's occupation.

**oc·cu·pa·tion·al ex·po·sure** (ok´yū-pā´shŭn-ăl eks-pō´zhŭr) Reasonably anticipated skin, eye, mucous membrane, or parenteral contact with blood, bodily fluids, or other potentially infectious material that may result from the performance of one's professional duties.

**Oc·cu·pa·tion·al Safe·ty and Health Ad·min·i·stra·tion (OSHA)** (ok´yū-pā´shŭn-ăl sāf´tē helth ad-min´i-strā´shŭn) A division of the U.S. Department of Labor, responsible for establishing and enforcing safety and health standards in the workplace.

**OCD** Abbreviation for obsessive-compulsive disorder.

**oc·ta·pres·sin** (ok´tă-pres´in) SYN felypressin.

**oc·ta·vus** (ok-tā´vŭs) SYN vestibulocochlear nerve [CN VIII]. [L.]

**oc·ul·ar a·prax·i·a** (ok´yū-lăr ă-prak´sē-ă) Inability to fixate on certain points in the peripheral visual field despite intact eye movements.

**oc·u·lar bob·bing** (ok´yū-lăr bob´ing) Sudden conjugate downward deviation of eyes with slow return to normal position.

**oc·u·lar cic·a·tri·cial pem·phi·goid** (ok´yū-lăr sik´ă-trish´ăl pem´fi-goyd) SYN benign mucous membrane pemphigoid.

**oc·u·lar hy·per·tel·or·ism** (ok´yū-lăr hī´pĕr-tel´ŏr-izm) Increased width between the eyes due to an enlarged sphenoid bone; other congenital anomalies and mental retardation may be associated. SYN Greig syndrome, Opitz BBB syndrome, Opitz G syndrome.

**oc·u·lar mo·tor a·prax·i·a** (ok´yū-lăr mō´tŏr ă-prak´sē-ă) Congenital inability to initiate horizontal saccades.

**oc·u·lo·au·ric·u·lo·ver·te·bral dys·pla·si·a** (ok´yū-lō-awr-ik´yū-lō-vĕr´tĕ-brăl dis-plā´zē-ă) Syndrome characterized by epibulbar dermoids, preauricular appendages, micrognathia, and vertebral and other anomalies.

**oc·u·lo·den·to·dig·i·tal** (ok´yū-lō-den´tō-dij´i-tăl) Relating to eyes, teeth, and fingers.

**oc·u·lo·den·to·dig·i·tal dys·pla·si·a (ODD)** (ok´yū-lō-den´tō-dij´i-tăl dis-plā´zē-ă) Microphthalmia, coloboma, or anomalies of iris associated with malformed and malpositioned teeth and with anomalies of the fingers.

**oc·ul·o·fa·cial pa·ral·y·sis** (ok´yū-lō-fā´shăl păr-al´i-sis) SYN Moebius syndrome.

**oc·u·lo·man·dib·u·lo·dys·ceph·a·ly** (ok´yū-lō-man-dib´yū-lō-dis-sef´ă-lē) SYN dyscephalia mandibulooculofacialis.

**oc·u·lo·man·dib·u·lo·fa·cial syn·drome** (ok´yū-lō-man-dib´yū-lō-fā´shăl sin´drōm) SYN dyscephalia mandibulooculofacialis.

**oc·u·lo·mo·tor nerve [CN III]** (ok´yū-lō-mō´tŏr nĕrv) [TA] Third cranial nerve; supplies all extrinsic muscles of eye, except lateral rectus and superior oblique. SYN nervus oculomotorius [CN III], third cranial nerve [CN III].

**oc·u·lo·mo·tor re·sponse** (ok´yū-lō-mō´tŏr rĕ-spons´) Widespread myogenic potential evoked by visual stimuli.

**oc·u·lo·pha·ryn·ge·al syn·drome** (ok´yū-lō-fă-rin´jē-ăl sin´drōm) Myopathic disorder with a slowly progressive blepharoptosis and dysphagia, beginning late in life.

**oc·u·lo·ver·te·bral dys·pla·si·a** (ok´yū-lō-vĕr´tĕ-brăl dis-plā´zē-ă) Microphthalmia, colobomas, or anophthalmia with small orbit, twisted face due to unilateral dysplasia of maxilla, macrostomia with malformed teeth and malocclusion, vertebral malformations, and branched and hypoplastic ribs.

**o.d.** Abbreviation for L. *omni die*, every day.

**OD** Abbreviation for drug overdose.

**ODD** Abbreviation for oculodentodigital dysplasia.

✿ **odont-, odonto-** Combining forms meaning a tooth, teeth. [G. *odous* (*odont-*)]

**o·don·tag·ra** (ō´don-tag´ră) Obsolescent term for toothache thought to be of gouty origin. [*odonto-* + G. *agra,* seizure]

**o·don·tal·gi·a** (ō´don-tal´jē-ă) SYN toothache. [*odont-* + G. *algos,* pain]

**o·don·tal·gi·a den·ta·lis** (ō´don-tal´jē-ă den-tā´lis) Reflex auricular pain due to dental disease, usually along auriculotemporal nerve.

**o·don·tal·gic** (ō´don-tal´jik) Relating to or marked by toothache.

**o·don·tec·to·my** (ō′don-tek′tŏ-mē) Removal of teeth by reflection of a mucoperiosteal flap and excision of bone from around root or roots before application of force to effect tooth removal. [*odont-* + G. *ektomē*, excision]

**o·don·ter·ism** (ō-don′tĕr-izm) Chattering of teeth. [*odont-* + G. *erismos*, quarrel]

**o·don·ti·a·sis** (ō′don-tī′ă-sis) SYN teething. [G. *odontiaō*, to cut teeth]

**o·don·ti·noid** (ō-don′ti-noyd) **1.** Resembling dentin. **2.** A small excrescence from a tooth, most common on root or neck. **3.** Toothlike.

**o·don·ti·tis** (ō′don-tī′tis) SYN pulpitis.

**o·don·to·am·e·lo·blas·to·ma** (ō-don′tō-am′ĕ-lō-blas-tō′mă) See page A16. SYN ameloblastic odontoma.

**o·don·to·blast** (ō-don′tō-blast) One of the dentin-forming cells, derived from mesenchyme of neural crest origin, lining pulp cavity of teeth; arranged in a peripheral layer in dental pulp, each with an odontoblastic process extending part way into dentinal tubules; cells generally are columnar in the coronal pulp but more cuboidal in radicular area and adjacent to tertiary dentin. [*odonto-* + G. *blastos*, sprout, germ]

**o·don·to·blas·tic lay·er** (ō-don′tō-blast′ik lā′ĕr) Layer of odontoblasts at periphery of dental pulp of tooth.

**o·don·to·blas·tic pro·ces·ses** (ō-don′tō-blast′ik pro′ses-ĕz) See this page. SYN dentinal fibers.

**o·don·to·blas·tic zone** (ō-don′tō-blast′ik zōn) Most peripheral zone of pulp; composed of odontoblasts, cells responsible for dentinogenesis; cell bodies of the odontoblasts adjoin the cell-free zone and their odontoblastic processes enter the dentinal tubules.

**o·don·to·blas·to·ma** (ō-don′tō-blas-tō′mă) **1.** Tumor composed of neoplastic epithelial and mesenchymal cells that may differentiate into cells able to produce calcified tooth substances. **2.** An odontoma in its early formative stage. [*odontoblast* + G. *-oma*, tumor]

**o·don·to·clast** (ō-don′tō-klast) One of the cells believed to produce resorption of roots of deciduous teeth. [*odonto-* + G. *klastos*, broken]

**o·don·to·dyn·i·a** (ō-don′tō-din′ē-ă) SYN toothache. [*odonto-* + G. *odynē*, pain]

**o·don·to·dys·pla·si·a** (ō-don′tō-dis-plā′zē-ă) Developmental disturbance of one or several adjacent teeth, of unknown etiology, characterized by deficient formation of enamel and dentin, which results in an abnormally large pulp chamber and imparts a ghostlike radiographic image to affected teeth; such teeth erupt into oral cavity late. See page 412.

**o·don·to·gen·e·sis** (ō-don′tō-jen′ĕ-sis) Process of development of teeth. [*odonto-* + G. *genesis*, production]

**o·don·to·gen·ic cyst** (ō-don′tō-jen′ik sist) Lesion derived from odontogenic epithelium. [*odont-* + G. *genos*, birth, origin, + suffix *-ic*, pertaining to]

**op**

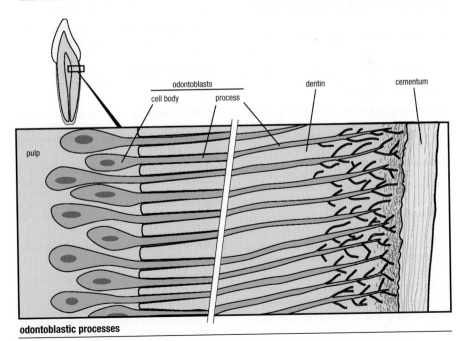

odontoblasts
cell body     process
dentin     cementum
pulp

**odontoblastic processes**

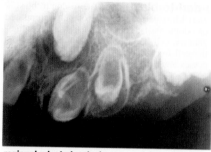

regional odontodysplasia

**☐o·don·to·gen·ic ker·a·to·cyst** (ō-don′ tō-jen′ik ker′ă-tō-sist) Lesion of dental lamina origin with a high recurrence rate and well-defined histologic criteria of corrugated parakeratin surface, uniformly thin epithelium, and a palisaded basal layer. One manifestation of the basal cell nevus syndrome. See this page.

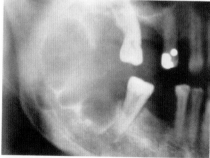

**odontogenic keratocyst:** multilocular and recurrent

**o·don·to·gen·ic myx·o·ma** (ō-don′tō-jen′ik mik-sō′mă) Benign, expansile, multilocular radiolucent neoplasm of jaws consisting of myxomatous fibrous connective tissue; presumably derived from mesenchymal components of odontogenic apparatus.

**o·don·to·glyph·ics** (ō-don′tō-glif′iks) Method of classification of molar grooves defined in an individually distinctive pattern like that of fingerprints. [odonto- + G. glyphē, carving]

**o·don·toid** (ō-don′toyd) **1.** Shaped like a tooth. SYN dentoid. **2.** Relating to the toothlike odontoid process of second cervical vertebra. [odont- + G. eidos, resemblance]

**o·don·toid pro·cess** (ō-don′toyd pro′ses) SYN dens (2).

**o·don·toid pro·cess of ep·i·stro·phe·us** (ō-don′toyd pro′ses ep′i-strō′fē-ŭs) SYN dens (2).

**o·don·tol·o·gy** (ō′don-tol′ŏ-jē) SYN dentistry. [donto- + G. logos, study]

**o·don·tol·y·sis** (ō′don-tol′i-sis) SYN erosion (1).

**o·don·to·ma** (ō′don-tō′mă) **1.** Tumor of odontogenic origin. **2.** Hamartomatous odontogenic tumor composed of enamel, dentin, cementum, and pulp tissue that may or may not be arranged in the form of a tooth. [odonto- + G. -oma, tumor]

**o·don·to·neu·ral·gi·a** (ō-don′tō-nūr-al′jē-ă) Facial neuralgia caused by a carious tooth.

**o·don·ton·o·my** (ō′don-ton′ŏ-mē) Dental nomenclature. [odonto- + G. onoma, name]

**o·don·to·no·sol·o·gy** (ō-don′tō-nō-sol′ŏ-jē) SYN dentistry. [odonto- + G. nosos, disease, + logos, study]

**o·don·to·par·al·lax·is** (ō-don′tō-par′ă-lak′sis) Irregularity of teeth. [odonto- + G. parallax, alternately]

**o·don·top·a·thy** (ō′don-top′ă-thē) Any disease of teeth or their sockets. [odonto- + G. pathos, suffering]

**o·don·to·pho·bi·a** (ō-don′tō-fō′bē-ă) Morbid fear of teeth. [odonto- + G. phobos, fear]

**o·don·to·plas·ty** (ō-don′tō-plas-tē) Surgical contouring of tooth surface to enhance plaque control and gingival morphology. [odonto- + G. plassō, to mold]

**o·don·top·ri·sis** (ō′don-top′ri-sis) Grinding together of teeth.

**o·don·top·to·sis** (ō′don-top-tō′sis, -tō-tō′sis) Downward movement of an upper tooth due to loss of its lower antagonist(s). SEE ALSO supereruption. [odonto- + G. ptōsis, a falling]

**o·don·tor·rha·gi·a** (ō-don′tō-rā′jē-ă) Profuse bleeding from socket after tooth extraction. [odonto- + G. rhēgnymi, to burst forth]

**o·don·to·schism** (ō-don′tō-skizm, -sizm) Fissure of a tooth. [odonto- + G. schisma, a cleft]

**o·don·to·scope** (ō-don′tō-skōp) Optic device, similar to a closed circuit television system, which projects a view of oral cavity onto a screen for multiple viewing.

**o·don·tos·co·py** (ō′don-tos′kŏ-pē) **1.** Examination of oral cavity with an odontoscope. **2.** Examination of markings in prints of cutting edges of teeth; used, like fingerprints, as a method of personal identification. [odonto- + G. skopeō, to view]

**o·don·to·ther·a·py** (ō-don′tō-ther′ă-pē) Treatment of diseases of teeth.

**o·don·tot·o·my** (ō′don-tot′ŏ-mē) Cutting into a tooth crown. [odonto- + G. tomē, incision]

**o·dor** (ō′dŏr) Emanation from any substance that stimulates the olfactory cells in the organ of smell. SYN smell. [L.]

**oedema** [Br.] SYN edema.

**oenomania** [Br.] SYN delirium tremens.

**oesophageal** [Br.] SYN esophageal.

**oesophageal achalasia** [Br.] SYN esophageal achalasia.

**oesophageal reflux** [Br.] SYN esophageal reflux.

**oesophageal varices** [Br.] SYN esophageal varices.

**oesophagitis** [Br.] SYN esophagitis.

**oesophagogastric junction** [Br.] SYN esophagogastric junction.

**oesophagospasm** [Br.] SYN esophagospasm.

**oesophagus** [Br.] SYN esophagus.

**oestrogen** [Br.] SYN estrogen.

**OFD** Abbreviation for orofaciodigital syndrome.

**of·fic·i·nal** (ŏ-fis′i-năl) Denoting a chemical or pharmaceutical preparation kept in stock.

**off-la·bel in·di·ca·tion** (awf-lā′bĕl in′di-kā′shŭn) Use of a medication for a clinical purpose other than that approved by the U.S. Food and Drug Administration.

**off·set blade** (awf′set blād) Blade of an instrument such as a Gracey curette, in which the lower shank is at a 70-degree angle to the face of the blade.

**OHI** Abbreviation for Oral Hygiene Index.

**OHI-S** Abbreviation for Simplified Oral Hygiene Index.

**oil** (oyl) An inflammable liquid, of fatty consistency and unctuous feel, which is insoluble in water, soluble or insoluble in alcohol, and freely soluble in ether.

**oil of clove** (oyl klōv) Volatile oil used in dentistry as a local anesthetic and component of temporary teeth fillings. Also used to flavor foods; has a strong, pungent odor.

**oil of lem·on** (oyl lem′ŏn) Volatile oil expressed from fresh peel of *Citrus limonum;* used for flavoring pharmaceuticals.

**oil of pep·per·mint** (oyl pep′ĕr-mint) Volatile oil used as a pharmaceutical aid (flavor).

**oil of spear·mint** (oyl spēr′mint) Volatile oil from flowering tops of *Mentha spicata;* pharmaceutical aid (flavor) and a carminative.

**oint·ment** (oynt′mĕnt) Semisolid preparation usually containing medicinal substances, intended for external application. [O. Fr. *oignement;* L. *unguo,* pp. *unctus,* to smear]

**o·le·ag·i·nous** (ō′lē-aj′i-nŭs) Oily or greasy. [L. *oleagineus,* pertaining to *olea,* the olive tree]

**o·le·ate** (ō′lē-āt) **1.** A salt of oleic acid. **2.** A pharmacopeial preparation consisting of a combination or solution of an alkaloid or metallic base in oleic acid, used as an inunction.

**o·le·ic ac·id** (ō-lē′ik as′id) A fatty acid used commercially in preparation of oleates and lotions, and as a pharmaceutical solvent. [L. *oleum,* oil]

**o·le·o·ther·a·py** (ō′lē-ō-ther′ă-pē) Treatment of disease by an oil given internally or applied externally. [*oleo-* + G. *therapeia,* therapy]

**ol·fac·tion** (ōl-fak′shŭn) **1.** Sense of smell. **2.** Act of smelling. [L. *ol-facio,* pp. *-factus,* to smell]

**ol·fac·to·ry bulb** (ōl-fak′tŏr-ē bŭlb) [TA] The grayish expanded rostral extremity of the olfactory tract, lying on the cribriform plate of the ethmoid and receiving the olfactory filaments. SYN bulbus olfactorius [TA].

**ol·fac·to·ry nerve [CN I]** (ōl-fak′tŏr-ē nĕrv) [TA] Collective term denoting numerous olfactory filaments. SYN first cranial nerve [CN I], nervus olfactorii [CN I].

**oligaemia** [Br.] SYN oligemia.

**ol·i·ge·mi·a** (ol′i-jē′mē-ă) Deficiency in amount of blood in body or any organ or tissue. SYN oligaemia.

**oligo-** Combining form meaning **1.** A few, a little; too little, too few. **2.** In chemistry, used in contrast to "poly-" in describing polymers; e.g., oligosaccharide. [G. *oligos,* few]

**ol·i·go·dip·si·a** (ol′i-gō-dip′sē-ă) Abnormal lack of thirst. [*oligo-* + G. *dipsa,* thirst]

**ol·i·go·don·ti·a** (ol′i-gō-don′shē-ă) SYN hypodontia. [*oligo-* + G. *odous,* tooth]

**ol·i·go·dy·nam·ic** (ol′i-gō-dī-nam′ik) Active in very small quantity.

**ol·i·go·men·or·rhe·a** (ol′i-gō-men-ōr-ē′ă) Scanty menstruation. SYN oligomenorrhoea.

**oligomenorrhoea** [Br.] SYN oligomenorrhea.

**ol·i·go·mer** (ol′i-gō-mĕr) A polymer containing fewer than 20 repeating units.

**ol·i·go·nu·cle·o·tide** (ol′i-gō-nū′klē-ō-tīd) A compound made up of the condensation of a small number of nucleotides.

**ol·i·go·sac·cha·ride** (ol′i-gō-sak′ă-rīd) A compound made up of the condensation of a small number of monosaccharide units.

**ol·i·go·tro·phi·a, ol·i·got·ro·phy** (ol′i-

op

gō-trō′fē-ă, -got′rŏ-fē) Deficient nutrition. [*ol-igo-* + G. *trophē,* nourishment]

**ol·i·gu·ri·a** (ol′i-gyūr′ē-ă) Scant urine production. [*oligo-* + G. *ouron,* urine]

**o·lym·pi·an fore·head** (ō-lim′pē-ăn fōr′hed) Abnormally prominent, high, and broad forehead associated with hereditary syphilis.

**OM** Abbreviation for otitis media.

**o·mis·sion** (ō-mish′ŭn) PHARMACY drug error in which requisite dose is wrongly missed.

**omn. hor.** Abbreviation for L. *omni hora,* every hour.

**o·mo·hy·oid mus·cle** (ō′mō-hī′oyd mŭs′ĕl) Formed of two bellies attached to intermediate tendon; *origin,* by inferior belly from upper border of scapula between superior angle and notch; *insertion,* by superior belly into hyoid bone; *action,* depresses hyoid; *nerve supply,* upper cervical spinal nerves through ansa cervicalis. SYN musculus omohyoideus [TA].

***On·cho·cer·ca*** (ong′kō-ser′kă) A genus of elongated filariform nematodes that inhabit host's connective tissue, usually within firm nodules in which these parasites are coiled and entangled. SYN *Oncocerca.* [G. *onkos,* a barb, + *kerkos,* tail]

**on·co·cy·to·ma** (ong′kō-sī-tō′mă) A glandular tumor composed of large cells with cytoplasm that is granular and eosinophilic because of the presence of abundant mitochondria; occurs uncommonly in the kidney and salivary and endocrine glands.

**on·co·gene** (ong′kō-jēn) Any of a family of genes that normally encodes proteins involved in cell growth or regulation but may foster malignant processes if mutated or activated by contact with retroviruses. [*onco-* + gene]

**on·col·o·gy** (on-kol′ŏ-jē) Study or science dealing with physical, chemical, and biologic properties and features of neoplasms, including causation, pathogenesis, and treatment.

**on·lay** (on′lā) Cast restoration (porcelain, pressed ceramic, metal) of occlusal surface of a posterior tooth or lingual surface of an anterior tooth, the entire surface of which is in dentin without side walls; retention in anterior tooth involves pins and in the posterior pins and/or boxes in retentive grooves in buccal and lingual walls.

**on·to·gen·e·sis** (on′tō-jen′ĕ-sis) SYN ontogeny.

**on·tog·e·ny** (on-toj′ĕ-nē) Development of the individual. SYN ontogenesis. [G. *ōn,* being, + *genesis,* origin]

**on·y·choph·a·gy, on·y·cho·pha·gi·a** (on′i-kof′ă-jē, -kō-fā′jē-ă) Habitual nail-biting. [*onycho-* + G. *phagō,* to eat]

**o·o·cyte** (ō′ō-sīt) Female gamete or sex cell. [G. *ōon,* egg, + *kytos,* a hollow (cell)]

**o·pac·i·fi·ca·tion** (ō-pas′i-fi-kā′shŭn) **1.** The process of making opaque. **2.** The formation of opacities. [L. *opacus,* shady]

**o·pac·i·ty** (ō-pas′i-tē) **1.** On a radiograph, a more transparent area is interpreted as an opacity to x-rays in the body. **2.** A lack of transparency. [L. *opacitas,* shadiness]

**o·pa·les·cent** (ō′pă-les′ĕnt) Resembling an opal in the display of various colors. [Fr. fr. L. *opalus,* opal]

**o·pal·es·cent den·tin** (ō′pă-les′ĕnt den′tin) Dentin usually associated with dentinogenesis imperfecta that gives an unusual opalescent or translucent appearance to the teeth. SYN hereditary opalescent dentin (2).

**o·paque** (ō-pāk′) Impervious to light; not translucent or only slightly so. Cf. radiopaque. [Fr. fr. L. *opacus,* shady]

**o·pen bite** (ō′pĕn bīt) **1.** SYN large interarch distance. **2.** SYN apertognathia.

**o·pen con·tact** (ō′pĕn kon′takt) Lack of contact between adjacent teeth that would normally touch each other on their proximal sides. May be due to tooth position, absence of a tooth or faulty restoration(s).

**o·pen frac·ture** (ō′pĕn frak′shŭr) Break in which the skin is perforated and there is an open wound down to the fracture. SYN compound fracture.

**o·pen·ing ax·is** (ō′pĕn-ing ak′sis) Imaginary line around which mandibular condyles may rotate during opening and closing.

**o·pen·ing move·ment** (ō′pĕn-ing mūv′mĕnt) In dentistry, movement of mandible executed during jaw separation.

**o·pen·ing of ves·tib·u·lar ca·nal·ic·u·lus** (ō′pĕn-ing ves-tib′yū-lăr kan′ă-lik′yū-lŭs) [TA] External opening of the vestibular aqueduct on the posterior surface of the petrous part of the temporal bone near the groove for the sigmoid sinus. SYN external aperture of vestibular aqueduct.

**o·pen·ings of ca·rot·id ca·nal** (ō′pĕn-ingz kă-rot′id kă-nal′) [TA] The orifice at each extremity of the carotid canal in the pyramidal petrous part of the temporal bone. SYN carotid foramen.

**o·pen-packed po·si·tion** (ō′pĕn-pakt pŏ-zish′ŏn) **1.** Joint position in which contact between the articulating structures is minimal. **2.** SYN flexion.

**o·pen scal·ing and root plan·ing** (ō′pĕn skăl′ing rūt plăn′ing) Instrumentation performed after the operative area has been exposed by tissue removal or by the tissue's having been separated and laid back as a flap; visibility and accessibility thus afforded allow more thorough treatment.

**o·pen tu·ber·cu·lo·sis** (ō′pĕn tū-bĕr′kyū-lō′sis) Pulmonary tuberculosis, tuberculous ulceration, or another form in which tubercle bacilli are in excretions or secretions.

**op·er·ant con·di·tion·ing** (op′ĕr-ănt kŏn-dish′ŭn-ing) Type of conditioning in which an experimenter waits for target response (e.g., head scratching) to be conditioned to occur (emitted) spontaneously, immediately after which organism is given a reinforcer reward.

**op·er·ate** (op′ĕr-āt) 1. To work on the body manually or with an instrument. 2. To perform a surgical procedure. 3. Used to describe the action of using an instrument to achieve a diagnostic or therapeutic endpoint.

**op·er·a·ted cleft** (op′ĕr-ā-tĕd kleft) A gap that has been repaired surgically. SYN postoperative cleft.

**op·er·a·ting room (OR)** (op′ĕr-āt-ing rūm) An area in a health care facility used to perform nonemergency surgical interventions.

**op·er·a·tion** (op-ĕr-ā′shŭn) 1. Any surgical procedure. 2. Act, manner, or process of functioning.

**op·er·a·tive den·tis·try** (op′ĕr-ă-tiv den′tis-trē) Individual restoration of teeth using metallic or nonmetallic materials.

**o·per·cu·li·tis** (ō-per′kyū-lī′tis) A pericoronitis originating under an operculum. [L. operculum, cover or lid, + G. -itis, inflammation]

**o·per·cu·lum,** pl. **o·per·cu·la** (ō-pĕr′kyū-lŭm, -lă) [TA] 1. [TA] The mucosal flap partially or completely covering an unerupted tooth. 2. Anything resembling a lid or cover. [L. cover or lid, fr. operio, pp. opertus, to cover]

**op·er·on** (op′ĕr-on) A genetic functional unit that controls production of a messenger RNA.

**oph·ry·o·sis** (of′rē-ō′sis) Spasmodic twitching of upper portion of orbicularis palpebrarum muscle causing eyebrow wrinkling. [G. ophrys, eyebrow, + -osis, condition]

**oph·thal·mic nerve [CN V1]** (of-thal′mik nĕrv) [TA] Branch of trigeminal nerve that passes forward from trigeminal ganglion in lateral wall of cavernous sinus, entering the orbit through the superior orbital fissure. SYN nervus ophthalmicus [CN V1].

**oph·thal·mol·o·gy** (of′thăl-mol′ŏ-jē) The medical specialty concerned with the eye, its diseases, and refractive errors. [ophthalmo- + G. logos, study]

**oph·thal·mo·man·dib·u·lo·mel·ic dys·pla·si·a** (of-thal′mō-man-dib′yū-lō-mel′ik dis-

plā′zē-ă) Disorder with corneal clouding and multiple abnormalities of mandible and limbs.

**oph·thal·mop·a·thy** (of′thăl-mop′ă-thē) Any ocular disease. [ophthalmo- + G. pathos, suffering]

**oph·thal·mo·ple·gi·a** (of-thal′mō-plē′jē-ă) Paralysis of one or more of the ocular muscles. [ophthalmo- + G. plēgē, stroke]

**oph·thal·mo·scope** (of-thal′mŏ-skōp) A device for studying the interior of the eyeball through the pupil. SYN funduscope. [ophthalmo- + G. skopeō, to examine]

**o·pi·ate** (ō′pē-ăt) Any preparation or derivative of opium.

**o·pi·ate re·cep·tors** (ō′pē-ăt rĕ-sep′tŏrz) Brain regions with capacity to bind morphine.

**o·pi·oid** (ō′pē-oyd) Originally, synthetic narcotics resembling opiates but increasingly used to refer to both opiates and synthetic narcotics.

**o·pi·oid an·tag·o·nists** (ō′pē-oyd an-tag′ŏ-nists) Agents with a high affinity for opiate receptors but do not activate them.

**o·pis·thi·on** (ō-pis′thē-on) [TA] The middle point on the posterior margin of the foramen magnum, opposite the basion. [G. opisthios, posterior]

**o·pi·um** (ō′pē-ŭm) The air-dried milky exudation obtained by incising the unripe capsules of *Papaver somniferum* or the variant, *P. album;* used as an analgesic, hypnotic, and diaphoretic, and to treat diarrhea and spasmodic conditions. [L. fr. G. opion, poppy-juice]

**op·por·tu·nis·tic in·fec·tion** (op′ōr-tū-nis′tik in-fek′shŭn) Infection occurs in a systemically or locally impaired host.

**op·por·tu·nis·tic path·o·gen** (op′ōr-tū-nis′tik path′ŏ-jen) Pathogen capable of causing disease only when the host's resistance is lowered.

**op·po·site arch ful·crum** (op′ŏ-zit ahrch ful′krŭm) Advanced intraoral stabilizing point in which the finger rest is established on the opposite arch from the treatment area.

**op·tic chi·asm** (op′tik kī′azm) [TA] A flattened quadrangular body in front of the tuber cinereum and infundibulum, the point of crossing or decussation of the fibers of the optic nerves. SYN optic decussation.

**op·tic de·cus·sa·tion** (op′tik dē-kŭs-ā′shŭn) SYN optic chiasm.

**op·tic nerve [CN II]** (op′tik nĕrv) [TA] Although classified as a cranial nerve, it is actually an extension of the forebrain; conveys afferent fibers from the ganglion cells of the retina and passes out of orbit through optic canal to the

**op**

chiasm. SYN nervus opticus [CN II], second cranial nerve [CN II].

**op·tic neu·ri·tis** (op′tik nūr-ī′tis) Inflammation of the optic nerve.

**op·tics** (op′tiks) The science concerned with the properties of light, its refraction and absorption, and the refracting media of the eye in that relation. [G. *optikos,* fr. *ōps,* eye]

**op·ti·mal dose** (op′ti-măl dōs) Dose of drug or radiation that will produce desired effect with least likelihood of undesirable symptoms.

**op·tom·e·try** (op-tom′ĕ-trē) The profession concerned with the examination of the eyes and related structures to determine the presence of vision problems and eye disorders, and with the prescription and adaptation of lenses and other optic aids or the use of visual training for maximum visual efficiency.

**OR** Abbreviation for operating room.

**o·ra,** pl. **o·rae** (ō′ră, -rē) An edge or a margin. [Plural of L. *os,* the mouth.]

**or·ad** (ōr′ad) In a direction toward the mouth. [L. *os,* mouth, + *ad,* to]

**or·al** (ōr′ăl) Relating to the mouth. [L. *os (or-),* mouth]

**or·al and max·il·lo·fa·cial sur·ge·ry** (ōr′al mak′sil-ō-fā′shăl sŭr′jĕr-ē) Dental specialty that includes surgical correction of injuries and malformations of the midface, jaws, and dentition. Cf. oral surgery.

**or·al a·ware·ness** (ōr′ăl ă-wār′nĕs) Perception by someone of structures or conditions within the person's own mouth.

**or·al bi·ol·o·gy** (ōr′ăl bī-ol′ŏ-jē) Aspect of biology devoted to study of biologic phenomena associated with oral cavity in health and disease (e.g., dental caries, mastication, periodontal disease).

**or·al brush bi·op·sy** (ōr′ăl brŭsh bī′op-sē) SEE ALSO biopsy. SYN brush biopsy.

**or·al can·cer** (ōr′ăl kan′sĕr) Cancer affecting lips, tongue, floor of the mouth, palate, gingiva, alveolar mucosa, buccal mucosa, and oropharynx.

**⬛or·al cav·i·ty** (ōr′ăl kav′i-tē) [TA] Region consisting of the narrow cleft between the lips and cheeks, and the teeth and gums, as well as any related structure. See page 417. SYN cavum oris, mouth (1).

**or·al cav·i·ty prop·er** (ōr′ăl kav′i-tē prop′ĕr) [TA] Space between dental arches, limited posteriorly by isthmus of fauces (palatoglossal arch).

**o·ra·le** (ō-rā′lē) Point at lingual side of alveolar termination of premaxillary suture. [Mod. L. *punctum orale,* oral point, fr. L. *os (or-),* mouth]

**or·al ep·i·the·li·al ne·vus** (ōr′ăl ep′i-thē′lē-ăl nē′vŭs) SYN white sponge nevus.

**or·al (e·ro·sive) li·chen pla·nus** (ōr′ăl ē-rō′siv lī′kĕn plā′nŭs) Manifestations of lichen planus characterized orally by white striae of oral mucous membrane and sometimes associated with ulceration; patients may not exhibit a history of cutaneous lichen planus.

**or·al e·vac·u·a·tion** (ōr′ăl ĕ-vak′yū-ā′shŭn) Clearing oral cavity of saliva, blood, fluids, and debris to maintain a clear operative field during a dental procedure.

**or·al fis·sure** (ōr′ăl fish′ŭr) [TA] Horizontal opening between the lips leading into oral vestibule; aperture of mouth. SYN oral opening.

**o·ral flor·a** (ōr′ăl flōr′ă) Bacteria and other microorganisms that normally inhabit the oral cavity.

**or·al fo·cal mu·ci·no·sis** (ōr′ăl fō′kăl myū′si-nō′sis) Area of myxomatous connective tissue.

**or·al hy·giene** (ōr′ăl hī′jēn) Cleaning mouth by brushing, flossing, irrigating, massaging, or use of other devices.

**Or·al Hy·giene In·dex (OHI)** (ōr′ăl hī′jēn in′deks) Measurement used in epidemiologic studies of dental disease to evaluate dental plaque and dental calculus separately.

**or·al ir·ri·ga·tion** (ōr′ăl ir′i-gā′shŭn) Targeted delivery of water or solution to specific oral locations.

**or·al mem·brane** (ōr′ăl mem′brān) SYN buccopharyngeal membrane.

**or·al mu·co·sa** (ōr′ăl myū-kō′să) [TA] SYN mucosa of mouth.

**or·al open·ing** (ōr′ăl ō′pĕn-ing) SYN oral fissure.

**or·al par·es·the·si·a** (ōr′ăl par′es-thē′zē-ă) Abnormal spontaneous or evoked oral sensations. SEE ALSO dysesthesia.

**or·al pa·thol·o·gy** (ōr′ăl pă-thol′ŏ-jē) Branch of dental science dealing wih study, diagnosis, and causes of oral disease and the changes they produce. SYN dental pathology.

**or·al phar·ynx** (ōr′ăl far′ingks) SYN oropharynx.

**or·al phys·i·ol·o·gy** (ōr′ăl fiz′ē-ol′ō-jē) Science of the function of the oral structures.

**or·al phys·i·o·ther·a·py** (ōr′ăl fiz′ē-ō-thār′ă-pē) Use of a toothbrush, interdental stimulator, floss, irrigating device, or other adjunct aid to maintain oral health; also includes active (e.g., jaw manipulation, jaw exercises) and pas-

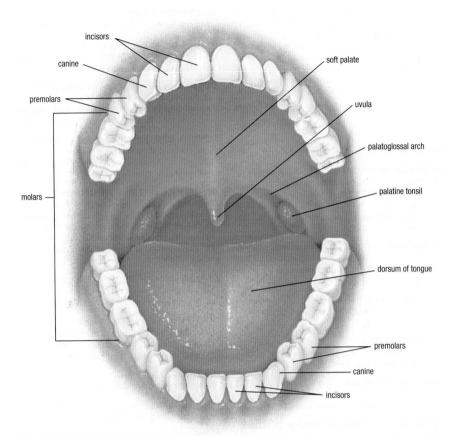

incisors
canine
premolars
molars
soft palate
uvula
palatoglossal arch
palatine tonsil
dorsum of tongue
premolars
canine
incisors

**oral cavity:** anterior view

op

sive (e.g., laser, ultrasound, thermal therapy) physical therapy modalities to improve jaw function and reduce pain with musculoskeletal disorders.

**or·al plate** (ōr´ăl plāt) Circumscribed area of fusion of foregut endoderm and stomodeal ectoderm in the embryo that ruptures early in development to establish oral opening. SEE ALSO buccopharyngeal membrane.

**or·al re·gi·on** (ōr´ăl rē´jŏn) [TA] Facial area comprising lips and mouth.

**or·al shields** (ōr´ăl shēldz) Removable appliances used in orthodontic treatment, usually placed between labial and buccal mucosa and teeth.

**or·al sub·mu·cous fi·bro·sis** (ōr´ăl sŭb-myū´kŭs fī-brō´sis) Precancerous condition of oral mucosa and upper aerodigestive tract characteristically found in residents of India.

**or·al sur·ge·ry** (ōr´ăl sŭr´jĕr-ē) Branch of dentistry concerned with diagnosis, surgery and adjunctive treatment of diseases, injuries, and deformities of oral and maxillofacial regions.

**or·al symp·toms of men·o·pause** (ōr´ăl simp´tŏmz men´ŏ-pawz) Constellation of findings including a burning sensation and dryness of the oral cavity.

**or·al teeth** (ōr´ăl tēth) SYN anterior tooth.

**or·al ves·ti·bule** (ōr´ăl ves´ti-byūl) [TA] Mouth area bounded anteriorly and laterally by lips and cheeks, posteriorly and medially by teeth and/or gums, and above and below by reflections of mucosa from lips and cheeks to gums. SYN buccal cavity.

**or·ange stain** (ōr´ănj stān) Anterior dental discoloration likely due to chromogenic bacteria.

**or·ange wood** (ōr´ănj wūd) Soft wood used in dentistry for placement of bridges, crowns, and other structures to assess biting pressure and as a burnishing point.

**or·bic·u·la·ris oc·u·li re·flex** (ōr-bik-yū-lā´ris ok´yū-lī rē´fleks) Contraction of the orbicularis oculi muscles on tapping the margin of the orbit, or the bridge or tip of the nose.

**or·bi·cu·la·ris o·ris mus·cle** (ōr-bik´yū-lā′ris ō′ris mŭs′ĕl) *Origin,* by nasolabial band from septum of the nose, by superior incisive bundle from incisor fossa of maxilla, by inferior incisive bundle from lower jaw each side of symphysis; *insertion,* fibers surround mouth between skin and mucous membrane of lips and cheeks, and are blended with other muscles; *action,* closes lips; *nerve supply,* facial. SYN musculus orbicularis oris [TA].

**or·bit** (ōr′bit) [TA] Bony cavity containing eyeball and its adnexa.

**or·bi·tal** (ōr′bi-tăl) Relating to the orbits.

**or·bi·tal branch·es of max·il·lar·y nerve** (ōr′bi-tăl branch′ĕz mak′si-lar-ē nĕrv) [TA] Branches of pterygopalatine ganglion traversing inferior orbital fissure, distributed in orbit to periorbita and mucosa of ethmoidal and sphenoidal sinuses.

**or·bi·ta·le** (ōr-bi-tā′lē) CEPHALOMETRICS the lowermost point in the lower margin of the bony orbit that may be felt under the skin. [L. of an orbit]

**or·bi·tal ex·en·ter·a·tion** (ōr′bi-tăl eks-en′tĕr-ā′shŭn) Surgical removal of orbital contents.

**or·bi·tal plane** (ōr′bi-tăl plān) Orbital surface of maxilla, lying perpendicular to orbitomeatal plane at the orbitale.

**or·bi·tal sur·face** (ōr′bi-tăl sŭr′făs) [TA] The surface of a bone that contributes to the walls of the orbit. SYN facies orbitalis.

**or·bi·tal sur·face of bod·y of max·il·la** (ōr′bi-tăl sŭr′făs bod′ē mak-sil′ă) Smooth, triangular, slightly concave plate of bone extending posteriorly from the body of the maxilla to form most of the floor of the orbit. SYN facies orbitalis maxillae.

**or·bi·tal sur·face of great·er wing of sphe·noid bone** (ōr′bi-tăl sŭr′făs grā′tĕr wing sfē′noyd bōn) The roughly quadrilateral plate formed by the greater wing of the sphenoid bone that makes up most of the lateral wall of the orbit. SYN facies orbitalis alaris majoris ossis sphenoidalis.

**or·bit·ing con·dyle** (ōr′bit-ing kon′dīl) SYN nonworking side condyle.

**or·bi·to·me·a·tal line** (ōr′bi-tō-mē-ā′tăl līn) SYN baseline.

**or·bi·to·me·a·tal plane** (ōr′bi-tō-mē-ā′tăl plān) A line approximating the base of the cranium, passing from the infraorbital ridge to the midline of the occiput, intersecting the superior margin of the external auditory meatus; the cranium is in the anatomic position when the base line lies in the horizontal plane and right and left sides are level.

**or·bi·to·sphe·noid** (ōr′bi-tō-sfē′noyd) Relating to orbit and sphenoid bone.

**or·chi·op·a·thy** (ōr′kē-op′ă-thē) Disease of a testis. [*orchio-* + G. *pathos,* suffering]

**or·der** (ōr′dĕr) In biologic classification, division just below class (or subclass) and above family. [L. *ordo,* regular arrangement]

**or·gan** (ōr′găn) [TA] A differentiated structure or part of a system of the body; composed of tissues and cells. SYN organum [TA], organon. [L. *organum,* fr. G. *organon,* a tool, instrument]

**or·gan·elle** (ōr′gă-nel′) One of the specialized parts of a protozoan or tissue cell. SYN organoid (3). [G. *organon,* organ, + Fr. *-elle,* dim. suffix, fr. L. *-ella*]

**or·gan·ic brain syn·drome** (ōr-gan′ik brān sin′drōm) Constellation of behavioral or psychological signs and symptoms including problems with attention, concentration, memory, confusion, anxiety, and depression caused by transient or permanent dysfunction of the brain.

**or·gan·ic den·tal ce·ment** (ōr-gan′ik den′tăl sĕ-ment′) Fixative agent consisting mainly of synthetic polymers.

**or·gan·ic dis·ease** (ōr-gan′ik di-zēz′) Disorder in which anatomic or pathophysiologic changes occur in some bodily tissue or organ, in contrast to a functional disorder.

**or·gan·ic mur·mur** (ōr-gan′ik mŭr′mŭr) A murmur caused by structural change.

**or·ga·nism** (ōr′gă-nizm) Any living individual, considered as a whole.

**or·ga·ni·za·tion** (ōr′găn-ī-zā′shŭn) Conversion of coagulated blood, exudate, or dead tissue into fibrous tissue.

♻ **organo-** Combining form denoting organ; organic. [G. *organon*]

**or·gan·o·gen·e·sis** (ōr′gă-nō-jen′ĕ-sis) Formation of organs during development. [*organo-* + G. *genesis,* origin]

**or·ga·noid** (ōr′gă-noyd) **1.** Resembling in superficial appearance or in structure any of the organs or glands of the body. **2.** Composed of glandular or organic elements, and not of a single tissue. **3.** SYN organelle. [*organo-* + G. *eidos,* resemblance]

**or·ga·non** (ōr′gă-non) SYN organ.

**or·ga·nop·a·thy** (ōr′gă-nop′ă-thē) Any disease that especially affects one organ of the body. [*organo-* + G. *pathos,* suffering]

**or·ga·no·ther·a·py** (ōr′gă-nō-thār′ă-pē) Treatment of disease by preparations made from animal organs; now frequently by synthetic preparations instead of natural extracts of a gland.

**or·ga·num** (ōr-gă′nŭm) SYN organ.

**or·i·en·ta·tion** (ōr′ē-ĕn-tā′shŭn) Recognition

of one's temporal, spatial, and personal relationships and environment.

**or·i·fice** (ōr′i-fis) [TA] Any aperture or opening. [L. *orificium*]

**Orn** Abbreviation for ornithine.

**or·ni·thine (Orn)** (ōr′ni-thēn) Amino acid formed when L-arginine is hydrolyzed by arginase; important intermediate in the urea cycle.

**oro-** Prefix meaning mouth (its archaic alternative spelling is ortho-). [L. *os, oris,* mouth]

**or·o·an·tral fis·tu·la** (ōr′ō-an′trăl fis′tyū-lă) Pathologic communication between the oral cavity and maxillary sinus, most commonly a complication of maxillary premolar molar tooth extraction.

**or·o·dig·i·to·fa·cial** (ōr′ō-dij′i-tō-fā′shăl) Relating to mouth, fingers, and face.

**or·o·dig·i·to·fa·cial dy·so·sto·sis** (ōr′ō-dij′i-tō-fā′shăl dis′os-tō′sis) SYN orofaciodigital syndrome.

**or·o·fa·cial** (ōr′ō-fā′shăl) Relating to mouth and face.

**or·o·fa·cial fis·tu·la** (ōr′ō-fā′shăl fis′tyū-lă) Pathologic communication between oral cavity and face.

**or·o·fa·ci·o·dig·i·tal syn·drome (OFD)** (ōr′ō-fā′shē-ō-dij′i-tăl sin′drōm) Inherited syndrome, lethal in males, with varying combinations of defects of oral cavity, face, and hands, including lobulated or bifid tongue, cleft or pseudocleft palate, tongue tumors, and missing or malpositioned teeth. SYN orodigitofacial dysostosis.

**or·o·lin·gual** (ōr′ō-ling′gwăl) Relating to mouth and tongue.

**or·o·na·sal** (ōr′ō-nā′zăl) Relating to mouth and nose.

**or·o·na·sal fis·tu·la** (ōr′ō-nā′zăl fis′tyū-lă) Pathologic communication between oral and nasal cavity.

**or·o·na·sal mem·brane** (ōr′ō-nā′zăl mem′brān) SYN bucconasal membrane.

**or·o·pha·ryn·ge·al** (ōr′ō-fă-rin′jē-ăl) Relating to oropharynx.

**or·o·pha·ryn·ge·al mem·brane** (ōr′ō-fă-rin′jē-ăl mem′brān) SYN buccopharyngeal membrane.

**or·o·phar·ynx** (ōr′ō-far′ingks) [TA] Portion of pharynx that lies posterior to mouth; continuous above with nasopharynx via pharyngeal

isthmus and below with laryngopharynx. See this page. SYN oral pharynx.

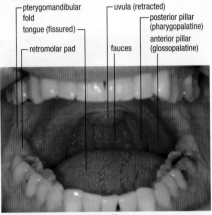

**oropharynx and tonsillar pillars**

**or·phan prod·ucts** (ōr′făn prod′ŭkts) Drugs, biologicals, and medical devices that may be useful in either common or rare diseases but not considered commercially viable.

**ortho-, orth-** Combining forms meaning straight, normal, in proper order.

**or·tho·den·tin** (ōr′thŏ-den′tin) Straight tubed dentin seen in mammalian teeth.

**or·tho·don·ti·a** (ōr′thŏ-don′shē-ă) SYN orthodontics.

**or·tho·don·tic and den·to·fa·ci·al or·tho·ped·ics** (ōr′thŏ-don′tic den′tō-fā′shăl ōr′thŏ-pē′diks) Specialty area of dentistry concerned with diagnosis, supervision, guidance, and treatment of growing and mature dentofacial structures; includes conditions that require movement of teeth and the treatment of malrelationships and malformations of the craniofacial complex.

**or·tho·don·tic ap·pli·ance** (ōr′thŏ-don′tik ă-plī′ăns) Mechanism for application of force to teeth and their supporting tissues to change relationship of teeth and/or related osseous structures. See page 420.

**or·tho·don·tic band** (ōr′thŏ-don′tik band) Thin strip of metal or plastic closely adapted to tooth crown to which wires may be attached for tooth movement.

**or·tho·don·tic e·las·tic** (ōr′thŏ-don′tik ĕ-las′tic) Thin band of pliant material attached to a tooth or an orthodontic appliance and used to apply force or traction to teeth to elicit orthodontic movement.

**or·tho·don·tics** (ōr′thŏ-don′tiks) Branch of dentistry concerned with correction and prevention of irregularities and malocclusion of the

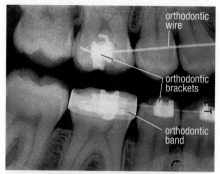

**orthodontic appliance:** radiograph showing bands, brackets, and wires

---

teeth. SYN dental orthopedics, orthodontia. [*ortho-* + G. *odous,* tooth]

**or·tho·don·tic space main·tain·er** (ōr´thŏ-don´tik spās mān-tā´nĕr) A fixed or removable device used to maintain or regain space in the dental arch to allow for subsequent eruption of teeth.

**or·tho·don·tic ther·a·py** (ōr´thŏ-don´tik thār´ă-pē) SEE orthodontics.

**or·tho·dont·ist** (ōr´thŏ-don´tist) A dental specialist who practices orthodontics.

**or·thog·nath·i·a, or·thog·nath·ism** (ōr´thog-nath´ē-ă, ōr-thog´nă-thizm) Study of causes and treatment of conditions related to malposition of jaw bones. [*ortho-* + G. *gnathos,* jaw]

**or·thog·nath·ic, or·thog·na·thous** (ōr´thog-nath´ik, ōr-thog´nă-thŭs) **1.** Relating to orthognathia. **2.** Having a face without projecting jaw. [*ortho-* + G. *gnathos,* jaw]

**or·thog·nath·ic sur·ger·y** (ōr´thog-nath´ik sŭr´jĕr-ē) Operative intervention to alter relationships of the dental arches and/or supporting bone.

**Or·tho·myx·o·vir·i·dae** (ōr´thō-mik´sō-vir´i-dē) The family of viruses that comprises the three groups of influenza viruses, types A, B, and C. The only recognized genus is *Influenzavirus* (q.v.), which comprises the strains of virus types A and B, both of which are subject to mutation resulting in epidemics.

**or·tho·pae·dic** [Br.] SYN orthopedic.

**or·tho·pan·to·mog·ra·phy** (ōr´thō-pan´tŏ-mog´ră-fē) A radiographic process that takes into account the jawline; by doing so, teeth in proximity of tissues can be readily visualized.

**or·tho·pe·dic** (ōr´thŏ-pē´dik) Relating to orthopedics. SYN orthopaedic.

**or·tho·pe·dic ap·pli·ance** (ōr´thŏ-pē´dik ă-plī´ăns) Device used to influence growth and/or position of bones.

**or·tho·pe·dics, or·tho·pae·dics** (ōr´thŏ-pē´diks) The medical specialty concerned with the preservation, restoration, and development of form and function of the musculoskeletal system, extremities, spine, and associated structures by medical, surgical, and physical methods. [*ortho-* + G. *pais* (*paid-*), child]

**or·thop·ne·a** (ōr-thop´nē´ă) Discomfort in breathing that is brought on or aggravated by lying flat. SYN orthopnoea. [*ortho-* + G. *pnoē,* a breathing]

**orthopnoea** [Br.] SYN orthopnea.

**or·tho·pros·the·sis** (ōr´thō-pros-thē´sis) Appliance used to manage prosthetic problems related to tooth alignment.

**or·tho·stat·ic hy·po·ten·sion** (ōr-thŏ-stat´ik hī´pō-ten´shŭn) A form of low blood pressure that occurs in a standing patient. SYN postural hypotension.

**or·thot·ic** (ōr-thot´ik) **1.** Pertaining to orthotics. **2.** An orthotic appliance.

**Os** Symbol for osmium.

**OSAP** (ō´sap) Acronym for Organization for Safety and Asepsis Procedures, a nonprofit organization that promotes infection control and health and safety practices; membership consists of dental and other health care professionals.

**OSHA** Abbreviation for Occupational Safety and Health Administration.

**os in·ci·si·vum** (os in´si-sī´vŭm) [TA] Anterior and inner maxillary parts, which in the fetus and sometimes in the adult is a separate bone; incisive suture runs from incisive canal between lateral incisor and canine tooth.

**os in·ter·max·il·la·re** (os in´tĕr-mak´si-lā´rē) SYN incisive bone.

**Os·ler dis·ease** (ōs´lĕr di-zēz´) SYN polycythemia vera.

**os·mi·um (Os)** (oz´mē-ŭm) A metallic element of the platinum group.

**os·mo·lar** (os-mō´lăr) SYN osmotic.

**os·mo·sis** (os-mō´sis) Process by which solvent tends to move through a semipermeable membrane from a solution of lower to a solution of higher osmolal concentration of solutes to which membrane is relatively impermeable. [G. *ōsmos,* a thrusting, an impulsion]

**os·mot·ic** (os-mot´ik) Relating to osmosis. SYN osmolar.

**os·mot·ic pres·sure (Π)** (os-mot´ik presh´ŭr) The pressure that must be applied to a solution to prevent the passage into it of solvent when solution and pure solvent are separated by a membrane permeable only to the solvent.

**os pre·max·il·la·re** (os prē´mak-si-lā´rē) SYN incisive bone.

**os·se·o·in·te·gra·tion** (os´ē-ō-in´tĕ-grā´shŭn) SYN osseous integration.

**os·se·ous** (os´ē-ŭs) Bony, of bonelike consistency or structure. [L. *osseus*]

**os·se·ous de·fect** (os´ē-ŭs dē´fekt) Any imperfection or absence of bony structures.

**os·se·ous in·teg·ra·tion** (os´ē-ŭs in´tĕ-grā´shŭn) Apparent direct attachment or connection of osseous tissue to an inert alloplastic material without intervening connective tissue, as with dental implants. SYN osseointegration.

**os·si·cle** (os´i-kĕl) [TA] Small bone; specifically, a bone of tympanic cavity or middle ear. [L. *ossiculum*, dim. of *os*, bone]

**os·sic·u·la men·ta·li·a** (ŏ-sik´yū-lă men-tā´lē-ă) Small nodules of bone that appear at mandibular symphysis shortly before birth and fuse with mandible after birth.

**os·sif·ic** (ŏ-sif´ik) Relating to a change into, or formation of, bone.

**os·si·fi·ca·tion** (os´i-fi-kā´shŭn) 1. The formation of bone. 2. A change into bone. [L. *ossificatio*, fr. *os*, bone, + *facio*, to make]

**os·si·fy** (os´i-fī) To form bone or convert into bone. [*ossi-* + L. *facio*, to make]

**os·tec·to·my** (os-tek´tŏ-mē) 1. DENTISTRY resection of supporting osseous structure to eliminate periodontal pockets. 2. Surgical removal of bone. [*osteo-* + G. *ektomē*, excision]

▣ **os·te·i·tis** (os´tē-ī´tis) Inflammation of bone. See page A6. [*osteo-* + G. *-itis*, inflammation]

**os·te·i·tis de·for·mans** (os´tē-ī´tis dĕ-fōr´manz) SYN Paget disease (1).

♻ **osteo-** Combining form meaning bone. [G. *osteon*]

**os·te·o·an·a·gen·e·sis** (os´tē-ō-an-ă-jen´ĕ-sis) Regeneration of bone. [*osteo-* + G. *ana*, again, + *genesis*, generation]

**os·te·o·ar·thri·tis** (os´tē-ō-ahr-thrī´tis) Arthritis characterized by erosion of articular cartilage, either primary or secondary to trauma or other conditions, which becomes soft, frayed, and thinned with eburnation of subchondral bone and outgrowths of marginal osteophytes; pain and loss of function result. SYN arthrosis (2).

**os·te·o·blast** (os´tē-ō-blast) A bone-forming cell derived from mesenchymal osteoprognitor cells that forms an osseous matrix in which it becomes enclosed as an osteocyte. [*osteo-* + G. *blastos*, germ]

**os·te·o·blas·tic** (os´tē-ō-blas´tik) Relating to osteoblasts; describes any region of increased radiographic bone density.

**os·te·o·cal·cin** (os´tē-ō-kal´sin) Protein found in osteoblasts and dentin.

**os·te·o·chon·dri·tis** (os´tē-ō-kon-drī´tis) Inflammation of a bone and its articular cartilage. [*osteo-* + G. *chondros*, cartilage, + *-itis*, inflammation]

**os·te·o·clast** (os´tē-ō-klast) 1. Large multinucleated cell, with abundant acidophilic cytoplasm, functioning in absorption and removal of osseous tissue. 2. An instrument used to fracture bone to correct a deformity.

**os·te·o·clas·to·ma** (os´tē-ō-klas-tō´mă) SYN giant cell tumor of bone.

**os·te·o·cyte** (os´tē-ō-sīt) Cell of osseous tissue that occupies a lacuna and has cytoplasmic processes that extend into canaliculi. [*osteo-* + G. *kytos*, cell]

**os·te·o·dys·plas·ty** (os´tē-ō-dis-plas´tē) SYN Melnick-Needles osteodysplasty. [*osteo-* + G. *dys-*, bad, + *plastos*, formed]

**os·te·o·dys·tro·phy** (os´tē-ō-dis´trŏ-fē) Defective formation of bone. [*osteo-* + G. *dys*, difficult, imperfect, + *trophē*, nourishment]

**os·te·o·fi·bro·ma** (os´tē-ō-fī-brō´mă) A benign lesion of bone, probably not a true neoplasm, consisting of connective tissue with a small foci of osteogenesis.

**os·te·o·gen·e·sis** (os´tē-ō-jen´ĕ-sis) The formation of bone. [*osteo-* + G. *genesis*, production]

**os·te·o·gen·e·sis im·per·fec·ta** (os´tē-ō-jen´ĕ-sis im-pĕr-fek´tă) Group of connective tissue disorders of type I collagen, characterized by bone fragility, fractures on trivial trauma, skeletal deformity, blue sclerae, and hearing loss.

**os·te·o·gen·e·sis im·per·fec·ta con·gen·i·ta** (os´tē-ō-jen´ĕ-sis im´pĕr-fek´tă kŏn-jen´i-tă) Severe form with fractures occurring before or at birth.

**os·te·o·gen·e·sis im·per·fec·ta tar·da** (os´tē-ō-jen´ĕ-sis im´pĕr-fek´tă tahr´dă) Less severe form of the disorder, with fractures occurring later in childhood.

**os·te·o·gen·e·sis im·per·fec·ta type I** (os´tē-ō-jen´ĕ-sis im-pĕr-fek´tă tīp) Mild form characterized by hearing loss, easy bruising, prepubertal bone fragility, and short stature.

**os·te·o·gen·e·sis im·per·fec·ta type II** (os´tē-ō-jen´ĕ-sis im-pĕr-fek´tă tīp) Perinatal lethal form associated with stillbirth or lifespan less than 1 year.

**os·te·o·gen·e·sis im·per·fec·ta type III** (os´tē-ō-jen´ĕ-sis im-pĕr-fek´tă tīp) Progressive deforming form with severe bone fragility, easy fractures, triangular facies with relative macrocephaly, skeletal deformities with sco-

**op**

liosis, pectus and bowing of limbs, dwarfism, and radiographic findings of metaphysial flaring of long bones with sutural bone formation.

**os·te·o·gen·e·sis im·per·fec·ta type IV** (os′tē-ō-jen′ĕ-sis im-pĕr-fek′tă tīp) Moderately severe form, characterized by short stature, bone fragility, preambulatory fractures, and bowing of long bones.

**os·te·o·gen·ic, os·te·o·ge·net·ic** (os′tē-ō-jen′ik, -jĕ-net′ik) Relating to osteogenesis.

**os·te·o·gen·ic sar·co·ma** (os′tē-ō-jen′ik sahr-kō′mă) Most common and malignant of bone sarcomas, which arises from bone-forming cells and affects chiefly ends of long bones. SYN osteosarcoma.

**os·te·oid** (os′tē-oyd) **1.** Relating to or resembling bone. **2.** Newly formed organic bone matrix before calcification. SYN osteosarcoma. [*osteo-* + G. *eidos*, resemblance]

**os·te·oid os·te·o·ma** (os′tē-oyd os′tē-ō′mă) Painful but benign neoplasm that usually originates in one of bones of lower extremities, especially femur or tibia of adolescent and young adults; characterized by a nidus that consists of osteoid material, vascularized osteogenic stroma, and poorly formed bone.

**os·te·ol·o·gy** (os′tē-ol′ŏ-jē) The anatomy and science concerned with the bones and their structure.

**os·te·ol·y·sis** (os′tē-ol′i-sis) Softening, absorption, and destruction of bony tissue, a function of the osteoclasts. [*osteo-* + G. *lysis*, dissolution]

▣ **os·te·o·ma** (os′tē-ō′mă) Benign, slow-growing mass of mature, predominantly lamellar bone, usually arising from the cranium or mandible. See this page. [*osteo-* + G. *-oma*, tumor]

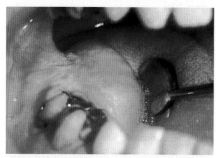

**mandibular osteoma:** bony mass located lingual to the mandibular molars

**os·te·o·ma·la·ci·a** (os′tē-ō-mă-lā′shē-ă) Disease in adults characterized by a gradual softening and bending of bones with varying severity of pain. SYN adult rickets. [*osteo-* + G. *malakia*, softness]

**os·te·o·my·e·li·tis** (os′tē-ō-mī-ĕ-lī′tis) Inflammation of the bone marrow and adjacent bone. SYN central osteitis (1). [*osteo-* + G. *myelos*, marrow, + *-itis*, inflammation]

**os·te·on, os·te·one** (os′tē-on, -ōn) A central canal containing blood capillaries and the concentric osseous lamellae around it occurring in compact bone. SYN haversian system. [G. *osteon*, bone]

**os·te·o·ne·cro·sis** (os′tē-ō-nĕ-krō′sis) Extensive death of bone, as distinguished from caries ("molecular death"). [*osteo-* + G. *nekrōsis*, death]

**os·te·o·nec·tin** (os′tē-ō-nek′tin) A protein found in bone and nonmineralized tissues.

**os·te·op·a·thy** (os′tē-op′ă-thē) **1.** Any disease of bone. **2.** School of medicine based on a concept of the normal body as a vital machine capable, when in correct adjustment, of making its own remedies against infections and other toxic conditions.

**os·te·o·pe·ni·a** (os′tē-ō-pē′nē-ă) **1.** Decreased calcification or density of bone; a descriptive term applicable to all skeletal systems in which such a condition is noted; carries no implication about causality. **2.** Reduced bone mass due to inadequate osteoid synthesis. [*osteo-* + G. *penia*, poverty]

**os·te·o·pe·tro·sis** (os′tē-ō-pĕ-trō′sis) Excessive formation of dense trabecular bone and calcified cartilage, especially in long bones, leading to obliteration of marrow spaces and to anemia with myeloid metaplasia and hepatosplenomegaly beginning in infancy. [*osteo-* + G. *petra*, stone, + *-osis*, condition]

**os·te·o·plas·ty** (os′tē-ō-plas-tē) **1.** In dentistry, resection of osseous structures to achieve acceptable gingival contour. **2.** Bone grafting; reparative or plastic surgery of bones. [*osteo-* + G. *plastos*, formed]

**os·te·o·pon·in** (os′tē-ō-pon′in) A protein produced by osteoblasts of unknown function.

**os·te·o·po·ro·sis** (os′tē-ō-pŏr-ō′sis) Reduction in the quantity of bone or atrophy of skeletal tissue; a widespread age-related disorder characterized by decreased bone mass and loss of normal skeletal microarchitecture, leading to increased susceptibility to fractures. [*osteo-* + G. *poros*, pore, + *-osis*, condition]

**os·te·o·po·rot·ic** (os′tē-ō-pŏr-ot′ik) Pertaining to a porous condition of bones.

**os·te·o·po·ro·tic mar·row de·fect** (os′tē-pŏr-ot′ik mar′ō dē′fekt) Focal osteoporotic bone marrow defect of jaw.

**os·te·o·ra·di·o·ne·cro·sis** (os′tē-ō-rā′dē-ō-nĕ-krō′sis) Necrosis of bone produced by ionizing radiation. [G. *osteon*, bone, + L. *radius*, ray, + G. *nekrōsis*, death, fr. *nekros*, dead]

**os·te·o·sar·co·ma** (os'tē-ō-sahr-kō'mă) See page A6. SYN osteogenic sarcoma.

**os·te·o·scle·ro·sis** (os'tē-ō-skler-ō'sis) Abnormal hardening or eburnation of bone. [*osteo-* + G. *sklērōsis,* hardness]

**os·te·o·syn·the·sis** (os'tē-ō-sin'thĕ-sis) Internal fixation of a fracture by means of a mechanical device (e.g., pin, screw, rod, or plate).

**os·te·o·tome** (os'tē-ō-tōm) Surgical instrument for use in cutting bone. [*osteo-* + G. *tomē,* incision]

**os·te·ot·o·my** (os'tē-ot'ŏ-mē) Cutting a bone. [*osteo-* + G. *tomē,* incision]

**os·ti·um,** pl. **os·ti·a** (os'tē-ŭm, -ă) [TA] Small opening, especially one of entrance into a hollow organ or canal. SEE ALSO orifice, mouth (2). [L. door, entrance, mouth]

**OTC** Abbreviation for over-the-counter (drug).

**o·tic gan·gli·on** (ō'tik gang'glē-ŏn) [TA] An autonomic ganglion situated inferior to the foramen ovale medial to the mandibular nerve. SYN auricular ganglion.

**o·ti·tic ab·scess** (ō-tit'ik ab'ses) Brain abscess, usually involving temporal lobe or cerebellar hemisphere, secondary to suppuration of the middle ear.

**o·ti·tis** (ō-tī'tis) Inflammation of the ear.

**o·ti·tis ex·ter·na** (ō-tī'tis eks-ter'nă) Inflammation of the external auditory canal, usually due to bacterial or fungal infection; swimming, cerumen accumulation, foreign body, and trauma may all be predisposing factors.

**o·ti·tis me·di·a (OM)** (ō-tī'tis mē'dē-ă) Inflammation of the middle ear, or tympanum.

**o·to·lar·yn·gol·o·gist** (ō'tō-lar-in-gol'ŏ-jist) A physician who specializes in otolaryngology.

**o·to·lith·ic** (ō'tō-lith'ik) Pertaining to otoliths.

**o·tol·o·gist** (ō-tol'ŏ-jist) A specialist in otology.

**o·tol·o·gy** (ō-tol'ŏ-jē) The branch of medical science concerned with the study, diagnosis, and treatment of diseases of the ear and related structures. [G. *oto-* [ous] ear, + G. *logos,* study]

**o·to·man·dib·u·lar dys·os·to·sis** (ō'tō-man'dib'yū-lăr dis'os-tō'sis) Hypoplasia of mandible, often with malformation of temporomandibular joint.

**o·to·neu·ral·gi·a** (ō'tō-nū-ral'jē-ă) Earache of neuralgic origin, not caused by inflammation. [*oto-* + G. *neuron,* nerve, + *algos,* pain]

**o·to·pal·a·to·dig·i·tal syn·drome** (ō'tō-pal'ă-tō-dij'i-tăl sin'drōm) Conductive hearing impairment, cleft palate, broad nasal root, frontal bossing, wide spacing of toes, broad thumbs

and great toes, and often other signs of generalized bone dysplasia.

**o·to·pha·ryn·ge·al** (ō'tō-fă-rin'jē-ăl) Relating to middle ear and pharynx.

**o·tor·rhe·a** (ō'tō-rē'ă) Discharge from the ear. SYN otorrhoea. [*oto-* + G. *rhoia,* flow]

**otorrhoea** [Br.] SYN otorrhea.

**o·to·scope** (ō'tō-skōp) An instrument for examining the drum membrane or auscultating the ear. [*oto-* + G. *skopeō,* to view]

**o·tos·co·py** (ō-tos'kŏ-pē) Inspection of the ear. [*oto-* + G. *skopeō,* to view]

**ounce (oz.)** (owns) A weight containing 480 g, or 1/12 pound troy and apothecaries' weight, or 437.5 g, 1/16 pound avoirdupois. [L. *uncia,* the twelfth part (of a pound or foot) hence also inch]

**out·line form** (owt'līn fōrm) Shape of tooth surface area included within cavosurface margins of cavity preparation of a dental restoration.

**out·pa·tient** (owt'pā'shĕnt) Patient treated in a hospital dispensary or clinic instead of in an overnight room or ward.

**out·put** (owt'put) The quantity produced, ejected, or excreted of a specific entity in a specified period of time or per unit time, e.g., urinary sodium output; the opposite of intake or input.

**o·val·o·cy·to·sis** (ō-val'ō-sī-tō'sis) SYN elliptocytosis.

**o·va·ry** (ō'vă-rē) [TA] One of the paired female reproductive glands containing the oocytes or germ cells. [Mod. L. *ovarium,* fr. *ovum,* egg]

**o·ver·bite** (ō'vĕr-bīt) SYN vertical overlap.

**o·ver·clo·sure** (ō'vĕr-klō'zhŭr) Decrease in occlusal vertical dimension.

**o·ver con·tour** (ō'vĕr kon'tūr) An excess of restorative material such that it alters the normal anatomic form.

**o·ver·cor·rec·tion** (ō'vĕr-kŏ-rek'shŭn) Correction of tooth positioning beyond what would be optimal at that moment to prevent relapse to an abnormal position in response to growth changes in tissues.

**o·ver·den·ture** (ō'vĕr-den'chŭr) SYN overlay denture.

**o·ver·e·rup·tion** (ō'vĕr-ĕ-rŭp'shŭn) Occlusal tooth projection beyond line of occlusion.

**o·ver·hang** (ō'vĕr-hang-ing) Excess of dental

op

filling material beyond cavity margin or normal tooth contour. See this page.

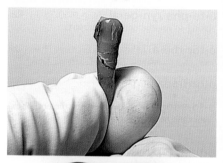

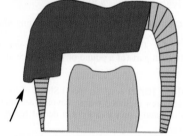

**amalgam overhang:** improperly contoured restoration with overhang that may lead to increased risk of caries and periodontal disease

**o·ver·hang·ing res·tor·a·tion** (ō'vĕr-hang-ing res'tŏr-ā'shŭn) Restoration with excessive material at junction of restoration margin and tooth.

**o·ver·hang re·mo·val** (ō'vĕr-hang rĕ-mū'văl) Recontouring procedures that correct defective margins of restorations to provide a smooth surface to deter bacterial accumulation. If a minor amalgam overhang is acting as a plaque trap and preventing effective plaque control, the excess amalgam can be removed using a specialized powered instrument tip for this purpose.

**o·ver·jet, o·ver·jut** (ō'vĕr-jĕt, -jŭt) See this page. SYN horizontal overlap.

**o·ver·lap** (ō'vĕr-lap) **1.** Suturing of a layer of tissue above or under another to gain strength. **2.** Extension or projection of one tissue over another.

**o·ver·lay** (ō'vĕr-lā) An addition to an already existing condition.

**o·ver·lay den·ture** (ō'vĕr-lā den'chŭr) Complete denture supported by both soft tissue and natural teeth that have been altered to permit denture to fit over them. Altered teeth may have been fitted with short or long copings, locking devices, or connecting bars. SYN bar joint denture, hybrid prosthesis, overdenture, telescopic denture.

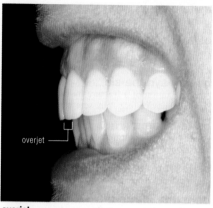

**overjet**

**o·ver-the-coun·ter (drug) (OTC)** (ō'vĕr kown'tĕr) Denotes drugs or therapeutic aids sold to the consumer without the necessity of prescription provided by a health care professional.

**o·void** (ō'voyd) Oval or egg-shaped form.

**o·vum,** pl. **o·va** (ō'vŭm, -vă) Term is imprecise because it has been variously applied to various stages from the primary oocyte to the implanting blastocyst. SEE oocyte. [L. egg]

**Ow·en lines** (ō'ĕn līnz) Accentuated incremental lines in dentin thought to be due to disturbances in mineralization.

**Ow·ren dis·ease** (ō'ren di-zēz') A congenital deficiency of factor V, resulting in prolongation of prothrombin time; bleeding and clotting times are consistently prolonged.

**ox·a·cil·lin so·di·um** (ok'să-sil'in sō'dē-ŭm) Semisynthetic penicillin used in oral therapy of penicillin-resistant staphylococcal infections.

**ox·a·late** (ok'să-lāt) A salt of oxalic acid.

**ox·al·ic ac·id** (ok-sal'ik as'id) Acid found in many plants and vegetables; toxic in elevated levels when ingested by humans; also used in the removal of ink and other stains, and as a general reducing agent.

**ox·a·lu·ri·a** (ok'să-lyūr'ē-ă) SYN hyperoxaluria. [oxalate + G. ouron, urine]

**Ox·ford u·nit** (oks'fŏrd yū'nit) Minimal amount of penicillin that will prevent growth of *Staphylococcus aureus* over an area 26 mm in diameter in a standard culture medium.

**ox·i·dant** (ok'si-dănt) The substance that is reduced and that, therefore, oxidizes the other component of an oxidation-reduction system.

**ox·i·da·tion** (ok'si-dā'shŭn) Combination with oxygen; increasing the valence of an atom or ion by the loss from it of hydrogen or of one or more electrons.

**ox·i·da·tive** (ok'si-dā'tiv) Having the power to oxidize.

**ox·ide** (ok'sīd) A compound of oxygen with another element or a radical.

**ox·im·e·try** (ok-sim'ă-trē) Measurement with an oximeter of the oxygen saturation of hemoglobin in a sample of blood.

**OXT** Abbreviation for oxytocin.

**ox·y·ceph·a·ly** (ok'sē-sef'ă-lē) A type of craniosynostosis in which there is premature closure of the lambdoid and coronal sutures, resulting in an abnormally high, peaked, or cone-shaped cranium. SYN acrocephaly, acrocephalia. [G. *oxys*, pointed, + *kephalē*, head]

**ox·y·co·done** (ok'sē-kō'dōn) A narcotic analgesic often prepared with aspirin or acetaminophen.

**ox·y·gen** (ok'si-jĕn) Abundant and widely distributed gaseous chemical element, which combines with most other elements to form oxides and is essential to animal and plant life. [G. *oxys*, sharp, acid and *genes*, forming]

**ox·y·gen·ate** (ok'si-jĕ-nāt) To accomplish oxygenation.

**ox·y·gen·a·tion** (ok'si-jĕ-nā'shŭn) **1.** Addition of oxygen to any chemical or physical sys-

tem. **2.** Specifically used to describe interventions that provide greater oxygen supply to lungs and thus the circulation.

**ox·y·gen ther·a·py** (oks'i-jĕn thār'ă-pē) Treatment in which an increased concentration of oxygen is made available for breathing, through a nasal catheter, tent, chamber, or mask.

**oxyhaemoglobin** [Br.] SYN oxyhemoglobin.

**ox·y·he·mo·glo·bin** (ok'sē-hē'mŏ-glō'bin) Hemoglobin in combination with oxygen; the form of hemoglobin present in arterial blood. SYN oxyhaemoglobin.

**ox·y·phil, ox·y·phile** (ok'sē-fil, -fīl) **1.** Oxyphil *cell.* **2.** SYN eosinophilic leukocyte. **3.** SYN oxyphilic. [G. *oxys*, sour, acid, + *philos*, fond]

**oxyphilic** SYN oxyphil, oxyphile.

**ox·y·phil·ic leu·ko·cyte** (ok'sē-fil'ik lū' kō-sīt) SYN eosinophilic leukocyte.

**ox·y·to·cin (OXT)** (ok'si-tō'sin) Nonapeptide neurohypophysial hormone that causes myometrial contractions at term and promotes milk release during lactation.

**oz.** Abbreviation for ounce.

**o·zo·sto·mi·a** (ō'zō-stō'mē-ă) SYN halitosis. [G. *ozō*, to smell, + *stoma*, mouth]

**op**

# P

**II** Abbreviation for osmotic pressure.

**P** Abbreviation for pressure.

**PA** Abbreviation for physician assistant; posteroanterior.

**pace·mak·er** (pās′mā-kĕr) **1.** Biologically, any rhythmic center that establishes a pace of activity. **2.** An artificial regulator of rate activity. [L. *passus,* step, pace]

**pach·y·glos·si·a** (pak′ē-glos′ē-ă) An enlarged thick tongue. [G. *pachy-,* thick + G. *glōssa,* tongue]

**pa·chyg·na·thous** (pă-kig′nă-thŭs) Characterized by a large or thick jaw. [G. *pachy-,* thick + G. *gnathos,* jaw]

**pach·y·men·in·gi·tis** (pak′ē-men-in-jī′tis) Inflammation of the dura mater.

**pack** (pak) **1.** To fill, stuff, or tampon. **2.** To enwrap or envelop body in a sheet, blanket, or other covering. **3.** To apply a dressing or covering to a surgical site. **4.** Items used for wound dressing. [M.E. *pak,* fr. Germanic]

**pack·er** (pak′ĕr) **1.** Instrument for tamponing. **2.** SYN plugger.

**pack·ing** (pak′ing) **1.** Filling a natural cavity, wound, or mold with some material. **2.** The material so used. **3.** The application of a pack.

**pack·ing pro·cess** (pak′ing pro′ses) Method of placing denture base material in a flask for processing.

**pac·li·tax·el** (pak′li-taks′ĕl) Antitumor agent that promotes microtubule assembly by preventing depolymerization; currently used in salvage therapy for metastatic carcinoma of ovary and other cancers.

**PACU** Abbreviation for postanesthesia care unit.

**pad** (pad) **1.** Portion of finger that rests on dental instrument. **2.** Soft material forming a cushion, used in applying or relieving pressure on a part, or in filling a depression so that dressings can fit snugly. **3.** More or less encapsulated body of fat or some other tissue serving to fill a space or act as a cushion in the body (e.g., heel pad).

**pad-to-pad pinch** (pad pad pinch) OCCUPATIONAL THERAPY a grip between the thumb pad and the index finger pad distal to the distal interphalangeal joint.

**paediatric dentist** [Br.] SYN pediatric dentist.

**paediatric dentistry** [Br.] SYN pediatric dentistry.

**paediatrician** [Br.] SYN pediatrician.

**paediatrics** [Br.] SYN pediatrics.

**paedodontia** [Br.] SYN pedodontia.

**paedodontics** [Br.] SYN pedodontics.

**paedodontist** [Br.] SYN pedodontist.

**pain** (pān) Variably unpleasant sensation associated with tissue damage and mediated by specific nerve fibers to brain where its conscious appreciation is modified. [L. *poena,* a fine, a penalty]

**Pa·get dis·ease** (paj′ĕt di-zēz′) **1.** A generalized skeletal disease, frequently familial, of older people in which bone resorption and formation are both increased, leading to thickening and softening of bones (e.g., the skull), and bending of weight-bearing bones. SYN osteitis deformans. **2.** A disease of elderly women, characterized by an infiltrated, somewhat eczematous lesion surrounding and involving the nipple and areola, and associated with subjacent intraductal cancer of the breast and infiltration of the lower epidermis by malignant cells.

**pain dis·or·der** (pān dis-ōr′dĕr) Somatoform disorder in which pain is the predominant presenting symptom.

**pain·ful an·es·the·si·a** (pān′fŭl an′es-thē′zē-ă) SYN anesthesia dolorosa.

**pain re·ac·tion** (pān rē-ak′shŭn) Dilation of pupil or other involuntary act in response to a stimulus causing sharp pain anywhere.

**pain thresh·old** (pān thresh′ōld) Lowest intensity of a painful stimulus at which subject perceives pain.

**pain tol·er·ance** (pān tol′ĕr-ăns) Highest intensity of painful stimulation that a tested subject is able to tolerate.

**pair·ed work·ing-end** (pārd wŏrk′ing-end) Double-ended instrument with working-ends that are exact mirror images of each other.

**pal·a·tal** (pal′ă-tăl) Relating to palate or palate bone. SYN palatine.

**pal·a·tal ab·scess** (pal′ă-tăl ab′ses) **1.** Lateral periodontal abscess associated with lingual surface of a maxillary tooth. **2.** Alveolar abscess that has eroded cortical plate, allowing extension into palatal soft tissues.

**pal·a·tal bar** (pal′ă-tăl bahr) Major connector that crosses palate and unites two or more parts of a maxillary removable partial denture. SYN palatal bar connector.

**pal·a·tal bar con·nec·tor** (pal′ă-tăl bahr kŏ-nek′tŏr) SYN palatal bar.

**pal·a·tal cross·bite** (pal′ă-tăl kraws′bīt) Displacement of maxillary teeth as related to the opposing teeth.

**pal·a·tal nys·tag·mus** (pal′ă-tăl nis-tag′mŭs) Clonic spasm of the levator palati muscle, causing an audible click.

**pal·a·tal plate** (pal′ă-tăl plāt) Major connector of a removable maxillary prosthesis that covers part of palate.

**pal·a·tal re·flex, pal·a·tine re·flex** (pal′ă-tăl rē′fleks, pal′ă-tīn) Swallowing reflex induced by stimulation of palate.

**pal·a·tal seal** (pal′ă-tăl sēl) SYN posterior palatal seal.

**pal·a·tal shelves** (pal′ă-tăl shelvz) SYN lateral palatine processes.

**pal·a·tal trem·or** (pal′ă-tăl trem′ŏr) Involuntary, persistent, rapid regular tremor of the soft palate, face, and diaphragm related to lesions of the olivocerebellar pathway.

**pal·a·tal tri·an·gle** (pal′ă-tăl trī′ang-gĕl) Area bounded by greatest transverse diameter of palate and by lines converging from its extremities to alveolar point.

**pal·ate** (pal′ăt) [TA] Bony and muscular partition between oral and nasal cavities. See this page. SYN roof of mouth. [L. *palatum,* palate]

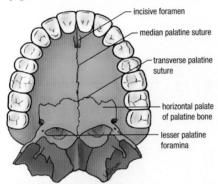

incisive foramen
median palatine suture
transverse palatine suture
horizontal palate of palatine bone
lesser palatine foramina

**osseous structures of palate:** inferior view

**pa·lat·i·form** (pă-lat′i-fōrm) Palate-shaped; resembling the palate.

**pal·a·tine** (pal′ă-tīn) SYN palatal.

**pal·a·tine ap·o·neu·ro·sis** (pal′ă-tīn ap′ō-nūr-ō′sis) [TA] Expanded interlacing tendons of tensor veli palatini muscles in anterior two thirds of soft palate to which other palatine muscles attach.

**pal·a·tine bone** (pal′ă-tīn bōn) [TA] Irregularly shaped bone posterior to maxilla, which enters into formation of nasal cavity, orbit, and hard palate; articulates with maxilla, inferior nasal concha, sphenoid, and ethmoid bones, vomer and its fellow of the opposite side.

**pal·a·tine crest of hor·i·zon·tal pro·cess of pal·a·tine bone** (pal′ă-tīn krest hōr′i-zon′tăl pro′ses pal′ă-tīn bōn) [TA] Transverse ridge near posterior border of bony palate, located on inferior surface of horizontal plate of palatine bone. SYN crista palatina.

**pal·a·tine glands** (pal′ă-tīn glandz) [TA] Racemose mucous glands in posterior half of submucous tissue covering hard palate, soft palate, and uvula.

**pal·a·tine grooves** (pal′ă-tīn grūvz) [TA] Grooves on lower surface of palatine process of maxilla in which palatine vessels and nerves lie.

**pal·a·tine pro·cess of max·il·la** (pal′ă-tīn pro′ses mak-sil′ă) [TA] Medially directed shelves from maxillae that, with horizontal plate of palatine bone, form bony palate.

**pal·a·tine ra·phe** (pal′ă-tīn rā′fē) [TA] Low narrow elevation in center of hard palate that extends from incisive papilla posteriorly over entire length of mucosa of hard palate. See page 428.

**pal·a·tine spines** (pal′ă-tīn spīnz) [TA] Longitudinal ridges along palatine grooves on inferior surface of palatine process of maxilla.

**pal·a·tine sur·face of hor·i·zon·tal plate of pal·a·tine bone** (pal′ă-tīn sŭr′făs hōr′i-zon′tăl plăt pal′ă-tīn bōn) [TA] Inferior surface of palatine bone. SYN facies palatina laminae horizontalis ossis palatini.

**pal·a·tine sur·face of tooth** (pal′ă-tīn sŭr′făs tūth) [TA] Oral surface of a maxillary tooth, directed toward palate. SYN facies palatina dentis.

**pal·a·tine ton·sil** (pal′ă-tīn ton′sil) [TA] Large oval mass of lymphoid tissue embedded in lateral wall of oral pharynx on either side between the pillars of the fauces. SYN tonsil (2), tonsilla palatina, tonsilla.

**pal·a·tine to·rus, to·rus pal·a·ti·nus** (pal′ă-tīn tōr′ŭs, pal′ă-tī′nŭs) Exostosis protruding from midline of hard palate.

**pal·a·tine uv·u·la** (pal′ă-tīn yū′vyū-lă) A conic projection from the posterior edge of the middle of the soft palate, composed of connective tissue containing several racemose glands, and some muscular fibers (musculus uvulae).

**pal·a·ti·tis** (pal′ă-tī′tis) Inflammation of palate.

**palato-** Combining form meaning palate. [L. *palatum,* palate]

**pal·a·to·eth·moi·dal su·ture** (pal′ă-tō-eth-moy′dăl sū′chŭr) [TA] Line of junction of orbital process of palatine bone and orbital plate of ethmoid.

**pal·a·to·glos·sal** (pal′ă-tō-glos′ăl) Relating to palate and tongue or to palatoglossus muscle.

**pal·a·to·glos·sal arch** (pal′ă-tō-glos′ăl ahrch) [TA] One of a pair of ridges of mucous membrane passing from soft palate to side of tongue; encloses palatoglossus muscle and forms anterior margin of tonsillar fossa. SYN anterior palatine arch, anterior pillar of fauces.

**pal·a·to·glos·sus (mus·cle)** (pal′ă-tō-glos′ŭs mŭs′ĕl) [TA] Palatine muscle that forms anterior pillar of tonsillar fossa.

**pal·a·to·gram** (pal′ă-tō-gram) Registration of tongue action against palate made by placing soft wax or powder on a baseplate.

**pal·a·to·graph** (pal′ă-tō-graf) Instrument

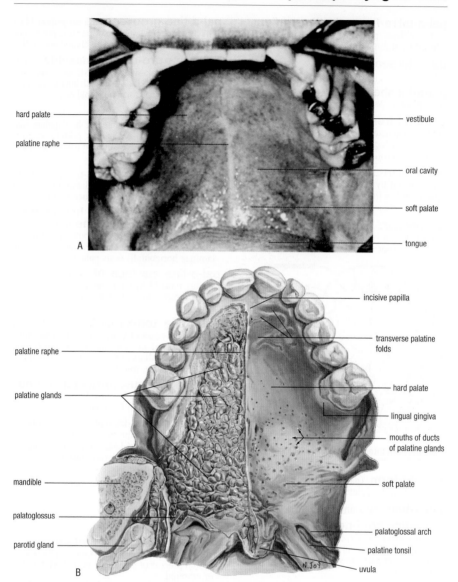

**maxillary teeth and palate:** (A) anterior view of maxillary teeth and mucosa covering hard palate (bony palate) in a patient; (B) inferior view of mucous membrane and glands of palate

used to record movements of soft palate in speaking and during respiration.

**pal·a·to·max·il·lar·y** (pal′ă-tō-mak′si-lar-ē) Relating to palate and maxilla.

**pal·a·to·max·il·lar·y in·dex** (pal′ă-tō-mak′si-lar-ē in′deks) Relation of palatomaxillary width, measured between outer borders of alveolar arch just above middle of second molar tooth, and palatomaxillary length.

**pal·a·to·max·il·lar·y su·ture** (pal′ă-tō-mak′si-lar-ē sū′chŭr) [TA] Line of union, in

floor of orbit, between orbital process of palatine bone and orbital surface of maxilla.

**pal·a·to·na·sal** (pal′ă-tō-nā′zăl) Relating to palate and nasal cavity.

**pal·a·to·pha·ryn·ge·al** (pal′ă-tō-fă-rin′jē-ăl) Relating to palate and pharynx.

**pal·a·to·pha·ryn·ge·al (mus·cle)** (pal′ă-tō-fă-rin′jē-ăl mŭs′el) SYN palatopharyngeus (muscle).

**pal·a·to·pha·ryn·ge·al arch** (pal′ă-tō-fă-rin′jē-ăl ahrch) [TA] Type of ridge of mucous membrane that passes downward from posterior margin of soft palate to lateral wall of pharynx.

**pal·a·to·pha·ryn·ge·al ridge** (pal´ă-tō-fă-rin´jē-ăl rij) Prominence on posterior wall of nasopharynx formed by contraction of superior constrictor muscle of pharynx during swallowing. Also called Passavant bar, cushion, pad, and ridge. SYN crista palatopharyngea.

**pal·a·to·pha·ryn·ge·al sphinc·ter** (pal´ă-tō-fă-rin´jē-ăl sfingk´tĕr) SYN posterior fascicle of palatopharyngeus muscle.

**pal·a·to·pha·ryn·ge·us (mus·cle)** (pal´ă-tō-fă-rin´jē-us mŭs´ĕl) [TA] *Origin*, soft palate; forms the posterior pillar of the fauces or tonsillar fossa; *insertion*, posterior border of thyroid cartilage and aponeurosis of pharynx; *action*, narrows fauces, depresses soft palate, elevates pharynx and larynx; *nerve supply*, pharyngeal plexus (cranial root of accessory nerve). SYN musculus palatopharyngeus [TA].

**pal·a·to·plas·ty** (pal´ă-tō-plas-tē) Surgery of palate to restore form and function. [*palato-* + G. *plassō*, to form]

**pal·a·to·ple·gi·a** (pal´ă-tō-plē´jē-ă) Paralysis of muscles of soft palate.

**pal·a·tor·rha·phy** (pal´ă-tōr´ă-fē) Suture of a cleft palate. [*palato-* + G. *rhaphē*, suture]

**pa·li·nop·si·a** (pal´i-nop´sē-ă) Abnormal recurring visual hallucinations. [G. *palin*, again, + *opsis*, vision]

**pal·la·di·um (Pd)** (pă-lā´dē-ŭm) A metallic element resembling platinum.

**pallaesthesia** [Br.] SYN pallesthesia.

**pallanaesthesia** [Br.] SYN pallanesthesia.

**pal·lan·es·the·si·a** (pal´an-es-thē´zē-ă) Absence of pallesthesia. SYN apallesthesia, pallanaesthesia. [G. *pallō*, to quiver, + *anaisthēsia*, insensibility]

**pal·les·the·si·a** (pal´es-thē´zē-ă) Appreciation of vibration. SYN pallaesthesia. [G. *pallō*, to quiver, + *aisthēsis*, sensation]

**pal·li·ate** (pal´ē-āt) To reduce severity of something; to relieve slightly. SYN mitigate. [L. *palliatus* (adj.), dressed in a *pallium*, cloaked]

**pal·li·a·tive** (pal´ē-ă-tiv) Reducing the severity of pain or discomfort.

**pal·li·a·tive treat·ment** (pal´ē-ă-tiv trēt´mĕnt) Treatment to alleviate symptoms without curing the disease.

**pal·li·dot·o·my** (pal´i-dot´ŏ-mē) A destructive operation on the globus pallidus. [*pallidum* + G. *tomē*, incision]

**pal·lor** (pal´ŏr) Paleness, as of the skin. [L.]

**Pal·mer den·tal no·men·cla·ture** (pahl´mĕr den´tăl nō´mĕn-klā-chŭr) **1.** System of identifying permanent teeth by use of a number indicating sequential position of a tooth distally from the midline; number is bracketed with a right angle to identify the tooth's dental quadrant. **2.** System for deciduous teeth analogous to permanent tooth with letters substituted for numbers (A through E or a through e). SYN Zsigmondy dental nomenclature.

**palm grasp** (pahlm grasp) Mode of holding in which instrument handle is held in the palm of the hand with all four fingers securely gripping it; employed in dentistry for forceps and the air-water syringe.

**pal·mic** (pahl´mik) Beating; throbbing; relating to a palmus.

**pal·mit·ic ac·id** (pal-mit´ik as´id) A common saturated fatty acid in palm oil and olive oil.

**pal·mo·men·tal re·flex** (pal´mō-men´tăl rē´fleks) Unilateral (sometimes bilateral) contraction of mentalis and orbicularis oris muscles caused by a brisk scratch made on palm of ipsilateral hand.

**pal·mo·plan·tar ker·a·to·der·ma** (pal´mō-plan´tăr ker´ă-tō-dĕr´mă) Symmetric diffuse or patchy areas of hypertrophy of horny layer of epidermis on the palms and soles.

**pal·mus**, pl. **pal·mi** (pahl´mŭs, -mī) **1.** SYN facial tic. **2.** Rhythmic fibrillary contractions in a muscle.

**pal·pa·ble** (pal´pă-bĕl) **1.** Perceptible to touch. **2.** Evident; plain.

**pal·pate** (pal´pāt) To examine by feeling and pressing with palms of hands and fingers.

**pal·pa·tion** (pal-pā´shŭn) Examination with hands, feeling for organs, masses, or infiltration of a body part, feeling the heart or pulse beat, or chest vibrations.

**pal·pa·to·per·cus·sion** (pal´pă-tō-pĕr-kŭsh´ŭn) Examination using palpation and percussion.

**pal·pa·to·ry per·cus·sion** (pal´pă-tōr´ē pĕr-kŭsh´ŭn) Digital percussion in which attention is focused on tissue resistance and reverberation and under finger.

**pal·pi·ta·tion** (pal´pi-tā´shŭn) Forcible or irregular pulsation of the heart, perceptible to the patient, usually with an increase in frequency or force, with or without irregularity in rhythm. SYN trepidatio cordis. [L. *palpito*, to throb]

**pal·sy** (pawl´zē) Paralysis or paresis.

**pan·a·ce·a** (pan´ă-sē´ă) A cure-all; remedy claimed to be curative of all diseases.

**pan·cre·a·tin** (pan´krē-ă-tin) A combination of specific digestive (pancreatic) enzymes obtained from swine or cattle; used medicinally in various ways. [G. *pankreas*, pancreas]

**pan·cre·a·ti·tis** (pan´krē-ă-tī´tis) Inflammation of pancreas.

op

**pan·cre·at·o·gen·ic, pan·cre·at·og·e·nous** (pan′krē-ă-tō-jen′ik, -toj′ĕ-nŭs) Of pancreatic origin. [*pancreato-* + G. *genesis,* origin]

**pan·cre·a·top·a·thy, pan·cre·op·a·thy** (pan′krē-ă-top′ă-thē, -krē-op′ă-thē) Any disease of the pancreas. [*pancreato-* + G. *pathos,* suffering]

**pan·cre·li·pase** (pan′krē-lip′ās) A concentrate of pancreatic enzymes standardized for lipase content.

**pan·cy·to·pe·ni·a** (pan′sī-tō-pē′nē-ă) Pronounced reduction in number of erythrocytes, all types of leukocytes, and blood platelets in the circulating blood. [G. *pan-,* all + G. *kytos,* cell, + *penia,* poverty]

**pan·dem·ic** (pan-dem′ik) Denoting a disease affecting or attacking the population of an extensive region, country, continent; extensively epidemic. [*pan-* + G. *dēmos,* the people]

**pang** (pang) A sudden sharp, brief pain.

**pan·hy·po·pi·tu·i·tar·ism** (pan-hī′pō-pi-tū′i-tă-rizm) A state in which secretion of all anterior pituitary hormones is diminished. SYN hypophysial cachexia.

**pan·ic** (pan′ik) Extreme and unreasoning anxiety and fear. [fr. G. myth. char., *Pan*]

**pan·ic at·tack** (pan′ik ă-tak′) Sudden onset of intense apprehension, fear, terror, or impending doom accompanied by increased autonomic nervous system activity and by various constitutional disturbances.

**pan·ic dis·or·der** (pan′ik dis-ōr′dĕr) Recurrent panic attacks that occur unpredictably.

**pan·my·e·loph·thi·sis** (pan′mī-ĕ-lof′thi-sis) SYN myelophthisis (2).

**pan·o·ram·ic ra·di·o·graph** (pan′ŏ-ram′ik rā′dē-ō-graf) Radiographic view of maxillae and mandible extending from left to right glenoid fossae. See this page.

**pan·o·ram·ic ro·tat·ing ma·chine** (pan′ŏr-am′ik rō′tāt-ing mă-shēn′) X-ray machine using a reciprocating motion of tube and extraoral film to produce a radiograph of all teeth and surrounding structures.

**pan·o·ram·ic x-ray film** (pan′ŏ-ram′ik eks′ rā film) In dentistry, radiograph taken to give a panoramic view of the entire upper and lower dental arch and the temporomandibular joints.

**pan·si·nu·si·tis** (pan′sī-nŭ-sī′tis) Inflammation involving all the paranasal sinuses.

**pan·to·graph** (pan′tō-graf) In dentistry, instrument used to record mandibular border movements that may be transferred to make equivalent settings on an articulator. [*panto-* + G. *graphō,* to record]

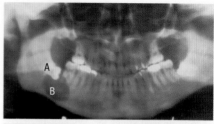
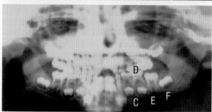

panoramic radiograph, adult dentition (top): unerupted mandibular third molar (A) and a large cyst in mandibular bone around crown of molar (B); panoramic radiograph, mixed dentition (bottom): partially formed permanent mandibular molars (C) erupting below deciduous molars (D); erupted permanent first molar with incompletely formed roots (E); crown of incompletely formed, unerupted, second permanent molar (F)

**pan·to·graph·ic trac·ing** (pan′tō-graf′ik trās′ing) Graphic recording of mandibular movements in various planes.

**pan·to·mo·gram** (pan′tō-mŏ-gram) Panoramic radiographic record of maxillary and mandibular dental arches and their associated structures, obtained by a pantomograph. [*pan-* + *tomogram*]

**pan·to·mo·graph** (pan′tō-mŏ-graf) Panoramic radiographic instrument that permits visualization of entire dentition, alveolar bone, and contiguous structures on a single extraoral film.

**pan·to·mog·ra·phy** (pan′tŏ-mog′ră-fē) Method of radiography by which a radiograph (pantomogram) of maxillary and mandibular dental arches and their contiguous structures may be obtained on a single film.

**pan·to·then·ic ac·id** (pan′tŏ-then′ik as′id) The β-alanine amide of pantoic acid. A growth substance widely distributed in plant and animal tissues, and essential for growth of a number of organisms; deficiency in diet causes a dermatitis in chicks and rats and achromotrichia in the latter; a precursor to coenzyme A.

**pa·pa·in, pa·pa·in·ase** (pă-pā′in, -ās) A cysteine endopeptidase, or a crude extract containing it, obtained from papaya latex. It has esterase, thiolase, transamidase, and transesterase activities; is used as a protein digestant, meat tenderizer, and to prevent adhesions.

**pa·pav·er·ine** (pă-pav′ĕr-ēn) Mild analgesic and powerful spasmolytic. [L. *papaver,* poppy]

**pa·pa·yo·tin** (pah′pah′yō-tin) SYN papain.

**pa·per** (pā′pĕr) A square of paper folded over so as to form an envelope containing a dose of any medicinal powder.

**pa·per points** (pā′pĕr poynts) SYN absorbent points.

**pa·pil·la,** pl. **pa·pil·lae** (pă-pil′ă, -ē) [TA] Any small, nipplelike process. See this page. [L. a nipple, dim. of *papula,* a pimple]

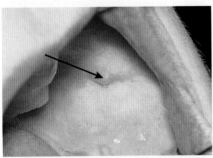
**parotid papilla (adjacent to maxillary first molar)**

**pa·pil·lae of tongue** (pă-pil′ē tŭng) [TA] Projections of mucous membrane of dorsum of tongue; includes filiform, foliate, fungiform, and vallate papillae.

**pap·il·lar·y, pap·il·late** (pap′i-lar-ē, -i-lāt) Relating to, resembling, or provided with papillae.

**pa·pil·le·de·ma** (pap′il-ĕ-dē′mă) Edema of the optic disc. SYN choked disc, papilloedema. [*papilla* + *edema*]

**papilloedema** [Br.] SYN papilledema.

**pap·il·lo·ma** (pap′i-lō′mă) Circumscribed, benign epithelial neoplasm consisting of villous or arborescent outgrowths of fibrovascular stroma covered by neoplastic cells. See this page. [*papilla* + G. *-oma,* tumor]

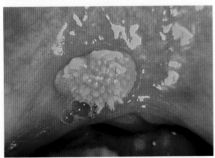
**papilloma:** note fingerlike projections

**Pa·pil·lon-Le·fèv·re syn·drome** (pap′ ē-ōn[h] lĕ-fev′ sin′drōm) Congenital hyperkeratosis of palms and soles, with progessive destruction of alveolar bone about deciduous and permanent teeth beginning as early as 2 years of age, and premature exfoliation of teeth and calcification of falx cerebri.

**Pa·po·va·vir·i·dae** (pă-pō′vă-vir′i-dē) A family of small antigenically distinct viruses that replicate in nuclei of infected cells; most have oncogenic properties. The family includes the genera *Papillomavirus* and *Polyomavirus.* [*pa*-pilloma + *po*lyoma + *va*cuolating]

**pap·ule** (pap′yūl) A circumscribed, solid elevation on the skin; may be pedunculated, sessile, or filiform. See this page. [L. *papula,* pimple]

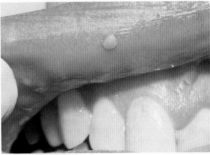
**papule:** fibroepithelial polyp due to chronic irritation

🜚 **para-** *Do not confuse this prefix with pari- or peri-.* **1.** Prefix denoting a departure from the normal. **2.** Prefix denoting involvement of two like parts or a pair. **3.** Prefix denoting adjacent, alongside, near. [G. alongside, near]

**par·a·chlor·o·phe·nol** (par′ă-klōr′ō-fē′nol) A disinfectant effective against most gram-negative organisms.

**par·ac·mas·tic** (par′ak-mas′tik) Relating to the paracme.

**par·ac·me** (par-ak′mē) **1.** Stage of subsidence of a fever. **2.** Period of life beyond its prime. [G. the point at which the prime is past; fr. *para,* beyond, + *akmē,* highest point, prime]

**par·a·coc·cid·i·oi·do·my·co·sis** (par′ ă-kok-sid′ē-oy′dō-mī-kō′sis) Chronic mycosis characterized by primary pulmonary lesions with dissemination to many visceral organs, conspicuous ulcerative granulomas of buccal and nasal mucosa with extensions to skin, and generalized lymphangitis; caused by *Paracoccidioides brasiliensis.*

**par·a·cone** (par′ă-kōn) Mesiobuccal cusp of upper molar tooth. [*para-* + G. *kōnos,* cone]

**par·a·co·nid** (par′ă-kō′nid) Mesiobuccal cusp of a lower molar tooth.

op

**par·a·cu·sis, par·a·cu·si·a, par·a·cou·sis** (par'ă-kyū'sis, -zē-ă, -sis) **1.** Impaired hearing. **2.** Auditory illusions or hallucinations. [*para-* + G. *akousis*, hearing]

**par·a·den·tal** (par'ă-den'tăl) SYN periodontal.

**par·a·den·ti·um** (par'ă-den'tē-ŭm) SYN periodontium.

**par·a·dip·si·a** (par'ă-dip'sē-ă) A perverted appetite for fluids, ingested without relation to bodily need. [*para-* + G. *dipsa*, thirst]

**par·a·don·to·sis** (par'ă-don-tō'sis) Older usage for degenerative disease of the peridontium but without clinical evidence of inflammation; today term has in some sense been replaced by periodontosis (q.v.).

**par·a·dox** (par'ă-doks) That which is apparently, although not actually, inconsistent with or opposed to known facts in any case. [G. *paradoxos*, incredible, beyond belief, fr. *doxa*, belief]

**par·a·dox·ic pu·pil·lar·y re·flex** (par'ă-doks'ik pyū'pi-lar-ē rē'fleks) Constriction of pupils in darkness, the reverse of that expected.

**par·a·dox·ic re·flex** (par'ă-doks'ik rē'fleks) Any reflex in which usual response is reversed or does not conform to characteristic pattern.

**paraesthesia** [Br.] SYN paresthesia.

**par·af·fin** (par'ă-fin) SYN hard paraffin. [L. *parum*, little, + *affinis*, neighboring, akin]

**par·af·fin bath** (par'ă-fin bath) Warmed paraffin wax and mineral oil mixture used to coat a body part, causing heat to penetrate into the tissues; used to treat joint inflammation.

**par·af·fin wax** (par'ă-fin waks) Wax derived from petroleum.

**par·a·for·mal·de·hyde** (par'ă-fōr-mal'dĕ-hīd) A disinfectant agent.

**par·a·func·tion** (par'ă-fŭngk'shŭn) **1.** In dentistry, movements of mandible that are outside normal function (e.g., bruxism). **2.** Abnormal or disordered function.

**pa·ra·func·tion·al** (par'ă-fungk'shŭn-ăl) Denotes in dentistry abnormal or deviated function.

**par·a·gan·gli·o·ma** (par'ă-gang-glē-ō'mă) A neoplasm usually derived from the chromoreceptor tissue of a paraganglion or the medulla of the suprarenal gland.

**par·a·glot·tic space** (par'ă-glot'ik spās) Area on each side of glottis bounded laterally by perichondrium of thyroid cartilage and cricothyroid membrane and posteriorly by mucous membrane of pyriform sinus.

**pa·rag·na·thus** (pă-rag'nă-thŭs) Developmental defect resulting in a child with an accessory lower jaw. [*para-* + G. *gnathos*, jaw]

**par·a·gon·i·mi·a·sis** (par'ă-gon'i-mī'ă-sis) Infection with a worm of the genus *Paragonimus*, especially *P. westermani*.

**par·a·ker·a·to·sis** (par'ă-ker'ă-tō'sis) Retention of nuclei in the cells of the stratum corneum of the epidermis, observed in many scaling dermatoses such as psoriasis and subacute or chronic dermatitis.

**par·al·ge·si·a** (par'al-jē'zē-ă) Painful paresthesia; any disorder or abnormality of the sense of pain. [*para-* + G. *algēsis*, the sense of pain]

**par·al·lax** (par'ă-laks) The apparent displacement of an object that follows a change in the position from which it is viewed. [G. alternately, fr. *par-allassō*, to make alternate, fr. *allos*, other]

**par·al·lel cop·ing** (par'ă-lel kōp'ing) Casting placed over an abutment tooth or implant to make it parallel to another abutment.

**par·al·le·ling tec·hnique** (par'ă-lel-ing tek-nēk') Radiographic modality in which the incident beam is perpendicular to the long axis of the tooth and the plane of the film.

**par·al·lel·ism** (par'ă-lel-izm) State of being structurally parallel. [*para-* + G. *allēlōn*, of one another, fr. *allos*, other]

**par·al·lel·om·e·ter** (par'ă-lel-om'ĕ-tĕr) Apparatus used for paralleling attachments and abutments for fixed or removable partial dentures.

**par·al·lel o·pen·ing** (par'ă-lel ō'pĕn-ing) Casting placed over an abutment tooth or implant to make it parallel to another abutment.

**pa·ral·y·sis,** pl. **pa·ral·y·ses** (păr-al'i-sis, -sēz) **1.** Loss of power of voluntary movement in a muscle through injury or disease of it or its nerve supply. **2.** Loss of any function. [G. fr. *para-* + *lysis*, a loosening]

**par·a·lyze** (par'ă-līz) To render incapable of movement.

**par·a·med·ic** (par'ă-med'ik) A person trained and certified to provide emergency care.

**par·a·med·i·cal** (par'ă-med'i-kăl) Related to medical profession in an adjunctive capacity.

**pa·ram·e·ter** (pă-ram'ĕ-tĕr) One of many dimensions or ways of measuring or describing an object or evaluating a subject. [*para-* + G. *metron*, measure]

**par·a·mo·lar** (par'ă-mō'lăr) Supernumerary tooth lying among, lingual to, or buccal to maxillary or mandibular molars.

**par·am·y·loi·do·sis** (par-am'i-loy-dō'sis) Deposition in tissues of an amyloidlike protein resembling light chains of immunoglobulins in primary amyloidosis or in atypical amyloidosis of multiple myeloma.

**Par·a·myx·o·vir·i·dae** (par′ă-mik-sō-vir′i-dē) RNA-containing viruses. Three genera are recognized: *Paramyxovirus*, *Morbillivirus*, and *Pneumovirus*, all cause cell fusion and produce cytoplasmic eosinophilic inclusions.

**paranaesthesia** [Br.] SYN paranesthesia.

**par·an·al·ge·si·a** (par′an-ăl-jē′zē-ă) Analgesia of the lower half of the body.

**par·a·na·sal** (par′ă-nā′zăl) Adjacent to the nose. [*para-* + L. *nasus*, nose]

**☐par·a·na·sal si·nus·es** (par′ă-nā′zăl sī′nŭs-ĕz) [TA] Paired air-filled cavities in bones of face lined by mucous membrane continuous with that of the nasal cavity; frontal, sphenoidal, maxillary, and ethmoidal. See this page.

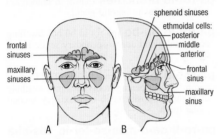

sphenoid sinuses
ethmoidal cells:
posterior
middle
anterior
frontal sinus
maxillary sinus

frontal sinuses

maxillary sinuses

A     B

**paranasal sinuses:** (A) anterior and (B) lateral views of head

**par·a·ne·o·plas·tic syn·drome** (par′ă-nē-ō-plas′tik sin′drōm) Syndrome directly resulting from a malignant neoplasm, but not resulting from presence of tumor cells.

**par·an·es·the·si·a** (par′an-es-thē′zē-ă) Loss of feeling or sensation (anesthesia) in the lower half of the body. SYN paranaesthesia.

**par·a·noi·a** (par′ă-noy′ă) Severe but relatively rare mental disorder characterized by systematized delusions, often of a persecutory character involving being followed, or harmed by other means. [G. derangement, madness, fr. *para-* + *noeō*, to think]

**par·a·noid per·son·al·i·ty dis·or·der** (par′ă-noyd pĕr-sŏ-nal′i-tē dis-ōr′dĕr) Personality disorder less debilitating than paranoid or delusional paranoid disorder.

**par·a·o·ral** (par′ă-ōr′ăl) Adjacent to mouth. [*para-* + L. *os* (*or-*), mouth]

**par·a·pa·re·sis** (par′ă-pă-rē′sis) Weakness affecting lower extremities.

**par·a·pe·de·sis** (par′ă-pĕ-dē′sis) Excretion or secretion through an abnormal channel. [*para-* + G. *pēdēsis*, a bending, deflection]

**par·a·phil·i·a** (par′ă-fil′ē-ă) A mental disorder with obsession with socially proscribed sexual practices. [*para-* + G. *philos*, fond]

**par·a·ple·gi·a** (par′ă-plē′jē-ă) Paralysis of both lower extremities and, generally, lower trunk. [*para-* + *plēgē*, a stroke]

**par·a·pso·ri·a·sis** (par′ă-sōr-ī′ă-sis) A heterogenous group of skin disorders including pityriasis lichenoides.

**par·a·site** (par′ă-sīt) An organism that lives on or in another and draws its nourishment therefrom. [G. *parasitos*, a guest, fr. *para*, beside, + *sitos*, food]

**par·a·sym·pa·thet·ic** (par′ă-sim′pă-thet′ik) Pertaining to a division of the autonomic nervous system.

**par·a·sym·pa·thet·ic ner·vous sys·tem** (par′ă-sim′pă-thet′ik nĕr′vŭs sis′tĕm) Branch of the autonomic nervous system that sends motor signals to glandular smooth muscle, and cardiac tissue, during recovery from threat.

**par·a·sym·pa·thet·ic root of pter·y·go·pal·a·tine gan·gli·on** (par′ă-sim′pă-thet′ik rūt ter′i-gō-pal′ă-tīn gang′glē-ŏn) SYN greater petrosal nerve.

**par·a·sym·path·o·lyt·ic** (par′ă-sim′pă-thō-lit′ik) Relating to agent that annuls or antagonizes effects of parasympathetic nervous system; e.g., atropine.

**par·a·sym·pa·tho·mi·met·ic** (par′ă-sim′pă-thō-mi-met′ik) Relating to drugs or chemicals having an action resembling that caused by stimulation of the parasympathetic nervous system. [*para-* + G. *sympatheia*, sympathy, + *mimētikos*, imitative]

**par·a·thy·roid·ec·to·my** (par′ă-thī-roy-dek′tŏ-mē) Excision of the parathyroid glands. [*parathyroid* + G. *ektomē*, excision]

**par·a·thy·roid hor·mone** (par′ă-thī′royd hōr′mōn) Peptide hormone formed by parathyroid glands.

**par·a·thy·roid tet·a·ny** (par′ă-thī′royd tet′ă-nē) Tetany due to lack of parathyroid function.

**par·a·tri·gem·i·nal syn·drome** (par′ă-trī-jem′i-năl sin′drōm) A transitory condition, usually in males, associated with interruption of sympathetic pathways in a trigeminal nerve; characterized by unilateral ptosis and deep facial pain. SYN incomplete Horner syndrome, Raeder syndrome.

**par·a·ty·phoid fe·ver, par·a·ty·phoid** (par′ă-tī′foyd fē′vĕr) Acute infectious disease with symptoms and lesions resembling those of typhoid fever, although milder in character.

**parch·ment crack·ling** (pahrch′mĕnt krak′ling) Sensation as of crackling of stiff paper or parchment, noted on palpation of cranium in cases of craniotabes.

op

**par·e·gor·ic** (par'ĕ-gōr'ik) Camphorated opium tincture, an antiperistaltic agent. [G. *parēgorikos*, soothing]

**par·en·ceph·a·li·tis** (par'en-sef'ă-lī'tis) Inflammation of the cerebellum. [*parencephalon* + G. *-itis*, inflammation]

**pa·ren·ter·al** (pă-ren'tĕr-ăl) By some other means than through the gastrointestinal tract; referring particularly to the introduction of substances into an organism by intravenous, subcutaneous, intramuscular, or intramedullary injection. [*para-* + G. *enteron*, intestine]

**pa·ren·ter·al ab·sorp·tion** (pă-ren'tĕr-ăl ăb-sōrp'shŭn) Absorption by any route other than through alimentary tract.

**pa·ren·ter·al nu·tri·tion (PN)** (pă-ren' tĕr-ăl nū-trish'ŭn) Providing the body with nutrition intravenously. SYN intravenous alimentation.

**pa·re·sis** (pă-rē'sis) Partial or incomplete paralysis. [G. a letting go, slackening, paralysis, fr. *paritēmi*, to let go]

**par·es·the·si·a** (par'es-thē'zē-ă) *Avoid the jargonistic use of the plural of this abstract noun to mean 'episodes or zones of paresthesia.'* In dentistry, a temporary or permanent condition of prolonged numbness after effects of an injected local anesthetic have ceased; may be caused by trauma to nerve sheath during injection, hemorrhage about that sheath, or administration of contaminated anesthetic. SYN paraesthesia. [*para-* + G. *aisthēsis*, sensation]

**pa·ri·e·tal bone** (pă-rī'ĕ-tăl bōn) [TA] A flat, curved bone of irregular quadrangular shape, at either side of the vault of the cranium.

**Pa·ri·naud syn·drome, Pa·ri·naud oph·thal·mo·ple·gi·a** (pah-rī-nō' sin'drōm, ofthal'mō-plē'jē-ă) Paralysis of conjugate upward gaze with a lesion at level of superior colliculi; Bell phenomenon is present.

**par·i·ty** (par'i-tē) The condition of having given birth to an infant or infants, alive or dead; a multiple birth is considered as a single parous experience. [L. *pario*, to bear]

**Par·kin·son dis·ease** (pahr'kin-sŏn di-zēz') SYN parkinsonism (1).

**Par·kin·son fa·ci·es** (pahr'kin-sŏn fā'shēēz) Expressionless or masklike facies characteristic of parkinsonism (1).

**par·kin·son·ism** (pahr'kin-sŏn-izm) Neurologic syndrome usually resulting from deficiency of neurotransmitter dopamine as consequence of degenerative, vascular, or inflammatory changes in basal ganglia; characterized by rhythmic muscular tremors, rigidity of movement, festination, droopy posture, and masklike facies. SYN Parkinson disease. [J. *Parkinson*]

**pa·rot·id** (pă-rot'id) Situated near the ear; denoting several structures in this area. [G. *parōtis* (*parōtid-*), the gland beside the ear, fr. *para*, beside, + *ous* (*ōt-*), ear]

**pa·rot·id bed** (pă-rot'id bed) Structures that surround and are in contact with the parotid gland, forming boundaries of parotid space: anteriorly, ramus of the mandible flanked by masseter and medial pterygoid muscles; medially, pharyngeal wall, carotid sheath and structures originating from the styloid process; posteriorly, mastoid process, sternocleidomastoid muscle, and posterior belly of digastric muscle; superiorly, temporomandibular joint and tympanic bone and cartilaginous portion of external acoustic meatus.

**pa·rot·id branch·es** (pă-rot'id branch'ĕz) [TA] Branches to parotid gland.

**pa·rot·id bu·bo** (pă-rot'id bū'bō) Swelling of parotid gland due to secondary septic infection.

**pa·rot·id duct** (pă-rot'id dŭkt) [TA] Duct of parotid gland opening from cheek into vestibule of mouth opposite neck of maxillary second molar tooth.

**pa·ro·ti·de·o·mas·se·ter·ic fas·ci·a** (pă-rot'i-dē-ō-mas'ĕ-ter'ik fash'ē-ă) Dense membrane covering both lateral and medial surfaces of parotid gland, continuous anteriorly with fascia covering masseter muscle.

**pa·rot·id fas·ci·a** (pă-rot'id fash'ē-ă) [TA] Part of investing cervical fascia that ensheaths parotid gland and is fixed above to zygomatic arch.

**pa·rot·id gland** (pă-rot'id gland) [TA] Largest of salivary glands, one of the bilateral compound acinous glands situated in the parotid bed, inferior and anterior to the ear, on either side, extending from angle of jaw inferiorly, to zygomatic arch superiorly, posteriorly to sternocleidomastoid muscle, and medially into infratemporal fossa, deep to ramus of mandible. See page 435. SYN external salivary gland.

**pa·rot·id notch** (pă-rot'id noch) Space between ramus of the mandible and the mastoid process of the temporal bone.

**pa·ro·ti·do·au·ri·cu·la·ris** (pă-rot'i-dō-awrik'yū-lā'ris) **1.** Occasional band of muscle fibers passing from parotid gland surface to auricle. **2.** Relating to parotid gland and the external ear.

**pa·rot·id plex·us of fa·ci·al nerve** (părot'id pleks'ŭs fā'shăl nĕrv) [TA] Diverging branches of facial nerve passing through parotid gland substance, connected by numerous looped anastomoses.

**pa·rot·id space** (pă-rot'id spās) Deep hollow on side of face flanking posterior aspect of

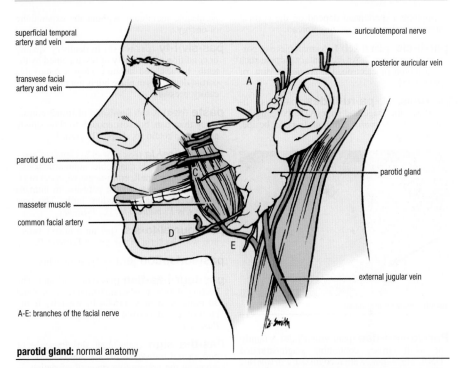

superficial temporal artery and vein

auriculotemporal nerve

posterior auricular vein

transvese facial artery and vein

A

B

parotid duct

C

parotid gland

masseter muscle

common facial artery

D

E

external jugular vein

A-E: branches of the facial nerve

*J. Smith*

**parotid gland:** normal anatomy

ramus of mandible with its attached muscles that is occupied by parotid gland.

**pa·rot·id veins** (pă-rot′id vānz) [TA] Branches draining part of parotid gland and emptying into retromandibular vein.

**par·o·tin** (par′ō-tin) A globulin obtained from parotid glands that causes hypocalcemia, and promotes calcification of dentin.

**par·o·ti·tis** (par′ō-tī′tis) Inflammation of parotid gland.

**par·ox·ysm** (par′ok-sizm) **1.** Sharp spasm or convulsion. **2.** Sudden onset of symptom or disease, especially one with recurrent manifestations. [G. *paroxysmos*, fr. *paroxynō*, to sharpen, irritate, fr. *oxys*, sharp]

**par·ox·ys·mal** (par′ok-siz′măl) *Avoid the mispronunciation parox′ysmal.* Relating to or occurring in paroxysms.

**par·rot jaw** (par′ŏt jaw) Condition caused by protruding incisor teeth.

**pars,** pl. **par·tes** (pahrz, pahr′tēz) [TA] SYN part. [L. *pars* (*part-*) a part]

**part** (pahrt) [TA] A portion. SYN pars [TA].

**part. aeq.** Abbreviation for L. *partes aequales*, in equal parts (amounts).

**par·tial a·no·don·ti·a** (pahr′shăl an′ō-don′shē-ă) Congenital absence of one or more teeth.

Third molars, maxillary lateral incisors, and second premolars most frequently fail to develop.

**par·tial an·ti·gen** (pahr′shăl an′ti-jen) SYN hapten.

**par·tial crown** (pahr′shăl krown) Artificial crown that coverts part, but not all, of the anatomic crown of a tooth; often defined by amount of tooth structure covered (e.g., three-quarter crown).

**par·tial den·ture, dis·tal ex·ten·sion** (pahr′shăl den′chŭr, dis′tăl ek-sten′shŭn) Dental prosthesis that restores one or more, but not all, natural teeth or associated parts and is supported by teeth or mucosa; may be removable or fixed; part of functional load carried by residual ridge. SYN bridgework.

**par·tial den·ture im·pres·sion** (pahr′shăl den′chŭr im-presh′ŭn) Negative copy of all or a part of partially edentulous dental arch or area, made to design or construct a partial denture.

**par·tial den·ture re·ten·tion** (pahr′shăl den′chŭr rē-ten′shŭn) Fixation of a removable appliance with clasps, indirect retainers, or precision attachments.

**par·tial pres·sure** (pahr′shăl presh′ŭr) The pressure exerted by a single component of a mixture of gases, commonly expressed in mm/ Hg or torr.

**par·tial sei·zure** (pahr′shăl sē′zhŭr) Seizure characterized by localized cerebral ictal onset;

symptoms experienced depend on the cortical area of ictal onset or seizure spread.

**par·ti·cle** (pahr′ti-kĕl) **1.** A small piece or portion of anything. **2.** An elementary particle such as a proton or electron. [L. *particula,* dim. of *pars,* part]

**pa·ru·lis,** pl. **pa·ru·li·des** (pă-rū′lis, -li-dēz) See this page and page A15. SYN gingival abscess. [G. *paroulis,* gumboil, fr. *para,* beside, + *oulon,* gum]

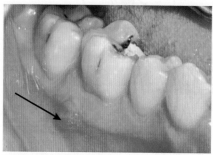

parulis: nonvital first molar

**Par·vo·vir·i·dae** (pahr′vō-vir′i-dē) A family of small viruses containing single-stranded DNA. Three genera are recognized: *Parvovirus, Densovirus,* and *Dependovirus,* which includes the adenoassociated satellite virus.

**PAS** Abbreviation for periodic acid–Schiff stain.

**pas·sive** (pas′iv) Not active; submissive. [L. *passivus,* fr. *patior,* to endure]

**pas·sive-ag·gres·sive be·ha·vi·or** (pas′iv-ă-gres′iv bĕ-hā′vyŏr) Apparently compliant behavior, with intrinsic obstructive or stubborn qualities, to cover deeply held aggressive feelings that cannot be more directly expressed.

**pas·sive dif·fu·sion** (pas′iv di-fyū′zhŭn) Passage of molecules across a semipermeable membrane without expenditure of energy.

**pas·sive e·rup·tion** (pas′iv ē-rŭp′shŭn) Continued tooth eruption; actually results from regression of gingivae and crestal bone.

**pas·sive im·mu·ni·ty** (pas′iv i-myūn′i-tē) SEE acquired immunity.

**pas·sive range of mo·tion (PROM)** (pas′iv rānj mō′shŭn) Amount of motion at a given joint when the joint is moved by an external force or therapist.

**pas·sive smoke** (pas′iv smōk) Cigarette, cigar, or pipe smoke inhaled unintentionally by non-smokers. May have negative health implications if inhaled over a long period of time. Also called second-hand smoke.

**pas·sive trans·port** (pas′iv trans′pōrt) The movement of particles or ions across a semi-permeable membrane without the expenditure of energy.

**pas·siv·i·ty** (pas-iv′i-tē) In dentistry, quality or condition of inactivity or rest assumed by the teeth, tissues, and denture when a removable partial denture is in place but is not under masticatory pressure.

**paste** (pāst) A soft semisolid of firmer consistency than pap, but soft enough to flow slowly and not to retain its shape. [L. *pasta*]

***Pas·teu·rel·la*** (pas′tyŭr-el′ă) Genus of aerobic to facultatively anaerobic, nonmotile bacteria containing small, gram-negative, cocci or ellipsoid-to-elongated rods; parasitic in humans and other animals, including birds. The type species is *P. multocida.* [L. *Pasteur*]

**pas·teur·el·lo·sis** (pas′tur-e-lō′sis) Infection with bacteria of the genus *Pasteurella.*

**pasteurisation** [Br.] SYN pasteurization.

**pas·teur·i·za·tion** (pas′tyŭr-ī-zā′shŭn) The heating of milk, wines, and fruit juices, for about 30 minutes at 68°C (154.4°F) whereby living bacteria are destroyed. SYN pasteurisation. [L. *Pasteur*]

**Pas·ti·a sign** (pahs′tē-ah sīn) Presence of pink or red transverse lines at the bend of the elbow in the preeruptive stage of scarlatina.

**patch** (pach) **1.** A small circumscribed area differing in color or structure from the surrounding surface. **2.** In dermatology, a flat area larger than 1 cm in diameter. See this page.

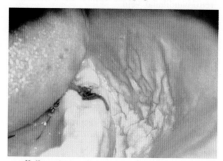

snuff dipper's patch: mucobuccal fold

**patch test** (pach test) A test of skin sensitivity; a small piece of paper, tape, or a cup, wet with a dilute solution or suspension of test material, is applied to skin of the upper back or upper outer arm, and after 48 hours the area previously covered is compared with the uncovered surface; an erythematous reaction with vesicles occurs if the substance causes contact allergy.

**pa·tent** (pā′tĕnt) Open or exposed. [L. *patens,* pres. p. of *pateo,* to lie open]

**pa·tent duc·tus ar·te·ri·o·sus** (pā′tĕnt dŭk′tŭs ahr-tēr′ē-ō′sŭs) A condition in which the normal channel between the pulmonary artery and the aorta fails to close at birth.

**pa·tent med·i·cine** (pat′ĕnt med′i-sin) Medicine originally patented, advertised to the public and colloquially, although in somewhat dated usage, available without prescription.

**path** (path) 1. A road or way. 2. Course taken by an electrical current or by nervous impulses. [A.S. *paeth*]

**pa·thet·ic nerve** (pă-thet′ik nĕrv) SYN trochlear nerve [CN IV].

**path·find·er** (path′fīnd-ĕr) A filiform bougie introduced through a narrow stricture that serves as a guide for the passage of a larger sound or catheter.

**path·ic** (path′ik) Denotes a person who assumes a passive role during sexual activity. [G. *pathikos*, remaining passive]

♲ **patho-** Combining form meaning disease. [G. *pathos*, feeling, suffering, disease]

**path·o·don·ti·a** (path′ō-don′shē-ă) Science concerned with tooth diseases. [*patho-* + G. *odous*, tooth]

**path of clo·sure** (path klō′zhŭr) Direction taken by mandible during mouth closure.

**path of in·ser·tion** (path in-sĕr′shŭn) Trajectory during insertion of a prosthesis that correctly positions it in relation to the adjacent oral tissues. SYN path of placement.

**path·o·for·mic** (path′ō-fōr′mik) Relating to beginning of disease; denoting especially some symptoms occurring in transition between normal and diseased states. [*patho-* + L. *formo*, to form]

**path of place·ment** (path plās′mĕnt) SYN path of insertion.

**path·o·gen** (path′ō-jĕn) Any virus, microorganism, or other substance causing disease. [*patho-* + G. *-gen*, to produce]

**path·o·gen·e·sis** (path′ō-jen′ĕ-sis) The pathologic, physiologic, or biochemical mechanism resulting in development of disease or morbidity. [*patho-* + G. *genesis*, production]

**path·o·gen·ic, path·o·ge·net·ic** (path′ō-jen′ik, -jĕ-net′ik) Causing disease or abnormality.

**path·o·gen·ic oc·clu·sion** (path′ō-jen′ik ō-klū′zhŭn) Occlusal relationship capable of producing pathologic changes in the supporting tissues.

**path·og·no·mon·ic** (path′og-nō-mon′ik) Characteristic or indicative of a given disease; denoting especially one or more typical symptoms, findings, or pattern of abnormalities specific for a given disease and not any others.

**path·og·no·mon·ic symp·tom** (path′og-nō-mon′ik simp′tŏm) Symptom that, when present, definitely points to presence of a given disease.

**path·o·log·ic ab·sorp·tion** (path′ō-loj′ik ăb-sōrp′shŭn) Parenteral absorption of any pathologic material into bloodstream.

**path·o·log·ic mi·gra·tion** (path′ō-loj′ik mī-grā′shŭn) Movement of a tooth out of its natural position as a result of periodontal infection.

**path·o·log·ic phys·i·ol·o·gy** (path′ō-loj′ik fiz′ē-ol′ō-jē) Area of science of disease concerned with disordered function, as distinguished from anatomic lesions.

**path·o·log·ic star·tle syn·dromes** (path′ō-loj′ik stahr′tĕl sin′drōmz) Disorders characterized by markedly exaggerated startle reflex and other exaggerated stimulus-induced responses.

**pa·thol·o·gy** (pă-thol′ō-jē) *Avoid the jargonistic use of this word in the sense of 'disease' or 'abnormality.'* Form of medical science and specialty practice concerned with all aspects of disease, but with special reference to the essential nature, causes, and development of abnormal conditions and structural and functional changes that result from disease. [*patho-* + G. *logos*, study, treatise]

**path·o·met·ric** (path′ō-met′rik) Relating to pathometry.

**path·o·mi·o·sis** (path′ō-mī-ō′sis) Attitude that leads a patient to minimize his or her disease. [*patho-* + G. *meiōsis*, a lessening]

**path·o·phys·i·ol·o·gy** (path′ō-fiz-ē-ol′ō-jē) Derangement of function seen in disease.

**path·way** (path′wā) 1. Collection of axons establishing conduction route for nerve impulses from one group of nerve cells to another or to an effector organ composed of muscle or gland cells. 2. Any sequence of chemical reactions leading from one compound to another.

**pa·tient** (pā′shĕnt) Any person suffering from any disease or behavioral disorder and undergoing treatment for it. Cf. case. [L. *patiens*, pres. p. of *patior*, to suffer]

**pa·tient-con·trolled an·al·ge·si·a, pa·tient-con·trolled an·es·the·si·a (PCA)** (pā′shĕnt kŏn-trōld′ an′ăl-jē′zē-ă, an′es-thē′zē-ă) Method for control of pain using a pump for constant intravenous or epidural infusion of a dilute narcotic solution that includes a mechanism for self-administration at predetermined intervals.

**pa·tient ed·u·ca·tion** (pā′shĕnt ed′yū-kā′shŭn) NURSING teaching of the patient; pro-

**op**

cess of assisting the patient to gain knowledge related to a health problem.

**pa·tient re·call in·ter·val** (pā'shĕnt rē' kawl in'tĕr-văl) SYN recare.

**pa·tient sat·is·fac·tion** (pā'shĕnt sat'is-fak'shŭn) Patient's opinion of care received.

**Pa·tient's Bill of Rights** (pā'shĕnts bil rīts) Developed in 1973 by the American Hospital Association to affirm the rights of patients. Key elements are the right to respectful and considerate care, privacy, information about treatment, prognosis, right to refuse treatment.

**pat·tern** (pat'ĕrn) **1.** In dentistry, form used in making a mold, as for an inlay or partial denture framework. **2.** A design; often refers to chest radiographic findings.

**pat·u·lous** (patch'yū-lŭs) SYN patent.

**pause** (pawz) Temporary stop. [G. *pausis,* cessation]

**PB** Abbreviation for pyridostigmine bromide.

**p.c.** Abbreviation for *post cibum* (*L.* after meals).

**PCA** Abbreviation for patient-controlled analgesia.

**PCP** Abbreviation for phencyclidine.

**PCR** Abbreviation for polymerase chain reaction.

**Pd** Abbreviation for palladium.

**PDGF** Abbreviation for platelet-derived growth factor.

**PDI** Abbreviation for Periodontal Disease Index.

**PDL** Abbreviation for periodontal ligament.

**peak** (pēk) The top or upper limit of a graphic tracing or of any variable. [M.E. *peke, pike,* fr. Sp. *pico,* beak, fr. L. *picus,* magpie]

**peak ex·pi·ra·to·ry flow** (pēk ek-spīr'ă-tōr-ē flō) Maximum flow at outset of forced expiration, which is reduced in proportion to severity of airway obstruction, as in asthma.

**pearl** (pĕrl) SYN enameloma.

**pear-shap·ed a·re·a** (per'shāpt ar'ē-ă) SYN retromolar pad.

**pear-shap·ed pad** (pār shāpt pad) SYN retromolar pad.

**pec·cant** (pek'ănt) Unhealthy. [L. *peccans* (*-ant-*), pres. p. of *pecco,* to sin]

**pec·tin** (pek'tin) Broad generic term for what are now more correctly called pectic substances or materials; specifically, a gelatinous substance, which is extracted from fruits where it is presumed to exist as protopectin (pectose).

**pec·ti·nate line** (pek'ti-nāt līn) [TA] The line between the simple columnar epithelium of the rectum and the stratified epithelium of the anal canal, usually defined as being at the level of the anal valves at the bases of the anal columns. SYN dentate line.

**pe·di·at·ric den·tist** (pē'dē-at'rik den'tist) A health care professional concerned with dental care and treatment of children. SYN pedodontist, paediatric dentist.

**pe·di·at·ric den·tis·try** (pē'dē-at'rik den'tis-trē) Branch of practice concerned with diagnosis, management, and treatment of dental and orofacial conditions in children. SYN pedodontia, pedodontics, paediatric dentistry.

**pe·di·a·tric·ian** (pē'dē-ă-trish'ăn) A specialist in pediatrics. SYN paediatrician.

**pe·di·at·rics** (pē'dē-at'riks) Medical specialty concerned with treatment of children in health and disease through adolescence. SYN paediatrics. [G. *pais* (*paid-*), child, + *iatreia,* medical treatment]

**pe·di·at·ric speech aid pros·the·sis** (pē'dē-at'rik spēch ād pros'thē'sis) Temporary device used to close a defect in the hard and/or soft palate.

**ped·i·cle flap** (ped'i-kĕl flap) In periodontal surgery, flap used to increase width of attached gingiva, or cover a root surface, by moving attached gingiva, which remains joined at one side, to an adjacent position and suturing free end.

**pe·do·don·ti·a** (pē'dō-don'shē-ă) SYN pediatric dentistry, paedodontia.

**pe·do·don·tics** (pē'dō-don'tiks) SYN pediatric dentistry, paedodontics. [G. *pais,* child, + *odous,* tooth]

**pe·do·don·tist** (pē'dō-don'tist) SYN pediatric dentist, paedodontist.

**peer re·view** (pēr rĕ-vyū') Assessment of research proposals, manuscripts submitted for publication, or a physician's clinical practice by other physicians or scientists in the same field.

**PEG** Abbreviation for polyethylene glycols.

**peg·ged tooth** (pegd tūth) Conic tooth with a convergence from cervical to incisal regions.

**peg lat·e·ral** (peg lat'ĕr-ăl) Lateral incisor tooth that has a conic deformity by which the tooth surfaces taper toward the incisal edge.

**peg third mo·lar** (peg thĭrd mō'lăr) Third molar tooth that has a conic form in which tooth surfaces taper toward the occlusal surface.

**pel·lag·ra** (pĕ-lag'ră) Disease characterized by gastrointestinal disturbances, erythema (particularly of exposed areas) followed by desquamation, and by nervous and mental disorders;

may occur due to poor diet, alcoholism, or some other disease impairing nutrition. [It. *pelle*, skin, + *agra*, rough]

**pel·let** (pel′ĕt) A pilule, or very small pill. [Fr. *pelote*; L. *pila*, a ball]

**pel·let im·plan·ta·tion** (pel′ĕt im′plan-tā′shŭn) Intramuscular or subcutaneous insertion of an active therapeutic agent in such form to provide protracted absorption at rate slower than subcutaneous or intramuscular injection and to provide sustained therapeutic effect.

**pel·li·cle** (pel′i-kĕl) Any thin skin or film, but in dentistry, especially that which forms in the oral cavity. [L. *pellicula*, dim of *pellis*, skin]

**pel·vis**, pl. **pel·ves** (pel′vis, -vēz) [TA] Massive cup-shaped ring of bone, with its ligaments, at inferior end of the trunk, formed of hip bone (pubic bone, ilium, and ischium) on either side and in front of sacrum and coccyx, posteriorly. [L. basin]

**pem·phi·goid** (pem′fi-goyd) 1. Resembling pemphigus. 2. A disease resembling pemphigus but significantly distinguishable histologically and clinically. [G. *pemphix*, blister, + *eidos*, resemblance]

**pem·phi·gus** (pem′fi-gŭs) Autoimmune bullous diseases with acantholysis: pemphigus vulgaris, pemphigus foliaceus, pemphigus erythematosus, or pemphigus vegetans. See page A11. [G. *pemphix*, a blister]

**pen·e·tra·tion** (pen′ĕ-trā′shŭn) 1. A piercing or entering. 2. Mental acumen. 3. SYN focal depth. [L. *penetratio*, fr. *penetro*, pp. -*atus*, to enter]

**pen·e·trom·e·ter** (pen′ĕ-trom′ĕ-tĕr) SYN step wedge. [penetration + G. *metron*, measure]

**pen·i·cil·la·mine** (pen′i-sil′ă-mēn) Degradation product of penicillin used to treat lead poisoning, hepatolenticular degeneration, and cystinuria.

**pen·i·cil·lic ac·id** (pen′i-sil′ik as′id) Antibiotic active against gram-positive and gram-negative bacteria but toxic to animal tissues.

**pen·i·cil·lin** (pen′i-sil′in) One of a family of natural or synthetic variants of penicillic acid; mainly bactericidal, are especially active against gram-positive organisms, and, with the exception of hypersensitivity reactions, show a particularly low toxic action on animal tissue.

**pen·i·cil·li·nase** (pen′i-sil′i-nās) SYN beta-lactamase.

**pen·i·cil·li·nate** (pen′i-sil′i-nāt) A salt of a penicillic acid (i.e., of a penicillin).

**pen·i·cil·lin B** (pen′i-sil′in) SYN phenethicillin potassium.

**pen·i·cil·lin G** (pen′i-sil′in) Common penicillin compound used orally and parenterally in dentistry and general medicine, primarily active against gram-positive staphylococci and streptococci. SYN benzylpenicillin.

**pen·i·cil·lin G ben·za·thine** (pen′i-sil′in benz′ă-thēn) Relatively insoluble parenteral penicillin preparation that may remain in the body for 1–2 weeks.

**pen·i·cil·lin V** (pen′i-sil′in) Penicillin derivative that resists destruction by gastric juice; potassium salt is used orally.

**Pen·i·cil·li·um** (pen′i-sil′ē-ŭm) Fungal genus; some species yield various antibiotic substances and biologicals.

**Pen·rose drain** (pen′rōz drān) A soft, tube-shaped rubber drain.

**pe·num·bra** (pĕ-nŭm′bră) 1. RADIOLOGY the blurred margin of an image. 2. RADIATION PHYSICS the region at the edges of a radiation beam over which a rapid change in dosage rate occurs. SYN geometric unsharpness. [Mod. L., fr. L. *paene*, almost, + *umbra*, shadow]

**pep·per·mint** (pep′ĕr-mint) Dried leaves and flowering tops of *Mentha piperita;* carminative and antiemetic.

**pep pills** (pep pilz) Colloquialism for tablets containing central nervous system stimulants.

**pep·tic, pep·sic** (pep′tik, -sik) Relating to stomach, to gastric digestion, or to pepsin A. [G. *peptikos*, fr. *peptō*, to digest]

**pep·tic ul·cer** (pep′tik ŭl′sĕr) A lesion of the alimentary mucosa or which has been exposed to acid gastric secretion.

**pep·tide** (pep′tīd) Compound of two or more amino acids in which a carboxyl group of one is united with an amino group of another, with the elimination of a molecule of water, thus forming a peptide bond.

**pep·tide bond** (pep′tīd bond) The common link (—CO—NH—) between amino acids in proteins.

**Pep·to·strep·to·coc·cus** (pep′tō-strep-tō-kok′ŭs) A genus of nonmotile, anaerobic, chemoorganotrophic bacteria found in normal and pathologic female genital tracts and blood in puerperal fever, in respiratory and intestinal tracts of normal humans and other animals, in the oral cavity, and in pyogenic infections, and appendicitis; may be pathogenic. [G. *peptō*, to digest, + *streptos*, curved, + *kokkos*, berry]

**PER** Abbreviation for protein efficiency ratio.

**per·a·cute** (per′ă-kyūt′) Very acute; said of a disease. [L. *peracutus*, very sharp]

**per·cen·tile** (pĕr-sen'tīl) Rank position of an individual in a serial array of data, stated in terms of what percentage of the group the individual equals or exceeds.

**per·cep·tion** (pĕr-sep'shŭn) The mental process of becoming aware of or recognizing an object or idea.

**per·co·la·tion** (pĕr'kŏ-lā'shŭn) 1. Passage of saliva or other fluids into interface between tooth structure and restoration. 2. SYN filtration. [L. *percolatio,* fr. *per- + col,* to strain]

**per·cus·sion** (pĕr-kŭsh'ŭn) Diagnostic procedure designed to determine density of a body part by sound produced by tapping surface with finger or plessor. [L. *percussio,* fr. *per-cutio,* pp. *-cussus,* to beat, fr. *quatio,* to shake, beat]

**per·cus·sion sound** (pĕr-kŭsh'ŭn sownd) Sound elicited on percussing a body cavity.

**per·cus·sion test** (pĕr-kŭsh'ŭn test) Assessment involving striking tissue or tooth with an instrument and then listening for the resulting sound or observing the patient's reaction; used to determine tooth sensitivity.

**per·cu·ta·ne·ous** (pĕr'kyū-tā'nē-ŭs) Denoting passage of substances through unbroken skin, as in absorption by inunction; also passage through the skin by needle puncture.

**per·cu·ta·ne·ous trans·lu·mi·nal cor·o·nar·y an·gi·o·plas·ty (PTCA)** (pĕr' kyū-tā'nē-ŭs trans-lū'mi-năl kōr'ŏ-nar-ē an'jē-ō-plas'tē) Surgical operation for enlarging the narrowed lumen of a coronary artery by inflating and withdrawing through the stenotic region a balloon on the tip of an angiographic catheter.

**per·fo·rat·ing fi·bers** (pĕr'fŏr-āt-ing fī'bĕrz) SYN Sharpey fibers.

**per·fo·ra·tion** (pĕr'fŏr-ā'shŭn) Abnormal opening in a hollow organ or viscus. SYN tresis.

**per·fu·sion** (pĕr-fyū'zhŭn) Flow of blood or other perfusate per unit volume of tissue.

♻ **peri-** *Do not confuse this prefix with para-, pari-, or per-.* Combining form meaning around, about, near. [G. around]

**per·i·ad·e·ni·tis mu·co·sa ne·cro·ti·ca re·cur·rens** (per'ē-ad-ĕ-nī'tis myū-kō'să ne-krot'i-kă rē-kŭr'enz) A severe form of aphthae characterized by unusually numerous, large, deep, and frequent ulcers; healing may take as long as 6 weeks and produce scarring. SYN aphthae major, Mikulicz aphthae, recurrent scarring aphthae, recurring scarring aphthae, Sutton disease.

**per·i·al·ve·o·lar wir·ing** (per'ē-al-vē'ŏ-lăr wīr'ing) Wiring that passes through the maxillary alveolar process from buccal to lingual surface to affix a splint to the maxilla.

**per·i·a·pex** (per'ē-ā'peks) Periapical structures (e.g., periodontal membrane, adjacent bone).

**per·i·ap·i·cal** (per'ē-ap'i-kăl) 1. At or around apex of a tooth root. 2. Denoting the periapex.

▊**per·i·ap·i·cal ab·scess** (per'ē-ap'i-kăl ab'ses) Inflammation of tissues and collection of pus around a tooth apex; may result from pulp infection due to carious lesion or pulp necrosis resulting from injury. See this page. SYN apical abscess, apical periodontal abscess.

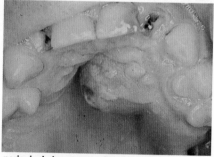

**periapical abscess:** nonvital lateral incisor

▊**per·i·ap·i·cal ce·ment·al dys·pla·si·a** (per'ē-ap'i-kăl sĕ-men'tăl dis-plā'zē-ă) Benign, painless, nonneoplastic condition of jaws that occurs almost exclusively in middle-aged black women; lesions are usually multiple, most frequently involve vital mandibular anterior teeth, surround root apices, and are initially radiolucent (becoming more opaque as they mature). See page A16.

**per·i·ap·i·cal cu·ret·tage** (per'ē-ap'i-kăl kŭr'ĕ-tahzh') 1. Removal of a cyst or granuloma from its pathologic bony crypt, using a curette. 2. Removal of tooth fragments and debris from sockets at time of extraction or subsequent removal of bone sequestra.

**per·i·ap·i·cal cyst** (per'ē-ap'i-kăl sist) SYN apical periodontal cyst.

**per·i·ap·i·cal film** (per'ē-ap'i-kăl film) Intraoral radiographic projection taken to include tooth apices and surrounding alveolar bone.

**per·i·ap·i·cal gran·u·lo·ma** (per'ē-ap'i-kăl gran'yū-lō'mă) Slowly proliferating chronic inflammatory tissue enclosed within a fibrous capsule continuous with periodontal ligament at tooth apex. Often results from necrotic pulp. SYN apical granuloma, dental granuloma, root end granuloma.

▊**per·i·ap·i·cal ra·di·o·graph** (per'ē-ap'i-kăl rā'dē-ō-graf) Radiograph demonstrating tooth apices and surrounding structures in a particular intraoral area. See this page.

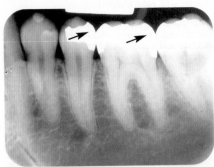

**mandibular molars and premolars (periapical radiograph):** radiopaque areas (arrows) indicate metallic restorations

**per·i·ap·i·cal ra·di·o·graph·ic sur·vey** (per´ē-ap´i-kăl rā´dē-ō-graf´ik sŭr´vā) Series of periapical intraoral dental films necessary for accurate diagnosis and dental treatment plan.

**per·i·ap·i·cal tis·sue** (per´ē-ap´i-kăl tish´ū) Collection of cells around periapical area of a tooth; responsible for maintaining integrity and vitality of this oral region.

**per·i·ar·te·ri·al plex·us of lin·gual ar·te·ry** (per´ē-ahr-tēr´ē-ăl pleks´ŭs ling´gwăl ahr´tĕr-ē) Autonomic plexus on the lingual artery, derived from the external carotid plexus. SYN lingual plexus.

**per·i·ar·te·ri·al plex·us of max·il·lar·y ar·te·ry** (per´ē-ahr-tēr´ē-ăl pleks´ŭs mak´si-lar-ē ahr´tĕr-ē) An autonomic plexus on the maxillary artery derived from the external carotid plexus. SYN maxillary plexus.

**per·i·au·ric·u·lar** (per´ē-aw-rik´yū-lăr) 1. SYN periconchal. 2. Around the external ear.

**per·i·buc·cal** (per´i-bŭk´ăl) Surrounding the cheek.

**per·i·car·di·tis** (per´i-kahr-dī´tis) Inflammation of the pericardium.

**per·i·car·di·um,** pl. **per·i·car·di·a** (per´i-kahr´dē-ŭm, -ă) [TA] The fibroserous membrane, consisting of mesothelium and submesothelial connective tissue, covering the heart and beginning of the great vessels. [L. fr. G. *pericardion*, the membrane around the heart]

**per·i·ce·men·tal** (per´i-sĕ-men´tăl) SYN periodontal.

**per·i·ce·men·tal ab·scess** (per´i-sĕ-men´tăl ab´ses) SYN lateral alveolar abscess.

**per·i·ce·men·tal at·tach·ment** (per´i-

sĕ-men´tăl ă-tach´mĕnt) Tissues surrounding tooth cementum.

**per·i·ce·men·ti·tis** (per´i-sĕ-men-tī´tis) Inflammation of the periodontal ligament.

**per·i·con·chal** (per´i-kong´kăl) Surrounding the concha of the auricle. SYN periauricular (1).

**per·i·cor·o·nal** (per´i-kōr´ŏ-năl) Around a tooth crown.

**per·i·cor·o·nal ab·scess** (per´i-kōr´ŏ-năl ab´ses) Lesion developing in inflamed dental follicular tissue overlying crown of a partially erupted tooth.

**per·i·cor·o·nal flap** (per´i-kōr´ŏ-năl flap) Flap of gingiva covering an unerupted tooth, especially lower third molar.

**per·i·cor·o·ni·tis** (per´i-kōr-ŏ-nī´tis) Acute or chronic inflammation of the gingiva around the crown of a partially erupted tooth, usually the third molar. See this page. [*peri-* + L. *corona*, crown, + G. *-itis*, inflammation]

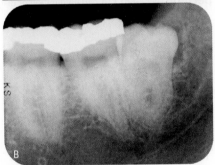
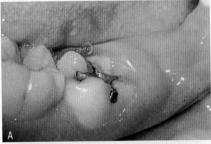

**pericoronitis:** (A) distal to partially erupted molar; (B) radiolucency distal to crown of third molar

**per·i·dens** (per´i-denz) Supernumerary tooth appearing elsewhere than midline of the dental arch. [*peri-* + L. *dens*, tooth]

**per·i·den·tal** (per´i-den´tăl) SYN periodontal.

**per·i·den·tal mem·brane** (per´i-den´tăl mem´brăn) SYN periodontium.

**per·i·glot·tic** (per´i-glot´ik) Around the tongue, especially around base of tongue and epiglottis,

op

or around glottis. [*peri-* + G. *glōssa* or *glōtta,* tongue]

**per·i·glot·tis** (per′i-glot′is) Mucous membrane of tongue.

**per·i·im·plan·ti·tis** (per′ē-im-plan-tī′tis) Inflammation of tissue around a dental implant.

**per·i·im·plan·to·cla·si·a** (per′ē-im-plan′tō-klā′zē-ă) In dentistry, general term implying disease of supporting bone involving an implant. [*peri-* + L. *im,* in, + *planto,* to plant, + G. *klasis,* breaking up]

**per·i·ky·ma·ta** (per′i-kī′mă-tă) Transverse ridges and grooves on tooth enamel surface. [*peri-* + G. *kyma,* wave]

**per·i·mol·y·sis, per·i·my·lo·ly·sis** (per′i-mol′i-sis, -mī-lol′i-sis) Decalcification of teeth from exposure to gastric acid in people with chronic vomiting. [fr. *peri-* + G. *mylos,* molar + *lysis,* loosening, dissolving, fr. *luō,* to loosen]

**per·i·mu·co·sal (bi·o·log·ic) seal** (per′i-myū-kō′sĕl bī′ō-lij′ik sēl) Unbroken junction between soft tissue and implant abutment surface that maintains periimplant tissue health.

**per·i·na·tal** (per′i-nā′tăl) Occurring during, or pertaining to, the periods before, during, or after the time of birth. [*peri-* + L. *natus,* pp. of *nascor,* to be born]

**per·i·neu·ri·tis** (per′i-nūr-ī′tis) Inflammation of the perineurium.

**per·i·od** (pēr′ē-ŏd) **1.** A certain duration or division of time. **2.** One of the stages of a disease. [G. *periodos,* a way round, a cycle, fr. *peri,* around, + *hodos,* way]

**per·i·od·ic ac·id–Schiff stain (PAS)** (pēr′ē-od′ik as′id shif stān) A clinical tissue-staining procedure.

**per·i·od·ic dis·ease** (pēr′ē-od′ik di-zēz′) Condition or disorder in which episodes tend to recur at regular intervals.

**per·i·o·di·ci·ty** (pēr′ē-ŏ-dis′i-tē) Tendency to recur at regular intervals.

**per·i·od·ic mi·grain·ous neu·ral·gi·a** (pēr′ē-od′ik mī′gră-nŭs nūr-al′jē-ă) Recurrent facial pain and headache, more common in men.

**per·i·od·ic neu·tro·pe·ni·a** (pēr′ē-od′ik nū′trō-pē′nē-ă) Neutropenia recurring at regular intervals (14–45 days), in association with various infectious diseases (e.g., stomatitis). SYN cyclic neutropenia.

**per·i·od·ic si·al·or·rhe·a** (pēr′ē-od′ik sī′ă-lōr-ē′ă) Episodic sialorrhea that may be result from salivary gland infection.

**per·i·o·don·tal** (per′ē-ō-don′tăl ) Around a tooth. SYN paradental, pericemental, peridental. [*peri-* + G. *odous,* tooth]

**⬚per·i·o·don·tal ab·scess** (per′ē-ō-don′tăl ab′ses) Localized area of inflammation of tissues and collection of pus within the periodontal space alongside the root of the tooth; usually caused by periodontitis. See this page.

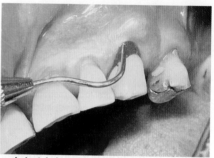

**periodontal abscess:** 12-mm pocket

**per·i·o·don·tal an·es·the·si·a** (per′ē-ō-don′tăl an′es-thē′zē-ă) Anesthesia of periodontal ligament, produced by local injection of anesthetic.

**per·i·o·don·tal as·sess·ment** (per′ē-ō-don′tăl ă-ses′mĕnt) Fact-gathering process designed to provide a complete picture of a patient's periodontal health.

**per·i·o·don·tal a·tro·phy** (per′ē-ō-don′tăl at′rŏ-fē) Decrease in size and/or cellular elements of periodontium after it has reached normal maturity.

**⬚per·i·o·don·tal at·tach·ment sys·tem** (per′ē-ō-don′tăl ă-tach′mĕnt sis′tĕm) Group of structures that work together to attach teeth to cranium; composed of the junctional epithelium, fibers of the gingiva, periodontal ligament fibers, and alveolar bone. See page 443.

**per·i·o·don·tal cyst** (per′ē-ō-don′tăl sist) An epithelium-lined fluid-filled sac at the apex of a tooth with impaired pulp. SYN dental cyst, dental root cyst, dentoalveolar cyst.

**per·i·o·don·tal dé·bride·ment** (per′ē-ō-don′tăl dā-brēd-mon[h]′) Dental procedure that includes therapeutic interventions such as scaling to remove calculus and all soft deposits, root planing to eliminate subgingival calculus and smooth the tooth surface, and root débridement to eliminate subgingival biofilm and lightly mineralized deposits.

**⬚per·i·o·don·tal dis·ease** (per′ē-ō-don′tăl di-zēz′) Chronic bacterial infection of gingivae and surrounding periodontal tissue; caused predominantly by bacterial plaque and calculus; worsened by smoking, smokeless tobacco, genetic predisposition, pregnancy, puberty, stress,

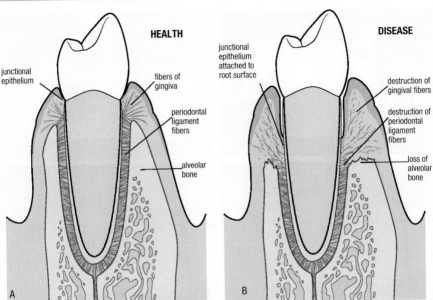

**cross-section of periodontal attachment system:** (A) healthy patient; (B) destruction of periodontal attachment system in patient with periodontal disease

**op**

poor nutrition, diabetes mellitus, and other systemic diseases. Immunologic reactions are also involved. When limited to inflammation of the gingival tissues termed gingivitis (q.v.); when gingiva, periodontal ligament, bone, and cementum involved termed periodontitis (q.v.). See this page.

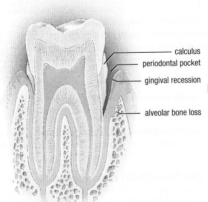

**periodontal disease:** inflammation of supporting tissues of the tooth and loss of connective tissue attachment, gingival recession and bone loss resulting in a periodontal pocket

**Per·i·o·don·tal Dis·ease In·dex (PDI)**
(per′ē-ō-don′tăl di-zēz′ in′deks) Measurement used to estimate degree of periodontal disease

based on measurement of six representative teeth for gingival inflammation, pocket depth, calculus and plaque, attrition, mobility, and lack of contact.

**per·i·o·don·tal dres·sing** (per′ē-ō-don′tăl dres′ing) Hard or soft dressing applied over a periodontal surgical site to promote regeneration of tissue and to enhance healing; provides patient comfort and mechanical protection, maintains the initial clot and prevents postoperative bleeding, supports mobile teeth, and helps in molding newly formed tissue. See page 444.

**per·i·o·don·tal fi·ber** (per′ē-ō-don′tăl fī′bĕr) SYN desmodentium.

**per·i·o·don·tal file** (per′ē-ō-don′tăl fīl) Instrument with a series of ridges or points arranged in rows on its surface, used for scaling or removing dental calculus from the teeth. See page 444.

**per·i·o·don·tal flap** (per′ē-ŏ-don′tăl flap) Procedure in which a portion of periodontal tissue is partially removed to allow access to alveolar bone and tooth root surface for deposit removal or for rearranging the soft tissue.

**Per·i·o·don·tal In·dex (PI)** (per′ē-ō-don′tăl in′deks) Index for epidemiologic classification of periodontal disease.

**per·i·o·don·tal lig·a·ment (PDL)** (per′ē-ō-don′tăl lig′ă-mĕnt) Investing and supporting connective tissue structure by which a tooth and tooth root are anchored within its alveolus; consists of bands of collagen fibers connecting

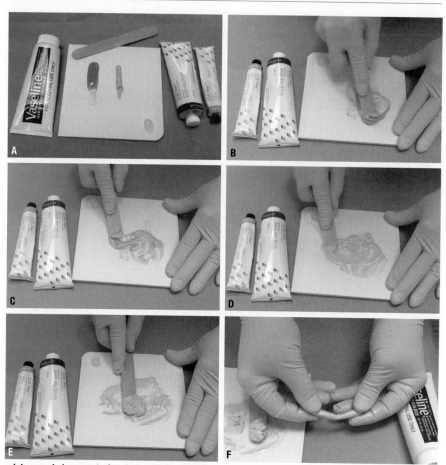

**mixture and placement of periodontal dressings:** (A) equal lengths of base and accelerator are dispensed onto mixing pad; (B, C, D) base and accelerator are combined on mixing pad until color is uniform; (E) mixture is gathered into a compact mass; (F) when mixture ceases to be tacky, it is formed into a rope

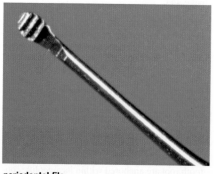

**periodontal file**

tooth cementum to both gingival and alveolar bone and to cementum of adjacent teeth.

**per·i·o·don·tal main·te·nance** (per´ē-ō-don´tăl mānt´ĕ-năns) SYN supportive periodontal treatment.

**per·i·o·don·tal mem·brane** (per´ē-ō-don´tăl mem´brān) Developmental stage of periodontal ligament, i.e., the transitional stage between dental sac (dental follicle) and periodontal ligament.

**per·i·o·don·tal pack** (per´ē-ō-don´tăl pak) SEE periodontal dressing.

**per·i·o·don·tal pock·et** (per´ē-ō-don´tăl pok´ĕt) Pathologic deepening of gingival sulcus resulting from detachment of gingiva from tooth.

**per·i·o·don·tal probe** (per´ē-ō-don´tăl prōb) Calibrated instrument used to measure periodontal pocket depth and provide assessment of bone loss and periodontal health. See this page.

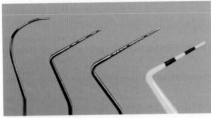

**periodontal probes**

**per·i·o·don·tal pros·the·sis** (per´ē-ō-don´tăl pros-thē´sis) Device used as a therapeutic adjunct in periodontal disease (e.g., fixed bridge used to splint mobile teeth together).

**Per·i·o·don·tal Screen·ing and Re·cord·ing (PSR)** (per´ē-ō-don´tăl skrēn´ing rĕ-kōrd´ing) An examination with standards established by the American Dental Association to evaluate a patient's periodontal status through inspection of all oral sites to detect early signs of disease and determine whether a more thorough periodontal examination is needed.

**Per·i·o·don·tal Screen·ing Re·cord (PSR)** (per´ē-ō-don´tăl skrēn´ing rek´ōrd) A modified version of the Community Periodontal Index of Treatment Needs used primarily in the United States (q.v.).

**per·i·o·don·tal ther·a·py** (per´ē-ō-don´tăl thār´ă-pē) Care intended to preserve natural dentition, periodontium, and preimplant tissues and to maintain and improve the health of these tissues.

**per·i·o·don·tal treat·ment plan·ning** (per´ē-ō-don´tăl trēt´mĕnt plan´ing) Therapeutic plan intended to stop or slow periodontal disease progression. Generally, it includes medical consultation as needed; periodontal procedures to be performed; consideration of interdisciplinary treatment; reevaluation schedule; chemotherapeutic agent adjunctive treatment; genetic, microbiologic, and biochemical testing; and a periodontal maintenance program.

**per·i·o·don·ti·a** (per´ē-ō-don´shē-ă) Plural of periodontium.

**per·i·o·don·tics** (per´ē-ŏ-don´tiks) Branch of dentistry concerned with study of normal tissues and treatment of abnormal conditions of tissues immediately about teeth. [peri- + G. odous, tooth]

**per·i·o·don·tist** (per´ē-ō-don´tist) Dentist who specializes in periodontics.

**per·i·o·don·ti·tis** (per´ē-ō-don-tī´tis) Inflammatory disease of periodontium occurring in response to bacterial plaque on adjacent teeth; characterized by gingivitis, destruction of alveolar bone and periodontal ligament, apical migration of the epithelial attachment resulting in formation of periodontal pockets, and ultimately loosening and exfoliation of teeth. See this page and pages A2–A3. [periodontium + G. -itis, inflammation]

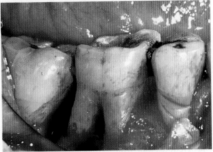

**moderate periodontitis:** class II furcation involvement

**per·i·o·don·ti·tis com·plex** (per´ē-ō-don-tī´tis kom´pleks) Vertical resorption of alveolar process with pockets of uneven depth on adjacent teeth, and with traumatic occlusion as a factor.

**per·i·o·don·ti·tis sim·plex** (per´ē-ō-don-tī´tis sim´pleks) Horizontal resorption of alveolar process with pockets of even depth on adjacent teeth; traumatic occlusion is not a factor.

**per·i·o·don·ti·um, per·i·den·ti·um,** pl. **per·i·o·don·ti·a, per·i·den·ti·a** (per´ē-ō-don´shē-ŭm, -den´shē-ŭm, -don´shē-ă, -den´shē-ă) [TA] Connective tissue that surrounds tooth root and attaches it to its bony socket; consists of fibers anchored in cementum and extending into alveolar bone; tissues that surround and support teeth, including gingivae, cementum, desmodentium, periodontal fibers, and alveolar and supporting bone. See page 446. SYN alveolar periosteum, alveolodental membrane, gingivodental ligament, paradentium, peridental membrane. [L. fr. peri- + G. odous, tooth]

**per·i·o·don·to·cla·si·a, per·i·o·don·to·ly·sis** (per´ē-ō-don´tō-klā´zē-ă, -don-tol´i-sis) Destruction of periodontal tissues, gingiva, pericementum, alveolar bone, and cementum. [periodontium + klasis, breaking]

**per·i·o·don·tol·o·gy** (per´ē-ō-don-tol´ŏ-jē) Science and study of the periodontium and its characteristics, functions, and disorders.

**per·i·o·don·tom·e·ter** (per´ē-ō-don-tom´ĕ-tĕr) Instrument used to measure and assess the severity of periodontal disease. The term commonly denotes an instrument measuring dental mobility, but sometimes is also used for an instrument that measures pocket depth.

**per·i·o·don·to·path·ic** (per´ē-ō-don´tō-path´

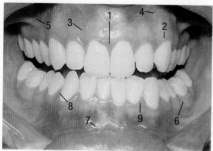

**healthy periodontium:** anterior view, (1) interdental gingivae or papillae; (2) gingival margin (marginal gingiva); (3) attached gingiva; (4) alveolar mucosa; (5) buccal frenum (frenulum); (6) mandibular vestibule; (7) labial mucosa; (8) gingiva; (9) mucogingival junction

ik) Denotes that which causes pathologic states in the peridontium. It typically describes bacteria that cause periodontal disease.

**per·i·o·don·to·sis** (per'ē-ō-don-tō'sis) SYN juvenile periodontitis. [*periodontium* + G. *-osis*, condition]

**per·i·o·ral** (per'ē-ō'răl) Around the mouth.

**per·i·os·te·al el·e·va·tor** (per'ē-os'tē-ăl el'ĕ-vā-tŏr) A surgical instrument used to reflect the attached periosteum from the underlying alveolar bone.

**per·i·os·te·al re·flex** (per'ē-os'tē-ăl rē'fleks) Reflex muscle contraction mistakenly assumed to result from tapping various long bones; misnomer because these are actually deep tendon reflexes, in that bone itself has no receptors to initiate such muscle action.

**per·i·os·te·um,** pl. **per·i·os·ti·a** (per'ē-os'tē-ŭm, -ă) [TA] Thick, fibrous membrane covering entire surface of a bone except its articular cartilage and areas where it attaches to tendons and ligaments.

**per·i·os·ti·tis, per·i·os·te·i·tis** (per'ē-os-tī'tis, -tē-ī'tis) Inflammation of the periosteum.

**pe·riph·er·al ner·vous sys·tem (PNS)** (pĕr-if'ĕr-ăl nĕr'vŭs sis'tĕm) [TA] The peripheral part of the nervous system external to the brain and spinal cord from their roots to their peripheral terminations.

**pe·riph·er·al os·si·fy·ing fi·bro·ma** (pĕr-if'ĕr-ăl os'i-fī-ing fī-brō'mă) Reactive focal gingival overgrowth derived histogenetically from cells of periodontal ligament and usually developing in response to local irritants (e.g., plaque, calculus) on associated teeth; consists microscopically of a hyperplastic cellular fibrous stroma supporting deposits of bone, cementum, or dystrophic calcification.

**pe·ri·pher·al vas·cu·lar dis·ease (PVD)** (pĕr-if'ĕr-ăl vas'kyū-lăr di-zēz') Noncardiac-centered disease of blood vessels.

**pe·riph·e·ry** (pĕr-if'ĕr-ē) **1.** SYN denture border. **2.** The part of a body away from the center. [G. *periphereia*, fr. *peri*, around, + *pherō*, to carry]

**per·i·ra·dic·u·lar** (per'i-ră-dik'yū-lăr) Denotes areas near or around the tooth root.

**per·i·rhi·nal** (per'i-rī'năl) Around nose or nasal cavity. [*peri-* + G. *rhis*, nose]

**per·i·rhi·zo·cla·si·a** (per'i-rī-zō-klă'zē-ă) Inflammatory destruction of tissues immediately around tooth root, i.e., pericementum, cementum, and approximating layers of alveolar bone. [*peri-* + G. *rhiza*, root, + *klasis*, destruction]

**per·i·ton·sil·lar** (per'i-ton'si-lăr) Denotes area near or around the tonsils. [*peri-*, + L. *tonsilla*, + *-ar*, adj. suffix]

**per·i·ton·sil·lar ab·scess** (per'i-ton'si-lăr ab'ses) Extension of tonsillar infection beyond the tonsillar capsule with abscess formation between the capsule and the musculature of the tonsillar fossa; frequent complication of tonsillitis.

**per·i·tu·bu·lar den·tin** (per'i-tū'byū-lăr den'tin) Electron-dense layer of dentin observed adjacent to odontoblastic process.

**per·i·tu·bu·lar zone** (per'i-tū'byū-lăr zōn) Dentinal matrix surrounding odontoblastic process; more highly calcified and contains finer collagen fibers than the rest of dentinal matrix.

**per·i·typh·li·tis** (per'i-tif-lī'tis) Inflammation of the peritoneum surrounding the cecum.

**per·kin·ism** (pĕr'kin-izm) A form of quackery purporting to treat disease by applying metals with magnetic and purportedly magic properties.

**per·lèche** (pĕr-lesh') SYN angular cheilitis. [Fr. *per*, intensive, + *lécher*, to lick]

**per·lin·gual** (per-ling'gwăl) Through or by way of tongue, denoting method of medication. [L. *per*, through, + *lingua*, tongue]

**per·ma·nent den·ti·tion** (pĕr'mă-nĕnt den-tish'ŭn) Adult dentition of 32 teeth, consisting in each quadrant of two incisors, one canine, two premolars, and three molars, in that order, from the midline.

**per·ma·nent res·tor·a·tion** (pĕr'mă-nĕnt res'tŏr-ā'shŭn) Definitive restoration, in contradistinction to a temporary or provisional restoration.

**per·ma·nent tooth** (per'mă-nĕnt tūth) [TA] One of 32 teeth belonging to the second, or permanent, dentition; eruption of permanent teeth begins from the fifth to the seventh year, and is not completed until the 17th–23rd year, when the last of the third molars appears. See this page. SYN dens permanens [TA], dens succedaneus, second tooth, secondary dentition, succedaneous dentition.

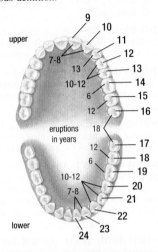

upper

7-8
9
10
11
12
13
13
10-12
14
6
15
12
16

eruptions in years
18

17
12
18
6
19
10-12
20
7-8
21
22
lower
23
24

**Key**

| | |
|---|---|
| central incisor 9, 24 | second bicuspid 13, 20 |
| lateral incisor 10, 23 | First molar 14, 19 |
| canine 11, 22 | second molar 15, 18 |
| first bicuspid 12, 21 | third molar 16, 17 |

**permanent teeth with approximate age of eruption**

**per·me·a·bil·i·ty** (pĕr′mē-ă-bil′i-tē) The property of being penetrable.

**per·mu·co·sal** (pĕr′myu-kō′săl) Denotes by way of, or through, a mucous membrane.

**per·mu·co·sal (bi·o·log·ic) seal** (pĕr′ myu-kō′săl bī′ŏ-loj′ik sēl) Unbroken junction between soft tissue and implant abutment surface that maintains periimplant health.

**per·mu·co·sal route** (pĕr′myu-kō′săl rūt) Pathway taken by infectious organisms across the mucosa to infect a host.

**per·ni·ci·ous** (pĕr-nish′ŭs) Destructive; denoting a disease of severe character and usually fatal without appropriate treatment. [L. *perniciosus*, destructive, fr. *pernicies*, destruction]

**per·ni·cious a·ne·mi·a** (pĕr-nish′ŭs ă-nē′ mē-ă) Chronic progressive anemia of older adults (occurring more frequently during the fifth and later decades, rarely before 30 years of age), due to failure of absorption of vitamin B12, usually resulting from a defect of the stomach accompanied by mucosal atrophy and associated with lack of secretion of ''intrinsic'' factor. SYN Addison anemia, Addison-Biermer disease, addisonian anemia.

**per·o·ral** (pĕr-ō′răl) Through the mouth, de-

noting method of medication or approach. [L. *per*, through, + *os* (*or-*), mouth]

**per·o·ral en·dos·co·py** (pĕr-ōr′ăl en-dos′ kŏ-pē) Visual examination of interior sections of the body by introduction of an instrument (e.g., an endoscope) through the mouth; examples include esophagoscopy, gastroscopy, and bronchoscopy.

**per os (PO)** (pĕr os) By or through the mouth, denoting method of delivering medication. [L.]

**pe·rox·ide** (pĕr-ok′sīd) That oxide of any series that contains the greatest number of oxygen atoms.

**per·pet·u·al·ly grow·ing tooth** (pĕr-pet′yū-ă-lē grōw′ing tūth) Physiologic phenomenon whereby tooth continually or constantly grows, calcifies, and erupts; e.g., the incisor tooth in rats.

**per rec·tum** (pĕr rek′tŭm) By or through the rectum, denoting a method of delivering medication. [L.]

**per·sis·tent gen·er·al·ized lymph·ad·e·nop·a·thy** (pĕr-sis′tĕnt jen′ĕr-ăl-īzd lim-fad′ĕ-nop′ă-thē) Chronic, persistent swellings in the lymph nodes associated with HIV infection and AIDS.

**per·sis·tent ve·ge·ta·tive state** (pĕr-sis′tĕnt vej′ĕ-tā-tiv stāt) Condition of a patient of prolonged duration (defined in different sources as duration of longer than 1 month, 1 year, or 2 years); usually permanent.

**per·son·al·i·ty** (pĕr′sŏn-al′i-tē) Unique self, totality of someone's conscious and unconscious cognition and interpersonal behavior and related emotional responses.

**per·son·al·i·ty dis·or·der** (pĕr′sŏn-al′i-tē dis-ōr′dĕr) General term for a group of behavioral disorders characterized by usually lifelong ingrained maladaptive patterns of subjective internal experience and deviant behavior, lifestyle, and social adjustment.

**per·son·al·i·ty test** (pĕr′sŏn-al′i-tē test) Form of psychological assessment designed to test characteristics of personality, emotional status, mental disorder.

**per·son·al space** (pĕr′sŏn-ăl spās) Term used in the behavioral sciences to denote physical area immediately surrounding a person who is in proximity to one or more others, whether known or unknown; serves as a body buffer zone in such interpersonal transactions. Measurement of space determined as appropriate varies among ethnic groups and cultures.

**per·son-years** (per′sŏn yērz) Product of number of years times number of members of a population who have been affected by a certain condition (e.g., years of treatment with a given drug).

**op**

**pers·pi·ra·tion** (pĕrs'pir-ā'shŭn) **1.** The excretion of fluid by the sweat glands of the skin. SYN diaphoresis, sudation, sweating. **2.** All fluid loss through normal skin, whether by sweat gland secretion or by diffusion through other skin structures. SYN sudor. SEE ALSO sweat (2), sweat (1). [L. *per-spiro*, pp. *-atus*, to breathe everywhere]

**per tu·bam** (pĕr tū'băm) Through a tube. [L.]

**per·tus·sis** (pĕr-tŭs'is) Acute infectious inflammation of larynx, trachea, and bronchi caused by *Bordetella pertussis*. SYN whooping cough. [L. *per*, very (intensive), + *tussis*, cough]

**per·va·sive de·vel·op·men·tal dis·or·der** (pĕr-vā'siv dĕ-vel'ŏp-men'tăl dis-ōr'dĕr) Any of a group of mental disorders of infancy, childhood, or adolescence characterized by distortions in the acquisition of the multiple basic psychological funtions necessary for the elaboration of social skills, language skills, and imagination.

**pes·tle** (pes'tĕl) Rodlike instrument with one rounded and weighted extremity, used for grinding and mixing substances in a mortar. [L. *pistillum*, fr. *pinso*, or *piso*, to pound]

**PET** Abbreviation for positron emission tomography.

**pe·te·chi·ae** (pĕ-tē'kē-ē) Minute punctate hemorrhagic spots on mucosa or skin that do not blanch even when pressed. See this page. [Mod. L. form of It. *petecchie*]

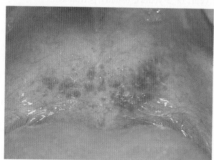

**petechiae:** on the soft palate, due to viral infection and associated cough

**pe·tro·la·tum** (pet'rō-lā'tŭm) Soft yellowish mixture application to burns and abrasions of the skin; usually called petroleum jelly.

**Peutz-Jeg·hers syn·drome** (pŭts jā'gĕrz sin'drōm) Inherited intestinal polyposis syndrome in which polyps are hamartomatous and thus do not transform to malignancy. Small macular pigmentations may appear around mouth. See page A14.

**phaeochromocytoma** [Br.] SYN pheochromocytoma.

**phage** (fāj) SYN bacteriophage.

**phago-** Combining form meaning eating, devouring. [G. *phagō*, to eat]

**phag·o·cyte** (fag'ō-sīt) Cell that can ingest bacteria, foreign particles, and other cells. [*phago-* + G. *kytos*, cell]

**phag·o·cy·to·sis** (fāg'ō-sī-tō'sis) Process of ingestion and digestion by cells of solid substances. [*phagocyte* + G. *-osis*, condition]

**phag·o·dy·na·mom·e·ter** (fag'ō-dī'nă-mom'ĕ-tĕr) Device for measuring force required to chew various foods. [*phago-* + G. *dynamis*, force, + *metron*, measure]

**phan·er·o·gen·ic** (fan'ĕr-ō-jen'ik) Denoting a disease, the etiology of which is manifest. [G. *phanero-*, visible + G. *genesis*, origin]

**phan·tom** (fan'tŏm) **1.** A model, especially a transparent one, of the human body or its parts. **2.** RADIOLOGY mechanical or computer-generated model for predicting irradiation dosage deep in the body. [G. *phantasma*, an appearance]

**phan·tom limb pain** (fan'tŏm lim pān) Painful sensations experienced in an amputated (phantom) limb, most often an upper limb.

**phan·tom o·don·tal·gi·a** (fan'tŏm ō'don-tal'jē-ă) Pain in an area from which a tooth has been lost. Also called ghost pain.

**phar·ma·ceu·tic, phar·ma·ceu·ti·cal** (fahr'mă-sū'tik, -ăl) Relating to pharmacy or pharmaceutics. [G. *pharmakeutikos*, relating to drugs]

**phar·ma·ceu·tic chem·is·try** (fahr'mă-sū'tik kem'is-trē) Medicinal chemistry in its application to analysis, development, preparation, and manufacture of drugs.

**phar·ma·cist** (fahr'mă-sist) One who is licensed to prepare and dispense drugs and compounds. [G. *pharmakon*, a drug]

**pharmaco-** Combining form meaning drugs. [G. *pharmakon*, medicine]

**phar·ma·co·di·ag·no·sis** (fahr'mă-kō-dī'ăg-nō'sis) Use of drugs in diagnosis.

**phar·ma·co·dy·nam·ics** (fahr'mă-kō-dī-nam'iks) Study of uptake, movement, binding, and interactions of pharmacologically active molecules at their tissue site(s) of action. [*pharmaco-* + G. *dynamis*, force]

**phar·ma·cog·no·sy** (fahr'mă-kog'nŏ-sē) Branch of pharmacology concerned with physical characteristics and sources of crude drugs. [*pharmaco-* + G. *gnōsis*, knowledge]

**phar·ma·cog·ra·phy** (fahr'mă-kog'ră-fē) A treatise on or description of drugs. [*pharmaco-* + G. *graphē*, description]

**phar·ma·co·ki·net·ic** (fahr'mă-kō-ki-net'ik)

Relating to disposition of drugs in body (i.e., absorption, distribution, metabolism).

**phar·ma·co·ki·net·ics** (fahr′mă-kō-ki-net′ iks) Movements of drugs within biologic systems; particularly rates of such movements. [*pharmaco-* + G. *kinēsis,* movement]

**phar·ma·co·log·ic, phar·ma·co·log·i·cal** (fahr′mă-kŏ-loj′ik, -i-kăl) Relating to pharmacology or drugs.

**phar·ma·col·o·gy** (fahr′mă-kol′ŏ-jē) Science concerned with drugs, their sources, appearance, chemistry, actions, and uses. [*pharmaco-* + G. *logos,* study]

*Phar·ma·co·pe·i·a, Phar·ma·co·poe·i·a* (fahr′mă-kō-pē′ă) A work containing monographs of therapeutic agents, standards for their strength and purity, and their formulations. Various national pharmacopeias are referred to by abbreviations, of which the following are the most frequently encountered: *USP,* the Pharmacopeia of the United States of America (United States Pharmacopeia); *BP,* British Pharmacopoeia; *Codex medicamentarius,* French Pharmacopeia; *I.C. Add.* (or *BA*), the Indian and Colonial Addendum to the BP; *IP,* International Pharmacopeia; *Österreichisches Arzneibuch,* Austrian Pharmacopeia; *Pharmacopoea Germanica,* German Pharmacopeia (D.A.B.); and *Pharmacopeia Helvetica,* Swiss Pharmacopeia. [G. *pharmakopoiia,* fr. *pharmakon,* a medicine, + *poieo,* to make]

**phar·ma·co·ther·a·py** (fahr′mă-kō-thār′ă-pē) Treatment of disease with drugs. SEE ALSO chemotherapy.

**phar·ma·cy** (fahr′mă-sē) **1.** Practice of preparing and dispensing drugs. **2.** A drugstore. [G. *pharmakon,* drug]

**pha·ryn·ge·al** (făr-in′jē-ăl) Relating to pharynx. [Mod. L. *pharyngeus*]

**pha·ryn·ge·al arch car·ti·lage** (făr-in′jē-ăl ahrch kahr′ti-lăj) A cartilage bar in the mandibular arch that forms a temporary supporting structure in the embryonic mandible. SYN mandibular cartilage.

**pha·ryn·ge·al arch·es** (făr-in′jē-al ahrch′ĕz) Obliquely disposed, rounded ridges on either side of the head and neck of human embryos during fourth and fifth gestational weeks, which contribute to formation of face and neck.

**pha·ryn·ge·al flap** (făr-in′jē-ăl flap) Flap of mucosa and muscle raised from posterior wall of pharynx and attached to soft palate, used to obturate velopharyngeal passage and thereby correct nasal air escape during speech.

**pha·ryn·ge·al glands** (făr-in′jē-ăl glandz) [TA] Racemose mucous glands under mucous membrane of pharynx.

**pha·ryn·ge·al lym·phat·ic ring** (făr-in′jē-ăl lim-fat′ik ring) [TA] Broken ring of lymphoid tissue, formed of the lingual, faucial, and pharyngeal tonsils. SYN tonsillar ring.

**pha·ryn·ge·al mem·branes** (făr-in′jē-ăl mem′brănz) Thin sheets, which separate pharyngeal pouches from overlying pharyngeal grooves in the early embryo.

**pha·ryn·ge·al mes·o·derm** (făr-in′jē-ăl mez′ō-dĕrm) Mesoderm surrounding primordial stomodeum and pharynx that contributes to mesenchymal cores of pharyngeal arches.

**pha·ryn·ge·al mus·cles** (făr-in′jē-ăl mŭs′ĕlz) [TA] Muscular layer of pharyngeal wall; has outer circular and inner longitudinal layers.

**pha·ryn·ge·al nerve** (făr-in′jē-ăl nĕrv) [TA] Branch of pterygopalatine ganglion passing posteriorly through pharyngeal canal to supply postsynaptic parasympathetic fibers to mucous glands of nasopharynx.

**pha·ryn·ge·al re·flex** (făr-in′jē-ăl rē′fleks) **1.** SYN swallowing reflex. **2.** SYN vomiting reflex.

**pha·ryn·ge·al ton·sil** (făr-in′jē-ăl ton′sil) A collection of more or less closely aggregated lymphoid nodules on the posterior wall and roof of the nasopharynx.

**pha·ryn·ge·al veins** (făr-in′jē-ăl vānz) [TA] Several veins from pharyngeal venous plexus emptying into internal jugular vein.

**phar·yn·gis·mus** (far′in-jiz′mŭs) Spasm of pharynx muscles.

**phar·yn·gi·tis** (far′in-jī′tis) Inflammation of mucous membrane and underlying parts of pharynx. [Mod. L. fr. G. *pharynx* throat + G. *-itis,* inflammation]

**pha·ryn·go·con·junc·ti·val fe·ver vi·rus** (făr-ing′gō-kŏn-jŭngk′ti-văl fē′vĕr vī′rŭs) One of several types of adenoviruses associated with outbreaks of fever and pharyngitis, sometimes with conjunctivitis.

**pha·ryn·go·plas·ty** (fă-ring′gō-plas-tē) Surgical repair of the pharynx. [*pharyngo-* + G. *plastos,* formed]

**pha·ryn·go·ple·gi·a** (fă-ring′gō-plē′jē-ă) Paralysis of pharynx muscles. [*pharyngo-* + G. *plēgē,* stroke]

**phar·yn·got·o·my** (far′ing-got′ŏ-mē) Any cutting operation on the pharynx. [*pharyngo-* + G. *tomē,* incision]

**pha·ryn·go·tym·pan·ic (aud·i·tor·y) tube** (fă-ring′gō-tim-pan′ik aw′di-tōr-ē tūb) [TA] A tube leading from the tympanic cavity to the nasopharynx. SYN auditory tube.

**phar·ynx,** pl. **pha·ryn·ges** (far′ingks, fă-rin′jēz) [TA] Superior expanded portion of ali-

op

mentary tract, between mouth and nasal cavities (superiorly and anteriorly) and esophagus (inferiorly); consisting of nasopharynx, oropharynx, and laryngopharynx.

**phase** (fāz) **1.** Stage in course of change or development. **2.** Homogeneous, physically distinct, and separable portion of a heterogeneous system. **3.** Time relationship between two or more events. **4.** Particular part of a recurring time pattern or wave form. [G. *phasis,* an appearance]

**phat·nor·rha·gi·a** (fat′nōr-ā′jē-ă) Dental alveolar hemorrhage. [G. *phatnōma,* manger (*alveolus*), + G. *rhēgnymi,* to burst forth]

**phen·cy·cli·dine (PCP)** (fen-sī′kli-dēn) Substance of abuse, used for its hallucinogenic properties, which can produce profound psychological and behavioral disturbances.

**phe·neth·i·cil·lin po·tas·si·um** (fĕ-neth′-i-sil′in pŏ-tas′ē-ŭm) A penicillin preparation that is stable in gastric juice and is rapidly but only partially absorbed from gastrointestinal tract. SYN penicillin B.

**phe·no·bar·bi·tal** (fē′nō-bahr′bi-tahl) A long-acting oral or parenteral sedative, anticonvulsant, and hypnotic.

**phe·nol** (fē′nol) Hydroxybenzene; an antiseptic, anesthetic, and disinfectant.

**phe·no·lat·ed** (fē′nō-lāt′ĕd) Impregnated or mixed with phenol. SYN carbolated.

**phe·nol co·ef·fi·cient** (fē′nol kō′ĕ-fish′ ĕnt) SYN Rideal-Walker coefficient.

**phe·nol·ic com·pound** (fē-nol′ik kom′ pownd) Chemical disinfectant containing phenol or phenollike chemicals.

**phe·nom·e·non,** pl. **phe·nom·e·na** (fĕ-nom′ē-non, -ă) A symptom; an occurrence of any sort, whether ordinary or extraordinary, in relation to a disease. [G. *phainomenon,* fr. *phainō,* to cause to appear]

**phe·no·type** (fē′nō-tīp) Observable characteristics, at physical, morphologic, or biochemical levels of an organism. [G. *phainō,* to display, + *typos,* model]

**phen·yl·al·a·nine (F)** (fen′il-al′ă-nēn) One of the common amino acids in proteins; a nutritionally essential amino acid.

**phen·yl·ke·to·nu·ri·a (PKU)** (fen′il-kē′tō-nyūr′ē-ă) Inborn error of metabolism of phenylalanine characterized by deficiency of phenylalanine hydroxylase. [*phenyl + ketone* + G. *ouron,* urine]

**phen·y·to·in** (fĕ-nit′ō-in) Anticonvulsant used to treat generalized tonic clonic and complex partial epilepsy.

**phe·o·chro·mo·cy·to·ma** (fē′ō-krō′mō-

sī-tō′mă) A functional chromaffinoma characterized by secretion of catecholamines, resulting in hypertension. SYN phaeochromocytoma. [G. *pheo* + G. *chrōm,* color; *-oma* - tumor]

**phil·o·pro·gen·i·tive** (fil′ō-prō-jen′i-tiv) Procreative, producing offspring. [*philo-* + L. *progenies,* offspring, progeny]

**phil·trum,** pl. **phil·tra** (fil′trŭm, -tră) [TA] [NA] Infranasal indention or groove on upper lip. [L., fr. G. *philtron,* a love-charm, depression on upper lip, fr. *phileō,* to love]

**phleb·ec·ta·si·a** (fleb′ek-tā′zē-ă) Dilation of the veins. SYN venectasia. [G. *phlebo,* vein + G. *ektasis,* a stretching]

**phle·bi·tis** (flĕ-bī′tis) Inflammation of a vein. [G. *phlebo,* vein + G. *-itis,* inflammation]

**phleb·o·lith** (fleb′ō-lith) Calcific deposit in a venous wall or thrombus. [G. *phlebo,* vein + G. *lithos,* stone]

**phle·bol·o·gy** (flĕ-bol′ŏ-jē) Medical science concerned with anatomy and diseases of veins. [G. *phlebo,* vein + G. *logos,* study]

**phle·bot·o·mize** (flĕ-bot′ō-mīz) To draw blood from.

**phlegm** (flem) Abnormal amounts of mucus. [G. *phlegma,* inflammation]

**PHN** Abbreviation for public health nurse.

**pho·bi·a** (fō′bē-ă) Any objectively unfounded morbid dread or fear that arouses a state of panic; used as a combining form in many terms expressing the object that inspires the fear. [G. *phobos,* fear]

**pho·nac·o·scope** (fō-nak′ŏ-skōp) An instrument for increasing the intensity of the percussion note or of the voice sounds. [*phon-* G. *phōnē* voice + G. *akouō,* to listen, + *skopeō,* to view]

**pho·na·tion** (fō-nā′shŭn) The utterance of sounds by means of vocal folds. [G. *phōnē,* voice]

**pho·neme** (fō′nēm) The smallest sound unit that, in terms of the phonetic sequences of sound, controls meaning. [G. *phōnēma,* a voice]

**pho·net·ics** (fō-net′iks) Science of speech and pronunciation. Phonetic tests are used to determine vertical dimensions of occlusion (e.g., in sounding 'ch,' 'j,' and 's,' anterior teeth are brought closer together).

**pho·no·my·oc·lo·nus** (fō′nō′mī-ok′lŏ-nŭs) Clonic spasms of muscles in response to aural stimuli. [*phono-* G. *phōne,* voice + G. *mys,* muscle, + *klonos,* tumult]

**pho·re·sis** (fŏr-ē′sis) **1.** SYN electrophoresis. **2.** A biologic association in which one organism is transported by another. [G. *phorēsis,* a being borne]

**phose** (fōz) Subjective visual sensation (e.g., light). [G. *phōs,* light]

**phos·pha·tase** (fos'fă-tās) Any of a group of enzymes (EC sub-subclass 3.1.3) that liberate inorganic phosphate from phosphoric esters.

**phos·pho·lip·ase** (fos'fō-lip'ās) An enzyme that catalyzes the hydrolysis of a phospholipid. SYN lecithinase.

**phos·pho·lip·id** (fos'fō-lip'id) A lipid containing phosphorus; basic constituent of biomembranes.

**phos·pho·ne·cro·sis** (fos'fō-nĕ-krō'sis) Necrosis of jaw bone, due to poisoning by inhalation of phosphorus fumes. [*phosphorus* + G. *nekrōsis,* death (necrosis)]

**phos·pho·pro·tein** (fos'fō-prō'tēn) A protein containing phosphoryl groups attached directly to the side chains of some of its constituent amino acids.

**phos·pho·res·cence** (fos'fŏr-es'ĕns) The quality or property of emitting light with neither active combustion nor production of heat, generally as the result of prior exposure to radiation, which persists after the inciting cause is removed. [G. *phōs,* light, + *phoros,* bearing]

**phos·phor·ic ac·id** (fos-fōr'ik as'id) Orthophosphoric acid. In dentistry, it constitutes about 60% of the liquid used in zinc phosphate and silicate cements; solutions in varying concentrations are used to etch enamel and dentin surfaces to improve mechanical bonds before application of various types of resins. Sometimes used as a component in zinc phosphate cement.

**phos·phor plate** (fos'fŏr plāt) Coated plate used in place of a radiographic film cassette in a computed radiography system.

**phos·pho·rus** (fos'fŏr-ŭs) A nonmetallic chemical element, occurring extensively in nature; the elemental form is extremely poisonous, causing intense inflammation and fatty degeneration; repeated inhalation of phosphorus fumes may cause necrosis of the jaw (phosphonecrosis). [G. *phosphoros,* fr. *phōs,* light, + *phoros,* bearing]

**phos·pho·rus 32** (fos'fŏr-ŭs) Radioactive phosphorus isotope; used as tracer in metabolic studies and to treat some diseases of the osseous and hematopoietic systems.

**phos·phor·y·la·tion** (fos'fŏr-i-lā'shŭn) Addition of phosphate to an organic compound, such as glucose to produce glucose monophosphate, through the action of a phosphotransferase (phosphorylase) or kinase.

**phos·pho·tung·stic ac·id (PTA)** (fos'fō-tŭng'stik as'id) A mixture of phosphoric and tungstic acids; a protein precipitant and reagent for arginine, lysine, histidine, and cystine; used with hematoxylin for nuclear and muscle staining; also used in electron microscopy as a stain for collagen and as a negative stain.

**phos·pho·vi·tin** (fos'fō-vī'tin) SYN phosvitin.

**phos·sy jaw** (fos'ē jaw) Phosphorus necrosis of the jaw, caused by overexposure of white phosphorus, which was used in the manufacture of matches until the early 20th century; agent is still used for signaling, filtering, and incendiary purposes.

**phos·vi·tin** (fos-vī'tin) A phosphated protein used as an anticoagulant. SYN phosphovitin.

**pho·tom·e·try** (fō-tom'ĕ-trē) The measurement of the intensity of light.

**pho·ton (γ)** (fō'ton) In physics, corpuscle of energy or particle of light; a quantum of light or other electromagnetic radiation.

**pho·to-patch test** (fō'tō pach test) A test of contact photosensitization: After application of a patch with the suspected sensitizer for 48 hours to two sites, if there is no reaction, one area is exposed to a weak erythema dose of sunlight or ultraviolet light; if positive, a more severe reaction with vesiculation develops at the exposed patch area than the nonexposed skin patch site.

**pho·to·pol·y·mer·i·sa·tion** [Br.] SYN photopolymerization.

**pho·to·pol·y·mer·i·za·tion** (fō'tō-pol'ĭ-mĕr-ī-zā'shŭn) Polymerization with the use of an external light source. SYN photopolymerisation.

**pho·to·ptar·mo·sis** (fō-top'tahr-mō'sis) Sneezing on looking at light, especially sunlight. [*photo-* + G. *ptarmos,* a sneezing, + *-osis,* condition]

**phren·o·ple·gi·a** (fren'ō-plē'jē-ă) Paralysis of diaphragm. [*phreno-* G. phren, diaphragm + G. *plēgē,* stroke]

**phren·o·trop·ic** (fren'ō-trō'pik) Affecting or working through the mind or brain. [*phreno-* G. phren, diaphragm + G. *tropē,* a turning]

**PHS** Abbreviation for Public Health Service.

**phyl·lo·quin·one** (fil'ō-kwin'ōn) Major form of vitamin K found in plants isolated from alfalfa. SYN vitamin K1.

**phy·sa·lop·ter·i·a·sis** (fī'să-lop'tĕr-ī'ă-sis) Infection of animals and humans with nematodes of the genus *Physaloptera.*

**phys·i·a·try** (fi-zī'ă-trē, fiz'e-at'rē) SYN physical medicine.

**phys·i·cal** (fiz'i-kăl) Relating to the body, as

op

distinguished from the mind. [Mod. L. *physicalis,* fr. G. *physikos*]

**phys·i·cal di·ag·no·sis** (fiz′i-kăl dī′ăg-nō′sis) **1.** Diagnosis made by means of physical examination of the patient. **2.** Process of a physical examination.

**phys·i·cal ex·am·i·na·tion** (fiz′i-kăl eg-zam′i-nā′shŭn) Examination by means such as visual inspection, palpation, and auscultation to collect information for diagnosis.

**phys·i·cal fit·ness** (fiz′i-kăl fit′nĕs) A set of attributes relating to one's ability to perform physical activity.

**phys·i·cal med·i·cine** (fiz′i-kăl med′i-sin) The study and treatment of disease mainly by mechanical and other physical methods. SYN physiatry.

**phys·i·cal sign** (fiz′i-kăl sīn) Sign observed or elicited by inspection, palpation, percussion, or auscultation.

**phys·i·cal ther·a·pist** (fiz′i-kăl thăr′ă-pist) A practitioner of physical therapy. SYN physiotherapist.

**phys·i·cal ther·a·py (PT)** (fiz′i-kăl thăr′ă-pē) **1.** Treatment of pain, disease, or injury by physical means. **2.** Profession concerned with promotion of health, with prevention of physical disabilities, with evaluation and rehabilitation of patients disabled by pain, disease, or injury, and with treatment by physical therapeutic measures.

**phy·si·cian** (fi-zish′ŭn) A doctor; a person who has been educated, trained, and licensed to practice the art and science of medicine. [Fr. *physicien,* a natural philosopher]

**phy·si·cian as·sis·tant (PA)** (fi-zish′ŭn ă-sis′tănt) One trained, certified, and licensed to perform history taking, physical examination, diagnosis, and treatment of commonly encountered medical problems, and some technical skills, under the supervision of a licensed physician, and who thereby extends the physician's capacity to provide medical care.

**phys·ics** (fiz′iks) The branch of science concerned with the phenomena of matter and energy and their interactions.

⟁**physio-** Combining form meaning **1.** Physical, physiologic. **2.** Natural, relating to physics. [G. *physis,* nature]

**phys·i·og·no·my** (fiz′ē-og′nŏ-mē) Physical appearance of one's face, countenance, or habitus, especially regarded as an indication of character. [*physio-* + G. *gnōmōn,* a judge]

**phys·i·og·no·sis** (fiz′ē-og-nō′sis) Diagnosis of disease based on study of facial appearance or bodily habitus. [*physio-* + G. *gnōsis,* knowledge]

**phys·i·o·log·ic, phys·i·o·log·ic·al** (fiz′ē-ŏ-loj′ik, -ăl) **1.** Relating to physiology. **2.** Normal, as opposed to pathologic. **3.** Denoting something apparent from its functional effects rather than from its anatomic structure.

**phys·i·o·log·i·cal·ly bal·anced oc·clu·sion** (fiz′ē-ŏ-loj′ik-ă-lē bal′ănst ŏ-klū′zhŭn) One in harmony with the temporomandibular joints and the neuromuscular system.

**phys·i·o·log·i·c chem·i·stry** (fiz′ē-ŏ-loj′ik kem′is-trē) SYN biochemistry.

**phys·i·o·log·ic dead space** (fiz′ē-ŏ-loj′ik ded spās) The sum of anatomic and alveolar dead space.

**phys·i·o·log·ic oc·clu·sion** (fiz′ē-ŏ-loj′ik ŏ-klū′zhŭn) Dental occlusion that functions in harmony with the masticatory system.

**phys·i·o·log·ic rest po·sit·ion** (fiz′ē-ŏ-loj′ik rest pŏ-zish′ŭn) Position of the mandible, with the head resting comfortably in an upright position and the person resting comfortably, and the masticatory muscles in equilibrium with minimal tonic activity.

**phys·i·ol·o·gy** (fiz′ē-ol′ŏ-jē) Science concerned with normal vital processes of organisms, especially as to how things normally function in living organism rather than to their anatomic structure. [L. or G. *physiologia,* fr. G. *physis,* nature, + *logos,* study]

**phys·i·o·ther·a·pist** (fiz′ē-ō-thăr′ă-pist) SYN physical therapist.

**phy·so·stig·mine** (fī′sō-stig′mēn) Alkaloid used as a cholinergic agent, and experimentally to enhance action of acetylcholine at any of its sites of liberation.

**phy·to·sis** (fī-tō′sis) Disease process caused by infection with a vegetable organism, such as a fungus.

**PI** Abbreviation for Periodontal Index.

**pI** Abbreviation for isoelectric point.

**pi, π** (pī) **1.** The 16th letter of the Greek alphabet. **2.** (Π). Symbol for osmotic pressure; in mathematics, symbol for the product of a series.

**pi·ca** (pī′kă) Perverted appetite for substances not fit as food or of no nutritional value; e.g., clay, dried paint, starch, ice. [L. *pica,* magpie]

**pick·ling** (pik′ling) In dentistry, process of cleansing metallic surfaces of products of oxidation and impurities by immersion in acid.

**pick·ling so·lu·tion** (pik′ling sŏ-lū′shŭn) An acid bath used to remove impurities and oxidation products from metallic surfaces.

**pick·up im·pres·sion** (pik′ŭp im-presh′ŭn) Technique used to obtain accurate imprint of implant abutments and surrounding soft tissue. Before doing it, the implant superstructure is placed in situ and then picked up in impression material.

**PICO** (pī'kō) An acronym used in formulating patient-centered questions. What is the *P*atient, *P*opulation, or *P*roblem? Which *I*ntervention is being considered? What *C*omparator to this intervention will be used? What *O*utcome will be measured?

**Pi·cor·na·vir·i·dae** (pi-kōr'nă-vir'i-dē) A family of very small viruses having a core of single-stranded RNA. Numerous species (including the polioviruses, coxsackieviruses, and echoviruses) are included in the family. [It. *piccolo*, very small, + *RNA* + *-viridae*]

**pic·ric ac·id** (pik'rik as'id) Agent used as an application in burns, eczema, erysipelas, and pruritus. [G. *pikros*, bitter]

**PID** Abbreviation for position-indicating device.

**Pi·erre Rob·in syn·drome** (pē-yār' rō-ban[h]' sin'drōm) Complex of congenital anomalies including micrognathia and abnormal smallness of tongue, often with cleft palate. Intelligence of those affected is usually normal.

**pi·e·zo·e·lec·tric ul·tra·son·ic de·vice** (pē-ā'zō-ĕ-lek'trik ŭl'tră-son'ik dĕ-vīs') Electronically powered tool that uses rapid energy vibrations of a powered instrument tip to fracture calculus from tooth surfaces and clean environment of periodontal pocket; consists of a portable electronic generator, a handpiece, and instrument inserts.

**pig·ment** (pig'mĕnt) 1. Any coloring matter, such as that in the red blood cells, hair, or iris, or in the stains used in histologic or bacteriologic work, or that in paint. 2. A medicinal preparation for external use, applied to the skin like paint. [L. *pigmentum,* paint]

**pig·ment·ed ne·vus** (pig'men-tĕd nē'vŭs) Any congenital skin lesion containing melanin; a birthmark.

**pig·tail ex·plo·rer** (pig'tāl eks-plōr'ĕr) Instrument with a sharp, pointed, curved end used to check the integrity of margins of restorations and to detect carious lesions in enamel and cementum surfaces.

**pill** (pil) *A pill is spheric. Avoid referring to tablets and capsules as pills.* A small globular mass of some coherent, but soluble, substance containing a medicinal substance to be swallowed. [L. *pilula;* dim. of *pila,* ball]

**pill-roll·ing** (pil'rōl-ing) Circular movement of opposed tips of thumb and index finger appearing as a form of tremor in paralysis agitans.

**pi·lo·car·pine** (pī'lō-kahr'pēn) An alkaloid used experimentally to induce seizures externally as a miotic and to treat glaucoma. [G. *pilos,* a felt hat, + *karpos,* fruit]

**pi·lo·mo·tor re·flex** (pī'lō-mō'tŏr rē'fleks) Contraction of smooth muscle of skin resulting in "gooseflesh" caused by mild application of a tactile stimulus or local cooling.

**pim·e·lor·thop·ne·a** (pim'ĕ-lōr-thop'nē-ă) Orthopnea; difficulty breathing when not upright, due to obesity. [*pimelo-* G. *pimēlē,* soft fat + G. *orthos,* straight, + *pnoē,* breath]

**pin** (pin) A metallic implant used in surgical treatment of bone fractures. SEE ALSO nail. [O.E. *pinn,* fr. L. *pinna,* feather]

**pin a·mal·gam** (pin ă-mal'găm) Amalgam restoration held in place largely by small metal rods protruding from holes drilled into tooth structure.

**pin·cer grasp** (pin'sĕr grasp) A grasp pattern emerging in the 10th–12th month whereby a small object is held between the distal pads of the opposed thumb and index or middle finger.

**pinch** (pinch) OCCUPATIONAL THERAPY a grip between the fingers at the most distal joints.

**pin·do·lol** (pin'dō-lol) A β-adrenergic blocking agent used in the treatment of hypertension; also possesses intrinsic sympathomimetic activity.

**pin im·plant** (pin im'plant) Dental implant usually rod-shaped, used in the area of maxillary sinuses.

**pink dis·ease** (pingk di-zēz') SYN acrodynia (2).

**pink tooth** (pingk tūth) Roseate tooth indicating internal resorption of the dentin.

**pin·ledge** (pin'lej) Cast metal dental restoration that employs parallel pins as part of casting to increase retention of restoration.

**pin·na,** pl. **pin·nae** (pin'ă, -ē) 1. SYN auricle (1). 2. A feather, wing, or fin. [L. *pinna* or *penna,* a feather, in pl. a wing]

**pin·o·cy·to·sis** (pin'ō-sī-tō'sis) The cellular process of actively engulfing liquid, a phenomenon in which minute incuppings or invaginations are formed in the surface of the cell membrane and close to form fluid-filled vesicles. [*pinocyte* + G. *-osis,* condition]

**pi·per·a·cil·lin so·di·um** (pi-per'ă-sil'in sō'dē-ŭm) Semisynthetic extended spectrum penicillin active against many gram-positive and gram-negative bacteria.

**pi·per·a·zine** (pī-per'ă-zēn, -zin) A veterinary anthelmintic and filaricide. SYN diethylenediamine.

**pi·pette, pi·pet** (pī-pet') A graduated tube (marked in mL) used to transport a definite volume of a gas or liquid in laboratory work. [Fr. dim. of *pipe,* pipe]

**op**

**pir·i·form, pyr·i·form** (pir´i-fōrm) Pear-shaped. [L. *pirum,* pear, + *forma,* form]

**pi·ri·form ap·er·ture** (pir´i-fōrm ap´ĕr-chŭr) [TA] Common, pear-shaped anterior nasal opening in cranium.

**pir·i·form fos·sa** (pir´i-fōrm fos´ă) [TA] Recess in anterolateral wall of nasopharynx on each side of vestibule of the larynx separated from it by aryepiglottic folds.

**pir·i·for·mis fas·ci·a** (pir´i-fōrm´is fash´ē-ă) [TA] Fascia surrounding piriformis muscle.

**pit** (pit) **1.** Sharp-pointed depression in enamel tooth surface, due to faulty or incomplete calcification or formed at confluent point of two or more lobes of enamel. **2.** SYN fovea. **3.** Pinhead-sized depressed scar that develops after pustule of acne, chickenpox, or smallpox (pockmark).

**pit and fis·sure ca·ries** (pit fish´ŭr kar´ēz) Caries initiated in areas where developmental pits and fissures are located on tooth surfaces.

**pit and fis·sure cav·i·ty** (pit fish´ŭr kav´i-tē) Carious lesion within the pits and fissures of the occlusal surface of a tooth. Typically it occurs in areas with steep morphology that are difficult to reach with oral hygiene products.

**pit and fis·sure seal·ant** (pit fish´ŭr sēl´ănt) Preventive resin material applied to pit and fissure dental areas to prevent caries.

**pit ca·ries** (pit kar´ēz) Carious lesion, usually small, beginning in a pit on labial, buccal, lingual, or occlusal tooth surface.

**pit·ting** (pit´ing) In dentistry, formation of well-defined, relatively deep depressions in a surface, usually used in describing defects in surfaces (often golds, solder joints, or amalgam).

**pit·ting e·de·ma** (pit´ing ĕ-dē´mă) Area of swelling that retains for a time the indentation produced by pressure.

**pi·tu·i·tar·y** (pi-tū´i-tar-ē) Relating to the pituitary gland (hypophysis). [L. *pituita,* phlegm]

**pi·tu·i·tar·y ap·o·plex·y** (pi-tū´i-tar-ē ap´ŏ-plek-sē) Syndrome of abrupt onset, consisting of impaired consciousness, retroorbital pain, meningism, ophthalmoplegia, and rapidly progressive visual loss resulting from infarction of pituitary gland.

**pi·tu·i·tar·y ca·chex·i·a** (pi-tū´i-tar-ē kă-kek´sē-ă) SYN Simmonds disease.

**pi·tu·i·tar·y gland** (pi-tū´i-tar-ē gland) [TA] Unpaired compound gland suspended from base of the hypothalamus by a short extension of infundibulum; the infundibular or pituitary stalk. SYN hypophysis [TA].

**pi·tyr·i·a·sis ro·se·a** (pit´i-rī´ă-sis rō-zē´ă) A self-limited eruption of macules or papules involving the trunk and, less frequently, extremities, scalp, and face; the lesions are usually oval and follow the crease lines of the skin.

**piv·ot** (piv´ŏt) A post on which something hinges or turns.

**piv·ot·ing** (piv´ŏt-ing) A swinging motion of the hand and arm carried out by balancing on the fulcrum finger during periodontal scaling. The hand pivot is used to assist in maintaining adaptation of the working-end of the scaling instrument.

**pix·el** (piks´ĕl) Contraction for picture element, two-dimensional representation of a volume element (voxel) in the display of the computed tomographic or magnetic resonance image, usually $512 \times 512$ or $256 \times 256$ pixels, respectively.

**PK** Abbreviation for pyruvate kinase.

**PKU** Abbreviation for phenylketonuria.

**pla·ce·bo** (plă-sē´bō) Inert substance given as a medicine for its suggestive effect. SYN active placebo. [L. I will please, future of *placeo*]

**pla·ce·bo ef·fect** (plă-sē´bō e-fekt´) A response when a treatment or medication with no known therapeutic value is administered to a patient and the patient's symptoms improve due to their belief that the treatment is effective.

**place·ment** (plās´mĕnt) In dentistry, typically used to denote the insertion of a prosthesis.

**place·ment stroke** (plās´mĕnt strōk) Instrumentation stroke used to position the working-end of a scaling instrument apical to a calculus deposit or at the base of a sulcus or pocket.

**pla·cen·ta** (plă-sen´tă) Fetomaternal organ of metabolic interchange between embryo or fetus and mother. [L. a flat cake]

**pla·gi·o·ceph·a·ly** (plā´jē-ō-sef´ă-lē) An asymmetric craniostenosis due to premature closure of the lambdoid and coronal sutures on one side; characterized by an oblique deformity of the cranium. SYN asynclitism of the skull. [G. *plagios,* oblique, + *kephalē,* head]

**plague** (plāg) Widely prevalent disease or one causing excessive mortality. [G. *plege,* a stroke, a wound; L. *plaga,* a stroke, injury]

**plan** (plan) **1.** A program or method for the achievement of an objective. **2.** A picture or diagram showing a structure or arrangement of parts. [Fr. *plant,* ground plan, fr. L. *planta,* sole of the foot]

**Planck the·o·ry** (plahngk thē´ŏr-ē) SYN quantum theory.

**plane** (plān) [TA] **1.** Two-dimensional flat surface. **2.** Imaginary surface formed by extension of a point through any axis or two definite points, in reference especially to craniometry and to pelvimetry. [L. *planus,* flat]

**planes of ref·er·ence** (plānz ref´ĕr-ĕns) Planes that guide to the location of other planes.

**pla·nig·ra·phy** (plă-nig´ră-fē) SYN tomography. [L. *planum,* plane, + G. *graphē,* a writing]

**pla·nim·e·ter** (plă-nim´ĕ-tĕr) An instrument formed of jointed levers with a recording index used for measuring the area of any surface, by tracing its boundaries. [L. *planum,* plane, + G. *metron,* measure]

**plan of care** (plan kār) SYN care plan.

**pla·nog·ra·phy** (plă-nog´ră-fē) SYN tomography.

**plaque, placque** (plak) **1.** SEE dental plaque. **2.** Patch or small, differentiated area on body surface (e.g., skin, mucosa, or arterial endothelium) or on cut surface of an organ. **3.** An area of clearing in a flat, confluent growth of bacteria or tissue cells. [Fr. a plate]

**plaque bi·o·film** (plak bī´ō-film) Well-organized community of bacteria that adheres tenaciously to tooth surfaces, restorations, and prosthetic appliances; has been determined the primary cause of most periodontal disease.

**plaque in·dex** (plak in´deks) Measure for estimating status of oral hygiene by measuring dental plaque that occurs in areas adjacent to gingival margin.

**plaque re·ten·tive fac·tors** (plak rĕ-ten´ tiv fak´tŏrz) Conditions that foster establishment and growth of plaque biofilms (e.g., calculus deposits, overhanging restorations).

**plas·ma** (plaz´mă) Proteinaceous fluid (noncellular) portion of circulating blood, as distinguished from the serum obtained after coagulation. [G. something formed]

**plas·ma ac·cel·er·a·tor glob·u·lin** (plaz´ mă ak-sel´ĕ-rā-tŏr glob´yū-lin) SYN factor V.

**plas·ma cell** (plaz´mă sel) Ovoid cell with an eccentric nucleus; derived from B lymphocytes and active in formation and secretion of antibodies.

**plas·ma cell gin·gi·vi·tis** (plaz´mă sel jin´ji-vī´tis) Intense hyperemic edema and inflammation of gingiva resulting from a hypersensitivity reaction. A dense plasma cell infiltrate is seen in the lamina propria. SYN atypical gingivitis.

**plas·ma cell my·e·lo·ma** (plaz´mă sel mī´ĕ-lō´mă) **1.** SYN multiple myeloma. **2.** Plasmacytoma of bone, which is usually a solitary lesion and not associated with the occurrence of Bence Jones protein or other disturbances in the metabolism of protein.

**plas·ma·crit** (plaz´mă-krit) A measure of the percentage of the volume of blood occupied by plasma. [*plasma* + G. *krinō,* to separate]

**plas·ma·cy·to·ma** (plaz´mă-sī-tō´mă) A discrete, presumably solitary mass of neoplastic plasma cells in bone or in one of various extramedullary sites; in humans, such lesions are probably the initial phase of developing plasma cell myeloma. [*plasmacyte* + G. *-oma,* tumor]

**plas·ma·lem·ma** (plaz´mă-lem´ă) SYN cell membrane. [*plasma* + G. *lemma,* husk]

**plas·ma mem·brane** (plaz´mă mem´brān) SYN cell membrane.

**plas·ma throm·bo·plas·tin an·te·ce·dent (PTA)** (plaz´mă throm´bō-plas´tin an´ti-sē´dĕnt) SYN factor XI.

**plas·ma throm·bo·plas·tin com·po·nent (PTC)** (plaz´mă throm´bō-plas´tin kŏm-pō´nĕnt) SYN factor IX.

**plas·mid** (plaz´mid) Genetic particle physically separate from chromosome of host cell (chiefly bacterial), which can function and replicate stably and usually confer some advantage to the host cell. [cyto*plasm* + *-id*]

**plas·min** (plaz´min) An enzyme responsible for the dissolution of blood clots. SYN fibrinase (2), fibrinolysin.

**plas·min·o·gen** (plaz-min´ŏ-jen) A precursor of plasmin; may promote thrombosis.

**plas·min·o·gen ac·ti·va·tor** (plaz-min´ ŏ-jen ak´ti-vā-tŏr) A proteinase that converts plasminogen to plasmin and prevents formation of fibron clots. SYN urokinase.

***Plas·mo·di·um*** (plaz-mō´dē-ŭm) A genus of the protozoan family Plasmodidae blood parasites of vertebrates; includes the causal agents of malaria in humans and other animals, with an asexual cycle occurring in liver and red blood cells of vertebrates. [Mod. L. from G. *plasma,* something formed, + *eidos,* appearance]

***Plas·mo·di·um fal·cip·a·rum*** (plaz-mō´ dē-ŭm fal´si-pā´rŭm) *Laverania falcipara,* a species that is the causal agent of falciparum (malignant tertian) malaria.

***Plas·mo·di·um ma·lar·i·ae*** (plaz-mō´ dē-ŭm mă-lar´ē-ē) Protozoan species that is the causal agent of quartan malaria.

***Plas·mo·di·um o·va·le*** (plaz-mō´dē-ŭm ō-vā´lē) Protozoan species that is the agent of the least common form of human malaria.

***Plas·mo·di·um vi·vax*** (plaz-mō´dē-ŭm vī´ vaks) Protozoan species that is the most common malarial parasite of humans.

**plas·ter** (plas´tĕr) **1.** In dentistry, general term for calcined gypsum products used to fabricate dental casts and products used to attach casts to articulators. Principal constituent is calcium

**op**

sulfate hemihydrate. **2.** A solid preparation that can be spread when heated and becomes adhesive at body temperature; used to keep wound edges in apposition, to protect raw surfaces, and, when medicated, to redden or blister skin, as in mustard plaster, or to apply drugs to the surface to obtain their systemic effects. [L. *emplastrum;* G. *emplastron,* plaster or mold]

**plas·ter of Par·is** (plas′tĕr par′is) Exsiccated calcium sulfate from which water of crystallization has been expelled by heat, but which, when mixed with water, forms a paste that then sets. [L. *plastrum,* plaster + *Paris,* France]

**plas·tic** (plas′tik) **1.** Capable of being formed or molded. **2.** A material that can be shaped by pressure or heat to the form of a cavity or mold. [G. *plastikos,* relating to molding]

**plas·tic in·stru·ments** (plas′tik in′strŭ-mĕnts) Those devices made of plastic used to assess and débride implant teeth.

**plas·tic·i·ty** (plas-tis′i-tē) Capability of being formed or molded; quality of being plastic.

**plas·tic ma·trix** (plas′tik mā′triks) SYN matrix (1).

**plas·tic res·to·ra·tion ma·te·ri·al** (plas′tik res′tŏr-ā′shŭn mă-tēr′ē-ăl) In dentistry, any material that may be shaped directly to the tooth cavity, such as amalgam, cement, or resin.

**plas·tic strip** (plas′tik strip) SYN separating strip.

**plas·tic sur·ge·ry** (plas′tik sŭr′jĕr-ē) The surgical specialty or procedure concerned with the restoration, construction, reconstruction, or improvement in the shape and appearance of body structures.

**plas·tic teeth** (plas′tik tēth) Artificial teeth constructed of synthetic resins.

**plate** (plāt) **1.** [TA] In anatomy, thin, relatively flat, structure. SYN lamina [TA]. **2.** A metal bar perforated for screws applied to a fractured bone to maintain the ends in apposition. **3.** Agar layer within a Petri dish or similar vessel. **4.** To form a thin layer of a bacterial culture by streaking it on the surface of an agar plate (usually within a Petri dish) to isolate individual organisms from which a colonial clone will develop. [O.Fr. *plat,* a flat object, fr. G. *platys,* flat, broad]

**plate·let** (plāt′lĕt) An irregularly shaped, disclike, cytoplasmic fragment of a megakaryocyte that is shed in the marrow sinus and subsequently found in the peripheral blood, where it functions in clotting. SYN blood disc, elementary particle (1), thrombocyte, thromboplastid (1).

**plate·let-de·rived growth fac·tor (PDGF)** (plāt′lĕt-dĕ-rīvd′ grōth fak′tŏr) Factor mitogenic for cells at wound site.

**plat·i·num** (plat′i-nŭm) A metallic element used for making small parts for chemical apparatus because of its resistance to acids; its powdered form (**platinum black**) is an important

catalyst in hydrogenation. Some salts have been used to treat syphilis; one derivative, cisplatin, is used as an antineoplastic agent. [Mod. L., originally *platina,* fr. Sp. *plata,* silver]

**plat·i·num foil** (plat′i-nŭm foyl) Pure platinum rolled into extremely thin sheets; its high fusing point makes it suitable as a matrix for various soldering procedures and also suitable for providing internal form to porcelain restorations during their fabrication.

***Plat·y·hel·min·thes*** (plat′i-hel-min′thēz) A phylum of flatworms that are bilaterally symmetric, flattened, and acelomate.

**pla·typ·ne·a** (plă-tip′nē-ă) Difficulty in breathing when upright, which is relieved by recumbency. Cf. orthopnea. SYN platypnoea.

**platypnoea** [Br.] SYN platypnea.

**pla·tys·ma,** pl. **pla·tys·mas,** pl. **pla·tys·ma·ta** (plă-tiz′mă, -măz, -mă-tă) [TA] SYN platysma muscle. [G. *platysma,* a flatplate]

**pla·tys·ma mus·cle** (plă-tiz′mă mŭs′ĕl) *Origin,* subcutaneous layer and fascia covering pectoralis major and deltoid at level of first or second rib; *insertion,* lower border of mandible, risorius, and platysma of opposite side; *action,* depresses lower lip, forms ridges in skin of neck and upper chest when jaws are "clenched," denoting stress, anger; *nerve supply,* cervical branch of facial. SYN platysma [TA].

**Plea·sure curve** (plezh′ŭr kŭrv) Arc of occlusion that when viewed in sagittal section conforms to a line that is convex upward except for the last molars.

**pled·get** (plej′ĕt) A tuft of wool, cotton, or lint.

**ple·o·mor·phic ad·e·no·ma** (plē′ō-mōr′fik ad′ĕ-nō′mă) A benign neoplasm composed of salivary gland epithelial and mesodermal elements. See this page.

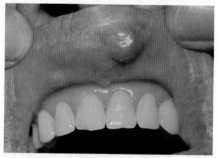

**pleomorphic adenoma:** firm bluish nodule

**ple·o·mor·phism** (plē′ō-mōr′fizm) SYN polymorphism. [*pleo-* + G. *morphē,* form]

**ples·sor** (ples′ŏr) A small hammer, usually

with soft rubber head, used to tap a body part. [G. *plēssō*, to strike]

**pleth·o·ra** (pleth'ŏr-ă) **1.** SYN hypervolemia. **2.** An excess of any of the body fluids. SYN repletion (2). [G. *plēthōrē*, fullness, fr. *plēthō*, to become full]

**pleur·al ef·fu·sion** (plūr'ăl ĕ-fyū'zhŭn) Increased fluid in pleural space; can cause shortness of breath by compression of the lung and/or increased intrathoracic pressure resulting in mediastinal shift and increased work of breathing.

**pleur·i·sy** (plūr'i-sē) Inflammation of the pleura. [L. *pleurisis*, fr. G. *pleuritis*]

**plex·us**, pl. **plex·us** (plek'sŭs) [TA] A network or interjoining of nerves and blood vessels or of lymphatic vessels. [L. a braid]

**pli·ca fim·bri·a·ta** (plī'kă fim'brē-ā'tă) Fringelike projections located on the fold of tissue on ventral surface of tongue.

**plo·sive** (plō'siv) Speech sound made by impounding the air stream for a moment and then suddenly releasing it.

**plug** (plŭg) Any mass filling a hole or closing an orifice.

**plug·ger** (plŭg'ĕr) Dental instrument used to condense gold (foil), amalgam, or any plastic material in a cavity; operated by hand or by mechanical methods. SYN packer (2), plugging instrument.

**plug·ging in·stru·ment** (plŭg'ing in'strŭ-mĕnt) SYN plugger.

**plum·bic** (plŭm'bik) Relating to or containing lead. [L. *plumbum*, lead]

**plum·bism** (plŭm'bizm) SYN lead poisoning. [L. *plumbum*, lead]

**Plum·mer-Vin·son syn·drome** (plŭm'ĕr vin'sŏn sin'drōm) Iron deficiency anemia, dysphagia, esophageal web, and atrophic glossitis.

**plun·ger cusp** (plŭn'jĕr kŭsp) Cusp with a postion such as to force food into interproximal areas.

**plur·i·cau·sal** (plūr'i-kaw'zăl) Having two or more causes; used in reference to disease etiology.

**plur·i·glan·du·lar** (plūr'i-glan'dyū-lăr) Denoting several glands or their secretions.

**PMA in·dex** (in'deks) The first (1947) epidemiologic assay for gingivitis that evaluated the three morphologic gingival compartments given in the abbreviated title (*p*apillae, *m*arginal, or *a*ttached [gingivae]).

**PMS** Abbreviation for premenstrual syndrome.

**PN** Abbreviation for parenteral nutrition.

**pne·o·pne·ic re·flex** (nē'op-nē'ik rē'fleks) Modification of respiratory rhythm caused by inhalation of an irritating vapor.

**pneu·mo·car·di·al** (nū'mō-kahr'dē-ăl) SYN cardiopulmonary.

**pneu·mo·coc·cal em·py·e·ma** (nū'mō kŏk'ăl em'pī-ē'mă) Infection of pleural cavity by *Streptococcus pneumoniae*, with pus formation.

**pneu·mo·coc·cus**, pl. **pneu·mo·coc·ci** (nū'mō-kok'ŭs, -sī) SYN *Streptococcus pneumoniae*. [G. *pneumōn*, lung, + *kokkos*, berry (coccus)]

**pneu·mo·co·lon** (nū'mō-kō'lŏn) Gas in colon or interstitial gas in colon wall. [G. *pneuma*, air, + *kolon*, colon]

**pneu·mo·co·ni·o·sis, pneu·mo·no·co·ni·o·sis, pneu·mo·ko·ni·o·sis,** pl. **pneu·mo·co·ni·o·ses, pneu·mo·no·co·ni·o·ses, pneu·mo·no·ko·ni·o·ses** (nū'mō-kō-nē-ō'sis, nū'mō-nō-, nū'mō-kō-, -sēz) Inflammation commonly leading to lung fibrosis caused by inhalation of dust incident to various occupations; characterized by chest pain, cough with little or no expectoration, dyspnea, reduced thoracic excursion, sometimes cyanosis, and fatigue after slight exertion. [G. *pneumōn*, lung, + *konis*, dust, + *-osis*, condition]

**Pneu·mo·cys·tis ji·ro·ve·ci pneu·mo·ni·a** (nū-mō-sis'tis jī-rō-vē'chē nū-mō'nē-ă) Pneumonia resulting from infection with *Pneumocystis jiroveci*, frequently seen in the immunologically compromised, such as people with AIDS, or those treated with steroids, the elderly, or premature or debilitated babies during their first 3 months. Formerly, causative agent was known as *Pneumocystis carinii*.

**pneu·mo·em·py·e·ma** (nū'mō-em'pī-ē'mă) A rarely used term for pyopneumothorax.

**pneu·mo·gas·tric** (nū'mō-gas'trik) Relating to lungs and stomach. [G. *pneumōn*, lung, + *gastēr*, stomach]

**pneu·mo·ni·a** (nū-mō'nē-ă) Inflammation of lung parenchyma characterized by consolidation of affected part, alveolar air spaces being filled with exudate, inflammatory cells, and fibrin. [G. fr. *pneumōn*, lung, + *-ia*, condition]

**pneu·mo·ni·tis** (nū'mō-nī'tis) Inflammation of the lungs. SEE ALSO pneumonia. SYN pulmonitis. [G. *pneumōn*, lung, + *-itis*, inflammation]

**pneu·mo·nop·a·thy** (nū'mō-nop'ă-thē) Disease of the lung.

**pneu·mo·thor·ax** (nū'mō-thōr'aks) Presence of free air or gas in pleural cavity. [G. *pneuma*, air, + thorax]

op

**PNS** Abbreviation for peripheral nervous system.

**PO** Abbreviation for *per os.* [L. by mouth].

**pock·et** (pok′ĕt) **1.** Diseased gingival attachment; space between inflamed gum and tooth surface, limited apically by an epithelial attachment. **2.** Cul-de-sac or pouchlike cavity. [Fr. *poche*]

**pock·et depth** (pok′ĕt depth) Measurement in millimeters of the depth from the gingival margin to the epithelial attachment in unhealthy gingival tissue; usually consists of depths greater than 3 mm. pocket

**pock·et ep·i·the·li·um** (pok′ĕt ep′i-thē′lē-ŭm) Epithelium that lines the wall of the periodontal pocket.

**po·di·a·try** (pŏ-dī′ă-trē) The health care specialty concerned with the human foot. SYN chiropody.

**POEMS syn·drome** (pō′ĕmz sin′drōm) Condition characterized by *p*olyneuropathy, *o*rganomegaly, *e*ndocrinopathy, *m*onoclonal gammopathy, and *s*kin changes.

**po·go·ni·on** (pō-gō′nē-on) In craniometry, most anterior point on mandible in the midline. [G. dim. of *pōgōn*, beard]

♻ **-poietin** Suffix used with words to indicate an agent with a stimulatory effect on growth or multiplication of cells, such as erythropoietin, among others. [G. *poietēs*, maker, + *-in*]

**poikilocythaemia** [Br.] SYN poikilocythemia.

**poi·ki·lo·cy·the·mi·a** (poy′ki-lō-sī-thē′mē-ă) SYN poikilocytosis, poikilocythaemia. [*poikilocyte* + G. *haima*, blood]

**poi·ki·lo·cy·to·sis** (poy′ki-lō-sī-tō′sis) The presence of poikilocytes in the peripheral blood. SYN poikilocythemia. [*poikilocyte* + G. *-osis*, condition]

**poi·ki·lo·den·to·sis** (poy′ki-lō-den-tō′sis) Hypoplastic defects or mottling of enamel due to excessive fluoride in the water supply. [*poikilo-* G. *poikilos*, irregular + L. *dens*, tooth, + G. *-osis*, condition]

**poi·ki·lo·der·ma** (poy′ki-lō-dĕr′mă) Variegated hyperpigmentation and telangiectasia of the skin, followed by atrophy. [*poikilo-* G. *poikilos*, irregular + G. *derma*, skin]

**point** (poynt) **1.** SYN punctum. **2.** Sharp end or apex. **3.** Slight projection. **4.** To become ready to open, said of an abscess or boil, the wall of which is thin and about to rupture. [Fr.; L. *punctum*, fr. *pungo*, pp. *punctus*, to pierce]

**point A** (poynt) SYN subspinale.

**point an·gle** (poynt ang′gĕl) Junction of three surfaces of tooth crown, or of cavity walls.

**point B** (poynt) SYN supramentale.

**point·ing** (poynt′ing) Preparing to open spontaneously, said of an abscess or a boil. See this page.

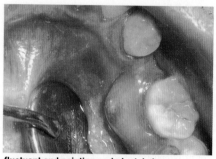

fluctuant and pointing periodontal abscess

**point of prox·i·mal con·tact** (poynt prok′si-măl kon′takt) SYN contact area.

**poi·son** (poy′zŏn) Any substance, either taken internally or applied externally, injurious to health or dangerous to life. [Fr., fr. L. *potio*, potion, draught]

**poi·son·ing** (poy′zŏn-ing) **1.** Administering of poison. **2.** State of being poisoned.

**po·li·o·en·ceph·a·li·tis** (pō′lē-ō-en-sef′ă-lī′tis) Inflammation of gray matter of brain. [G. *polion*, gray matter + G. *enkephalos*, brain, + *-tis*, inflammation]

**po·li·o·my·e·li·tis** (pō′lē-ō-mī′ĕ-lī′tis) Inflammatory process involving gray matter of spinal cord. [G. *polion*, gray matter + G. *myelos*, marrow, + *-itis*, inflammation]

**pol·ish** (pol′ish) To make a tooth or dental restoration smoother and glossier, usually by the action of friction.

**pol·ish·ing** (pol′ish-ing) **1.** Cosmetic dental procedure to remove stains from enamel surfaces of teeth, a nonessential cosmetic procedure. **2.** Act or process of making a dental restoration smoother and glossy. SYN coronal polishing.

**pol·ish·ing a·gent** (pol′ish-ing ā′jĕnt) An abrasive used to achieve a smooth, lustrous finish to a tooth surface.

**pol·ish·ing brush** (pol′ish-ing brŭsh) In dentistry, brush, usually mounted in a rotating instrument, used to polish teeth or artificial replacements. See page 459.

**pol·ish·ing strip** (pol′ish-ing strip) A piece of plastic or linen, with or without abrasive, used to buff proximal surfaces of dental restoration. SEE ALSO linen strip.

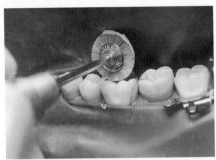
**wheel brush used in polishing**

**pol·len** (pol'ĕn) Microspores of seed plants carried by wind or insects prior to fertilization; important in the etiology of hay fever and other allergies. [L. fine dust, fine flour]

♻ **poly-** 1. Prefix denoting many; multiplicity. 2. In chemistry, prefix meaning "polymer of," as in polypeptide, polysaccharide, polynucleotide; often used with symbols, as in poly(A) for poly (adenylic acid), poly(Lys) for poly(L-lysine). [G. *polys,* much, many]

**pol·y·ad·e·ni·tis** (pol'ē-ad'ĕ-nī'tis) Inflammation of many lymph nodes, especially with reference to the cervical group.

**pol·y·an·gi·i·tis** (pol'ē-an'jē-ī'tis) Inflammation of multiple blood vessels involving more than one type of vessel.

**pol·y·an·ti·bi·ot·ic** (pol'ē-an'tē-bī-ot'ik) Combination of two or more antibiotics.

**pol·y·car·box·y·late ce·ment** (pol'ē-kahr-bok'si-lāt sĕ-ment') Powder containing primarily zinc oxide mixed with a liquid containing polyacrylic acid that reacts to form a hard crystalline mass on standing; when used to lute metal castings to teeth, has potential to bond to calcium contained in tooth structure as well as to any base metals contained in casting. SYN zinc polycarbonate cement.

**pol·y·chro·ma·to·phil·i·a** (pol'ē-krō'mă-tō-fil'ē-ă) A tendency of certain cells, such as the red blood cells in pernicious anemia, to stain with basic and also acidic dyes.

**polycythaemia** [Br.] SYN polycythemia.

**polycythaemia rubra** [Br.] SYN polycythemia rubra.

**pol·y·cy·the·mi·a** (pol'ē-sī-thē'mē-ă) An abnormal increase in the number of red blood cells. SYN erythrocythemia, polycythaemia. [poly- + G. *kytos,* cell, + *haima,* blood]

**pol·y·cy·the·mi·a ru·bra** (pol'ē-sī-thē'mē-ă rū'bră) SYN polycythemia vera, polycythaemia rubra.

**pol·y·cy·the·mi·a ve·ra** (pol'ē-sī-thē'mē-

ă vēr'ă) Chronic form of polycythemia of unknown cause. SYN polycythemia rubra.

**pol·y·dac·ty·ly** (pol'ē-dak'ti-lē) Presence of more than five digits on hand or foot. [poly- + G. *daktylos,* finger]

**pol·y·dip·si·a** (pol'ē-dip'sē-ă) Excessive prolonged thirst. [poly- + G. *dipsa,* thirst]

**pol·y·en·do·crin·op·a·thy** (pol'ē-en'dō-kri-nop'ă-thē) A disease usually caused by insufficiency of multiple endocrine glands.

**pol·y·eth·y·lene gly·cols (PEG)** (pol'ē-eth'i-lēn glī'kolz) Condensation polymers of ethylene oxide and water used as pharmaceutic aids.

**pol·y·mer** (pol'i-mĕr) Substance of high molecular weight, made up of a chain of repeated units sometimes called "mers."

**pol·ym·er·ase chain re·ac·tion (PCR)** (pŏ-lim'ĕr-ās chān rē-ăk'shŭn) An enzymatic method for the repeated copying and amplification of the two strands of DNA of a particular gene sequence.

**polymerisation** [Br.] SYN polymerization.

**po·lym·er·i·za·tion** (pol'i-mĕr'ī-zā'shŭn) A reaction in which a high molecular weight product is produced by successive additions to or condensations of a simpler compound. SYN polymerisation.

**pol·y·mor·phism** (pol'ē-mōr'fizm) Occurrence in more than one form; existence in same species or other natural group of more than one morphologic type. SYN pleomorphism.

**pol·y·mor·pho·nu·cle·ar leu·ko·cyte, pol·y·nu·cle·ar leu·ko·cyte** (pol'ē-mōr' fō-nū'klē-ăr lū'kō-sīt, pol'ē-nū'klē-ăr) Common term for granulocyte or granulocytic leukocyte; includes basophilic, eosinophilic, and neutrophilic leukocytes, but generally used with special reference to the neutrophilic leukocytes.

**pol·y·myx·in** (pol'ē-mik'sin) A mixture of antibiotic substances obtained from cultures of *Bacillus polymyxa* (*B. serosporus*).

**pol·y·neu·rop·a·thy** (pol'ē-nūr-op'ă-thē) 1. Disease process involving several peripheral nerves (literal sense). 2. Nontraumatic generalized disorder of peripheral nerves, affecting distal fibers most severely, with proximal shading. [poly- + G. *neuron,* nerve, + *pathos,* disease]

**pol·y·o·don·ti·a, pol·y·den·ti·a** (pol'ē-ō-don'shē-ă, -den'shē-ă) Presence of supernumerary teeth. [poly- + G. *odous,* tooth]

**pol·y·os·tot·ic** (pol'ē-os-tot'ik) Involving more than one bone. [poly- + G. *osteon,* bone]

**pol·yp** (pol'ip) General descriptive term used with reference to any mass of tissue that bulges or projects outward or upward from normal sur-

**op**

face level; may be neoplasms, foci of inflammation, degenerative lesions, or malformations. [L. *polypus;* G. *polypous,* contr. fr. G. *polys,* many, + *pous,* foot]

**pol·y·pap·il·lo·ma** (pol′ē-pap′i-lō′mă) Multiple papillomas.

**pol·y·path·i·a** (pol′ē-path′ē-ă) Multiplicity of diseases or disorders. [*poly-* + G. *pathos,* disease]

**pol·y·pha·gi·a** (pol′ē-fā′jē-ă) Excessive eating; gluttony. [*poly-* + G. *phagō,* to eat]

**pol·y·phar·ma·cy** (pol′ē-fahr′mă-sē) Administration of multiple drugs simultaneously.

**pol·y·phy·o·dont** (pol′ē-fī′ō-dont) Having several sets of teeth formed in succession throughout life. [*poly-* + G. *phyō,* to produce, + *odous* (*odont-*), tooth]

**pol·yp·ne·a** (pŏ-lip′nē′ă) SYN tachypnea, polypnoea. [*poly-* + G. *pnoia,* breath]

**polypnoea** [Br.] SYN polypnea.

**pol·y·po·sis** (pol′i-pō′sis) Presence of several polyps. [*polyp* + G. *-osis,* condition]

**pol·y·ra·dic·u·lop·a·thy** (pol′ē-ră-dik′yū-lop′ă-thē) Diffuse root involvement; seen with, among other disorders, diabetic neuropathy (diabetic polyradiculopathy).

**pol·yr·rhe·a** (pol′i-rē′ă) Profuse discharge of serous or other fluid. [*poly-* + G. *rhoia,* a flow]

**pol·y·sac·char·ide** (pol′ē-sak′ă-rīd) A carbohydrate containing a large number of saccharide groups (e.g., starch). SYN glycan.

**pol·y·sub·stance de·pen·dence** (pol′ē-sŭb′stăns dĕ-pen′dĕns) Addiction to at least three categories of psychoactive substances or agents (*not* including nicotine or caffeine) but one in which no simple psychoactive substance predominates.

**pol·y·sul·fide rub·ber** (pol′ē-sŭl′fīd rŭb′ĕr) Synthetic elastic material used to make dental impressions.

**pol·y·tro·phic** (pol′ē-trō′fik) Exhibiting an attraction, trophism, for multiple organs.

**pol·y·u·ri·a** (pol′ē-yūr′ē-ă) Excessive excretion of urine resulting in profuse and frequent micturition. [*poly-* + G. *ouron,* urine]

**pol·y·va·lent vac·cine** (pol′ē-vā′lĕnt vak-sēn′) Vaccine prepared from cultures of two or more strains of same species or microorganism.

**pol·y·vi·nyl chlo·ride** (pol′ē-vī′nil klōr′īd) Polymer plastic used as rubber substitute in many industrial applications; suspected of being carcinogenic.

**pons,** pl. **pon·tes** (ponz, pon′tēz) Any bridge-like formation connecting two more-or-less disjoined parts of the same structure or organ. [L. bridge]

**pon·tic** (pon′tik) Artificial tooth on a fixed partial denture; replaces lost natural tooth, restores its functions, and usually occupies space previously occupied by natural crown.

**pool** (pūl) Collection of blood or other fluid in any body region; blood pooling results from dilation and retardation of circulation in capillaries and veins of the region. [A.S. *pōl*]

**pop·u·la·tion** (pop′yū-lā′shŭn) Statistical term denoting all the objects, events, or subjects in a class. [L. *populus,* a people, nation]

**POR** Abbreviation for problem-oriented record.

**por·ce·lain** (pōr′sĕ-lin) Powder composed of clay, silica, and a flux that, when mixed with water, forms a paste that is molded to form artificial teeth, inlays, jacket crowns, and dentures. When heated, materials fuse to form a ceramic.

**▣ por·ce·lain fused to met·al crown** (pōr′sĕ-lin fyūzd met′ăl krown) See this page. SYN veneer crown.

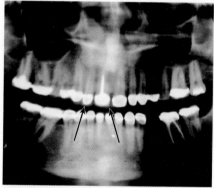

**porcelain fused to metal crown:** numerous porcelain fused to metal crowns visible on panoramic radiograph; radiolucent shadow at the incisal (#6-11) and occlusal (#2, 3, 14) surfaces is the radiolucent porcelain (arrows point to porcelain)

**por·ce·lain in·lay** (pōr′sĕ-lin in′lā) Fused composition restoration luted in a cavity prepared in a tooth.

**por·ce·lain ve·neer crown** (pōr′sĕ-lin vĕ-nēr′ krown) SYN veneer crown.

**por·i·on,** pl. **po·ri·a** (pōr′ē-on, -ă) Central point on upper margin of external auditory meatus. [G. *poros,* a passage]

**po·ro·sis,** pl. **po·ro·ses** (pōr-ō′sis, -sēz) A porous condition. SYN porosity (1). [L. *porosus,* porous]

**po·ros·i·ty** (pōr-os′i-tē) **1.** SYN porosis. **2.** A perforation. [G. *poros,* pore]

**po·rot·ic den·tin** (pōr-ot´ik den´tin) A condition in which the dentin of a tooth becomes very porous; commonly seen with a vitamin C deficiency.

**porphin** SYN porphyrin.

**por·phy·rin** (pōr´fi-rin) SYN porphin.

**por·phy·rin·o·gens** (pōr´fir-in´ō-jenz) Intermediates in the biosynthesis of heme.

**por·phyr·in·op·a·thy** (por´fir-in-op´ă-thē) Syndrome that results from abnormal porphyrin metabolism (e.g., acute porphyria). [*porphyrin* + G. *pathos*, disease]

**por·tal** (pōr´tăl) **1.** Relating to any porta or hilus, specifically to the porta hepatis and the portal vein. **2.** The point of entry into the body of a pathogenic microorganism. **3.** SYN field size. [L. *portalis*, pertaining to a *porta* (gate)]

**por·tal hy·per·ten·sion** (pōr´tăl hī´pĕr-ten´shŭn) Elevation of pressure in the hepatic portal circulation due to cirrhosis or other fibrotic change in liver tissue.

**por·tal of en·try** (pōr´tăl en´trē) Refers to the process whereby a pathogen enters the body, gains access to susceptible tissues, and causes disease or infection.

**po·si·tion** (pŏ-zish´ŏn) **1.** An attitude, posture, or place occupied. **2.** Posture or attitude assumed by a patient for comfort and to facilitate the performance of diagnostic, surgical, or therapeutic procedures. [L. *positio*, a placing, position, fr. *pono*, to place]

**po·si·tion·er** (pŏ-zish´ŏn-ĕr) Resilient elastoplastic or rubber removable appliance fitting over occlusal tooth surface to limit tooth movement or provide stabilization, generally used at end of orthodontic treatment.

**po·si·tion-in·di·ca·ting de·vice (PID)** (pŏ-zish´ŭn-in´di-kāt-ing dĕ-vīs´) The lead-lined cone or cylinder that directs the x-ray beam during a radiographic exposure. SYN beam-indicating device.

**po·si·tion of the in·stru·ment face** (pŏ-zish´ŭn in´strŭ-ment fās) Denotes placement the face of an instrument is put in to sharpen it.

**pos·i·tive** (poz´i-tiv) **1.** Affirmative; definite; not negative. **2.** Denoting a response, the occurrence of a reaction, or the existence of the entity or condition in question. [L. *positivus*, settled by arbitrary agreement, fr. *pono*, pp. *positus*, to set, place]

**pos·i·tive ni·tro·gen bal·ance** (poz´i-tiv nī´trŏ-jen bal´ăns) Nitrogen intake exceeds the sum of all nitrogen excretion.

**pos·i·tron e·mis·sion tom·og·ra·phy (PET)** (poz´i-tron ĕ-mish´ŭn tŏ-mog´ră-fē) Tomographic images formed by computer analysis of photons detected from annihilation of positrons emitted by radionuclides incorporated into biochemical substances.

**po·sol·o·gy** (pŏ-sol´ŏ-jē) Branch of pharmacology and therapeutics concerned with determination of doses of remedies; the science of dosage. [G. *posos*, how much, + *logos*, study]

**post** (pōst) In dentistry, dowel or pin inserted into root canal of a natural tooth as an attachment for an artificial crown.

**post·an·es·the·si·a care u·nit (PACU)** (pōst´an-es-thē´zē-ă kār yū´nit) Room(s) with special personnel and equipment designated for recovery of patients.

**post·an·es·thet·ic** (pōst´an-es-thet´ik) Occurring after anesthesia.

**post·au·ric·u·lar** (pōst´awr-ik´yū-lăr) Denotes area located behind the auricle (external part of the ear).

**post ci·bum (p.c.)** (pōst sī´bŭm) Latin expression meaning "after meals."

**post·crown** (pōst-krown´) Crown, replacing natural crown, which is retained on the stump of tooth root from which pulp has been removed, by a post or pin integral with crown and sealed in the treated root canal with a cement. SYN dowel crown.

**post·dam ar·e·a** (pōst-dam ar´ē-ă) Portion of palate where a maxillary denture ends on soft palate.

**pos·ter·i·or** (pos-tēr´ē-ŏr) **1.** After, in relation to time or space. **2.** HUMAN ANATOMY denoting the back surface of the body. Often used to indicate the position of one structure relative to another, i.e., nearer the back of the body. SYN dorsal (2). [L. comparative of *posterus*, following]

**pos·te·ri·or ar·ti·cu·lar fa·cet of dens** (pos-tēr´ē-ŏr ahr-tik´yū-lăr fas´ĕt denz) [TA] Facet on posterior surface of dens of axis that articulates with the transverse ligament of the atlas. SYN facies articularis posterior dentis.

**pos·te·ri·or bor·der po·si·tion** (pos-tēr´ē-ŏr bōr´dĕr pŏ-zish´ŭn) Posteriormost position of the mandible at any specific vertical relation. These positions make up part of the border envelope of jaw movement.

**pos·te·ri·or cross·bite** (pos-tēr´ē-ŏr kraws´ bīt) Abnormal placement in which the posterior teeth occlude in an abnormal buccolingual relationship with the opposing teeth.

**pos·te·ri·or fas·ci·cle of pal·a·to·pha·ryn·ge·us mus·cle** (pos-tēr´ē-ŏr fas´i-kĕl pal´ă-tō-fă-rin´jē-ŭs mŭs´ĕl) [TA] Thinner portion of the muscle of the palatopharyngeal arch. SYN palatopharyngeal sphincter.

**pos·ter·i·or na·sal spine** (pos-tēr´ē-ŏr

**op**

nā′zăl spīn) The sharp posterior extremity of the nasal crest of the hard palate.

**pos·te·ri·or oc·clu·sion** (pos-tēr′ē-ŏr ŏ-klū′zhŭn) Most effective contact of molar and premolar teeth of maxillae and mandible that allows for all natural movements essential to normal mastication and closure.

**pos·te·ri·or pal·a·tal bar** (pos-tēr′ē-ŏr pal′ă-tăl bahr) That portion of a removable partial denture framework that lies against the posterior part of the palate.

**pos·te·ri·or pal·a·tal seal** (pos-tēr′ē-ŏr pal′ă-tăl sēl) Seal at posterior border of a denture. SYN palatal seal.

**pos·te·ri·or pal·a·tal seal a·re·a** (pos-tēr′ē-ŏr pal′ă-tăl sēl ar′ē-ă) Soft tissues along junction of hard and soft palates on which pressure within the physiologic limits of the tissues can be applied by a denture to aid its retention.

**pos·te·ri·or tooth** (pos-tēr′ē-ŏr tūth) Premolar or molar tooth; these teeth are organs of mastication located in back part of the jaws.

**pos·te·ri·or tooth form** (pos-tēr′ē-ŏr tūth fōrm) Distinguishing contours of occlusal surface of various posterior teeth.

**pos·ter·o·an·ter·i·or (PA)** (pos′tĕr-ō-an-tēr′ē-ŏr) A term denoting direction of view or progression, from posterior to anterior, through a part.

**pos·ter·o·lat·er·al** (pos′tĕr-ō-lat′ĕr-ăl) Behind and to one side.

**pos·ter·o·me·di·al** (pos′tĕr-ō-mē′dē-ăl) Behind and to inner side.

**post·feb·rile** (pōst-feb′ril) Occurring after a fever. SYN metapyretic.

**post·gan·gli·on·ic** (pōst′gang-glē-on′ik) Distal to or beyond a ganglion; referring to unmyelinated nerve fibers originating from cells in an autonomic ganglion.

**post·he·pat·ic jaun·dice** (pōst′he-pat′ik jawn′dis) Liver disease caused by complete or partial obstruction of flow in cystic bile ducts.

**post·ic·tal** (pōst-ik′tăl) Following a seizure, e.g., epileptic.

**post im·plant** (pōst im′plant) Portion of a dental implant substructure that protrudes through mucosa to connect with restoration.

**post·in·flu·en·zal** (post′in-flū-en′zăl) Occurring as a sequel to influenza.

**post·ma·lar·i·al** (pōst′mă-lar′ē-ăl) Occurring as a sequel to malaria.

**post·men·o·pau·sal at·ro·phy** (pōst-men′ō-pawz′ăl at′rŏ-fē) Thinning of the oral mucosa seen in postmenopausal women.

**post·mor·tem ri·gi·di·ty** (pōst-mōr′tĕm ri-jid′i-tē) SYN rigor mortis.

**post·na·sal** (pōst-nā′zăl) Posterior to the nasal cavity.

**post·op·er·a·tive cleft** (pōst′op′ĕr-ā-tĭv kleft) SYN operated cleft.

**post·pal·a·tal seal** (pōst-pal′ă-tăl sēl) Slightly raised area on the posterior border of a maxillary removable dental prosthesis that slightly displaces soft tissue so as to facilitate retention of the prosthesis.

**post·pal·a·tal seal a·re·a** (pōst-pal′ă-tăl sēl ar′ē-ă) Soft tissue area in the region of the soft palate on which physiologic pressure from a removable complete prosthesis will aid its retention.

**post·par·a·lyt·ic** (pōst′par-ă-lit′ik) Following or consequent to paralysis.

**post·par·tum** (pōst-pahr′tŭm) After childbirth. Cf. antepartum, intrapartum. [L. *partus,* birth (noun), fr. *pario,* pp. *partus,* to bring forth]

**post·par·tum blues** (pōst-pahr′tŭm blūz) Mood disturbance (including insomnia, tearfulness, depression, anxiety, and irritability) experienced by up to 50% of women the first week after birth.

**post·pran·di·al pain** (pōst-pran′dē-ăl pān) Pain occurring after eating, typical of malignancy in esophagus or stomach.

**post·pu·bes·cent** (pōst′pyū-bes′ĕnt) Subsequent to the period of puberty.

**post·trau·mat·ic** (pōst′traw-mat′ik) Occurring after trauma and, by implication, caused by it.

**post·trau·mat·ic neck syn·drome** (post′traw-mat′ik nek sin′drōm) Constellation of neck pain, tenderness, and spasm, often associated with ill-defined symptoms (e.g., dizziness, blurred vision), resulting from neck trauma, most often ''whiplash.''

**post·trau·mat·ic stress dis·or·der (PTSD)** (pōst′traw-mat′ik stres dis-ōr′dĕr) Development of characteristic long-term symptoms following a psychologically harmful event that is generally outside range of usual human experience; symptoms include persistently reexperiencing event and attempting to avoid stimuli reminiscent of the trauma, numbed responsiveness to environmental stimuli, autonomic and cognitive dysfunctions, and dysphoria.

**pos·tur·al hy·po·ten·sion** (pos′chŭr-ăl hī′pō-tĕn′shŭn) SYN orthostatic hypotension.

**pos·tur·al po·si·tion, pos·tur·al rest·ing po·si·tion** (pos′chŭr-ăl pŏ-zish′ŏn, rest′ing) SYN rest position.

**pos·tur·al syn·co·pe** (pos′chŭr-ăl sing′kŏ-pē) Syncope on assuming an upright position; due to orthostatic hypotension.

**pos·tur·ing** (pos′chŭr-ing) Placement of body, head, and limbs such that in some cases may be indicative of or diagnostic for a condition, disease, or disorder.

**po·ta·ble** (pō′tă-bĕl) Drinkable; fit to drink. [L. *potabilis,* fr. *poto,* to drink]

**po·ta·ble wa·ter** (pō′tă-bĕl waw′tĕr) Water fit for drinking, being free from contamination and not containing a sufficient quantity of saline material to be regarded as a mineral water.

**po·tas·si·um** (pŏ-tas′ē-ŭm) An alkaline metallic element, occurring abundantly in nature but always in combination; its salts are used medicinally. [Mod. L., fr. Eng. *potash* (fr. pot + ashes) + *-ium*]

**po·tas·si·um bi·car·bon·ate** (pŏ-tas′ē-ŭm bī-kahr′bŏ-nāt) Agent used as diuretic to decrease acidity of urine.

**po·tas·si·um chlo·ride** (pŏ-tas′ē-ŭm klōr′īd) Agent used to correct potassium deficiency.

**po·ten·cy** (pō′tĕn-sē) Power, force, or strength; the condition or quality of being potent. [L. *potentia,* power, potency]

**po·ten·tial** (pŏ-ten′shăl) Capable of doing or being, although not yet in course of doing or being; possible, but not actual. [L. *potentia,* power, potency]

**po·ten·ti·a·tion** (pŏ-ten′shē-ā′shŭn) Interaction between two or more drugs or agents resulting in a pharmacologic response greater than the sum of individual responses to each drug or agent.

**po·tion** (pō′shŭn) A draft or large dose of liquid medicine. [L. *potio,* fr. *poto,* to drink]

**Pott dis·ease** (pot di-zēz′) SYN tuberculous spondylitis.

**Pot·ter-Buck·y di·a·phragm** (pot′ĕr-bŭk′ē dī′ă-fram) SYN Bucky diaphragm.

**pouch** (powch) Pocket or cul-de-sac.

**poul·tice** (pōl′tis) Soft magma or mush prepared by wetting various powders or other absorbent substances with oily or watery fluids, sometimes medicated, and usually applied to surface while hot. [L. *puls* (*pult-*), a thick pap; G. *poltos*]

**pound** (pownd) Unit of weight, containing 12 ounces, apothecaries' weight, or 16 ounces, avoirdupois. [A.S. *pund;* L. *pondus,* weight]

**po·vi·done** (pō′vi-dōn) Synthetic polymer used as a dispersing and suspending agent.

**po·vi·done i·o·dine** (pō′vi-dōn ī′ŏ-dīn) Agent used as an antiseptic solution or ointment

to clean and disinfect skin, prepare skin preoperatively, and treat infections susceptible to it.

**pow·der** (pow′dĕr) **1.** A dry mass of minute separate particles of any substance. **2.** In pharmaceutics, a homogeneous dispersion of finely divided, relatively dry, particulate matter consisting of one or more substances. [Fr. *poudre;* L. *pulvis*]

**pow·der·ed gold** (pow′dĕrd gōld) Gold formed by atomizing or by chemical precipitation, lightly precondensed, and wrapped with gold foil to form pellets.

**pow·er point** (pow′ĕr poynt) In dentistry, vertical dimension at which greatest masticatory force may be registered.

**pow·er tooth·brush** (pow′ĕr tūth′brŭsh) Oral health care device driven by electricity or battery; also called power-assisted, automatic, electric, or mechanical (in contrast with manual).

**pox** (poks) An eruptive disease, usually qualified by a descriptive prefix; e.g., smallpox, cowpox, chickenpox. [var. of pl. *pocks*]

**PP** Abbreviation for pyrophosphate.

**PPO** Abbreviation for preferred provider organization.

**prac·tice** (prak′tis) Exercise of the profession of dentistry, medicine, or one of the allied health professions. [Mediev. L. *practica,* business, G. *praktikos,* pertaining to action]

**prac·tice guide·lines** (prak′tis gīd′līnz) Recommendations developed by groups of clinicians for delivery of care.

**prac·ti·tion·er** (prak-tish′ŭn-ĕr) A person who practices dentistry, medicine, or one of the allied health care professions.

**Pra·der-Wil·li syn·drome** (prah′dĕr-vē′lē sin′drōm) A congenital syndrome characterized by severe obesity, mental retardation, small hands and feet, and small genitalia.

**praecordial** [Br.] SYN precordial.

**pran·di·al** (pran′dē-ăl) Relating to a meal. [L. *prandium,* breakfast]

**prax·i·ol·o·gy** (prak′sē-ol′ŏ-jē) The science or study of behavior. [G. *praxis,* action, + *logos,* study]

**prax·is** (prak′sis) The performance of an action. [G. *praxis,* action]

♻ **pre-** Combining form meaning anterior; before (in time or space). [L. *prae*]

**pre·ag·o·nal** (prē-ag′ŏ-năl) Immediately preceding death. [*pre-* + G. *agōn,* struggle (agony)]

**preanaesthetic** [Br.] SYN preanesthetic.

**op**

**pre·an·es·thet·ic** (prē′an-es-thet′ik) **1.** Before anesthesia. **2.** A medication given as an agent to and before a primary anesthetic. SYN preanaesthetic.

**pre·an·es·thet·ic med·i·ca·tion** (prē′an-es-thet′ik med′i-kā′shŭn) Drugs administered before an anesthetic to decrease anxiety and obtain smoother induction of, maintenance of, and emergence from anesthesia. SYN premedication.

**pre·au·ric·u·lar** (prē′aw-rik′yū-lăr) Anterior to the auricle of the ear; denoting lymphatic nodes so situated.

**pre·au·ric·u·lar deep pa·rot·id lymph nodes** (prē′awr-ik′yū-lăr dēp pă-rot′id limf nōdz) [TA] Small lymph nodes located deep to the parotid fascia and in front of the ear.

**pre·auth·or·i·za·tion** (prē′awth′ŏr-ī-zā′shun) In the U.S., authorization of medical necessity by a primary care physician before a health care service is performed. A referring health care provider must be able to document why the procedure is needed. It *still* does not guarantee coverage.

**pre·can·cer·ous** (prē-kan′sĕr-ŭs) Pertaining to any lesion that is interpreted as precancer. SYN premalignant.

**pre·cer·ti·fi·ca·tion** (prē′sĕr-ti-fi-kā′shŭn) Verification of a procedure as a covered benefit for a third-party payer before a health care service is performed. It *still* does not guarantee coverage.

**pre·cip·i·tate** (prē-sip′i-tāt, -tăt) **1.** To cause a substance in solution to separate out as a solid. **2.** A solid separated out from a solution or suspension; a floc or clump, such as that resulting from mixture of a specific antigen and its antibody. [L. *praecipito,* pp. *-atus,* to cast headlong]

**pre·cip·i·tat·ing cause** (prē-sip′i-tāt-ing kawz) Factor that initiates onset of manifestations of a disease process.

**pre·ci·sion at·tach·ment** (prē-si′zhŭn ă-tach′mĕnt) **1.** Frictional or mechanically retained unit used in fixed or removable prosthodontics, consisting of closely fitting male and female parts. The receptacle (matrix) is typically contained within the abutment crown with the precision fitting extension (patrix) attached to the pontic or removable prosthesis. **2.** Attachment that may be rigid in function or may incorporate a movable stress control unit to reduce torque on the abutment. SYN internal attachment, key attachment, keyway attachment.

**pre·ci·sion rest** (prē-si′zhŭn rest) Rigid metallic extension (patrix) of closely interlocking parts in a fixed or removable prosthesis that fits precisely into a receptacle (matrix) of a precision attachment within a restoration.

**pre·co·cious** (prē-kō′shŭs) Developing unusually early or rapidly. [L. *praecox,* premature]

**pre·co·cious pseu·do·pu·ber·ty** (prē-kō′shŭs sū′dō-pyū′bĕr-tē) Development of pseudopuberty in very young children.

**pre·co·cious pu·ber·ty** (prē-kō′shŭs pyū′bĕr-tē) Condition in which pubertal changes begin unexpectedly early.

**pre·cog·ni·tion** (prē′kog-nish′ŭn) Advance knowledge, by means other than the normal senses, of a future event; a form of extrasensory perception. [L. *praecogito,* to ponder before]

**pre·crit·i·cal** (prē-krit′i-kăl) Relating to the phase before a crisis.

**pre·cur·sor** (prē′kŭrs-ŏr) That which precedes another or from which another is derived. [L. *praecursor,* fr. *prae-,* pre- + *curro,* to run]

**pre·den·tin** (prē-den′tin) Organic fibrillar matrix of dentin before its calcification.

**pre·de·ter·mi·na·tion** (prē′dĕ-tĕr′mi-nā′shŭn) Determination of the reimbursement amount from a third-party payor before a health care service is performed. It *still* does not guarantee coverage.

**pre·dis·pose** (prē′dis-pōz′) To render susceptible.

**pre·dis·pos·ing fac·tors** (prē′dis-pōz′ing fak′tŏrz) Genetic, attitudinal, personality, and environmental factors associated with health, or lack of it, in a person.

**pre·dis·po·si·tion** (prē-dis′pŏ-zish′ŭn) A condition of special susceptibility to a disease.

**pred·nis·o·lone** (pred-nis′ŏ-lōn) A dehydrogenated analogue of cortisol with the same actions and uses.

**pred·ni·sone** (pred′ni-sōn) A dehydrogenated analogue of cortisone with the same actions and uses; must be converted to prednisolone before active.

**pre·e·rup·tive** (prē′ē-rŭp′tiv) Denoting the stage of an exanthematous disease preceding the eruption.

**pre·ex·is·ting con·di·tion** (prē′eg-zist′ing kŏn-dish′ŭn) A health problem that existed or for which treatment was received before the effective date of a new insurance policy.

**pre·ex·trac·tion rec·ord** (prē′eks-trak′shŭn rek′ŏrd) SYN preoperative record.

**pre·fer·red pro·vid·er or·gan·i·za·tion (PPO)** (prē-fĕrd′ prŏ-vī′dĕr ŏr′gă-nī-zā′shŭn) A U.S. health care organization that negotiates set rates of reimbursement with participating health care providers for services to insured clients. This is a type of prospective payment or managed care system.

**preg·nan·cy** (preg′năn-sē) State of a female after conception and until termination of gestation. [L. *praegnans* (*praegnant-*), pregnant, fr. *prae*, before, + *gnascor*, pp. *natus*, to be born]

**preg·nan·cy gin·gi·vi·tis** (preg′năn-sē jin′ji-vī′tis) SYN hormonal gingivitis.

**preg·nan·cy tu·mor** (preg′năn-sē tū′mŏr) See page A15. SYN granuloma gravidarum.

**pre·hor·mone** (prē-hōr′mōn) A glandular secretory product, having little or no inherent biologic potency, which is converted peripherally to an active hormone. Cf. prohormone.

**pre·ic·tal** (prē-ik′tăl) Occurring before a seizure or stroke. [*pre-* + L. *ictus*, a stroke]

**pre·kal·li·kre·in** (prē′kal-i-krē′in) A plasma glycoprotein that in complex with kininogen serves as a cofactor in the activation of factor XII; also serves as the proenzyme for plasma kallikrein. SYN Fletcher factor.

**pre·lim·i·nar·y im·pres·sion** (prē-lim′i-nar-ē im-presh′ŭn) In dentistry, impression made for purpose of diagnosis or construction of a tray. SYN primary impression.

**pre·load** (prē′lōd) 1. The load to which a muscle is subjected before shortening. 2. SYN ventricular preload.

**pre·ma·lig·nant** (prē′mă-lig′nănt) SYN precancerous.

**pre·ma·ture** (prē′mă-chŭr′) 1. Occurring before the usual or expected time. 2. Denoting an infant born at a gestational age of less than 37 weeks. [L. *praematurus*, too early, fr. *prae-*, pre- + *maturus*, ripe (mature)]

**pre·ma·ture birth** (prē′mă-chŭr′ bĭrth) Birth of an infant after viability has been achieved with gestation of at least 20 weeks or birth weight of at least 500 g, but before 37 weeks.

**pre·ma·ture con·tact** (prē′mă-chŭr′ kon′takt) SYN deflective occlusal contact.

**pre·ma·ture ven·tri·cu·lar con·trac·tion (PVC)** (prē′mă-chŭr′ ven-trik′yū-lăr kŏn-trak′shŭn) Compression within the lower cardiac chambers.

**pre·max·il·la** (prē′mak-sil′ă) 1. SYN incisive bone. 2. Central isolated bony part in a complete bilateral cleft of the lip. [*pre-* + L. *maxilla*, jawbone]

**pre·max·il·lar·y** (prē-mak′si-lar′ē) 1. Anterior to the maxilla. 2. Denoting the premaxilla.

**pre·max·il·lar·y bone** (prē-maks′i-lar′ē bōn) SYN incisive bone.

**pre·max·il·lar·y su·ture** (prē-mak′si-lar′ē sū′chŭr) SYN incisive suture.

**pre·med·i·ca·tion** (prē′med-i-kā′shŭn) SYN preanesthetic medication.

**pre·men·stru·al** (prē-men′strū-ăl) Relating to the period of time preceding menstruation.

**pre·men·stru·al dys·phor·ic dis·or·der** (prē-men′strū-ăl dis-fōr′ik dis-ōr′dĕr) Pervasive pattern occurring during last week of luteal phase in most menstrual cycles for at least 1 year and remitting within a few days of onset of follicular phase, with some combination of depressed mood, mood lability, marked anxiety, or irritability.

**pre·men·stru·al syn·drome (PMS)** (prē-men′strū-ăl sin′drōm) In women of reproductive age, constellation of emotional, behavioral, and physical symptoms that occur in luteal (premenstrual) phase of the menstrual cycle and subside with onset of menstruation; characterized by swelling and weight gain due to fluid retention, breast tenderness, and many other symptoms.

**pre·mi·um** (prē′mē-ŭm) The amount that must be paid to the insurer to maintain the desired health insurance coverage.

**pre·mo·lar** (prē-mō′lăr) 1. Anterior to a molar tooth. 2. Denotes permanent teeth that replace the deciduous molars.

**pre·mo·lar tooth** (prē-mō′lăr tūth) [TA] Tooth usually with two tubercles or cusps on grinding surface and a flattened root, single in lower jaw and upper second premolar, and furrowed in upper first premolar. There are four premolars in each jaw, two on either side between the canine and the molars; there are no premolars in deciduous dentition. SYN dens premolaris [TA], bicuspid tooth, dens bicuspidus.

**pre·mor·bid** (prē-mōr′bid) Preceding occurrence of disease. [*pre-* + L. *morbidus*, ill, fr. *morbus*, disease]

**pre·op·er·a·tive rec·ord** (prē-op′ĕr-ă-tiv rek′ŏrd) In dentistry, any note or file made for purpose of study or treatment planning. SEE ALSO diagnostic cast. SYN preextraction record.

**pre·o·ral** (prē-ō′răl) In front of the mouth. [*pre-* + L. *os* (*or-*), mouth]

**pre·ox·y·gen·a·tion** (prē′ok-si-jĕ-nā′shŭn) Denitrogenation with 100% oxygen before induction of general anesthesia.

**prep** (prep) Colloquially, to prepare skin or other body surface for an operative procedure, usually by applying antiseptic solutions.

**pre·pal·a·tal** (prē-pal′ă-tăl) Relating to anterior part of palate, or anterior to palate bone.

**prep·a·ra·tion** (prep′ă-rā′shŭn) 1. The act of making or getting ready. 2. Something made ready, e.g., medicine. [L. *praeparatio*, fr. *prae*, before, + *paro*, pp. *-atus*, to get ready]

**pre·pro·ce·dur·al rinse** (prē′prō-sē′jŭr-ăl rins) Antimicrobial or antiseptic mouth rinse used before a treatment procedure begins to reduce the number of bacteria introduced into the patient's bloodstream and to control aerosols released into the surrounding environment.

**pre·pu·ber·al, pre·pu·ber·tal** (prē-pyū′bĕr-ăl, -tăl) Before puberty.

**pre·pu·bes·cent** (prē′pyū-bes′ĕnt) Immediately before commencement of puberty.

**pres·by·cu·sis** (prez′bē-kyū′sis) A usually gradual, frequently bilateral sensorineural or conductive hearing loss often related to the middle ear that gradually occurs in most people as they age; usually more pronounced for high-pitched sounds. [G. *presbys,* old man, + *akousis,* hearing]

**pres·by·o·pi·a** (prez′bē-ō′pē-ă) The physiologic loss of accommodation in the eyes in advancing age. [*presby-* + G. *ōps,* eye]

**pre·scribe** (prĕ-skrīb′) To give directions, either orally or in writing, for preparation and administration of a remedy to be used to treat any disease. [L. *prae-scribo,* pp. *-scriptus,* to write before]

**pre·scrip·tion** (prĕ-skrip′shŭn) Written formula for the preparation and administration of any remedy.

**pre·se·ni·um** (prē-sē′nē-ŭm) The period preceding old age.

**pre·sent** (prĕ-zent′) To appear for examination or treatment, said of a patient.

**pre·sent·ing symp·tom** (prĕ-zent′ing simp′tŏm) Complaint offered by patient as the main reason for seeking dental care; usually synonymous with chief complaint.

**pre·ser·va·tive** (prĕ-zĕr′vă-tiv) Substance added to food products or organic solutions to prevent chemical change or bacterial action.

**pres·so·re·cep·tive** (pres′ō-rĕ-sep′tiv) Capable of receiving as stimuli changes in pressure, especially changes of blood pressure.

**pres·so·re·cep·tor** (pres′ō-rĕ-sep′tŏr) SYN baroreceptor.

**pres·so·re·cep·tor sys·tem** (pres′ō-rĕ-sep′tŏr sis′tĕm) Pressoreceptive areas that, with their afferent fibers and connections with autonomic nervous system, react to a rise in arterial blood pressure and serve to buffer it by inhibiting heart rate and vascular tone.

**pres·sure (P)** (presh′ŭr) Stress or force acting in any direction against resistance. [L. *pressura,* fr. *premo,* pp. *pressus,* to press]

**pres·sure an·es·the·si·a** (presh′ŭr an′es-thē′zē-ă) Loss of sensation produced by pressure applied to a nerve.

**pres·sure a·re·a** (presh′ŭr ar′ē-ă) Mucosal region that is subjected to nonphysiologic pressure from a prosthesis.

**pres·sure a·tro·phy** (presh′ŭr at′rŏ-fē) Damage and wasting of hard or soft tissue resulting from excessive pressure applied to tissue by a denture base.

**pres·sure dress·ing** (presh′ŭr dres′ing) A dressing by which pressure is exerted on the covered area to prevent the collection of fluids in the underlying tissues.

**pres·sure-in·di·ca·tor paste** (presh′ŭr in′di-kā′tŏr pāst) Fixative applied to tissue side of a complete or partial denture to check for pressure spots or high spots where the prosthesis contacts tissue when seated in the oral cavity. Pressure spots indicated by smudging of the paste on the prosthesis are adjusted to relieve tissue irritation.

**pres·sure pa·ral·y·sis** (presh′ŭr păr-al′i-sis) Paralysis due to compression of a nerve, nerve trunk, plexus, or spinal cord.

**pres·sure point** (presh′ŭr poynt) Cutaneous locus with pressure-sensitive elements that, when compressed, yield a sensation of pressure.

**pres·sure sense** (presh′ŭr sens) Faculty of discriminating various degrees of pressure on the surface.

**pres·sure sore** (presh′ŭr sōr) SYN decubitus ulcer.

**pres·sure ul·cer** (presh′ŭr ŭl′sĕr) SYN decubitus ulcer.

**prev·a·lence** (prev′ă-lĕns) Number of cases of a disease existing in a given population at a specific period of time or at a particular moment in time.

**pre·ven·tive** (prĕ-ven′tiv) SYN prophylactic (1). [L. *prae-venio,* pp. *-ventus,* to come before, prevent]

**pre·ven·tive den·tal hy·giene** (prĕ-ven′tiv den′tăl hī′jēn) Aggregate efforts to promote, restore, and maintain oral health.

**pre·ven·tive den·tis·try** (prĕ-ven′tiv den′tis-trē) Philosophy and method of dental practice that seek to prevent initiation, progression, and recurrence of dental disease.

**pre·ven·tive dose** (prĕ-ven′tiv dōs) Smallest amount of any substance that prevents occurrence of symptoms of a disease or consequences of lack of a particular dietary factor.

**pre·ven·tive main·te·nance** (prĕ-ven′tiv mān′tĕn-ăns) SYN supportive periodontal treatment.

**pre·ven·tive med·i·cine** (prĕ-ven′tiv med′i-sin) The branch of medical science concerned with the prevention of disease and with promotion of physical and mental health, through study of the etiology and epidemiology of disease processes.

**Pre·vo·tel·la** (prev′ō-tel′ă) Bacterial genus of gram-negative, nonmotile, non-spore-forming, obligately anaerobic, chemoorganotrophic, and pleomorphic rods; includes many species previously classified in the genus *Bacteroides.*

**Pre·vo·tel·la den·ti·co·la** (prev′ō-tel′ă den-tik′ō-lă) Bacterial species found in the human mouth; cause of infections of oral cavity and adjacent structures.

**Pre·vo·tel·la hep·a·ri·no·lyt·ic·a** (prev′ō-tel′ă hep′ă-rin′ō-lit′i-kă) Bacterial species associated with human periodontal disease.

**Pre·vo·tel·la in·ter·me·di·a** (prev′ō-tel′ă in-tĕr-mē′dē-ă) Bacterial species found in gingival crevices, especially associated with gingivitis and other oral infections.

**Prev·o·tel·la mel·a·nin·o·gen·ic·a** (prev′ō-tel′ă mel′ă-nin-ō-jen′i-kă) Bacterial species found in the mouth, feces, soft tissue, and the respiratory, urogenital, and intestinal tracts; implicated in periodontal disease. Type species of *Pretovella.*

**Prev·o·tel·la o·ra·lis** (prev′ō-tel′ă ō-rā′lis) Bacterial species found in gingival crevice of humans and in infections of oral cavity and upper respiratory and genital tracts.

**pri·mar·y** (prī′mar-ē) The first or foremost, as in a disease or symptoms to which others may be secondary or occur as complications. [L. *primarius,* fr. *primus,* first]

**pri·mar·y ae·ro·don·tal·gi·a** (prī′mar-ē ar′ō-don-tal′jē-ă) Dental pain associated with expansion of trapped gases within a tooth, as under a filling or in an infected pulp.

**pri·mar·y al·dos·te·ron·ism** (prī′mar-ē al-dos′tĕr-ōn-izm) An adrenocortical disorder caused by excessive secretion of aldosterone. SYN Conn syndrome, idiopathic aldosteronism.

**pri·mar·y a·my·loid·o·sis** (prī′mar-ē am′i-loy-dō′sis) Form of the disorder not associated with other recognized disease; tends to involve arterial walls and mesenchymal tissues in the tongue, lungs, intestinal tract, skin, skeletal muscle, and myocardium.

**pri·mar·y an·es·thet·ic** (prī′mar-ē an′es-thet′ik) Compound that contributes most to loss of sensation when a mixture is administered.

**pri·mar·y care** (prī′mar-ē kār) Continuing, comprehensive, and preventive health care services that are the first point of health care for a patient in an ambulatory setting.

**pri·mar·y ca·ries** (prī′mar-ē kar′ēz) Initial lesions produced by direct extension from an external surface.

**pri·mar·y ce·ment** (prī′mar-ē sĕ-ment′) Cementum that has no cementocytes; may cover entire tooth root but is often missing on apical third of the root.

**pri·ma·ry cil·i·ar·y dys·ki·ne·si·a** (prī′mar-ē sil′ē-ar-ē dis′ki-nē′zē-ă) Disorder in which mucus clearance is sluggish and bronchiectasis is prevalent and intractable.

**pri·mar·y cu·ti·cle** (prī′mar-ē kyū′ti-kĕl) SYN enamel cuticle.

**pri·mar·y den·tal lam·i·na** (prī′mar-ē den′tăl lam′i-nă) SYN dental ledge.

**pri·mar·y den·tin** (prī′mar-ē den′tin) Dentin formed during normal tooth development until root is completed.

🔲**pri·mar·y den·ti·tion** (prī′mar-ē den-tish′ŭn) See this page. SYN deciduous tooth.

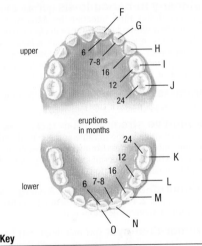

Key

central incisor F, O     lateral incisor G, N
canine H, M     second molar I, L     first molar J, K

**primary teeth with approximate age of eruption**

**pri·mar·y dis·ease** (prī′mar-ē di-zēz′) Disorder that arises spontaneously and is not associated with or caused by a previous disease, but may lead to a secondary disease.

🔲**pri·ma·ry her·pet·ic gin·gi·vo·sto·ma·ti·tis** (prī′mar-ē hĕr-pet′ik jin′ji-vō-stō′mă-tī′tis) See page A12. SYN acute primary herpetic gingivostomatitis.

**pri·mar·y her·pet·ic sto·ma·ti·tis** (prī′mar-ē hĕr-pet′ik stō′mă-tī′tis) Initial infection of oral tissues with herpes simplex virus; characterized by gingival inflammation, vesicles, and ulcers.

**pri·mar·y hy·per·ten·sion** (prī′mar-ē hī′pĕr-ten′shŭn) SYN essential hypertension.

**pri·mar·y im·pres·sion** (prī′mar-ē im-presh′ŭn) SYN preliminary impression.

**pri·mar·y med·i·cal care** (prī′mar-ē med′i-kăl kār) Patient care by member of health care system who has initial contact with patient.

**pri·mar·y pal·ate** (prī′măr-ē pal′ăt) In the early embryo, the shelf, formed from median palatine processes, which anteriorly separates oral cavity below from primordial nasal cavities above.

**pri·mar·y pre·ven·tive nurs·ing** (prī′mar-ē prē-ven′tiv nŭrs′ing) Nursing interventions and care directed at health promotion. The focus of primary preventive care includes promotion of a healthy lifestyle and reduction of major risk factors of health.

**pri·mar·y syph·i·lis** (prī′mar-ē sif′i-lis) The first stage of syphilis.

**pri·mar·y tu·ber·cu·lo·sis** (prī′mar-ē tū-bĕr′kyū-lō′sis) First infection by *Mycobacterium tuberculosis*, typically seen in children but also occurs in adults, characterized in lungs by formation of a primary complex consisting of small peripheral pulmonary focus with spread to hilar or paratracheal lymph nodes.

**pri·mate** (prī′māt) An individual of the order Primates. [L. *primus*, first]

**prim·i·tive streak** (prim′i-tiv strēk) An ectodermal ridge in the midline at the caudal end of the embryonic disc from which arises the intraembryonic mesoderm; achieved by inward and then lateral migration of cells.

**pri·mor·di·al** (prī-mōr′dē-ăl) 1. Relating to a primordium. 2. Relating to a structure in its first or earliest stage of development.

**pri·mor·di·al cyst** (prī-mōr′dē-ăl sist) Lesion that develops in place of a tooth through cystic degeneration of enamel organ before formation of calcified odontogenic tissue.

**pri·mor·di·um**, pl. **pri·mor·di·a** (prī-mōr′dē-ŭm, -ă) An aggregation of cells in the embryo indicating the first trace of an organ or structure. SYN anlage. [L. origin, fr. *primus*, first, + *ordior*, to begin]

**prin·ci·ple** (prin′si-pĕl) 1. A general or fundamental doctrine or tenet. 2. Essential ingredient in a substance. [L. *principium*, a beginning, fr. *princeps*, chief]

**pris·ma·ta ad·a·man·ti·na** (priz′mă-tă ad′ă-man-tī′nă) Calcified, microscopic, keyhole-shaped rods radiating from the dentinoenamel junction, forming the substance of tooth enamel. SYN enamel fibers, enamel prisms, enamel rods.

**pris·on fe·ver ty·phus** (priz′ŏn fē′vĕr tī′fŭs) SYN epidemic typhus.

**pri·va·cy** (prī′vă-sē) 1. Being apart from oth-

ers; seclusion; secrecy. 2. Especially in psychiatry and clinical psychology, but also in all fields of dentistry and health care, respect for confidential nature of the clinician-patient relationship.

**PRN** Abbreviation for *pro re nata* (L. as needed).

**Pro** Abbreviation for proline.

**pro-** 1. Prefix denoting before, forward. 2. In chemistry, prefix indicating precursor of. [L. and G. *pro*]

**pro·ac·cel·er·in** (prō′ak-sel′ĕr-in) SYN factor V.

**pro·ac·tive in·hib·i·tion** (prō-ak′tiv in′hi-bish′ŭn) Type of interference or negative transfer, observed in memory experiments and other learning situations, when something learned previously impedes present learning or recall.

**prob·a·bil·i·ty** (prob′ă-bil′i-tē) A measure, ranging from 0–1, of the degree of belief in a hypothesis or statement.

**prob·a·bil·i·ty curve** (prob′ă-bil′i-tē kŭrv) Graph of the gaussian (normal) distribution representing relative probabilities.

**probe** (prōb) A slender rod of rigid or flexible material, with a blunt bulbous tip, used for exploring sinuses, fistulae, or wounds. [L. *probo*, to test]

**pro·ben·e·cid** (prō-ben′ĕ-sid) A uricosuric agent.

**prob·ing** (prōb′ing) Act of "walking" the tip of a probe along the junctional epithelium within a sulcus to assess the condition of the periodontal tissues.

**prob·ing depth** (prōb′ing depth) Measurement of the depth of a sulcus or periodontal pocket determined by measuring distance from a gingival margin to the base of the sulcus or pocket with a calibrated periodontal probe. See this page.

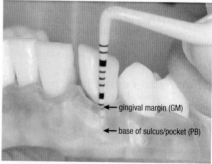

gingival margin (GM)

base of sulcus/pocket (PB)

**probing depth:** distance in millimeters from gingival margin (GM) to base of sulcus or periodontal pocket (PB) as measured with a calibrated probe

**prob·lem-o·ri·ent·ed re·cord (POR)** (prob'lĕm-ōr'ē-ĕn-tĕd rek'ŏrd) System of record keeping in which a list of patient's problems is made and all history, physical findings, and laboratory data, and other factors pertinent to each problem are placed under that heading.

**pro·cain·a·mide hy·dro·chlor·ide** (pro-kān'ă-mīd hī'drŏ-klōr'īd) Potent antiarrhythmic agent used to treat atrial fibrillation and other cardiac disorders.

**pro·caine hy·dro·chlor·ide** (prō'kān hī'drŏ-klōr'īd) Local anesthetic for infiltration and spinal use, although it lacks activity when used topically.

**pro·car·ba·zine hy·dro·chlor·ide** (prō-kahr'bă-zēn hī'drŏ-klōr'īd) An antineoplastic agent.

**pro·ce·dure** (prŏ-sē'jŭr) Act or conduct of diagnosis, treatment, or operation.

**pro·cess** (pros'es) **1.** In dentistry, series of operations that convert a wax pattern, such as that of a denture base, into a solid denture base of another material. SEE dental curing. **2.** In anatomy, a projection or outgrowth. **3.** A pathologic condition or disease.

**pro·cess·ing** (pros'es-ing) The activity of effecting a series of changes in something so as to achieve a particular result.

**pro·chei·li·a, pro·chi·li·a** (prō-kī'lē-ă) Protruding lips. [*pro-* + G. *cheilos*, lip]

**pro·ci·den·ti·a** (pros'i-den'shē-ă) A sinking down or prolapse of any organ or part. [L. a falling forward, fr. *procido*, to fall forward]

**pro·con·ver·tin** (prō'kŏn-vĕr'tin) SYN factor VII.

**proc·ti·tis** (prok-tī'tis) Inflammation of the mucous membrane of the rectum. SYN rectitis. [*proct-* + G. *-itis*, inflammation]

**pro·dro·mal pe·ri·od** (prō-drō'măl pēr'ē-ŏd) Time during which a disease process has begun but is not yet clinically manifest.

**pro·dro·mal stage** (prō-drō'măl stāj) Early stage or symptoms of disease before characteristic symptoms appear.

**pro·drome** (prō'drōm) Early or premonitory symptom of a disease.

**pro·drug** (prō'drŭg) A class of drugs, the pharmacologic action of which results from conversion by metabolic processes within the body.

**pro·es·tro·gen** (prō-es'trŏ-jen) Substance that acts as an estrogen only after it has been metabolized in the body to an active compound.

**Pro·fes·sion·al Eth·ics Stan·dards Re·view Or·gan·i·za·tion (PSRO)** (prŏ-fesh'ŭn-ăl eth'iks stan'dārdz rĕ-vyū' ŏr'gă-nī-zā'shŭn) U.S. federal agency formed to determine the quality and appropriateness of health care services paid for, in whole or part, under the Social Security Act.

**pro·file** (prō'fīl) **1.** Outline or contour, especially one representing a side view of the human head. **2.** A summary, brief account, or record. [It. *profilo*, fr. L. *pro*, forward, + *filum*, thread, line (contour)]

**pro·fi·lom·e·ter** (prō'fi-lom'ĕ-tĕr) An instrument for measuring surface roughness (e.g., teeth).

**pro·ge·ri·a** (prō-jēr'ē-ă) A condition of precocious aging with onset at birth or early childhood. [*pro-* + G. *gēras*, old age]

**pro·ges·ta·tion·al hor·mone** (prō'jes-tā'shŭn-ăl hōr'mōn) SYN progesterone.

**pro·ges·ter·one** (prŏ-jes'tĕr-ōn) Antiestrogenic steroid, believed to be the active principle of corpus luteum, isolated from corpus luteum and placenta or synthetically prepared; used to correct abnormalities of the menstrual cycle, as a contraceptive, and to control habitual abortion. SYN progestational hormone.

**pro·ges·tin** (prō-jes'tin) **1.** Hormone of corpus luteum. **2.** Generic term for any substance, natural or synthetic, which effects some or all biologic changes produced by progesterone. [*pro-* + *gest*ation + *-in*]

**pro·ges·to·gen** (prŏ-jes'tō-jen) Any agent capable of producing biologic effects similar to those of progesterone; most are steroids, such as natural hormones. [*pro-* + *gest*ation + G. *-gen*, producing]

**prog·nath·ic** (prog-nath'ik) **1.** Having a projecting jaw. **2.** Denoting a forward projection of either or both jaws relative to craniofacial skeleton. [*pro-* + G. *gnathos*, jaw]

**prog·na·thism** (prog'nă-thizm) Condition of being prognathic; abnormal forward projection of one or both jaws beyond established normal relationship with cranial base; mandibular condyles are in their normal rest relationship to the temporomandibular joints.

**prog·no·sis** (prog-nō'sis) Forecast of probable course and/or outcome of a disease. [G. *prognōsis*, fr. *pro*, before, + *gignōskō*, to know]

**pro·gram·med cell death** (prō'gramd sel deth) SYN apoptosis.

**pro·gram·ming** (prō'gram-ing) Sequential instruction; a method of training in discrete segments.

**pro·gress** (prog'res, prŏ-gres') **1.** An advance; disease course. **2.** To advance; go forward; said of a disease, especially, when unqualified, of one taking an unfavorable course. [L. *pro-gredior*, pp. *-gressus*, to go forth, fr. *gradior*, to step, go, fr. *gradus*, a step]

op

**pro·gres·sive bul·bar pal·sy** (prŏ-gres´ iv bŭl´bahr pawl´zē) One of the subgroups of motor neuron disease. Tongue weakness and wasting are usually evident. Often fasciculation potentials are present in the tongue and facial muscles. SYN glossolabiolaryngeal paralysis, glossopharyngeolabial paralysis.

**pro·hor·mone** (pro-hōr´mōn) Intraglandular precursor of a hormone; e.g., proinsulin.

**pro·jec·tile vom·i·ting** (prŏ-jek´tĭl vom´it- ing) Oral expulsion of stomach contents with great force.

**pro·jec·tion** (prŏ-jek´shŭn) **1.** [TA] A push- ing out; an outgrowth or protuberance. **2.** The referring of a sensation to the object producing it. **3.** System or systems of nerve fibers (projec- tion fibers [TA]) by which a group of nerve cells discharges its nerve impulses (''projects'') to one or more other cell groups. **4.** In radiography, standardized views of parts of body, described by body part position or direction of the x-ray beam through body part. [L. *projectio;* fr. *pro- jicio,* pp. *-jectus,* to throw before]

**pro·la·bi·al** (pro-lā´bē-ăl) Denoting isolated central soft-tissue segment of upper lip in em- bryonic state and in an unrepaired bilateral cleft lip and palate.

**pro·la·bi·um** (pro-lā´bē-ŭm) **1.** Exposed car- mine lip margin. **2.** Isolated central soft-tissue segment of upper lip in embryonic state and in an unrepaired bilateral cleft lip and palate. [*pro- + L. labium,* lip]

**pro·lac·tin** (pro-lak´tin) Protein hormone of anterior lobe of hypophysis that stimulates se- cretion of milk and possibly, during pregnancy, breast growth. [*pro- + L. lac, lact-,* milk, *+ -in*]

**pro·lapse** (pro´laps) **1.** To sink down; said of an organ or other part. **2.** A sinking of an organ or other part, especially its appearance at a natu- ral or artificial orifice. [L. *prolapsus,* a falling]

**pro·lep·sis** (pro-lep´sis) Recurrence of pa- roxysm of a periodic disease at regularly short- ening intervals. [G. *prolēpsis,* anticipation]

**pro·lif·er·ate** (pro-lif´ĕr-āt) To grow and in- crease in number by reproduction of similar forms. [L. *proles,* offspring, *+ fero,* to bear]

**pro·lif·er·a·tion** (pro-lif´ĕr-ā´shŭn) Growth and reproduction of similar cells.

**pro·lif·er·a·tive gin·gi·vi·tis** (pro-lif´ĕr- ă-tiv jin´ji-vī´tis) Inflammatory changes in gin- giva characterized by proliferation of gingival components.

**pro·line (Pro)** (pro´lēn) An amino acid found in proteins, especially the collagens.

**pro·lo·ther·a·py** (pro´lō-thār´ă-pē) Use of inflammation-inducing injections in periarticu- lar soft tissue intended to strengthen ligaments and tendons; an unproven therapy.

**PROM** Abbreviation for premature rupture of membranes; passive range of motion.

**prom·i·nence** (prom´i-nĕns) [TA] ANATOMY tissues or parts that project beyond a surface. [L. *prominentia*]

**pro·mo·tion** (prŏ-mō´shŭn) Stimulation of tumor induction, following initiation, by a pro- moting agent which may be noncarcinogenic.

**pro·na·si·on** (pro-nā´zē-on) Point of angle between nasal septum and surface of upper lip, found at point where a tangent applied to nasal septum meets upper lip. [pro- + L. *nasus,* nose]

**prone** (prōn) **1.** The body when lying face downward. **2.** Pronation of forearm or foot. [L. *pronus,* bending down or forward]

**pro·ot·ic** (pro-ō´tik) In front of the ear. [*pro- + G. ous,* ear]

**prop·a·gate** (prop´ă-gāt) **1.** To reproduce; to generate. **2.** To move along a fiber, e.g., propa- gation of the nerve impulse. [L. *propago,* pp. *-atus,* to generate, reproduce]

**prop·a·ga·tion** (prop´ă-gā´shŭn) The act of propagating.

**pro·phy** (pro´fē) Colloq. jargon for prophy- laxis.

**pro·phy·lac·tic** (pro´fi-lak´tik) **1.** Preventing disease; relating to prophylaxis. SYN preventive. **2.** Agent that acts to prevent disease. e.g., a con- dom [G. *prophylaktikos;* see etymology of pro- phylaxis]

**pro·phy·lac·tic an·ti·bi·ot·ic** (pro´fi- lak´tik an´tē-bī-ot´ik) Medication given to pre- vent an infection; may be administered before dental procedures to patients with cardiac valvu- lar disease or implanted prostheses. SYN antibi- otic prophylaxis.

**pro·phy·lac·tic o·don·tot·o·my** (pro´fi- lak´tik ō´don-tot´ŏ-mē) Preventive dental opera- tion in which imperfectly formed developmental grooves, pits, and fissures are opened up with a bur and filled to obviate future decay.

**pro·phy·lax·is,** pl. **pro·phy·lax·es** (pro´ fi-lak´sis, -sēz) Removal of dental plaque, ex- trinsic stains, and coronal polish. [Mod. L. fr. G. *pro-phylassō,* to guard before, take precaution]

**pro·phy·lax·is an·gle** (pro´fi-lak´sis ang´ gĕl) A dental instrument, available in disposable and reusable (i.e., sterilizable) form, which is usually attached to a dental handpiece, into which are fitted various devices intended for specific cleaning and scaling of teeth. See page 471.

**pro·phy·lax·is paste** (pro-fi-lak´sis pāst) Compound containing a mild abrasive (and sometimes fluoride), used professionally to re- move dental plaque and extrinsic stains, polish teeth, and to minimize plaque accumulation and retention.

**pro·po·fol** (pro´pō-fōl) A hypnotic with rapid

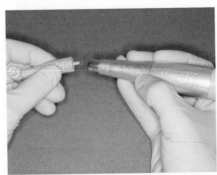

**dental handpiece with disposable prophylaxis angle**

onset and short duration of action; used intravenously for induction and maintenance of general anesthesia. SYN 2, 6-diisopropyl phenol.

**pro·pos·i·tus,** pl. **pro·po·si·ti** (prō-poz′i-tŭs, -tī) **1.** Proband, usually referring to the first index case to be ascertained. **2.** A premise; an argument. [L. fr. *propono,* pp. *-positus,* to lay out, propound]

**pro·pox·y·phene hy·dro·chlo·ride** (prō-pok′si-fēn hī′drŏ-klōr′īd) A nonantipyretic, orally effective weak narcotic analgesic used to relieve mild to moderate pain; less effective than codeine.

**pro·pri·e·tar·y med·i·cine** (prŏ-prī′ĕ-tar-ē med′i-sin) Medicinal compound, the formula and mode of manufacture of which are the property of the maker.

**pro·pri·e·tar·y name** (prŏ-prī′ĕ-tar-ē nām) Protected brand name or trademark, registered with the U.S. Patent Office (or other governmental authority), under which a manufacturer markets its product. It is written with a capital initial letter and is often further distinguished by a superscript R in a circle (®). [L. *proprietas,* ownership]

**pro·pri·o·cep·tive** (prō′prē-ō-sep′tiv) Capable of receiving stimuli originating in muscles, tendons, and other internal tissues. [L. *proprius,* one's own, + *capio,* to take]

**prop·to·sis** (prop-tō′sis) SYN exophthalmos. [G. *proptōsis,* a falling forward]

**pro·pul·sion** (prŏ-pŭl′shŭn) Tendency to fall forward. [G. *pro-pello,* pp. *-pulsus,* to drive forth]

**pro·pyl·thi·o·u·ra·cil** (prō′pil-thī′ō-yūr′ă-sil) An agent used to treat hyperthyroidism; a goitrogen.

**pro rat. aet.** Abbreviation for L. *pro ratione aetatis,* according to (patient's) age.

**pro re na·ta (PRN)** (prō rā nā′tă) As the occasion arises; as necessary. [L.]

**pros·ta·cy·clin** (pros′tă-sī′klin) A potent natural inhibitor of platelet aggregation and a powerful vasodilator.

**pros·ta·glan·din** (pros′tă-glan′din) Any of a class of physiologically active substances present in many tissues, with effects such as vasodilation, vasoconstriction, stimulation of intestinal or bronchial smooth muscle, uterine stimulation, and antagonism to hormones influencing lipid metabolism.

**pros·ta·glan·din E₁** (pros′tă-glan′din) SYN alprostadil.

**pros·ta·ta** (pros′tă-tă) SYN prostate.

**pros·tate** (pros′tāt) [TA] A chestnut-shaped body, surrounding the beginning of the urethra in the male. The secretion of the glands is a milky fluid that is discharged by excretory ducts into the prostatic urethra at the time of the emission of semen. USAGE NOTE Often mispronounced as *prostrate,* and so misspelled.

**pros·tate gland** (pros′tāt gland) SYN prostate.

**pros·ta·ti·tis** (pros′tă-tī′tis) Inflammation of the prostate. [*prostat-* + G. *-itis,* inflammation]

**pros·the·sis,** pl. **pros·the·ses** (pros-thē′sis, -sēz) Fabricated substitute used to assist a damaged or replace a missing body part. [G. an addition]

**pros·the·sis-in·duced fi·brous hy·per·pla·si·a** (pros-thē′sis in-dūst′ fī′brŭs hī′pĕr-plā′zē-ă) Fibrous tissue proliferation associated with poorly fitted denture resulting from alveolar bone resorption.

**pros·thet·ics** (pros-thet′iks) The art and science of making and adjusting artificial parts of the human body.

**pros·the·tist** (pros′thĕ-tist) One skilled in constructing and fitting prostheses.

**pros·thi·on** (pros′thē-on) The most anterior point on the maxillary alveolar process in the midline. SYN alveolar point. [G. ntr. of *prosthios,* foremost]

**pros·tho·don·ti·a** (pros′thŏ-don′shē-ă) SYN prosthodontics. [L.]

**pros·tho·don·tics** (pros′thŏ-don′tiks) Science of providing suitable substitutes for coronal portions of teeth, or for one or more lost or missing teeth and their associated parts, so that impaired function, appearance, and comfort, may be restored. SYN dental prosthetics, prosthodontia. [L. *prosthodontia,* fr. G. *prosthesis* + *odous* (*odont-*), tooth]

**pros·tho·don·tic ther·a·py** (pros′thŏ-don′tik thār′ă-pē) Treatment that uses dental prostheses to restore the form and function of missing teeth.

op

**pros·tho·don·tist** (pros´thŏ-don´tist) A dentist engaged in the practice of prosthodontics.

**pro·ta·no·pi·a, pro·ta·nop·si·a** (prō´tă-nō´pē-ă, -nop´sē-ă) Ocular disorder that is form of dichromatism. [G. *prōtos,* first, + *a-* priv. + *ōps* (*ōp-*) eye]

**pro·te·ase in·hib·i·tor** (prō´tē-ās in-hib´i-tŏr) Class of synthetic drug used to treat human immunodeficiency virus (HIV-1) infection.

**pro·tec·ted health in·for·ma·tion** (prŏ-tek´tĕd helth in´fŏr-mā´shŭn) An umbrella term embracing all data collected and stored in any medium relating to the health of the individual patient. Legal construct forbids passing along such information to a third party without the express permission of the patient or the patient's deputy.

**pro·tec·tive bar·ri·er tech·ni·ques** (prŏ-tek´tiv bar´ē-ĕr tek-nēks´) Use of disposable barrier covers on dental operatory surfaces to protect surfaces from contamination; such barriers are discarded and replaced between patients.

**pro·tec·tive base** (prŏ-tek´tiv bās) SYN liner.

**pro·tec·tive dress·ing** (prŏ-tek´tiv dres´ing) A covering to shield an area from injury or trauma.

**⬛pro·tec·tive eye·wear** (prŏ-tek´tiv ī´wār) Safety-type spectacles with side shields necessary for the dental team and patients to prevent ocular injuries and infections during dental procedures. See this page.

**pro·tec·tive la·ryn·ge·al re·flex** (prŏ-tek´tiv lă-rin´jē-ăl rē´fleks) Glottal closure to prevent entry of foreign substances into respiratory tract.

**pro·tein** (prō´tēn) Macromolecules consisting of long sequences of α-amino acids; represents three fourths of dry weight of most cell matter; involved in structures, hormones, enzymes, muscle contraction, immunologic response, and essential life functions. [G. *prōtos,* first, + *-in*]

**pro·tein ef·fi·cien·cy ra·ti·o (PER)** (prō´tēn ĕ-fish´ĕn-sē rā´shē-ō) Weight gain in grams divided by protein intake in grams.

**pro·tein mal·nu·tri·tion** (prō´tēn mal´nū-trish´ŭn) Undernutrition resulting from inadequate intake of protein; characteristic manifestations include nutritional edema.

**pro·tein me·ta·bo·lism** (prō´tēn mĕ-tab´ŏ-lizm) Decomposition and synthesis of protein in tissues.

**pro·tein·o·sis** (prō´tē-nō´sis) A state characterized by disordered protein formation and distribution, particularly as manifested by deposition of abnormal proteins in tissues. [*protein* + G. *-osis,* condition]

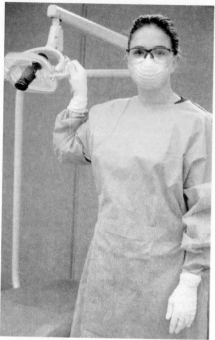

**protective eyewear:** personal protective equipment (PPE) includes eyeware, gloves, mask and gown

**pro·tei·nu·ri·a** (prō´tē-nyūr´ē-ă) Presence of urinary protein in amounts exceeding 0.3 g in a 24-hour urine collection or in concentrations more than 1 g per liter (1+ to 2+ by standard turbidometric methods) in a random urine collection on two or more occasions at least 6 hours apart; specimens must be clean, voided midstream, or obtained by catheterization. [*protein* + G. *ouron,* urine]

**pro·te·o·lyt·ic** (prō´tē-ō-lit´ik) Relating to or effecting proteolysis.

***Pro·te·us*** (prō´tē-ŭs) A genus of motile, peritrichous, non-spore-forming, aerobic to facultatively anaerobic bacteria found primarily in fecal matter and in putrefying materials. [G. *Proteus,* a sea god, who had the power to change his form]

**pro·throm·bin** (prō-throm´bin) A glycoprotein, formed and stored in the parenchymal cells of the liver and present in blood in a concentration of approximately 20 mg/100 mL; deficiency leads to impaired blood coagulation.

**pro·throm·bi·nase** (prō-throm´bi-nās) SYN factor X.

**pro·throm·bi·no·gen** (prō-throm´bi-nō-jen) SYN factor VII.

**pro·throm·bin time (PT)** (prō-throm´bin tīm) Time required for clotting after thromboplastin and calcium are added in optimal amounts to blood of normal fibrinogen content; if prothrombin is diminished, clotting time increases.

**pro·throm·bo·ki·nase** (prō'throm-bō-kī'nās) SYN factor V, factor VIII.

**pro·to·cone** (prō'tō-kōn) Mesiolingual cusp of mammalian upper molar tooth. [*proto-* + G. *kōnos,* cone]

**pro·to·co·nid** (prō'tō-kon'id) Mesiolingual cusp of mammalian lower molar tooth. [*proto-cone* + *-id*]

**pro·ton** (prō'ton) The positively charged unit of the nuclear mass; protons form part (or in hydrogen 1, the whole) of the nucleus of the atom around which the negative electrons revolve. [G. ntr. of *prōtos,* first]

**pro·ton pump in·hib·i·tor** (prō'ton pŭmp in-hib'i-tŏr) Agent that blocks transport of hydrogen ions into stomach and hence are useful in treatment of gastric hyperacidity.

**pro·to·plasm** (prō'tō-plazm) **1.** Living matter, the substance of which animal and vegetable cells are formed. **2.** Total cell material, including cell organelles. [*proto-* + G. *plasma,* thing formed]

**pro·to·sty·lid** (prō'tō-stī'lid) Accessory cusp found on buccal surface of mesiobuccal cusp of lower molars, ranging from a small groove to a cusp rivaling the mesiobuccal cusp in size. [*proto-* + G. *stylis, -idos,* mast, spar]

**pro·trac·tion** (prō-trak'shŭn) In dentistry, extension of teeth or other maxillary or mandibular structures into a position anterior to normal.

**pro·trud·ing teeth** (prō-trŭd'ing tēth) Teeth extending beyond normal contour of dental arches; usually in an anterior direction.

**pro·tru·sion** (prō-trū'zhŭn) **1.** In dentistry, position of mandible forward from centric relation. **2.** The state of being thrust forward or projected. [L. *protrusio*]

**pro·tru·sive ex·cur·sion** (prō-trū'siv eks-kŭr'zhŭn) Movement of mandible to a position forward of centric position.

**pro·tru·sive in·ter·oc·clu·sal rec·ord** (prō-trū'siv in-tĕr-ok-klū'zăl rek'ŏrd) SYN protrusive checkbite.

**pro·tru·sive jaw re·la·tion** (prō-trū'siv jaw rĕ-lā'shŭn) One resulting from protrusion of mandible.

**pro·tru·sive oc·clu·sion** (prō-trū'siv ŏ-klū'zhŭn) Occlusion that results when mandible is protruded forward from centric position.

**pro·tru·sive po·si·tion** (prō-trū'siv pŏ-zish'ŭn) Forward position of mandible produced by muscular effort.

**pro·tru·sive rec·ord** (prō-trū'siv rek'ŏrd) Registration of a forward position of mandible with reference to maxillae.

**pro·tru·sive re·la·tion** (prō-trū'siv rĕ-lā'shŭn) Relation of mandible to maxillae when lower jaw is thrust forward.

**pro·tu·ber·ance** (prō-tū'bĕr-ăns) [TA] A swelling, protruding, or knoblike outgrowth. [Mod. L. *protuberantia*]

***Prov·i·den·ci·a*** (prov-i-den'sē-ă) A genus of motile, peritrichous, non-spore-forming bacteria that occur in urinary tract infections.

**pro·vid·er** (prō-vī'dĕr) A person or agency that supplies goods or services, particularly medical or paramedical services. [L. *pro-videre*]

**pro·vi·rus** (prō-vī'rŭs) The precursor of an animal virus; theoretically analogous to the prophage in bacteria, the provirus being integrated into the nucleus of infected cells.

**pro·vi·sion·al pros·the·sis** (prō-vizh'ŭn-ăl pros-thē'sis) Interim dental prosthesis worn for varying periods of time. SYN interim prosthesis.

**pro·vi·sion·al res·tor·a·tion** (prō-vizh'ŏn-ăl res'tŏr-ā'shŭn) SYN temporary restoration.

**pro·vi·sion·al treat·ment plan** (prō-vizh'ŭn-ăl trēt'mĕnt plan) Program of treatment that may be modified depending on the outcome of initial stages of therapy.

**pro·vi·ta·min** (prō'vī'tă-min) An inactive form of a vitamin that needs activation before it can be used by the body.

**pro·voc·a·tive test** (prŏ-vok'ă-tiv test) Any procedure in which a suspected pathophysiologic abnormality is deliberately induced by manipulating conditions known to provoke that abnormality.

**prox·i·mad** (prok'si-mad) In a direction toward a proximal part, or toward the center; not distad. [L. *proximus,* nearest, next, + *ad,* to]

**prox·i·mal** (prok'si-măl) DENTAL ANATOMY denoting tooth surface in relation to its neighbor, whether mesial or distal, i.e., nearer to or farther from anteroposterior median plane. [Mod. L. *proximalis,* fr. L. *proximus,* nearest, next]

**prox·i·mal ca·ries** (prok'si-măl kar'ēz) Caries occurring in proximal surface, either distal or mesial, of a tooth.

**prox·i·mo·buc·cal** (prok'si-mō-bŭk'ăl) Relating to proximal and buccal tooth surfaces; denoting angle formed by their junction.

**prox·i·mo·la·bi·al** (prok'si-mō-lā'bē-ăl) Relating to proximal and labial tooth surfacesl denoting angle formed by their junction.

**prox·i·mo·lin·gual** (prok'si-mō-ling'gwăl)

op

Relating to proximal and lingual tooth surfaces; denoting angle formed by their junction.

**prune-juice spu·tum** (prūn'jūs spyū'tŭm) Thin reddish expectoration, characteristic of necrosis of lung tissue, usually by infection; sometimes seen with lung tumors.

**pru·ri·tus** (prū-rī'tŭs) SYN itch (1). [L. an itching, fr. *prurio,* to itch]

**Prus·sian blue** (prŭsh'ăn blū) [CI 77510] SYN Berlin blue.

**pseu·dan·ky·lo·sis** (sūd'ang-ki-lō'sis) SYN fibrous ankylosis.

**pseu·dar·thro·sis** (sūd'ahr-thrō'sis) A false joint arising at the site of an ununited fracture. SYN false joint. [*pseud-* + G. *arthrōsis,* a joint]

⚙ **pseudo-** *Do not confuse this prefix with the combining form sudor-. False (often used about a deceptive resemblance).* [G. *pseudēs*]

**pseu·do·an·o·don·ti·a** (sū'dō-an'ō-don'shē-ă) Clinical absence of teeth due to a failure in eruption. [*pseudo-* + G. *an-* priv. + *odous,* tooth]

**pseu·do·ar·thro·sis** (sū'dō-ahr-thrō'sis) SYN pseudarthrosis.

**pseu·do·cho·lin·es·ter·ase de·fi·cien·cy** (sū'dō-kō'lin-es'tĕr-ās dĕ-fish'ĕn-sē) Disorder with exaggerated responses to drugs ordinarily hydrolyzed by serum pseudocholinesterase.

**pseu·do·geu·si·a** (sū'dō-gū'sē-ă) Subjective taste sensation not produced by an external stimulus. [*pseudo-* + G. *geusis,* taste]

**pseu·do-Grae·fe sign** (sū'dō grā'fĕ sīn) Lid retraction phenomenon similar to Graefe sign, but due to aberrant regeneration of fibers of the oculomotor nerve.

**pseu·do·mem·brane** (sū'dō-mem'brān) SYN false membrane.

*Pseu·do·mo·nas* (sū'dō-mō'năs) A genus of motile, polar-flagellate, non-spore-forming bacteria that occur commonly in soil and in fresh-water and marine environments. Some species that are involved in human infections. The type species is *P. aeruginosa.* [*pseudo-* + G. *monas,* unit, monad]

**pseu·do·pa·re·sis** (sū'dō-păr-ē'sis) Condition marked by pupillary changes, tremors, and speech disturbances suggestive of early paretic neurosyphilis.

**pseu·do·pock·et** (sū'dō-pok'ĕt) A pocket, adjacent to a tooth, resulting from gingival hyperplasia and edema but without apical migration of the epithelial attachment.

**pseu·do·prog·na·thism** (sū'dō-prog'năthizm) Acquired projection of mandible due to occlusal disharmonies that force it forward;

mandibular condyles are forward of their expected functional position.

**pseu·do·rick·ets** (sū'dō-rik'ĕts) SYN renal rickets.

**pseu·do·strat·i·fied ep·i·the·li·um** (sū'dō-strat'i-fīd ep'i-thē'lē-ŭm) An epithelium that gives a superficial appearance of being stratified because the cell nuclei are at different levels, but in which all cells reach the basement membrane.

**pseu·do·vom·i·ting** (sū'dō-vom'it-ing) Regurgitation of matter from esophagus or stomach without expulsive effort.

**psi·lo·sis** (sī-lō'sis) Losing one's hair. [G. *psilōsis,* a stripping, fr. *psilos,* bare]

**pso·ri·a·sis** (sōr-ī'ă-sis) A common inherited condition characterized by the eruption of reddish, silvery-scaled maculopapules, predominantly on the elbows, knees, scalp, and trunk. [G. *psōriasis,* fr. *psōra,* an itch]

**PSR** Abbreviation for Periodontal Screening and Recording; Periodontal Screening Record.

**PSRO** Abbreviation for Professional Ethics Standards Review Organization.

**psy·chal·gi·a, psy·chal·ga·li·a** (sī-kal'jē-ă sī'kal-gā'lē-ă) **1.** Distress attending a mental effort. **2.** SYN psychogenic pain. [*psych-* + G. *algos,* pain]

**psy·chi·a·try, psy·chi·at·rics** (sī-kī'ă-trē, sī'kē-at'riks) Medical specialty concerned with diagnosis and treatment of mental disorders. [*psych-* + G. *iatreia,* medical treatment]

**psy·chic** (sī'kik) Relating to the phenomena of consciousness, mind, or soul. [G. *psychikos*]

⚙ **psycho-** *Do not confuse this combining form with psychro-. Although p in the diphthong ps is normally silent only at the beginning of a word, by long tradition the p usually remains silent even within a word when it occurs in the combining form psych-, as in antipsychotic and neuropsychiatric.* The mind; mental; psychological. [G. *psychē,* soul, mind]

**psy·cho·ac·tive** (sī'kō-ak'tiv) Possessing ability to alter mood, anxiety, behavior, cognitive processes, or mental tension.

**psy·cho·ac·tive drug** (sī'kō-ak'tiv drŭg) Pharmacotherapeutic agent that possesses action to alter mood, behavior, cognitive processes, or mental stress.

**psy·cho·dy·nam·ics** (sī'kō-dī-nam'iks) Systematized study and theory of psychological forces that underlie human behavior, emphasizing interplay between unconscious and conscious motivation. [*psycho-* + G. *dynamis,* force]

**psy·cho·gen·e·tic** (sī-kō-gĕ-net'ik) Refers

to the interplay between genetic variability and psychological and psychiatric phenomena.

**psy·cho·gen·ic** (sī′kō-jen′ik) **1.** Of mental origin or causation. **2.** Relating to emotional and related psychological development or to psychogenesis.

**psy·cho·gen·ic pain** (sī′kō-jen′ik pān) Somatoform pain that associated or correlated with a psychological, emotional, or behavioral stimulus. SYN psychalgia (2), somatoform pain.

**psy·cho·gen·ic pain dis·or·der** (sī′kō-jen′ik pān dis-ōr′děr) Condition in which principal complaint is pain that is out of proportion to objective findings and is related to psychological factors.

**psy·cho·gen·ic tor·ti·col·lis** (sī′kō-jen′ik tōr′ti-kol′is) Spasmodic contractions of neck muscles.

**psy·cho·gen·ic vom·it·ing** (sī′kō-jen′ik vom′it-ing) Regurgitation associated with emotional distress and anxiety.

**psy·cho·geu·sic** (sī′kō-gyū′sik) Pertaining to mental perception and interpretation of taste. [*psycho-* + G. *geusis*, taste]

**psy·cho·lin·guis·tics** (sī′kō-ling-gwis′tiks) Study of psychological factors associated with speech, including voice, attitudes, emotions, and grammatical rules. [*psycho-* + L. *lingua*, tongue]

**psy·cho·log·i·cal tests** (sī′kŏ-loj′i-kăl tests) Measures designed to assess a person's achievements, intelligence, neuropsychological functions, skills, personality, or individual and occupational characteristics or potentialities.

**psy·chol·o·gist** (sī-kol′ŏ-jist) A specialist in psychology licensed to practice.

**psy·chol·o·gy** (sī-kol′ŏ-jē) The profession (e.g., clinical psychology), scholarly discipline (academic psychology), and science (research psychology) concerned with the behavior of humans and animals, and related mental and physiologic processes. [*psycho-* + G. *logos*, study]

**psy·cho·mo·tor** (sī′kō-mō′tŏr) Relating to psychological processes associated with muscular movement and to production of voluntary movements. [*psycho-* + L. *motor*, mover]

**psy·cho·mo·tor goals** (sī′kō-mō′tŏr gōlz) Goals that reflect a patient's skill development.

**psy·cho·neu·ro·im·mu·nol·o·gy** (sī′kō-nū′rō-im′yū-nol′ŏ-jē) Area of study that focuses on emotional and other psychological states that affect the immune system, rendering the patient less or more susceptible to disease.

**psy·cho·neu·ro·sis** (sī′kō-nūr-ō′sis) Mental or behavioral disorder of mild or moderate severity. [*psycho-* + G. *neuron*, nerve, + -*osis*, condition]

**psy·cho·pa·thol·o·gy** (sī′kō-pă-thol′ŏ-jē) **1.** Science concerned with pathology of mind and behavior. **2.** Science of mental and behavioral disorders. [*psycho-* + G. *pathos*, disease, + *logos*, study]

**psy·cho·phar·ma·ceu·tics** (sī′kō-fahr′mă-sū′tiks) Drugs used to treat emotional disorders.

**psy·cho·phar·ma·col·o·gy** (sī′kō-fahr′mă-kol′ŏ-jē) **1.** Use of drugs to treat mental and psychological disorders. **2.** Science of drug-behavior relationships. [*psycho-* + G. *pharmakon*, drug, + *logos*, study]

**psy·cho·phys·i·cal** (sī′kō-fiz′i-kăl) Relating to mental perception of physical stimuli.

**psy·cho·phys·ics** (sī′kō-fiz′iks) Science of relation between physical attributes of a stimulus and measured quantitative attributes of mental perception of that stimulus.

**psy·cho·phys·i·o·log·ic man·i·fes·ta·tion** (sī′kō-fiz′ē-ŏ-loj′ik man′i-fes-tā′shŭn) Sign characterized by visceral expression of affect, symptoms due to a chronic and exaggerated state of physiologic expression of emotion with feeling repressed; characteristic of psychosomatic disorders.

**psy·cho·sis,** pl. **psy·cho·ses** (sī-kō′sis, -sēz) A mental and behavioral disorder causing gross distortion or disorganization of a person's mental capacity, affective response, and capacity to recognize reality, communicate, and relate to others to degree of interfering with that person's capacity to cope with the ordinary demands of everyday life. [G. an animating]

**psy·cho·so·mat·ic** (sī′kō-sŏ-mat′ik) Refers to influence of mind or psychological functioning of brain on physiologic functions of body relative to bodily disorders or disease and reciprocal impact of disease on psychological functioning. [*psycho-* + G. *sōma*, body]

**psy·cho·so·mat·ic med·i·cine** (sī′kō-sŏ-mat′ik med′i-sin) Study and treatment of diseases, disorders, or abnormal states in which psychologic processes resulting in physiologic reactions are believed to play a prominent role.

**psy·cho·so·mat·ic meth·od** (sī′kō-sŏ-mat′ik meth′ŏd) Any nonpharmacologic technique that reduces anxiety and improves pain control.

**psy·cho·stim·u·lant** (sī′kō-stim′yū-lănt) Agent with antidepressant or mood-elevating properties.

**psy·cho·sur·ger·y** (sī′kō-sŭr′jěr-ē) Treatment of mental disorders by surgical operation on the brain, e.g., lobotomy.

**psy·cho·ther·a·pist** (sī′kō-thār′ă-pist) A person, usually a psychiatrist or clinical psychologist, professionally trained and engaged

op

in psychotherapy. Currently, also applied to social workers, nurses, and others whose state-licensed practice activities include psychotherapy.

**psy·cho·ther·a·py** (sī'kō-thār'ă-pē) Treatment of emotional, behavioral, personality, and psychiatric disorders based primarily on verbal or nonverbal communication and interventions with the patient, in contrast to treatments using chemical and physical measures. [*psycho-* + G. *therapeia,* treatment]

**psy·cho·tro·phic** (sī'kō-trō'pik) Denotes a pharmacotherapeutic agent that affects brain function, usually used in the context of drugs. [G. *psychros,* cold, + *trophē,* growth, nourishment, + *-ic,* adj. suffix]

**PT** Abbreviation for prothrombin time; physical therapy.

**PTA** Abbreviation for phosphotungstic acid; plasma thromboplastin antecedent.

**PTC** Abbreviation for plasma thromboplastin component.

**PTCA** Abbreviation for percutaneous transluminal coronary angioplasty.

**pte·ryg·i·um** (tĕr-ij'ē-ŭm) **1.** Triangular patch of hypertrophied bulbar subconjunctival tissue, extending from medial angle or canthus of eye to border of cornea or beyond, with apex pointing toward pupil. **2.** Forward growth of the cuticle over the nail plate, seen most commonly in lichen planus. [G. *pterygion,* anything like a wing, a disease of the eye, dim. of *pteryx,* wing]

**pte·ryg·i·um col·li** (tĕr-ij'ē-ŭm kol'ī) Congenital, usually bilateral, web or tight band of skin of the neck extending from acromion to mastoid process.

**pter·y·goid pro·cess of sphe·noid bone** (ter'i-goyd pro'ses sfē'noyd bōn) [TA] A long process extending downward from the junction of the body and greater wing of the sphenoid bone on either side.

**pter·y·goid ve·nous plex·us** (ter'i-goyd vē'nŭs pleks'ŭs) [TA] A venous plexus occupying the infratemporal fossa receiving veins accompanying the branches of the maxillary artery, and terminating posteriorly in the maxillary vein.

**pte·ry·go·max·il·la·re** (ter'i-gō-mak'si-lar'ē) The point at which the pterygoid process of sphenoid bone and pterygoid process of maxilla begin to form the pterygomaxillary fissure.

**pter·y·go·max·il·lar·y** (ter'i-gō-mak'si-lar'ē) Relating to the pterygoid process and the maxilla.

**pto·sis,** pl. **pto·ses** (tō'sis, -sēz) **1.** A sinking down or prolapse of an organ. **2.** SYN blepharoptosis. [G. *ptōsis,* a falling]

**PTSD** Abbreviation for posttraumatic stress disorder.

**pty·a·lec·ta·sis** (tī'ă-lek'tă-sis) SYN sialectasis. [*ptyal-* + G. *ektasis,* a stretching out]

**pty·a·lism** (tī'ăl-izm) SYN sialism. [G. *ptyalismos,* spitting]

**pu·ber·ty** (pyu'bĕr-tē) Sequence of events during which a child becomes a young adult, characterized by beginning of gonadotropin secretion, gametogenesis, secretion of gonadal hormones, development of secondary sexual characteristics and reproductive functions; sexual dimorphism is accentuated. [L. *pubertas,* fr. *puber,* grown up]

**pu·bes·cence, pu·bes·cen·cy** (pyū-bes'ĕns, -ē) **1.** Approach of age of puberty or sexual maturity. **2.** Presence of downy or fine, short hair. [L. *pubesco,* to attain puberty]

**pub·lic health** (pub'lik helth) Art and science of community health, concerned with statistics, epidemiology, hygiene, and prevention and eradication of epidemic diseases.

**pub·lic health den·tis·try** (pŭb'lik helth-den'tis-trē) That specialty of dentistry concerned with prevention and control of dental diseases and promotion of oral health through organized community efforts.

**pub·lic health nurse (PHN)** (pŭb'lik helth nŭrs) Nurse who provides care to individual patients or groups in a community outside institutions through the auspices of a state or city health department. SYN community nurse.

**pu·er·per·al** (pyū-er'pĕr-ăl) Relating to the puerperium, or period after childbirth. SYN puerperant (1).

**pu·er·pe·rant** (pyū-er'pĕr-ant) SYN puerperal.

**pull stroke ac·tion** (pul strōk ak'shŭn) Movement of the dental instrument in the direction of the clinician.

**pul·mo·nar·y an·thrax** (pul'mŏ-nar-ē an'thraks) Form of anthrax acquired by inhalation of dust containing *Bacillus anthracis.*

**pul·mo·nar·y cir·cu·la·tion** (pul'mŏ-nar-ē sir'kyū-lā'shŭn) Passage of blood from right ventricle through pulmonary artery to lungs and back through pulmonary veins to left atrium.

**pul·mo·nar·y e·de·ma** (pul'mŏ-nar-ē ĕ-dē'mă) Accumulation of extravascular fluid in lung tissues and alveoli usually resulting from mitral stenosis or left ventricular failure.

**pul·mo·nar·y em·bo·lism** (pul'mŏ-nar-ē em'bŏ-lizm) Embolism of pulmonary arteries, most frequently by detached fragments of thrombus from a leg or pelvic vein.

**pul·mo·ni·tis** (pul'mō-nī'tis) SYN pneumonitis.

**pulp** (pŭlp) Highly innervated and vascular component of tooth. Primary sensation signaled by pulp is pain, because it is extremely sensitive (touching exposed pulp with even a wisp of cotton is severely painful). Dental innervation has neurotrophic-interactive and autonomic components. [L. *pulpa*, flesh]

**pulp ab·scess** (pŭlp ab´ses) Abscess involving soft tissue within pulp chamber of a tooth, usually sequela of caries or less frequently of trauma.

**pul·pal** (pŭl´păl) Relating to the pulp.

**pul·pal·gi·a** (pŭlp-al´jē-ă) Pain arising from dental pulp. [L. *pulpa*, pulp, + G. *algos*, pain]

**pulp am·pu·ta·tion** (pŭlp am´pyū-tā´shŭn) SYN pulpotomy.

**pulp at·ro·phy** (pŭlp at´rŏ-fē) Diminution in size and/or cellular elements of dental pulp due to interference with the blood supply.

**pulp cal·ci·fi·ca·tion** (pŭlp kal´si-fi-kā´shŭn) SYN endolith.

**pulp cal·cu·lus** (pŭlp kal´kyū-lŭs) SYN endolith.

**pulp ca·nal** (pŭlp kă-nal´) SYN root canal of tooth.

**pulp cap** (pŭlp kap) A covering or dressing, usually containing a sedative in nature, placed over exposed dental pulp.

**pulp cav·i·ty** (pŭlp kav´i-tē) [TA] Central hollow of tooth consisting of pulp cavity of crown and root canal; contains fibrovascular dental pulp and is lined throughout by odontoblasts. SYN cavitas dentis [TA], cavity of tooth, cavum dentis.

**pulp cav·i·ty of crown** (pŭlp kav´i-tē krown) [TA] Space (part of pulp cavity) within tooth crown continuous with root canal. SYN crown cavity.

**pulp cham·ber** (pŭlp chăm´bĕr) That portion of the pulp cavity contained in the crown or body of the tooth. SEE ALSO dental pulp.

**pulp·ec·to·my** (pŭl-pek´tŏ-mē) Removal of tooth's entire pulp structure, including root pulp tissue. [L. *pulpa*, pulp, + G. *ektomē*, excision]

**pulp horn** (pŭlp hōrn) Prolongation of pulp extending toward tooth cusp.

**pulp in·volve·ment** (pŭlp in-volv´mĕnt) Colloq. for dental decay, trauma, or instrumentation that extends into the pulpal portion of the tooth. Penetration into the dental pulp is known as a pulp exposure.

**pul·pi·tis** (pŭl-pī´tis) Inflammation of tooth pulp. SYN odontitis. [L. *pulpa*, pulp, + G. *-itis*, inflammation]

**pulp·less** (pŭlp´lĕs) **1.** Denoting tooth in which pulp has died or from which pulp has been removed. **2.** Denoting a tooth that gives no response to an electric pulp or thermal test.

**pulp·less tooth** (pŭlp´lĕs tūth) Tooth with a nonvital or necrotic pulp, or one from which pulp has been extirpated.

**pulp nod·ule** (pŭlp nod´yūl) SYN endolith.

**pulp·o·don·ti·a** (pŭlp´ŏ-don´shē-ă) Science of root canal therapy. [L. *pulpa*, pulp, + G. *odous*, tooth]

**pulp·ot·o·my** (pŭl-pot´ŏ-mē) Removal of portion of tooth's pulp structure, usually the coronal portion. SYN pulp amputation. [L. *pulpa*, pulp, + G. *tomē*, incision]

**pulp pol·yp** (pŭlp pol´ip) SYN hyperplastic pulpitis.

**pulp pres·sure** (pŭlp presh´ŭr) Pressure in dental pulp cavity associated with extracellular fluid pressure, but showing pulsatile variations during cardiac cycle because of encasement of pulp within tooth.

**pulp stones** (pŭlp stōnz) Calcifications found in the pulp chamber or pulp canals of teeth. SEE ALSO pulp calcification, endolith.

**pulp test** (pŭlp test) SYN vitality test.

**pulse** (pŭls) Rhythmic dilation of an artery, produced by increased volume of blood thrown into vessel by contraction of heart. [L. *pulsus*]

**pulse pres·sure** (pŭls presh´ŭr) Variation in blood pressure occurring in an artery during cardiac cycle.

**pulse ther·a·py** (pŭls thār´ă-pē) Short, intensive course of pharmacotherapy, usually given at intervals such as weekly or monthly.

**pul·sus al·ter·nans** (pŭl´sŭs awl´tĕr-nanz) Heartbeats that alternate between strong and weak. SYN alternating pulse.

**pum·ice** (pŭm´is) Volcanic cinders ground to particles of varying sizes; used in dentistry for polishing restorations or teeth; an abrasive. [L. *pumex* (*pumic-*), a pumice stone]

**pump** (pŭmp) **1.** Apparatus for forcing gas or liquid from or to any part. **2.** Any mechanism for using metabolic energy to accomplish active transport of a substance.

**punch bi·op·sy** (pŭnch bī´op-sē) Any method that removes a small cylindric specimen for biopsy by means of a special instrument that pierces the organ directly or through the skin or a small incision in the skin.

**punc·tum,** pl. **punc·ta** (pŭngk´tŭm, -tă) [TA] **1.** Tip or end of a sharp process. **2.** Minute round spot differing in color or otherwise in appearance from the surrounding tissues. SYN point

op

(1). [L. a prick, point, pp. ntr. of *pungo,* to prick, used as noun]

**pu·pil** (pyū'pil) [TA] Circular orifice in center of iris, through which light rays enter eye. [L. *pupilla*]

**pure** (pyūr) Unadulterated; free from admixture or contamination with any extraneous matter. [L. *purus*]

**pur·ga·tive** (pŭr'gă-tiv) An agent used for purging the bowels. [L. *purgativus,* purging]

**purge** (pŭrj) **1.** To cause a copious evacuation of the bowels. **2.** A cathartic remedy. [L. *purgo,* to cleanse, fr. *purus,* pure, + *ago,* to do]

**pu·ri·fied wa·ter** (pyūr'ĭ-fīd waw'tĕr) Water obtained by distillation or deionization.

**pur·i·ty** (pyūr'ĭ-tē) The state of being pure, free from contaminants or pollutants. [L. *puritas,* fr. *purus,* clean, undefiled]

**pur·pu·ra** (pŭr'pyūr-ă) A condition characterized by hemorrhage into skin. Appearance of lesions varies with type of purpura, duration of lesions, and acuteness of onset. [L. fr. G. *porphyra,* purple]

**pur·pu·ra hem·or·rha·gi·ca** (pŭr'pyūr-ă hem-ō-raj'i-kă) SYN idiopathic thrombocytopenic purpura.

**pur·sed lips breath·ing** (pŭrst lips brēdh'ing) Technique in which air is inhaled slowly through nose and mouth and exhaled slowly through pursed lips; used by patients with chronic obstructive pulmonary disease to improve their breathing by increasing resistance to air flow, thus forcibly dilating small bronchi.

**purse-string su·ture** (pŭrs'string sū'chŭr) A continuous suture placed in a circular manner either for inversion or closure.

**pur·u·lent in·flam·ma·tion** (pyūr'ŭ-lĕnt in'flă-mā'shŭn) Acute exudative inflammation in which accumulation of polymorphonuclear leukocytes is sufficiently great that their enzymes cause liquefaction of affected tissues, focally or diffusely; this exudate is frequently termed pus; it consists of plasma and its constituents, end products of enzymatic digestion of tissue, degenerated and necrotic cells, debris, polymorphonuclear leukocytes and other white blood cells, and causal agent of the inflammation.

**pus** (pŭs) Fluid product of inflammation, consisting of liquid containing leukocytes and debris of dead cells and tissue elements liquefied by proteolytic and histolytic enzymes (e.g., leukoprotease) that are elaborated by polymorphonuclear leukocytes. [L.]

**pus ba·sin** (pŭs bā'sin) Receptacle curved to fit closely the surface to which it is applied, used to receive pus from wounds during drainage, cleansing, and/or redressing.

**push stroke ac·tion** (push strōk ak'shŭn) Movement of the dental instrument away from the clinician.

**pus·tule** (pŭs'tyūl) A circumscribed, superficial elevation of the skin, up to 1 cm in diameter, containing purulent material. See this page. [L. *pustula*]

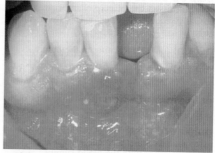

pustule: periodontal abscess during pointing stage

**pu·tre·fac·tion** (pyū'trĕ-fak'shŭn) Decomposition or rotting, breakdown of organic matter usually by bacterial action, resulting in formation of other substances of less complex constitution with evolution of ammonia or its derivatives and hydrogen sulfide; characterized usually by presence of toxic or malodorous products. SYN decay (3). [L. *putre-facio,* pp. *-factus,* to make rotten]

**pu·tres·cent pulp** (pyū-tres'ĕnt pŭlp) Decomposed tooth pulp, often infected.

**pu·tres·cine** (pyū-tres'ēn) A poisonous polyamine formed from the amino acid arginine during putrefaction; found in urine and feces.

**PVC** Abbreviation for premature ventricular contraction.

**PVD** Abbreviation for peripheral vascular disease.

**pyaemia** [Br.] SYN pyemia.

**py·em·e·sis** (pī-em'ĕ-sis) Vomiting of pus. [G. *pyon,* pus, + *emesis,* vomiting]

**py·e·mi·a** (pī-ē'mē-ă) Septicemia due to pyogenic organisms causing multiple abscesses. SYN pyaemia. [G. *pyon,* pus, + *haima,* blood]

**py·e·sis** (pī-ē'sis) SYN suppuration. [G. *pyon,* pus, + *-esis,* condition or process]

**pyk·nic** (pik'nik) Denoting a constitutional body type characterized by well-rounded external contours and ample body cavities; virtually synonymous with endomorphic. [G. *pyknos,* thick]

**pyk·no·sis** (pik-nō'sis) A thickening or condensation; specifically, a condensation and reduction in the size of the cell or its nucleus, usually associated with hyperchromatosis. [*pykno-* + G. *-osis,* condition]

**py·lor·ic in·com·pe·tence** (pī-lōr´ik in-kom´pĕ-tĕns) Patulous state or want of tone of pylorus that allows passage of food into intestine before gastric digestion is completed.

**py·lor·ic in·suf·fi·cien·cy** (pī-lōr´ik in´ sŭ-fish´ĕn-sē) Patulousness of pyloric outlet of stomach, allowing regurgitation of duodenal contents into stomach.

♲ **pyo-** *Do not confuse this combining form with pyelo-.* Suppuration, accumulation of pus. [G. *pyon,* pus]

**py·o·gen** (pī´ŏ-jen) Agent that causes pus formation. [*pyo-* + G. *-gen,* producing]

**py·o·gen·e·sis** (pī´ŏ-jen´ĕ-sis) SYN suppuration. [*pyo-* + G. *genesis,* production]

**py·o·gen·ic, py·o·ge·net·ic, py·og·e·nous** (pī´ŏ-jen´ik, -jĕ-net´ik, pī-oj´ĕ-nŭs) Pus-forming; relating to pus formation.

▣ **py·o·gen·ic gran·u·lo·ma, gran·u·lo·ma py·o·gen·i·cum** (pī´ŏ-jen´ik gran´yū-lō´mă, pī-ō-jen´i-kŭm) Acquired small rounded mass of highly vascular granulation tissue, frequently with an ulcerated surface, projecting from skin, especially facial, or oral mucosa. See this page and page A15.

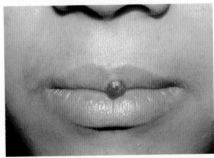

**pyogenic granuloma**

**py·o·gen·ic in·fec·tion** (pī´ŏ-jen´ik in-fek´shŭn) Infection characterized by severe local inflammation, usually with pus formation, generally caused by pyogenic bacteria.

**py·o·my·o·si·tis** (pī´ō-mī´ŏ-sī´tis) Abscesses, carbuncles, or infected sinuses lying deep in muscles. [*pyo-* + G. *mys,* muscle, + *-itis,* inflammation]

**py·o·poi·e·sis** (pī´ō-poy-ē´sis) SYN suppuration. [*pyo-* + G. *poiēsis,* a making]

**py·or·rhe·a** (pī´ŏ-rē´ă) Purulent discharge. [*pyo-* + G. *rhoia,* a flow]

**pyorrhoea** [Br.] SYN pyorrhea.

**py·o·sis** (pī-ō´sis) SYN suppuration. [G.]

**py·o·stat·ic** (pī´ŏ-stat´ik) Arresting formation of pus. [*pyo-* + G. *statikos,* causing to stand]

**py·ram·i·dal** (pir-am´i-dăl) **1.** Of the shape of a pyramid. **2.** Relating to any anatomic structure called a pyramid.

**py·ram·i·dal frac·ture** (pir-am´i-dăl frak´ shŭr) A fracture of the midfacial skeleton with the principal fracture lines meeting at an apex at or near the superior aspect of the nasal bones.

**pyr·a·mid sign** (pir´ă-mid sīn) Any symptoms or signs indicative of damage of pyramidal tracts, such as the Babinski or Gordon sign, spastic spinal paralysis, foot clonus, and others.

**py·raz·o·lone** (pi-raz´ŏ-lōn) A class of non-steroidal anti-inflammatory agents used to treat arthritic conditions.

**py·rec·tic, py·ret·ic** (pī-rek´tik, -ret´ik) SYN febrile.

**py·rex·i·a** (pī-rek´sē-ă) SYN fever. [G. *pyrexis,* feverishness]

**py·rex·i·a of un·known or·i·gin** (pī-rek´sē-ă ŭn´nōn ōr´i-jin) SYN fever of unknown origin.

♲ **pyro-** **1.** Combining form denoting fire, heat, or fever. **2.** In chemistry, combining form denoting derivatives formed by removal of water (usually by heat) to form anhydrides. [G. *pyr,* fire]

**py·ro·gen** (pī´rō-jen) Fever-inducing agent; produced by bacteria, molds, viruses, and yeasts. [*pyro-* + G. *-gen,* producing]

**py·rol·y·sis** (pī-rol´i-sis) Decomposition of a substance by heat. [*pyro-* + G. *lysis,* dissolution]

**py·ro·phos·pha·tase** (pī´rō-fos´fă-tās) Any enzyme cleaving a pyrophosphate bond between two phosphoric groups. SYN diphosphatase.

**py·ro·phos·phate (PP)** (pī´rō-fos´fāt) A salt of pyrophosphoric acid; accumulates in cases of hypophosphatasia.

**py·ro·sis** (pī-rō´sis) Substernal pain or burning sensation, usually associated with regurgitation of acid-peptic gastric juice into the esophagus. [G. a burning]

**py·ru·vate ki·nase (PK)** (pī´rū-vāt kī´nās) A phosphotransferase catalyzing the transfer of phosphate from phosphoenolpyruvate to adenosine diphosphate, forming adenosine triphosphate and pyruvate; other nucleoside phosphates can participate in the reaction; a key step in glycolysis; pyruvate kinase deficiency leads to hemolytic anemia.

**py·u·ri·a** (pī-yūr´ē-ă) Presence of pus in the urine when voided. [G. *pyon,* pus, + *ouron,* urine]

**op**

# Q

**Q** Abbreviation for quaternary.

**QA** Abbreviation for quality assurance.

**QC** Abbreviation for quality control.

**q.d** *The JCAHO directs that daily or every day be written in full, because q.d. can easily be misread as q.i.d. or q.o.d. Abbreviation for L. quaque die, every day.*

**q.h.** Abbreviation for L. *quaque hora*, every hour.

**q.h.s.** *The JCAHO directs that (nightly) at bedtime be written in full to avoid misreading of this abbreviation as q.h., every hour.* Abbreviation for L. *quaque hora somni*, every bedtime.

**q.i.d.** Abbreviation for L. *quater in die*, four times a day.

**q.o.d.** *The JCAHO directs that every other day be written in full, because q.o.d. can easily be misread as q.i.d. Every other day.*

**Q.O.L.** Abbreviation for quality of life.

**q.s.** Abbreviation for L. *quantum sufficiat* or *satis*, as much as suffices.

**quack** (kwak) SYN charlatan. [Abbreviation of quacksalver, Dutch *quack*, to boast + *salf*, cream]

**quad·rant** (kwahd'rănt) **1.** In dentistry, one quarter of combined dental arches; there are two maxillary and two mandibular quadrants. **2.** One quarter of a circle; various anatomic structures are described as having quadrants. [L. *quadrans*, a quarter]

**qua·dri·cus·pid** (kwah'dri-kŭs'pid) SYN tetracuspid.

**quad·ri·ple·gi·a** (kwahd'ri-plē'jē-ă) Paralysis of all four limbs. [L. *quadrus*, four + G. *plēgē*, stroke]

**quad·ri·tu·ber·cu·lar** (kwahd'ri-tū-bĕr'kyū-lăr) Having four tubercles or cusps, as a molar tooth. [L. *quadrus*, four + L. *tuberculum*, tubercle]

**qua·li·ty** (kwahl'i-tē) **1.** A property or trait inherent in the nature of anything. **2.** A degree of superiority. [L. *qualitas*]

**qual·i·ty as·sur·ance (QA)** (kwahl'i-tē ă-shŭr'ĕns) An institutional program designed to assess the success of the total organization in achieving its goals and to ensure that quality standards are met. SEE ALSO quality control.

**qual·i·ty con·trol (QC)** (kwahl'i-tē kŏn-trōl') Control of laboratory analytic error by the monitoring of analytic performance with control sera and maintenance of error within established limits around the mean control values, most commonly ±2 standard deviations. SEE ALSO quality assurance.

**qual·i·ty of life (Q.O.L.)** (kwah'li-tē līf) An overall assessment of a person's well-being, which may include physical, emotional, and social dimensions, as well as stress level, sexual function, and self-perceived health status.

**quan·tum,** pl. **quan·ta** (kwahn'tŭm, -tă) Unit of radiant energy (Q) varying by frequency (*v*) of radiation. [L. how much]

**quan·tum the·o·ry** (kwahn'tŭm thē'ŏr-ē) That energy can be emitted, transmitted, and absorbed only in discrete quantities (quanta), so that atoms and subatomic particles can exist only in certain energy states. SYN Planck theory.

**quar·an·tine** (kwōr'ăn-tēn) **1.** Isolation of a person with a known or possible contagious disease. **2.** A period (originally 40 days) of detention of vessels and their passengers coming from an area where an infectious disease prevails. **3.** A place where such vessels and their passengers are detained. [It. *quarantina* fr. L. *quadraginta*, forty]

**quar·an·tine pe·ri·od** (kwōr'ăn-tēn pēr'ē-ŏd) Time during which an infected individual or an area is kept isolated, avoiding contact with uninfected people; can be any period of time, varying with possible disease. The term is derived from the Italian word for 40, because the period of isolation for people suspected of having plague in the medieval period was 40 days.

**quart** (kwōrt) **1.** Measure of fluid capacity; fourth part of a gallon; equivalent of 0.9468 liter. An imperial quart contains about 20% more than the ordinary quart, or 1.1359 liters. **2.** A dry measure holding a little more than the fluid measure. [L. *quartus*, fourth]

**quar·tan** (kwōr'tăn) Recurring every fourth day, including the first day of an episode in computation, i.e., after a free interval of 2 days. [L. *quartanus*, relating to a fourth (thing)]

**quar·te·nar·y am·mo·ni·um com·pound** (kwah'tĕr-nar-ē ă-mō'nē-ŭm kom' pownd) A substance used as a mouth freshening agent in over-the-counter mouth rinse.

**quartz** (kwōrts) A crystalline form of silicon dioxide used in chemical apparatus and in optic and electrical instruments.

**qua·ter·nar·y (Q)** (kwah'tĕr-nar-ē) **1.** Denoting a chemical compound containing four elements. **2.** Fourth in a series. **3.** Relating to organic compounds in which some central atom is attached to four functional groups.

**quench·ing** (kwench'ing) **1.** The process of extinguishing, removing, or diminishing a physical property such as heat or light. **2.** Process of stopping a chemical reaction. [M. E. *quenchen*, fr. O.E. *ācwencan*]

**quick** (kwik) A sensitive part, painful to touch. [A.S. *cwic*, living]

**Quin·cke dis·ease** (kving′kĕ di-zēz′) Disorder that may involve deeper skin layers and subcutaneous tissues as well as mucosal surfaces of upper respiratory and gastrointestinal tracts. SYN angioedema (2), angioneurotic edema (2).

**qui·nine** (kwī′nīn, kwin′ēn) An agent effective against the asexual and erythrocytic forms of malaria but with no effect on the exoerythrocytic (tissue) forms; does not effect a radical cure of malaria, but is used to treat cerebral malaria and other severe outbreaks of malignant tertian malaria and in malaria produced by chloroquine-resistant strains of *P. falciparum.*

**quin·o·lones** (kwin′ō-lōnz) Synthetic broad-spectrum antibacterial agents with bactericidal action.

**quin·que·tu·ber·cu·lar** (kwin′kwĕ-tū-ber′ kyū-lăr) Having five tubercles or cusps, as in some molar teeth. [L. *quinque,* five, + *tuberculum,* tubercle, dim. of *tuber,* a swelling]

**quin·sy** (kwin′zē) SYN peritonsillar abscess.

**quin·tu·plet** (kwin-tŭp′lĕt) One of five children born during one birth. [L. *quintuplex,* fivefold]

**quo·tid·i·an** (kwō-tid′ē-ăn) Daily; occurring every day.

**quo·tient** (kwō′shĕnt) Number of times one amount is contained in another; ratio of two numbers. [L. *quoties,* how often]

qr

# R

**Ra** Symbol for radium.

**rab·id** (rab'id) Relating to or suffering from rabies. [L. *rabidus,* raving, mad]

**ra·bies** (rā'bēz) Highly fatal infectious disease that may affect all species of warm-blooded animals, including humans; transmitted by the bite of infected animals and caused by a neurotropic species of *Lyssavirus.* SYN hydrophobia.

**rac·coon eyes** (rak-ūn' īz) Bilateral ecchymosis in periorbital region; suggests basilar skull fracture or neuroblastoma. SYN raccoon sign.

**ra·ce·mic** (rā-sē'mik) Denoting mixture of compounds that is itself optically inactive, being composed of an equal number of dextrorotatory and levorotatory substances.

**ra·chit·ic** (ră-kit'ik) Relating to rickets.

**rad** (rad) The unit for the dose absorbed from ionizing radiation, equivalent to 100 ergs per gram of tissue; 100 rad = 1 Gy.

**ra·dec·to·my** (rā-dek'tŏ-mē) SYN root amputation. [L. *radix,* root, + G. *ektomē,* excision]

**ra·di·al ker·a·tot·o·my** (rā'dē-ăl ker'ă-tot'ŏ-mē) A form of refractive keratoplasty used in the treatment of myopia.

**ra·di·al pulse** (rā'dē-ăl pŭls) A palpable rhythmic expansion of the radial artery on the volar aspect of the wrist over the distal radius.

**ra·di·al tun·nel syn·drome** (rā'dē-ăl tŭn'ĕl sin'drōm) Pain in lateral aspect of elbow and forearm without motor or sensory deficits.

**ra·di·ate** (rā'dē-āt) 1. To spread out in all directions from a center. 2. To emit radiation. [L. *radio,* pp. *-atus,* to shine]

**ra·di·a·tion** (rā'dē-ā'shŭn) 1. Sending forth light, short radio waves, ultraviolet rays or x-rays, or any other rays for treatment, diagnosis, or another purpose. 2. Act or condition of diverging in all directions from a center. [L. *radiatio,* fr. *radius,* ray, beam]

**ra·di·a·tion a·ne·mi·a** (rā'dē-ā'shŭn ă-nē'mē-ă) Hypoplastic anemia sometimes occurring after high-level acute or low-level chronic exposure to ionizing radiation.

**ra·di·a·tion burn** (rā'dē-ā'shŭn bŭrn) Burn caused by exposure to atomic energy in any form and kindred modalities.

**ra·di·a·tion car·ies** (rā'dē-ā'shŭn kar'ēz) Caries of cervical regions of teeth, incisal edges, and cusp tips due to xerostomia induced by radiation therapy.

**ra·di·a·tion der·ma·ti·tis** (rā'dē-ā'shŭn dĕr'mă-tī'tis) An acute or chronic inflammation of the skin caused by exposure to ionizing radiation, typically as part of cancer radiation therapy; can range from erythema to wet desquamation of the skin (tissue sloughing) in acute form; tissue atrophy, fibrosis, and permanent scarring in chronic form. Permanent changes in skin pigmentation can also occur.

**ra·di·a·tion do·sim·e·ter** (rā'dē-ā'shŭn dō-sim'ĕ-tĕr) SYN film badge.

**ra·di·a·tion my·e·lop·a·thy** (rā'dē-ā'shŭn mī'ĕ-lop'ă-thē) Spinal cord damage from exposure to x-rays or other high-energy radiation; most often affects the cervical segments.

**ra·di·a·tion ne·cro·sis** (rā'dē-ā'shŭn nĕ-krō'sis) Death of cells or tissues resulting from the effects of radiation exposure.

**ra·di·a·tion on·col·o·gy** (rā'dē-ā'shŭn on-kol'ŏ-jē) 1. Medical specialty concerned with use of ionizing radiation in treatment of disease. 2. Use of radiation in the treatment of neoplasms.

**ra·di·a·tion sick·ness** (rā'dē-ā'shŭn sik'nĕs) Systemic condition caused by substantial whole-body irradiation, seen after nuclear explosions or accidents, but rarely after radiotherapy. Manifestations depend on dosage.

**ra·di·a·tion ther·a·py, ra·di·o·ther·a·py** (rā'dē-ā'shŭn thār'ă-pē, rā'dē-ō-thār'ă-pē) Treatment with x-rays or radionuclides.

**rad·i·cal** (rad'i-kăl) 1. In chemistry, a group of elements or atoms usually passing intact from one compound to another, but usually incapable of prolonged existence in a free state (e.g., methyl, $CH_3$). 2. Thorough or extensive; relating or directed to the extirpation of the root or cause of a morbid process. 3. Denoting treatment by extreme, drastic, or innovative, as opposed to conservative, measures. [L. *radix* (*radic-*), root]

**rad·i·cal neck dis·sec·tion** (rad'i-kăl nek di-sek'shŭn) An operation for the removal of metastases to the lymph nodes of the neck in which all tissue is removed between the superficial and the deep cervical fascia from the mandible to the clavicle.

**rad·i·cle** (rad'i-kĕl) A rootlet or structure resembling one, as the radicle of a vein or the radicle of a nerve, i.e, a nerve fiber that joins others to form a nerve; the smallest branches of a vessel or nerve. [L. *radicula,* dim. of *radix,* root]

**ra·dic·u·la** (ră-dik'yū-lă) Spinal nerve root. [L. dim of *radix,* root]

**ra·dic·u·lar** (ră-dik'yū-lăr) 1. Pertaining to a tooth root. 2. Relating to a radicle.

**ra·dic·u·lar ab·scess** (ră-dik'yū-lăr ab'ses) Abscess around a tooth root.

**ra·dic·u·lar cyst** (ră-dik'yū-lăr sist) SYN apical periodontal cyst.

**ra·dic·u·lar per·for·a·tion** (ră-dik′yū-lăr pĕr-fōr-ā′shŭn) Abnormal penetration of the root of a tooth during root canal therapy.

**ra·dic·u·lo·gang·li·on·i·tis** (ră-dik′yū-lō-gang′glē-ŏ-nī′tis) Involvement of roots and ganglia.

**ra·dic·u·lop·a·thy** (ră-dik′yū-lop′ă-thē) Disorder of spinal nerve roots.

♻ **radio-** Combining form meaning relation, chiefly (in medicine) gamma or x-ray. [L. *radius*, ray]

**ra·di·o·ac·tive i·so·topes** (rā′dē-ō-ak′tiv ī′sŏ-tōps) An isotope with an unstable nuclear composition; used as tracers, and as radiation and energy sources.

**ra·di·o·ac·tiv·i·ty** (rā′dē-ō-ak-tiv′i-tē) The property of some atomic nuclei of spontaneously emitting gamma rays or subatomic particles (alpha and beta rays).

**ra·di·o·al·ler·go·sor·bent test (RAST)** (rā′dē-ō-al′ĕr-gō-sōr′bĕnt test) A radioimmunoassay-based procedure to detect IgE-bound allergens responsible for tissue hypersensitivity.

**ra·di·o·au·tog·ra·phy** (rā′dē-ō-aw-tog′ră-fē) SYN autoradiography.

**ra·di·o·bi·ol·o·gy** (rā′dē-ō-bī-ol′ŏ-jē) The study of the biologic effects of ionizing radiation on living tissue. Cf. radiopathology.

**ra·di·o·graph** (rā′dē-ō-graf) A negative image on photographic film made by exposure to x-rays or gamma rays. SYN x-ray (3). [*radio-* + G. *graphō*, to write]

**ra·di·og·ra·pher** (rā′dē-og′ră-fĕr) A technician trained to position patients and take radiographs or perform other radiodiagnostic procedures.

**ra·di·o·graph·ic an·gu·la·tion** (rā′dē-ō-graf′ik ang′yū-lā′shŭn) The angle between the central beam of x-rays and the surface of the film or sensor.

**ra·di·o·graph·ic con·trast** (rā′dē-ō-graf′ik kon′trast) The variation of the light and dark areas on a radiograph.

**ra·di·o·graph·ic con·trast me·di·um** (rā′dē-ō-graf′ik kon′trast mē′dē-ŭm) Any internally administered substance with different opacity from soft tissue on radiography or computed tomography (e.g., barium).

**ra·di·o·graph·ic den·si·ty** (rā′dē-ō-graf′ik den′si-tē) The amount of blackening on an x-ray film produced by the interaction of silver halide crystals with developing agents.

**ra·di·o·graph·ic film** (rā′dē-ō-graf′ik film) Thin, transparent sheet of cellulose acetate coated with radiation-sensitive emulsions of silver bromide, silver halide, and silver iodide crystals that are suspended in a gelatinous component; sealed in a moisture-resistant, lightproof protective packet when used for intraoral dental radiographs.

**ra·di·o·graph·ic in·ter·pre·ta·tion** (rā′dē-ō-graf′ik in-tĕr′prĕ-tā′shŭn) Examination and study of a diagnostic radiograph to identify and explain findings viewed.

**ra·di·o·graph·ic lo·cal·i·za·tion** (rā′dē-ō-graf′ik lō′kăl-ī-zā′shŭn) In dentistry, a technique used to determine the position of teeth or other foreign objects in the jaw by correct positioning and angulation of the x-ray beam.

**ra·di·o·graph·ic ter·mi·nus** (rā′dē-ō-graf′ik tĕr′mi-nŭs) Apex of root canal where it exits from the tooth as determined by radiographic findings.

**ra·di·og·ra·phy** (rā′dē-og′ră-fē) Examination of any body part for diagnostic purposes with x-rays with the record of the findings exposed onto photographic film.

**ra·di·o·i·so·tope** (rā′dē-ō-ī′sŏ-tōp) An isotope that changes to a more stable state by emitting radiation.

**ra·di·o·log·ic ex·po·sure** (rā-dō-ō-loj′ĭk eks-pō′zhŭr) Measurement of ionization produced in air by x-radiation.

**ra·di·o·log·ic health** (ra′dē-ō-loj′ik helth) Art and science of protecting human beings from injury by accidental exposure to radiation, as well as of promoting better health through beneficial applications of radiation.

**ra·di·ol·o·gist** (rā′dē-ol′ō-jist) Physician trained in diagnostic and/or therapeutic use of x-rays and radionuclides, radiation physics, and biology.

**ra·di·ol·o·gy** (rā′dē-ol′ŏ-jē) **1.** Science of high-energy radiation and of sources and chemical, physical, and biologic effects of such radiation. **2.** Scientific discipline of medical imaging. SYN diagnostic radiology. [*radio-* + G. *logos*, study]

**ra·di·o·lu·cen·cy** (rā′dē-ō-lū′sĕn-sē) Region of a radiograph showing increased exposure, either because of greater transradiancy of corresponding portion of subject or because of inhomogeneity in source of radiation, such as off-center positioning.

**ra·di·o·lu·cent** (rā′dē-ō-lū′sĕnt) Relatively penetrable by x-rays or other forms of radiation. See page 484. [*radio-* + L. *lucens*, shining]

**ra·di·o·neu·ri·tis** (rā′dē-ō-nūr-ī′tis) Neuritis caused by prolonged or repeated exposure to x-rays or radium.

**ra·di·o·nu·clide** (rā′dē-ō-nū′klīd) An isotope of artificial or natural origin that exhibits radioactivity. Radionuclides are used in diagnostic imaging and cancer therapy.

qr

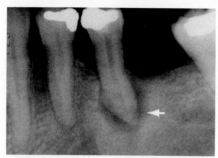

**radiolucent area** (arrow) around root of mandibular premolar indicating pathological process

**ra·di·o·nu·clide gen·er·a·tor** (rā′dē-ō-nū′klīd jen′ĕr-ā-tŏr) A column containing a large amount of a particular radionuclide (mother radionuclide) that decays to a second radionuclide with shorter physical half-life.

**ra·di·o·pac·i·ty** (rā′dē-ō-pas′i-tē) X-ray shadow of a radiopaque object.

**ra·di·o·paque** (rā′dē-ō-pāk′) Exhibiting relative opacity to, or impenetrability by, x-rays or any other form of radiation. Cf. radiolucent. [*radio-* + Fr. *opaque* fr. L. *opacus,* shady]

**ra·di·o·pa·thol·o·gy** (rā′dē-ō-pă-thol′ŏ-jē) Branch of radiology or pathology concerned with effects of radiation on cells and tissues.

**ra·di·o·re·cep·tor** (rā′dē-ō-rĕ-sep′tŏr) **1.** A receptor that normally responds to radiant energy such as light or heat. **2.** A receptor used as a binding agent for unlabeled and radiolabeled analyte in a type of competitive binding assay called radioreceptor assay.

**ra·di·o·sen·si·tiv·i·ty** (rā′dē-ō-sen′si-tiv′i-tē) The condition of being readily affected by radiant energy.

**ra·di·o·sen·si·ti·za·tion** (rā′dē-ō-sen′si-tī-zā′shŭn) Use of chemotherapy that increase sensitivity of tissue to radiation therapy.

**ra·di·o·ther·a·py** (rā′dē-ō-thār′ă-pē) The medical specialty concerned with the use of electromagnetic or particulate radiation in the treatment of disease.

**ra·di·o·tox·e·mi·a** (rā′dē-ō-tok-sē′mē-ă) Radiation sickness caused by products of disintegration produced by action of x-rays or other forms of radioactivity and by depletion of some cells and enzyme systems from organism. [*radio-* + G. *toxikon,* poison, + *haima,* blood]

**ra·di·sec·to·my** (rā′dē-sek′tŏ-mē) SYN root amputation. [L. *radix,* root, + G. *ektomē,* excision]

**ra·di·um (Ra)** (rā′dē-ŭm) A metallic element, extracted in minute quantities from pitchblende;

properties similar to those of barium with therapeutic action similar to that of x-rays. [L. *radius,* ray]

**ra·di·us,** pl. **ra·di·i** (rā′dē-ŭs, -ī) **1.** [TA] Lateral and shorter of two bones of forearm. **2.** Straight line passing from center to periphery of a circle. [L. spoke of a wheel, rod, ray]

**ra·don** (rā′don) A gaseous radioactive element, resulting from breakdown of radium; some isotopes used to treat malignancies. Poorly ventilated homes in some parts of the U.S. have accumulated a dangerous amount of naturally occurring radon gas.

**Rae·der syn·drome** (rā′dĕr sin′drōm) SYN paratrigeminal syndrome.

**rale** (rahl) Term for a sound heard on auscultation of breath sounds; used by some to denote rhonchus and by others crepitation.

**ral·ox·i·fene** (răl-ox′i-fēn) Selective estrogen receptor modulator with estrogen-agonistic effects on bone and lipid metabolism.

**ram·i·fi·ca·tion** (ram′i-fi-kā′shŭn) Process of dividing into a branchlike pattern.

**ram·i·fy** (ram′i-fī) To split into a branchlike pattern. [L. *ramus,* branch, + *facio,* to make]

**ram·pant car·ies** (ramp′ănt kar′ēz) Rapidly progressive caries in many teeth simultaneously.

**ra·mus,** pl. **ra·mi** (rā′mŭs, -mī) **1.** SYN branch. **2.** A primary division of a nerve or blood vessel. **3.** A part of an irregularly shaped bone that forms an angle with the main body. **4.** A primary division of a cerebral sulcus. [L.]

**ran·dom** (ran′dŏm) Governed by chance; denotes a process in which outcome is indeterminate. [M.E. *randon,* speed, errancy, fr. O. Fr. *randir,* to run, fr. Germanic]

**ran·dom sam·ple** (ran′dŏm samp′ĕl) Selection on basis of chance of individuals or items in a population for research.

**ran·dom waves** (ran′dŏm wāvz) Waves in electroencephalograms that occur paroxysmally and asynchronously.

**range** (rānj) Statistical measure of dispersion or variation of values determined by endpoint values themselves or the difference between them. [O.Fr. *rang,* line, fr. Germanic]

**range of mo·tion (ROM)** (rānj mō′shŭn) The measured beginning and terminal angles and total degrees of motion, traversed by a joint moved by active muscle contraction or by passive movement.

**ra·nine** (rā′nīn) Relating to the undersurface of the tongue.

**ra·nine an·as·to·mo·sis** (rā´nīn ă-nas´tŏ-mō´sis) Anastomosis between right and left end-branches of deep lingual artery.

**Ran·ke an·gle** (rahn´kĕ ang´gĕl) Area formed by horizontal plane of head and a line passing from center of margin of alveolar arch of maxilla, below nasal spine to center of frontonasal suture. [J. *Ranke*]

**ran·u·la** (ran´yū-lă) Any cystic tumor of the undersurface of the tongue or floor of the mouth. See this page and page A5. SYN sialocele. [L. tadpole, dim. of *rana*, frog]

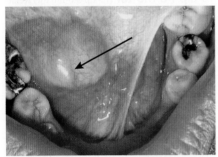

**ranula:** size, color, and translucency typical

**ra·phe, rha·phe** (rā´fē) [TA] Line of union of two contiguous, bilaterally symmetric structures. [G. *rhaphē*, suture, seam]

**rap·id eye move·ments (REM)** (rap´id ī mūv´mĕnts) Symmetric quick scanning movements of eyes occurring many times during sleep in clusters for 5–60 minutes; associated with dreaming.

**rap·id heat-trans·fer ster·i·li·zer** (rap´id hēt´trans-fĕr ster´i-lī-zĕr) SYN forced-air sterilizer.

**rap·port** (rap-ōr´) Conscious feeling of harmonious accord, trust, and mutual responsiveness between two or more people (e.g., dentist and patient) that fosters the therapeutic process. [Fr.]

**rash** (rash) Colloquial term for a cutaneous eruption.

**RAST** Abbreviation for radioallergosorbent test.

**rate** (rāt) **1.** Record of measurement of an event or process in terms of its relation to some fixed standard; expressed as ratio of one quantity to another or concentration formed per unit time. **2.** Measure of frequency of an event in a defined population. [L. *ratum*, a reckoning]

**Rath·ke pouch tu·mor** (raht´kĕ powch tū´mŏr) SYN craniopharyngioma.

**ra·ti·o** (rā´shē-ō) Expression of relation of one quantity to another (e.g., of a proportion or rate). [L. *ratio* (*ration-*) a reckoning, reason, fr. *reor*, pp. *ratus*, to reckon, compute]

**ra·tion·al·i·za·tion** (rash´ŭn-ăl-ī-zā´shŭn) Postulated psychoanalytic defense mechanism through which irrational behavior or feelings are made to appear reasonable. [L. *ratio*, reason]

**ra·ti·o of de·cay·ed and fill·ed sur·fac·es (RDFS)** (rā´shē-ō dĕ-kād´ fild sŭr´făs-ĕz) Index of such permanent surfaces per person, per full complement of 122 tooth surfaces.

**ra·ti·o of de·cay·ed and fill·ed teeth (RDFT)** (rā´shē-ō dĕ-kād´ fild tēth) Index of such permanent teeth per person, per full complement of 28 teeth.

**ray** (rā) **1.** Beam of light, heat, or other form of radiation. **2.** A part or branch that extends radially from a structure. [L. *radius*]

**Ray·naud phe·nom·e·non** (rā-nō´ fĕ-nom´ĕ-non) Spasm of the digital arteries, with blanching and numbness or pain of the fingers, often precipitated by cold. Fingers are variably colored red, white, and blue.

**RBC, rbc** Abbreviation for red blood cell.

**RDA** Abbreviation for relative dentin abrasivity index.

**RDFS** Abbreviation for ratio of decayed and filled surfaces.

**RDFT** Abbreviation for ratio of decayed and filled teeth.

**RDH** Abbreviation for registered dental hygienist.

**re·ac·tant** (rē-ak´tănt) A substance taking part in a chemical reaction.

**re·ac·tion** (rē-ak´shŭn) **1.** Response of a muscle or other living tissue or organism to a stimulus. **2.** Color change effected in litmus and other organic pigments by contact with substances. [L. *re-*, again, backward, + *actio*, action]

**re·ac·tion time** (rē-ak´shŭn tīm) Interval between presentation of a stimulus and responsive reaction to it.

**re·ac·ti·va·tion tu·ber·cu·lo·sis** (rē-ak´ti-vā´shŭn tū-bĕr´kyū-lō´sis) SYN secondary tuberculosis.

**re·ac·tive hy·po·gly·ce·mi·a** (rē-ak´tiv hī´pō-glī-sē´mē-ă) After eating a high carbohydrate meal, the affected subject overreacts and produces too much insulin in response to the food so that the glucose level decreases rapidly.

**re·ac·tive le·sion** (rē-ak´tiv lē´zhŭn) Painless production of hyperplastic tissue resulting from a repair response.

**re·a·gent** (rē-ā´jĕnt) Any substance added to a solution of another substance to participate in a chemical reaction. [Mod. L. *reagens*]

**re·a·gin** (rē-ā´jin) **1.** Wolff-Eisner term for antibody. **2.** Antibodies that mediate immediate hypersensitivity reactions (IgE in humans). **3.** SYN homocytotropic antibody.

qr

**ream·er** (rē′mĕr) Rotating finishing or drilling tool used to shape or enlarge a hole in bone or a tooth. [A.S. *ryman,* to widen]

**re·as·sign·ment** (rē′ă-sīn′mĕnt) Redirection of attributes or properties; transfer of patients from one care provider or facility to another.

**re·at·tach·ment** (rē′ă-tach′mĕnt) New epithelial or connective tissue attachment to tooth surface that was surgically detached and not exposed to oral environment.

**re·base** (rē′bās) In dentistry, to refit a denture by replacing the denture base material without changing the occlusal relationship of the teeth. SEE ALSO reline.

**re·bound** (rē′bownd) Act or condition of recovery or improvement in a patient.

**re·breath·ing** (rē-brēdh′ing) Inhalation of part or all of gases previously exhaled.

**re·breath·ing an·es·the·si·a** (rē-brēdh′ing an′es-thē′zē-ă) Technique for inhalation anesthesia in which some or all exhaled gases are subsequently inhaled.

**re·cal·ci·fi·ca·tion** (rē-kal′si-fi-kā′shŭn) Restoration of lost calcium salts to tissues.

**re·care** (rē′kār) Schedule of appointments for long-term maintenance phase of dental therapy. SYN patient recall interval.

**re·cep·tor** (rē-sep′tŏr) **1.** A structural protein molecule on cell surface or within cytoplasm that binds to a specific factor. **2.** Any sensory nerve endings in the skin or elsewhere.

**re·cess** (rē′ses) [TA] A small hollow or indentation. [L. *recessus*]

▮**re·ces·sion** (rē-sesh′ŭn) SEE gingival recession. See this page.

**re·ces·sive** (rĕ-ses′iv) Drawing away; receding.

**re·cid·i·va·tion** (rĕ-sid′i-vā′shŭn) Relapse of a disease or behavioral pattern. [L. *recidivus,* falling back, recurring, fr. *recido,* to fall back]

**rec·i·pe** (res′i-pē) Superscription of a prescription, usually indicated by the sign ℞. [L. imperative *recipio,* to receive]

**re·cip·i·ent** (rē-sip′ē-ĕnt) SYN beneficiary. [L. *recipiens,* fr. *recipio,* to receive]

**re·cip·i·o·mo·tor** (rē-sip′ē-ō-mō′tŏr) Relating to reception of motor stimuli. [L. *recipio,* to receive, + *motor,* mover]

**re·cip·ro·cal an·chor·age** (rĕ-sip′rŏ-kăl ang′kŏr-ăj) Anchorage in which movement of one tooth (or more) is balanced against movement of one or more opposing teeth.

**re·cip·ro·cal arm** (rĕ-sip′rŏ-kăl ahrm) Clasp arm or other extension used on a removable partial denture to oppose action of some other part or parts of the appliance.

**re·cip·ro·cal clasp** (rĕ-sip′rŏ-kăl klasp) Component of gripping device specifically intended to counter force of an opposing component by engaging a reciprocal guiding plane on same tooth during insertion and removal of partial denture clinically.

**re·cip·ro·cal forces** (rĕ-sip′rŏ-kăl fōr′sĕz) In dentistry, forces whereby resistance of one or more teeth is used to move one or more opposing teeth.

**re·cip·ro·ca·tion** (rĕ-sip′rŏ-kā′shŭn) In prosthodontics, means by which one part of an appliance is made to counter the effect created by another part. [L. *reciprocare,* pp. *reciprocatus,* to move back and forth]

**rec·og·ni·tion time** (rek′ŏg-nish′ŭn tīm) Interval between the application of a stimulus and recognition of its nature.

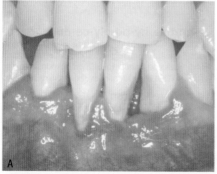 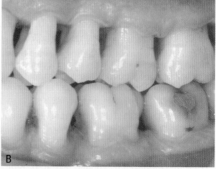

**recession:** gingival margin is significantly apical to cementoenamel junction, which leads to exposure of root surface; (A) gingival recession on facial aspect of three teeth; (B) gingival recession on the facial aspect of posterior teeth

**re·com·bi·nant** (rē-kom′bi-nănt) **1.** Cell or organism that has received genes from different parental strains. **2.** Pertaining to or denoting such organisms.

**re·com·bi·nant de·ox·y·ri·bo·nu·cle·ic ac·id** (rē-kom′bi-nănt dē-oks′ē-rī′bō-nū-klē′ik as′id) Altered DNA resulting from insertion into the chain, by chemical, enzymatic, or biologic means, of a sequence (a whole or partial chain of DNA) not originally (biologically) present in that chain.

**re·com·bi·nant vec·tor** (rē-kom′bi-nănt vek′tŏr) A vector into which foreign DNA has been inserted. SYN vector (5).

**re·con·tour** (rē-kon′tūr) Reshaping a tooth or a restoration to remove marginal excess and to restore natural anatomic form.

**re·con·tour·ing** (rē-kon′tūr-ing) Process of removing metal from the back and toe to restore the curved surfaces of a curette's working-end.

**re·cord** (rek′ŏrd) **1.** In dentistry or medicine, written account that includes a patient's initial complaint(s) and medical history, physical findings, tests results, any therapeutic medicines or procedures or treatment, and subsequent developments during illness. SYN medical record. **2.** In dentistry, registration of desired jaw relations in a plastic material or on a device to permit these relationships to be transferred to an articulator.

**re·cord base** (rek′ŏrd bās) SYN baseplate.

**re·cord·ing** (rē-kōrd′ing) Preserving the results of a study.

**re·cord rim** (rek′ŏrd rim) SYN occlusion rim.

**re·cov·er·y** (rē-kŏv′ĕr-ē) **1.** Recuperation. **2.** Emergence from general anesthesia.

**re·cru·des·cence** (rē′krū-des′ĕns) Resumption of morbid process or symptoms after remission.

**re·crys·tal·li·za·tion tem·per·a·ture** (rē-kris′tăl-ī-zā′shŭn tem′pĕr-ă-chŭr) The lowest level of heat at which the distorted grain structure of a metal is replaced by a strain-free grain structure.

**rec·ti·fi·er** (rek′ti-fī′ĕr) An electronic device for converting alternating to direct voltage, part of the circuitry of an x-ray machine.

**rec·ti·fy** (rek′ti-fī) **1.** To correct. **2.** To purify or refine by distillation; usually implies repeated distillations. [L. *rectus*, right, straight]

**rec·ti·tis** (rek-tī′tis) SYN proctitis.

**rec·to·la·ryn·ge·al re·flex** (rek′tō-lă-rin′jē-ăl rē′fleks) Laryngeal spasm precipitated by stretching the anal sphincter.

**re·cum·bent** (rē-kŭm′bĕnt) Leaning; reclin-

ing; lying down. [L. *recumbo*, to lie back, recline, fr. *re-*, back, + *cubo*, to lie]

**re·cu·per·ate** (rĕ-kū′pĕr-āt) To undergo recovery of or restoration to normal state of health and function. [L. *recupero* (or *recip-*), pp. *-atus*, to take again, recover]

**re·cu·per·a·tion** (rĕ-kū′pĕr-ā′shŭn) Recovery of or restoration to the normal state of health and function.

**re·cur·rence** (rĕ-kŭr′ĕns) **1.** Return of symptoms (recurrent fever). **2.** SYN relapse. [L. *recurro*, to run back, recur]

**re·cur·rent** (rĕ-kŭr′ĕnt) **1.** In anatomy, turning back on itself. **2.** Denoting symptoms or lesions reappearing after remission.

**re·cur·rent aph·thous sto·ma·ti·tis** (rĕ-kŭr′ĕnt af′thŭs stō′mă-tī′tis) SYN aphtha (2).

**re·cur·rent aph·thous ul·cers** (rĕ-kŭr′ĕnt af′thŭs ŭl′sĕrz) SYN aphtha (2).

**▮re·cur·rent ca·ries** (rĕ-kŭr′ĕnt kar′ēz) Caries returning to an area due to inadequate removal of initial decay, usually around or beneath a restoration or new decay at a site where caries has previously occurred. See this page. SYN recurrent decay.

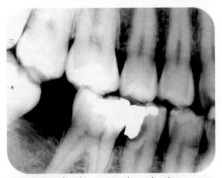

**recurrent caries:** lower premolar and molar

**▮re·cur·rent de·cay** (rĕ-kŭr′ĕnt dĕ-kā′) See this page.

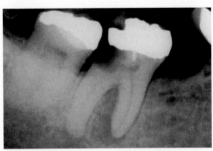

**recurrent decay:** under a metal restoration in a molar

qr

**re·cur·rent her·pet·ic sto·ma·ti·tis** (rĕ-kŭr´ĕnt hĕr-pet´ĭk stō´mă-tī´tis) Reactivation of herpes simplex virus infection, characterized by vesicles and ulceration limited to hard palate and attached gingiva.

**re·cur·rent in·fec·tion** (rĕ-kŭr´ĕnt in-fek´shŭn) Symptomatic reactivation of a latent infection.

**re·cur·rent scar·ring aph·thae** (rĕ-kŭr´ĕnt skahr´ing af´thē) SYN periadenitis mucosa necrotica recurrens.

**re·cur·rent ul·cer·a·tive sto·ma·ti·tis** (rĕ-kŭr´ĕnt ŭl´sĕr-ă-tiv stō´mă-tī´tis) SYN aphtha (2).

**re·cur·ring scar·ring aph·thae** (rĕ-kŭr´ing skahr´ing af´thē) SYN periadenitis mucosa necrotica recurrens.

**red blood cell (RBC, rbc)** (red blŭd sel) SYN erythrocyte.

**red blood cell count** (red blŭd sel kownt) The concentration of erythrocytes in a specimen of whole blood; varies with age, time of day, environmental temperature, and altitude. SYN erythrocyte count.

**red cell** (red sel) SYN erythrocyte.

**red cor·pus·cle** (red kōr´pŭs-ĕl) SYN erythrocyte.

**re·din·te·gra·tion** (rē´din-tĕ-grā´shŭn) **1.** The restoration of lost or injured parts. **2.** Restoration to health. [L. red-integro, pp. -atus, to make whole again, renew, fr. integer, untouched, entire]

**re·dress·ment** (rē-dres´mĕnt) A renewed dressing of a wound.

**re·duced he·ma·tin** (rē-dūst´ hē´mă-tin) SYN heme.

**re·duced in·ter·arch dis·tance** (rē-dūst´ in´tĕr-ahrch´ dis´tăns) Occluding vertical dimension that results in an excessive interocclusal distance when mandible is in rest position, and in a reduced interridge distance when teeth are in contact.

**re·duc·tion de·for·mi·ty** (rē-dŭk´shŭn dĕ-fōrm´i-tē) Congenital absence or attenuation of one or more body parts.

**re·du·pli·ca·tion** (rē-dū´pli-kā´shŭn) **1.** A duplication or doubling, as of the sounds of the heart in certain morbid states. **2.** A fold or duplicature. [L. reduplicatio, fr. re-, again, + duplico, to double, fr. duplex, two-fold]

**re·fec·tion** (rē-fek´shŭn) Restoration to the normal state. [L. refectio, fr. reficere, to restore, fr. re- + facio, to do]

**re·fer·ral** (rĕ-fĕr´ăl) Any health care services that are ordered or arranged.

**re·fer·red pain** (rĕ-fĕrd´ pān) **1.** Pain from deep structures perceived as arising from a surface area remote from its actual origin. **2.** Area where pain is appreciated is innervated by the same spinal segment(s) as the deep structure.

**re·fer·red sen·sa·tion** (rĕ-fĕrd´ sen-sā´shŭn) Sensation perceived in one place in response to a stimulus applied in another.

**re·fine** (rē-fīn´) To free from impurities.

**re·flect** (rē-flekt´) **1.** To bend back. **2.** To throw back, as of radiant energy from a surface. **3.** To meditate; to think over a matter. **4.** To send back a motor impulse in response to a sensory stimulus. [L. re-flecto, pp. -flexus, to bend back]

**re·flec·tion** (rē-flek´shŭn) **1.** The act of reflecting. **2.** That which is reflected. [L. reflexio, a bending back]

**re·flex** (rē´fleks) Involuntary reaction to a stimulus applied to periphery and transmitted to nervous centers in brain or spinal cord. [L. reflexus, pp. of reflecto, to bend back]

**re·flex arc** (rē´fleks ahrk) **1.** Route followed by nerve impulses in production of a reflex act, from peripheral receptor organ through afferent nerve to central nervous system synapse and then through efferent nerve to effector organ. **2.** Neural pathway that involes both peripheral and central nervous systems.

**re·flex ep·i·lep·sy** (rē´fleks ep´i-lep´sē) Seizures that are induced by peripheral stimulation. SYN sensory precipitated epilepsy.

**re·flex·om·e·ter** (rē´fleks-om´ĕ-tĕr) Instrument for measuring force necessary to excite a reflex. [reflex + G. metron, measure]

**re·flex symp·tom** (rē´fleks simp´tŏm) Disturbance of sensation or function in an organ or part more or less remote from morbid condition giving rise to it.

**re·flux** (rē´flŭks) Backward flow of a substance. [L. re-, back, + fluxus, a flow]

**re·flux e·soph·a·gi·tis, pep·tic e·soph·a·gi·tis** (rē´flŭks ĕ-sof´ă-jī´tis, pep´tik) Inflammation of lower esophagus due to regurgitation of acid gastric contents, usually due to malfunction of lower esophageal sphincter; symptoms include substernal pain, "heartburn," and regurgitation of acid.

**re·frac·to·ry** (rĕ-frak´tŏr-ē) Resistant to treatment, as of a disease. [L. refractarius, fr. refringo, pp. -fractus, to break in pieces]

**re·frac·to·ry cast** (rĕ-frak´tŏr-ē kast) Cast made of material that will withstand high temperatures of metal casting or soldering without disintegrating. SYN investment cast.

**re·frac·to·ry flask** (rĕ-frak´tŏr-ē flask) Metal tube in which a refractory mold is made for casting metal dental restorations or appliances.

**re·frac·to·ry in·vest·ment** (rĕ-frak´tŏr-ē in-vest´mĕnt) Investment material that can withstand high temperatures used in soldering or casting.

**re·frac·to·ry pe·ri·od** (rē-frak´tŏr-ē pēr´ē-ŏd) Duration following effective stimulation, during which excitable tissue fails to respond to a stimulus.

**re·frac·to·ry per·i·o·don·ti·tis** (rĕ-frak´ tŏr-ē per´ē-ō-don-tī´tis) Clinical attachment loss despite optimal subgingival débridement and performance of acceptable oral hygiene.

**re·frac·to·ry state** (rĕ-frak´tŏr-ē stāt) Subnormal excitability immediately following response to previous excitation; divided into absolute and relative phases.

**re·frig·er·ant** (rĕ-frij´ĕr-ănt) 1. Cooling; reducing slight fever. 2. Agent that gives a sensation of coolness or relieves feverishness.

**re·gain·er** (rē-gān´ĕr) Appliance used to attempt to regain space in dental arches.

**re·gen·er·a·tion** (rē-jen´ĕr-ā´shŭn) Reproduction or reconstitution of a lost or injured part. [L. *regeneratio*]

**reg·i·men** (rej´i-mĕn) A program, including pharmacotherapy, which regulates aspects of one's lifestyle for a hygienic or therapeutic purpose; a program of treatment. [L. direction, rule]

**re·gion** (rē´jŭn) [TA] 1. An often arbitrarily limited portion of a body surface. 2. Portion of body with special nervous or vascular supply, or organ part with special function. SEE ALSO area, space, zone. [L. *regio*]

**re·gion·al** (rē´jŭn-ăl) Relating to a region.

**re·gion·al an·es·the·si·a** (rē´jŭn-ăl an´es-thē´zē-ă) Use of local anesthetic solution(s) to produce circumscribed areas of loss of sensation.

**re·gion·al per·fu·sion** (rē´jŏn-ăl pĕr-fyū´zhŭn) Perfusion of a body part, especially a limb, and particularly with chemotherapeutic agents, to treat a primary, recurrent, or metastatic malignant tumor.

**reg·is·ter·ed den·tal hy·gien·ist (RDH)** (rej´i-stĕrd den´tăl hī-jē´nist) Health care professional who specializes in the cleaning and care of the oral cavity.

**reg·is·ter·ed nurse (RN)** (rej´i-stĕrd nŭrs) A health care professional who has graduated from an accredited nursing program and been licensed by public authority to practice nursing.

**reg·is·tra·tion** (rej´is-trā´shŭn) In dentistry, a record.

**re·gres·sion** (rĕ-gresh´ŭn) 1. Subsidence of symptoms. 2. Relapse; return of symptoms. 3. Any retrograde movement or action. [L. *regredior*, pp. *-gressus*, to go back]

**re·gres·sion a·nal·y·sis** (rĕ-gresh´ŭn ă-nal´i-sis) The statistical method of finding the "best" mathematic model to describe one variable as a function of another.

**reg·u·la·ted waste** (reg´yū-lā-tĕd wāst) Refuse, often contaminated with infectious materials, which must be discarded according to specified regulations and guidelines.

**re·gur·gi·tate** (rē-gŭr´ji-tāt) 1. To flow backward. 2. To expel stomach contents in small amounts, short of vomiting. [L. *re-*, back, + *gurgito*, pp. *-atus*, to flood, fr. *gurges* (gurgit-), a whirlpool]

**re·gur·gi·ta·tion** (rē-gŭr´ji-tā´shŭn) 1. A backward flow. 2. Return of gas or small amounts of food from the stomach. [L. *regurgitatio*]

**re·ha·bil·i·ta·tion** (rē´hă-bil´i-tā´shŭn) Restoration, following disease, illness, or injury, of the ability to function in a normal or near-normal manner. [L. *rehabilitare*, pp. *-tatus*, to make fit, fr. *re-* + *habilitas*, ability]

**Rei·chert car·ti·lage** (rī´kĕrt kahr´ti-lăj) SYN second pharyngeal arch cartilage.

**re·in·forced an·chor·age** (rē´in-fōrst´ ang´kŏr-ăj) SYN multiple anchorage.

**qr**

**re·in·force·ment** (rē´in-fōrs´mĕnt) In dentistry, structural addition or inclusion used to give additional strength in function; e.g., bars in plastic denture base.

**Rei·ter syn·drome** (rī´ter sin´drōm) The association of urethritis, iridocyclitis, mucocutaneous lesions, and arthritis, sometimes with diarrhe; thought to represent an abnormal host response to infectious agents.

**re·lapse** (rē´laps) Return of disease manifestations after improvement. SYN recurrence (2). [L. *re-labor*, pp. *-lapsus*, to slide back]

**re·lap·sing fe·brile nod·u·lar non·sup·pur·a·tive pan·ni·cu·li·tis** (rē-lap´ sing feb´ril nod´yū-lăr non´sŭp´yŭr-ă-tiv pă-nik´ yū-lī´tis) Nodular fat necrosis of a variety of possible causes. SYN Christian disease (2), Christian syndrome, Weber-Christian disease.

**re·la·tion** (rĕ-lā´shŭn) In dentistry, the mode of contact of teeth or the positional relationship of oral structures. [L. *relatio*, a bringing back]

**re·la·tion·al thresh·old** (rĕ-lā´shŭn-ăl thresh´ōld) Smallest degree of difference between two stimuli that permits them to be perceived as different.

**re·la·tion·ship** (rĕ-lā´shŭn-ship) The state of being related, associated, or connected.

**rel·a·tive den·tin a·bra·siv·i·ty in·dex (RDA)** (rel´ă-tiv den´tin ă-brā-siv´ĭ-tē in´deks) A scale that is used to assess the abrasivity of a dentifrice.

**rel·a·tive hu·mid·i·ty** (rel´ă-tiv hyū-mid´ĭ-tē) Actual amount of water vapor present in air or gas, divided by amount necessary for saturation at same temperature and pressure; expressed as a percentage.

**rel·a·tive mo·lec·u·lar mass** (rel´ă-tiv mŏ-lek´yū-lăr mas) SYN molecular weight.

**rel·a·tive pol·y·cy·the·mi·a** (rel´ă-tiv pol´ē-sī-thē´mē-ă) A relative increase in the number of red blood cells as a result of loss of the fluid portion of the blood.

**re·lax·ant** (rĕ-lak´sănt) 1. Relaxing; reducing tension. 2. An agent that reduces muscular tension or produces skeletal muscle paralysis.

**re·lax·a·tion** (rē´lak-sā´shŭn) Loosening, lengthening, or lessening of tension in a muscle.

**re·li·a·bil·i·ty** (rĕ-lī´ă-bil´i-tē) Degree of stability exhibited when a measurement is repeated under identical conditions. SEE correlation coefficient. [M.E. *relien,* fr. O.Fr. *relier,* fr. L. *religo,* to bind]

**re·lief** (rĕ-lēf´) 1. In dentistry, reduction or elimination of pressure from a specific area under a denture base. 2. Removal of pain or distress, physical or mental.

**re·lief a·re·a** (rĕ-lēf´ ar´ē-ă) In dentistry, portion of denture-bearing area over which denture base is altered to reduce functional pressure.

**re·lief cham·ber** (rĕ-lēf´ chăm´bĕr) Recess in impression surface of a denture to reduce pressure from that oral area.

**re·lieve** (rĕ-lēv´) To free wholly or partly from pain or discomfort, either physical or mental. [through O. Fr. fr. L. *re-levo,* to lift up, lighten]

**re·line** (rē´līn) In dentistry, to resurface tissue side of a denture with new base material to make it fit more accurately. SEE ALSO rebase.

**REM** Acronym for rapid eye movements; reticular erythematous mucinosis.

**rem** Abbreviation for roentgen-equivalent-man.

**re·me·di·a·ble** (rĕ-mē´dē-ă-bĕl) Curable. [L. *remediabilis,* fr. *remedio,* to cure]

**re·me·di·al** (rĕ-mē´dē-ăl) Curative; acting to cure disease or alleviate symptoms.

**re·min·er·al·i·za·tion** (rē-min´ĕr-ăl-ī-zā´shŭn) 1. In dentistry, process enhanced by presence of fluoride whereby partially decalcified enamel, dentin, and cementum become recalcified by mineral replacement. 2. Return to body or area of necessary mineral constituents lost through disease or dietary deficiencies.

**re·mis·sion** (rĕ-mish´ŭn) 1. Abatement or lessening in severity of disease symptoms. 2. Period during which such abatement occurs. [L. *remissio,* fr. *re-mitto,* pp. *-missus,* to send back, slacken, relax]

**re·mit** (rē-mit´) To become less severe for a time without absolutely ceasing.

**re·mit·tent** (rĕ-mit´ĕnt) Characterized by temporary periods of abatement of the symptoms of a disease.

**re·mov·a·ble bridge** (rē-mūv´ă-bĕl brij) SYN removable partial denture.

🔲**re·mov·a·ble par·tial den·ture** (rĕ-mūv´ă-bĕl pahr´shăl den´chŭr) Appliance that supplies teeth and associated structures on a partially edentulous jaw and that can be readily removed from the mouth. See this page. SYN removable bridge.

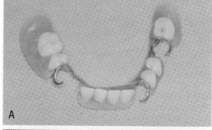

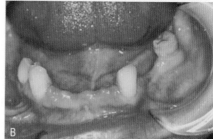

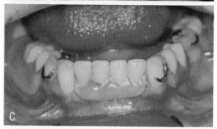

**removable partial denture:** (A) removable partial denture; (B) patient without denture in place; (C) with denture in place

**re·mov·a·ble space main·tain·er** (rĕ-mūv´ă-bĕl spās mān-tā´nĕr) Any such device easily removable by the patient.

**re·nal** (rē´năl) SYN nephric.

**re·nal col·ic** (rē'năl kol'ik) Severe colicky pain caused by impaction or passage of dental calculus in the ureter or renal pelvis.

**re·nal fail·ure** (rē'năl fāl'yŭr) Impairment of renal function, either acute or chronic, with retention of urea, creatinine, and other waste products. SYN kidney failure.

**re·nal rick·ets** (rē'năl rik'ĕts) Form in children due to renal disease with hyperphosphatemia. SYN pseudorickets.

**Re·o·vi·rus** (rē'ō-vī'rŭs) A genus of viruses recovered from children suffering mild fever and sometimes diarrhea but also from children with no apparent infection; a causative relationship to illness has not been proven.

**re·pair** (rē-pār') Restoration of diseased or damaged tissues naturally, by healing processes, or artificially, as by surgical means. [M.E., fr. O.Fr., fr. L. *re-paro*, fr. *re-*, back, again, + *paro*, prepare, put in order]

**re·par·a·tive den·tin** (rep'ăr-ă-tiv den'tin) SYN tertiary dentin.

**re·pe·ti·tive strain dis·or·der** (rĕ-pet'i-tiv strān dis-ōr'dĕr) SYN cumulative trauma disorder.

**re·place·ment ther·a·py** (rē-plās'mĕnt thār'ă-pē) Treatment designed to compensate for lack or deficiency arising from inadequate nutrition, from dysfunctions or losses.

**re·plan·ta·tion** (rē'plan-tā'shŭn) Replacement of an organ or part in its original site. [L. *re-*, again, + *planto*, pp. *-atus*, to plant, fr. *planta*, a sprout, slip]

**re·ple·tion** (rē-plē'shŭn) 1. SYN hypervolemia. 2. SYN plethora (2). [L. *repletio*, fr. *re-pleo*, pp. *-pletus*, to fill up]

**rep·li·cate** (rep'li-kăt, -kāt) 1. One of several identical processes or observations. 2. To repeat; to produce an exact copy.

**re·port·a·ble dis·ease** (rē-pōrt'ă-bĕl di-zēz') SYN notifiable disease.

**re·press·ed** (rē-prest') Subjected to repression.

**re·pres·sion** (rē-presh'ŭn) 1. In psychotherapy, the active process or defense mechanism of keeping out and ejecting and banishing from consciousness those ideas or impulses that are unacceptable to the ego or superego. 2. Decreased expression of some gene product. [L. *re-primo*, pp. *-pressus*, to press back, repress]

**re·pres·sor** (rē-pres'ŏr) The product of a regulator or repressor gene.

**re·pres·sor gene** (rē-pres'ŏr jēn) Gene that prevents a nonallele from being transcribed.

**re·pro·duc·tion** (rē'prō-dŭk'shŭn) 1. The total process by which organisms produce offspring. 2. The recall and presentation in the mind of the elements of a former impression. [L. *re-*, again, + *pro-duco*, pp. *-ductus*, to lead forth, produce]

**re·pro·duc·tive as·sim·i·la·tion** (rē'prŏ-dŭk'tiv ă-sim'i-lā'shŭn) In sensorimotor theory, an active cognitive process by which past experience is applied to novel situations.

**re·pul·sion** (rĕ-pŭl'shŭn) 1. The act of repelling or driving apart, in contrast to attraction. 2. Strong dislike; aversion; repugnance. 3. Coupling phase of genes at linked loci that are borne on opposite chromosomes. [L. *re-pello*, pp. *-pulsus*, to drive back]

**re·quired arch length** (rĕ-kwīrd' ahrch length) Sum of the mesiodistal widths of the permanent teeth from first permanent molar to first permanent molar.

**res·cue breath·ing** (res'kyū brēdh'ing) SYN head-tilt/chin-lift maneuver.

**re·search** (rē'sĕrch, rē-sĕrch') 1. The organized quest for new knowledge and better understanding. 2. To conduct a scientific inquiry.

**re·sec·tion** (rē-sek'shŭn) 1. A procedure performed for the specific purpose of removal of a significant part of an organ or bodily structure; may be partial or complete. 2. To remove a part. 3. SYN excision (1).

**re·serve** (rē-zĕrv') Something available but held back for later use.

**re·serve air** (rē-zĕrv' ār) SYN expiratory reserve volume.

**re·serve tooth germ** (rē-zĕrv' tūth jĕrm) Enamel organ and papilla of a permanent tooth.

**res·er·voir bag** (rez'ĕr-vwahr bag) SYN breathing bag.

**res·i·dent** (rez'i-dĕnt) A house officer attached to a hospital for clinical training. SYN resident physician. [L. *resideo*, to reside]

**re·sid·u·al** (rē-zid'yū-ăl) Relating to or of the nature of a residue.

**re·sid·u·al ca·pa·ci·ty** (rē-zid'yū-ăl kă-pas'i-tē) SYN residual volume.

**re·si·du·al cyst** (rē-zid'yū-ăl sist) Persistence of an apical periodontal cyst that remains after tooth extraction.

**re·sid·u·al ridge** (rē-zid'yū-ăl rij) Remnant of the alveolar ridge after tooth extraction; resorbs over time in the absence of teeth.

**re·sid·u·al vol·ume (RV)** (rē-zid'yū-ăl vol' yūm) The volume of air remaining in the lungs after a maximal expiration. SYN residual capacity.

**res·i·due** (rez'i-dū) That which remains after

removal of one or more substances. [L. *re-siduum*]

**re·sil·i·ence** (rē-zil'yĕns) 1. Springiness or elasticity. 2. Energy (per unit of volume) released on unloading. [L. *resilio,* to spring back, rebound]

**res·in** (rez'in) 1. An amorphous, brittle substance consisting of hardened secretion of various plants, probably derived from a volatile oil and similar to a stearoptene. 2. Broad term for organic substances insoluble in water. 3. A precipitate formed by the addition of water to certain tinctures. [L. *resina*]

**re·sin ce·ment** (rez'in sĕ-ment') Monomer or monomer/polymer system used as a dental luting agent; used in cementation of restorations or orthodontic brackets to teeth.

**res·in·ous** (rez'i-nŭs) Relating to or derived from a resin.

**res ip·sa lo·qui·tur** (res ip'să lō'kwi-tŭr) Latin meaning the thing speaks for itself. [L.]

**re·sis·tance** (rĕ-zis'tăns) 1. Force exerted in opposition to an active force. 2. Opposition to flow of a fluid through one or more passageways. 3. Ability of an organism to maintain its immunity to or to oppose effects of an antagonistic agent. [L. *re-sisto,* to stand back, withstand]

**re·sis·tance form** (rĕ-zis'tăns fōrm) Shape given to a cavity preparation that enables dental restoration to withstand masticatory forces.

**re·sis·tin** (rē-zis'tin) Cytokine secreted by adipocytes into the circulation; causes resistance of peripheral tissues to insulin; possible link between obesity and Type 2 diabetes mellitus.

**res·o·lu·tion** (rez'ŏ-lū'shŭn) 1. The arrest of an inflammatory process without suppuration. 2. The optic ability to distinguish detail. SYN resolving power (3). [L. *resolutio,* a slackening, fr. *re-solvo* pp. *-solutus,* to loosen, relax]

**re·solv·ing pow·er** (re'-zolv'ing pow'ĕr) 1. Definition of a lens. 2. SYN resolution (2).

**res·o·nance** (rez'ŏ-năns) 1. In chemistry, the manner in which electrons or electric charges are distributed among the atoms in compounds. 2. Sympathetic or forced vibration of air in cavities above, below, in front of, or behind a source of sound. 3. Sound obtained on percussion of a body part. 4. Intensification and hollow character of voice sound obtained on auscultation over a cavity. [L. *resonantia,* echo, fr. *re-sono,* to resound, to echo]

**re·sor·ci·nol** (rē-zōr'si-nol) A dermal antiseptic.

**re·sorp·tion** (rē-sōrp'shŭn) Loss of substance by lysis, or by physiologic or pathologic means.

**re·sorp·tion la·cu·na,** pl. **re·sorp·tion la·cu·nae** (rē-sōrp'shŭn lă-kū'nă, -nē) SYN Howship lacuna.

**res·pir·a·ble** (res'pir-ă-bĕl) Capable of being breathed.

**re·spir·a·ble aer·o·sols** (res'pir-ă-bĕl ar'ŏ-solz) Aerosols with an aerodynamic size less than 10 mcm.

**res·pi·ra·tion** (res'pir-ā'shŭn) 1. Fundamental process of life, characteristic of both plants and animals, in which oxygen is used to oxidize organic fuel molecules, providing a source of energy as well as carbon dioxide and water. In green plants, photosynthesis is not considered respiration 2. SYN ventilation (2). [L. *respiratio,* fr. *re spiro,* pp. *-atus,* to exhale, breathe]

**res·pi·ra·tor** (res'pir-ā'tŏr) 1. An apparatus for administering artificial respiration in cases of respiratory failure. SYN ventilator. 2. An appliance fitting over the mouth and nose, used to exclude dust, smoke, or other irritants, or of otherwise altering air before it enters respiratory passages. SYN inhaler (1).

**res·pi·ra·to·ry** (res'pir-ă-tōr-ē) Relating to respiration.

**res·pi·ra·to·ry ac·i·do·sis** (res'pir-ă-tōr-ē as'i-dō'sis) Acidosis caused by retention of carbon dioxide. SYN hypercapnic acidosis.

**res·pi·ra·to·ry al·ka·lo·sis** (res'pir-ă-tōr-ē al'kă-lō'sis) Alkalosis resulting from an abnormal loss of $CO_2$ produced by hyperventilation, either active or passive, with concomitant reduction in arterial bicarbonate concentration.

**res·pi·ra·to·ry ca·pac·i·ty** (res'pir-ă-tōr-ē kă-pas'i-tē) SYN vital capacity.

**res·pi·ra·to·ry care** (res'pir-ă-tōr-ē kār) Adjunctive form of health care intended to maintain or restore optimal respiratory function through the use of appropriate devices and techniques; includes diagnostic testing and monitoring, patient education, therapy, and rehabilitation.

**res·pi·ra·to·ry dis·turb·ance in·dex** (res'pir-ă-tōr-ē dis-tŭr'băns in'deks) A calculation of the average number of incidents of hypopnea and apnea per hour of sleep, as measured by polysomnography. SYN apnea-hypopnea index.

**res·pi·ra·tory fail·ure** (res'pir-ă-tōr-ē fāl'yŭr) Loss of pulmonary function, either acute or chronic; final common pathway for myriad respiratory disorders.

**res·pi·ra·to·ry fre·quen·cy** (res'pir-ă-tōr-ē frē'kwĕn-sē) Number of breaths per minute.

**res·pi·ra·to·ry in·suf·fi·cien·cy** (res'pir-ă-tōr-ē in-sŭ-fish'ĕn-sē) Failure to provide adequate oxygen to cells of body and to remove excess carbon dioxide from them.

**res·pi·ra·to·ry pause** (res′pir-ă-tōr-ē pawz) Cessation of air flow for less than 10 seconds.

**res·pi·ra·tory rate** (res′pir-ă-tōr-ē rāt) Frequency of breathing, recorded as number of breaths per minute.

**res·pi·ra·to·ry ther·a·py** (res′pir-ă-tōr-ē thār′ă-pē) SEE respiratory care.

**res·pi·ra·to·ry tract** (res′pir-ă-tōr-ē trakt) The air passages from the nose to the pulmonary alveoli.

**re·spire** (rĕ-spīr′) 1. To breathe. 2. To consume oxygen and produce carbon dioxide by metabolism. [L. *respiro,* to breathe]

**res·pi·rom·e·ter** (res′pir-om′ĕ-tŏr) 1. An instrument for measuring extent of respiratory movements. 2. An instrument to gauge oxygen consumption or carbon dioxide production. [L. *respiro,* to breathe, + G. *metron,* measure]

**re·sponse** (rĕ-spons′) 1. Reaction of a muscle, nerve, gland, or other excitable tissue to a stimulus. 2. Any act or behavior or its constituents that a living organism is capable of emitting. [L. *responsus,* an answer]

**re·sponse di·ag·no·sis** (rĕ-spons′ dī-ăg-nō′sis) Diagnosis made at a reevaluation at some point after treatment.

**rest** (rest) Rigid stabilizing occlusion of fixed or removable partial denture that contacts remaining tooth or teeth; prevents movement toward mucosa and transmits functional forces to teeth. [A.S. *raest*]

**rest a·re·a** (rest ar′ē-ă) Portion of tooth structure or restoration in a tooth that is prepared to receive positive seating of metallic occlusal, incisal, lingual, or cingulum rest of a removable prosthesis.

**rest bite** (rest bīt) Misnomer for physiologic rest position of mandible (q.v.).

**rest·ing en·er·gy ex·pen·di·ture** (rest′ing en′ĕr-jē eks-pen′di-chŭr) Energy expenditure measured under resting, although not necessarily basal conditions. Cf. basal metabolic rate.

**rest·ing sa·li·va** (rest′ing să-lī′vă) Saliva found in mouth in intervals of food consumption and mastication.

**rest·less legs syn·drome** (rest′lĕs legz sin′drōm) Combined uneasiness, twitching, aching, or agitation that occurs in the legs after going to bed, frequently leading to insomnia, which may be relieved temporarily by walking about.

■**res·to·ra·tion** (res′tŏr-ā′shŭn) 1. In dentistry, prosthetic restoration or appliance; broad term applied to any inlay, crown, bridge, partial denture, or complete denture that restores or replaces lost tooth structure, teeth, or oral tissues.

2. A plug or stopper; any substance (e.g., gold, amalgam) used for restoring missing portion of a tooth as a result of removing decay in tooth. See page 494. [L. *restauro,* pp. *-atus,* to restore, to repair]

**re·stor·a·tive** (rĕ-stōr′ă-tiv) Colloq. term for restorative dentistry, pertaining to placement of restorative materials into cavity preparations to return the affected tooth to good health and restore proper function. [L. *restauro,* to restore]

**re·stor·a·tive den·tal ma·te·ri·als** (rĕ-stōr′ă-tiv den′tăl mă-tēr′ē-ălz) Materials used to replace oral tissues in dentistry; e.g., amalgam, gold alloys, cements, porcelain, plastics, and denture materials.

**re·stor·a·tive den·tis·try** (rĕ-stōr′ă-tiv den′tis-trē) Individual restoration of teeth by means of amalgam, synthetic porcelainlike materials, resins, or inlays.

**rest po·si·tion** (rest pŏ-zish′ŏn) The usual position of the mandible when the patient is resting comfortably in an upright position and the condyles are in a neutral, unstrained position in the mandibular fossa. SYN physiologic rest position, postural position, postural resting position.

**re·strain·ed beam** (rĕ-strānd′ bēm) In dentistry, beam with two or more supports, at least one of which permits some freedom of rotation to point of support but not as much as if it were a free support.

**rest re·la·tion** (rest rĕ-lā′shŭn) Postural relation of mandible to maxillae when patient is resting comfortably in upright position and condyles are in a neutral unstrained position in glenoid fossa. SYN unstrained jaw relation.

**rest ver·ti·cal di·men·sion** (rest vĕr′ti-kăl di-men′shŭn) Facial measurement with jaws in rest relation; a *decrease* may or may not accompany decrease in occlusal vertical dimension; may occur without a decrease in occlusal vertical dimension in patients with a preponderant activity of jaw-closing musculature, as in patients with muscular hypertenseness or in long-term gum chewers; *increase* may or may not accompany an increase in occlusal vertical dimension; sometimes occurs after removal of remaining occlusal contacts, perhaps as a result of the removal of noxious reflex stimuli.

■**re·tain·er** (rē-tā′nĕr) 1. Any type of clasp, attachment, or device used to fixate or stabilize a prosthesis. 2. Appliance used to prevent shifting of teeth after orthodontic treatment. See page 494.

**re·tar·da·tion** (rē′tahr-dā′shŭn) 1. Slowness or limitation of development. 2. An impairment associated with cognitive development.

**re·tard·ed den·ti·tion** (rĕ-tahrd′ĕd den-tish′ŭn) Dentition in which growth phenomena such as calcification, elongation, and eruption occur later than average range of normal varia-

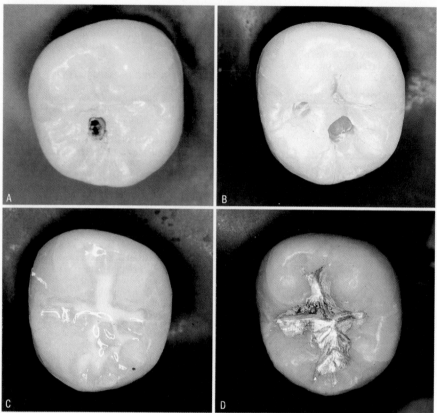

**caries:** (A) molar with decay in several pits; (B) decay removed and central groove opened; (C) restoration using preventive resin; (D) preventive resin restoration has been removed and restored with conventional cavity preparation and amalgam; note amount of tooth structure conserved by preventive resin restoration

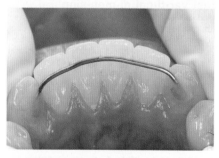

**orthodontic fixed lingual retainer**

tion due to some systemic metabolic dysfunction (e.g., hypothyroidism).

**re·tard·er** (rĕ-tahr´dĕr) An agent used to slow chemical hardening of gypsum, resins, or impression materials used in dentistry.

**retch·ing** (rech´ing) Gastric and esophageal movements of vomiting without expulsion of vomitus. SYN vomiturition.

**re·ten·tion** (rē-ten´shŭn) **1.** In dentistry, passive period following treatment when a patient is wearing an appliance or appliances to maintain or stabilize teeth in the new position into which they have been moved. **2.** Resistance to dislodgement. [L. *retentio,* a holding back]

**re·ten·tion a·re·a** (rē-ten´shŭn ar´ē-ă) Tooth area provided during its preparation for restoration that will aid in holding restoration in place.

**re·ten·tion arm** (rē-ten´shŭn ahrm) Portion of a removable partial denture clasp that engages a retentive area of the tooth and provides resistance to displacement of the prosthesis. SYN retentive arm.

**re·ten·tion form** (rē-ten´shŭn fōrm) Shape of a cavity preparation that prevents displacement of dental restoration by lateral or tipping forces as well as masticatory forces.

**re·ten·tion groove** (rē-ten´shŭn grūv) Striatum forming opposing vertical constrictions in a tooth to aid in retention of a dental restoration.

**re·ten·tion jaun·dice** (rē-ten´shŭn jawn´

dis) Hepatic disorder due to insufficiency of liver function or to an excess of bile pigment production.

**re·ten·tion pin** (rē-ten′shŭn pin) One or more metal pins projecting from a cast restoration to enhance retention by being inserted in one or more parallel holes in dentin.

**re·ten·tion point** (rē-ten′shŭn poynt) Provision made within a tooth cavity preparation to hold in place the first pieces of gold when placing a direct gold restoration.

**re·ten·tive arm** (rē-ten′tiv ahrm) Flexible segment of a removable partial denture that engages an undercut on an abutment and is designed to retain denture. SYN retention arm.

**re·ten·tive cir·cum·fer·en·tial clasp arm** (rē-ten′tiv sĭr-kŭm′fĕr-en′shăl klasp ahrm) Arm that is flexible and that engages infrabulge at terminal end of itself.

**re·ten·tive clasp** (rē-ten′tiv klasp) Gripping device on a removable partial denture with a flexible segment to engage undercuts of abutment tooth to help retain prosthesis.

**re·ten·tive ful·crum line** (rē-ten′tiv ful′ krŭm līn) 1. Imaginary line connecting retentive points of clasp arms on retaining teeth adjacent to mucosa-borne denture bases. 2. Imaginary line connecting retentive points of clasp arms, around which line the denture tends to rotate when subjected to forces such as the pull of sticky foods.

**re·ten·tive un·der·cut** (rē-ten′tiv ŭn′dĕr-kŭt) The area of an abutment tooth surface suitable for placing a clasp to retain a removable prosthesis.

**re·tic·u·lat·ed bone** (rĕ-tik′yū-lāt′ĕd bōn) SYN woven bone.

**re·tic·u·lo·cyte** (rĕ-tik′yū-lō-sīt) A young erythrocyte that contains no nucleus but has residual RNA. [reticulo- + G. kytos, cell]

**re·tic·u·lo·cyte pro·duc·tion in·dex** (rĕ-tik′yū-lō-sīt prŏ-dŭk′shŭn in′deks) A calculated value that indicates bone marrow response in anemia.

**re·tic·u·lo·sis** (rĕ-tik′yū-lō′sis) An increase in histiocytes, monocytes, or other reticuloendothelial elements. [reticulo- + G. -osis, condition]

**ret·i·na** (ret′i-nă) [TA] Grossly, section of eye that consists of three parts: optic, ciliary, and iridial. The optic part, the physiologic portion that receives the visual light rays, is further divided into two parts, the pigmented part (pigment epithelium) and the nervous part. [Mediev. L. prob. fr. L. rete, a net]

**ret·i·nal de·tach·ment, de·tach·ment of ret·i·na** (ret′i-năl dĕ-tach′mĕnt, ret′i-nă) Loss of apposition between the sensory retina and the retinal pigment epithelium.

**ret·i·ni·tis** (ret′i-nī′tis) Inflammation of retina. [retina + G. -itis, inflammation]

**ret·i·no·blas·to·ma** (ret′i-nō-blas-tō′mă) Malignant ocular neoplasm of childhood. [retino- + G. blastos, germ, + -oma, tumor]

**ret·i·no·ic ac·id** (ret′i-nō′ik as′id) Agent used topically to treat acne. SYN vitamin A1 acid.

**ret·i·noids** (ret′i-noydz) Keratolytic drugs used to treat severe acne and psoriasis.

**ret·i·nop·a·thy** (ret′i-nop′ă-thē) Noninflammatory degenerative disease of the retina. [Med. L. fr. L. rete, net + G. pathos, suffering]

**re·trac·tion** (rĕ-trak′shŭn) 1. Posterior movement of teeth, usually with aid of an orthodontic appliance. 2. A shrinking, drawing back, or pulling apart. See this page. [L. retractio, a drawing back]

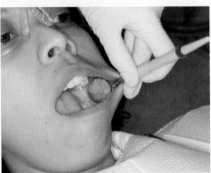

**retraction:** dental mirror is used to retract buccal mucosa away from facial surface of maxillary left posterior teeth and also to view tooth surfaces indirectly

**re·trac·tor** (rē-trak′tŏr) 1. An instrument for drawing aside wound edges or holding back structures adjacent to operative field. 2. Muscle that draws a body part backward, e.g., middle part of trapezius muscle is a retractor of the scapula; horizontal fibers of temporalis muscle serve to retract the mandible.

**re·trad** (rē′trad) Backward; toward back part; directed posteriorly. [L. retro, backward, + ad, to]

**ret·ro·buc·cal** (ret′rō-buk′ăl) Relating to back part of, or behind, cheek.

**ret·ro·bul·bar neu·ri·tis** (ret′rō-bŭl′bahr nūr-ī′tis) Optic neuritis without swelling of optic disc.

**ret·ro·ces·sion** (ret′rō-sesh′ŭn) 1. A going back; relapse. 2. Cessation of external symptoms of disease followed by signs of involvement of some internal organ or part. [L. retrocedo, pp. -cessus, to go back, retire]

**ret·ro·cli·na·tion** (ret′rō-kli-nā′shŭn) The long axis orientation of teeth such that they are

qr

angled posteriorly and the incisal edge is posterior to the root apex.

**ret·ro·co·chle·ar hear·ing loss** (ret′rō-kok′lē-ăr hĕr′ing laws) Term for sensorineural hearing impairment.

**ret·ro·col·lic** (ret′rō-kol′ik) Relating to back of neck; drawing back the head. [*retro-* + L. *collum,* neck]

■**ret·ro·cus·pid pa·pil·la** (ret′rō-kŭs′pid pă-pil′ă) Small tissue tag located on mandibular gingiva lingual to cuspid teeth; usually occurs bilaterally, is more commonly identified in children, and is considered a normal anatomic structure. See this page.

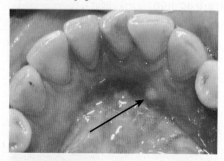

retrocuspid papilla

**ret·ro·fill·ing** (ret′rō-fil′ing) Putting sealant into apical foramen of dental root from apical end.

**ret·ro·gnath·ic** (ret′rog-nath′ik) Denoting a state in which mandible is located behind its normal position in relation to maxillae.

**ret·ro·gnath·ism** (ret-rog′nă-thizm) Condition of facial disharmony in which one or both jaws are posterior to normal in their craniofacial relationships. [*retro-,* back + G. *gnathos,* jaw]

**ret·ro·grade** (ret′rō-grād) 1. Moving backward. 2. Degenerating; reversing the normal order of growth and development. [L. *retrogradus,* fr. *retro-,* back + *gradior,* to go]

**ret·ro·lin·gual** (ret′rō-ling′gwăl) Relating to back part of tongue; posterior to tongue. [*retro-,* back + L. *lingua,* tongue]

**ret·ro·man·dib·u·lar** (ret′rō-man-dib′yū-lăr) Posterior to lower jaw. [*retro-,* back + L. *mandibula,* lower jaw]

**ret·ro·man·dib·u·lar fos·sa** (ret′rō-man-dib′yū-lăr fos′ă) Depression inferior to auricle and posterior to ramus and angle of mandible.

**ret·ro·man·dib·u·lar vein** (ret′rō-man-dib′yū-lăr vān) [TA] Vein formed by union of superficial temporal and maxillary veins in front of ear; runs posterior to ramus of mandible through parotid gland, and unites with posterior auricular vein to form external jugular vein; usually has a large communicating branch with the facial vein.

**ret·ro·mas·toid** (ret′rō-mas′toyd) Posterior to mastoid process.

**ret·ro·mo·lar** (ret′rō-mō′lăr) Distal (or posterior) to last erupted (or present) molar tooth.

**ret·ro·mo·lar fos·sa** (ret′rō-mō′lăr fos′ă) [TA] Triangular depression in mandible posterior to third molar tooth.

**ret·ro·mo·lar pad** (ret′rō-mō′lăr pad) Tissue mass, posterior to prior location of third molars on mandible; posterior limit of removable denture. SYN pear-shaped area, pear-shaped pad.

**ret·ro·mo·lar tri·an·gle** (ret′rō-mō′lăr trī′ang-gĕl) [TA] Three-cornered area posterior to third mandibular molar tooth.

**ret·ro·my·lo·hy·oid space** (ret′rō-mī-lō-hī′oyd spās) Sulcus at posterior end of the mylohyoid line.

**ret·ro·na·sal** (ret′rō-nā′zăl) Posterior nasal; relating to posterior nares.

**ret·ro·pha·ryn·ge·al** (ret′rō-fă-rin′jē-ăl) Posterior to pharynx.

**ret·ro·pha·ryn·ge·al lymph nodes** (ret′rō-fă-rin′jē-ăl limf nōdz) [TA] Three groups of lymph nodes located between pharynx and prevertebral layer of cervical fascia.

**ret·ro·pha·ryn·ge·al space** (re′trō-fă-rin′jē-ăl spās) [TA] Part of peripharyngeal spatium located posterior to pharynx.

**ret·ro·phar·ynx** (ret′rō-far′ingks) Posterior part of pharynx.

**ret·ro·ver·sion** (ret′rō-vĕr′zhŭn) Condition in which the teeth are located in a more posterior position than normal. [*retro-,* back + L. *verto,* pp. *versus,* to turn]

**ret·ro·vi·rus** (ret′rō-vī′rŭs) Any virus of the family Retroviridae. A virus with RNA core genetic material; requires the enzyme reverse transcriptase to convert its RNA into proviral DNA.

**re·trud·ed con·tact po·si·tion** (rĕ-trū′dĕd kon′takt pŏ-zish′ŭn) Guided position of the teeth in which the mandible is located with the condyles in the most retruded position in the fossae.

**re·tru·sion** (rĕ-trū′zhŭn) 1. Retraction of mandible from any given point. 2. Backward movement of mandible. [L. *re-trudo,* pp. *-trusus,* to push back]

**re·tru·sive ex·cur·sion** (rĕ-trū′siv eks-kŭr′zhŭn) Slight backward and return movement of mandible between position of closure and a slightly posterior position.

**re·tru·sive oc·clu·sion** (rĕ-trū'siv ŏ-klū' zhŭn) **1.** Biting relationship in which mandible is forcefully or habitually placed more distally than the patient's centric occlusion. **2.** SYN distal occlusion (1).

**Ret·zi·us stri·ae** (ret'zē-ŭs strī'ē) Dark, concentric lines crossing enamel prisms of teeth seen in axial cross-sections of enamel. SYN brown striae.

**re·vas·cu·lar·i·za·tion** (rē-vas'kyū-lăr-ī-zā'shŭn) Reestablishment of blood supply to a body part.

**re·verse ar·tic·u·la·tion** (rĕ-vĕrs' ahr-tik'yū-lā'shŭn) SYN cross-bite.

**re·verse bev·el** (rĕ-vĕrs' bev'ĕl) Sloping edge of a cutting instrument.

**re·verse con·den·ser** (rĕ-vĕrs' kŏn-den'sĕr) SYN back-action condenser.

**re·verse curve** (rĕ-vĕrs' kŭrv) Denotes an occlusion, in which, when viewed in the sagittal plane, the mandibular cusp tips and incisal edges form a convex curve.

**re·verse plug·ger** (rĕ-vĕrs' plŭg'ĕr) SYN back-action condenser.

**re·verse trans·crip·tase** (rĕ-vĕrs' tran-skrip'tās) RNA-dependent DNA polymerase, present in virions of RNA tumor viruses.

**re·ver·si·ble** (rĕ-vĕr'si-bĕl) Capable of reversal; said of diseases or chemical reactions.

**re·ver·si·ble cal·ci·no·sis** (rĕ-vĕr'si-bĕl kal'si-nō'sis) Build-up of calcium salts that can be stopped.

**re·ver·si·ble hy·dro·col·loid** (rĕ-vĕrs'ĭ-bĕl hī'drŏ-kol'oyd) A hydrocolloid composed of a base substance the physical state of which may be changed from a solid or semisolid to a liquid by the application of heat and then changed to that of an elastic gel by cooling.

**re·vers·i·ble pul·pi·tis** (rĕ-vĕrs'ĭ-bĕl pŭlp-ī'tis) Minor inflammation from which pulp is able to recover; characterized clinically by pain that disappears rapidly on removal of thermal stimulation.

**re·viv·i·fi·ca·tion** (rē-viv'i-fi-kā'shŭn) Refreshening edges of a wound by paring or scraping to promote healing. [L. re-, again, + vivo, to live, + facio, to make]

**Rh** Symbol for rhodium.

**rhab·do·my·o·ma** (rab'dō-mī-ō'mă) A benign neoplasm derived from striated muscle. [rhabdo- + G. mys, muscle, + -oma, tumor]

**rhab·do·my·o·sar·co·ma, rhab·do·sar·co·ma** (rab'dō-mī-ō-sahr-kō'mă, rab'dō-sahr-) Malignant neoplasm derived from skeletal (striated) muscle, occurring in children or, less commonly, in adults. [rhabdo- + G. mys, muscle, + sarkōma, sarcoma]

**Rhab·do·vir·i·dae** (rab'dō-vir'i-dē) Rod-shaped or bullet-shaped viruses of vertebrates, insects, and plants, including rabies virus.

**rhag·a·des** (rag'ă-dēz) Cracks or fissures occurring at mucocutaneous junctions. [G. rhagas, pl. rhagades, a crack]

**rhe·ol·o·gy** (rē-ol'ŏ-jē) The study of the deformation and flow of materials. [rheo- + G. logos, study]

**rhe·o·stat** (rē'ō-stat) A variable resistor used to adjust current in an electrical circuit. [rheo- + G. statos, stationary]

**rheu·mat·ic fe·ver** (rū-mat'ik fē'vĕr) An inflammatory disease with pyrexia following infection of the throat with group A beta-hemolytic streptococci, occurring primarily in children and young adults.

**rheu·mat·ic heart dis·ease** (rū-mat'ik hahrt di-zēz') Cardiac disorder resulting from rheumatic fever, chiefly manifested by abnormalities of the valves.

**rheu·ma·tism** (rū'mă-tizm) Indefinite term applied to various conditions with pain or other symptoms of articular origin or related to other elements of musculoskeletal system. [G. rheumatismos, rheuma, a flux]

**rheu·ma·toid ar·thri·tis** (rū'mă-toyd ahr-thrī'tis) Generalized disease, more common in women, which primarily affects connective tissue. SYN arthritis deformans.

**rheu·ma·tol·o·gy** (rū'mă-tol'ŏ-jē) Medical specialty concerned with study, diagnosis, and treatment of rheumatic conditions. [G. rheuma, flux, + logos, study]

**Rh fac·tor** (fak'tŏr) A protein substance present in the red blood cells of most people (85%), capable of inducing intense antigenic reactions. A person who has the protein substance is called Rh positive and a person who does not have the protein substance is called Rh negative.

**rhin-** Combining form meaning the nose. [G. rhis]

**rhi·ni·tis** (rī-nī'tis) Inflammation of nasal mucous membrane. [rhin- + G. -itis, inflammation]

**rhi·no·cele** (rī'nō-sēl) Cavity (ventricle) of rhinencephalon, primitive olfactory part of telencephalon. [rhino- + G. koilia, a hollow]

**rhi·no·ceph·a·ly, rhi·no·ce·pha·li·a** (rī'nō-sef'ă-lē, -sĕ-fā'lē-ă) Form of cyclopia in which nose is represented by a fleshy proboscislike protuberance arising above slitlike orbits. [rhino- + G. kephalē, head]

**rhi·no·dym·i·a** (rī'nō-dim'ē-ă) Duplication of the nose on an otherwise normal face. [rhino- + G. -dymos, fold]

**rhi·no·la·li·a** (rī′nō-lā′lē-ă) Nasalized speech. [*rhino-* + G. *lalia*, talking]

**rhi·no·pha·ryn·ge·al** (rī′nō-fă-rin′jē-ăl) **1.** SYN nasopharyngeal. **2.** Relating to the rhinopharynx.

**rhi·no·phar·ynx** (rī′nō-far′ingks) SYN nasopharynx.

**rhi·no·plas·ty** (rī′nō-plas-tē) **1.** Repair of a defect of the nose with tissue taken from elsewhere. **2.** Plastic surgery to change the shape or size of the nose. [*rhino-* + G. *plastos*, formed]

**rhi·nor·rhe·a** (rī′nōr-ē′ă) Discharge from nose. SYN rhinorrhoea. [*rhino-* + G. *rhoia*, flow]

**rhinorrhoea** [Br.] SYN rhinorrhea.

*Rhi·no·vi·rus* (rī′nō-vī′rŭs) A genus of acid-labile viruses associated with the common cold.

**rho·da·nate** (rō′dă-nāt) SYN thiocyanate.

*Rho·do·coc·cus* (rō′dō-kok′ŭs) A genus of rod-shaped, gram-positive, partially acid-fast, aerobic bacteria found in soil and in the feces of herbivores. Some species are pathogenic for animals and humans.

**rho·dop·sin** (rō-dop′sin) A red thermolabile protein found in the rods of the retina. SYN visual purple.

**rhon·chal frem·i·tus** (rong′kăl frem′i-tŭs) Fremitus produced by vibrations from passage of air in bronchial tubes partially obstructed by mucous secretion.

**rhon·chus, so·no·rous rhon·chus, sib·i·lant rhon·chus,** pl. **rhon·chi** (rong′kŭs, son′ŏr-ŭs, sib′i-lănt, rong′kī) Added sound with musical pitch occurring during inspiration or expiration, heard on chest auscultation and caused by air passing through bronchi narrowed by inflammation, spasm of smooth muscle, or presence of mucus in lumen. [L. fr. G. *rhenchos*, a snoring]

**rhythm** (ridh′ŭm) Measured time or motion; the regular alternation of two or more different or opposite states. [G. *rhythmos*]

**rhyt·i·do·sis** (rit′i-dō′sis) **1.** Facial wrinkling disproportionate to age. **2.** Corneal laxity and wrinkling, an indication of approaching death. [G. a wrinkling, fr. *rhytis*, a wrinkle, + *-osis*, condition]

**rib·bon arch** (rib′ŏn ahrch) Thin, ribbon-shaped, rectangular orthodontic arch wire applied to dental arches so that its widest dimension is parallel to the labial or buccal tooth surfaces.

**rib·bon arch ap·pli·ance** (rib′ŏn ahrch ă-plī′ăns) Appliance consisting of a rectangular wire inserted into a specially designed bracket attached to labial and buccal tooth surfaces.

**rib [I–XII]** (rib) One of 24 elongated curved bones forming main portion of bony chest wall. [A.S. *ribb*]

**ri·bo·fla·vin** (rī′bō-flā′vin) Heat-stable factor of vitamin B complex with isoalloxazine nucleotides that are coenzymes of the flavodehydrogenases; dietary sources for this vitamin include green vegetables, liver, kidneys, wheat germ, milk, eggs, cheese, and fish. SYN flavin (1), vitamin B2.

**ri·bo·nu·cle·ase** (rī′bō-nū′klē-ās) Transferase or phosphodiesterase that catalyzes hydrolysis of ribonucleic acid.

**ri·bo·nu·cle·ic ac·id (RNA)** (rī′bō-nū-klē′ik as′id) Macromolecule consisting of ribonucleoside residues connected by phosphate from the 3′-hydroxyl of one to the 5′-hydroxyl of the next nucleoside; found in all cells, in both nuclei and cytoplasm and in particulate and nonparticulate form, and also in many viruses. Various RNA fractions are identified by location, form, or function.

**ri·bose** (rī′bōs) The pentose present in ribonucleic acid.

**ri·bo·so·mal DNA** (rī′bō-sō′măl) Species of DNA present in ribosomes, where it participates in protein synthesis, rather than in nucleus.

**rice dis·ease** (rīs di-zēz′) Beriberi; its original outbreaks were caused by feeding people dehusked rice, which decreased rice's vitamin B1 content.

**ri·cin** (rī′sin) A highly toxic lectin and hemagglutinin that occurs in castor beans (the seeds of the castor oil plant, *Ricinus communis*); if ingested, acts as a violent irritant with possibly fatal results, on the respiratory and gastrointestinal mucosa. [L. *ricinus*, castor oil plant]

**rick·ets** (rik′ĕts) Disease due to vitamin D deficiency, characterized by overproduction and deficient calcification of osteoid tissue, with associated skeletal deformities, disturbances in growth, hypocalcemia, and sometimes tetany; usually accompanied by irritability, listlessness, and generalized muscular weakness; fractures are frequent. [E. *wrick*, to twist]

*Rick·ett·si·a* (ri-ket′sē-ă) Genus of bacteria that usually occur intracytoplasmically in lice, fleas, ticks, and mites; pathogenic species infect humans and other animals, causing epidemic, murine, or endemic typhus, Rocky Mountain spotted fever other diseases.

**ric·kett·si·o·sis** (ri-ket′sē-ō′sis) Infection with rickettsiae.

**Rick·les test** (rik′ĕlz test) *Avoid the incorrect forms Rickle and Rickle's.* Colorimetric assessment for predicting dental caries activity by incubating saliva in sucrose and determining pH changes.

**Rid·e·al-Walk·er co·ef·fi·cient** (rid′ē-ăl waw′kĕr kō′ĕ-fish′ĕnt) A figure expressing the disinfecting power of any substance. SYN phenol coefficient.

**ridge** (rij) [TA] **1.** Linear elevation, usually rough. SEE ALSO crest. **2.** In dentistry, any linear elevation on tooth surface. **3.** Remainder of alveolar process and its soft tissue covering after teeth are removed. [A. S. *hyrcg,* back, spine]

**ridge aug·men·ta·tion** (rij awg′mĕn-tā′shŭn) Addition of bone to the alveolar ridge to increase its height and thickness; fills in defects and facilitates retention of implants and prostheses.

**ridge ex·ten·sion** (rij ek-sten′shŭn) Intraoral surgical operation for deepening labial, buccal, or lingual sulci; performed to increase intraoral height of alveolar ridge to assist denture retention.

**ridge re·la·tion** (rij rĕ-lā′shŭn) Positional relation of mandibular ridge to maxillary ridge.

**ridge re·sorp·tion** (rij rĕ-sōrp′shŭn) Loss in volume and size of alveolar portion of mandible or maxilla.

**Rie·ger syn·drome** (rē′ger sin′drōm) Iridocorneal mesenchymal dysgenesis combined with hypodontia or anodontia and maxillary hypoplasia.

**Ri·ga-Fe·de dis·ease** (rē′gah fā′dā di-zēz′) Ulceration of lingual frenum in teething infants, related to abrasion of tissue.

**right-hand·ed** (rīt-hand′ĕd) Denoting habitual or more skillful use of right hand for writing and most manual activity.

**right ven·tric·u·lar fail·ure** (rīt ven-trik′ yū-lăr fāl′yŭr) Congestive heart failure manifested by distention of the neck veins, enlargement of the liver, and dependent edema.

**ri·gid con·nec·tor** (rij′id kŏ-nek′tŏr) Connector that is solid or rigid, as a soldered joint.

**ri·gid·i·ty** (ri-jid′i-tē) Stiffness or inflexibility. [L. *rigidus,* rigid, inflexible]

**rig·id shank** (rij′id shank) Larger diameter instrument shank to withstand pressure needed to remove heavy calculus deposits.

**rig·or mor·tis** (rig′ŏr mōr′tis) Stiffening of the body, from 1–7 hours after death, due to hardening of the muscular tissues in consequence of the coagulation of the myosinogen and paramyosinogen. SYN postmortem rigidity.

**rim** (rim) Margin, border, or edge, usually circular.

**ri·ma,** pl. **ri·mae** (rī′mă, -mē) [TA] Slit or fissure, or narrow elongated opening between two symmetric parts. [L. a slit]

**ri·mose** (rī′mōs) Fissured; in all directions. [L. *rimosus,* fr. *rima,* a fissure]

**rim·u·la** (rim′yū-lă) Minute slit or fissure. [L. dim. of *rima*]

**ring** (ring) [TA] **1.** Circular band surrounding a wide central opening; anular or circular structure surrounding an opening or level area.

**Ring·er so·lu·tion** (ring′ĕr sŏ-lū′shŭn) **1.** Solution resembling blood serum in its salt constituents; used as a fluid and electrolyte replenisher by intravenous infusion. **2.** Salt solution usually used in combination with naturally occuring body substances and more complex chemically defined nutritive solutions for culturing animal cells.

**ring·worm** (ring′wŏrm) SYN tinea.

**risk** (risk) Probability that an event will occur.

**risk as·sess·ment** (risk ă-ses′mĕnt) Determination of possible future disease by identifying risk factors in comparison with possible protective factors.

**risk fac·tor** (risk fak′tŏr) Characteristic statistically associated with, although not necessarily causally related to, an increased danger of morbidity or mortality.

**ri·so·ri·us (mus·cle)** (ri-sō′rē-ŭs mŭs′ĕl) [TA] Facial muscle of mouth; *origin,* from platysma and fascia of masseter; *insertion,* orbicularis oris and skin at corner of mouth; *action,* draws angle of mouth laterally, lenghthening rima oris; *nerve supply,* facial. [L. *risor,* one who laughs, fr. *rideo,* pp. *risus,* to laugh]

**RN** Abbreviation for registered nurse.

**Rn** Symbol for radon.

**RNA** Abbreviation for ribonucleic acid.

**RNA splic·ing** (splīs′ing) SYN splicing (2).

**Roach clasp** (rōch klasp) SYN bar clasp.

**Rob·erts syn·drome** (rob′ĕrts sin′drōm) Phocomelia or lesser degrees of hypomelia, microbrachycephaly, midfacial defect, prenatal growth deficiency, and cryptorchidism.

**Rob·i·now syn·drome** (rob′i-now sin′drōm) Skeletal dysplasia characterized by bulging forehead, hypertelorism, depressed nasal bridge (so-called fetal face), and wide mouth.

**Rob·in syn·drome** (rō-ban[h]′ sin′drōm) SYN Pierre Robin syndrome.

**Rock·well hard·ness test** (rok′wel hahrd′nĕs test) Common dental assessment to determine hardness of ductile materials using a hard-

qr

ened steel ball or diamond point; hardness is related to depth of penetration and measured directly by the instrument. SEE ALSO Brinell hardness test.

**Rock·y Moun·tain spot·ted fe·ver** (rok'ē mown'tăn spot'ĕd fē'vĕr) Acute infectious disease of high mortality, characterized by frontal and occipital headache, intense lumbar pain, malaise, moderately high continuous fever, and rash on wrists, palms, ankles, and soles from the second to the fifth day, later spreading to all parts of body; occurs in spring of the year primarily in the southeastern U.S. and the Rocky Mountain region, although it is also endemic elsewhere in the U.S., in parts of Canada, in Mexico, and in South America.

**rod** (rod) **1.** A straight, slender, cylindric structure or device. **2.** The photosensitive, outward-directed process of a rhodopsin-containing rod cell in the external granular layer of the retina. [A.S. *rōd*]

**rod cell** SYN rod.

**ro·dent ul·cer** (rō'dĕnt ŭl'sĕr) A slowly enlarging ulcerated basal cell carcinoma, usually on the face.

**roent·gen-e·quiv·a·lent-man (rem)** (rent'gen ē-kwiv'ă-lĕnt-man) A unit of dose-equivalent quantity of ionizing radiation of any type that produces in human subjects the same biologic effect as one rad of x-rays or gamma rays; the number of rems is equal to the absorbed dose, measured in rads, multiplied by the quality factor of the radiation in question. 100 rem = 1 Sv.

**roent·gen·o·gram** (rent'gen-ŏ-gram') SYN radiograph.

**roent·gen·o·graph** (rent'gen-ŏ-graf') SYN radiograph.

**roent·gen·og·ra·phy** (rent'gen-og'ră-fē) SYN radiography.

**roent·gen ray** (rent'gen rā) SYN x-ray.

**Rog·er An·der·son pin fix·a·tion ap·pli·ance** (roj'ĕr an'dĕr-sŏn pin fiks-ā'shŭn ă-plī'ăns) Appliance used in extraoral fixation of mandibular fractures and prognathic corrections in which pins placed in bone segments are joined by metal connecting rods.

**role** (rōl) Pattern of behavior that a person exhibits in relationship to significant others in his or her life. [Fr.]

**ROM** Abbreviation for range of motion.

**Rom·berg sign** (rom'berg sīn) With feet approximated, the patient stands with eyes open and then closed; if closing the eyes increases the unsteadiness, a loss of proprioceptive control is indicated, and the sign is present.

**ron·geur** (rōn[h]-zhur') A strong, biting forceps for nipping away bone. [Fr. *ronger,* to gnaw]

**roof** (rūf) Covering or rooflike structure; e.g., tectorium, tectum, tegmen, tegmentum, integument. [A.S. *hrōf*]

**roof of mouth** (rūf mowth) SYN palate.

**roof of or·bit** (rūf ōr'bit) [TA] Formed by orbital plate of frontal bone and lesser wing of sphenoid bone.

**root** (rūt) [TA] **1.** Primary or beginning portion of any part, as of a nerve at its origin from the brainstem or spinal cord. **2.** SYN root of tooth. **3.** Loosely used to denote the etiology of a process, event, or conflict requiring solutions to allow mitigation. [A.S. *rot*]

**root ab·scess** (rūt ab'ses) SYN alveolar abscess.

**root am·pu·ta·tion** (rūt amp'yū-tā'shŭn) Surgical removal of one or more roots of a multirooted tooth; remaining root canal(s) are usually treated endodontically. SYN radectomy, radisectomy.

**root a·pex** (rūt ā'peks) [TA] Conic tip of tooth root, that part farthest from incisal or occlusal side. SYN apex radicis dentis, root tip.

**root a·vul·sion** (rūt ă-vŭl'shŭn) Tearing away of anterior and posterior primary nerve roots from spinal cord, as a result of severe traction; most often, the C5 through T1 roots are affected.

**root ca·nal file** (rūt kă-nal' fīl) Pointed, flexible, steel intracanal instrument used in rasping canal walls.

**root ca·nal of tooth** (rūt kă-nal' tūth) [TA] Chamber of the dental pulp lying within root portion of tooth. SYN marrow canal, pulp canal.

**root ca·nal or·i·fice** (rūt kă-nal' ōr'i-fis) Opening in pulp chamber leading to the root canal.

**root ca·nal plug·ger** (rūt kă-nal' plŭg'ĕr) **1.** Fine-tapered root canal instrument, blunt at the tip, used for pressing or forcing a gutta percha cone into a root canal. **2.** SYN condenser.

**root ca·nal res·tor·a·tion** (rūt kă-nal' res'tŏr-ā'shŭn) Gutta-percha, silver, or plastic cone that has been carried into a root canal, either alone or in conjunction with a cement, paste, or solvent, to obturate canal space.

**root ca·nal spread·er** (rūt kă-nal' spred'ĕr) Tapered instrument used for condensing root filling materials laterally.

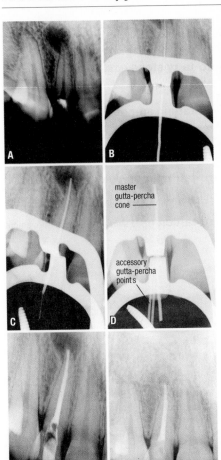

**root canal therapy (radiographs):** (A) initial state with periapical radiolucency; (B) initial working file; (C) master apical file; (D) master cone and several accessory gutta-percha points; (E) completed therapy; (F) one-year follow-up

(labels within image: master gutta-percha cone; accessory gutta-percha points)

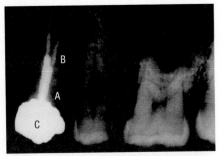

**root canal filling** (A), posts for retention (B) for metal-lined replacement crown (C)

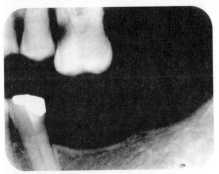

**root caries:** extruded molar

defect in area of cementoenamel junction. See this page.

**root car·ies in·dex** (rūt kar´ēz in´deks) Ratio of the number of teeth with carious lesions of root, and/or restorations of root, to number of teeth with exposed root surfaces.

**root cause a·nal·y·sis** (rūt kawz ă-nal´i-sis) Measure used in medical quality management whereby obvious or elusive causes that may lead to adverse outcomes or patterns of suboptimal outcomes are sought and analyzed to correct faulty processes.

**root con·cav·i·ty** (rūt kŏn-kav´i-tē) Linear developmental depression in the root surface; commonly occur on the proximal surfaces of anterior and posterior teeth and the facial and lingual surfaces of molar teeth. In healthy patients, it is covered with alveolar bone and thus help to secure tooth in bone.

**root dé·bride·ment stroke** (rūt dā-brēd-mo[h]´ strōk) Instrumentation stroke to remove residual calculus deposits, bacterial plaque, and by-products from root surfaces.

**root de·his·cence** (rūt dē-his´ĕns) Loss of buccal or lingual bone overlaying root portion of tooth, leaving that area covered by soft tissue only.

**root end cyst** (rūt end sist) SYN apical periodontal cyst.

**root ca·nal ther·a·py** (rūt kă-nal´ thār´ă-pē) See this page. SYN root canal treatment.

**root ca·nal treat·ment** (rūt kă-nal´ trēt´mĕnt) **1.** Means by which painful or diseased teeth, in which pulp is involved, are restored to a healthy state. **2.** Removal of a normal, diseased, or dead pulp by biochemical and mechanical means, enlargement and sterilization of the root canal, followed by filling the canal, to effect healing of diseased periapical tissues. **3.** Diagnosis and treatment of diseases of dental pulp and their sequelae. See this page. SYN endodontic treatment, root canal therapy.

**root car·ies** (rūt kar´ēz) Caries of root surface of a tooth, usually appearing as a broad shallow

**qr**

**root end gran·u·lo·ma** (rūt end gran′yū-lō′mă) SYN periapical granuloma.

**root for·a·men** (rūt fōr-ā′měn) SYN apical foramen of tooth.

**root-form im·plant** (rūt′fōrm im′plant) An implant shaped like the root of a tooth.

**root of tongue** (rūt tŭng) [TA] Posterior attached portion of tongue. SYN base of tongue.

**root of tooth** (rūt tūth) [TA] That part of a tooth below its neck, covered by cementum rather than enamel, and attached by periodontal ligament to alveolar bone. SYN root (2) [TA].

**root plan·ing** (rūt plān′ing) In dentistry, abrading of rough root surfaces to achieve a smooth surface. See this page.

small, closely aggregated patches of rose-red color caused by human herpesvirus-6. [Mod. L. dim. of L. *roseus,* rosy]

**ro·ta·ry stone** (rō′tă-rē stōn) Honing implement mounted on a metal mandrel for use in a dental hand piece.

**ro·tat·ing an·ode** (rō′tāt-ing an′ōd) In diagnostic radiography, modern x-ray tubes that have a mushroom-shaped anode that rotates rapidly to avoid local heat buildup from electron impact during x-ray generation.

**ro·tat·ing con·dyle** (rō′tāt-ing kon′dīl) Condyle on the side where a bolus of food is chewed; braces and rotates during mastication.

**ro·ta·tion** (rō-tā′shŭn) Turning or movement

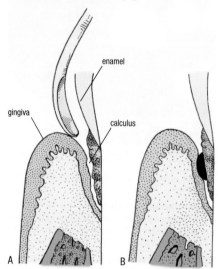
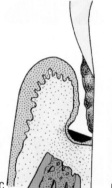
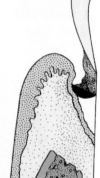

**subgingival scaling and root planing:** (A) curette is inserted gently under gingival margin; (B) with a placement stroke blade is passed over the surface of tooth or calculus, note 0° angle of curette face with the calculus; (C) curette is lowered to base of pocket until tension of soft tissue is felt with rounded back of curette, curette is then positioned at 70°–80° angle with tooth surface beneath calculus deposit; (D) blade is moved along root surface in a scaling stroke to remove calculus

**root re·sec·tion** (rūt rē-sek′shŭn) SYN apicoectomy.

**root re·sorp·tion** (rūt rĕ-sōrp′shŭn) Dissolution of tooth root; either external, with loss or blunting of apical portion, or internal, with loss of dentin from inside (pulpal) part of root area.

**root tip** (rūt tip) SYN root apex.

**ro·sa·ce·a** (rō-sā′shē-ă) Chronic vascular and follicular dilation involving the nose and contiguous portions of the cheeks with erythema, hyperplasia of sebaceous glands, deep-seated papules and pustules, and telangiectasia. SYN acne erythematosa, acne rosacea. [L. *rosaceus,* rosy]

**ro·se·o·la** (rō′zē-ō′lă) Symmetric eruption of

of a body around its axis. [L. *rotatio,* fr. *roto,* pp. *rotatus,* to revolve, rotate]

**ro·ta·tion·al ax·is** (rō-tā′shŭn-ăl ak′sis) SYN fulcrum line.

***Ro·ta·vi·rus*** (rō′tă-vī′rŭs) A genus of RNA viruses that includes the human gastroenteritis viruses. SYN gastroenteritis virus type B. [L. *rota,* wheel, + *virus*]

**rough·age** (rŭf′ăj) Anything in the diet that may stimulate intestinal peristalsis.

**round bur** (rownd bŭr) Dental bur with the cutting blades spherically arranged.

**round win·dow** (rownd win′dō) [TA] Opening on medial wall of middle ear leading into cochlea, closed in life by the secondary tympanic membrane. SYN fenestra of the cochlea.

**round·worm** (rownd′wŏrm) A nematode member of the phylum Nematoda.

**rub·ber-bulb sy·ringe** (rŭb′bĕr-bŭlb′ sir-inj′) Device with a hollow rubber bulb and cannula provided with a check valve, used to obtain a jet of air or water.

**rub·ber cup pol·ish·ing** (rŭb′ĕr kŭp pol′ish-ing) Technique that uses an abrasive polishing agent and a slowly revolving polishing cup to abrade stain from the surfaces.

**rub·ber dam** (rŭb′ĕr dam) **1.** Thin sheet of rubber with holes that is placed over teeth to isolate them from oral cavity. **2.** In surgery, thin strips of rubber used as a surgical drain or barrier.

**rub·ber dam clamp** (rŭb′ĕr dam klamp) SYN dental dam clamp.

**rub·ber dam clamp for·ceps** (rŭb′bĕr dam klamp fŏr′seps) SYN clamp forceps.

**rub·bing al·co·hol** (rŭb′ing al′kŏ-hol) Alcoholic mixture intended for external use; used as a rubefacient for muscle and joint aches and pains.

**ru·be·fa·cient** (rū′bĕ-fā′shĕnt) **1.** Causing a reddening of the skin. **2.** A counterirritant that produces erythema when applied to the skin surface. [L. *rubi-facio,* fr. *ruber,* red, + *facio,* to make]

**ru·bel·la** (rū-bel′ă) An acute but mild exanthematous disease caused by rubella virus, with enlargement of lymph nodes, but usually with little fever or constitutional reaction. SYN German measles. [L. *rubellus,* fem. -*a,* reddish, dim. of *ruber,* red]

**ru·be·o·la** (rū′bē-ō′lă) A term used for measles; not to be confused with rubella among English speakers. [Mod. L. dim. of *ruber,* red, reddish]

**ru·bor** (rū′bōr) Redness, as one of the four signs of inflammation (the others are calor, dolor, tumor) enunciated by Celsus. [L.]

**ru·di·ment** (rū′di-mĕnt) Organ or structure that is incompletely developed. [L. *rudimentum,* a beginning, fr. *rudis,* unformed]

**ru·di·men·tar·y** (rū′di-men′tăr-ē) Relating to a rudiment. SYN abortive (2).

**ru·gi·tus** (rū-jī′tŭs) Rumbling sound in the intestines. [L. a roaring, fr. *rugio,* to roar]

**rule** (rūl) Principle, criterion, standard, or guideline, applied to procedures or situations in which accumulated observation is considered relevant. [O. Fr. *reule,* fr. L. *regula,* a guide, pattern]

**Rum·pel-Leede phe·nom·e·non** (rūmp′ĕl lēd′ fĕ-nom′ĕ-nŏn) Appearance of petechiae in an area following application of vascular constriction, such as by a tourniquet.

**Rum·pel-Leede test** (rūmp′ĕl lēd′ test) SYN capillary fragility test.

**ru·pi·a** (rū′pē-ă) Ulcers of late secondary syphilis, covered with yellowish or brown crusts that have been compared in their appearance with oyster shells. [G. *rhypos,* filth]

**rup·ture** (rŭp′shŭr) **1.** SYN hernia. **2.** A solution of continuity or a tear; a break of any organ or other of the soft parts. [L. *ruptura,* a fracture (of limb or vein), fr. *rumpo,* pp. *ruptus,* to break]

**Rush·ton bod·ies** (rŭsh′tŏn bod′ēz) Linear or curved hyaline bodies, presumably of hematogenous origin, found in epithelial lining of odontogenic cysts.

**Rus·sell Per·i·o·don·tal In·dex** (rŭs′ĕl per′ē-ŏ-don′tăl in′deks) Assessment tool that estimates degree of periodontal disease present in the mouth by measuring both bone loss around teeth and gingival inflammation; used frequently in epidemiologic investigation of periodontal disease.

**Rus·sell sign** (rŭs′ĕl sīn) Abrasions and scars on the back of the hands of patients with bulimia nervosa, usually due to manual attempts to induce vomiting.

**rust·y spu·tum** (rŭs′tē spyū′tŭm) Reddish brown, blood-stained expectoration characteristic of lobar pneumonococcal pneumonia.

**RV** Abbreviation for residual volume.

**qr**

# S

**S** Abbreviation for sulfur; signature; sinister; stready state.

**ŝ** Abbreviation for L. sine, without.

**Sa·bin vac·cine** (sā′bin vak-sēn′) Orally administered vaccine containing live attenuated strains of poliovirus.

**sa·bur·ra** (să-bŭr′ă) Foulness of stomach or mouth due to decomposed food. [L. sand]

**sac** (sak) 1. Encysted abscess at the root of a tooth. 2. Pouch or bursa. 3. Capsule of a tumor, or envelope of a cyst. [L. *saccus*, a bag]

**sac·cha·rides** (sak′ă-rīdz) A group of carbohydrates that includes the sugars.

**sac·cha·rin** (sak′ă-rin) Noncaloric sweetening agent (sugar substitute).

**sac·cha·rine** (sak′ă-rēn, -rin) Relating to sugar; sweet.

**sac·cha·ro·me·tab·o·lism** (sak′ăr-ō-mĕ-tab′ŏ-lizm) Metabolism of sugar; process of use of sugar in cells.

**Sac·cha·ro·my·ces** (sak′ă-rō-mī′sēz) Genus of budding yeasts used to produce brewer's yeast and ethanol.

**sac·cu·lar nerve** (sak′yū-lăr nĕrv) [TA] Branch of inferior part of vestibular nerve going to macula of sacculus.

**sac·cule** (sak′yūl) 1. [TA] Smaller of two membranous sacs in vestibule of labyrinth, lying in spheric recess; connected with cochlear duct by a short tube, the ductus reuniens, and with utriculus by beginning of endolymphatic sac and the utriculosaccularis duct that joins it. 2. Immense bag-shaped structure formed by peptidoglycans as part of the cell wall of some microorganisms. [L. *sacculus*]

**sac·cule of lar·ynx** (sak′yūl lar′ingks) SYN laryngeal saccule.

**sac·cu·lo·co·chle·ar** (sak′yū-lō-kok′lē-ăr) Relating to sacculus and membranous cochlea.

**sa·cro·il·i·ac joint** (sā′krō-il′ē-ak joynt) [TA] The synovial joint between the sacrum and the ilium.

**SAD** Abbreviation for seasonal affective disorder.

**sad·dle** (sad′ĕl) 1. SYN denture base. 2. A structure shaped like, or suggestive of, a seat or saddle used in horseback riding.

**sad·dle a·re·a** (sad′ĕl ar′ē-ă) SYN denture foundation area.

**sad·dle con·nec·tor** (sad′ĕl kŏ-nek′tŏr) Metal plate or bar that joins units on one side of a removable partial denture to those on the other.

**safe·light** (sāf′līt) Illumination permitted in a darkroom during processing.

**sag·it·tal** (saj′i-tăl) [TA] Resembling an arrow; in line of an arrow shot from a bow, i.e., in an anteroposterior direction. [L. *sagitta*, an arrow]

**sag·it·tal ax·is** (saj′i-tăl ak′sis) In dentistry, line in frontal plane around which working side condyle rotates during mandibular movement.

**sag·it·tal plane** (saj′i-tăl plān) [TA] Plane parallel to median plane; i.e., vertical planes in the anatomic position.

**sag·it·tal sec·tion** (saj′i-tăl sek′shŭn) Cross-section obtained by slicing, actually or through imaging techniques, the body or any body part, or any anatomic structure in sagittal plane.

**sag·it·tal split man·dib·u·lar os·te·ot·o·my** (saj′i-tăl split man-dib′yū-lăr os′tē-ot′ŏ-mē) Intraoral surgical procedure for correction of retrognathism, apertognathia, and prognathism; mandibular rami and posterior body are sectioned in the sagittal plane.

**sal·i·cyl·am·ide (SA)** (sal′i-sil′ă-mīd) An analgesic, antipyretic, and antiarthritic, similar in action to that of aspirin.

**sa·lic·y·late** (să-lis′i-lāt) A salt or ester of salicylic acid.

**sal·i·cyl·ism** (sal′i-sil′izm) Poisoning by salicylic acid or any of its compounds.

**sal·i·cyl·sal·i·cyl·ic ac·id** (sal′i-sil-sal′i-sil′ik as′id) SYN salsalate.

**sa·line** (sā′lēn) 1. Relating to, of the nature of, or containing salt; salty. 2. Salt solution, usually sodium chloride. [L. *salinus*, salty, fr. *sal*, salt]

**sa·li·va** (să-lī′vă) Clear, tasteless, odorless, slightly acidic (pH 6.8) viscid fluid, consisting of secretion from the parotid, sublingual, and submandibular salivary glands and the mucous glands of oral cavity; its function is to keep mucous membrane of mouth moist, to lubricate food during mastication, and, in some measure, to convert starch into maltose. [L. akin to G. *sialon*]

**sa·li·va e·jec·tor** (să-lī′vă ē-jek′tŏr) Hollow perforated suction tube used in the evacuation of saliva or liquid debris from oral cavity. SYN dental pump.

**sal·i·vant** (sal′i-vănt) 1. Causing saliva flow. 2. Agent that increases flow of saliva. SYN salivator.

**sal·i·var·y** (sal′i-var-ē) Relating to saliva. SYN sialic, sialine. [L. *salivarius*]

**sal·i·var·y cal·cu·lus** (sal´i-var-ē kal´kyū-lŭs) Calculus in a salivary duct or gland.

**sal·i·var·y di·ges·tion** (sal´i-var-ē di-jes´chŭn) Conversion of starch into sugar by salivary amylase.

**sal·i·var·y fis·tu·la** (sal´i-var-ē fis´tyū-lă) Pathologic communication between a salivary duct or gland and the cutaneous surface or between oral cavity, pharynx, or esophagus to cutaneous surface of neck as a complication of head and neck cancer surgery.

**sal·i·var·y gland** (sal´i-var-ē gland) [TA] Any of the saliva-secreting exocrine glands of oral cavity. SEE ALSO major salivary glands, minor salivary glands. See this page.

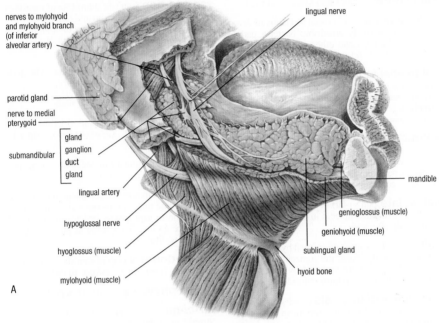

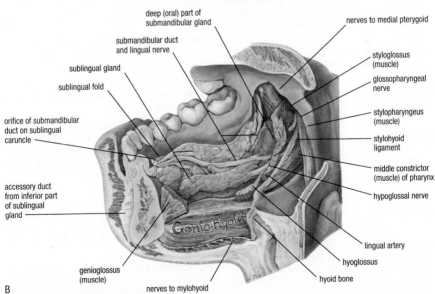

**parotid, submandibular, and sublingual salivary glands:** (A) lateral right view, body and parts of ramus of mandible have been removed; (B) medial view of right lower jaw and floor of mouth; tongue has been excised

st

**sal·i·var·y pel·li·cle** (sal´i-var-ē pel´i-kĕl) Thin nonbacterial salivary film that quickly forms after teeth are cleaned; covers teeth and serves as a medium for plaque formation.

**sal·i·vate** (sal´i-vāt) To cause an excessive flow of saliva.

**sal·i·va·tion** (sal´i-vā´shŭn) SYN sialism.

**sal·i·va·tor** (sal´i-vā-tŏr) SYN salivant (2).

*Sal·mo·nel·la* (sal´mō-nel´ă) Genus of aerobic to facultatively anaerobic bacteria pathogenic for humans and other animals. The type species is *S. choleraesuis.*

**sal·mo·nel·la food poi·son·ing** (sal´mō-nel´ă fūd poy´zŏn-ing) Gastroenteritis caused by various strains of *Salmonella* that multiply freely in gastrointestinal tract but do not produce septicemia.

**sal·mo·nel·lo·sis** (sal´mō-nĕl-ō´sis) Infection with *Salmonella* bacteria. Patients with sickle cell anemia or compromised immune systems are particularly susceptible. [*Salmonella* + G. -*osis*, condition]

**sal·sa·late** (sal´să-lāt) A combination of two molecules of salicylic acid in ester linkage. SYN salicylsalicylic acid.

**salt** (sawlt) 1. Compound formed by interaction of an acid and a base, the ionizable hydrogen atoms of the acid are replaced by the positive ion of the base. 2. Sodium chloride. [L. *sal*]

**salt-de·ple·tion cri·sis** (sawlt dĕ-plē´shŭn krī´sis) Severe illness resulting from loss of sodium chloride, usually in urine (i.e., salt-losing nephritis), in sweat following severe exercise in hot weather, or in intestinal secretions, as in cholera.

**salt e·de·ma** (sawlt ĕ-dē´mă) Swelling due to excessive intake or retention of sodium chloride.

**Sal·ter in·cre·men·tal lines** (sawl´tĕr in´ kră-ment´ăl līnz) Transverse lines sometimes seen in dentin, due to improper calcification.

**sam·ple** (sam´pĕl) 1. Specimen of a whole entity small enough to involve no threat or damage to the whole; an aliquot. 2. Selected subset of a population; may be random or nonrandom (haphazard), representative or nonrepresentative. [M.E. *ensample*, fr. L. *exemplum*, example]

**san·a·tive** (san´ă-tiv) Having a tendency to heal. [L. *sano*, to cure, heal]

**san·a·to·ri·um** (san´ă-tōr´ē-ŭm) Institution for treatment of chronic disorders and a place for recuperation under medical supervision. [Mod. L. neuter of *sanatorius*, curative, fr. *sano*, to cure, heal]

**sand·pa·per discs** (sand´pā-pĕr disks) Paper coated with various grits of silica; used to abrade or smooth surface of teeth or dental materials.

**san·gui·na·rine** (sang´gwi-nār´ēn) Alkaloid used to treat and remove dental plaque.

**san·i·tar·y** (san´i-tar-ē) Healthful; conducive to health; usually in reference to a clean environment. [L. *sanitas*, health]

**san·i·ta·tion** (san´i-tā´shŭn) Use of measures designed to promote health and prevent disease; development and establishment of conditions in the environment favorable to health. [L. *sanitas*, health]

**san·i·ti·za·tion** (san´i-tī-zā´shŭn) The process of making something sanitary.

**SA node** (nōd) SEE sinuatrial node.

**sa·pon·i·fi·ca·tion** (să-pon´i-fi-kā´shŭn) Conversion into soap. [L. *sapo-* (*sapon-*), soap + L. *facio*, to make]

**sapro-** Combining form meaning rotten, putrid, decayed. [G. *sapros*]

**sap·robe** (sap´rōb) An organism that lives on dead organic material. USAGE NOTE This term is preferable to saprophyte, because bacteria and fungi are no longer regarded as plants. [*sapro-* + G. *bios*, life]

**sap·ro·don·ti·a** (sap´rō-don´shē-ă) SYN dental caries. [*sapro-* + G. *odous*, tooth]

**sap·ro·phyte** (sap´rŏ-fīt) SEE saprobe.

*Sar·ci·na* (sahr´si-nă) A genus of nonmotile, strictly anaerobic bacteria containing gram-positive cocci involved in dental disease. [L. *sarcina*, a pack, bundle, fr. *sarcio*, to mend, patch]

**sar·co·car·ci·no·ma** (sahr´kō-kahr´si-nō´ mă) A malignant neoplasm that contains elements of carcinoma and sarcoma.

*Sar·co·di·na* (sahr´kō-dī´nă) The amebae. Most species are free living. [Mod. L. fr. G. *sarx*, flesh]

**sar·coi·do·sis** (sahr´koy-dō´sis) Systemic granulomatous disease of unknown cause, especially involving lungs with resulting interstitial fibrosis, but also involving lymph nodes, skin, liver, spleen, eyes, phalangeal bones, and parotid glands. [*sarcoid* + G. -*osis*, condition]

**sar·co·ma** (sahr-kō´mă) Connective tissue neoplasm, usually highly malignant, formed by proliferation of mesodermal cells. [G. *sarkōma*, a fleshy excrescence, fr. *sarx*, flesh, + -*oma*, tumor]

**Sar·co·mas·ti·goph·o·ra** (sahr´kō-mas´ ti-gof´ŏr-ă) A phylum of the subkingdom Protozoa characterized by flagella, pseudopodia, or both types of locomotory organelles; includes both flagellates and amebae. [*sarco-* + G. *mastix* (*mastig-*), whip, + *phoros*, to bear]

**SARS** Abbreviation for severe acute respiratory syndrome.

**sat·u·rat·ed fat·ty ac·id** (sach'ŭr-āt'ĕd fat'ē as'id) A fatty acid, the carbon chain of which contains no ethylenic or other unsaturated linkages between carbon atoms (e.g., stearic acid and palmitic acid); called saturated because it is incapable of absorbing any more hydrogen.

**sat·u·rat·ed so·lu·tion** (sach'ŭr-āt'ĕd sŏ-lū'shŭn) Solution in which the solvent contains the maximum amount of solute possible without its precipitating out.

**sat·u·ra·tion** (sach'ŭr-ā'shŭn) **1.** Impregnation of one substance by another to the greatest possible extent. **2.** Neutralization, as of an acid by an alkali. **3.** That concentration of a dissolved substance that cannot be exceeded. [L. *saturatio,* fr. *saturo,* to fill, fr. *satis,* enough]

**sat·u·ra·tion in·dex** (sach'ŭr-ā'shŭn in' deks) An indication of the relative concentration of hemoglobin in the red blood cells.

**sau·cer·i·za·tion** (saw'sĕr-ī-zā'shŭn) Excavation of tissue to form a shallow depression, performed in wound treatment to facilitate drainage from infected areas.

**saw** (saw) A metal operating instrument having an edge of sharp, toothlike projections, for dividing bone, cartilage, or plaster; edges may be attached to a rigid band, a flexible wire or chain, or a motorized oscillator. [A.S. *saga*]

**S-BP line** (līn) Line connecting sella with Bolton point; indicates posterior portion of cranial base in cephalometrics.

**SBS** Abbreviation for shaken baby syndrome.

**SC** Abbreviation for subcutaneous.

**Sc** Symbol for scandium.

**sca·bies** (skā'bēz) A dermal eruption producing a vesicular eruption with intense pruritus between the fingers, on the male or female genitalia, on the buttocks, and elsewhere. [L. *scabo,* to scratch]

**scald·ed mouth syn·drome** (skawld'ĕd mowth sin'drōm) Syndrome in which patient complains of a burning sensation of tongue, lips, throat, or palate, likened to scalding caused by hot liquids; clinically, tissues appear normal.

**scald·ing** (skawld'ing) In medical terms, burning pain experienced during urinating.

**scale** (skāl) To remove tartar from the teeth. **2.** To desquamate. [L. *scala,* a stairway]

**scal·er** (skā'lĕr) An instrument for removing calculus from teeth.

**scal·ing** (skāl'ing) In dentistry, removal of accretions from crowns and roots of teeth by use of special instruments.

**scal·ing stroke ac·tion** (skāl'ing strōk ak' shŭn) Movement of dental tool so as to dislodge and remove calculus deposits.

**scal·pel** (skalp'ĕl) A knife used in surgical dissection. [L. *scalpellum;* dim. of *scalprum,* a knife]

**scan** (skan) **1.** To survey by traversing with an active or passive sensing device. **2.** Image, record, or data obtained by scanning, usually identified by technology or device employed.

**scan·di·um (Sc)** (skan'dē-ŭm) A metallic element used in endodontics.

**scan·ning** (skan'ing) Act of imaging by traversing with an active or passive sensing device, often identified by technology or device employed.

**scan·ning e·lec·tron mi·cro·scope** (skan'ing ĕ-lek'tron mī'krŏ-skōp) A microscope in which the object in a vacuum is scanned in a raster pattern by a slender electron beam, generating reflected and secondary electrons from the specimen surface that are used to modulate the image on a synchronously scanned cathode ray tube; with this method a three-dimensional image is obtained, with both high resolution and great depth of focus.

**scap·u·la,** pl. **scap·u·lae** (skap'yū-lă, -lē) [TA] Large triangular flattened bone lying over the ribs, posteriorly on either side, articulating laterally with clavicle at the acromioclavicular joint and humerus at the glenohumeral joint. [L. *scapulae,* the shoulder blades]

**scar** (skahr) Fibrous tissue replacing normal tissues destroyed by injury or disease or divided after an incision. See this page. [G. *eschara,* scab]

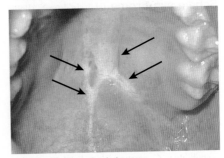

scar: fibrotic tissue due to trauma

**scar·i·fy** (skahr'i-fī) To produce scarification by cutting the skin.

**scar·la·ti·na** (skahr'lă-tē'nă) Acute exanthematous disease, caused by infection with streptococcal organisms producing an erythrogenic toxin, marked by fever and other constitutional disturbances; mucous membrane of mouth and fauces is usually also involved. SYN scarlet fever. [through It. fr. Mediev. L. *scarlatum,* scarlet, a scarlet cloth]

**scar·la·ti·na hem·or·rha·gi·ca** (skahr´ lă-tē´nă hem´ŏr-raj´i-kă) Form of scarlatina in which blood extravasates into skin and mucous membranes, giving eruption a dusky hue; frequent bleeding from the nose and into the intestine also occurs.

**scar·la·ti·ni·form** (skahr´lă-tē´ni-fōrm) Resembling scarlatina, denoting a rash.

**scar·let fe·ver** (skahr´lĕt fē´vĕr) SYN scarlatina.

**scat·ter** (skat´ĕr) 1. Change in direction of a photon or subatomic particle due to collision or interaction. 2. Secondary radiation due to interaction of primary radiation with matter.

**scat·tered ra·di·a·tion** (skat´ĕrd rā´dē-ā´ shŭn) Radiation that has been deflected from its path by impact with matter. This form of secondary radiation is emitted diffusely by the tissues of the patient during exposure to x-radiation.

**scav·eng·ing de·vice** (skav´ĕn-jing dĕ-vīs´) That part of nitrous oxide equipment that collects exhaled nitrous oxide and removes it; main component is the scavenging nasal hood.

**ScD** Abbreviation for Doctor of Science.

**sched·ule** (sked´jūl) A procedural plan for a proposed objective (e.g., dental care), especially sequence and time allotted for each item or operation required for its completion. [L. *scheda,* fr. *scida,* a strip of papyrus, leaf of paper]

**sched·uled drug** (sked´jūld drŭg) SEE controlled substance.

**Scheie syn·drome** (shā sin´drōm) Allelic to Hurler syndrome but with a milder phenotype; characterized by α-L-iduronidase deficiency, corneal clouding, deformity of hands, aortic valve involvement, and normal intelligence.

**sche·mat·ic** (skĕ-mat´ik) Made after a definite type of formula; representing in general, but not with absolute exactness; denoting an anatomic drawing or model. [G. *schēmatikos,* in outward show, fr. *schēma,* shape, form]

**Schick test** (shik test) An assessment for susceptibility to *Corynebacterium diphtheriae* toxin.

**schis·to·glos·si·a** (skis´tō-glos´ē-ă) Congenital fissure or cleft of tongue. [G. *schistron,* split + G. *glōssa,* tongue]

**Schis·to·so·ma** (skis´tō-sō´mă) Genus of digenetic trematodes, which cause schistosomiasis. [G. *schiston,* split + G. *sōma,* body]

**schis·to·so·mi·a·sis** (skis´tō-sō-mī´ă-sis) Infection with a species of *Schistosoma* can

elicit portal hypertension and esophageal varices, as well as liver damage leading to cirrhosis.

**schiz·o·af·fec·tive dis·or·der** (skit´sō-a-fek´tiv dis-ōr´dĕr) Illness manifested by an enduring major depressive, manic, or mixed episode along with delusions, hallucinations, disorganized speech and behavior, and negative symptoms of schizophrenia.

**schiz·oid** (skits´oyd) Socially isolated, having few (if any) friends or social relationships.

**schiz·oid per·son·al·i·ty dis·or·der** (skits´oyd pĕr´sŏ-nal´i-tē dis-ōr´dĕr) Enduring and pervasive pattern of behavior in adulthood characterized by social withdrawal, emotional coldness, aloofness, and indifference to others.

**schiz·o·phre·ni·a** (skits´ō-frē´nē-ă) A common type of psychosis, characterized by abnormalities in perception, content of thought, and thought processes. [G. *schizō,* split + G. *phrēn,* mind]

**Schmidt syn·drome** (shmit sin´drōm) Unilateral paralysis of soft palate, trapezius, and sternocleidomastoid.

**school nurse** (skūl nŭrs) Nurse, usually an R.N., working in an educational institution.

**Schult·ze sign** (shūlt´sĕ sīn) In latent tetany, tapping tongue causes its depression with a concave dorsum. SYN tongue phenomenon.

**schwan·no·ma** (shwah-nō´mă) A benign, encapsulated neoplasm in which the fundamental component is structurally identical to a syncytium of Schwann cells. SYN neurilemmoma.

**sci·at·i·ca** (sī-at´i-kă) Pain in lower back and hip radiating down back of thigh into leg, due to herniated lumbar discs compressing a nerve root, most commonly L5 or S1.

**SCID** Abbreviation for severe combined immunodeficiency.

**scin·til·lat·ing sco·to·ma** (sin´ti-lāt´ing skō-tō´mă) Localized area of blindness edged by brilliantly colored shimmering lights; usually prodromal symptom of migraine.

**scin·til·la·tion count·er** (sin´ti-lā´shŭn kown´tĕr) An instrument used for the detection and measurement of radioactivity.

**scis·sor-bite** (siz´ŏr bīt) Malocclusion that is present when one or more adjacent posterior teeth are positioned either completely buccal or lingual to the opposing (i.e., antagonistic) teeth.

**scis·su·ra,** pl. **scis·su·rae** (shi-sūr´ă, -ē) 1. Cleft or fissure. 2. A splitting. [L.]

**scle·ra,** pl. **scle·ras,** pl. **scler·ae** (skler´ă, -ăz, -ē) [TA] Portion of fibrous layer forming outer envelope of eyeball, except for its anterior sixth, which is the cornea. [Mod. L. fr. G. *sklēros,* hard]

**scle·ro·dac·ty·ly, scle·ro·dac·tyl·i·a** (sklĕr′ō-dak′ti-lē, -dak-til′ē-ă) SYN acrosclerosis. [*sclero-* + G. *daktylos,* finger or toe]

**scle·ro·der·ma** (sklĕr′ō-dĕr′mă) Thickening and induration of skin caused by new collagen formation, with atrophy of pilosebaceous follicles. [*sclero-* + G. *derma,* skin]

**scle·ro·sis,** pl. **scle·ro·ses** (skler-ō′sis, -sēz) **1.** SYN induration (2). **2.** In neuropathy, induration of nervous and other structures by a hyperplasia of the interstitial connective tissue. See page A6. [G. *sklērōsis,* hardness]

**scle·ro·ther·a·py** (skler′ō-thār′ă-pē) Treatment involving the injection of a sclerosing solution into vessels or tissues.

**scle·rot·ic ce·ment·al mass** (skler-ot′ik sĕ-men′tăl mas) Benign fibroosseous jaw lesions of unknown etiology, occurring predominantly in middle-aged black women; lesions present as large painless radiopaque masses usually involving several quadrants of the jaw.

**scle·rot·ic den·tin** (skler-ot′ik den′tin) Dentin characterized by calcification of dentinal tubules due to injury or normal aging. SYN transparent dentin.

**scle·rot·ic teeth** (skler-ot′ik tēth) Naturally hard teeth that are resistant to caries.

**sco·li·o·sis** (skō′lē-ō′sis) [TA] Abnormal lateral curvature of the vertebral column. [G. *skoliōsis,* a crookedness]

**scoop tech·nique** (skūp tek-nēk′) Method for capping needles that involves placing the needle cover on a flat surface, then inserting the needle into it without touching needle or cover; intended to prevent accidental needle-stick.

**sco·pol·a·mine** (skō-pol′ă-mēn, -min) An alkaloid found in the leaves and seeds of various plants; exerts anticholinergic actions similar to that of atropine, but is thought to have greater central nervous system effects; useful in preventing motion sickness. SYN hyoscine.

**scor·bu·tic** (skor-byū′tik) Relating to, suffering from, or resembling scurvy (scorbutus).

**scor·di·ne·ma** (skōr′di-nē′mă) Heaviness of head with yawning and stretching, occurring as a prodrome of an infectious disease. [G. *skordinēma,* yawning]

**sco·to·ma,** pl. **sco·to·ma·ta** (skō-tō′mă, -mă-tă) An isolated area of varying size and shape, within visual field, in which vision is absent or depressed. [G. *skotōma,* vertigo, fr. *skotos,* darkness]

**scratch test** (skrach test) A form of skin test

in which antigen is applied through a scratch in the skin.

**screen** (skrēn) **1.** A sheet of any substance used to shield an object from any influence, such as heat, light, or x-rays. **2.** A sheet on which an image is projected. **3.** To examine, evaluate; to process a group to select or separate some individuals from it. SYN screening (1). [Fr. *écran*]

**screen·ing** (skrēn′ing) **1.** To screen (4) SYN Screen (3). **2.** Examination of a group of usually asymptomatic people to detect those with a high probability of having a given disease, typically by means of an inexpensive diagnostic test.

**screw** (skrū) Helically grooved cylinder for attaching two objects or adjusting position of an object resting on one end of screw.

**screw·driv·er teeth** (skrū′drī-vĕr tēth) SYN Hutchinson teeth.

**screw el·e·va·tor** (skrū el′ĕ-vā-tŏr) Dental instrument with a threaded extremity used to extract a broken tooth root.

**scribe** (skrīb) **1.** To write, trace, or mark by making a line with a marker or pointed instrument, as in surveying a dental cast for a removable prosthesis. **2.** To form, by instrumentation, negative areas within a master cast to provide a positive beading in framework of a removable partial denture, or posterior palatal seal area for a complete denture. [L. *scribo,* pp. *scripto,* to write]

**scrub nurse** (skrŭb nŭrs) Nurse who has cleaned arms and hands, donned sterile gloves and, usually, a sterile gown, to assist an operating surgeon, primarily by passing instruments.

**scru·ple** (skrū′pĕl) An apothecaries' weight of 20 grains or one third of a dram.

**scur·vy** (skŭr′vē) Disease marked by inanition, debility, anemia, and edema of dependent parts; sometimes causes gum ulceration and loss of teeth; due to a diet lacking vitamin C. [fr. A.S. *scurf*]

**SD** Abbreviation for standard deviation; streptodornase.

**seal** (sēl) **1.** Tight closure. **2.** To effect a tight closure.

**seal·ant** (sēl′ănt) **1.** Material used to effect an airtight closure. **2.** Substance applied to a damaged organ to affect homeostasis, to curtail other leakage, or to facilitate prolonged drug delivery to a limited area. **3.** Composite material applied to dental pits and fissures to prevent decay.

**seal·ant re·ten·tion** (sēl′ănt rĕ-ten′shŭn) The ability of a dental sealant material to be retained in or on a tooth surface.

**sea·son·al af·fec·tive dis·or·der (SAD)** (sē′zŏn-ăl a-fek′tiv dis-ōr′dĕr) Depres-

st

sive mood disorder that occurs at approximately the same time each year and spontaneously remits at the same time each year. Most common type is winter depression characterized by morning hypersomnia, low energy, increased appetite, weight gain, and a craving for carbohydrates, all of which findings remit in the spring.

**seat** (sēt) A surface against which an object may rest to gain support.

**Seb·i·leau hol·low** (seb-i-lō´ hol´ō) Depression between inferior aspect of tongue and sublingual glands.

**seb·or·rhe·a** (seb´ōr-ē´ă) Overactivity of the sebaceous glands, resulting in an excessive amount of sebum. SYN seborrhoea.

**seb·or·rhe·ic der·ma·ti·tis, der·ma·ti·tis seb·or·rhe·i·ca** (seb´ōr-ē´ik dĕr´mă-tī´tis, seb-ōr-ē´i-kă) A common scaly macular eruption that occurs primarily on the face, scalp (dandruff), and other areas of increased sebaceous gland secretion. SYN dyssebacia, dyssebacea, Unna disease.

**seb·or·rhe·ic der·ma·to·sis** (seb´ōr-ē´ik dĕr´mă-tō´sis) SYN seborrheic dermatitis, dermatitis seborrheica.

**seb·or·rhe·ic ker·a·to·sis, ker·a·to·sis seb·or·rhe·i·ca** (seb´ōr-ē´ik ker´ă-tō´sis, seb-ōr-ē´i-kă) Superficial, benign, verrucous, often pigmented, greasy lesions consisting of proliferating epidermal cells, resembling basal cells, enclosing horn cysts; usually occur after the third decade. SYN basal cell papilloma.

**seb·or·rhe·ic ver·ru·ca** (seb´ōr-ē´ik vĕr-ū´kă) SYN seborrheic keratosis, keratosis seborrheica.

**seborrhoea** [Br.] SYN seborrhea.

**sec·on·dary** (sek´ŏn-dar-ē) **1.** Second in order. **2.** Caused by another condition (e.g., a secondary infection caused by antibiotic treatment for a primary infection).

**sec·on·dar·y ae·ro·don·tal·gia** (sek´ŏn-dar-ē ar´ō-don-tal´jē-ă) Pain referred to dental area from area affected by aerosinusitis.

**sec·on·dary am·y·loid·o·sis** (sek´ŏn-dar-ē am´i-loy-dō´sis) Amyloidosis occurring in association with another chronic inflammatory disease; organs chiefly involved are the liver, spleen, and kidneys.

**sec·on·dary a·nes·thet·ic** (sek´ŏn-dar-ē an´es-thet´ik) Compound that contributes to, but is not primarily responsible for, loss of sensation when two or more anesthetics are simultaneously administered.

**sec·on·dary car·ies** (sek´ŏn-dar-ē kar´ēz) Caries of enamel beginning at dentoenamel junction due to a rapid lateral spread of decay from the original site of decay.

**sec·on·dary den·tin** (sek´ŏn-dar-ē den´tin) Dentin formed by normal pulp function after root end formation is complete.

**sec·on·dary den·ti·tion** (sek´ŏn-dar-ē den-tish´ŭn) See this page. SYN permanent tooth.

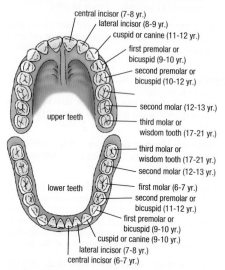

central incisor (7-8 yr.)
lateral incisor (8-9 yr.)
cuspid or canine (11-12 yr.)
first premolar or bicuspid (9-10 yr.)
second premolar or bicuspid (10-12 yr.)
second molar (12-13 yr.)
upper teeth
third molar or wisdom tooth (17-21 yr.)
third molar or wisdom tooth (17-21 yr.)
second molar (12-13 yr.)
lower teeth
first molar (6-7 yr.)
second premolar or bicuspid (11-12 yr.)
first premolar or bicuspid (9-10 yr.)
cuspid or canine (9-10 yr.)
lateral incisor (7-8 yr.)
central incisor (6-7 yr.)

**permanent secondary dentition: adult**

**sec·on·dar·y fail·ure** (sek´ŏn-dar-ē fāl´yŭr) **1.** Failure of function of an organ as a result of antecedent pathology elsewhere. **2.** Decreasing responsiveness to a drug after an initial satisfactory response, usually occurring several months after initiation of treatment.

**sec·on·dary hem·or·rhage** (sek´ŏn-dar-ē hem´ŏr-ăj) Hemorrhage at an interval after an injury or an operation.

**sec·on·dar·y hy·per·par·a·thy·roid·ism** (sek´ŏn-dar-ē hī´pĕr-par´ă-thī´royd-izm) Disorder that occurs as a complication of renal disease that affects all four parathyroid glands.

**sec·on·dar·y lin·gual bar** (sek´ŏn-dār-ē ling´gwăl bahr) SYN continuous clasp.

**sec·on·dar·y nu·tri·tion·al de·fic·ien·cy** (sek´ŏn-dar-ē nū-trish´ŭn-ăl de-fish´ĕn-sē) The interference of ingestions, absorption, digestion, and use of nutrients resulting from a systemic disorder.

**sec·on·dar·y pal·ate** (sek´ŏn-dar-ē pal´ăt) Portion of embryonic palate, posterior to primary palate that forms from lateral palatine processes of the embryonic maxilla. See page 511.

**sec·on·dar·y ra·di·a·tion** (sek´ŏn-dar-ē rā´dē-ā´shŭn) SYN scattered radiation.

**sec·on·dary syph·il·is** (sek´ŏn-dar-ē sif´i-lis) The second stage of syphilis.

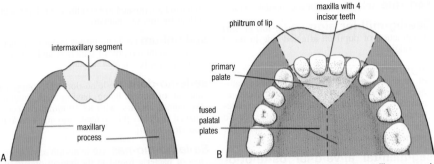

**secondary palate development:** (A) intermaxillary segment and maxillary processes; (B) intermaxillary segment giving rise to philtrum of upper lip, median part of maxillary bone with its four incisor teeth, and triangular primary palate

**sec·on·dar·y tu·ber·cu·lo·sis** (sek′ŏn-dar-ē tū-bĕr′kyū-lō′sis) Tuberculosis found in adults characterized by lesions near the apex of an upper lobe, which may cavitate or heal with scarring without spreading to lymph nodes. SYN reactivation tuberculosis.

**sec·ond cra·ni·al nerve [CN II]** (sek′ ŏnd krā′nē-ăl nĕrv) SYN optic nerve [CN II].

**sec·ond gas effect** (sek′ŏnd gas ĕ-fekt′) When a constant concentration of an anesthetic such as halothane is inspired, increase in alveolar concentration is accelerated by concomitant administration of nitrous oxide, because alveolar uptake of latter creates a potential subatmospheric intrapulmonary pressure that leads to increased tracheal inflow.

**sec·ond in·ci·sor** (sek′ŏnd in-sī′zŏr) Second maxillary or mandibular permanent or deciduous tooth on either side of midsagittal cranial plane. SYN lateral incisor.

**sec·ond mo·lar** (sek′ŏnd mō′lăr) Seventh permanent or fifth deciduous tooth in maxilla and mandible on either side of midsagittal cranial plane following arch form.

**sec·ond pha·ryn·ge·al arch car·ti·lage** (sek′ŏnd făr-in′jē-ăl ahrch kahr′ti-lăj) A cartilage in the mesenchyme of the second pharyngeal arch in the embryo, from which develop the stapes, styloid process, stylohyoid ligament, and lesser cornu (horn). SYN Reichert cartilage.

**sec·ond tooth** (sek′ŏnd tūth) SYN permanent tooth.

**se·cre·ta·gogue, se·cre·to·gogue** (sĕ-krē′tă-gog, -tŏ-gog) Agent that promotes secretion. [*secreta* + G. *agōgos*, drawing forth]

**se·crete** (sĕ-krēt′) To elaborate or produce some physiologically active substance (e.g., enzyme, hormone, metabolite) by a cell and deliver it into blood, body cavity, or sap, either by direct diffusion, cellular exocytosis, or by means of a duct. [L. *se-cerno*, pp. *-cretus*, to separate]

**se·cre·tin** (sĕ-krē′tin) Hormone formed by epithelial cells of duodenum under stimulus of acid contents from stomach, which incites secretion of pancreatic juice.

**se·cre·tion** (sĕ-krē′shŭn) **1.** Production by a cell or aggregation of cells (a gland) of a physiologically active substance and its movement out of cell or organ in which formed. **2.** Solid, liquid, or gaseous product of cellular or glandular activity stored in or used by organism in which it is produced. [L. *se-cerno,* pp. *-cretus,* to separate]

**se·cre·to·mo·tor, se·cre·to·mo·to·ry** (sĕ-krē′tō-mō′tŏr, -ē) Stimulating secretion. [*se-crete* + *motor,* mover]

**se·cre·to·ry** (sĕ-krē′tŏr-ē) Relating to secretion or the secretions.

**sec·tion·al im·pres·sion** (sek′shŭn-ăl im-presh′ŭn) Negative likeness that is made in sections then reassembled to provide a full contour cast.

**sec·tor·i·al tooth** (sek-tōr′ē-ăl tūth) SYN carnassial tooth.

**se·da·tion** (sĕ-dā′shŭn) The act of calming, especially with a sedative. [L. *sedatio,* to calm, allay]

**sed·a·tive** (sed′ă-tiv) **1.** Calming; quieting. **2.** Drug that quiets nervous excitement; designated according to organ or system on which specific action is exerted.

**sed·i·ment** (sed′i-mĕnt) **1.** Insoluble material that tends to sink to the bottom of a liquid, as in hypostasis. **2.** To cause the formation of a sediment or deposit. SYN sedimentate. [L. *sedimentum,* a settling, fr. *sedeo,* to sit, settle down]

**sed·i·men·tate** (sed′i-men′tāt) SYN sediment.

**sed·i·men·ta·tion rate (sed. rate)** (sed′i-mĕn-tā′shŭn rāt) The sinking velocity of blood cells; used to detect and monitor inflammatory processes in the body.

st

**sed. rate** Abbreviation for sedimentation rate.

**See·lig·mül·ler sign** (zā´lig-mil´er sīn) Contraction of pupil on affected side in facial neuralgia.

**seg·ment** (seg´měnt) [TA] **1.** A section; part of an organ or other structure delimited naturally, artificially, or by invagination from remainder. **2.** Territory of an organ having independent function, supply, or drainage. **3.** To divide and redivide into minute equal parts. [L. *segmentum,* fr. *seco,* to cut]

**seg·men·tal al·ve·o·lar os·te·ot·o·my** (seg-men´tăl al-vē´ŏ-lăr os´tē-ot´ŏ-mē) Intraoral surgical procedure in which segments of alveolar bone containing teeth are sectioned between, and apically to, teeth for repositioning of alveolus and teeth; may be maxillary or mandibular and may be combined with ostectomy.

**seg·men·tal an·es·the·si·a** (seg-men´tăl an´es-thē´zē-ă) Loss of sensation limited to area supplied by one or more spinal nerve roots.

**seg·men·tal neu·ri·tis** (seg-men´tăl nūr-ī´tis) Inflammation occurring at several points along course of a nerve.

**seg·men·ta·tion** (seg´měn-tā´shŭn) Act of dividing into segments.

**sei·zure** (sē´zhŭr) **1.** An attack; sudden onset of disease or some symptoms. **2.** An epileptic attack. SYN convulsion (2). [O. Fr. *seisir,* to grasp, fr. Germanic]

**se·lec·tion** (sĕ-lek´shŭn) The combined effect of the causes and consequences of genetic factors that determine the average number of progeny of a species that attain sexual maturity. [L. *se-ligo,* to separate, select, fr. *se,* apart, + *lego,* to pick out]

**se·lec·tive grind·ing** (sĕ-lek´tiv grīnd´ing) Removal of structure from occlusal surfaces of the teeth to improve intercuspal contacts and reduce dental interference during jaw movements. This irreversible procedure is carried out according to a plan or at selected places marked by articulating ribbon or paper.

**se·lec·tive nor·ep·i·neph·rine re·up·take in·hib·i·tor** (sĕ-lek´tiv nōr-ep´i-nef´rin rē-ŭp´tāk in-hib´i-tŏr) Class of chemical compounds that selectively, to varying degrees, inhibit reuptake of norepinephrine.

**se·lec·tive pol·ish·ing** (sĕ-lek´tiv pol´ish-ing) Cleaning only aesthetically objectionable tooth surfaces; stresses daily patient self-care for the removal of plaque biofilms.

**se·lec·tive ser·o·to·nin re·up·take in·hib·i·tor (SSRI)** (sĕ-lek´tiv ser´ŏ-tō´nin rē-ŭp´tāk in-hib´i-tŏr) Class of chemical compounds that selectively, to varying degrees, inhibit reuptake of serotonin by presynaptic neu-

rons and are posited to exert their antidepressant effect by this mechanism.

**se·le·ni·um** (sĕ-lē´nē-ŭm) A metallic element used in scintography of pancreas and parathyroid glands. [G. *selēnē,* moon]

**se·le·no·dont** (sĕ-lē´nō-dont) Denoting an animal, or human being, having teeth, such as the human molars, with longitudinal crescent-shaped ridges. [G. *selēnē,* moon, + *odous (odont-),* tooth]

*Se·le·no·mo·nas* (sĕ-lē´nō-mō´nas) A genus of bacteria found in the human oral vestibule. [G. *selēnē,* moon, + *monas,* single (unit)]

**self-a·nal·y·sis (SA)** (self´ă-nal´i-sis) SYN autoanalysis.

**self-an·gu·la·ted cu·rette** (self-ang´gyū-lā-těd kyūr-et´) Device in which the face is tilted in relation to the lower shank (e.g., area-specific curette). Tilted face causes one cutting edge to be lower than the other on a working-end, which positions the working cutting edge in correct angulation to the root surface.

**self-con·cept** (self kon´sept) Individual's sense of self, including self-definition in various social roles.

**self-con·trol** (self´kŏn-trōl´) **1.** Self-regulation of one's behavior in accordance with personal beliefs, goals, attitudes, and societal expectations. **2.** A person's use of active coping strategies to deal with problem situations.

**self-cur·ing res·in** (self´kyūr´ing rez´in) SYN autopolymer resin.

**self-ef·fi·ca·cy** (self-ef´i-kă-sē) Person's estimate or personal judgment of his or her own ability to succeed in reaching a specific or more general goal.

**self-lim·it·ed dis·ease** (self-lim´i-těd di-zēz´) Disease process that resolves spontaneously with or without specific treatment.

**self-reg·u·la·tion** (self´reg-yū-lā´shŭn) Three-stage strategy patients are taught to use to end risky health-associated behaviors such as smoking and overeating: stage 1: self-monitoring (self-observation), the first stage in self-regulation involves the person's deliberately attending to and recording his or her own behavior; stage 2: self-evaluation, in which the person assesses what was learned by self-monitoring, such as how often and where smoking occurred, and uses those observational data to establish health goals or criteria; and stage 3: self-reinforcement, in which the person rewards herself or himself for each behavioral success on the road to that goal, thereby enhancing the chance of reaching it.

**self-stim·u·la·tion** (self´stim-yū-lā´shŭn) A technique for electrical stimulation of peripheral nerves, spinal cord, or brain by the patient to relieve pain.

**self-thread·ing pin** (self-thred´ing pin) Cylindric metal pin used for retention of a dental restoration that is screwed into dentin.

**sel·la tur·ci·ca** (sel´ă tŭr´si-kă) [TA] Saddlelike bony prominence on the upper surface of the body of the sphenoid bone, constituting the middle part of the butterfly-shaped middle cranial fossa.

**sem·i·ca·nal** (sem´ē-kă-nal´) A half canal; a deep groove on the edge of a bone that, uniting with a similar groove or part of an adjoining bone, forms a complete canal.

**sem·i·cir·cu·lar ca·nals (of bon·y lab·y·rinth)** (sem´ē-sĭr´kyū-lăr kă-nalz´ bō´nē lab´ĭ-rinth) [TA] Organ of balance; three bony tubes of labyrinth of inner ear within which membranous semicircular ducts are located; lie in planes at right angles to each other and are known as anterior semicircular canal [TA] posterior semicircular canal [TA], and lateral semicircular canal [TA].

**sem·i·cir·cu·lar ducts** (sem´ē-sĭr´kyū-lăr dŭkts) [TA] Three small membranous tubes of the vestibular labyrinth within the bony semicircular canals of the bony labyrinth that form loops of about two thirds of a circle.

**sem·i·closed cir·cle** (sem´ē-klōzd´ sĭr´kĕl) Circuit for administration of an inhalation anesthetic in which partial rebreathing with carbon dioxide absorption is combined with loss from circuit of a portion of respired gases through valves.

**sem·i·co·ma·tose** (sem´ē-kō´mă-tōs) Imprecise term for a state of drowsiness and inaction, in which more than ordinary stimulation may be required to evoke a response.

**sem·i·con·duc·tor** (sem´ē-kŏn-dŭk´tŏr) A metalloid that conducts electricity more easily than a true nonmetal but less easily than a metal.

**sem·i·cris·ta** (sem´ē-kris´tă) Small or imperfect ridge or crest. [semi- + L. crista, crest, tuft]

**sem·i·lu·nar hi·a·tus** (sem´ē-lū´năr hī-ā´tŭs) [TA] Deep, narrow groove in lateral wall of middle meatus of nasal cavity, into which maxillary sinus, frontonasal duct, and middle ethmoid cells open.

**sem·i·per·me·a·ble** (sem´ē-pĕr´mē-ă-bĕl) Freely permeable to water (or other solvent) but relatively impermeable to solutes.

**sem·i·re·cum·bant** (sem´ē-rē-kŭm´bănt) SYN semisupine position.

**sem·i·su·pine po·si·tion** (sem´ē-sū´pīn pŏ-zish´ŭn) SYN semirecumbent.

**sem·i·syn·thet·ic** (sem´ē-sin-thet´ik) Describing process of synthesizing a particular chemical using a naturally occurring chemical as a starting material, thus obviating part of a total synthesis, e.g., conversion of cholesterol into a corticosteroid.

**sem·i·sys·te·mat·ic name** (sem´ē-sis´tĕ-mat´ik nām) Name of a chemical of which at least one part is systematic and at least one part is not (i.e., is trivial).

**se·nes·cence** (sĕ-nes´ĕns) The state of being old. [L. senesco, to grow old, fr. senex, old]

**se·nile** (sen´il) Negative or pejorative connotations of this word may render it offensive in some contexts. Relating to or characteristic of old age. [L. senilis]

**se·nile at·ro·phy** (sen´il at´rŏ-fē) Wasting of tissues and organs with advancing age from decreased catabolic or anabolic processes, at times due to endocrine changes, decreased use, or ischemia.

**se·nile de·men·ti·a** (sen´il dĕ-men´shē-ă) Dementia of Alzheimer disease developing after age 65.

**se·nile den·tal car·ies** (sen´il den´tăl kar´ēz) Caries occurring in old age, usually interproximally and in the cementum.

**se·nile ker·a·to·sis** (sen´il ker´ă-tō´sis) Benign flat, raised, or pedunculated lesions, colored yellow to dark brown; more usual on the trunk and increase in incidence after 40 years of age; may be known as basal cell papillomas because of their cells of origin but are not neoplastic. SYN seborrheic keratosis (2). [L. senilis, old age, + G. keras, horn, + -osis, condition]

**se·nile mem·or·y** (sen´il mem´ŏr-ē) Memory that is better for remote than current events; seen in aged or demented people.

**se·nile psy·cho·sis** (sen´il sī-kō´sis) Mental disturbance occurring in old age related to degenerative cerebral processes.

**se·nile trem·or** (sen´il trem´ŏr) Essential tremor that becomes symptomatic in old people.

**se·nil·i·ty** (sĕ-nil´i-tē) Negative and pejorative connotations of this word may render it offensive in some contexts. 1. Old age. 2. General term for a variety of organic disorders, both physical and mental, occurring in old age.

**sen·sate** (sen´sāt) Able to perceive touch and other sensations.

**sen·sa·tion** (sen-sā´shŭn) A feeling; translation into consciousness of effects of a stimulus exciting any of the organs of sense. [L. sensatio, perception, feeling, fr. sentio, to perceive, feel]

**sense** (sens) Faculty of perceiving any stimulus. [L. sentio, pp. sensus, to feel, to perceive]

**sense of e·qui·lib·ri·um** (sens ē´kwi-lib´

**st**

rē-ŭm) Sense that makes possible a normal physiologic posture.

**sen·sim·e·ter** (sen-sim'ĕ-ter) Instrument that measures degrees of cutaneous sensation. [L. *sensus,* sense, + G. *metron,* measure]

**sen·si·tive** (sen'si-tiv) **1.** Capable of perceiving sensations. **2.** Responsive to a stimulus. **3.** Acutely perceptive of interpersonal situations. **4.** Readily undergoing a chemical change, with but slight change in environmental conditions.

**sen·si·tiv·i·ty** (sen'si-tiv'i-tē) **1.** Ability to appreciate by one or more senses. **2.** State of being sensitive. SYN esthesia. **3.** In clinical pathology and medical screening, proportion of affected patients who give a positive test result for disease test is intended to reveal, i.e., true-positive results divided by total true-positive and false-negative results, usually expressed as a percentage. [L. *sentio,* pp. *sensus,* to feel]

**sen·si·ti·za·tion** (sen'si-tī-zā'shŭn) **1.** Immunization, especially with reference to antigens (immunogens) not associated with infection; induction of acquired sensitivity or of allergy. **2.** In substance use/abuse parlance, increased response seen to subsequent administration of the substance.

**sen·si·tiz·ing in·jec·tion** (sen'si-tīz-ing in-jek'shŭn) Injection that sensitizes a person so that subsequent exposure to the antigen (allergen) evokes an allergic response.

**sen·sor** (sen'sŏr) In digital radiography, detector placed intraorally to capture an image. SEE sense.

**sen·so·ri·al** (sen-sōr'ē-ăl) Relating to the sensorium.

**sen·so·ri·glan·du·lar** (sen'sŏr-ē-glan'dyū-lăr) Relating to glandular secretion excited by stimulation of sensory nerves.

**sen·so·ri·mo·tor, sen·so·mo·tor** (sen'sŏr-ē-mō'tŏr, sen'sō-) Both sensory and motor; denoting a mixed nerve with afferent and efferent fibers.

**sen·so·ri·mus·cu·lar** (sen'sŏr-ē-mŭs'kyū-lăr) Denoting muscular contraction in response to a sensory stimulus.

**sen·sor·i·neu·ral hear·ing loss** (sen'sŏr-ē-nūr'ăl hēr'ing laws) A form of auditory problem due to a lesion of the auditory division of the vestibulocochlear nerve or the inner ear.

**sen·so·ri·um,** pl. **sen·so·ri·a,** pl. **sen·so·ri·ums** (sen-sōr'ē-ŭm, -ă, -ŭmz) **1.** Organ of sensation. **2.** The hypothetic "seat of sensation." **3.** In human biology and psychology, consciousness; sometimes used as a generic term for the intellectual and cognitive functions. [Late L.]

**sen·so·ri·vas·o·mo·tor** (sen'sŏr-ē-vā'sō-

mō'tŏr) Denoting contraction or dilation of the blood vessels occurring as a sensory reflex.

**sen·so·ry** (sen'sŏr-ē) Relating to sensation. [L. *sensorius,* fr. *sensus,* sense]

**sen·so·ry ep·i·lep·sy** (sen'sŏr-ē ep'i-lep'sē) Focal epilepsy initiated by a somatosensory phenomenon.

**sen·so·ry im·age** (sen'sŏr-ē im'ăj) Image based on one or more types of sensation.

**sen·so·ry phan·tom** (sen'sŏr-ē fan'tŏm) Perceived sensation unrelated to or distinct from any actual stimulus, which can occur in any of the senses.

**sen·so·ry pre·cip·i·tat·ed ep·i·lep·sy** (sen'sŏr-ē prĕ-sip'i-tā-tĕd ep'i-lep-sē) SYN reflex epilepsy.

**sen·su·al** (sen'shū-ăl) **1.** Relating to the body and the senses, as distinguished from the intellect or spirit. **2.** Denoting bodily or sensory pleasure, not necessarily sexual. [L. *sensualis,* endowed with feeling]

**sep·a·rat·ing me·di·um** (sep'ăr-āt-ing mē'dē-ŭm) **1.** In dentistry, material usually applied to a cast to facilitate separation from the resin denture base after curing; coating on impressions to facilitate cast removal. **2.** Any coating that serves to prevent one surface from adhering to another.

**sep·a·rat·ing strip** (sep'ăr-āt-ing strip) A piece of plastic or metal used to prevent restorative resin from bonding to the tooth adjacent to the one being restored. SYN plastic strip.

**sep·a·rat·ing wire** (sep'ăr-āt-ing wīr) Wire, usually soft brass, used to gain separation between teeth. SEE ALSO separation (2).

**sep·a·ra·tion** (sep'ăr-ā'shŭn) In dentistry, process of gaining slight spaces between teeth preparatory to treatment.

**sep·a·ra·tion of teeth** (sep'ăr-ā'shŭn tēth) **1.** Loss of proximal contact of teeth. **2.** In orthodontics, creation of interproximal spaces to fit an appliance.

**sep·a·ra·tor** (sep'ăr-ā-tŏr) **1.** In dentistry, instrument for forcing two teeth apart, so as to gain access to adjacent proximal walls. **2.** That which divides or keeps apart two or more substances. [L. *se-paro,* pp. *-atus,* to separate, fr. *se,* apart, + *paro,* to prepare]

**sep·sis,** pl. **sep·ses** (sep'sis, -sēz) Presence of various pathogenic organisms, or their toxins, in blood or tissues. [G. *sēpsis,* putrefaction]

**sep·sis syn·drome** (sep'sis sin'drōm) Clinical evidence of acute infection with hyperthermia or hypothermia, tachycardia, tachypnea, and evidence of inadequate organ function.

**sep·ta** (sep'tă) Plural of septum. [L.]

**sep·tal** (sep′tăl) Relating to a septum.

**sep·tal ar·te·ry** (sep′tăl ahr′tĕr-ē) Branch of superior labial artery that supplies lower part of nasal septum.

**sep·tal gin·gi·va** (sep′tăl jin′ji-vă) Portion of gingiva that covers interdental septum.

**sep·ti·ce·mi·a** (sep′ti-sē′mē-ă) Systemic disease caused by the spread of microorganisms and their toxins through circulating blood; formerly called "blood poisoning." [G. *sēpsis*, putrefaction, + *haima*, blood]

**sep·tic shock** (sep′tik shok) **1.** Shock associated with infection that has released large enough quantities of toxins or vasoactive substances including cytokines, to be associated with hypotension. **2.** Shock associated with septicemia caused by gram-negative bacteria.

**sep·to·na·sal** (sep′tō-nā′zăl) Relating to nasal septum.

**sep·to·op·tic dys·pla·si·a** (sep′tō-op′tik dis-plā′zē-ă) Congenital optic nerve hypoplasia associated with midline cerebral anomalies.

**sep·tum,** pl. **sep·ta** (sep′tŭm, -tă) *Avoid the incorrect plurals septi and septae.* **1.** [TA] Thin wall dividing two cavities or masses of softer tissue. **2.** In nasal anatomy, sagittal partition dividing nasal airways. [L. *saeptum*, a partition]

**se·que·la,** pl. **se·que·lae** (sĕ-kwel′ă, -lē) A condition following as a consequence of a disease. [L. *sequela*, a sequel, fr. *sequor*, to follow]

**se·quence** (sē′kwĕns) **1.** Succession, or following, of one thing, process, or event after another. **2.** Imposition of a particular order on several items. [L. *sequor*, to follow]

**se·ques·tra·tion** (sē′kwes-trā′shŭn) **1.** Formation of a sequestrum. **2.** Loss of blood or of its fluid content into body spaces so that it is withdrawn from the circulating volume, resulting in hemodynamic impairment, hypovolemia, hypotension, and reduced venous return to heart. [L. *sequestratio*, fr. *sequestro*, pp. *-atus*, to lay aside]

**se·ques·trum,** pl. **se·ques·tra** (sē-kwes′trŭm, -tră) Piece of necrotic tissue, usually bone, which has become separated from the surrounding healthy tissue. [Mod. L. use of Mediev. L. *sequestrum*, something laid aside, fr. L. *sequestro*, to lay aside, separate]

**ser·en·dip·i·ty** (ser-en-dip′i-tē) A knack for discovery involving combined accident and wisdom while pursuing something else.

**se·ri·al ex·trac·tion** (sēr′ē-ăl ek-strak′shŭn) Selective extraction of some deciduous or permanent teeth, or both, during early years of dental development, usually with eventual extraction of first, or occasionally second, premolars, to encourage autonomous adjustment of moderate to severe crowding of anterior teeth; may or may not require subsequent orthodontic treatment.

**ser·ies,** pl. **ser·ies** (sēr′ēz) **1.** Succession of similar objects following one another in space or time. **2.** In diagnostic medicine, denotes a group of related tests leading to examination to either establish or rule out a given diagnosis. [L. fr. *sero*, to *join* together]

**ser·ine** (sĕr′ēn) One of the amino acids occurring in proteins.

**se·ro·con·ver·sion** (sēr′ō-kŏn-vĕr′zhŭn) Development of detectable specific antibodies in the serum due to infection.

**se·ro·di·ag·no·sis** (sēr′ō-dī′ăg-nō′sis) Diagnosis by means of serologic reactions using blood serum or other serous body fluids.

**se·ro·ep·i·de·mi·ol·o·gy** (sēr′ō-ep′i-dē′mē-ol′ŏ-jē) Epidemiologic study based on the detection of infection by serologic testing.

**se·ro·lo·gic di·ag·no·sis** (sēr′ō-loj′ik dī′ăg-nō′sis) Identification and diagnosis of disease based on findings of serum markers specific to that condition.

**se·ro·lo·gic test** (sēr′ō-loj′ik test) Any diagnostic test in which serum (blood) is used.

**se·ro·mu·cous gland** (sēr′ō-myū′kŭs gland) **1.** Gland in which some secretory cells are serous and some mucous. **2.** Gland with cells that secrete a fluid intermediate varying between watery and a more viscous mucoid substances.

**se·ro·neg·a·tive** (sēr′ō-neg′ă-tiv) Lacking an antibody of a specific type in serum.

**se·ro·pos·i·tive** (sēr′ō-poz′i-tiv) Containing antibody of a specific type in serum.

**se·ro·pus** (sēr′ō-pŭs) Purulent serum, i.e., pus largely diluted with serum.

**se·ro·sa** (sēr-ō′să) [TA] Outermost coat or serous layer of visceral structure that lies in body cavities of abdomen or thorax. SYN serous membrane. [fem. of Mod. L. *serosus*, serous]

**se·ro·ther·a·py** (sēr′ō-thār′ă-pē) Treatment of infectious disease by injection of antitoxin or serum containing specific antibody.

**ser·o·to·nin** (ser′ō-tō′nin) A vasoconstrictor, liberated by platelets; inhibits gastric secretion and stimulates smooth muscle; also acts as a neurotransmitter; present in the central nervous system, many peripheral tissues and cells, and carcinoid tumors. SYN 5-hydroxytryptamine. [L. *serum* + G. *tonos*, tone, tension, + *-in*]

**ser·o·to·nin nor·ep·i·neph·rine re·up·take in·hib·i·tor** (ser′ō-tō′nin nōr-ep′i-nef′rin rē-ŭp′tăk in-hib′i-tŏr) Class of antidepressant drugs the action of which is thought

**st**

to result from inhibition of presynaptic reuptake of serotonin and norepinephrine.

**se·rous** (sēr'ŭs) Relating to, containing, or producing serum or a substance having a watery consistency.

**se·rous cell** (sēr'ŭs sel) A cell, especially of the salivary gland, which secretes a watery albuminous fluid.

**se·rous di·ar·rhe·a** (sēr'ŭs dī'ă-rē'ă) Diarrhea characterized by watery stools.

**se·rous gland** (sēr'ŭs gland) Gland that secretes a watery substance that may or may not contain an enzyme.

**se·rous mem·brane** (sēr'ŭs mem'brān) SYN serosa.

**ser·pig·i·nous cor·ne·al ul·cer** (sĕr-pij'i-nŭs kōr'nē-ăl ŭl'sĕr) Corneal serpentine ulceration, due to infection, most often with *Streptococcus pneumoniae.*

**ser·rate su·ture** (sĕr'āt sū'chŭr) [TA] One with opposing margins that present deep sawlike indentations, as with most of the sagittal suture. SYN dentate suture.

***Ser·ra·ti·a*** (sĕ-rā'shē-ă) A genus of motile, peritrichous, aerobic to facultatively anaerobic bacteria that cause infection in humans. [Serafino *Serrati,* 18th-century Italian physicist]

**se·rum,** pl. **se·ra,** pl. **se·rums** (sēr'ŭm, -ă, -ŭmz ) *Avoid the colloquial or jargonistic use of this word in the sense of 'any biologic agent' ("allergy serum") or 'any injected drug' ("truth serum").* **1.** Clear, watery fluid, especially that moistening the surface of serous membranes, or exuded in inflammation of any of those membranes. **2.** Fluid portion of blood obtained after removal of fibrin clot and blood cells. [L. whey]

**se·rum ac·cel·er·a·tor** (sēr'ŭm ak-sel'ĕr-ā-tŏr) SYN factor VII.

**se·rum ac·cel·er·a·tor glob·u·lin** (sēr'ŭm ak-sel'ĕr-ā-tŏr glob'yū-lin) A substance in serum that accelerates the conversion of prothrombin to thrombin in the presence of thromboplastin and calcium.

**se·rum ac·ci·dent** (sēr'ŭm ak'si-dĕnt) Anaphylactic shock resulting from injection of serum of a different species for therapeutic purposes.

**se·rum·al cal·cu·lus** (sēr'ŭm kal'kyū-lŭs) **1.** Greenish or dark brown calcareous tooth deposit, usually apical to gingival margin. **2.** SYN subgingival calculus.

**se·rum mark·er** (sēr'ŭm mahr'kĕr) Specific component in the blood.

**se·rum pro·throm·bin con·ver·sion ac·cel·er·a·tor (SPCA)** (sēr'ŭm prō-

throm'bin kŏn-vĕr'zhŭn ăk-sel'ĕr-ā-tŏr) SYN factor VII.

**se·rum sick·ness** (sēr'ŭm sik'nĕs) Immune complex disease appearing some days (usually 7–14) after injection of foreign serum or serum protein, with local and systemic reactions such as urticaria, fever, general lymphadenopathy, edema, and arthritis.

**ser·vice** (sĕr'vis) A firm or agency that provides on-scene response, assessment, stabilization, initial treatment as directed, and transport to the appropriate receiving facility (i.e., trauma center or hospital) for medical emergency or trauma patients. [L. *servio,* to serve, fr. *servus,* slave]

**set** (set) **1.** Readiness to perceive or respond in some way; attitude that facilitates or predetermines an outcome, e.g., prejudice or bigotry as a set to respond negatively, independently of merits of the stimulus. **2.** To reduce a fracture, i.e., to bring bones back into a normal position or alignment. **3.** Defined group of events, objects, data, distinguishable from other groups. [M.E. *sette,* fr. O.Fr., fr. Med. L. *secta,* course, fr. *sequor,* to follow]

**set·back** (set'bak) Surgical treatment of bilateral cleft of the palate in which premaxilla is moved posteriorly.

**set·ting** (set'ing) Hardening, as of amalgam.

**set·ting ex·pan·si·on** (set'ing eks-pan'shŭn) Dimensional increase that occurs concurrently with hardening of various materials, such as plaster of Paris.

**set·ting time** (set'ing tīm) Duration required for a dental material (e.g., amalgam) to harden into its permanent state.

**set-up** (set'ŭp) **1.** Arrangement of teeth on a trial denture base. **2.** Procedure in dental case analysis involving cutting off and repositioning teeth in desired positions on a plaster cast.

**sev·enth cra·ni·al nerve [CN VII]** (sev'ĕnth krā'nē-ăl nĕrv) SYN facial nerve [CN VII].

**se·vere a·cute res·pi·ra·tory syn·drome (SARS)** (sĕ-vēr' ă-kyūt' res'pir-ă-tōr-ē sin'drōm) Disorder that usually begins with a fever often accompanied by other symptoms such as headache, malaise, myalgia, or diarrhea. Following this prodrome by approximately 3–7 days, the patient develops cough (not usually productive) and shortness of breath.

**se·vere com·bined im·mu·no·de·fi·cien·cy (SCID)** (sĕ-vēr' kŏm-bīnd' im'yū-nō-dĕ-fish'ĕn-sē) Immunodeficiency with absence of both humoral and cellular immunity with lymphopenia (of both B-type and T-type lymphocytes); characterized by thymus atrophy, lack of delayed hypersensitivity, and marked susceptibility to infections by bacteria, viruses, fungi, protozoa, and live vaccines.

**sex** (seks) **1.** Biologic character or quality that distinguishes male and female from one another as expressed by analysis of person's gonadal, morphologic (internal and external), chromosomal, and hormonal characteristics. **2.** Physiologic and psychological processes within a person that prompt behavior related to procreation or erotic pleasure. [L. *sexus*]

**sex cell** (seks sel) Sperm or oocyte. SYN germ cell.

**sex chro·mo·somes** (seks krō'mŏ-sōmz) The pair of chromosomes responsible for sex determination. In humans and most animals, the sex chromosomes are designated X and Y; females have two X chromosomes, males have one X and one Y chromosome.

**sex hor·mones** (seks hōr'mōnz) General term covering those steroid hormones formed by testicular, ovarian, and adrenocortical tissues: androgens, estrogens, or progestins.

**sex-in·flu·enced** (seks-in'flū-ĕnst) Denoting a class of genetic disorders in which the same genotype has differing manifestations in two sexes; variation may be rational (e.g., breast cancer occurs less frequently in males) or have only empiric support (e.g., pattern baldness behaves as a dominant trait in male and as a recessive trait in female).

**sex-in·flu·enced in·her·i·tance** (seks-in'flū-ĕnst in-her'i-tăns) Autosomal inheritance that has a different intensity of expression in two sexes, e.g., male pattern baldness.

**sex link·age, sex-link·ed** (seks lingk'ăj, seks-lingkt) Inheritance of trait, a sex chromosome, or gonosome. A man receives all his sex-linked genes from his mother and transmits them all to his daughters but not to his sons; recessive sex-linked character is much more likely to be expressed in the male.

**sex-link·ed cha·rac·ter** (seks'lingkt kar'ăk-tĕr) Inherited character determined by a gene on a gonosome.

**sex-link·ed in·her·i·tance** (seks'lingkt in-her'i-tăns) Pattern of inheritance that may result from a mutant gene located on either X or Y chromosomes.

**sex·tant** (seks'tănt) One of six divisions of dentition; teeth of upper and lower jaws are divided into right posterior, left posterior, and anterior. [L. *sextus*, sixth]

**sex·u·al di·morph·ism** (sek'shū-ăl dī-mōr'fizm) Somatic differences within species between male and female individuals that arise as a consequence of sexual maturation.

**sex·u·al dis·or·ders** (sek'shū-ăl dis-ōr'dĕrz) Group of behavioral and psychophysio-

logic disorders with symptomatic variability in sexual functioning, including eroticized behavior associated with sexual activity.

**sex·u·al·i·ty** (sek'shū-al'i-tē) **1.** Sum of a person's sexual behaviors and tendencies, and strength of such tendencies. **2.** One's degree of sexual attractiveness. **3.** Quality of having sexual functions or implications.

**sex·u·al·i·za·tion** (sek'shū-ăl-ī-zā'shŭn) **1.** State characterized by the presence of sexual energy or drive. **2.** Act of acquiring sexual energy or drive. **3.** Act of imputing a sexual meaning or quality to people or behaviors.

**sex·u·al·ly trans·mit·ted dis·ease (STD)** (sek'shū-ă-lē tranz-mit'ĕd di-zēz') Contagious disease acquired during sexual contact (e.g., syphilis, gonorrhea, chancroid). SYN venereal disease, sexually transmitted infection.

**sex·u·al·ly trans·mit·ted infection (STI)** (sek'shū-ăl-ē tranz-mit'ĕd in-fek'shŭn) SYN sexually transmitted disease.

**shad·ow** (shad'ō) Surface area defined by interception of light or x-rays by a body.

**shaft** (shaft) [TA] An elongated rodlike structure. SYN diaphysis [TA]. [A.S. *sceaft*]

**shak·en ba·by syn·drome (SBS)** (shā'kĕn bā'bē sin'drōm) A syndrome of neurologic and other injuries, of variable presentation, induced by the violent shaking of an infant.

**shakes** (shāks) Colloquial term for paroxysm associated with an intermittent fever and with tremor associated with alcohol (and other substance) withdrawal.

**shal·low breath·ing** (shal'ō brēdh'ing) Respiration with abnormally low tidal volume.

**sham-move·ment ver·ti·go** (sham-mūv'mĕnt vĕr'ti-gō) Dizziness accompanied by an impression that body is rotating or objects are rotating around it.

**shank** (shangk) The portion of an instrument that connects the cutting or functional portion to a handle; with rotary tools, such as burs and drills, the end that fits into the chuck. [A.S. *sceanca*]

**sharp cut·ting edge** (shahrp kŭt'ing ej) Fine line formed by pointed junction of instrument face and lateral surface.

**shar·pen·ing** (shahrp'ĕn-ing) Dental preparatory procedure in which a cutting-edge is honed or replaced on a dental tool (e.g., calculus-removal instrument).

**shar·pen·ing stone** (shahrp'ĕn-ing stōn) Natural or synthetic stone composed of abrasive particles used to restore a sharp cutting edge on a calculus removal instrument.

**shar·pen·ing tech·nique** (shahr'pĕn-ing

**st**

tek-nēk´) Procedure used to maintain the sharpness of a cutting edge on an instrument that is used for scaling. There are two versions: stationary and moving techniques.

**shar·pen·ing test stick** (shahrp´ĕn-ing test stik) Plastic or acrylic rod used to evaluate sharpness of a cutting edge.

**Shar·pey fi·bers** (shahr´pē fī´bĕrz) Bundles of collagenous fibers that pass into the outer circumferential lamellae of bone, alveolar bone proper of the alveolus of teeth, or the cementum of teeth. SYN perforating fibers.

**sharps** (shahrps) Medical instruments that are sharp or may produce sharp pieces; should be disposed of in a biohazard sharps container.

**sharps con·tain·er** (shahrps kŏn-tān´ĕr) A puncture-resistant and leak-proof container with a one-way top used to dispose of sharps.

**shave bi·op·sy** (shāv bī´op-sē) A biopsy technique performed with a surgical blade or a razorblade; used for lesions that are elevated above the skin level or confined to the epidermis and upper dermis, or to protrusions of lesions from internal sites.

**shear** (shēr) Distortion of a body by two oppositely directed parallel forces; consists of a sliding over one another of imaginary planes (within body) parallel to planes of forces. [A.S.]

**shear·ing edge** (shēr´ing ej) SYN incisal margin.

**sheath** (shēth) 1. Tube used as an orthodontic appliance, usually on molars. 2. Any enveloping structure, such as membranous covering of a muscle, nerve, or blood vessel. 3. Specially designed tubular instrument through which special obturators or cutting instruments can be passed, or through which blood clots, tissue fragments, and calculi can be evacuated. [A.S. *scaeth*]

**sheath of Schwann** (shēth shwahn) SYN neurilemma.

**shed·ding** (shed´ing) SEE viral shedding.

**Shee·han syn·drome** (shē´an sin´drōm) Hypopituitarism developing postpartum due to pituitary necrosis.

**shelf life** (shelf līf) Stability of a product after it is prepared or manufactured; length of time any substance may be stored before changes occur that alter its chemical structure or make-up and degeneration ensues.

**shel·lac** (shĕ-lak´) A resinous excretion that softens at low temperature and has many non-medicinal uses and is also used to coat confections and tablets and in dental materials, e.g., impression compound and denture base plates.

**shel·lac base** (shĕ-lak´ bās) Resinous wafer adapted to maxillary or mandibular casts to form baseplates.

**shield** (shēld) A lead sheet to protect operator and patient from x-rays.

**shift to the left** (shift left) Marked increase in percentage of immature cells in circulating blood.

**shift to the right** (shift rīt) In a differential count of leukocytes in peripheral blood, absence of young and immature forms.

**Shi·gel·la** (shē-gel´lă) Genus of nonmotile, aerobic to facultatively anaerobic bacteria with habitat in the intestinal tract of humans and of higher apes; all species produce dysentery. [Kiyoshi *Shiga*]

**Shi·gel·la son·ne·i** (shē-gel´lă son´ē-ī) Bacterial species causing dysentery, sometimes milder than that caused by other species.

**shig·el·lo·sis** (shig´ĕ-lō´sis) Bacillary dysentery caused by bacteria of the genus *Shigella*, often occurring in epidemic patterns; opportunistic infection in people with AIDS.

**shin·gles** (shing´gĕlz) SYN herpes zoster. [L. *cingulum,* girdle]

**shock** (shok) 1. State in which cells of body receive inadequate amounts of oxygen secondary to changes in perfusion; most commonly due to blood loss or sepsis. 2. Sudden physical or biochemical disturbance that results in inadequate blood flow and oxygenation of an animal's vital organs. 3. State of profound mental and physical depression consequent to severe physical injury or to emotional disturbance. [Fr. *choc,* fr. Germanic]

**short-bow·el syn·drome** (shōrt bow´ĕl sin´drōm) Complex of symptoms that can result whenever the absorptive surface of the small bowel is reduced, as in massive or multiple small bowel resections. Symptoms include diarrhea, weight loss, malabsorption, anemia, and vitamin, mineral, and electrolyte abnormalities. SYN short-gut syndrome.

**short-cone tech·nique** (shōrt-kōn´ tek-nēk´) A radiographic method in dentistry wherein the cone used for alignment of the head of the radiographic machine with the film is about 20 cm (8 in) long.

**short-gut syndrome** SYN short-bowel syndrome.

**short-scale con·trast** (shōrt-skāl´ kon´trast) A radiographic image that shows areas mainly of black and white, and thus has high contrast.

**short·sight·ed·ness** (shōrt-sīt´ĕd-nĕs) SYN myopia.

**short-term mem·o·ry (STM)** (shōrt-tĕrm´ mem´ŏr-ē) Phase of memory process in which stimuli that have been recognized and registered are stored briefly; decay occurs rapidly, sometimes within seconds.

**shot-feel** (shot´fēl) Peculiar sensation as of a nervous discharge or electric shock passing rapidly from top of the head to feet, sometimes described as a sensation of the rolling of shot down the body, occurring in acromegaly.

**shot·gun pre·scrip·tion** (shot´gŭn prĕ-skrip´shŭn) Prescription containing many ingredients, some of which may be useless, in an attempt to cover all possible types of therapy that may be needed; a pejorative term.

**shoul·der** (shōl′dĕr) **1.** In dentistry, any step formed by junction of gingival and axial walls in extracoronal restorative preparations. **2.** Lateral portion of scapular region, where scapula joins with clavicle and humerus and is covered by rounded mass of the deltoid muscle. [A.S. *sculder*]

**sho·vel-shaped in·ci·sor** (shŏv′ĕl-shāpt in-sī′zŏr) Incisor in which lingual, and occasionally labial, marginal ridges are accentuated; more highly developed in people of Asian origin. See this page.

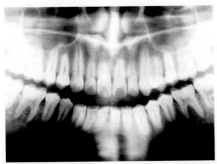

**shovel-shaped incisors:** (radiograph)

**shunt** (shŭnt) **1.** To bypass or divert. **2.** Bypass or diversion of fluid to another fluid-containing system by fistulation or a prosthetic device. [M.E. *shunten*, to flinch]

**Shwach·man syn·drome** (shwahk′măn sin′drōm) Disorder characterized by sinusitis, bronchiectasis, pancreatic insufficiency resulting in malabsorption, neutropenia with defect in neutrophile chemotaxis, short stature, and skeletal changes.

**SI** Abbreviation for International System of Units.

**Si** Symbol for silicon.

**SIADH** Abbreviation for syndrome of inappropriate secretion of antidiuretic hormone.

**si·al·a·den** (sī-al′ă-den) A salivary gland. [*sial-* + G. *adēn*, gland]

**si·al·ad·e·ni·tis, si·al·o·ad·e·ni·tis** (sī′al-ad′ĕ-nī′tis, sī′ă-lō-) Inflammation of a salivary gland. [*sial-* + G. *adēn*, gland, + *-itis*, inflammation]

**si·al·ad·e·no·trop·ic** (sī′ăl-ad′ĕ-nō-trō′pik) Having an influence on the salivary glands. [*sial-* + G. *adēn*, gland, + *tropē*, a turning]

**si·al·a·gogue, si·al·o·gogue** (sī-al′ă-gog, -ŏ-gog) **1.** Promoting saliva flow. **2.** Agent having this action (e.g., anticholinesterase agents). [*sial-* + G. *agōgos*, drawing forth]

**si·al·ec·ta·sis** (sī′ă-lek′tă-sis) Dilation of a salivary duct. [*sial-* + G. *ektasis*, a stretching]

**si·al·em·e·sis, si·al·e·me·si·a** (sī′al-ĕ-mē′sis, -ĕ-mē′zē-ă) Vomiting of saliva, or vomiting caused by or accompanying an excessive secretion of saliva. [*sial-* + G. *emesis*, vomiting]

**si·al·en·dos·co·py** (sī′ăl-en-dos′kŏ-pē) A method of visualization of the Wharton or Stensen duct to visualize sialolithiasis, stenosis, polyps, or sialodochitis.

**si·al·ic** (sī-al′ik) SYN salivary.

**si·a·line** (sī′ă-lēn) SYN salivary.

**si·a·lism, si·a·lis·mus** (sī′ă-lizm, -liz′mŭs) SYN sialorrhea. [G. *sialismos*]

○ **sialo-, sial-** Combining forms denoting saliva, salivary glands. [G. *sialon*]

**si·a·lo·ad·e·nec·to·my** (sī′ă-lō-ad′ĕ-nek′tŏ-mē) Excision of a salivary gland. [*sialo-* + G. *adēn*, gland, + *ektomē*, excision]

**si·a·lo·aer·oph·a·gy** (sī′ă-lō-ār-of′ă-jē) Habit of frequent swallowing whereby quantities of saliva and air are taken into the stomach. SYN aerosialophagy. [*sialo-* + G. *aēr*, air, + *phagō*, to eat]

**si·a·lo·an·gi·ec·ta·sis** (sī′ă-lō-an′jē-ek′tă-sis) Dilation of salivary ducts. [*sialo-* + G. *angeion*, vessel, + *ektasis*, a stretching]

**si·a·lo·an·gi·i·tis** (sī′ă-lō-an′jē-ī′tis) SYN sialodochitis. [*sialo-* + G. *angeion*, vessel, + *-itis*, inflammation]

**si·a·lo·cele** (sī′ă-lō-sēl) SYN ranula. [*sialo-* + G. *kēlē*, tumor]

**si·a·lo·do·chi·tis** (sī′ă-lō-dō-kī′tis) Inflammation of the duct of a salivary gland. SYN sialoangiitis. [*sialo-* + G. *dochē*, receptacle, + *-itis*, inflammation]

**si·a·lo·do·cho·plas·ty** (sī′ă-lō-dō′kō-plas′tē) Repair of a salivary duct. [*sialo-* + G. *dochē*, receptacle, + *plassō*, to fashion]

**si·al·o·gram** (sī-al′ō-gram) A radiograph using sialography. [*sialo-* + G. *gramma*, a writing]

**si·a·log·ra·phy** (sī′ă-log′ră-fē) Radiographic imaging of the salivary glands and ducts after the area of the oral cavity has been injected with a radiopaque dye to help the clinician visualize obstruction. [*sialo-* + G. *graphō*, to write]

**si·al·o·lith** (sī′ă-lō-lith) A salivary calculus. See page 520. [*sialo-* + G. *lithos*, stone]

st

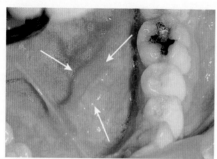

**salivary duct cyst:** caused by sialolith

**🖻 si·a·lo·li·thi·a·sis** (sī′ă-lō-li-thī′ă-sis) The formation or presence of a salivary calculus. See this page. [*sialolith* + G. *-iasis,* condition]

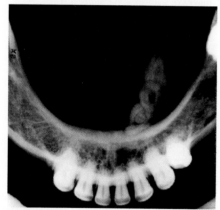

**sialolithiasis:** concentric laminations of multiple calculi

**si·a·lo·li·thot·o·my** (sī′ă-lō-li-thot′ŏ-mē) Incision of a salivary duct or gland to remove a calculus. [*sialolith* + G. *tome,* incision]

**si·a·lo·met·a·pla·si·a** (sī′ă-lō-met′ă-plā′zē-ă) Squamous cell metaplasia in the salivary ducts.

**si·a·lom·e·try** (sī′ă-lom′ĕ-trē) A measurement of salivary secretion, generally for a comparison of a denervated or diseased gland with its healthy counterpart. [*sialo-* + G. *metron,* measure]

**si·al·o·pro·tein** (sī′ă-lō-prō′tēn) Protein produced by salivary glands and thereby usually present in saliva.

**si·a·lor·rhe·a** (sī′ă-lōr-ē′ă) Hypersalivation that may be in response to intraoral pain and inflammation, and to neurologic and other systemic disorders. SYN sialism, sialismus, sialorrhoea. [*sialo-* + G. *rhoia,* a flow]

**sialorrhoea** [Br.] SYN sialorrhea.

**si·a·los·che·sis** (sī′ă-los′kĕ-sis) Suppression of the secretion of saliva. [*sialo-* + G. *schesis,* retention]

**si·a·lo·se·mi·ol·o·gy** (sī′ă-lō-sē′mē-ol′ō-jē) Study and analysis of saliva as an aid to diagnosis. [*sialo-* + G. *semeion,* sign, + *logos,* study]

**sib** (sib) SYN sibling.

**sib·i·lant** (sib′i-lănt) Hissing or whistling in character; denoting a form of rhonchus. [L. *sibilans* (*-ant-*), pres. p. of *sibilo,* to hiss]

**sib·i·lant rale** (sib′i-lănt rahl) Whistling sound caused by air moving through a viscid secretion narrowing lumen of a bronchus. SYN sibilus.

**sib·i·lus** (sib′i-lŭs) SYN sibilant rale. [L. a hissing]

**sib·ling** (sib′ling) SYN sib. [A. S. *sib,* relation, + *-ling,* diminutive]

**si·bu·tra·mine** (si-byū′tră-mēn) A serotonin and noradrenaline reuptake inhibitor used to reduce appetite to encourage weight loss.

**sic·ca com·plex** (sik′ă kom′pleks) Dryness of mucous membranes, as of eyes and mouth, in the absence of a connective tissue disease.

**sicklaemia** [Br.] SYN sicklemia.

**sick·le cell a·ne·mi·a** (sik′ĕl sel ă-nē′mē-ă) Blood disorder characterized by crescent- or sickle-shaped erythrocytes and accelerated hemolysis. Most common in people of African descent. Also called sickle cell disease.

**sick·le cell thal·as·se·mi·a dis·ease** (sik′ĕl sel thal′ă-sē′mē-ă di-zēz′) Anemia clinically resembling sickle cell anemia.

**sick·le·mi·a** (sik-lē′mē-ă) Presence of sickle- or crescent-shaped erythrocytes in peripheral blood; seen in sickle cell anemia and sickle cell trait. SYN sicklaemia.

**🖻 sick·le sca·ler** (sik′ĕl skā′lĕr) Periodontal instrument used to remove calculus deposits from tooth crowns. Its working-end has a pointed back, pointed tip, and appears triangular in cross section. See page 521.

**sick role** (sik rōl) In medical sociology, familially or culturally accepted behavior pattern or role that one is permitted to exhibit during illness or disability, including sanctioned absence from school or work and a submissive, dependent relationship to family, health care personnel, and significant others.

**side ef·fect** (sīd e-fekt′) SYN adverse effect.

**sid·er·a·tion** (sid′ĕr-ā′shŭn) Any sudden attack, as of apoplexy.

**side shift** (sīd shift) Mediolateral bodily movement (translation) of the mandible during lateral movements of the jaw. Such action typically oc-

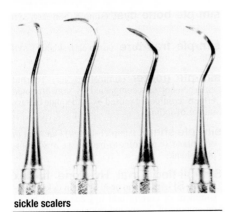

**sickle scalers**

curs in conjunction with horizontal plane rotation of the mandible; this mandibular shift can be programmed into some articulators.

**side·stream smoke** (sīd´strēm smōk) Aerosol emitted directly into the surrounding air from the lighted surface of a smoldering tobacco product; may be inhaled by the smoker or those in the vicinity.

**SIDS** Abbreviation for sudden infant death syndrome.

**sie·vert (Sv)** (sē´vĕrt) The SI unit of ionizing radiation effective dose.

**Sig, sig** Abbreviation for L. *signa*, label, write, or *signetur*, let it be labeled.

**sigh** (sī) **1.** An audible inspiration and expiration under the influence of some emotion. **2.** To perform such an act. [A.S. *sīcan*]

**sig·ma** (sig´mă) **1.** The 18th letter of the Greek alphabet (σ, Σ). **2.** (σ) reflection coefficient; standard deviation ; a factor in prokaryotic RNA initiation; surface tension. **3.** (Σ) Summation of a series.

**sig·moid** (sig´moyd) Resembling in outline the letter S or one of the forms of the Greek sigma σ or ç. [G. *sigma*, the letter S, + *eidos*, resemblance]

**sig·moid notch** (sig´moyd noch) SYN mandibular notch.

**sign** (sīn) Any abnormality indicative of disease, discoverable on examination of patient; objective indication of disease, in contrast to a symptom, which is a subjective indication of disease. [L. *signum*, mark]

**sig·na·ture (s)** (sig´nă-chŭr) Part of a prescription containing directions to the patient. [Mediev. L. *signatura*, fr. L. *signum*, a sign, mark]

**sign of the or·bic·u·la·ris** (sīn ōr-bik´yū-lā´ris) In hemiplegia, inability to voluntarily close the eye on paralyzed side except in conjunction with closure of the other eye.

**sil·den·a·fil** (sil-den´ă-fil) Agent that relaxes muscle in penis, resulting in greater blood flow and erection; used to treat male impotence; potentiates hypotensive effects of nitrates.

**si·lent** (sī´lĕnt) Producing no detectable signs or symptoms, said of certain diseases.

**si·lent a·re·a** (sī´lĕnt ar´ē-ă) Any area of cerebrum or cerebellum in which lesions cause no definite symptoms.

**si·lent pe·ri·od** (sī´lĕnt pēr´ē-ŏd) Time during which no electrical activity occurs in a muscle following its rapid unloading.

**sil·i·ca** (sil´i-kă) The chief constituent of sand, hence of glass. SYN silicon dioxide. [Mod. L. fr. L. *silex* (*silic*-), flint]

**sil·i·cate** (sil´i-kăt) **1.** Term sometimes applied to dental restorations made of synthetic porcelain. **2.** Salt of silicic acid.

**sil·i·cate ce·ment** (sil´i-kăt sĕ-ment´) Fixative used for anterior restorations; largely superseded in use by composite resins and glass ionomer cements.

**sil·i·cate re·stor·a·tion** (sil´i-kăt res´tŏr-ā´shŭn) Restoration of lost tooth structure made with silicate cement.

**sil·i·con di·ox·ide** (sil´i-kon dī-ok´sīd) SYN silica.

**sil·i·cone** (sil´i-kōn) Polymer of organic silicon oxides, which may be a liquid, gel, or solid, depending on extent of polymerization; used in surgical implants, in intracorporeal tubes to conduct fluids, as dental impression material, as a grease or sealing substance, as a coating on inside of glass vessels for blood collection, and in various ophthalmologic procedures.

**sil·i·co·phos·phate ce·ment** (sil´i-kō-fos´fāt sĕ-ment´) Adhesive that provides mechanical retention; fabricated from zinc phosphate and silicate cement.

**sil·i·co·sis** (sil´i-kō´sis) Form of pneumoconiosis resulting from occupational exposure to and inhalation of silica dust over a period of years. [L. *silex*, flint, + *-osis*, condition]

**si·li·qua o·li·vae** (sil´i-kwă ō-lī´vē) Arcuate fibers, which appear to encircle inferior olive in medulla oblongata.

**silk** (silk) The fibers or filaments obtained from the cocoon of the silkworm. [O.E. *sioloc*, fr. Chinese]

**silk su·ture** (silk sū´chŭr) SYN surgical silk.

**sil·ver** (sil´vĕr) L. *argentum;* a metallic element; many salts have clinical applications; used in dental amalgams and gold alloys. [A.S. *seolfor*]

**sil·ver a·mal·gam** (sil´vĕr ă-mal´găm) Alloy of silver, mercury, and other metals (e.g., tin, copper, zinc). The mercury is mixed with

**st**

the alloy powder resulting in a plastic material that can be condensed into a prepared tooth cavity and carved.

**sil·ver cone** (sil'vĕr kōn) Pure silver form with standard conic shape, used with cement to obturate dental root canals.

**sil·ver fil·ling** (sil'vĕr fil'ing) SYN amalgam restoration.

**sil·ver ni·trate** (sil'vĕr nī'trāt) Antiseptic and astringent.

**sil·ver point** (sil'vĕr poynt) Solid core cone of silver used to fill root canals in conjunction with cement or paste.

**sil·ver poi·son·ing** (sil'vĕr poy'zŏn-ing) SYN argyria.

**sil·ver sul·fa·di·a·zine** (sil'vĕr sŭl'fă-dī'ă-zēn) Silver derivative of sulfadiazine, used externally as a topical antibacterial agent.

**sil·ver-tin al·loy** (sil'vĕr-tin' al'oy) Any alloy of silver and tin; commonly 3 parts silver and 1 part tin, chief intermetallic compound in dental amalgam.

***si·mi·li·a si·mil·i·bus cur·an·tur*** (si-mil'ē-ă si-mil'i-bŭs kū-ran'tūr) Homeopathic concept expressing law of similars (literally, "likes are cured by likes"); doctrine that any drug capable of producing morbid symptoms in the healthy will remove similar symptoms occurring as an expression of disease. Another reading of the concept, employed by Hahnemann, the founder of homeopathy, is *similia similibus curentur*, "let likes be cured by likes." [L. likes are cured by likes]

**Sim·monds dis·ease** (sim'ŏndz di-zēz') Anterior pituitary insufficiency due to trauma, vascular lesions, or tumors. SYN hypophysial cachexia, pituitary cachexia.

**Si·mo·nart bands** (sē-mō-nahr' bandz) Web-like band of tissue partially filling gap between medial and lateral portions of a cleft lip.

**Si·mon clas·si·fi·ca·tion of mal·oc·clu·sion** (sī'mŏn klas'i-fi-kā'shŭn mal'ŏ-klū'zhŭn) System that relates tooth position to the Frankfurt horizontal, midsagittal, and orbital planes. Teeth are considered in attraction/distraction if too close or too far from the Frankfurt plane; in contraction/distraction if too close or too far from the midsagittal plane, and in protraction/retraction if too anterior or too posterior to the orbital plane.

**sim·ple an·chor·age** (simp'ĕl ang'kŏr-ăj) Anchorage in which resistance to movement of one or more teeth comes solely from resistance to tipping movement of anchorage unit.

**sim·ple beam** (simp'ĕl bēm) In dentistry, a straight beam that has only two supports, one at either end.

**sim·ple bone cyst** (simp'ĕl bōn sist) SYN solitary bone cyst.

**sim·ple frac·ture** (simp'ĕl frak'shŭr) SYN closed fracture.

**sim·ple goi·ter** (simp'ĕl goy'tĕr) Thyroid enlargement unaccompanied by constitutional effects, commonly caused by inadequate dietary intake of iodine.

**sim·ple shank** (simp'ĕl shangk) One bent in one plane (e.g., front-to-back). SEE ALSO complex shank.

**Sim·pli·fied Or·al Hy·giene In·dex (OHI-S)** (sim'pli-fīd ōr-ăl hī'jēn in'deks) Measurement of current oral hygiene status based on amount of debris and calculus occurring on six representative oral tooth surfaces; often used in field surveys of periodontal disease.

**sim·u·la·tion** (sim'yū-lā'shŭn) **1.** Imitation; said of a disease or symptom that resembles another, or of feigning of illness as in factitious illness or malingering. **2.** In radiation therapy, use of a geometrically similar radiographic system or computer to plan location of therapy ports. [L. *simulatio*, fr. *simulo*, pp. *-atus*, to imitate, fr. *similis*, like]

**sin·gle crys·tal sap·phire** (sing'gĕl kris'tăl saf'īr) Material composed of a crystalline aluminum oxide identical in structure to that of a sapphire gemstone; used as dental implant.

**sin·is·ter (s)** (sin-is'tĕr) [TA] Left. [L.]

**sin·is·trad** (sin'is-trad, si-nis'trad) Toward left side. [L. *sinister*, left, + *ad*, to]

**sin·is·tral** (sin'is-trăl) **1.** Relating to the left side. **2.** Denoting a left-handed person.

**si·no·pul·mo·nar·y** (sī'nō-pul'mŏ-nar-ē) Relating to paranasal sinuses and pulmonary airway.

**sin·ter** (sin'tĕr) To heat a powdered substance without thoroughly melting it, causing it to fuse into a solid but porous mass. [Ger. dross, slag]

**si·nu·a·tri·al node, si·no·a·tri·al node** (sin'yū-ā'trē-ăl nōd, sī'nō-) [TA] The mass of specialized cardiac muscle fibers that normally acts as the "pacemaker" of the cardiac conduction system; it lies under the epicardium at the upper end of the sulcus terminalis.

**si·nus,** pl. **si·nus,** pl. **si·nus·es** (sī'nŭs, -ĕz) *The plural of this word is sinus*, not *sini*. **1.** [TA] Channel for the passage of blood or lymph, without the coats of an ordinary vessel; e.g., blood passages in gravid uterus or those in cerebral meninges. **2.** [TA] Cavity or hollow space in bone or other tissue. **3.** Fistula or tract leading to a suppurating cavity. [L. *sinus*, cavity, channel, hollow]

**si·nus·i·tis** (sī'nŭ-sī'tis) Inflammation of the

lining membrane of any sinus, especially of one of the paranasal sinuses. [*sinus* + G. *-itis*, inflammation]

**si·nus tract** (sī′nŭs trakt) A channel that connects with an abscess or suppurating area. See this page.

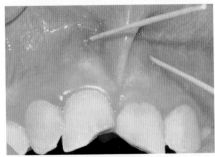

**sinus tracts:** exiting from nonvital incisors

**si op. sit. (s.o.s.)** Abbreviation for L. *si opus sit,* if needed.

**Sip·ple syn·drome** (sip′ĕl sin′drōm) Pheochromocytoma, medullary carcinoma of the thyroid, and parathyroid adenomas.

**site** (sīt) A place, location, or locus. [L. *situs*]

**sixth cra·ni·al nerve [CN VI]** (siksth krā′nē-ăl nĕrv) SYN abducent nerve [CN VI].

**sixth-year mo·lar** (siksth-yēr mō′lăr) First permanent molar tooth.

**Sjö·gren syn·drome** (shŏr′gren sin′drōm) Keratoconjunctivitis sicca, an autoimmune disease, involving dryness of mucous membranes, telangiectases, or purpuric spots on the face, and bilateral parotid enlargement; seen in menopausal women and often associated with rheumatoid arthritis, Raynaud phenomenon, and dental caries. [H.S.C. *Sjögren*]

**skel·e·ton** (skel′ĕ-tŏn) [TA] **1.** Bony body framework in vertebrates. **2.** All dry parts remaining after destruction and removal of soft parts; includes ligaments and cartilages as well as bones. **3.** All bones of body taken collectively. **4.** Rigid or semirigid nonosseous structure that functions as supporting framework of a particular structure. [G. *skeletos,* dried, ntr. *skeleton,* a mummy, a skeleton]

**skill** (skil) The ability to produce, efficiently and in a coordinated manner, movement or result on demand or desire repeatedly.

**skin** (skin) [TA] Membranous protective body covering, consisting of epidermis and dermis (corium). SYN cutis [TA]. [A.S. *scinn* ]

**skin dose** (skin dōs) The quantity of radiation delivered to the skin surface.

**skin of teeth** (skin tēth) SYN enamel cuticle.

**skin tag** (skin tag) Polypoid outgrowth of both epidermis and dermal fibrovascular tissue.

**skin test** (skin test) A method for determining induced sensitivity (allergy) by applying an antigen (allergen) to, or inoculating it into, the skin; induced sensitivity (allergy) to the specific antigen is indicated by an inflammatory reaction. SYN intradermal test.

**skull** (skŭl) SYN cranium. [Mid. Eng. *skulle,* a bowl]

**skull plate** (skŭl plāt) SYN cranial prosthesis.

**SL** Abbreviation for spinal length; sublingual.

**SLE** Abbreviation for systemic lupus erythematosus.

**sleep** (slēp) Physiologic state of relative unconsciousness and inaction of voluntary muscles, its need recurs periodically. [A.S. *slaep*]

**sleep ap·ne·a** (slēp ap′nē-ă) Central and peripheral breathing disorder during sleep, associated with frequent awakening and often with daytime sleepiness.

**sleep ap·ne·a syn·drome** (slēp ap′nē-ă sin′drōm) Disorder characterized by multiple episodes of partial or complete cessation of respiration during sleep.

**sleep def·i·cit** (slēp def′i-sit) Lack of sleep time or a relative lack of one of the stages of sleep as determined by a sleep study.

**sleep phase de·lay syn·drome** (slēp fāz dĕ-lā′ sin′drōm) A disorder in which the circadian rhythm of sleep and waking falls into a delayed but stable relationship with external time cues of day and night.

**SLE-like syn·drome** (līk sin′drōm) Disease with manifestations suggestive of systemic lupus erythematosus, without meeting diagnostic criteria for that disease.

**slid·ing flap** (slīd′ing flap) A rectangular area raised in an elastic area, with its free end adjacent to a defect; the defect is covered by stretching the flap longitudinally until the end comes over it.

**slid·ing hook** (slīd′ing huk) Movable attachment used on an orthodontic wire for application of elastic traction or headgear force.

**slid·ing ob·lique os·te·o·to·my** (slīd′ing ō-blēk′ os′tē-ot′ŏ-mē) Oral surgical procedure in which mandibular ramus is cut vertically from sigmoid notch to angle to facilitate posterior repositioning of mandible in correction of mandibular prognathism; may be performed extraorally or intraorally and is similar to vertical osteotomy.

**slim-di·am·e·ter in·stru·ment tip** (slim′ dī-am″ĕ-tĕr in′strŭ-mĕnt tip) Sonic or ultrasonic instrument tip smaller than the working-end of

**st**

a Gracey curette. SYN thin-diameter instrument tip.

**slime ma·trix or lay·er (gly·co·ca·lyx)** (slīm mā′triks lā′ĕr glī′kŏ-kā′liks) An amorphous mass of carbohydrate-based material made of lipopolysaccharides secreted by bacteria. It protects the biofilm colony.

**slope** (slōp) An inclination or slant.

**slough** (slŭf) 1. Necrosed tissue separated from the living structure. 2. To separate from the living tissue. [M.E. *slughe*]

**Slu·der neu·ral·gi·a** (slū′dĕr nūr-al′jē-ă) SYN sphenopalatine neuralgia.

**sluice·way** (slūs′wā) SYN spillway.

**slur·ry** (slŭr′ē) A thin semifluid suspension of a solid in a liquid.

**small in·ter·arch dis·tance** (smawl in′tĕr-ahrch′ dis′tăns) Narrow distance between maxillary and mandibular arches. SYN close bite.

**small·pox** (smawl′poks) An acute eruptive contagious disease caused by a poxvirus (variola); characterized by chills, fever, and an eruption of papules. [E. *small pocks,* or pustules]

**smear** (smēr) Thin specimen for examination; usually prepared by spreading material uniformly onto a glass slide, fixing it, and staining it before examination.

**smear lay·er** (smēr lā′ĕr) A layer of grinding debris that is burnished to tooth enamel or dentin when the tooth is cut.

**smear plug** (smēr plŭg) Plugs of grinding debris that extend 1–5 mcm into dentin tubules.

**smell** (smel) 1. To scent; to perceive an odor by means of the olfactory apparatus. 2. SYN odor.

**smoke·less to·bac·co** (smōk′lĕs tŏ-bak′ō) A form of the leaf of the plant meant to be chewed or otherwise ingested orally, rather than smoked. SYN chewing tobacco.

**smok·er's tongue** (smō′kĕrz tŭng) SYN leukoplakia.

**smooth broach** (smūdh brōch) Exploring instrument used in endodontic practice; a root canal tine.

**smooth mus·cle** (smūdh mŭs′ĕl) One of the muscle fibers of the internal organs, blood vessels, hair follicles.

**smooth mus·cle re·lax·ant** (smūdh mŭs′ĕl rē-lak′sănt) Pharmacologic agent, such as an antispasmodic, bronchodilator, or vasodilator, which reduces tension of smooth muscle.

**smooth sur·face** (smūdh sŭr′făs) Proximal, buccal, and lingual areas of teeth.

**smooth sur·face ca·ries** (smūdh sŭr′făs kar′ēz) Caries initiated on smooth surfaces of teeth.

**smooth tongue** (smūdh tŭng) SYN atrophic glossitis.

**SMX** Abbreviation for sulfamethoxazole.

**S-N-A an·gle** (ang′gĕl) In cephalometrics, an angle measuring anteroposterior relationship of maxillary basal arch on anterior cranial base; shows degree of maxillary prognathism.

**S-N-B an·gle** (ang′gĕl) Angle showing anterior limit of mandibular basal arch in relation to anterior cranial base.

**Sned·don syn·drome** (sned′ŏn sin′drōm) Cerebral arteriopathy of unknown etiology, characterized by noninflammatory intimal hyperplasia of medium-sized vessels associated with diffuse cutaneous livedo reticularis.

**sneeze** (snēz) 1. To expel air from nose and mouth by an involuntary spasmodic contraction of muscles of expiration. 2. Reflex excited by an irritation of the mucous membrane of nose or, sometimes, by a bright light striking the eye. [A.S. *fneōsan*]

**S-N line** (līn) Line connecting a point (S) representing center of sella turcica with frontonasal junction (N); denotes anterior portion of cranial base in cephalometrics.

**snout re·flex** (snowt rē′fleks) Pouting or pursing of lips induced by light tapping of closed lips in midline.

**snuff** (snŭf) 1. To inhale forcibly through the nose. 2. Finely powdered tobacco used by nasal inhalation or applied to the gums. 3. Any medicated powder applied by insufflation to the nasal mucous membrane.

**Sny·der test** (snī′dĕr test) Colorimetric measurement for determining dental caries activity or susceptibility based on rate of acid production by acidogenic oral microorganisms (e.g., lactobacillus) in a glucose medium, using bromcresol green as the indicator, and producing a color change from green to yellow.

**SOAP** (sōp) Acronym for *s*ubjective, *o*bjective, *a*ssessment, and *p*lan; used in problem-oriented records for organizing follow-up data, evaluation, and planning.

**soap** (sōp) Sodium or potassium salts of long-chain fatty acids; used as an emulsifier for cleansing purposes and as an excipient in making of pills and suppositories. [A.S. *sape,* L. *sapo,* G. *sapōn*]

**so·cial·ized med·i·cine** (sō′shăl-īzd med′i-sin) Organization and control of medical practice by a government agency, the practitioners being employed by the organization from which they receive standardized compensation for their services, and to which the public contributes usually in the form of taxation rather than fee-for-service.

**so·cial pho·bi·a** (sō′shăl fō′bē-ă) Persistent pattern of significant fear of a social or performance situation.

**so·ci·o·ac·u·sis** (sō′sē-ō-ă-kyū′sis) Hearing loss produced by exposure to nonoccupational noise. [L. *socius*, companion + G. *akousis*, hearing]

**so·ci·o·cen·trism** (sō′sē-ō-sen′trizm) Taking one's own social group as the standard against which others are measured.

**sock·et** (sok′ĕt) **1.** The hollow part of a joint. **2.** Any hollow or concavity into which another part fits. [thr. O. Fr. fr. L. *soccus*, a shoe, a sock]

**so·da** (sō′dă) SYN sodium carbonate. [It., possibly fr. Mediev. L. barilla plant]

**so·di·um bi·car·bon·ate** (sō′dē-ŭm bī-kahr′bŏ-nāt) Agent used as a gastric and systemic antacid, to alkalize urine, and for washes of body cavities. SYN baking soda.

**so·di·um bo·rate** (sō′dē-ŭm bōr′āt) Agent used in lotions, gargles, mouthwashes, and as a detergent. SYN borax.

**so·di·um car·bon·ate** (sō′dē-ŭm kahr′bŏ-nāt) Agent used to treat scaly skin diseases, but rarely used in medicine because of its irritant action. SYN soda.

**so·di·um chlo·ride** (sō′dē-ŭm klōr′īd) Chief ionic component of blood, urine, and other body fluids; used to make isotonic and physiologic saline solutions, in the treatment of salt depletion, and topically for inflammatory lesions. SYN common salt.

**so·di·um fluor·ide** (sō′dē-ŭm flōr′īd) Agent used in drinking water as a dental prophylactic against caries and topically as a 2% solution applied to teeth.

**so·di·um hex·a·flu·o·ro·sil·i·cate** (sō′dē-ŭm hek′să-flŏr′ō-sil′i-kăt) Agent used (in dilute solutions) as an antiseptic and deodorant, and for fluoridation of drinking water.

**so·di·um lau·ryl sul·fate** (sō′dē-ŭm lawr′il sŭl′fāt) Surface-active anionic agent used in toothpaste.

**so·di·um (Na)** (sō′dē-ŭm) A metallic element; an alkali metal oxidizing readily in air or water; its salts are found in natural biologic systems and are extensively used in medicine and industry. [Mod. L. fr. *soda*]

**so·di·um pump** (sō′dē-ŭm pŭmp) Biologic mechanism that uses metabolic energy from adenosine triphosphate to achieve active transport of sodium across a membrane.

**so·di·um thi·o·sul·fate** (sō′dē-ŭm thī′ō-sŭl′fāt) An injectable compound used immediately after injection of sodium nitrate in the antidotal treatment of cyanide poisoning in the U.S.

**soft chan·cre** (sawft shang′kĕr) SYN chancroid.

**soft di·et** (sawft dī′ĕt) Normal diet limited to soft foods for those who have difficulty chewing or swallowing; no restrictions made on seasoning or method of food preparation.

**soft pal·ate** (sawft pal′ăt) [TA] Posterior muscular portion of palate, forming an incomplete septum between mouth and oropharynx and between oropharynx and nasopharynx. SYN velum palatinum.

**soft tis·sue un·der·cut** (sawft tish′ū ŭn′dĕr-kŭt) Inward notching at the residual ridge or soft tissue of a dental arch that would influence the form of a removable denture.

**sol** Abbreviation for solution.

**so·lar chei·li·tis** (sō′lăr kī-lī′tis) Mucosal atrophy with drying and fissuring of the vermilion border of the lower lip in older fair-skinned people, resulting from chronic exposure to sunlight. SYN actinic cheilitis.

**sol·der** (sod′ĕr) **1.** A fusible alloy used to unite edges or surfaces of two pieces of metal of higher melting point; hard solders, usually containing gold or silver as their main constituent, are frequently used in dentistry to connect noble metal alloys. **2.** To join two pieces of metal with such an alloy. [L. *solido*, to make solid, through Fr., various forms]

**sol·der·ing** (sod′ĕr-ing) In dentistry, joining of two metals by fusion of intermediary alloys that have a lower melting temperature.

**sol·ip·sism** (sol′ip-sizm) A philosophic concept that whatever exists is a product of will and the ideas of the person making the perception. [L. *solus*, alone, + *ipse*, self]

**sol·i·tar·y bone cyst** (sol′i-tar-ē bōn sist) Unilocular cyst containing serous fluid and lined with a thin layer of connective tissue, occurring usually in the shaft of a long bone in a child. SYN simple bone cyst.

**soln** Abbreviation for solution.

**sol·u·bil·i·ty** (sol′yū-bil′i-tē) The property of being soluble.

**sol·u·ble lig·a·ture** (sol′yū-bĕl lig′ă-chŭr) Temporary ligature of material that can be absorbed by human tissues.

**sol·u·ble ma·te·ri·al** (sol′yŭ-bĕl mă-tēr′ē-ăl) Substance that dissolves in a liquid.

**sol·ute** (sol′yūt) The dissolved substance in a solution. [L. *solutus*, dissolved, pp. of *solvo*, to dissolve]

st

**so·lu·tion (soln, sol)** (sŏ-lū′shŭn) **1.** The incorporation of a solid, liquid, or gas into a liquid or noncrystalline solid resulting in a homogeneous single phase. **2.** Generally, an aqueous solution of a nonvolatile substance. **3.** The termination of a disease by crisis. **4.** A break, cut, or laceration of the solid tissues. [L. *solutio*]

**sol·vent** (sol′vĕnt) A liquid that holds another substance in solution, i.e., dissolves it. [L. *solvens*, pres. p. of *solvo*, to dissolve]

**so·ma** (sō′mă) **1.** Axial part of the body, i.e., head, neck, trunk, and tail, excluding limbs. **2.** All of an organism except germ cells. [G. *sōma*, body]

**so·ma·tal·gi·a** (sō′mă-tal′jē-ă) **1.** Body pain. **2.** Pain due to organic causes, as opposed to psychogenic pain. [*somat-* + G. *algos*, pain]

**so·ma·tas·the·ni·a** (sō′mat-as-thē′nē-ă) Chronic physical weakness and fatigability. [*somat-* + G. *astheneia*, weakness]

**so·mat·ic** (sō-mat′ik) **1.** Relating to soma or trunk, wall of the body cavity, or body in general. **2.** Relating to or involving the skeleton or skeletal muscle and innervation of the latter. [G. *sōmatikos*, bodily]

**so·mat·ic swal·low** (sō-mat′ik swahl′ō) Swallowing pattern with muscular contractions that appear to be under someone's control at a subconscious level.

**so·ma·ti·za·tion** (sō′mă-tī-zā′shŭn) Process by which psychological needs are expressed in physical symptoms; e.g., expression or conversion into physical symptoms of anxiety, or by a wish for material gain associated with legal action following an injury, or a related psychological need.

♻ **somato-** Combining form meaning the body, bodily. [G. *sōma*, body]

**so·ma·to·form dis·or·der** (sō′mă-tō-fōrm dis-ōr′dĕr) Group of disorders in which physical symptoms suggesting physical disorders for which no demonstrable organic findings or known physiologic mechanisms exist, and for which there is positive evidence, or a strong presumption that the symptoms are linked to psychological factors.

**so·ma·to·form pain** (sō′mă-tō-fōrm pān) SYN psychogenic pain.

**so·ma·to·gen·ic** (sō′mă-tō-jen′ik) **1.** Originating in soma or body under influence of external forces. **2.** Having origin in body cells. [*somato-* + G. *genesis*, origin]

**so·ma·to·lib·er·in** (sō′mă-tō-lib′ĕr-in) Decapeptide released by the hypothalamus, which induces the release of human growth hormone (somatotropin). [*somatotropin* + L. *libero*, to free, + *-in*]

**so·ma·to·mam·mo·tro·pin** (sō′mă-tō-mam′ō-trō′pin) Peptide hormone, closely related to somatotropin in its biologic properties. [*somato-* + L. *mamma*, breast, + G. *tropē*, a turning, + *-in*]

**so·ma·to·me·din** (sō′mă-tō-mē′din) One of several peptides; also called insulinlike growth factor II, is synthesized in the liver and probably kidney. [*somato*, tropin + *mediator* + *-in*]

**so·ma·to·pros·thet·ics** (sō′mă-tō-pros-thet′iks) Art and science of prosthetically replacing missing or deformed external body parts. [*somato-* + G. *prosthesis*, an addition]

**so·ma·to·psy·chic** (sō′mă-tō-sī′kik) Relating to body-mind relationship; study of effects of body on mind. [*somato-* + G. *psychē*, soul]

**so·ma·to·psy·cho·sis** (sō′mă-tō-sī-kō′sis) Emotional disorder associated with an organic disease. [*somato-* + G. *psychōsis*, an animating]

**so·ma·to·sen·so·ry** (sō′mă-tō-sen′sŏr-ē) Sensation relating to body's superficial and deep parts.

**so·ma·to·stat·in** (sō′mă-tō-stat′in) Tetradecapeptide capable of inhibiting release of somatotropin by anterior lobe of pituitary gland. [*somatotropin* + G. *stasis*, a standing still, + *-in*]

**so·ma·to·tro·pin, so·ma·to·tro·pic hor·mone** (sō′mă-tō-trō′pin, -trō′pik hōr′mōn) Protein hormone of anterior lobe of pituitary, produced by acidophil cells, which promotes body growth, fat mobilization, and inhibition of glucose use. SYN growth hormone. [fr. *somato-* + G. *trophē* nourishment; corrupted to *-tropin* and reanalyzed as fr. G. *tropē*, a turning]

**som·es·thet·ic sys·tem** (sō′mes-thet′ik sis′tĕm) Sensory data derived from skin, muscles, and body organs in contrast to those derived from the five special senses.

**so·mite** (sō′mīt) One of the paired, metamerically arranged cell masses formed in early embryonic paraxial mesoderm; develop in a caudal direction typically until 42 pairs are formed. [G. *sōma*, body, + *-ite*]

**som·nam·bu·lism, som·nam·bu·lance** (son-am′byū-lizm, -lăns) Sleep disorder involving complex motor acts. [L. *somnus*, sleep, + *ambulo*, to walk]

**som·ni·fa·cient** (som′ni-fā′shĕnt) SYN soporific. [L. *somnus*, sleep, + *facio*, to make]

**som·nif·er·ous** (som-nif′ĕr-ŭs) SYN soporific. [L. *somnus*, sleep, + *fero*, to bring]

**som·no·lence, som·no·len·cy** (som′nō-lĕns, -sē) **1.** An inclination to sleep. **2.** A condition of obtusion. [L. *somnolentia*]

**som·no·lent, som·no·les·cent** (som′nō-lĕnt, -les′ĕnt) **1.** Drowsy; sleepy; having an inclination to sleep. **2.** In a condition of incomplete sleep; semicomatose. [L. *somnus*, sleep]

**som·no·lism** (som'nō-lizm) SYN hypnotism (1).

**So·mog·yi ef·fect, So·mog·yi phe·no·me·non** (sō-mō'jē e-fekt', fē-nom'ĕ-non) In diabetes, a rebound phenomenon of reactive hyperglycemia in response to a preceding period of relative hypoglycemia that has increased secretion of hyperglycemic agents.

**son·ic de·vice** (son'ik dĕ-vīs') Electronically powered device that uses energy to vibrate tip to break calculus from the tooth surface; consist of a handpiece that attaches to the dental units high-speed handpiece tubing and interchangeable instrument tips. Its instrument tip vibrates between 3000 and 8000 cycles/sec (3–8 kHz).

**son·o·gram** (son'ō-gram) SYN ultrasonogram. [L. *sonus*, sound, + G. *gramma*, a drawing]

**son·o·graph** (son'ō-graf) SYN ultrasonograph. [L. *sonus*, sound, + G. *graphō*, to write]

**so·nog·ra·phy** (sŏ-nog'ră-fē) SYN ultrasonography. [L. *sonus*, sound. + G. *graphō*, to write]

**so·no·rous rale** (son'ŏr-ŭs rahl) Cooing or snoring sound often produced by vibration of a projecting mass of viscid secretion in a large bronchus.

**sop·o·rif·ic** (sop'ŏr-if'ik) Causing sleep. SYN somnifacient, somniferous. [L. *sopor*, deep sleep, + *facio*, to make]

**sor·bi·tol** (sōr'bi-tol) Reduction product of glucose and sorbose found in the berries of rowan/mountain ash, *Sorbus aucuparia*, and in many other fruits and seaweeds. Has many industrial and pharmaceutical uses.

**sor·des** (sōr'dēz) Dark brown or blackish crustlike collection on lips, teeth, and gums of a dehydrated person associated with chronic debilitating disease. [L. filth, fr. *sordeo*, to be foul]

**sore** (sōr) 1. A wound, ulcer, or any open skin lesion. 2. Painful; aching; tender. [A.S. *sār*]

**s.o.s.** Abbreviation for L. *si opus sit*, if needed.

**So·tos syn·drome** (sō'tōs sin'drōm) Cerebral gigantism and generalized large muscles in childhood.

**souf·fle** (sū'fĕl) Soft blowing sound heard on auscultation. [Fr. *souffler*, to blow]

**sound** (sownd) 1. Vibrations produced by a sounding body, transmitted in air or other medium, and perceived by internal ear. 2. An elongated cylindric, usually curved, metal instrument, used to explore bladder or other body cavities, to dilate strictures of the urethra, esophagus, or other canal, to calibrate lumen of body cavity, or to detect presence of a foreign body in a body cavity. 3. To explore or calibrate a cavity with a sound.

**source-film dis·tance** (sōrs-film' dis' tăns) SYN target-film distance.

**source-to-im·age dis·tance** (sōrs-im'ăj dis'tăns) SYN focal-film distance.

**South A·mer·i·can blas·to·my·co·sis** (sowth ă-mer'i-kăn blas'tō-mī-kō'sis) SYN paracoccidioidomycosis.

**South A·mer·i·can try·pan·o·so·mi·a·sis** (sowth ă-mer'i-kăn trī-pan'ō-sō-mī'ă-sis) Disease seen most frequently in young children, with swelling of the skin at the site of entry, most often the face, and regional lymph node enlargement. SYN Chagas disease, Chagas-Cruz disease, Cruz trypanosomiasis.

**space** (spās) [TA] Any demarcated body portion, either surface area, tissue segment, or cavity. SEE ALSO region. [L. *spatium*, room, space]

**spaced teeth** (spāst tēth) Teeth that have separated and lost proximal contact with adjacent teeth.

**space main·tain·er** (spās mān-tān'ĕr) Orthodontic appliance used to prevent loss of space or shifting of teeth following extraction or premature loss of teeth. SYN space retainer.

**space ob·tain·er** (spās ŏb-tā'nĕr) An appliance used to increase interdental interstices.

**space of Don·ders** (spās don'derz) Area between dorsum of the tongue and hard palate when mandible is in rest position after expiratory cycle of respiration.

**space re·gain·er** (spās rĕ-gā'nĕr) Appliance used to correct tooth displacement resulting from premature loss of one or more teeth in patients unable to procure space maintenance in a more timely manner.

**space re·tain·er** (spās rĕ-tā'nĕr) SYN space maintainer.

**spasm** (spazm) Sudden involuntary contraction of one or more muscles; includes cramps and contractures. [G. *spasmos*]

**spas·mod·ic tic** (spaz-mod'ik tik) Disorder in which sudden spasmodic coordinated movements of some muscles or groups of physiologically related muscles occur at irregular intervals.

**spas·mod·ic tor·ti·col·lis** (spaz-mod'ik tōr'ti-kol'is) Disorder of unknown cause, manifested as a restricted dystonia, localized to some neck muscles.

**spas·mol·y·sis** (spaz-mol'i-sis) Arrest of a spasm or convulsion. [*spasmo-* + G. *lysis*, dissolution]

**spas·mo·lyt·ic** (spaz'mō-lit'ik) 1. Relating to spasmolysis. 2. Denoting a chemical agent that relieves smooth muscle spasms.

st

**spas·mo·phil·ic di·a·the·sis** (spaz′mō-fil′ik dī-ath′ĕ-sis) Condition with abnormal excitability of motor nerves, shown by tendency to tetany, laryngeal spasm, or general convulsions.

**spas·mus nu·tans** (spaz′mŭs nū′tanz) Fine nystagmus, sometimes rotary, sometimes monocular, associated with head-nodding movements; appears in patients aged between 6 months and 3 years.

**spas·tic** (spas′tik) 1. SYN hypertonic (1). 2. Relating to spasm or to spasticity. [L. *spasticus,* fr. G. *spastikos,* drawing in]

**spas·tic a·pho·ni·a** (spas′tik ă-fō′nē-ă) Speech disorder due to spasmodic contraction of laryngeal adductor muscles.

**spas·tic di·ple·gi·a** (spas′tik dī-plē′jē-ă) Cerebral palsy with bilateral spasticity. SYN spastic spinal paralysis.

**spas·tic gait** (spas′tik gāt) SYN hemiplegic gait.

**spas·tic·i·ty** (spas-tis′i-tē) Type of increase in muscle tone at rest; characterized by increased resistance to passive stretch; velocity dependent and asymmetric about joints.

**spas·tic spi·nal pa·ral·y·sis** (spas′tik spī′năl păr-al′i-sis) SYN spastic diplegia.

**spa·ti·um sub·du·ra·le** (spā′shē-ŭm sŭb-dū-rā′lē) [TA] SYN subdural space.

**spat·u·la** (spach′yū-lă) A flat blade, like a knife blade but without a sharp edge, used in pharmacy for spreading plasters and ointments and as an aid in mixing ingredients with a mortar and pestle. [L. dim. of *spatha,* a broad, flat wooden instrument, fr. G. *spathē*]

**spat·u·late** (spach′yū-lăt, -lāt) 1. Shaped like a spatula. 2. To mix using a spatula. 3. To incise cut end of a tubular structure longitudinally and splay it open so as to allow creation of an elliptic anastomosis of greater circumference than would be possible with conventional transverse or oblique (beveled) end-to-end anastomoses.

**spat·u·la·tion** (spach′yū-lā′shŭn) Manipulation of material with a spatula.

**SPCA** Abbreviation for serum prothrombin conversion accelerator.

**spe·cial·ist** (spesh′ă-list) One who has developed professional expertise in a particular branch of dentistry or medicine.

**spe·cial·i·za·tion** (spesh′ă-lī-zā′shŭn) 1. Professional practice limited to a particular specialty or subject area. 2. SYN differentiation (1).

**spe·cial sense** (spesh′ăl sens) One of the five senses related respectively to the organs of sight, hearing, smell, taste, and touch.

**spe·cial·ty** (spesh′ăl-tē) The particular subject area or branch of dental or medical science to which one devotes professional attention. [L. *specialitas* fr. *specialis,* special]

**spe·cif·ic** (spĕ-sif′ik) 1. Relating to a species. 2. Relating to an individual infectious disease, one caused by a special microorganism. 3. Remedy with definite therapeutic action in relation to a particular disease or symptom, such as quinine in relation to malaria. [L. *specificus* fr. *species* + *facio,* to make]

**spe·cif·ic dis·ease** (spĕ-sif′ik di-zēz′) Disease produced by action of a given pathogenic microorganism.

**spe·cif·ic grav·i·ty** (spĕ-sif′ik grav′i-tē) The weight of any body compared with that of another body of equal volume regarded as the unit; usually the weight of a liquid compared with that of distilled water.

**spec·i·fic·i·ty** (spes′i-fis′i-tē) *Do not confuse this word with sensitivity.* 1. Condition or state of being specific, of having a fixed relation to a single cause or definite result; manifested in relation of disease to its pathogenic microorganism, of reaction to a chemical union, or an antibody to its antigen, or the reverse. 2. In clinical pathology and medical screening, proportion of those tested with negative test results for the disease the test is intended to reveal, i.e., true-negative results as a proportion of the total of true-negative and false-positive results.

**spe·ci·fic pho·bi·a** (spĕ-sif′ik fō′bē-ă) Persistent pattern of significant fear of specific objects or situations, manifesting in anxiety or panic on exposure to object or situation or in anticipation of them, which person realizes is unreasonable or excessive and significantly interferes with the person's functioning.

**spe·cif·ic ther·a·py** (spĕ-sif′ik thār′ă-pē) Treatment aimed at cause(s) of a disease process, as opposed to symptomatic therapy.

**spec·trum,** pl. **spec·trums,** pl. **spec·tra** (spek′trŭm, -trŭmz, -tră) 1. Range of colors presented when white light is resolved into its constituent colors by being passed through a prism or through a diffraction grating: red, orange, yellow, green, blue, indigo, and violet. 2. Range of pathogenic microorganisms against which an antibiotic or other antibacterial agent is active. [L. an image, fr. *specio,* to look at]

**spec·u·lum,** pl. **spec·u·la** (spek′yŭ-lŭm, -lă) *The correct plural of this word is specula, not speculae or speculi.* Instrument for exposing opening of any canal or cavity to facilitate inspection of its interior. [L. a mirror, fr. *specio,* to look at]

**speech aid** (spēch ād) Any therapy or form of mechanical or electronic implement intended to improve speech quality.

**speech aid pros·the·sis** (spēch ād pros-thē′sis) Removable device used to restore a defect of the soft palate, thus facilitating speech. SYN cleft palate prosthesis.

**speech bulb** (spēch bŭlb) Speech prosthesis used to close a cleft or other opening in hard or soft palate or to replace absent tissue necessary for the production of good speech.

**speech lan·guage path·ol·o·gy** (spēch lang′gwij pă-thol′ŏ-jē) Science concerned with functional and organic speech defects and disorders.

**speech read·ing** (spēch rēd′ing) Use, by people with hearing impairments, of nonauditory clues as to what is being said, acquired by observing the speaker's facial expressions and gestures. SYN lip reading.

**Spens syn·drome** (spents sin′drōm) SYN Adams-Stokes syndrome.

**sperm** (spĕrm) Male gamete or sex cell that contains the genetic information to be transmitted by the male, exhibits autokinesia, and is able to effect zygosis with an oocyte. [G. *sperma*, seed]

**sphe·noid** (sfē′noyd) [TA] 1. SYN sphenoidal. 2. SYN sphenoid bone. [G. *sphēnoeidēs*, fr. *sphēn*, wedge, + *eidos*, resemblance]

**sphe·noi·dal** (sfē-noy′dăl) SYN sphenoid.

**sphe·noi·dal an·gle of pa·ri·e·tal bone** (sfē-noyd′ăl ang′gĕl pă-rī′ĕ-tăl bōn) [TA] The anterior inferior angle of the parietal bone. SYN angulus sphenoidalis ossis parietalis.

**sphe·noi·da·le** (sfē′noy-dā′lē) Point of greatest convexity between anterior contour of sella turcica and jugum sphenoidale.

**sphe·noi·dal si·nus** (sfē-noy′dăl sī′nŭs) [TA] One of a pair of paranasal sinuses in body of sphenoid bone communicating with upper posterior nasal cavity.

**sphe·noid bone** (sfē′noyd bōn) A bone of irregular shape occupying the base of the skull. SYN sphenoid (2).

**sphe·no·man·dib·u·lar lig·a·ment** (sfē′nō-man-dib′yū-lăr lig′ă-mĕnt) [TA] Fibrous band that passes from spine of sphenoid bone to lingula of mandible; primary passive support of mandible serving as a "swinging axis," permitting depression and elevation around a transverse axis passing through the two lingulae, while at the same time permitting protraction and retraction.

**sphe·no·max·il·lar·y** (sfē′nō-mak′si-lar-ē) Relating to sphenoid bone and maxilla.

**sphe·no·max·il·lar·y su·ture** (sfē′nō-mak′si-lar-ē sū′chŭr) [TA] Inconstant suture between pterygoid process of sphenoid bone and body of maxilla.

**sphe·no·pal·a·tine** (sfē′nō-pal′ă-tīn) Relating to sphenoid and palatine bones.

**sphe·no·pal·a·tine neu·ral·gi·a** (sfēn′ō-pal′ă-tīn nūr-al′jē-ă) Pain related to the nervous system in the lower half of the face, with pain referred to the root of the nose, upper teeth, eyes, ears, mastoid, and occiput, in association with nasal congestion and rhinorrhea occurring in infection of the nasal sinuses, and produced by lesions of the sphenopalatine ganglion. SYN Sluder neuralgia.

**spher·ic a·mal·gam** (sfēr′ik ă-mal′găm) Alloy for dental amalgam composed of spheric particles instead of filings.

**spher·ic form of oc·clu·sion** (sfēr′ik fōrm ŏ-klū′zhŭn) Arrangement of teeth that places their occlusal surfaces on surface of an imaginary sphere (usually 8 inches in diameter) with its center above level of teeth.

**spher·o·cyt·ic a·ne·mi·a** (sfēr′ō-sit′ik ă-nē′mē-ă) SYN hereditary spherocytosis.

**sphe·ro·cy·to·sis** (sfēr′ō-sī-tō′sis) Presence of spheric red blood cells in blood. [*spherocyte* + G. *-osis*, condition]

**sphinc·ter** (sfingk′tĕr) [TA] Muscle that encircles a duct, tube, or orifice in such a way that its contraction constricts the lumen or orifice. [G. *sphinktēr*, a band or lace]

**sphin·go·lip·i·do·sis,** pl. **sphin·go·lip·i·do·ses, sphin·go·lip·o·dys·tro·phy** (sfing′gō-lip′i-dō′sis, -i-dō′sēz, -ō-dis′trŏ-fē) Collective designation for various diseases characterized by abnormal sphingolipid metabolism.

**sphyg·mo·ma·nom·e·ter** (sfig′mō-mă-nom′ĕ-tĕr) Dental instrument for measuring arterial blood pressure consisting of an inflatable cuff, inflating bulb, and a gauge showing the blood pressure. [G. *sphygmos*, pulsation, + *manos*, sparse, + *metron*, measure]

**spic·ule** (spik′yūl) A small, needle-shaped body. [L. *spiculum*, dim. of *spica*, or *spicum*, a point]

**spike** (spīk) Brief electrical event of 3–25 msec that gives appearance in electroencephalogram of a rising and falling vertical line.

**spill·way** (spil′wā) Groove or channel through which food may pass from occlusal surfaces of teeth during masticatory process. SYN sluice way.

**spi·na bi·fi·da** (spī′nă bif′i-dă) Embryologic failure of fusion of one or more vertebral arches.

**spi·nal an·es·the·si·a** (spī′năl an′es-thē′zē-ă) 1. Loss of sensation produced by injection of local anesthetic solution(s) into the spinal subarachnoid space. 2. Loss of sensation due to disease of the spinal cord.

**st**

**spi·nal an·es·thet·ic** (spī'năl an'es-thet'ik) Local anesthetic agent producing loss of sensation when injected into subarachnoid space.

**spi·nal a·tax·i·a** (spī'năl ă-tak'sē-ă) Ataxia due to spinal cord disease, as in tabes dorsalis.

**spi·nal block** (spī'năl blok) Obstruction to flow of cerebrospinal fluid in spinal subarachnoid space.

**spi·nal cord** (spī'năl kōrd) [TA] The elongated cylindric portion of the cerebrospinal axis, or central nervous system, which is contained in the spinal or vertebral canal. SYN medulla spinalis.

**spi·nal mus·cu·lar at·ro·phy** (spī'năl mŭs'kyū-lăr at'rŏ-fē) Heterogeneous group of degenerative diseases of anterior horn cells in spinal cord and motor nuclei of brainstem; all are characterized by weakness.

**spi·nal nerves** (spī'năl nĕrvz) [TA] The nerves emerging from the spinal cord; there are 31 pairs, each attached to the cord by two roots, anterior and posterior, or ventral and dorsal. SYN nervi spinales [TA].

**spi·nal pa·ral·y·sis** (spī'năl păr-al'i-sis) Loss of motor power due to spinal cord lesion.

**spi·nal shock** (spī'năl shok) Transient depression of reflex activity below level of an acute spinal cord injury or transection.

**spin·dle** (spin'dĕl) In anatomy and pathology, any fusiform cell or structure. [A.S.]

**spine** (spīn) [TA] A short, sharp, thornlike process of bone; a spinous process. [L. spina]

**spine of sphe·noid bone** (spīn sfē'noyd bōn) [TA] A posterior and downward projection from the greater wing of the sphenoid bone on either side, located posterolateral to the foramen spinosum, so named for its proximity to this spine; gives attachment to the sphenomandibular ligament. SYN alar spine.

**spi·no·cer·e·bel·lar a·tax·i·a** (spī'nō-ser'ĕ-bĕl'lăr ă-tak'sē-ă) Generic term now increasingly used to describe autosomal dominant-inherited ataxias that have a progressive course.

**spi·ral** (spī'răl) 1. Coiled; winding around a center like a watch spring; winding and ascending like a wire spring. 2. Structure in shape of a coil. [Mediev. L. spiralis, fr. G. speira, a coil]

**spi·ral lig·a·ment of coch·le·ar duct** (spīr'ăl lig'ă-mĕnt kok'lē-ăr dŭkt) [TA] Thickened periosteal lining of bony cochlea forming outer wall of cochlear duct to which basal lamina attaches.

**spi·ral or·gan** (spī'răl ōr'găn) [TA] Prominent ridge of highly specialized epithelium on floor of cochlear duct overlying basilar membrane of cochlea, containing one inner row and three outer rows of hair cells. SYN acoustic papilla.

**spi·ral prom·i·nence of coch·le·ar duct** (spīr'ăl prom'i-nĕns kok'lē-ăr dŭkt) [TA] Projecting portion of cochlear spiral ligament, bounding lower edge of stria vascularis and containing within it, the vas prominens.

**Spi·ril·lum** (spī-ril'ŭm) A genus of large, rigid, helical, gram-negative bacteria that are motile using bipolar fascicles of flagella. [Mod. L. dim. of L. spira, coil, fr. G. speira]

**spir·it** (spir'it) 1. An alcoholic liquor stronger than wine (i.e., 15%) obtained by distillation. 2. Any distilled liquid. 3. An alcoholic or hydroalcoholic solution of volatile substances. [L. spiritus, a breathing, life soul, fr. spiro, to breathe]

**spi·ro·chete** (spī'rō-kēt) A vernacular term used to refer to any organism resembling a Leptospira, Spirochaeta, or Treponema cell.

**spi·ro·graph** (spī'rō-graf) Device for representing depth and rapidity of respiratory movements graphically. [L. spiro, to breathe, + G. graphō, to write]

**spi·rom·e·ter** (spī-rom'ĕ-tĕr) In clinical practice and research, any device used for measuring flows and volumes. [L. spiro, to breathe, + G. metron, measure]

**spi·rom·e·try** (spī-rom'ĕ-trē) Making pulmonary measurements with a spirometer.

**spi·ro·no·lac·tone** (spī'rō-nō-lak'tōn) A diuretic agent that blocks the renal tubular actions of aldosterone.

**splat·ter** (splat'ĕr) Colloq. for airborne particles larger than 10 mcm in diameter. Unlike aerosols, splatter is often visible after it lands on objects (e.g., spectacles, protective eyewear, dental uniforms, skin, hair, or other surfaces).

**splay** (splā) To lay open the end of a tubular structure by making a longitudinal incision to increase its potential diameter.

**spleen** (splēn) [TA] Large, vascular lymphatic organ lying in upper part of abdominal cavity on left side, between stomach and diaphragm, composed of white and red pulp; blood-forming organ in early life and later a storage organ for red corpuscles and platelets. SYN lien. [G. splēn]

**splen·ic flex·ure syn·drome** (splen'ik flek'shŭr sin'drōm) Symptoms of pain, gas, bloating, and a sense of fullness experienced in the left upper abdominal quadrant, sometimes beneath the ribs, in some instances radiating upward, and in some instances producing anterior chest pain central or predominantly on the left.

**sple·no·meg·a·ly, sple·no·me·ga·li·a** (splē'nō-meg'ă-lē, -mĕ-gā'lē-ă) Enlargement of the spleen. [spleno- + G. megas (megal-), large]

**sple·nop·a·thy** (splē-nop'ă-thē) Any disease of the spleen. [*spleno-* + G. *pathos*, suffering]

**splic·ing** (splīs'ing) **1.** Attachment of one DNA molecule to another. SYN gene splicing. **2.** Removal of introns from mRNA precursors and the reattachment or annealing of exons. SYN RNA splicing.

**splint** (splint) **1.** An appliance for preventing movement of a joint or fixation of displaced or movable parts. **2.** The splint bone, or fibula. [M. Dutch *splinte*]

**splint·ed a·but·ment** (splint'ĕd ă-bŭt'mĕnt) Joining two or more teeth into a rigid unit by means of fixed restorations to form a single abutment with multiple roots.

**splint·ing** (splint'ing) **1.** In dentistry, joining of two or more teeth into a rigid unit by means of fixed or removable restorations or appliances. **2.** Application of a splint or treatment using a splint. **3.** Stiffening of a body part to avoid pain caused by movement of the part.

**split cast meth·od** (split kast meth'ŏd) **1.** Procedure for placing indexed casts on an articulator to facilitate their removal and replacement on the instrument. **2.** Procedure of checking ability of an articulator to receive or be adjusted to a maxillomandibular relation record.

**split cast mount·ing** (split kast mownt'ing) **1.** Cast with key grooves on its base, mounted on an articulator for easy removal and accurate replacement; split remounting metal plates may be used instead of grooves in casts. **2.** Means for testing accuracy of articulator adjustment.

**split-thick·ness flap** (split-thik'nĕs flap) Flap of portion of skin (i.e., epidermis and part of dermis), or of part of mucosa and submucosa, but not including the periosteum.

**split-thick·ness graft** (split-thik'nĕs graft) Graft of portions of skin (i.e., epidermis and part of dermis), or of part of mucosa and submucosa, but not including the periosteum.

**spon·dyl·ar·thri·tis** (spon'dil-ahr-thrī'tis) Inflammation of intervertebral articulations. [G. *spondylos*, vertebra + G. *arthron*, joint, + -*itis*, inflammation]

**spong·y bone** (spŏn'jē bōn) [TA] **1.** SYN substantia spongiosa. **2.** A turbinate bone.

**spon·ta·ne·ous** (spon-tā'nē-ŭs) Without apparent cause; said of disease processes or remissions. [L. *spontaneus*, voluntary, capricious]

**spo·rad·ic** (spōr-ad'ik) **1.** Denoting temporal pattern of disease occurrence in which the disease occurs only rarely and without regularity. **2.** Occurring irregularly, haphazardly. [G. *sporadikos*, scattered]

**spore** (spōr) **1.** The asexual or sexual reproductive body of fungi or sporozoan protozoa. **2.** A resistant form of some species of bacteria. [G. *sporos*, seed]

**spore test·ing** (spōr test'ing) Use of bacterial spores to determine the efficacy of a sterilizing device.

**spo·ri·cide** (spōr'i-sīd) An agent that kills spores.

**spo·ro·tri·cho·sis** (spōr'ō-tri-kō'sis) Chronic cutaneous mycosis spread by way of lymphatics; caused by inoculation of *Sporothrix schenckii*.

**sports med·i·cine** (spōrts med'i-sin) Field of medicine that uses a holistic, comprehensive, and multidisciplinary approach to health care for patients engaged in a sporting or recreational activity.

**spot** (spot) **1.** SYN macula. **2.** To lose a slight amount of blood through the vagina.

**sprain** (sprān) **1.** An injury to a ligament when the joint is carried through a range of motion greater than normal, but without dislocation or fracture. **2.** To cause a sprain of a joint.

**spray** (sprā) A jet of liquid in fine drops, coarser than a vapor; produced by forcing liquid through minute opening of an atomizer, mixing it with air.

**spread·er** (spred'ĕr) **1.** Instrument used to distribute a substance over a surface or area. **2.** Device for spacing or parting structures. **3.** Colloq. for condenser (q.v.).

**sprout** (sprowt) A structure resembling the sprout of a plant.

**sprue** (sprū) In dentistry, wax or metal used to form aperture(s) for molten metal to flow into a mold to make a casting; also, metal that later fills sprue hole(s). [D. *spruw*]

**sprue base** (sprū bās) SYN sprue-former.

**sprue-for·mer** (sprū-fōr'mĕr) Base to which sprue is attached while wax pattern is being invested in a refractory investment in a casting flask; sometimes called crucible-former. SYN sprue base.

**sprue pin** (sprū pin) A hollow or solid length of metal or wax used to attach a pattern or form to a sprue base during the laboratory fabrication of a cast metal restoration. Pin provides pathway for molten metal to pass through refractory investment into mold.

**spu·tum** (spyū'tŭm) **1.** Expectorated matter, especially mucus or mucopurulent matter expectorated in diseases of the air passages. **2.** An individual mass of such matter. [L. *sputum*, fr. *spuo*, pp. *sputus*, to spit]

**spu·tum aer·u·gi·no·sum** (spyū'tŭm ē-rū-ji-nō'sŭm) Green expectoration seen occa-

st

sionally in jaundice, due to staining of sputum by bile pigments. SYN green sputum.

**SQ** Abbreviation for subcutaneous.

**squa·mous cell car·ci·no·ma** (skwā′ mŭs sel kahr′si-nō′mă) A malignant neoplasm derived from stratified squamous epithelium, but that may also occur in sites such as bronchial mucosa where glandular or columnar epithelium is normally present. See this page and page A9.

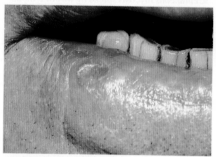

squamous cell carcinoma: indurated and raised

**squa·mous ep·i·the·li·um** (skwā′mŭs ep′i-thē′lē-ŭm) Epithelium consisting of a single layer of cells.

**squa·mous o·don·to·gen·ic tu·mor** (skwā′mŭs ō-don′tŏ-jen′ik tū′mŏr) Benign epithelial odontogenic tumor thought to arise from the epithelial cell rests of Malassez; appears clinically as a radiolucent lesion closely associated with tooth root and histologically as islands of squamous epithelium enclosed by a peripheral layer of flattened cells.

**squa·mous part of oc·cip·i·tal bone** (skwā′mŭs pahrt ok-sip′i-tăl bōn) [TA] Tabular or squamous portion of occipital bone. SYN frontal squama.

**squint** (skwint) SYN strabismus.

**Sr** Symbol for strontium.

**ss** Abbreviation for steady state.

**SSRI** Abbreviation for selective serotonin reuptake inhibitor.

**sta·bile** (stā′bīl, -bil) Steady; fixed. [L. stabilis]

**sta·bil·i·ty** (stă-bil′i-tē) The condition of being stable or resistant to change.

**sta·bi·li·za·tion** (stā′bi-lī-zā′shŭn) 1. In dentistry, preparing for instrumentation stroke by locking joints of ring finger and pressing fingertip against tooth surface to control instrumentation stroke. 2. SYN denture stability. 3. Accomplishment of a stable state.

**sta·bi·lized base·plate** (stā′běl-īzd bās′

plāt) Baseplate lined with plastic material to improve its fit and stability.

**sta·bi·liz·er** (stā′bi-līz′ĕr) 1. That which provides or maintains stability. 2. Part possessing quality of or creating rigidity when added to another part. 3. Agent that retards effect of an accelerator, thus preserving a chemical equilibrium.

**sta·bi·liz·ing cir·cum·fer·en·tial clasp arm** (stā′běl-īz-ing sĭr-kŭm′fĕr-en′shăl klasp ahrm) Relatively rigid arm that embraces height of tooth contour.

**sta·bi·liz·ing ful·crum line** (stā′běl-īz-ing ful′krŭm līn) Imaginary line connecting occlusal rests, around which denture tends to rotate under masticatory force.

**sta·ble** (stā′běl) Steady; not varying; resistant to change. SEE ALSO stabile.

**sta·ble i·so·tope** (stā′běl ī′sŏ-tōp) A nonradioactive nuclide; an isotope that shows no tendency to undergo radioactive decomposition.

**stack** (stak) To build up porcelain in the shape of a tooth in the fabrication of a tooth crown.

**staff** (staf) 1. A specific group of workers (e.g., reception, dental technicians, dentists). 2. SYN director (1). [A.S. staef]

**stage** (stāj) 1. Period in disease course; description of extent of involvement of a disease process or status of a patient with a specific disease, as of distribution and extent of dissemination of a malignant neoplastic disease; also, act of determining stage of a disease, especially cancer. 2. Part of a microscope on which microslide bears object to be examined. 3. A particular step, phase, or position in a developmental process. [M.E. thr. O. Fr. estage, standing-place, fr. L. sto, pp. status, to stand]

**stag·ing** (stāj′ing) 1. Determination or classification of distinct phases or periods in disease course or pathologic process. 2. Determination of specific extent of disease process in an individual patient.

**stain** (stān) 1. To discolor. 2. To color; to dye. 3. A discoloration. 4. A dye used in histologic and bacteriologic techniques 5. A procedure in which a dye or combination of dyes and reagents is used to color constituents of cells and tissues. [M.E. steinen]

**stain·ing** (stān′ing) 1. In dentistry, modification of the color of the tooth or denture base. 2. Act of applying a stain. SEE ALSO stain.

**stain·less steel crown** (stān′lĕs stēl krown) A preformed type, rather than one custom fit to an individual tooth; often used in interim restorations.

**stalk** (stawk) A narrowed connection with a structure or organ.

**stam·mer** (stam′ĕr) To hesitate in speech, halt, repeat, and mispronounce, by reason of embarrassment, agitation, unfamiliarity with the topic, or as yet unidentified physiologic causes. [A.S. *stamur*]

**stam·mer·ing** (stam′ĕr-ing) SYN stuttering.

**stamp cusp** (stamp kŭsp) A tooth cusp that, when the tooth is in occlusion, fits in the fossa of the antagonist in a mortar-and-pestle fashion.

**stan·dard** (stan′dărd) Something that serves as a basis for comparison; a technical specification or written report by experts. [M.E., fr. O.Fr. *estandard*, rallying place, fr. Frankish *standan*, to stand, + *hard*, hard, fast]

**stan·dard de·vi·a·tion (SD)** (stan′dărd dē′vē-ā′shŭn) 1. Statistical index of degree of deviation from central tendency, namely, of variability within a distribution; square root of average of squared deviations from mean. 2. Measure of dispersion or variation used to describe a characteristic of a frequency distribution.

**stan·dard er·ror of the mean** (stan′dărd er′ŏr mēn) Statistical index of probability that a given sample mean is representative of mean of the population from which the sample was drawn.

**stan·dard of care** (stan′dărd kār) The ordinary level of skill and care that any health care practitioner woud be expected to observe in caring for patients.

**stan·dard pre·cau·tions** (stan′dărd prē-kaw′shŭnz) Infection prevention practices that apply to all patients, regardless of diagnosis or presumed status in terms of infection. (This concept expands those provisions covered by the terms "universal precautions" and "body substance isolation.") It is based on the principle that all blood, body fluids, secretions, excretions (except sweat), nonintact skin, and mucous membranes may transmit infectious agents. It also includes hand hygiene, and depending on the anticipated exposure, use of gloves, gown, mask, eye protection, or face shield. Equipment or items in use around patients that are likely to have been contaminated with infectious fluids must be handled in such a manner so as to prevent transmission of infectious agents (i.e., should be regarded as infectious).

**stan·nic** (stan′ik) Relating to tin, especially when in combination in its higher valency. [L. *stannum*, tin]

**stan·nous** (stan′ŭs) Relating to tin, especially when in combination in its lower valency. [L. *stannum*, tin]

**stan·nous fluor·ide** (stan′ŭs flōr′īd) A preparation used in dentistry as a prophylactic against caries.

**sta·phyl·i·on** (stă-fil′ē-on) Midpoint of posterior edge of hard palate; craniometric point. [G. dim. of *staphylē*, a bunch of grapes]

♻ **staphylo-**Combining form meaning resemblance to a grape or a bunch of grapes, hence relating usually to staphylococci or, in older use, to the uvula palatina. [G. *staphyle*, a bunch of grapes]

**staph·y·lo·coc·cal pneu·mo·ni·a** (staf′i-lō-kok′ăl nū-mō′nē-ă) Pneumonia, usually caused by *Staphylococcus aureus*, usually commencing as a bronchopneumonia.

***Staph·y·lo·coc·cus***, pl. **staph·y·lo·coc·ci** (staf′i-lō-kok′ŭs, -kok′sī) A genus of nonmotile, non-spore-forming, aerobic to facultatively anaerobic bacteria that are found on the skin, in skin glands, on the nasal and other mucous membranes of warm-blooded animals, and in various food products. The type species is *S. aureus*. [*staphylo-* + G. *kokkos*, a berry]

***Staph·y·lo·coc·cus au·re·us*** (staf′i-lō-kok′ŭs aw′rē-ŭs) Common species found especially on nasal mucous membranes and skin (hair follicles); bacterial species that produces exotoxins including those that cause toxic shock syndrome, with resulting skin rash, and renal, hepatic, and central nervous system disease, and an enterotoxin associated with food poisoning; it causes furunculosis, cellulitis, pyemia, pneumonia, osteomyelitis, endocarditis, suppuration of wounds, other infections; also a cause of infection in burn patients; humans are the chief reservoir. The type species of the genus *Staphylococcus*.

***Staph·y·lo·coc·cus ep·i·der·mis*** (staf′i-lō-kok′ŭs ep′i-děr′mis) Species of bacteria, the most common of the coagulase-negative *Staphylococcus* group.

**staph·y·lo·phar·yn·gor·rha·phy** (staf′i-lō-far′in-gōr′ă-fē) Surgical repair of defects in uvula or soft palate and pharynx. [*staphylo-* + *pharynx* + G. *rhaphē*, suture]

**starch** (stahrch) High molecular weight polysaccharide made up of D-glucose residues consisting of 20% amylose and 80% amylopectin. SYN amylum. [A.S. *stearc*, strong]

**star·va·tion** (stahr-vā′shŭn) Lengthy and continuous deprivation of food.

**star·va·tion ac·id·o·sis** (stahr-vā′shŭn as′i-dō′sis) Ketoacidosis resulting from lack of food intake.

**star·va·tion di·a·be·tes** (stahr-vā′shŭn dī′ă-bē′tēz) After prolonged fasting, glycosuria following ingestion of carbohydrate or glucose because of reduced output of insulin and/or reduced rate of glucose metabolism with a reduced ability to form glycogen.

**starve** (stahrv) 1. To suffer from lack of food. 2. To deprive of food so as to cause suffering or death. [A.S. *steorfan*, to die]

**sta·sis** (stā′sis) Stagnation of the blood or other fluids. [G. a standing still]

**stat·ic-air ster·i·li·zer** (stat′ik ăr ster′i-lī-zĕr) A dry-heat disinfection device with heating coils in its bottom or sides. Hot air moves by natural convection.

**st**

**stat·ic pos·tion** (stat´ik pŏ-zish´ŏn) Holding the nondominant hand in a non-moving position during instrumentation.

**stat·ic re·la·tion** (stat´ik rē-lā´shŭn) Relationship between two parts that are not in motion.

**sta·tim (STAT, stat.)** (stā´tim) At once; immediately. [L.]

**sta·tion·ar·y an·chor·age** (stā´shŭn-ar-ē ang´kŏr-ăj) Anchorage in which resistance to movement of one or more teeth comes from resistance to bodily movement of anchorage unit; a questionable concept given that the selected teeth remain only relatively stable.

**sta·tis·tics** (stă-tis´tiks) A collection of numeric values, items of information, or other facts numerically grouped into definite classes and subject to analysis, particularly of the probability that resulting empiric findings are due to chance.

**stat·o·ki·net·ic re·flex** (stat´ō-ki-net´ik rē´fleks) Reflex that, through stimulation of receptors in neck muscles and semicircular canals, brings about movements of limbs and eyes appropriate to a given movement of head in space.

**STAT, stat.** Abbreviation for *statim.* [L. immediately]

**sta·tus** (stat´ŭs) *The correct plural of this word is status, not stati.* A state or condition. [L. a way of standing]

**sta·tus asth·mat·i·cus** (stā´tŭs az-mat´i-kŭs) Condition involving severe, prolonged asthma.

**sta·tus ep·i·lep·ti·cus** (stā´tŭs ep-i-lep´ti-kŭs) Repeated seizures or a seizure of at least 30 minutes.

**stau·ri·on** (stawr´ē-on) Craniometric point at intersection of median and transverse palatine sutures. [G. dim. of *stauros,* cross]

**STD** Abbreviation for sexually transmitted disease.

**stead·y state (s, ss)** (sted´ē stāt) **1.** A condition obtained in moderate muscular exercise when the removal of lactic acid by oxidation keeps pace with its production, the oxygen supply being adequate, and the muscles do not rely on energy from anaerobic sources. **2.** Any condition in which the formation or introduction of substances just keeps pace with their destruction or removal so that all volumes, concentrations, pressures, and flows remain constant. **3.** In enzyme kinetics, conditions such that the rate of change in the concentration of any enzyme species (e.g., free enzyme or the enzyme-substrate binary complex) is zero or much less than the rate of formation of product.

**steal** (stēl) Diversion of blood by alternate routes or reversed flow, from one vascular bed to another, often causing symptoms in organ from which blood flow has been diverted. [M.E. *stelen,* fr. A.S. *stelan*]

**steam-fit·ter's asth·ma** (stēm´fit-ĕrz az´mă) Breathing disorder associated with asbestosis acquired by exposure to asbestos-insulated heating and plumbing components.

**steg·no·sis** (steg-nō´sis) **1.** Stoppage of secretions or excretions. **2.** A constriction or stenosis. [G. stoppage]

**stel·late re·tic·u·lum** (stel´āt rĕ-tik´yū-lŭm) SYN enamel reticulum.

**stem cell** (stem sel) **1.** Any precursor cell. **2.** Cell with daughter cells that may differentiate into other cell types.

**sten·o·com·pres·sor** (sten´ō-kom-pres´ŏr) Instrument for compressing ducts of the parotid glands (Stensen duct) to keep back saliva during dental operations.

**ste·no·sis,** pl. **ste·no·ses** (stě-nō´sis, -sēz) Stricture of any canal or orifice. [G. *stenosis,* a narrowing]

**sten·o·ste·no·sis** (sten´ō-stě-nō´sis) Stricture of parotid duct (Stensen duct).

**sten·o·sto·mi·a** (sten´ō-stō´mē-ă) Narrowness of oral cavity. [G. *stenos,* narrow + G. *stoma,* mouth]

**Sten·sen duct** (sten´sen dŭkt) SYN parotid duct.

**stent** (stent) **1.** Device used to maintain a bodily orifice or cavity during skin grafting, or to immobilize a skin graft after placement. **2.** Slender thread, rod, or catheter, lying within the lumen of tubular structures, used to provide support during or after their anastomosis, or to ensure patency of an intact but contracted lumen. [C. Stent]

**step** (step) **1.** In dentistry, dove-tailed or similarly shaped projection of a cavity prepared in a tooth into a surface perpendicular to main part of cavity to prevent displacement of restoration (filling) by force of mastication. **2.** Change in direction resembling a stair-step in a line, surface, or construction of a solid body.

**step-down trans·form·er** (step´down trans-fōr´mer) Device used in radiology to decrease the voltage coming into the x-ray tube.

**step-up trans·form·er** (step´ŭp trans-fōr´mer) Device used in radiology to increase the voltage coming into an x-ray tube.

**step wedge** (step wej) Triangular aluminum device placed over a radiographic film during exposure to determine the penetrating ability of an x-ray beam. SYN penetrometer.

**ster·e·og·no·sis** (ster´ē-og-nō´sis) The appreciation of the form of an object by means of touch. [*stereo-,* solid + G. *gnōsis,* knowledge]

**ster·e·o·i·so·mer** (ster´ē-ō-ī´sŏ-mĕr) A molecule containing the same number and kind of atom groupings as another but in a different arrangement in space, in virtue of which it exhibits different optic properties. [G. *stereos,* solid + G. *isos,* equal, + *meros,* part]

**ster·e·o·scope** (ster′ē-ō-skōp) An instrument producing two horizontally separated images of the same object, providing a single image with an appearance of depth. [G. *stereos,* solid + G. *skopeō,* to view]

**ster·e·o·scop·ic mi·cro·scope** (ster′ē-ō-skop′ik mī′krŏ-skōp) A microscope having double eyepieces and objectives and thus independent light paths, giving a three-dimensional image.

**ster·e·o·scop·ic vi·sion** (ster′ē-ō-skop′ik vizh′ŭn) The single perception of a slightly different image from each eye.

**ster·e·o·ty·py** (ster′ē-ō-tī-pē) **1.** Maintenance of one attitude for a long period. **2.** Constant repetition of certain meaningless gestures or movements. [G. *stereos,* solid + G. *typos,* impression, type]

**ster·ile** (ster′il) Relating to or characterized by sterility. [L. *sterilis,* barren]

**ste·ril·i·ty** (stĕr-il′i-tē) Condition of being aseptic, or free from all living microorganisms. [L. *sterilitas*]

**ster·il·i·za·tion** (ster′i-lī-zā′shŭn) Destruction of all microorganisms in or about an object, such as by steam (flowing or pressurized), chemical agents (alcohol, phenol, heavy metals, ethylene oxide gas), high-velocity electron bombardment, heat, or ultraviolet light radiation.

**ster·no·clei·do·mas·toid** (stĕr′nō-klī′dō-mas′toyd) Relating to sternum, clavicle, and mastoid process.

**ster·no·thy·roid mus·cle** (ster′nō-thī′royd mŭs′ĕl) *Origin,* posterior surface of manubrium of sternum and first or second costal cartilage; *insertion,* oblique line of thyroid cartilage; *action,* depresses larynx; *nerve supply,* upper cervical via spinal nerves (ansa cervicalis). SYN musculus sternothyroideus [TA].

**ster·num,** pl. **ster·na** (stĕr′nŭm, -nă) [TA] A long, flat bone, articulating with the cartilages of the first seven ribs and with the clavicle, which forms the middle part of the anterior wall of the thorax. SYN breast bone. [Mod. L. fr. G. *sternon,* the chest]

**ster·oid** (ster′oyd) **1.** Pertaining to the steroids. **2.** One of the steroids (e.g., sterols, bile acids, cardiac glycosides, androgens, estrogens, corticosteroids, precursors of the D vitamins). [G. *stereos,* solid; solid lipids vs. oils]

**ster·oid hor·mones** (ster′oyd hor′mōnz) Those hormones possessing the steroid ring system (e.g., androgens, estrogens, adrenocortical hormones).

**ste·roid·o·gen·ic di·a·be·tes** (ster-oy′dō-jen′ik dī′ă-bē′tēz) Abnormal glucose tolerance, often frank diabetes mellitus (q.v.), induced by metabolic effects of adrenocortical steroid hormones such as cortisone or therapeutic analogues such as prednisone. Effect may be temporary, resolving when the steroid therapy is discontinued, or diabetes mellitus may persist.

**steth·o·scope** (steth′ŏ-skōp) An instrument used in auscultation of vascular or other sounds anywhere in body. [G. *stethos,* chest + G. *skopeō,* to view]

**Ste·vens-John·son syn·drome** (stē′vĕnz jon′sŏn sin′drōm) A bullous form of erythema multiforme that may be extensive, involving the mucous membranes and large areas of the body. See page A5.

**STI** Abbreviation for sexually transmitted infection.

**stiff neck** (stif nek) Nonspecific term for limited neck mobility, often due to muscle cramps and accompanied by pain.

**stiff·ness** (stif′nĕs) In dentistry, the reaction force exerted per unit area of the brush during deflection; used interchangeably with firmness in describing toothbrush bristles or filaments; depends primarily on length and diameter of filaments or bristles.

**stig·ma,** pl. **stig·ma·ta** (stig′mă, -mă-tă) **1.** Visible evidence of a disease. **2.** Any spot or blemish on skin. [G. a mark. fr. *stizō,* to prick]

**stilboestrol** [Br.] SYN diethylstilbestrol.

**still·born** (stil′bōrn) Born dead; denoting an infant dead at birth.

**Still·man clefts** (stil′măn klefts) Small fissures extending apically from midline of gingival margin; usually on vestibular surface.

**Still·man meth·od** (stil′măn meth′ŏd) Manual toothbrushing technique that angulates the toothbrush bristles at a 45-degree angle towards the apex of the tooth; bristles are placed partly on the cervical portion of the tooth and partly on the gingiva.

**stim·u·lant** (stim′yū-lănt) **1.** Stimulating; exciting to action. **2.** Agent that arouses organic activity, strengthens heart action, increases vitality, and promotes sense of well-being. SYN excitant. [L. *stimulans,* pres. p. of *stimulo,* pp. *-atus,* to goad, incite, fr. *stimulus,* a goad]

**stim·u·la·tion** (stim′yŭ-lā′shŭn) *Do not confuse this word with simulation.* **1.** Arousal of body or any of its parts or organs to increased functional activity. **2.** Condition of being stimulated.

**stim·u·lus,** pl. **stim·u·li** (stim′yū-lŭs, -lī) That which can elicit or evoke action (response) in a muscle, nerve, gland or other excitable tissue, or cause augmenting action on any function or metabolic process. [L. a goad]

**sting** (sting) Sharp momentary pain, most commonly produced by puncture of the skin by arthropods, including hexapods, myriapods, and

st

arachnids; can also be produced by jellyfish, sea urchins, sponges, mollusks, and several species of venomous fish, such as the stingray, toadfish, rabbitfish, and catfish.

**stip·pling** (stip′ling) 1. Orange peel appearance of attached gingiva. 2. Roughening of surfaces of a denture base to stimulate natural gingival stippling. 3. Speckling of a blood cell or other structure with fine dots when exposed to the action of a basic stain, due to presence of free basophil granules in cell protoplasm.

**stitch** (stich) 1. Sharp, sticking pain of momentary duration. 2. A single suture. 3. SYN suture (2). [A.S. *stice,* a pricking]

**St. John's wort** (sānt jonz wōrt) Shrubby perennial herb (*Hypericum perforatum*). Although widely used as an antidepressant, has not been shown, in clinical trials, to be superior to placebo in treatment of *major* depression.

**STM** Abbreviation for short-term memory.

**stock** (stok) All the populations of organisms derived from an isolate without any implication of homogeneity or characterization. [A.S. *stoc*]

**Stokes-Ad·ams syn·drome** (stōks ad′ ămz sin′drōm) SYN Adams-Stokes syndrome.

**sto·ma,** pl. **sto·mas,** pl. **sto·ma·ta** (stō′ mă, -măz, -mă-tă) 1. Minute opening or pore. 2. Artificial opening between two cavities or canals, or between such and body surface. [G. a mouth]

**stom·ach tooth** (stŏm′ăk tūth) One of the lower canine teeth.

**sto·ma·tal·gi·a** (stō′mă-tal′jē-ă) Pain in the mouth. SYN stomatodynia. [*stomat-* + G. *algos,* pain]

**sto·ma·ti·tis** (stō′mă-tī′tis) Inflammation of mucous membrane of mouth. [*stomat-* + G. *-itis,* inflammation]

**⊞sto·ma·ti·tis me·di·ca·men·to·sa** (stō′ mă-tī′tis med-i-kă-men-tō′să) Inflammatory alterations of oral mucosa associated with a systemic drug allergy; lesions may consist of erythema, vesicles, bullae, ulcerations, or angioedema. See page A8.

**♻ stomato-, stom-, stomat-** Combining forms denoting oral cavity. [G. *stoma*]

**sto·ma·to·dyn·i·a** (stō′mă-tō-din′ē-ă) SYN stomatalgia. [*stomato-* + G. *odynē,* pain]

**sto·ma·to·glos·si·tis** (stō′mă-tō-glos-ī′tis) Inflammation involving oral mucous membranes and the tongue. May be seen in association with nutritional disorders such as pellagra, beriberi, vitamin B complex deficiency, and various infections.

**sto·ma·tog·nath·ic sys·tem** (stō′mă-

tog-nath′ik sis′tĕm) All structures involved in speech and in reception, mastication, and deglutition of food. SYN masticatory apparatus (2).

**sto·ma·tol·o·gist** (stō′mă-tol′ŏ-jist) A specialist in diseases of oral cavity.

**sto·ma·tol·o·gy** (stō′mă-tol′ŏ-jē) Study of structure, function, and diseases of the mouth. [*stomato-* + G. *logos,* study]

**sto·ma·to·ma·la·ci·a** (stō′mă-tō-mă-lā′ shē-ă) Pathologic softening of any mouth structures. [*stomato-* + G. *malakia,* softness]

**sto·ma·to·my·co·sis** (stō′mă-tō-mī-kō′ sis) Disease of oral cavity due to a fungus. [*stomato-* + G. *mykēs,* fungus, + *-osis,* condition]

**⊞sto·ma·top·a·thy, sto·ma·to·sis** (stō′ mă-top′ă-thē, -tō′sis) Any disease of oral cavity. See this page. [*stomato-* + G. *pathos,* suffering]

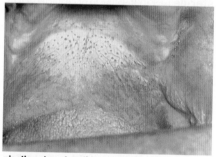

**nicotine stomatopathy:** prominent on soft palate

**sto·ma·tor·rha·gi·a** (stō′mă-tōr-ā′jē-ă) Bleeding from gums or another part of the oral cavity. [*stomato-* + G. *rhēgnymi,* to burst forth]

**sto·ma·to·scope** (stō′mă-tō-skōp) Apparatus for illuminating interior of mouth to facilitate dental examination. [*stomato-* + G. *skopeō,* to view]

**sto·mi·on** (stō′mē-on) Median point of oral slit with lips closed.

**sto·mo·ceph·a·lus** (stō′mō-sef′ă-lŭs) Malformed person with an undeveloped jaw and a snoutlike mouth; likely to be combined with an ethmocephalic type of cyclopia. [G. *stoma,* mouth, + *kephalē,* head]

**sto·mo·de·al** (stō′mō-dē′ăl) Relating to a stomodeum.

**sto·mo·de·um, sto·ma·to·de·um** (stō′ mō-dē′ŭm, -mă-tō-dē′ŭm) A midline ectodermal depression ventral to the embryonic brain and surrounded by the mandibular arch; when the buccopharyngeal membrane disappears, the stomodeum becomes continuous with the foregut and forms the mouth. [Mod. L. fr. G. *stoma,* mouth, + *hodaios,* on the way, fr. *hodos,* a way]

**stone** (stōn) 1. SYN calculus. 2. An abrading

instrument. **3.** A British unit of weight for the human body, equal to 14 pounds. [A.S. *stān*]

**stone an·gu·la·tion** (stōn ang′gyū-lā′shŭn) Camber of sharpening stone between 70 and 80 degrees to the instrument face during instrument sharpening.

**stone die** (stōn dī) Replica of a tooth composed of dental stone commonly used to fabricate a restoration (e.g., crown).

**stool** (stūl) **1.** A discharging of the bowels. **2.** The matter discharged at one movement of the bowels. SYN evacuation (2), movement (2). [A.S. *stōl,* seat]

**stop·ping** (stop′ing) Any material used to seal a dressing in a tooth.

**stops** (stops) Bends in, or wires soldered to, an archwire to limit passage through a bracket or tube.

**stor·age dis·ease** (stōr′ăj di-zēz′) Generic term that includes any accumulation of a specific substance within tissues.

**stor·age phos·phor im·ag·ing** (stōr″ăj fos′fŏr im″ăj-ing) Method of obtaining a radiographic image by recording it on phosphor-coated plates and then putting it in an electronic processor where a laser scans the plate and produces an image on a computer screen.

**storm** (stōrm) An exacerbation of symptoms or a crisis in the course of a disease.

**stra·bis·mus** (stră-biz′mŭs) A manifest lack of parallelism of the visual axes of the eyes. SYN crossed eyes, heterotropia, squint (1). [Mod. L., fr. G. *strabismos,* a squinting]

**straight shank** (strāt shangk) SYN complex shank.

**strain** (strān) **1.** Population of homogeneous organisms possessing a set of defined characteristics. **2.** Specific host cell(s) designed or selected to optimize production of recombinant products. **3.** To make an effort to the limit of one's strength. **4.** To injure by overuse or improper use (usually refers to a muscle tear). **5.** An act of straining. **6.** Injury resulting from strain or overuse. **7.** Change in shape that a body undergoes when acted on by an external force. **8.** To filter; to percolate. [A.S. *strēon,* progeny]

**stra·tig·ra·phy** (stră-tig′ră-fē) SYN tomography. [L. *stratum,* layer, + G. *graphē,* a writing]

**stra·tum,** pl. **stra·ta** (strā′tŭm, -tă) One of the layers of differentiated tissue, the aggregate of which forms any given structure.

**stra·tum ba·sa·le** (strā′tŭm bā-sā′lē) **1.** The outermost layer of the endometrium that undergoes only minimal changes during the menstrual cycle; SYN basal layer. **2.** SYN stratum basale epidermidis.

**stra·tum ba·sa·le ep·i·derm·i·dis** (strā′tŭm bā-sa′lē ep-i-děrm′i-dis) The deepest layer of the epidermis, composed of dividing stem cells and anchoring cells. SYN basal cell layer, stratum basale (2).

**stra·tum lu·ci·dum** (strā′tŭm lū′sid-ŭm) Layer of lightly staining corneocytes in the deepest level of the stratum corneum. SYN clear layer of epidermis.

**stra·tum spon·gi·o·sum** (strā′tŭm spon-jē-ō′sŭm) The middle spongy layer of the endometrium formed chiefly of dilated glandular structures.

**Straus sign** (strows sīn) In facial paralysis, if an injection of pilocarpine is followed by sweating on the affected side later than on the other, the lesion is peripheral.

**straw·ber·ry he·man·gi·o·ma** (straw′ber-ē hē-man′jē-ō′mă) Hyperproliferation of immature capillary vessels, usually on the head and neck, present at birth or within the first 2–3 months postnatally, which commonly regresses without scar formation.

**straw·ber·ry tongue** (straw′ber-ē tŭng) Tongue with a whitish coat through which enlarged fungiform papillae project as red points, characteristic of scarlet fever and of Kawasaki disease.

**streak** (strēk) A line, stria, or stripe, especially one that is indistinct or evanescent. [A.S. *strica*]

**stream** (strēm) SYN flumen.

**street drug** (strēt drŭg) Substance taken for nonmedical purposes; amphetamines, anesthetics, barbiturates, opiates, and psychoactive drugs.

**strength** (strengkth) **1.** The quality of being powerful. **2.** Degree of intensity. **3.** The property of materials by which they endure the application of force without yielding.

**strepto-** Combining form meaning curved or twisted (usually relating to organisms thus described). [G. *streptos,* twisted, fr. *strepho,* to twist]

**strep·to·coc·cal tox·ic shock syn·drome** (strep′tō-kok′ăl tok′sik shok sin′drŏm) Condition characterized by hypotension and signs and symptoms indicative of multiorgan failure including cerebral dysfunction, renal failure, acute respiratory distress syndrome, and hepatic dysfunction; usually precipitated by local infections of skin or soft tissue by streptococci.

***Strep·to·coc·cus*** (strep′tō-kok′ŭs) A genus of nonmotile non-spore-forming, aerobic to facultatively anaerobic bacteria containing gram-positive, spheric or ovoid cells that occur regularly in mouth and intestines of humans and in dairy and other food products, and in fermenting

**st**

plant juices. [*strepto-* + G. *kokkos,* berry (coccus)]

**Strep·to·coc·cus mil·ler·i** (strep′tō-kok′ ŭs mil′ler-ī) *Streptococcus intermedius* group found in human oral cavity and associated with infections including bacteremia, endocarditis, and central nervous system, oral, and thoracic infections.

**Strep·to·coc·cus mu·tans** (strep′tō-kok′ ŭs myū′tanz) A bacterial species associated with the production of dental caries in humans and with subacute endocarditis.

**Strep·to·coc·cus pneu·mo·ni·ae** (strep′ tō-kok′ŭs nū-mō′nē-ē) A bacterial species of gram-positive, lancet-shaped diplococci frequently occurring in pairs or chains. Normal inhabitants of the respiratory tract, and the cause of lobar pneumonia, otitis media, meningitis, sinusitis, and other infections. SYN pneumococcus.

**Strep·to·coc·cus py·og·e·nes** (strep′ tō-kok′ŭs pī-oj′ĕ-nēz) A bacterial species found in the human mouth, throat, and respiratory tract and in inflammatory exudates, bloodstream, and lesions in human diseases found in dust from sickrooms, hospital wards, schools, theaters, and other public places; causes formation of pus or even fatal septicemias.

**Strep·to·coc·cus sa·li·va·ri·us** (strep′ tŏ-kok′ŭs sal-var′ē-ŭs) Bacteria present in plaque biofilm that may result in endocarditis and dental decay.

**Strep·to·coc·cus vir·i·dans** (strep′tō-kok′ŭs vir′i-danz) SYN viridans streptococci.

**strep·to·dor·nase (SD)** (strep′tō-dōr′nās) A "dornase" (deoxyribonuclease) obtained from streptococci; used with streptokinase to facilitate drainage in septic surgical conditions.

**strep·to·ki·nase** (strep′tō-kī′nās) Extracellular protein produced by some streptococci that binds to plasminogen and activates its conversion to plasmin; no enzyme activity of its own.

**strep·to·ki·nase-strep·to·dor·nase** (strep′tō-kī′nās-strep′tō-dōr′nās) Purified mixture of streptokinase, streptodornase, and other proteolytic enzymes; used by topical application or by injection into body cavities to remove clotted blood and fibrinous and purulent accumulations of exudate.

**Strep·to·my·ces** (strep′tō-mī′sēz) Genus of nonmotile, aerobic, gram-positive bacteria that grows as a many-branched mycelium. [*strepto-* + G. *mykēs,* fungus]

**strep·to·my·cin** (strep′tō-mī′sin) An antibiotic agent obtained from *Streptomyces griseus* that is active against the tubercle bacillus and many gram-positive and gram-negative bacteria; also used in the form of dihydrostreptomycin; used almost exclusively in treatment of tuberculosis; toxicity includes eighth cranial nerve damage leading to deafness or vestibular dysfunction.

**stress** (stres) **1.** In dentistry, forces set up in teeth, their supporting structures, and structures restoring or replacing teeth due to force of mastication. **2.** Reactions of body to forces of a deleterious nature, infections, and various abnormal states that tend to disturb its normal physiologic equilibrium (homeostasis). [L. *strictus,* tight, fr. *stringo,* to draw together]

**stress-bear·ing a·re·a** (stres′ber-ing ar′ē-ă) **1.** SYN denture foundation area. **2.** Surfaces of oral structures that resist forces, strains, or pressures brought on them during function.

**stress break·er** (stres brā′kĕr) Device that relieves abutment teeth, to which a fixed or removable partial denture is attached, of all or part of the forces generated by occlusal function.

**stress frac·ture** (stres frak′shŭr) SYN fatigue fracture.

**stretch re·cep·tors** (strech rĕ-sep′tōrz) Receptors sensitive to elongation, especially those in Golgi tendon organs and muscle spindles, but also those found in visceral organs.

**stretch re·flex** (strech rē′fleks) SYN myotactic reflex.

**stri·a,** pl. **stri·ae** (strī′ă, -ē) [TA] Stripe, band, streak, or line, distinguished by color, texture, depression, or elevation from tissue in which it is found. [L. channel, furrow]

**stri·ae of Ret·zi·us** (strī′ē ret′zē-ŭs) Incremental growth lines in tooth enamel seen microscopically as dark bands.

**stri·at·ed duct** (strī′āt-ĕd dŭkt) A type of intralobular duct found in some salivary glands that modifies the secretory product.

**stri·at·ed mus·cle** (strī′āt-ĕd mŭs′ĕl) Skeletal or voluntary muscle in which cross-striations occur in the fibers as a result of regular overlapping of thick and thin myofilaments.

**stri·dent** (strī′dĕnt) Creaking; grating; harsh-sounding; denoting an auscultatory sound or rale. [L. *stridens,* pres. p. of *strideo,* to creak]

**stri·dor** (strī′dŏr) A high-pitched, noisy respiration; sign of respiratory obstruction. [L. a harsh, creaking sound]

**stri·dor den·ti·um** (strī′dŏr den′shē-ŭm) Grinding of the teeth.

**strip** (strip) **1.** In dentistry, to smooth or polish proximal surfaces of a restoration using a plastic or linen ribbon. SYN milk (4). **2.** Subcutaneous excision of a vein in its longitudinal axis, performed with a stripper. **3.** Any narrow piece, relatively long and of uniform width. [A.S. *strypan,* to rob]

**stripe** (strīp) **1.** In anatomy, a streak, line, band, or stria. **2.** In radiography, a linear opacity differing in density from adjacent parts of image; usually represents tangential image of a planar structure. [M.E.]

**strip·ping** (strip'ing) Removal, often of a covering.

**stroke** (strōk) **1.** Single unbroken movement of an instrument in the task it was designed to perform. **2.** To pass the hand or any instrument gently over a surface. **3.** A gliding movement over a surface. [A.S. *strāc*]

**stroke vol·ume** (strōk vol'yūm) The volume pumped out of one ventricle of the heart in a single beat.

**stro·ma,** pl. **stro·ma·ta** (strō'mă, -tă) Framework, usually of connective tissue, of an organ, gland, or other structure. [G. *strōma*, bed]

**stron·gy·loi·di·a·sis** (stron'ji-loy-dī'ă-sis) Infection with soil-borne nematodes of the genus *Strongyloides*, considered to be a parthenogenetic parasitic female. Autoreinfection also may develop in patients with AIDS.

**stron·ti·um (Sr)** (stron'shē-ŭm) A metallic element; one of the alkaline earth series and similar to calcium in chemical and biologic properties. [*Strontian,* a town in Scotland]

**stroph·o·ceph·a·ly** (strof'ō-sef'ă-lē) Condition characterized by a congenitally distorted head and face, with a tendency toward cyclopia and malformation of oral region. [G. *strophē,* a twist, + *kephalē,* head]

**struc·tur·al in·ter·face** (strŭk'shŭr-ăl in'tĕr-fās) In dentistry, a boundary between tooth and restorative material.

**struc·ture** (strŭk'shŭr) **1.** Arrangement of the details of a part; the manner of formation of a part. **2.** A tissue or formation made up of different but related parts. **3.** In chemistry, the specific connections of the atoms in a given molecule. [L. *structura,* fr. *struo,* pp. *structus,* to build]

**stru·ma,** pl. **stru·mae** (strū'mă, -mē) *Do not confuse this word with stroma.* **1.** SYN goiter. **2.** Formerly, any enlargement of tissue. [L. a scrofulous tumor, fr. *struo,* to pile up, build]

**stru·ma me·di·ca·men·to·sa** (strū'mă med'i-kă-men-tō'să) Goiter due to use of a therapeutic agent.

**Stry·ker-Hal·bei·sen syn·drome** (strī'kĕr hahl'bī-sĕn sin'drōm) Reddish, scaling, macular eruption on head and upper trunk due to vitamin B complex deficiency.

**Stu·art factor, Stu·art-Prow·er fac·tor** (stū'ărt fak'tŏr, prow'ĕr) SYN factor X.

**Stu·dent *t*-test** (stū'dĕnt test) Statistical significance measure for assessing difference between, or equality of, two or more population means.

**stud·y** (stŭd'ē) Research, detailed examination, and analysis of an organism, object, or phenomenon. [L. *studium,* study, inquiry]

**stud·y cast** (stŭd'ē kast) Positive reproduction of teeth and surrounding structures for the purpose of study and treatment planning; created by pouring to allow an impression in plaster or stone. SEE ALSO cast (1).

**stu·por** (stū'pŏr) Impaired consciousness in which patient shows a marked diminution in reactivity to environmental stimuli and can be aroused only by continual stimulation. [L. fr. *stupeo,* to be stunned]

**stu·por·ous** (stū'pŏr-ŭs) Relating to or marked by stupor.

**stu·por·ous ca·ta·to·ni·a** (stū'pŏr-ŭs kat'ă-tō'nē-ă) Catatonia in which the patient is subdued, mute, and negativistic.

**Sturge-Web·er syn·drome** (stŭrj vā'bĕr sin'drōm) In its complete form, triad of unilateral occurrence of congenital capillary malformation (flame nevus) in distribution of the trigeminal nerve; ipsilateral leptomeningeal vascular malformations with intracranial calcification and neurologic signs; and vascular malformation of the choroid plexus. See this page.

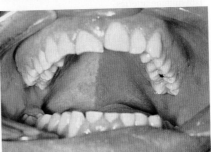

**Sturge-Weber angiomatosis:** to midline of palate

**stut·ter·ing** (stŭt'ĕr-ing) A phonatory or articulatory disorder, characteristically beginning in childhood, with intense anxiety about the efficiency of oral communications, and characterized by dysfluency.

**sty·lette, sty·let** (stī-let', stī'let) **1.** Flexible metallic rod inserted in lumen of flexible catheter to stiffen and give it form during its passage. **2.** Slender probe. [It. *stilletto,* a dagger; dim. of L. *stilus* or *stylus,* a stake, a pen]

**sty·lo·glos·sus mus·cle** (stī'lō-glos'ŭs mŭs'ĕl) *Action,* retracts tongue; *origin,* lower end of styloid process; *insertion,* side and undersurface of tongue; *nerve supply,* hypoglossal. SYN musculus styloglossus [TA].

**sty·lo·hy·oid lig·a·ment** (stī-lō-hī´oyd lig´ă-mĕnt) [TA] Ligament that connects the styloid process and the hyoid bone.

**sty·lo·hy·oid mus·cle** (stī´lō-hī´oyd mŭs´ĕl) *Origin*, styloid process of temporal bone; *insertion*, hyoid bone by two slips on either side of intermediate tendon of digastric; *action*, elevates hyoid bone; *nerve supply*, facial. SYN musculus stylohyoideus [TA].

**sty·lo·man·dib·u·lar** (stī´lō-man-dib´yū-lăr) Relating to styloid process of temporal bone and mandible; denoting stylomandibular ligament.

**sty·lo·man·dib·u·lar lig·a·ment** (stī´lō-man-dib´yū-lăr lig´ă-mĕnt) [TA] Condensation of deep cervical fascia extending from tip of styloid process of temporal bone to posterior border of angle of jaw; blends with (i.e., a thickening of) parotid sheath. SYN stylomaxillary ligament.

**sty·lo·mas·toid** (stī´lō-mas´toyd) Relating to styloid and mastoid processes of temporal bone.

**sty·lo·mas·toid ar·te·ry** (stī´lō-mas´toyd ahr´tĕr-ē) [TA] *Origin*, posterior auricular; *distribution*, external acoustic meatus, mastoid cells, semicircular canals, stapedius muscle, and vestibule; *anastomoses*, tympanic branches of internal carotid and ascending pharyngeal, and labyrinthine arteries.

**sty·lo·mas·toid for·a·men** (stī´lō-mas´toyd fōr-ā´mĕn) [TA] Distal or external opening of the facial canal on the inferior surface of the petrous portion of the temporal bone, between the styloid and mastoid processes; it transmits the facial nerve and stylomastoid artery.

**sty·lo·mas·toid vein** (stī´lō-mas´toyd vān) [TA] Drains the tympanic cavity, traverses the facial canal exiting via the stylomastoid foramen, and empties into the retromandibular vein.

**sty·lo·max·il·lar·y lig·a·ment** (stī´lō-mak´si-lar-ē lig´ă-mĕnt) SYN stylomandibular ligament.

**sty·lo·ra·di·al re·flex** (stī´lō-rā´dē-ăl rē´fleks) SYN brachioradial reflex.

**sty·lus** (stī´lŭs) Any pencil-shaped structure or pencil-shaped medicinal preparation for external application. [L. *stilus* or *stylus,* a stake or pen]

**sty·lus trac·ing** (stī´lŭs trās´ing) SYN intraoral tracing.

**styp·tic** (stip´tik) An astringent and hemostatic agent used topically to stop bleeding. [G. *styptikos,* astringent]

♻ **sub-** Prefix used in words formed from L. roots,

denoting beneath, less than the normal or typical, inferior. [L. *sub,* under]

**sub·a·cute** (sŭb´ă-kyūt´) Between acute and chronic; denoting course of a disease of moderate duration or severity.

**sub·a·cute in·flam·ma·tion** (sŭb´ă-kyūt´ in´flă-mā´shŭn) Inflammation intermediate in duration between acute inflammation and chronic inflammation.

**sub·al·i·men·ta·tion** (sŭb´al-i-men-tā´shŭn) Condition due to insufficient nourishment.

**subarachnoid haemorrhage** [Br.] SYN subarachnoid hemorrhage.

**sub·a·rach·noid hem·or·rhage** (sŭb´ă-rak´noyd hem´ŏr-ăj) Extravasation of blood into subarachnoid space. SYN subarachnoid haemmorhage.

**sub·au·ral** (sŭb-awr´ăl) Below the ear.

**sub·au·ric·u·lar** (sŭb´aw-rik´yū-lăr) Below an auricle; especially concha or pinna of ear.

**sub·cep·tion** (sŭb-sep´shŭn) Subliminal perception as in the reaction to a stimulus not fully perceived. [sub- + L. *-ceptum,* perceived]

**sub·cla·vi·an steal** (sŭb-klā´vē-ăn stēl) Obstruction of the subclavian artery proximal to origin of the vertebral artery.

**sub·clin·i·cal** (sŭb-klin´i-kăl) Denoting presence of a disease without manifest symptoms; may be an early stage in disease evolution.

**sub·clin·i·cal di·a·be·tes** (sŭb-klin´i-kăl dī´ă-bē´tēz) Diabetes mellitus clinically evident only under certain circumstances, such as pregnancy or extreme stress. *Term declared obsolete by American Diabetes Association.*

**sub·clin·i·cal sei·zure** (sŭb-klin´i-kăl sē´zhŭr) A seizure detected by electroencephalogram, which has no clinical correlate.

**sub·con·scious** (sŭb-kon´shŭs) 1. Not wholly conscious. 2. Denoting an idea or impression present in the mind, but of which there is at the time no conscious knowledge or realization.

**sub·con·scious·ness** (sŭb-kon´shŭs-nĕs) 1. Partial unconsciousness. 2. The state in which mental processes take place without conscious perception.

**sub·cos·tal·gi·a** (sŭb´kos-tal´jē-ă) Pain in the subcostal region. [subcostal + G. *algos,* pain]

**sub·crep·i·tant** (sŭb-krep´i-tănt) Nearly, but not frankly, crepitant; denoting a rale.

**sub·crep·i·tant rale** (sŭb-krep´i-tănt rahl) Fine crepitant rale.

**sub·crep·i·ta·tion** (sŭb′krep-i-tā′shŭn) 1. The presence of subcrepitant rales. 2. A sound approaching crepitation in character.

**sub·crest·al pock·et** (sŭb-krest′ăl pok′ĕt) SYN infrabony pocket.

**sub·cul·ture** (sŭb′kŭl-chŭr) 1. A culture made by transferring to a fresh medium microorganisms from a previous culture. 2. To make a fresh culture with material obtained from a previous one.

**sub·cur·a·tive** (sŭb-kyūr′ă-tiv) Denoting a dose of a pharmacotherapeutic agent lower than necessary for a curative effect.

**sub·cu·ta·ne·ous (SC, SQ)** (sŭb′kyū-tā′nē-ŭs) Beneath the skin. SYN hypodermic (1). [*sub-* + L. *cutis,* skin]

**sub·cu·ta·ne·ous wound** (sŭb′kyū-tā′nē-ŭs wūnd) Injury extending below skin into subcutaneous tissue, but not affecting underlying bones or organs.

**sub·den·tal** (sŭb-den′tăl) Beneath roots of the teeth.

**sub·du·ral** (sŭb-dūr′ăl) 1. Deep to the dura mater. SEE spatium subdurale. 2. Between the dura mater and the arachnoid mater.

**sub·du·ral he·ma·to·ma** (sŭb-dūr′ăl hē′mă-tō′mă) Extravasation of blood between dural and arachnoidal membranes; acute and chronic forms occur; chronic hematomas may become encapsulated by neomembranes. SYN subdural hemorrhage.

**sub·du·ral hem·or·rhage** (sŭb-dūr′ăl hem′ŏr-ăj) SYN subdural hematoma.

**sub·ep·i·the·li·al** (sŭb′ep-i-thē′lē-ăl) Below the epithelium.

**su·ber·o·sis** (sū′ber-ō′sis) Extrinsic allergic alveolitis caused by inhalation of mold spores from contaminated cork. [L. *suber,* cork, + G. *-osis,* condition]

**sub·gin·gi·val** (sŭb-jin′ji-văl) Below the gingival margin.

**sub·gin·gi·val cal·cu·lus** (sŭb-jin′ji-văl kal′kyū-lŭs) Calcareous dental deposit found apical to gingival margin. SYN serumal calculus (2).

**sub·gin·gi·val cu·ret·tage** (sŭb-jin′ji-văl kyūr′ĕ-tahzh′) Removal of subgingival calculus and ulcerated epithelial and granulation tissues found in periodontal pockets. SYN apoxesis.

**sub·gin·gi·val in·stru·men·ta·tion** (sŭb-jin′ji-văl in′strŭ-mĕn-tā′shŭn) Use of an instrument apical to (below) the gingival margin.

**sub·gin·gi·val ir·ri·ga·tion** (sŭb-jin′ji-văl ir′i-gā′shŭn) Point of delivery of irrigation

is placed in a sulcus or pocket and may reach the apical border.

**sub·gin·gi·val plaque** (sŭb-jin′ji-văl plak) Plaque on teeth below the gingival margin in gingival crevice and periodontal pockets.

**sub·ic·ter·us** (sŭb-ik′tĕr-ŭs) Slightly elevated levels of serum bilirubin without clinical evidence of jaundice. [*sub-* + G. *ikterikos,* jaundiced]

**sub·ja·cent** (sŭb-jā′sĕnt) Below or beneath another part. [L. *sub-jaceo,* to lie under]

**sub·ject** (sŭb′jekt) A person, animal, or organism that is an object of research, treatment, experimentation, or dissection. [L. *subjectus,* lying beneath]

**sub·jec·tive** (sŭb-jek′tiv) 1. Perceived only by patient and not evident to examiner. 2. Colored by personal beliefs and attitudes. [L. *subjectivus,* fr. *subjicio,* to throw under]

**sub·jec·tive da·ta col·lec·tion** (sŭb-jek′tiv dā′tă kŏ-lek′shŭn) Information given by the patient (or caretaker) describing the onset, course, and character of the presenting compaint.

**sub·jec·tive sign** (sŭb-jek′tiv sīn) One perceived only by patient, also said of symptoms.

**sub·jec·tive vi·sion** (sŭb-jek′tiv vizh′ŭn) Visual impressions that arise centrally and do not originate with ocular stimuli.

**subleukaemic leukaemia** [Br.] SYN subleukemic leukemia.

**sub·leu·ke·mic leu·ke·mi·a** (sŭb′lū-kē′mik lū-kē′mē-ă) Disorder when abnormal cells are present in the peripheral blood, but total leukocyte count is not elevated. SYN subleukaemic leukaemia.

**sub·li·mate** (sŭb′lim-āt) 1. To perform or accomplish sublimation. 2. Any substance submitted to sublimation. [L. *sublimo,* pp. *-atus,* to raise on high, fr. *sublimis,* high]

**sub·li·ma·tion** (sŭb′li-mā′shŭn) Process of converting a solid directly into a gas; analogous to distillation.

**sub·lim·i·nal** (sŭb-lim′i-năl) Below threshold of perception, excitation, or consciousness. [*sub-* + L. *limen* (*limin-*), threshold]

**sub·lin·gual (SL)** (sŭb-ling′gwăl) Beneath or below the tongue.

**sub·lin·gual bur·sa** (sŭb-ling′gwăl bŭr′să) Inconstant serous bursa at level of frenulum of tongue between surface of genioglossus muscle and mucous membrane of floor of mouth.

**sub·lin·gual ca·run·cu·la** (sŭb-ling′gwăl kă-rŭng′kyū-lă) [TA] Papilla on each side of

st

frenulum of tongue marking opening of sub-mandibular duct.

**sub·lin·gual cres·cent** (sŭb-ling´gwăl kres´ĕnt) Crescentic area on floor of mouth formed by lingual wall of mandible and adjacent part of floor of mouth.

**sub·lin·gual fold** (sŭb-ling´gwăl fōld) [TA] Elevation in floor of mouth beneath tongue, on either side, marking site of sublingual gland.

**sub·lin·gual fos·sa** (sŭb-ling´gwăl fos´ă) [TA] Shallow depression on either side of mental spine, on inner surface of body of mandible, lodging sublingual gland. SYN sublingual pit.

**sub·lin·gual gan·gli·on** (sŭb-ling´gwăl gang´glē-ŏn) [TA] Tiny parasympathetic ganglion occasionally found anterior to the submandibular ganglion.

**sub·lin·gual gland** (sŭb-ling´gwăl gland) [TA] One of two salivary glands in the floor of the mouth beneath the tongue, discharging through the sublingual ducts; most of the secretory units in the human gland secrete mucus. SYN sublingual salivary gland.

**sub·lin·gual med·i·ca·tion** (sŭb-ling´gwăl med´i-kā´shŭn) Form of drug dosage intended to be used by placement under tongue.

**sub·lin·gual nerve** (sŭb-ling´gwăl nĕrv) [TA] Branch of lingual to sublingual gland and mucosa of floor of mouth.

**sub·lin·gual pit** (sŭb-ling´gwăl pit) SYN sublingual fossa.

**sub·lin·gual sal·i·var·y gland** (sŭb-ling´gwăl sal´i-var-ē gland) SYN sublingual gland.

**sub·lin·gual tab·let** (sŭb-ling´gwăl tab´lĕt) Usually a small, flat form of medicine intended to be inserted beneath tongue, where the active ingredient is absorbed directly through oral mucosa; such a tablet (e.g., nitroglyerine) dissolves very promptly.

**sub·lin·gual vein** (sŭb-ling´gwăl vān) [TA] Vein that accompanies the sublingual artery in floor of mouth, lateral to hypoglossal nerve.

**sub·man·dib·u·lar** (sŭb´man-dib´yū-lăr) **1.** Beneath mandible or lower jaw. **2.** Denoting some ducts, fossae, ganglia, glands, lymph nodes, or a triangle of the neck, below the mandible. SYN inframandibular, submaxillary (2).

**sub·man·dib·u·lar car·un·cle** (sŭb´man-dib´yū-lăr kăr-ŭng´kĕl) Bilateral opening of submandibular duct into the oral cavity on a small papilla adjacent to the lingual frenum.

**sub·man·dib·u·lar duct** (sŭb´man-dib´yū-lăr dŭkt) [TA] Duct of submandibular salivary gland; opens at sublingual caruncle adjacent to inferior part of frenum of tongue. SYN ductus submandibularis, ductus submaxillaris, submaxillary duct.

**sub·man·dib·u·lar fos·sa** (sŭb´man-dib´yū-lăr fos´ă) [TA] Depression on medial surface of body of mandible inferior to mylohyoid line in which submandibular gland is lodged. SYN submaxillary fossa.

**sub·man·dib·u·lar gan·gli·on** (sŭb´man-dib´yū-lăr gang´glē-ŏn) [TA] Small parasympathetic ganglion suspended from lingual nerve. SYN submaxillary ganglion.

◾**sub·man·dib·u·lar gland** (sŭb´man-dib´yū-lăr gland) [TA] One of two salivary glands in the neck, located in space bounded by two bellies of digastric muscle and angle of mandible; discharges through submandibular duct; secretory units are predominantly serous, although a few mucous alveoli, some with serous demi-lunes, occur. See page 543. SYN maxillary gland, submaxillary gland.

**sub·man·dib·u·lar lymph nodes** (sŭb´man-dib´yū-lăr limf nōdz) [TA] Four or five lymph nodes that lie in relationship to mandible and submandibular gland.

**sub·man·dib·u·lar tri·an·gle** (sŭb´man-dib´yū-lăr trī´ang-gĕl) [TA] Area of neck bounded by mandible and two bellies of digastric muscle. SYN submaxillary triangle.

**sub·mar·gin·al** (sŭb-mahr´jin-ăl) In dentistry, area below margin of cavity preparation or restoration of tooth.

**sub·max·il·la** (sŭb´mak-sil´ă) SYN mandible.

**sub·max·il·lar·y** (sŭb-mak´si-lar-ē) **1.** SYN mandibular. **2.** SYN submandibular.

**sub·max·il·lar·y duct** (sŭb-mak´si-lar-ē dŭkt) SYN submandibular duct.

**sub·max·il·lar·y fos·sa** (sŭb-mak´si-lar-ē fos´ă) SYN submandibular fossa.

**sub·max·il·lar·y gan·gli·on** (sŭb-mak´si-lar-ē gang´glē-ŏn) SYN submandibular ganglion.

**sub·max·il·lar·y gland** (sŭb-mak´si-lar-ē gland) SYN submandibular gland.

**sub·max·il·lar·y tri·an·gle** (sŭb-mak´si-lar-ē trī´ang-gĕl) SYN submandibular triangle.

**sub·men·tal** (sŭb-men´tăl) **1.** Beneath the chin. **2.** Denoting artery, vein, or triangle of neck below the chin.

**sub·men·tal lymph nodes** (sŭb-men´tăl limf nōdz) [TA] The group of lymph nodes located beneath the chin. SEE ALSO lymph nodes.

**sub·merged** (sŭb-mĕrjd´) In dentistry, describing a field of operation covered by saliva.

**sub·mu·co·sa** (sŭb´myū-kō´să) [TA] Layer of tissue beneath mucous membrane; layer of

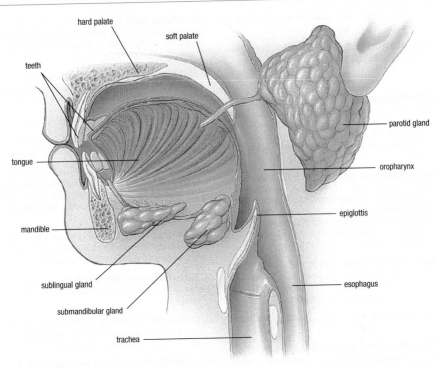

**oral cavity** (lateral view)

connective tissue beneath tunica mucosa. [TA lists submucosae of the following viscera: bronchi, esophagus, small and large intestines, pharynx, stomach, bladder.]

**sub·mu·co·sal im·plant** (sŭb-myū-kō′săl im′plant) Dental implant that rests beneath the mucosa.

**sub·mu·cous, sub·mu·co·sal** (sŭb-myū′kŭs, -myū-kō′săl) Beneath a mucous membrane.

**sub·mu·cous cleft** (sŭb-myū′kŭs kleft) SEE laryngotracheoesophageal cleft.

**sub·na·si·on** (sŭb-nā′zē-on) Point of angle between nasal septum and surface of upper lip.

**sub·nor·mal** (sŭb-nōr′măl) Below usual standard of some quality.

**sub·oc·clu·sal con·nec·tor** (sŭb′ŏ-klū′zăl kŏ-nek′tŏr) A nonrigid connector that fits gingiva to the occlusal plane.

**sub·oc·clu·sal sur·face** (sŭb′ŏ-klū′zăl sŭr′făs) Portion of occlusal tooth surface below level of occluding portion.

**sub·op·ti·mal** (sŭb-op′ti-măl) Below or less than the optimum.

**sub·per·i·os·te·al** (sŭb-per′ē-os′tē-ăl) Beneath the periosteum.

**sub·per·i·os·te·al ab·scess** (sŭb-per′ē-os′tē-ăl ab′ses) Lesion between periosteum and cortical plate of bone.

**sub·per·i·os·te·al im·plant** (sŭb-per′ē-os′tē-ăl im′plant) Artificial dental metal appliance made to conform to shape of a bone and placed on its surface beneath periosteum.

**sub·scrip·tion** (sŭb-skrip′shŭn) Part of prescription preceding signature, which has directions for compounding. [L. *subscriptio*, fr. *subscribo*, pp. *-scriptus*, to write under, subscribe]

**sub·sib·i·lant** (sŭb-sib′i-lănt) Denoting a rale with a quality of blowing or whistling.

**sub·spi·na·le** (sŭb′spī-nā′lē) In cephalometrics, most posterior midline point on premaxilla between anterior nasal spine and prosthion. SYN point A.

**sub·stance a·buse** (sŭb′stăns ă-byūs′) Maladaptive pattern of drug or alcohol use that may lead to social, occupational, psychological, or physical problems.

**sub·stance a·buse dis·or·ders** (sŭb′stăns ă-byūs′ dis-ōr′dĕrz) Mental disorders in which maladaptive behavioral and biologic changes are associated with regular use of alcohol, drugs, and related (usually chemical) substances that affect the central nervous system and result in failure to meet significant obliga-

**st**

tions in personal and social functioning and in physical and psychological problems.

**sub·stance de·pen·dence** (sŭb'stăns dĕ-pen'dĕns) Pattern of behavioral, physiologic, and cognitive symptoms that develop due to substance use or abuse.

**sub·stance P** (sŭb'stăns) Peptide neurotransmitter composed of eleven amino acyl residues (with the carboxyl group amidated), normally present in minute quantities in nervous system and intestines of humans and various animals.

**sub·stan·ti·a spon·gi·o·sa** (sŭb-stan' shē-ă spŭn-jē-ō'să) [TA] Bone in which the spicules or trabeculae form a three-dimensional latticework (cancellus), with the interstices filled with embryonal connective tissue or bone marrow. SYN cancellous bone, spongy bone (1), spongy substance, trabecular bone.

**sub·stan·tiv·i·ty** (sŭb'stăn-tiv'i-tē) Term comprising adherent qualities of a sunscreen and its ability to be retained after the skin is exposed to water and perspiration.

**sub·sti·tute** (sŭb'sti-tūt) Anything that takes the place of another.

**sub·sti·tu·ted phe·nol** (sŭb'sti-tū-tĕd fē' nol) Chemical disinfectant containing phenol with various chemical groups attached to the basic ring to enhance its disinfectant and detergent effects.

**sub·sti·tu·tion** (sŭb'sti-tū'shŭn) CHEMISTRY the replacement of an atom or group in a compound by another atom or group. [L. *substitutio*, to put in place of another]

**sub·strate** (sŭb'strāt) 1. Substance acted on and changed by an enzyme. 2. That on which an organism lives or grows (e.g., substrate on which microorganisms and cells grow in cell culture). [L. *sub-sterno*, pp. *-stratus*, to spread under]

**sub·struc·ture** (sŭb'strŭk-shŭr) A tissue or structure wholly or partly beneath the surface.

**sub·sur·face le·sion** (sŭb'sŭr'făs lē'zhŭn) Demineralized area below the surface of the enamel created by acid that has passed through micropores between enamel rods; subject to remineralization.

**sub·te·tan·ic** (sŭb'te-tan'ik) Denoting tonic muscular spasms or convulsions that are not entirely sustained but have brief remissions.

**sub·thresh·old stim·u·lus** (sŭb-thresh' ōld stim'yū-lŭs) Stimulus too weak to evoke a response.

**sub·vo·cal speech** (sŭb-vō'kăl spēch) Slight movements of muscles of speech related to thinking but producing no sound.

**suc·ce·da·ne·ous** (sŭk'sĕ-dā'nē-ŭs) 1. Relating to permanent or second teeth that replace deciduous or primary teeth. 2. Relating to a succedaneum. See this page.

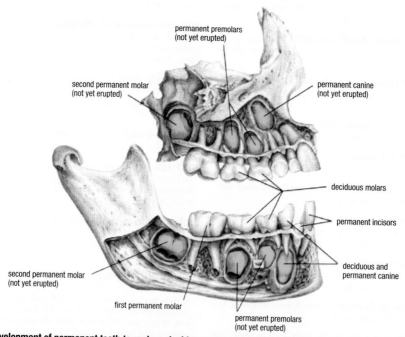

permanent premolars (not yet erupted)

second permanent molar (not yet erupted)

permanent canine (not yet erupted)

deciduous molars

permanent incisors

deciduous and permanent canine

second permanent molar (not yet erupted)

first permanent molar

permanent premolars (not yet erupted)

**development of permanent teeth to replace deciduous teeth in an 8-year-old child**

**suc·ce·da·ne·ous den·ti·tion** (sŭk´sĕ-dā´nē-ŭs den-tish´ŭn) SYN permanent tooth.

**suc·ce·da·ne·ous tooth** (sŭk´sĕ-dā´nē-ŭs tūth) SEE permanent dentition.

**suc·ce·da·ne·um** (sŭk´sĕ-dā´nē-ŭm) A substitute; a drug or any therapeutic agent that has the properties of and can be used in place of another.

**suc·ci·nyl·cho·line** (sŭk´si-nil-kō´lēn) A neuromuscular relaxant with short duration of action that characteristically first depolarizes the motor endplate (phase I block) but is often later associated with a curarelike, nondepolarizing neuromuscular block (phase II block).

**suc·ci·nyl·cho·line chlo·ride** (sŭk´si-nil-kō´lēn klōr´īd) Muscle relaxant used during dental surgery to reduce contractions.

**suc·cor·rhe·a** (sŭk´ōr-ē´ă) Abnormal increase in secretion of a digestive fluid. SYN succorrhoea. [L. *succus*, juice, + G. *rhoia*, a flow]

**succorrhoea** [Br.] SYN succorrhea.

**suc·cus·sion** (sŭ-kŭsh´ŭn) A diagnostic procedure involving shaking the body to elicit a splashing sound in a cavity containing both gas and fluid. [L. *sucussio*, fr. *suc-cutio* (*subc-*), pp. *-cussus*, to shake up, fr. *quatio*, to shake]

**su·cral·fate** (sū-kral´fāt) Sucrose octakis (hydrogen sulfate) aluminum complex; a polysaccharide with antipeptic activity, used to treat duodenal ulcers.

**su·crose** (sū´krōs) Common sweetener, used in pharmacy in manufacture of products such as syrup and confections.

**suc·tion** (sŭk´shŭn) The act or process of sucking. [L. *sugo*, pp. *suctus*, to suck]

**suc·tion plate** (sŭk´shŭn plāt) In dentistry, a plate held in place by atmospheric pressure.

**sud·den death** (sŭd´ĕn deth) Death occurring rapidly and generally unexpectedly.

**sud·den in·fant death syn·drome (SIDS)** (sŭd´ĕn in´fănt deth sin´drōm) Abrupt and inexplicable death of an apparently healthy infant; various theories have been advanced to explain such deaths (e.g., sleep-induced apnea, laryngospasm, overwhelming infectious disease), but none has been generally accepted or demonstrated at autopsy. SYN crib death.

**su·do·rif·ic** (sū´dŏr-if´ik) Causing sweat. [*sudor-* + L. *facio*, to make]

**su·fen·ta·nil cit·rate** (sū-fen´tă-nil sit´rāt) An injectable anesthetic and analgesic agent used in conjunction with general anesthesia.

**suf·fo·cate** (sŭf´ŏ-kāt) 1. To impede respiration; to asphyxiate. 2. To be unable to breathe.

**suf·fo·ca·tion** (sŭf´ŏ-kā´shŭn) The act or condition of suffocating or of asphyxiation.

**suf·fu·sion** (sŭ-fyū´zhŭn) 1. Pouring a fluid over the body. 2. Reddening of the surface.

**sug·ar** (shug´ăr) One of the sugars, e.g., confectioners' sugar. [G. *sakcharon;* L. *saccharum*]

**sug·gest·i·bil·i·ty** (sŭg-jes´ti-bil´i-tē) Responsiveness or susceptibility to a psychological process such as a hypnotic command whereby an idea is induced into a person without argument, command, or coercion.

**sug·ges·tion** (sŭg-jes´chŭn) Implanting an idea in mind of another by some word or act on one's part, subject's conduct or physical condition being influenced to some degree by implanted idea. [L. *sug-gero* (*subg-*), pp. *-gestus*, to bring under, supply]

**sug·ges·tive ther·a·peu·tics** (sŭg-jes´ tiv thār´ă-pyū´tiks) Treatment of disease or disorder by means of suggestion.

**su·i·cide** (sū´i-sīd) 1. The act of taking one's own life. 2. A person who commits such an act. [L. *sui*, self, + *caedo*, to kill]

**su·i·cide ges·ture** (sū´i-sīd jes´chŭr) Apparent attempt at suicide by someone wishing to attract attention, gain sympathy, or achieve some goal other than self-destruction.

**suit** (sūt) An outer garment designed for protection against specific environmental conditions.

**sul·bac·tam** (sŭl-bak´tam) A β-lactamase inhibitor with weak antibacterial action; when used with penicillins with little β-lactamase-inhibiting action, it greatly increases their effectiveness.

**sul·cu·lar brush·ing** (sŭl´kyū-lăr brŭsh´ ing) Method in which the end-rounded filament tips are activated at the gingival margin to remove dental biofilm from the gingival sulcus and tooth surface.

**sul·cus,** gen. and pl. **sul·ci** (sŭl´kŭs, -sī) 1. [TA] Groove or depression in oral cavity or on tooth surface. 2. [TA] One of the grooves or furrows on surface of brain, bounding several convolutions or gyri; a fissure. 3. [TA] Any long narrow groove, furrow, or slight depression. [L. a furrow or ditch]

**sul·fa** (sŭl´fă) Denoting the sulfa drugs or sulfonamides.

**sul·fa·di·a·zine** (sŭl´fă-dī´ă-zēn) Inhibitor of bacterial folic acid synthesis; highly effective against pneumococcal, staphylococcal, and streptococcal infections, against infections with *Escherichia coli* and *Klebsiella pneumoniae*.

**sul·fa·meth·ox·a·zole (SMX)** (sŭl´fă-methok´să-zōl) Sulfonamide related chemically to sulfisoxazole, with a similar antibacterial spec-

st

trum, but a slower rate of absorption from gastrointestinal tract and urinary excretion. Often used in combination with trimethoprim (i.e., SMX-TMP).

**sul·fa·sal·a·zine** (sŭl′fă-sal′ă-zēn) A sulfonamide (acid-azosulfa compound) with a marked affinity for connective tissues, especially for those rich in elastin, used in ulcerative colitis and rheumatoid arthritis.

**sul·fa·ti·do·sis** (sŭl′fă-ti-dō′sis) Disorder characterized by coarse facial features, ichthyosis, hepatosplenomegaly, and skeletal abnormalities.

**sul·fo·cy·a·nate** (sŭl′fō-sī′ă-nāt) SYN thiocyanate.

**sul·fon·a·mides** (sŭl-fon′ă-mīdz) Sulfa drugs, group of bacteriostatic drugs comprising sulfanilamide group (e.g., sulfanilamide, sulfapyridine).

**sul·fo·nyl·u·re·as** (sŭl′fō-nil-yūr′ē-ăz) Derivatives of isopropylthiodiazylsulfanilamide, chemically related to sulfonamides, which possess hypoglycemic action (e.g., acetohexamide, tolbutamide). SYN sulphonylureas.

**sul·fur (S)** (sŭl′fŭr) In oxide forms, added to water to make strong acids and used externally to treat skin diseases. SYN sulphur. [L. *sulfur*, brimstone, sulfur]

**sul·fur 35** (sŭl′fŭr) Radioactive sulfur isotope; used as a tracer in study of metabolism of cysteine. SYN sulphur 35.

**sulphate** [Br.] SYN sulfate.

**sulphonylureas** [Br.] SYN sulfonylureas.

**sulphur** [Br.] SYN sulfur.

**sulphur 35** [Br.] SYN sulfur 35.

**sum·ma·tion** (sŭ-mā′shŭn) Aggregation of several similar neural impulses or stimuli. [Mediev. L. *summatio*, fr. *summo*, pp. *-atus*, to sum up, fr. L. *summa*, sum]

**sum·ma·tion hy·per·path·i·a** (sŭ-mā′shŭn hī′pĕr-path′ē-ă) Exaggerated central pain response that occurs only when same area is stimulated simultaneously by two separate sensations or stimuli (i.e., light touch and pain).

**sum·mer asth·ma** (sŭm′ĕr az′mă) Asthma associated with hay fever or allergy to summer vegetation.

**sun·down·ing** (sŭn′down-ing) Exacerbation of delirium during evening or night with improvement or disappearance during the day; common in mid and later stages of dementing disorders, such as Alzheimer disease.

**su·per·a·cute** (sū′pĕr-ă-kyūt′) Denotes extreme severity of symptoms and rapid progress.

■ **su·per·e·rup·tion** (sū′pĕr-ē-rŭp′shŭn) Movement of a tooth beyond normal plane of occlusion due to loss of antagonist(s). See this page.

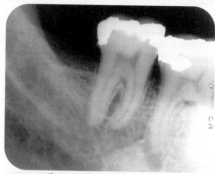

**supereruption:** mandibular second molar

**su·per·ex·ci·ta·tion** (sū′pĕr-ek′sī-tā′shŭn) **1.** The act of exciting or stimulating unduly. **2.** A condition of extreme excitement or stimulation.

**su·per·fi·cial** (sū′pĕr-fish′ăl) [TA] **1.** Situated nearer body surface in relation to specific reference point. **2.** Cursory; not thorough. [L. *superficialis*, fr. *superficies*, surface]

**su·per·fi·cial burn** (sū′pĕr-fish′ăl bŭrn) Epidermal burn causing erythema and edema without vesiculation. SYN first-degree burn.

**su·per·fi·cial re·flex** (sū′pĕr-fish′ăl rē′fleks) Reflex (e.g., the abdominal or cremasteric reflex, that is elicited by stimulation of skin).

**su·per·in·fec·tion** (sū′pĕr-in-fek′shŭn) A new infection in addition to one already present.

**su·per·i·or** (sŭ-pēr′ē-ŏr) [TA] **1.** Situated above or directed upward. **2.** HUMAN ANATOMY situated nearer the vertex of the head in relation to a specific reference point. SYN cranial (2). [L. comparative of *superus*, above]

**su·pe·ri·or al·ve·o·lar nerves** (sŭ-pēr′ē-ŏr al-vē′ŏ-lăr nĕrvz) [TA] Three branches of the maxillary nerve (or its continuation as the infraorbital nerve) that supply the mucosa of the maxillary sinuses, upper teeth, and gingiva.

**su·pe·ri·or as·pect** (sŭ-pēr′ē-ŏr as′pekt) Cranial surface viewed from above.

**su·pe·ri·or cer·e·bel·lar ar·te·ry syn·drome** (sŭ-pēr′ē-ŏr ser′ă-bel′ăr ahr′tĕr-ē sin′drōm) Disorder due to thrombosis of superior cerebellar artery that supplies spinothalamic tract and superior cerebellar peduncle; loss of pain and temperature senses on side of face and body opposite that of lesion.

**su·pe·ri·or den·tal arch** (sŭ-pēr′ē-ŏr den′tăl ahrch) SYN maxillary dental arcade.

**su·pe·ri·or den·tal branch·es (of su·pe·ri·or den·tal plex·us)** (sŭ-pēr′ē-ōr den′tăl branch′ĕz sŭ-pēr′ē-ŏr den′tăl pleks′ ŭs) [TA] Branches passing from superior dental plexus to roots of teeth of upper jaw.

**su·pe·ri·or den·tal (nerve) plex·us** (sŭ-pēr′ē-ŏr den′tăl nĕrv plek′ŭs) [TA] Formed by branches of the infraorbital nerve, gives off superior dental branches to upper and superior gingival branches to gums.

**su·pe·ri·or gin·gi·val branch·es (of su·pe·ri·or den·tal plex·us)** (sŭ-pēr′ē-ŏr jin′ji-văl branch′ĕz sŭ-pēr′ē-ŏr den′tăl pleks′ ŭs) [TA] Branches of superior dental plexus to gingiva of upper jaw.

**su·per·nu·mer·ar·y** (sū′pĕr-nū′mĕr-ar-ē) Exceeding normal number. SYN epactal. [L. *super-*, over + L. *numerus*, number]

🔲**su·per·nu·mer·ar·y root** (sū′pĕr-nū′mĕr-ar-ē rūt) Tooth root in excess of number usually present, taking into acount normal variability of a given tooth. See this page.

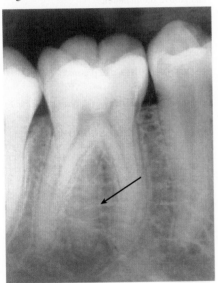

**supernumerary root:** first molar

**su·per·nu·mer·ar·y tooth** (sū′pĕr-nū′mĕr-ar-ē tūth) Any tooth in excess of 32; form may be normal or abnormal and may line inside or outside normal line of dental arch. SYN supplemental tooth.

**su·per·nu·tri·tion** (sū′pĕr-nū-trish′ŭn) Overeating leading to obesity.

**su·per·scrip·tion** (sū′pĕr-skrip′shŭn) Beginning of a prescription, consisting of injunction, *recipe*, take, usually denoted by sign ℞.

**su·per·struc·ture** (sū′pĕr-strŭk′shŭr) A structure above the surface.

**su·pine** (sū′pīn) 1. Denoting the body when

lying face upward. 2. Supination of the forearm or of the foot. [L. *supinus*]

**sup·ple·ment** (sŭp′lĕ-mĕnt) Agent or procedure added to complete, extend, or reinforce something. [L. *supplementum*, fr. *suppleo*, to fill, + *-mentum*, noun suffix]

**sup·ple·men·tal air** (sŭp′plĕ-men′tăl ār) SYN expiratory reserve volume.

**sup·ple·men·tal groove** (sŭp′plĕ-men′tăl grūv) Curvilinear depression on each side of a triangular ridge (crista triangularis).

**sup·ple·men·tal lobe** (sŭp′lĕ-men′tăl lōb) In dental anatomy, an extra lobe; one not included in typical tooth formation.

**sup·ple·men·tal ridge** (sŭp′lĕ-men′tăl rij) Ridge on tooth surface that is not normally present.

**sup·ple·men·tal tooth** (sŭp′lĕ-men′tăl tūth) SYN supernumerary tooth.

**sup·port** (sŭ-pōrt′) In dentistry, term used to denote resistance to vertical components of masticatory force. [L. *supporto*, to carry]

**sup·port beam** (sŭ-pōrt′ bēm) Descriptive term for the ring finger in the modified pen grasp, when it supports hands weight during instrumentation.

**sup·port·ing a·re·a** (sŭ-pōrt′ing ar′ē-ă) 1. Parts of maxillary and mandibular edentulous ridges considered best suited to carry forces of mastication when dentures are in function. 2. SYN denture foundation area.

**sup·port·ing cusp** (sŭ-pōr′ting kŭsp) Buccal cusp of lower posterior teeth and lingual cusp of upper posterior teeth.

**sup·por·tive per·i·o·don·tal treat·ment** (sŭ-pōr′tiv per′ē-ŏ-don′tăl trĕt′mĕnt) Extension of periodontal therapy that includes procedures performed at selected time intervals to review patients' general health history, reassess status of periodontal health, and provide preventive oral hygiene care. SYN periodontal maintenance, preventive maintenance.

**sup·pres·sion** (sŭ-presh′ŭn) 1. Deliberately excluding from conscious thought. 2. Arrest of the secretion of a fluid, such as urine or bile. Cf. retention (3). [L. *subprimo* (subp-), pp. *-pressus*, to press down]

**sup·pu·rate** (sŭp′yŭr-āt) To form pus. [L. *sup-puro* (subp-), pp. *-atus*, to form *pur*, pus]

**sup·pu·ra·tion** (sŭp′yŭr-ā′shŭn) The formation of pus. SYN pyesis, pyogenesis, pyopoiesis, pyosis. [L. *suppuratio*]

**sup·pu·ra·tive ar·thri·tis** (sŭp′yŭr-ă-tiv ahr-thrī′tis) Acute inflammation of synovial membranes, with purulent effusion into a joint, due to bacterial infection.

**st**

**sup·pu·ra·tive gin·gi·vi·tis** (sŭp′yŭr-ă-tiv jin′ji-vī′tis) Gingivitis in which a purulent exudate can be expressed from the gingival surface.

**sup·pu·ra·tive pe·ri·o·don·ti·tis** (sŭp′yŭr-ă-tiv per′ē-ō-don-tī′tis) Periodontitis accompanied by purulent exudate.

**sup·pu·ra·tive pneu·mo·ni·a** (sŭp′yŭr-ă-tiv nū-mō′nē-ă) Pneumonia associated with formation of pus and destruction of pulmonary tissue; abscess formation may occur.

❂ **supra-** Combining form meaning a position above the part indicated by the word to which it is joined; in this sense, the same as super-; opposite of infra-. [L. *supra*, on the upper side]

**su·pra·au·ric·u·lar** (sū′pră-aw-rik′yū-lăr) Above auricle or pinna of ear.

**su·pra·au·ric·u·lar point** (sū′pră-awr-ik′yū-lăr poynt) Craniometric point on posterior root of zygomatic process of temporal bone directly above auricular point.

**su·pra·bon·y pock·et** (sū′pră-bō′nē pok′ĕt) Periodontal opening extending apically by ending above adjacent alveolar bone crest.

**su·pra·buc·cal** (sū′pră-bŭk′ăl) Above the cheek.

**su·pra·bulge** (sū′pră-bŭlj) Tooth crown area that converges to tooth's occlusal surface.

**su·pra·cla·vic·u·lar lymph nodes** (sū′pră-klă-vik′yū-lăr limf nōdz) [TA] Deep cervical lymph nodes that are found along the length of the clavicle. SEE ALSO lymph node.

⬛ **su·pra·gin·gi·val cal·cu·lus** (sū′pră-jin′ji-văl kal′kyū-lŭs) Calcified plaques adherent to tooth surfaces coronal to the free gingival margin. See this page.

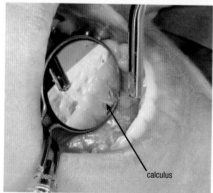

calculus

**detection of supragingival calculus deposits:** tooth surface should be visually examined while applying a continuous stream of air with a syringe

**su·pra·gin·gi·val in·stru·men·ta·tion** (sū′pră-jin′ji-văl in′strū-měn-tā′shŭn) Use of a dental instrument apical to (below) the gingival margin.

**su·pra·gin·gi·val ir·ri·ga·tion** (sū′pră-jin′ji-văl ir′i-gā′shŭn) Modality of therapy when point of delivery of irrigation is at, or coronal to, the free gingival margin.

**su·pra·gin·gi·val plaque** (sū′pră-jin′ji-văl plak) Plaque located on teeth below the gingival margin in the gingival crevice and periodontal pockets.

**su·pra·gin·gi·val scal·ing** (sū′pră-jin′ji-văl skāl′ing) Removal of hard and soft deposits above the gingival margin.

**su·pra·lim·i·nal** (sū′pră-lim′i-năl) More than just perceptible; above the threshhold for conscious awareness. [*supra-* + L. *limen*, threshold]

**su·pra·man·dib·u·lar** (sū′pră-man-dib′yū-lăr) Above the mandible.

**su·pra·mas·toid crest** (sū′pră-mas′toyd krest) [TA] The ridge that forms the posterior root of the zygomatic process of the temporal bone. SYN crista supramastoidea.

**su·pra·max·il·la** (sū′pră-mak-sil′ă) Obsolete term for maxilla.

**su·pra·max·il·lar·y** (sū′pră-mak′si-lar-ē) Above the maxilla.

**su·pra·max·i·mal stim·u·lus** (sū′pră-mak′si-mal stim′yu-lus) Stimulus with strength significantly above that required to activate all nerve or muscle fibers in contact with electrode; used when response of all fibers is desired.

**su·pra·men·ta·le** (sū′pră-men-tā′lē) In cephalometrics, most posterior midline point, above chin, on mandibula between infradentate and pogonion. SYN point B. [*supra-* + L. *mentum*, chin]

**su·pra·na·sal** (sū′pră-nā′zăl) Above the nose.

**su·pra·nu·cle·ar** (sū′pră-nū′klē-ăr) Above (i.e., cranial to) level of motor neurons of spinal or cranial nerves.

**su·pra·oc·clu·sion** (sū′pră-ŏ-klū′zhŭn) Occlusal relationship in which tooth extends beyond occlusal plane.

**su·pra·or·bi·tal nerve** (sū′pră-ōr′bit-ăl něrv) [TA] Branch of frontal nerve leaving orbit through supraorbital foramen or notch and dividing into branches distributed to forehead, scalp, upper eyelid, and frontal sinus.

**su·pra·or·bi·tal re·flex** (sū′pră-ōr′bi-tăl rē′fleks) Contraction of orbicularis oculi muscle induced by electrical or mechanical stimulation of supraorbital nerve.

**su·pra·per·i·os·te·al im·plant** (sū′prăper´ē-os´tē-al im´plant) Alloplastic graft inserted superficial to periosteum to change contour of an area.

**su·pra·re·nal gland** (sū´pră-rē´năl gland) [TA] A flattened, roughly triangular body positioned in relation to the superior end of each kidney but attached primarily to the diaphragmatic crura. SYN adrenal body, adrenal gland.

**su·pra·ten·to·ri·al** (sū´pră-ten-tōr´ē-ăl) Denoting cranial contents located above tentorium cerebelli; often used to describe functional symptoms.

**su·pra·troch·le·ar** (sū´pră-trok´lē-ăr) Above a trochlea, usually denoting a nerve.

**su·pra·troch·le·ar nerve** (sū´pră-trok´lē-ăr nĕrv) [TA] Branch of frontal nerve supplying medial part of upper eyelid, central part of skin of forehead, and nose root.

**su·pra·troch·le·ar veins** (sū´pră-trok´lē-ăr vānz) [TA] Veins that drain front part of scalp and unite with supraorbital vein to form the angular vein. SYN frontal veins (2).

**su·pra·ver·sion** (sū´pră-vĕr´zhŭn) In dentistry, position of a tooth when it is out of the line of occlusion in an occlusal direction; deep overbite. [supra- + L. verto, pp. versus, to turn]

**su·preme na·sal con·cha** (sŭ-prēm´ nā´zăl kong´kă) [TA] Small concha frequently present on posterosuperior part of lateral nasal wall; overlies supreme nasal meatus.

**sur·face** (sŭr´făs) [TA] Outer part of any solid or liquid at point of liquid-air interface. SYN face (3), facies (2). [F. fr. L. superficius]

**sur·face ep·i·the·li·um** (sŭr´făs ep´i-thē´lē-ŭm) 1. Layer of celomic epithelial cells covering gonadal ridges. 2. Mesothelial covering of definitive ovary.

**sur·face ther·mom·e·ter** (sŭr´făs thĕr-mom´ē-tĕr) Thermometer in the form of a disc or strip that indicates temperature of portion of skin to which it is applied.

**sur·fac·tant** (sŭr-fak´tănt) A surface-active agent, including substances commonly referred to as wetting agents, surface tension depressants, detergents, dispersing agents, and emulsifiers.

**sur·geon** (sŭr´jŏn) A physician who treats disease, injury, and deformity by operation or manipulation. [G. cheirougos; L. chirurgus]

**sur·ger·y** (sŭr´jĕr-ē) 1. Branch of medicine concerned with treatment of disease, injury, and deformity by physical operation or manipulation. 2. Performance or procedures of an operation. [L. chirurgia; G. cheir, hand, + ergon, work]

**sur·gi·cal an·es·the·si·a** (sŭr´ji-kăl an´es-thē´zē-ă) 1. Anesthesia administered to permit performance of an operative procedure. 2. Loss of sensation with muscle relaxation adequate for an operative procedure.

**sur·gi·cal ap·pli·ance** (sŭr´ji-kăl ă-plī´ăns) Metal or plastic appliance frequently constructed before or during an operation and used to immobilize or support tissue during postoperative period.

**sur·gi·cal cil·i·at·ed cyst** (sŭr´ji-kăl sil´ē-ā-tĕd sist) Lesion that arises from maxillary sinus epithelium implanted along a line of surgical entry.

**sur·gi·cal e·rup·tion** (sŭr´ji-kăl ē-rŭp´shŭn) Uncovering an unerupted tooth to permit its further eruption by surgically removing overlying soft tissue, bone, and sometimes teeth.

**sur·gi·cal li·ga·tion** (sŭr´ji-kăl lī-gā´shŭn) In dentistry, surgical exposure of an unerupted tooth so that a metal ligature can be placed around its cervix and fastened to an orthodontic appliance to facilitate eruption.

**sur·gi·cal or·tho·don·tics** (sŭr´ji-kăl ōr´thŏ-don´tiks) Correction of occlusal abnormalities by surgical repositioning of segments of mandible or maxillae containing one or more teeth or bodily repositioning of entire jaws to improve function and esthetics.

**sur·gi·cal path·ol·o·gy** (sŭr´ji-kăl pă-thol´ŏ-jē) Anatomic pathology concerned with examination of tissues removed from living patients to diagnose disease.

**sur·gi·cal pros·the·sis** (sŭr´ji-kăl pros-thē´sis) An appliance prepared as an aid or as a part of a surgical proceeding.

**sur·gi·cal scrub** (sŭr´ji-kăl skrŭb) Systematic handwashing of fingernails, hands, and forearms before undertaking a surgical procedure.

**sur·gi·cal silk** (sŭr´ji-kăl silk) Thread prepared in various sizes and used as suture material. SYN silk suture.

**sur·gi·cal splint** (sŭr´ji-kăl splint) General term for device used to maintain tissues in a new position following surgery.

**sur·gi·cal tem·plate** (sŭr´ji-kăl tem´plāt) 1. Thin, transparent, resin base shaped to duplicate form of impression surface of an immediate denture, used to guide surgical shaping of alveolar process to fit an immediate denture. 2. Guide for duplicating size and shape for an autogenic (free) gingival graft. 3. Guide to facilitate surgical placement of dental implants. 4. Guide in orthognathic surgery to establish occlusion.

**sur·ro·gate** (sŭr´ŏ-găt) Person who functions in another's life as a substitute for some third person. [L. surrogo, to put in another's place]

**sur·veil·lance** (sŭr-vā´lăns) 1. Collection, collation, analysis, and dissemination of data.

st

**2.** Ongoing scrutiny, generally using methods distinguished by practicability and rapidity, rather than complete accuracy. [Fr. *surveiller,* to watch over, fr. L. *super-* + *vigilo,* to watch]

**sur·vey** (sŭr′vā) **1.** A comprehensive examination or group of examinations to screen for one or more findings. **2.** An investigation in which information is systematically collected but in which the experimental method is not used. **3.** A series of questions administered to a sample of individuals in a population. See this page. [O.Fr. *surveeir,* fr. Mediev.L. *supervideo,* fr. *super,* over, + *video,* to see]

dissolved drugs dispersed in liquid vehicles for oral or parenteral use. [L. *suspensio,* fr. *suspendo,* pp. *-pensus,* to hang up, suspend]

**sus·tained ac·tion tab·let, sus·tained re·lease tab·let** (sŭ-stānd′ ak′shŭn tab′lĕt, rĕ-lēs′) Drug product that provides required dosage initially and then maintains it.

**sus·te·nance** (sŭs′tĕ-năns) Essential food or nutrients required to support or maintain life.

**Sut·ton dis·ease** (sŭt′ŏn di-zēz′) SYN periadenitis mucosa necrotica recurrens. [R. L. Sutton, Jr.]

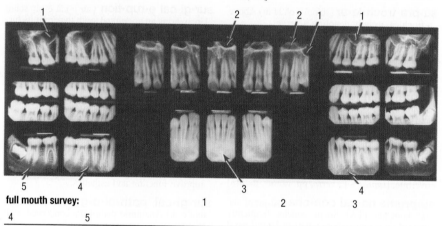

**full mouth survey:**

**sur·vey·ing** (sŭr-vā′ing) In dentistry, procedure of locating and delineating contour and position of abutment teeth and associated structures before designing a removable partial denture.

**sur·vey line** (sŭr′vā līn) **1.** Line scribed on an abutment tooth of a dental cast by means of a dental surveyor indicating height of tooth contour according to a specific path of insertion. **2.** Line that serves as a guide in proper location of various parts of a clasp assembly for a removable partial denture. SYN clasp guideline.

**sur·vey·or** (sŭr-vā′ŏr) In dentistry, instrument used in procedure of surveying.

**sur·viv·al time** (sŭr-vī′văl tīm) Period elapsing between completion or institution of any procedure and death.

**sus·cep·ti·ble** (sŭ-sep′ti-bĕl) Potential of a person to develop adverse effects from an external agent or influence.

**sus·pen·sion** (sŭs-pen′shŭn) **1.** Temporary interruption of any function. **2.** A hanging from a support, as used to treat spinal curvatures. **3.** Fixation of an organ to other tissue for support. **4.** Dispersion through a liquid of a solid in finely divided particles of a size large enough to be detected by purely optic means. **5.** Class of pharmacopoeial preparations of finely divided, un-

**su·ture** (sū′chŭr) [TA] **1.** Fibrous joint in which two bones formed in membrane are united by a fibrous membrane continuous with periosteum. **2.** To unite two surfaces by sewing. SYN stitch (3). **3.** The material (e.g., silk thread, wire, synthetic material) with which two surfaces are kept in apposition. See page 551. [L. *sutura,* a seam]

**su·ture ap·po·si·tion** (sū′chŭr ap′ŏ-zi′shŭn) Suture that holds margins of an incision tightly closed. SYN apposition suture.

**Sv** Abbreviation for sievert.

**swage** (swāj) **1.** To fuse suture thread to suture needles. **2.** To shape metal by hammering or adapting it onto a die. [Old F. *souage*]

**swal·low** (swahl′ō) To pass anything through fauces, pharynx, and esophagus into the stomach; to perform deglutition. [A.S. *swelgan*]

**swal·low·ing re·flex** (swahl′ō-ing rē′fleks) Act of swallowing (second stage) induced by stimulation of palate, fauces, or posterior pharyngeal wall. SYN pharyngeal reflex (1).

**swal·low·ing thresh·old** (swahl′ō-ing thresh′ōld) **1.** Moment that act of swallowing begins after mastication of food. **2.** Critical moment of reflex action initiated by minimum stimulation, before act of deglutition.

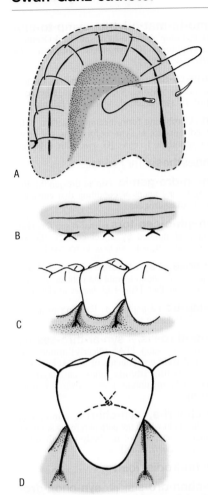

**types of sutures:** (A) blanket stitch; (B) interrupted, individual sutures; (C) interdental individual sutures; (D) sling or suspension suture tied on the lingual (*dotted line*)

**Swan-Ganz cath·e·ter** (swahn ganz kath′ ĕ-tĕr) A thin (5 Fr), flexible, flow-directed venous catheter using a balloon to carry it through the heart to a pulmonary artery. SYN pulmonary artery catheter.

**sweat** (swet) SYN perspiration (3). [ *A.S. swāt*]

**swell·ing** (swel′ing) Loosely used to describe the gross anatomic result of the inflammatory process.

**Swift dis·ease** (swift di-zēz′) SYN acrodynia (2).

**Syd·ney crease** (sid′nē krēs) Variation of the proximal transverse palmar flexion crease that reaches the ulnar side of the palm.

**sym·bal·lo·phone** (sim-bahl′ŏ-fōn) A steth-

oscope with two chest pieces. [G. *symballō*, to throw together, + *phōnē*, sound]

**sym·bi·on, sym·bi·ont** (sim′bē-on, -ont) Organism associated with another in symbiosis. [G. *symbion*, neut. of *symbiōs*, living together]

**sym·bi·o·sis** (sim′bē-ō′sis) **1.** Biologic association of two or more species. **2.** Mutual cooperation or interdependence of two people.

**sym·bi·ot·ic** (sim′bē-ot′ik) Relating to symbiosis.

**sym·bol** (sim′bŏl) **1.** A conventional sign serving as an abbreviation. **2.** In chemistry, abbreviation of name of an element, radical, or compound. [G. *symbolon*, a mark or sign, fr. *symballō*, to throw together]

**sym·me·try** (sim′ĕ-trē) Correspondence in form of parts distributed around center or axis, at extremities, or on opposite sides of any body.

♻ **sympath-** The sympathetic part of the autonomic nervous system.

**sym·pa·thec·to·my, sym·pa·the·tec·to·my, sym·pa·thi·cec·to·my** (sim′pă-thek′tŏ-mē, -thĕ-tek′tŏ-mē, -path′i-sek′tŏ-mē) Excision of segment of sympathetic nerve or one or more sympathetic ganglia.

**sym·pa·thet·ic** (sim′pă-thet′ik) **1.** Denoting the sympathetic part of the autonomic nervous system. **2.** Relating to or exhibiting sympathy. [G. *sympathētikos*, fr. *sympatheō*, to feel with, sympathize, fr. *syn*, with, + *pathos*, suffering]

**sym·pa·thet·ic block·ade** (sim′pă-thet′ ik blok-ād′) Interruption of transmission in sympathetic ganglia or conduction of impulses in preganglionic or postganglionic sympathetic nerve fibers.

**sym·pa·thet·ic hy·per·to·ni·a** (sim′pă-thet′ik hī′pĕr-tō′nē-ă) Overfunction of sympathetic nervous system.

**sym·pa·thet·ic ner·vous sys·tem** (sim′ pă-thet′ik nĕr′vŭs sis′tĕm) **1.** In earlier usage, the entire autonomic nervous system. **2.** The branch of the autonomic nervous system that supplies motor control to glands, smooth muscle, and cardiac tissue, specifically in response to perceived threat, danger, or to stress.

**sym·pa·thet·ic sa·li·va** (sim′pă-thet′ik să-lī′vă) Submaxillary saliva obtained by stimulation of sympathetic fibers innervating gland.

**sym·pa·tho·lyt·ic** (sim′pă-thō-lit′ik) Denoting antagonism to or inhibition of adrenergic nerve activity. [*sympatho-* + G. *lysis*, a loosening]

**sym·pa·tho·mi·met·ic** (sim′pă-thō-mi-met′ ik) Denoting mimicking of action of sympathetic system. [*sympatho-* + G. *mimikos*, imitating]

st

**sym·pa·tho·mi·met·ic a·mine** (sim'pă-thō-mi-met'ik ă-mēn') Agent that evokes responses similar to those produced by adrenergic nerve activity. SYN adrenergic amine, adrenomimetic amine.

**sym·pa·thy** (sim'pă-thē) *Do not confuse this word with empathy.* Mutual relation, physiologic or pathologic, between two organs, systems, or parts of body.

**sym·phal·an·gism, sym·pha·lan·gy** (sim-fal'ăn-jizm, -jē) **1.** SYN syndactyly. **2.** Ankylosis of the finger or toe joints. [*sym-* + *phalanx*]

**sym·phy·sis**, pl. **sym·phy·ses** (sim'fi-sis, -sēz) **1.** Form of cartilaginous joint in which union between two bones is effected with fibrocartilage. **2.** Union, meeting point, or commissure of any two structures. See this page. [G. a growing together]

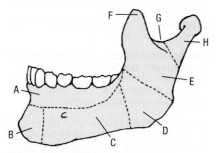

regions of the mandible: (A) alveolar process; (B) symphysis; (C) body; (D) angle; (E) ramus; (F) coronoid process; (G) mandibular notch; (H) condylar process

**symp·tom** (simp'tŏm) Any morbid departure from normal in structure or function experienced by patient and indicative of disease. [G. *symptōma*]

**symp·to·mat·ic** (simp'tŏ-mat'ik) Indicative; relating to or constituting aggregate of disease symptoms.

**symp·to·mat·ic head·ache** (simp'tŏ-mat'ik hed'āk) Headache secondary to another organic condition.

**symp·to·mat·ic pru·ri·tus** (simp'tŏ-mat'ik prūr-ī'tŭs) Itching occurring as a symptom of a systemic disease.

**symp·to·mat·ic treat·ment** (simp'tŏ-mat'ik trēt'mĕnt) Therapy aimed at relieving symptoms without necessarily affecting basic underlying cause(s) of the symptoms.

**symp·tom·a·tol·o·gy** (simp'tŏ-mă-tol'ŏ-jē) Science of disease symptoms, production, and indications. [G. *symptōma*, symptom + G. *logos*, study]

**symp·to·mat·o·lyt·ic, symp·to·mo·lyt·ic** (simp'tŏ-mat'ŏ-lit'ik, -mŏ-lit'ik) Removing symptoms. [G. *symptōma*, symptom + G. *lytikos*, dissolving]

**symp·to·sis** (simp-tō'sis) Localized or general bodily wasting. [G. a falling together, collapse, fr. *syn*, together, + *ptōsis*, a falling]

☆ **syn-** Combining form meaning together, with, joined; appears as sym- before b, p, ph, or m; corresponds to L. con-. [G. *syn*, with, together]

**synaesthesia** [Br.] SYN synesthesia.

**syn·an·dro·gen·ic** (sin'an-drō-jen'ik) Relating to any agent or condition that enhances effects of androgens.

**sy·naph·o·cep·tors** (si-naf'ō-sep'tŏrz) Receptors stimulated by direct contact. [G. *synaphe*, contact, + L. *recipio*, to receive]

**syn·apse**, pl. **syn·aps·es** (sin'aps, -ĕz) Functional membrane-to-membrane contact of nerve cell with another. [*syn-* + G. *hapto*, to clasp]

**sy·nap·tic** (si-nap'tik) **1.** Relating to a synapse. **2.** Relating to synapsis.

**syn·ar·thro·sis**, pl. **syn·ar·thro·ses** (sin'ahr-thrō'sis, -sēz) [TA] (Nearly) immovable union of rigid components of the skeletal system, including fibrous joints, cartilaginous joints, and bony unions. [*syn-* + *arthrōsis*, articulation]

**syn·chei·ri·a, syn·chi·ri·a** (sin-kī'rē-ă) Dyscheiria in which the patient refers a stimulus applied to one side of the body to both sides. [*syn-* + G. *cheir*, hand]

**synchodrodial joint** SYN sychondrosis.

**syn·chon·dro·sis**, pl. **syn·chon·dro·ses** (sin'kon-drō'sis, -sēz) [TA] A union between two bones formed either by hyaline cartilage or fibrocartilage. SYN synchondrodial joint. [*syn-* + *chondros*, cartilage, + *-osis*, condition]

**syn·chro·nism** (sing'krŏ-nizm) Occurrence of two or more events at same time; condition of being simultaneous. [*syn-* + G. *chronos*, time]

**syn·chro·nous** (sing'krŏ-nŭs) Occurring simultaneously. [G. *synchronos*]

**syn·co·pe** (sing'kŏ-pē) Loss of consciousness and postural tone due to diminished cerebral blood flow. [G. *synkopē*, cutting short]

**syn·dac·tyl·i·a, syn·dac·ty·lism** (sin'dak-til'ē-ă, sin-dak'ti-lizm) SYN syndactyly.

**syn·dac·ty·ly** (sin-dak'ti-lē) Any degree of webbing or fusion of fingers or toes. SYN symphalangism (1), syndactylia. [*syn-* + G. *daktylos*, finger or toe]

**syn·drome** (sin'drōm) Aggregate of symptoms and signs associated with any morbid process.

**syn·drome of in·ap·pro·pri·ate se·cre·tion of an·ti·di·u·ret·ic hor·mone (SIADH)** (sin'drōm in'ă-prō'prē-ăt sĕ-krē'shŭn an'tē-dī-yŭr-et'ik hōr'mŏn) Continued secretion of antidiuretic hormone despite low serum osmolality and expanded extracellular volume.

**syn·drom·ic** (sin-drō'mik) Relating to a syndrome.

**sy·ner·e·sis** (si-ner'ĕ-sis) The contraction of a gel, e.g., a blood clot, by which part of the dispersion medium is squeezed out. [G. *synairesis*, a taking or drawing together]

**syn·er·gism** (sin'ĕr-jizm) Coordinated or correlated action of two or more structures, agents, or physiologic processes so that combined action is greater than sum of each acting separately. SYN synergy. [G. *synergia*, fr. *syn*, together, + *ergon*, work]

**syn·er·gist** (sin'ĕr-jist) A structure, agent, or physiologic process that aids action of another.

**syn·er·gy** (sin'ĕr-jē) SYN synergism.

**syn·es·the·si·a** (sin'es-thē'zē-ă) A condition in which a stimulus, in addition to exciting usual and normally located sensation, gives rise to a subjective sensation of different character. SYN synaesthesia. [*syn-* + G. *aisthēsis*, sensation]

**syn·ge·ne·ic draft** (sin'jĕ-nē'ik draft) SYN syngraft.

**syn·gnath·i·a** (sin-gnath'ē-ă) Congenital adhesion of maxilla and mandible by fibrous bands. [*syn-* + G. *gnathos*, jaw]

**syn·graft** (sin'graft) A tissue or organ transplanted from one member of a species to another genetically identical member. SYN isograft, isogenic graft, isologous graft, isoplastic graft, syngeneic graft.

**syn·i·dro·sis** (sin'i-drō'sis) Condition in which excessive perspiration is part of clinical manifestation. [*syn-* + G. *hidrosis*, sweating]

**syn·os·to·sis, syn·os·te·o·sis** (sin-os'tō'sis, -tē-ō'sis) [TA] Osseous union between bones forming a joint. SYN bony ankylosis, true ankylosis.

**sy·no·vi·a** (si-nō'vē-ă) [TA] SYN synovial fluid. [*syn-* + *ōon* (L. *ovum*), egg]

**syn·o·vi·al flu·id** (si-nō'vē-ăl flū'id) [TA] A clear thixotropic fluid, the main function of which is to serve as a lubricant in a joint, tendon sheath, or bursa. SYN synovia [TA].

**syn·o·vi·al joint** (si-nō'vē-ăl joynt) [TA] A joint in which (1) the opposing bony surfaces are covered with a layer of hyaline cartilage or fibrocartilage, (2) there is a joint cavity containing synovial fluid, lined with synovial membrane and reinforced by a fibrous capsule and ligaments, and (3) there is some degree of free movement possible. SYN articulatio [TA], diarthrodial joint, diarthrosis, movable joint.

**syn·o·vi·tis** (sin'ŏ-vī'tis) Inflammation of a synovial membrane. [*synovia* + G. *-itis*, inflammation]

**syn·the·sis, pl. syn·the·ses** (sin'thĕ-sis, -sēz) 1. A composition. 2. In chemistry, formation of compounds by union of simpler compounds or elements. [*syn-* + *thesis*, a placing, arranging]

**syn·thet·ic** (sin-thet'ik) Relating to or made by synthesis.

**syn·tro·py** (sin'trŏ-pē) 1. Tendency sometimes seen in two diseases to coalesce. 2. In anatomy, number of similar structures inclined in one general direction. [*syn-* + G. *tropē*, a turning]

**syph·i·lid** (sif'i-lid) Any of the several kinds of cutaneous and mucous membrane lesions of secondary and tertiary syphilis. [*syphilis* + *-id*]

**syph·i·lis** (sif'i-lis) An acute and chronic infectious disease caused by the bacterium *Treponema pallidum* and transmitted by direct contact, usually sexual.

**syph·i·lit·ic** (sif'i-lit'ik) Relating to, caused by, or suffering from syphilis. SYN luetic.

**syph·i·lit·ic a·or·ti·tis** (sif'i-lit'ik ā'ōr-tī'tis) Common manifestation of tertiary syphilis, involving thoracic aorta, where destruction of elastic tissue in media results in dilation and aneurysm formation.

**syph·i·lit·ic teeth** (sif'i-lit'ik tēth) SYN Hutchinson teeth.

**sy·ringe** (sir-inj') An instrument used to inject or withdraw fluids, consisting of a barrel and plunger. [G. *syrinx*, pipe or tube]

**sy·rin·go·cys·to·ma** (si-ring'gō-sis-tō'mă) SYN hidrocystoma. [*syringo-* + *cystoma*]

**sy·rin·goid** (sĭ-ring'goyd) Resembling a tube or fistula. [*syringo-* + G. *eidos*, resemblance]

**sy·rin·go·my·el·ic dis·so·ci·a·tion** (si-ring'gō-mī-el'ik di-sō'sē-ā'shŭn) Loss of pain and temperature sensation with relative retention of tactile sensation, related to a cavity in central portion of cord interrupting decussation of nerve fibers.

**syr·up** (sir'ŭp) 1. Refined molasses. 2. Any sweet fluid; a solution of sugar in water in any proportion. 3. A liquid preparation of medicinal or flavoring substances in a concentrated aqueous solution of a sugar, usually sucrose; other polyols, such as glycerin or sorbitol, may be present to retard crystallization of sucrose or to increase the solubility of added ingredients.

**sys·tem** (sis'tĕm) 1. [TA] Consistent and complex whole made up of correlated and semiindependent parts or functionally related anatomic structures. 2. Entire organism seen as a complex organization of parts. 3. Any complex of struc-

st

tures anatomically or functionally related. **4.** Group of people, agencies, institutions, and activities or protocols that together deliver parts of overall health maintenance or intervention to mitigate injury or disease in the general public (i.e., systems of health care delivery). [G. *systēma*, an organized whole]

**sys·te·mat·ic de·sen·si·ti·za·tion** (sis´tĕ-mat´ik dē-sen´si-tī-zā´shŭn) Behavior therapy for eliminating phobias or anxieties.

**sys·te·mat·ic name** (sis´tĕ-mat´ik nām) As applied to chemical substances, composed of specially coined or selected words or syllables, each of which has a precisely defined chemical structural meaning, so that structure may be derived from the name. Water (trivial name) is hydrogen oxide (systematic).

**sys·tem·a·ti·za·tion** (sis´tĕ-mă-tī-zā´shŭn) Arrangement of ideas into orderly sequence.

**sys·tem·ic au·to·im·mune dis·eas·es** (sis-tem´ik aw´tō-i-myūn´ di-zēz´ĕz) Connective tissue diseases characterized by presence of autoantibodies responsible for immunopathologically mediated tissue lesions; systemic lupus erythematosus is the prototype.

**sys·tem·ic cir·cu·la·tion** (sis-tem´ik sĭr´kyū-lā´shŭn) Circulation of blood through arteries, capillaries, and veins of the general system, from left ventricle to right atrium.

**sys·tem·ic dis·ease** (sis-tem´ik di-zēz´) Conditionor disorder that affects the whole body or involves many organs (i.e. diabetes mellitus, systemic lupus erythematosus).

**sys·tem·ic lu·pus er·y·the·ma·to·sus (SLE)** (sis-tem´ik lū´pŭs ĕr-ith´ĕ-mă-tō´sŭs) Inflammatory connective tissue disease with variable features, frequently including fever, weakness and fatigability, joint pains or arthritis resembling rheumatoid arthritis, and diffuse erythematous skin lesions on the face, neck, or upper limbs.

**sys·to·le** (sis´tŏ-lē) Contraction of heart, especially of ventricles, by which blood is driven through aorta and pulmonary artery to traverse systemic and pulmonary circulations, respectively.

**sys·tol·ic pres·sure** (sis-tol´ik presh´ŭr) Intracardiac pressure during or resulting from systolic contraction of a cardiac chamber; highest arterial blood pressure reached during any given ventricular cycle. Also called systolic blood pressure.

# T

**T** Abbreviation for threonine.

**TA** Abbreviation for *Terminologia Anatomica*.

**Ta** Abbreviation for tantalum.

**tab** Abbreviation for tablet.

**ta·bes** (tā′bēz) Progressive wasting or emaciation. [L. a wasting away]

**ta·bes dor·sa·lis** (tā′bēz dōr-sā′lis) SYN tabetic neurosyphilis.

**ta·bet·ic ar·throp·a·thy** (tă-bet′ik ahr-throp′ă-thē) Neuropathic arthropathy that occurs with tabes dorsalis (tabetic neurosyphilis).

**ta·bet·ic neu·ro·syph·i·lis** (tă-bet′ik nūr′ō-sif′i-lis) Type of late tertiary syphilis, seen predominantly in men; its major clinical manifestations are ataxia, urinary incontinence, and brief lancinating pains ("lightning pains"), which can affect any portion of the body, but particularly the legs. SYN tabes dorsalis.

**ta·ble** (tā′běl) **1.** One of the two plates or laminae, separated by the diploë, into which the cranial bones are divided. **2.** A platform on which items (e.g., dental tools) can be placed. [L. *tabula*]

**ta·ble clin·ic** (tā′běl klin′ik) Educational display or demonstration on topic presented to small number of observers at one time.

**ta·ble·spoon** (tā′běl-spūn) A large spoon, used as a measure of the dose of a medicine, equivalent to about 4 fluidrams or 1/2 fluidounce or 15 mL.

**tab·let (tab)** (tab′lĕt) Solid dosage form containing medicinal substances with or without suitable diluents; may vary in shape, size, and weight. [Fr. *tablette*, L. *tabula*]

♻**tachy-** Combining form meaning rapid. [G. *tachys*, quick]

**tach·y·car·di·a** (tak′i-kahr′dē-ă) Rapid beating of heart, conventionally applied to rates over 90 beats per minute. [*tachy-* + G. *kardia*, heart]

**tach·y·gas·tri·a** (tak′i-gas′trē-ă) Increased rate of electrical pacemaker activity in stomach, defined as more than 4 cycles/minute for at least 1 minute. May be associated with nausea, gastroparesis, irritable bowel syndrome, and functional dyspepsia.

**tach·y·phy·lax·is** (tak′i-fī-lak′sis) Rapid appearance of progressive decrease in response to a given dose after repetitive administration of a pharmacologically or physiologically active substance. [*tachy-* + G. *phylaxis*, protection]

**tach·y·pne·a** (tak′ip-nē′ă) Rapid breathing. [*tachy-* + G. *pnoē* (*pnoiē*), breathing]

**tachypnoea** [Br.] SYN tachypnea.

**tac·rine** (tak′rēn) An anticholinesterase agent with nonspecific central nervous system stimulatory effects; used in early stages of Alzheimer disease.

**tac·tile** (tak′til) Relating to touch or sense of touch. [L. *tactilis*, fr. *tango*, pp. *tactus*, to touch]

**tac·tile cor·pus·cle** (tak′til kōr′pŭs-ĕl) One of numerous oval bodies found in the papillae of the skin, especially those of the fingers and toes. SYN Meissner corpuscle.

**tac·tile dis·crim·i·na·tion** (tak′til dis-krim′i-nā′shŭn) Clinicians' ability to distinguish relative degrees of roughness and smoothness, for example, on a tooth surface, using an instrument such as an explorer or a periodontal probe.

**tac·tile e·val·u·a·tion** (tak′til ĕ-val′yū-ā′shŭn) Method of assessing cutting edge sharpness by testing it against a plastic or acrylic rod called a sharpening test stick. A dull cutting edge will slide over the surface of the stick. A sharp cutting edge will scratch the surface of the test stick.

**tac·tile me·nis·cus** (tak′til mĕ-nis′kŭs) A specialized tactile sensory nerve ending in the epidermis. SYN Merkel corpuscle, Merkel tactile cell, Merkel tactile disc.

**tac·tile sen·si·tiv·i·ty** (tak′til sen′si-tiv′i-tē) Clinical ability to feel vibrations transmitted from instrument's working-end with his or her fingers as they rest on the shank and handle.

**tag** (tag) **1.** SEE tracer. **2.** Small outgrowth or polyp.

**tail** (tāl) [TA] Any taillike structure or tapering or elongated extremity. SYN cauda [TA]. [A.S. *taegl*]

**talc** (talk) Native hydrous magnesium silicate used in pharmacy as a filter aid, as a dusting powder, and in cosmetic preparations. Also called talcum. [Ar. *talq*]

**tal·on cusp** (tal′ŏn kŭsp) Anomalous cusp that projects lingually from cingulum of permanent incisors. See this page. [Eng. claw, heel, fr. O.Fr., fr. L. *talus*, ankle]

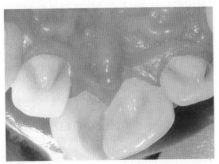

**talon cusps**

st

**tal·o·nid** (tal′ŏ-nid) Distal portion of human molar crown, consisting of hypoconid, hypoconulid, and entoconid.

**tam·pon** (tam′pon) A cylinder or ball of cotton-wool, gauze, or other loose substance; used as a plug or pack in a canal or cavity to restrain hemorrhage, absorb secretions, or maintain a displaced organ in position.

**tam·pon·ade, tam·pon·age** (tam′pŏ-nād′, -nazh′) **1.** Pathologic compression of an organ. **2.** Act of inserting a tampon.

**Tan·ner growth chart** (tan′ĕr grōth chahrt) Series of diagrams showing distribution of parameters of physical development, such as stature, growth curves, and skinfold thickness, for children by sex, age, and stages of puberty.

**tan·nin** (tan′in) Complex nonuniform plant constituent used in tanning, dyeing, photography, and as clarifying agents for beer and wine. Sometimes used synonymously with tannic acid.

**tan·ta·lum (Ta)** (tan′tă-lŭm) A heavy metal used in surgical prostheses because of its noncorrosive properties. [G. mythical king of Lydia, *Tantalus*]

**tan·trum** (tan′trŭm) A fit of bad temper, especially in children.

**tap** (tap) **1.** To withdraw fluid from a cavity by means of a hollow needle or catheter. **2.** To strike lightly with the finger in percussion or to elicit a reflex. [M.E. *tappe*, fr. A.S. *taeppa*]

**tape** (tāp) A thin, flat strip of fascia or tendon, or of synthetic material, used as a tie or suture. [A.S. *taeppe*]

**Ta·pi·a syn·drome** (tah′pē-ah sin′drōm) Unilateral paralysis of larynx, velum palati, and tongue, with atrophy of the last.

**ta·pir mouth** (tā′pĕr mowth) Protrusion of lips due to weakness of the orbicularis oris muscles; seen with some dystrophies. SYN bouche de tapir.

**tar·dive dys·ki·ne·si·a** (tahr′div dis′ki-nē′zē-ă) Involuntary movements of facial muscles and tongue, often persistent, which develop as a late complication of some neuroleptic therapy.

**tar·get** (tahr′gĕt) **1.** An object fixed as goal or point of examination. **2.** Anode of an x-ray tube. [It. *targhetta*, a small shield]

**tar·get cell** (tahr′gĕt sel) An erythrocyte in target cell anemia, with a dark center surrounded by a light band that again is encircled by a darker ring, thus resembling a target used in practice with firearms or archery; such cells also appear after splenectomy. SYN leptocyte, Mexican hat cell.

**tar·get-film dis·tance (TFD)** (tahr′gĕt-film′ dis′tăns) The space measured from the focal point of an x-ray tube to the film. SYN source-film distance.

**tar·get or·gan** (tahr′gĕt ōr′găn) Tissue or organ on which a hormone exerts its action.

**tar·get pop·u·la·tion** (tahr′gĕt pop′yū-lā′shŭn) Select group who share the same distinct set of qualities for epidemiologic purposes.

**tar·nish·ing** (tahr′nish-ing) Discoloration of the surface of a metal restoration, usually due to the action of sulfides.

**tar·tar** (tahr′tăr) A white, brown, or yellow-brown deposit at or below the gingival margin of teeth, chiefly hydroxyapatite in an organic matrix. SYN dental calculus (2).

**taste** (tāst) **1.** To perceive through gustatory system. **2.** Sensation produced by a suitable stimulus applied to taste buds. [It. *tastare;* L. *tango,* to touch]

**taste blind·ness** (tāst blīnd′nĕs) Inability to appreciate gustatory stimuli.

**taste bud** (tāst bŭd) Several flask-shaped cell nests located in epithelium of vallate, fungiform, and foliate papillae of tongue and also in soft palate, and elsewhere. There are five basic taste classifications, each exemplified by substance(s) in parenthesis after their types: bitter (quinine), salty (NaCl), sour (HCl), sweet (sugars and artificial sweeteners), and umami (glutamic acid).

**taste de·fi·cien·cy** (tāst dĕ-fish′ĕn-sē) Reduced or absent ability to detect a bitter taste in a group of compounds of which phenylthiocarbamide is prototype, due to homozygous state of common allele.

**taste pore** (tāst pōr) [TA] Minute opening of taste bud on surface of oral mucosa through which gustatory hairs of specialized neuroepithelial gustatory cells project.

**taste ridge** (tāst rij) One of the elevations surrounding vallate papillae of tongue.

**tau·ro·don·tism** (taw′rō-don′tizm) Developmental anomaly involving molar teeth in which bifurcation or trifurcation of the roots is very near the apex, resulting in an abnormally large and long pulp chamber with exceedingly short pulp canals. See this page. [L. *taurus,* bull, + G. *odous,* tooth]

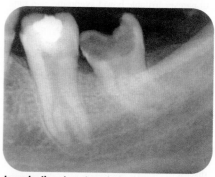

**taurodontism:** hypertaurodont

**tax·on·o·my** (taks-on'ŏ-mē) The systematic classification of living things or organisms. Kingdoms of living organisms are divided into groups (taxa) to show degrees of similarity or presumed evolutionary relationships, with the higher categories larger, more inclusive, and more broadly defined; the lower categories more restricted, with fewer species, and more closely related. The divisions below kingdom are, in descending order: phylum, class, order, family, genus, species, and subspecies (variety). [G. *taxis*, orderly arrangement, + *nomos*, law]

**Tay-Sachs dis·ease** (tā saks di-zēz') A lysosomal storage disease resulting from hexosaminidase-A deficiency.

**TB** Abbreviation for tuberculosis.

**TCA** Abbreviation for tricyclic antidepressant.

**T cell** (sel) SYN T lymphocyte.

**team prac·tice** (tēm prak'tis) Collaborative group of dental professionals who collaboratively manage patient care.

**tears** (tērz) SYN lacrimal fluid.

**tea·spoon** (tē'spūn) A small spoon, holding about 1 dram (or about 5 mL) of liquid; used as a measure in the dosage of fluid medicines.

**tech·nique** (tek-nēk') Manner of performance or details of any surgical operation, experiment, or mechanical act. [Fr., fr. G. *technikos*, relating to *technē*, art, skill]

**tech·nol·o·gist** (tek-nol'ŏ-jist) One trained in and using the techniques of a profession, art, or science.

**tech·nol·o·gy** (tĕk-nol'ŏ-jē) Knowledge and use of techniques of a profession, art, or science. [G. *technē*, an art, + *logos*, study]

**teeth** (tēth) Plural of tooth.

**teeth·ing** (tēdh'ing) Eruption or "cutting" of teeth, especially deciduous teeth. SYN odontiasis.

**tei·chop·si·a** (tī-kop'sē-ă) Jagged, shimmering visual sensation resembling fortifications of a walled medieval town; scintillating scotoma of migraine. [G. *teichos*, wall, + *opsis*, vision]

**tel·an·gi·ec·ta·si·a** (tel-an'jē-ek-tā'zē-ă) Dilation of previously existing small or terminal vessels of a part. See this page. [G. *telos*, end, + *angeion*, vessel, + *ektasis*, a stretching out]

**tel·an·gi·o·sis** (tel'an-jē-ō'sis) Any disease of capillaries and terminal arterioles.

**tel·e·di·ag·no·sis** (tel'ē-dī'ăg-nō'sis) Detection of disease by evaluation of data transmitted to a receiving station, a process normally involving patient-monitoring instruments and a

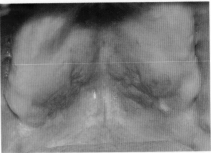

**primary lymphoma of palate:** telangiectasia

transfer link to a diagnostic center at some distance from the patient.

**te·lem·e·try** (tĕ-lem'ĕ-trē) Process of transmitting results using radio signals.

**tel·e·ra·di·og·ra·phy** (tel'ĕ-rā'dē-og'ră-fē) Radiography with the x-ray tube positioned about 2 meters from the film, thereby securing practical parallelism of the x-rays to minimize geometric distortion; the standard configuration for chest radiography. SYN teleroentgenography. [G. *tēle*, distant, + *radiography*]

**tel·e·roent·gen·og·ra·phy** (tel'ĕ-rent'gen-og'ră-fē) SYN teleradiography.

**tel·e·scop·ic den·ture** (tel'ĕ-skop'ik den' chŭr) SYN overlay denture.

**tem·per** (tem'pĕr) To treat metal by application of heat, as in annealing or quenching.

**tem·per·ance** (tem'pĕr-ăns) Moderation in all things; however, colloquially, usually abstinence from consumption of alcoholic beverages. [L. *temperantia*, moderation]

**tem·per·ate** (tem'pĕr-ăt) Moderate; restrained in the indulgence of any activity.

**tem·plate** (tem'plăt) 1. In dentistry, a curved or flat plate used as an aid in setting teeth. 2. An outline used to trace teeth, bones, or soft tissue to standardize their form. 3. A pattern or guide that determines the shape of a substance. [Fr. *templet*, temple of a loom, fr. L. *templum*, small timber]

**tem·po·ral** (tem'pŏr-ăl) 1. Relating to time; limited in time; temporary. 2. Relating to the temple. [L. *temporalis*, fr. *tempus* (*tempor-*), time, temple]

**tem·po·ral ar·ter·i·tis** (tem'pŏr-ăl ahr'tĕr-ī'tis) Subacute granulomatous arteritis involving the external carotid arteries, especially temporal artery; occurs in old people and may be manifested by constitutional symptoms, particularly severe headache.

st

**tem·po·ral bone** (tem′pŏr-ăl bōn) [TA] A large, irregular osseous formation situated in the base and side of the skull. SYN os temporale.

**tem·po·ral branch of fa·cial nerve** (tem′pŏr-ăl branch fā′shăl nĕrv) [TA] Branches of facial nerve innervating the superior portion of the orbicularis oculi muscle and other muscles of facial expression above the eye.

**tem·po·ra·lis mus·cle** (tem-pŏr-ā′lis mŭs′ĕl) *Origin*, temporal fossa; *insertion*, coronoid process of mandible and anterior border of ramus; *action*, elevates mandible (closes jaw); its posterior, nearly horizontally-oriented fibers are the primary retractors of the protruded mandible; *nerve supply*, deep temporal branches of mandibular division of trigeminal. SYN musculus temporalis [TA], temporal muscle.

**tem·po·ral lobe** (tem′pŏr-ăl lōb) [TA] The long and lowest of the major subdivisions of the cortical mantle, forming the posterior two thirds

Short-term artificial replacement for the natural crown of a tooth.

**tem·po·rar·y den·ture** (tem′pŏr-ar-ē den′chŭr) SYN interim denture.

**tem·po·rar·y pros·the·sis** (tem′pŏr-ar-ē pros-thē′sis) Short-term fixed or removable appliance used while a permanent replacement is being fabricated.

**tem·po·rar·y res·to·ra·tion** (tem′pŏr-ar-ē res′tŏr-ā′shŭn) Dental restoration to be used for a limited time, in contradistinction to a permanent restoration. SYN provisional restoration.

**tem·po·rar·y tooth** (tem′pŏr-ar-ē tŭth) SYN deciduous tooth.

**▣tem·po·ro·man·dib·u·lar** (tem′pŏr-ō-man-dib′yū-lăr) Relating to temporal bone and mandible; denoting joint of lower jaw. See this page. SYN temporomaxillary (2).

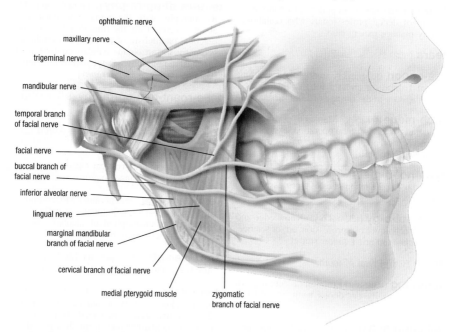

ophthalmic nerve

maxillary nerve

trigeminal nerve

mandibular nerve

temporal branch of facial nerve

facial nerve

buccal branch of facial nerve

inferior alveolar nerve

lingual nerve

marginal mandibular branch of facial nerve

cervical branch of facial nerve

medial pterygoid muscle

zygomatic branch of facial nerve

**nerves of the temporomandibular region**

of the ventral surface of the cerebral hemisphere, separated from the frontal and parietal lobes above it by the lateral sulcus arbitrarily delineated by an imaginary plane from the occipital lobe with which it is continuous posteriorly. SYN lobus temporalis [TA].

**tem·po·ral mus·cle** (tem′pŏr-ăl mŭs′ĕl) SYN temporalis muscle.

**tem·po·rar·y base** (tem′pŏr-ar-ē bās) SYN baseplate.

**tem·po·rar·y crown** (tem′pŏr-ar-ē krown)

**tem·po·ro·man·dib·u·lar ar·thro·sis** (tem′pŏr-ō-man-dib′yū-lăr ahr-thrō′sis) Noninfectious degenerative dysfunction of temporomandibular joint characterized by pain, cracking, and limited mandibular opening.

**tem·por·o·man·di·bu·lar dis·or·der** (tem′pŏr-ō-man-dib′yū-lăr dis-ōr′dĕr) An inclusive term for all functional disturbances of masticatory system including temporomandibular joint (TMJ) syndrome, myofacial pain–dysfunction syndrome, and temporomandibular pain-dysfunction syndrome.

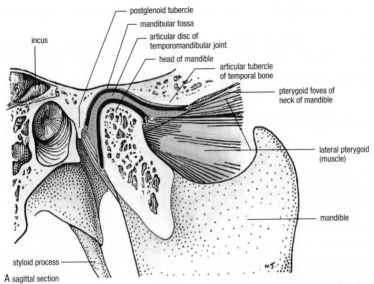

postglenoid tubercle
mandibular fossa
articular disc of temporomandibular joint
incus
head of mandible
articular tubercle of temporal bone
pterygoid fovea of neck of mandible
lateral pterygoid (muscle)
mandible
styloid process
A sagittal section

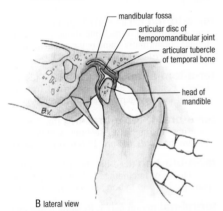

mandibular fossa
articular disc of temporomandibular joint
articular tubercle of temporal bone
head of mandible
B lateral view

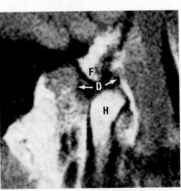

C sagittal view

**temporomandibular joint (TMJ):** (A) lateral view of sagittal section of right TMJ; (B) lateral view of sagittal section of TMJ with mouth open; (C) sagittal MRI of TMJ. D = articular disc; H = head of mandible; F = articular tubercle of temporal bone

st

**tem·po·ro·man·dib·u·lar joint** (tem′pŏr-ō-man-dib′yū-lăr joynt) [TA] Synovial articulation between head of mandible and mandibular fossa and articular tubercle of temporal bone; a fibrocartilaginous articular disc divides it into two cavities. See this page. SYN jaw joint, mandibular joint.

**tem·po·ro·man·dib·u·lar joint dys·func·tion (TMJ)** (tem′pŏr-ō-man-dib′yū-lăr joynt dis-fŭngk′shŭn) Impaired (sometimes long-term) function of temporomandibular articulation.

**tem·po·ro·man·dib·u·lar joint pain-dys·func·tion syn·drome (TMD syn·drome)** (tem′pŏr-ō-man-dib′yū-lăr joynt pān-dis-fŭngk′shŭn sin′drōm) SYN myofascial pain-dysfunction syndrome.

**tem·po·ro·man·dib·u·lar lig·a·ment** (tem′pŏr-ō-man-dib′yū-lăr lig′ă-mĕnt) SYN lateral ligament of temporomandibular joint.

**tem·po·ro·man·dib·u·lar nerve** (tem′pŏr-ō-man-dib′yū-lăr nĕrv) SYN zygomatic nerve.

**tem·po·ro·man·dib·u·lar syn·drome** (tem′pŏr-ō-man-dib′yū-lăr sin′drōm) Symptoms of discomfort and pain caused by loss of vertical dimension, lack of posterior occlusion, or other malocclusion, trismus, muscle tremor, or direct trauma to the temporomandibular joint.

**tem·po·ro·max·il·lar·y** (tem′pŏ-rō-mak′si-lar-ē) **1.** Relating to regions of temporal and maxillary bones. **2.** SYN temporomandibular.

**tem·po·ro·oc·cip·i·tal** (tem′pŏr-ō-ok-sip′

i-tăl) Relating to temporal and occipital bones or regions.

**ten·der** (ten'dĕr) Sensitive or painful due to pressure or contact insufficent to cause discomfort in normal tissues. [L. *tener,* soft, delicate]

**ten·di·ni·tis** (ten'di-nī'tis ) Inflammation of a tendon. SYN tendonitis, tenonitis (2), tenontitis, tenositis.

**ten·di·nous sy·no·vi·tis** (ten'di-nŭs sin'ō-vī'tis) SYN tenosynovitis.

♻ **tendo-** Combining form meaning a tendon.

**ten·don** (ten'dŏn) [TA] Nondistensible fibrous cord or band of variable length that is part of muscles (some authorities, however, consider it as part of the muscle complex), which connects fleshy (contractile) part of muscle with its bony attachment or other structure. [L. *tendo*]

**ten·don·i·tis** (ten'dŏ-nī'tis) SYN tendinitis.

**ten·don re·flex** (ten'dŏn rē'fleks) Myotatic or deep reflex in which muscle stretch receptors are stimulated by percussing muscle tendon.

**ten·do·syn·o·vi·tis** (ten'dō-sin'ō-vī'tis) SYN tenosynovitis.

♻ **teno-** Combining form meaning tendon. [G. *tenon*]

**ten·o·ni·tis** (ten'ŏ-nī'tis) SYN tendinitis.

**ten·o·si·tis** (ten'ŏ-sī'tis) SYN tendinitis.

**ten·sile stress** (ten'sil stres) Stress acting on a body per unit cross-sectional area so as to elongate the body.

**ten·sion** (ten'shŭn) **1.** Act of stretching. **2.** Condition of being stretched or tense, or a stretching or pulling force. [L. *tensio,* fr. *tendo,* pp. *tensus,* to stretch]

**ten·sion head·ache, ten·sion-type head·ache** (ten'shŭn hed'āk, ten'shŭn-tīp) Headache associated with nervous tension, anxiety, and other causes often related to chronic contraction of scalp muscles.

**ten·sion test** (ten'shŭn test) Application of stress at the mucogingival junction by retracting cheek, lip, and tongue to tighten the alveolar mucosa and determine the presence of attached gingiva; area of missing attached gingiva is revealed when the alveolar mucosa and frena are connected directly to the free gingiva.

**tent** (tent) **1.** Canopy used in various types of inhalation therapy to control humidity and concentration of oxygen in inspired air. **2.** Cylinder, usually absorbent, introduced into a canal or sinus to maintain its patency or to dilate it. **3.** To elevate or pick up a segment of skin, fascia, or tissue at a given point, giving it the appearance of a tent. [L. *tendo,* pp. *tensus,* to stretch]

**tenth cra·ni·al nerve [CN X]** (tĕnth krā'nē-ăl nĕrv) SYN vagus nerve [CN X].

♻ **terato-** Combining form meaning teras. [G. *teras,* monster]

**ter·a·to·gen** (ter'ă-tō-jen) Any substance that induces incidence of abnormal prenatal development. [*terato-* + G. *-gen,* producing]

**ter·a·to·gen·e·sis** (ter'ă-tō-jen'ĕ-sis) Disturbed growth processes involved in production of a malformed neonate.

**ter·a·to·gen·ic a·gent** (ter'ă-tō-jen'ik ā'jĕnt) Drug, virus, or irradiation that can cause malformation of the fetus. [*terato-* + *-genic,* producing, fr. *gennaō,* to produce, beget]

**ter·a·to·gen·ic ef·fect** (ter'ă-tō-jen'ik e-fekt') Appearance of anomalies and/or developmental defects due to exposure to a teratogenic agent during fetal development.

**ter·a·tol·o·gy** (ter'ă-tol'ŏ-jē) Embryologic science concerned with the production, development, anatomy, and classification of malformed embryos or fetuses. [*terato-* + G. *logos,* study]

**ter·a·to·ma** (ter'ă-tō'mă) Type of germ cell tumor composed of multiple tissues, including tissues not normally found in the organ in which it arises. [*terato-* + G. *-oma,* tumor]

**ter·a·tom·a·tous cyst** (ter'ă-tō'mă-tŭs sist) Lesion containing structures derived from all three of primary germ layers of the embryo.

**ter·e·brant, ter·e·brat·ing** (ter'ĕ-brănt, -brăt-ing) Boring into; stabbing; piercing. [L. *terebro,* pp. *-atus,* to bore, fr. *terebra,* an auger]

**ter·e·bra·tion** (ter'ĕ-brā'shŭn) **1.** Act of boring into, or of trephining. **2.** A boring, piercing pain. [L. *terebro,* to bore, fr. *terebra,* an auger]

**ter·mi·nal** (tĕr'mi-năl) **1.** Relating to the end; final. **2.** Relating to extremity or end of any body; e.g., end of a biopolymer. [L. *terminus,* a boundary, limit]

**ter·mi·nal hinge po·si·tion** (tĕr'mi-năl hinj pŏ-zish'ŏn) Mandibular hinge position from which further opening of mandible would produce translatory rather than hinge movement.

**ter·mi·nal ill·ness** (tĕr'mi-năl il'nĕs) Advanced disease state from which there is no expectation of recovery.

**ter·mi·nal jaw re·la·tion re·cord** (tĕr'mi-năl jaw rĕ-lā'shŭn rek'ŏrd) Measuring of relationship of mandible to maxillae made at vertical relation of occlusion and centric position.

**ter·mi·nal notch of au·ri·cle** (tĕr'mi-năl noch awr'i-kĕl) [TA] A deep notch separating the tragal lamina and cartilage of the external auditory meatus from the main auricular cartilage, the two being connected below by the isthmus. SYN auricular notch (2).

**ter·mi·nal plane** (tĕr´mi-năl plān) Primary second molars are in proper occlusal alignment.

**ter·mi·nal shank** (tĕr´mi-năl shangk) SYN lower shank.

**term in·fant** (tĕrm in´fănt) Neonate with gestational age between 37 completed weeks and 42 completed weeks.

**Ter·mi·no·lo·gi·a An·a·to·mi·ca (TA)** (tĕr´mi-nō-lō´jē-ă an´ă-tom´i-kă) A system of anatomic nomenclature, devised and approved by the International Federation of Associations of Anatomists (IFAA).

**Ter·mi·no·lo·gi·a Em·bry·o·log·ic·a** (tĕr´mi-nō-lō´jē-ă em´brē-ō-lō´ji-kă) Forthcoming list of Latin and English embryologic terms produced by the Federative International Committee on Anatomical Terminology.

**ter·ti·ar·y den·tin** (tĕr´shē-ă-rē den´tin) Morphologically irregular dentin formed in response to an irritant. SYN irregular dentin, reparative dentin.

**Tes·si·er clas·si·fi·ca·tion** (tes´yā klas´i-fi-kā´shŭn) Anatomic classification of facial, craniofacial, and laterofacial clefts that uses orbit as primary reference structure.

**test** (test) **1.** To prove; to try a substance; to determine chemical nature of a substance by means of reagents. **2.** Examination, to determine presence or absence of a definite disease or of some substance in bodily fluids, tissues, or excretions. [L. *testum*, an earthen vessel]

**test han·dle in·stru·ment** (test han´dĕl in´strŭ-mĕnt) Root canal instrument with a handle similar to that of a collet chuck; can be secured in position on root canal instrument to adjust its effective length.

**test·ing** (test´ing) Controlled analysis to determine specific findings.

**test·ing stick** (test´ing stik) A plastic 1/4-in. rod, about 3 in. long, used to test sharpness of a scaler or a curette.

**test meal** (test mēl) **1.** Toast and tea, or crackers and tea, or gruel or other bland food, given to stimulate gastric secretion before withdrawing gastric contents for analysis. **2.** Administration of food containing a substance thought responsible for symptoms, such as an allergic reaction.

**tes·tos·ter·one** (tes-tos´tĕ-rōn) Most potent naturally occurring androgen, formed in greatest quantities by interstitial cells of testes; used to treat some carcinomas, and other conditions.

**te·tan·ic** (te-tan´ik) Relating to or marked by sustained muscular contraction, as in tetanus. [G. *tetanikos*]

**tet·a·nig·e·nous** (tet´ă-nij´ĕ-nŭs) Causing tetanus. [*tetanus* + G. *-gen*, producing]

**tet·a·nize** (tet´ă-nīz) To stimulate a muscle by a rapid series of stimuli so that individual muscular responses (contractions) are fused into a sustained contraction.

**tet·a·nus** (tet´ă-nŭs) **1.** Disease marked by painful tonic muscular contractions, caused by the neurotropic toxin (tetanospasmin) of *Clostridium tetani* acting on central nervous system. **2.** Sustained muscular contraction caused by a series of nerve stimuli repeated so rapidly that individual muscular responses are fused, producing a sustained tetanic contraction. [L. fr. G. *tetanos*, convulsive tension]

**tet·a·ny** (tet´ă-nē) Clinical neurologic syndrome characterized by muscle twitches, cramps, and carpopedal spasm, and when severe, laryngospasm and seizures. Causes include hyperventilation, hypoparathyroidism, rickets, and uremia. [G. *tetanos*, tetanus]

**tet·ra·cus·pid** (tet´ră-kŭs´pid) Having four cusps. SYN quadricuspid.

**tet·ra·cy·cline** (tet´ră-sī´klēn, -klin) Broad-spectrum antibiotic; its fluorescence has been used in studies of growing tumors and calcium deposition in developing bones and teeth.

**tet·rad** (tet´rad) Collection of four things having something in common, such as a deformity with four features, e.g., tetralogy of Fallot. [G. *tetras* (*tetrad-*), the number four]

**te·tral·o·gy of Fal·lot** (te-tral´ŏ-jē fahl-ō´) A set of congenital cardiac defects including ventricular septal defect, pulmonic valve stenosis or infundibular stenosis, and dextroposition of the aorta such that it overrides the ventricular septum and receives venous as well as arterial blood.

**tet·ra·pa·re·sis** (tet´ră-pă-rē´sis) Weakness of all four limbs.

**TFD** Abbreviation for target-film distance.

**thal·a·mus**, pl. **thal·a·mi** (thal´ă-mŭs, -mī) [TA] The large, ovoid mass of gray matter that forms the larger dorsal subdivision of the diencephalon; it is placed medially to the internal capsule and the body and tail of the caudate nucleus. [G. *thalamos*, a bed, a bedroom]

**thalassaemia** [Br.] SYN thalassemia.

**thalassaemia major** [Br.] SYN thalassemia major.

**thalassaemia minor** [Br.] SYN thalassemia minor.

**thalassanaemia** [Br.] SYN thalassemia.

**thal·as·se·mi·a**, **thal·as·sa·ne·mi·a** (thal´ă-sē´mē-ă, -ă-să-nē´mē-ă) Any of a group of inherited disorders of hemoglobin metabolism with impaired synthesis of one or more polypeptide chains of globin; several genetic

**st**

types exist. SYN thalassaemia, thalassanaemia. [G. *thalassa*, the sea, + *haima*, blood]

**thal·as·se·mi·a ma·jor** (thal'ă-sē'mē-ă mā' jŏr) Syndrome of severe anemia resulting from homozygous state of one of the thalassemia genes or one of the hemoglobin Lepore genes with onset, in infancy or childhood, of pallor, icterus, weakness, splenomegaly, cardiac enlargement, thinning of inner and outer tables of skull, and other findings. SYN Cooley anemia, thalassaemia major.

**thal·as·se·mi·a mi·nor** (thal'ă-sē'mē-ă mī' nŏr) Heterozygous state of a thalassemia gene or a hemoglobin Lepore gene; usually asymptomatic and quite variable hematologically. SYN thalassaemia minor.

**tha·lid·o·mide** (thă-lid'ŏ-mīd) A hypnotic drug that, if taken in early pregnancy, may cause the birth of infants with phocomelia and other defects; approved for used in the treatment of erythema nodosum leprosum and is also under investigational use in other clinical areas.

**thal·lo·tox·i·co·sis** (thal'ō-tok'si-kō'sis) Poisoning by thallium; marked by stomatitis, gastroenteritis, peripheral and retrobulbar neuritis, endocrine disorders, and alopecia. [*thallium* + G. *toxikon*, poison, + *-osis*, condition]

**the·co·dont** (thē'kō-dont) Having teeth inserted in alveoli. [G. *thēkē*, box, + *odous* (*odont-*), tooth]

**the·in·ism, the·ism** (thē'i-nizm, thē'izm, -tē') Chronic poisoning due to immoderate levels of tea-drinking, marked by palpitation, insomnia, headache, and dyspepsia.

**the·oph·yl·line** (thē-of'i-lin) Alkaloid found with caffeine in tea leaves; shares chemical and pharmacologic properties with caffeine and theobromine.

**the·o·rem** (thē'ŏ-rĕm) Proposition that can be tested then and can be established as a law or principle.

**the·o·ry** (thē'ŏr-ē) Reasoned explanation of known facts or phenomena that serves as a basis of investigation by which to seek truth. [G. *theōria*, a beholding, speculation, theory, fr. *theōros*, a beholder]

**ther·a·peu·sis** (thār'ă-pyū'sis) 1. SYN therapeutics. 2. SYN therapy.

**ther·a·peu·tic** (thār'ă-pyū'tik) Relating to therapeutics or to treating, remediating, or curing a disorder or disease. [G. *therapeutikos*]

**ther·a·peu·tic dose** (ther'ă-pyū'tik dōs) Amount of medication required to produce the desired outcome. SEE ALSO dose.

**ther·a·peu·tic in·dex** (thār'ă-pyū'tik in' deks) Ratio of $LD_{50}$ to $ED_{50}$, used in quantitative comparison of drugs.

**ther·a·peu·tic ra·ti·o** (thār'ă-pyū'tik rā' shē-ō) Ratio of maximally tolerated dose of a drug to the minimal curative or effective dose; $LD_{50}$ divided by $ED_{50}$.

**ther·a·peu·tics** (thār'ă-pyū'tiks) Practical branch of medicine concerned with treatment of disease or disorder. SYN therapeusis (1). [G. *therapeutikē*, medical practice]

**ther·a·pist** (thār'ă-pist) One professionally trained in the practice of some type of therapy.

**ther·a·py** (thār'ă-pē) Treatment of disease or disorder by any method. SYN therapeusis (2). [G. *therapeia*, medical treatment]

**therm-** Heat. [G. *therme*, heat; *thermos*, warm or hot]

**ther·ma·co·gen·e·sis** (thĕr'mă-kō-jen'ē-sis) Elevation of body temperature by drug action. [G. *thermē*, heat, + *pharmakon*, drug, + *genesis*, production]

**ther·mal ex·pan·sion** (thĕr'măl eks-pan' shŭn) Enlargement caused by heat.

**ther·mal·ge·si·a** (thĕr'măl-jē'zē-ă) High sensibility to heat; pain caused by slight degree of heat. [*therm-* + G. *algēsis*, sense of pain]

**ther·mal·gi·a** (thĕr-mal'jē-ă) Burning pain. [*therm-* + G. *algos*, pain]

**thermanaesthesia** [Br.] SYN thermoanesthesia.

**ther·ma·tol·o·gy** (thĕr'mă-tol'ŏ-jē) Branch of therapeutics concerned with application of heat. [*therm-* + G. *logos*, study]

**ther·mi·on·ic e·mis·sion** (thĕr'mī-on'ik ē-mish'ŭn) Release of electrons that occurs when tungsten filament of a cathode is heated to incandescence.

**therm·is·tor** (thĕr'mis-tŏr) A device for determining temperature; also used to monitor control of temperature. [G. *thermē*, heat]

**thermoaesthesia** [Br.] SYN thermoesthesia.

**thermoanaesthesia** [Br.] SYN thermoanesthesia.

**ther·mo·an·es·the·si·a, therm·an·al·ge·si·a, therm·an·es·the·si·a** (thĕr'mō-an-es-thē'zē-ă, thĕrm'an-ăl-jē'zē-ă, -es-thē'zē-ă) Loss of temperature sense or ability to distinguish between heat and cold; insensibility to heat or to temperature changes. SYN thermoanaesthesia, thermanaesthesia. [*thermo-* + G. *an-* priv. + *aisthēsis*, sensation]

**ther·mo·co·ag·u·la·tion** (thĕr'mō-kō-ag' yū-lā'shŭn) Process of converting tissue into a gel by heat.

**ther·mo·cou·ple** (thĕr'mō-kŭp'ĕl) A device for measuring slight changes in temperature, consisting of two wires of different metals, one wire being kept at a given low temperature, the other in the tissue or other material with a temperature to be measured; a thermoelectric current setup is measured by a potentiometer.

**ther·mo·es·the·si·a, therm·es·the·si·a** (thĕr′mō-es-the̅′ze̅-ă, thĕrm′es-the̅′ze̅-ă) Ability to distinguish differences of temperature. SYN thermoaesthesia. [*thermo-* + G. *aisthēsis*, sensation]

**ther·mog·ra·phy** (thĕr-mog′ră-fe̅) The technique for making a thermogram.

**ther·mom·e·ter** (thĕr-mom′e̅-tĕr) An instrument for indicating temperature of any substance; often sealed vacuum tube containing mercury, which expands with heat and contracts with cold, its level accordingly rising or falling in the tube, with exact degree of variation of level being indicated by a scale, or, today, a device with an electronic sensor that displays temperature without use of mercury. [*thermo-* + G. *metron,* measure]

**ther·mo·phore** (thĕr′mō-fo̅r) Arrangement for applying heat to a body part; consists of a water heater, tube conveying hot water to a coil, and another tube conducting water back to heater. [*thermo-* + G. *phoros,* bearing]

**ther·mo·plas·tic** (ther′mō-plas′tik) Classification for materials that can be softened by application of heat and hardened on cooling.

**ther·mo·set** (ther′mō-set) Classification for materials that harden or cure on application of heat.

**ther·mo·ther·a·py** (thĕr′mō-thār′ă-pe̅) Treatment of disease by therapeutic application of heat. [*thermo-* + G. *therapeia,* treatment]

**the·roid** (the̅′royd) Resembling an animal in instincts or propensities. [G. *thēr,* a wild beast, + *eidos,* resemblance]

**thi·a·min** (thī′ă-min) Heat-labile and water-soluble vitamin contained in milk, yeast, and in the germ and husk of grains; essential for growth. Sometimes spelled thiamine. SYN vitamin B1. [*thia-* + *vitamin*]

**thi·mer·o·sal** (thī-mer′ŏ-săl) Antiseptic used topically and as a preservative.

**thin-di·am·e·ter in·stru·ment tip** (thin′ dī-am′e̅-tĕr in′stru̅-mĕnt tip) SYN slim-diameter instrument tip.

**thin ve·neer** (thin vĕn-e̅r′) Shallow, smooth coating of calculus on portion of root surface.

**thi·o·cy·a·nate** (thī′ō-sī′ă-nāt) A salt of thiocyanic acid. SYN rhodanate, sulfocyanate.

**thi·ol** (thī′ol) Mixture of sulfurated and sulfonated petroleum oils purified with ammonia; used to treat skin diseases.

**third cra·ni·al nerve [CN III]** (thĭrd kra̅′ne̅-ăl nĕrv) SYN oculomotor nerve [CN III].

**third-de·gree burn** (thĭrd-dĕ-gre̅′ bŭrn) SYN full-thickness burn.

**third mo·lar tooth** (thĭrd mō′lăr tu̅th) [TA] Eighth permanent tooth in maxilla and mandible on each side, making it most posterior tooth in human dentition; usually erupts between the 17th and 23rd years; roots are often fused, separation being marked only by grooves; because it tends to erupt in an anterosuperior direction, lower third molar often becomes impacted against lower second molar; common for one third molar (or more) to fail to develop. SYN dens molaris tertius [TA], dens sapientiae, dens serotinus, wisdom tooth.

**third oc·cip·i·tal nerve** (thĭrd ok-sip′i-tăl nĕrv) [TA] Medial branch of the dorsal primary ramus of the third cervical nerve.

**third-par·ty ad·min·is·tra·tor** (thĭrd-pahr′te̅ ad-min′i-stra̅′tŏr) SYN third-party payer.

**third-par·ty pay·er** (thĭrd-pahr′te̅ pā′ĕr) An institution or company that provides reimbursement to health care providers for services rendered to a third party (i.e., the patient). SYN third-party administrator.

**thirst** (thĭrst) Desire to drink associated with uncomfortable sensations in mouth and pharynx. [A.S. *thurst*]

**thix·o·tro·phic** (thiks′ŏ-trō′fik) SYN thixotrophic fluid. [G. *thixis,* a touching, + *tropē,* a turning, + *-ic* adj. suffix]

**thix·o·trop·ic flu·id** (thik′sŏ-trō′pik flu̅′id) Liquid that tends to turn into a gel when left standing, but that turns back into a liquid if agitated, as by vibrations or subjection to adequate shear. SYN thixotrophic.

**tho·ra·cal·gi·a** (thōr′ă-kal′je̅-ă) Pain in chest; thoracodynia. [*thoraco-* + G. *algos,* pain]

**tho·ra·co·my·o·dyn·i·a** (thōr′ă-kō-mī′ō-din′e̅-ă) Pain in muscles of chest wall. [*thoraco-* + G. *mys,* muscle, + *odynē,* pain]

**tho·ra·cos·to·my** (thōr′ă-kos′tŏ-me̅) Establishment of an opening into the chest cavity. [*thoraco-* + G. *stoma,* mouth]

**tho·rax,** pl. **tho·ra·ces** (thō′raks, thō-rā′ se̅z) [TA] Upper part of trunk between neck and abdomen; formed by 12 thoracic vertebrae, 12 pairs of ribs, sternum, and muscles and fasciae attached to these. [L. fr. G. *thōrax,* breastplate, the chest, fr. *thōrēssō,* to arm]

**Thr** Abbreviation for threonine.

**thread·ed im·plant** (thred′ĕd im′plant) Implant with screwlike threads that is either screwed into bone previously threaded by a tap,

**st**

or by self-tapping, implant cutting threads in bone as it is inserted into a predrilled hole.

**three-di·men·sion·al re·cord** (thrē´di-men´shŭn-ăl rek´ŏrd) Maxillomandibular record made at the occluding relation.

**thre·o·nine (T, Thr)** (thrē´ō-nēn) One of the naturally occurring amino acids, included in the structure of most proteins and nutritionally essential in the diet of humans and other mammals.

**thresh·old** (thresh´ōld) *Avoid the misspelling* threshhold. **1.** Point at which a stimulus first produces a sensation. **2.** Lower limit of perception of a stimulus. [A.S. *therxold*]

**thresh·old dose** (thresh´ōld dōs) Minimum dose that will result in the desired effect.

**thresh·old stim·u·lus** (thresh´ōld stim´yū-lŭs) Stimulus of threshold strength, i.e., one just strong enough to excite.

**thrill** (thril) Vibration accompanying a cardiac or vascular murmur that can be palpated.

**throat** (thrōt) **1.** The fauces and pharynx. **2.** Anterior aspect of neck. **3.** Any narrowed entrance into a hollow part. [A.S. *throtu*]

**throm·bas·the·ni·a** (throm´bas-thē´nē-ă) Abnormality of platelets. SYN thromboasthenia. [*thromb-* + G. *astheneia*, weakness]

**throm·bin** (throm´bin) **1.** An enzyme (proteinase), formed in shed blood, which converts fibrinogen into fibrin by hydrolyzing peptides (and amides and esters) of L-arginine; formed from prothrombin by the action of prothrombinase. **2.** A sterile protein substance prepared from prothrombin of bovine origin through interaction with thromboplastin in the presence of calcium; causes clotting; used as a topical hemostatic for capillary bleeding in general and plastic surgical procedures. SYN factor IIa.

♻ **thrombo-** Combining form meaning blood clot; coagulation; thrombin.

**thromboasthenia** SYN thrombasthenia.

**throm·bo·cyte** (throm´bō-sīt) SYN platelet. [G. *thrombos*, clot, + *kytos*, cell]

**thrombocythaemia** [Br.] SYN thrombocythemia.

**throm·bo·cy·the·mi·a** (throm´bō-sī-thē´mē-ă) SYN thrombocytosis, thrombocythaemia. [*thrombocyte* + G. *haima*, blood]

**throm·bo·cy·tin** (throm´bō-sī´tin) SYN serotonin.

**throm·bo·cy·to·pe·ni·a** (throm´bō-sī´tō-pē´nē-ă) A condition in which an abnormally small number of platelets is present in circulating blood. SYN thrombocythemia. [*thrombocyte* + G. *penia*, poverty]

**throm·bo·cy·to·pe·nic pur·pu·ra** (throm´bō-sī´tō-pēn´ik pŭr´pyŭr-ă) A systemic illness characterized by extensive ecchymoses and hemorrhages from mucous membranes and low platelet counts; resulting from platelet destruction by macrophages due to an antiplatelet factor.

**throm·bo·cy·to·sis, throm·bo·cy·the·mi·a** (throm´bō-sī-tō´sis, -sī-thē´mē-ă) An increase in the number of platelets in the circulating blood. SYN thrombocythaemia. [*thrombocyte* + G. *-osis*, condition]

**throm·bo·em·bo·lism** (throm´bō-em´bŏ-lizm) Embolism from a thrombus. [*thrombo-* + G. *embolismos*, embolism]

**throm·bo·gen** (throm´bō-jen) SYN prothrombin. [*thrombo-* + G. *-gen*, producing]

**throm·bo·gene** (throm´bō-jēn) SYN factor V.

**throm·bo·ki·nase** (throm´bō-kī´nās) SYN thromboplastin.

**throm·bop·a·thy** (throm-bop´ă-thē) General term applied to disorders of blood platelets resulting in defective thromboplastin. [*thrombo-* + G. *pathos*, disease]

**throm·bo·phle·bi·tis** (throm´bō-flĕ-bī´tis) Venous inflammation with thrombus formation. [*thrombo-* + G. *phleps*, vein, + *-itis*, inflammation]

**throm·bo·plas·tid** (throm´bō-plas´tid) **1.** SYN platelet. **2.** A nucleated spindle cell in submammalian blood. [*thrombo-* + G. *plastos*, formed]

**throm·bo·plas·tin** (throm´bō-plas´tin) A substance present in tissues, platelets, and leukocytes necessary for the coagulation of blood. SYN platelet tissue factor, thrombokinase.

**throm·bo·plas·tin·o·gen** (throm´bō-plas-tin´ō-jen) Obsolete term for factor VIII.

**throm·bo·sis, pl. throm·bo·ses** (throm-bō´sis, -sēz) **1.** Formation or presence of a thrombus. **2.** Clotting within a blood vessel that may cause infarction of tissues supplied by vessel. [G. *thrombōsis*, a clotting, fr. *thrombos*, clot]

**throm·bot·ic throm·bo·cy·to·pe·nic pur·pu·ra** (throm-bot´ik throm´bō-sī´tō-pē´nik pŭr´pyŭr-ă) A rapidly fatal or occasionally protracted disease with varied symptoms in addition to dermal hemorrhage, including signs of central nervous system involvement, due to formation of fibrin or platelet thrombi in arterioles and capillaries in many organs.

**throm·bus, pl. throm·bi** (throm´bŭs, -bī) A clot in the cardiovascular system formed during life from constituents of blood; it may be occlusive or attached to the vessel or heart wall without obstructing the lumen (mural thrombus). SYN blood clot. [L. fr. G. *thrombos*, a clot]

**thrush** (thrŭsh) Infection of the oral tissues with *Candida albicans;* often an opportunistic infection in patients with AIDS or other disorders that depress the immune system. [fr. the thrush fungus, *Candida albicans*]

**thumb for·ceps** (thŭm fōr′seps) A spring forceps used by compressing with thumb and forefinger.

**thun·der·clap head·ache** (thŭn′dĕr-klap hed′āk) Sudden severe nonlocalizing head pain not associated with any abnormal neurologic findings; of varied etiology.

**thy·mol** (thī′mol) Phenol present in thyme; used externally as an antiseptic and deodorizer, and internally as a specific for ancylostomiasis.

**thy·mo·ma** (thī-mō′mă) A usually benign neoplasm in the anterior mediastinum; occasionally invasive, but metastases are rare. [*thymus* + G. *-oma,* tumor]

**thy·mus,** pl. **thy·mi,** pl. **thy·mus·es** (thī′ mŭs, -mī, -mŭs-ĕz) [TA] A primary lymphoid organ, located in the superior mediastinum and lower part of the neck, which is necessary in early life for the normal development of immunologic function. [G. *thymos,* excrescence, sweetbread]

**thy·ro·a·pla·si·a** (thī′rō-ă-plā′zē-ă) Anomalies observed in patients with congenital defects of the thyroid gland and deficiency of its secretion. [*thyro-* + G. *a-* priv. + *plasis,* a molding]

**thy·ro·cele** (thī′rō-sēl) Tumor of thyroid gland, such as goiter. [*thyro-* + G. *kēlē,* tumor]

**thy·ro·hy·oid mus·cle** (thī′rō-hī′oyd mŭs′ ĕl) Apparently a continuation of the sternothyroid; *origin,* oblique line of thyroid cartilage; *insertion,* body of hyoid bone; *action,* approximates hyoid bone to the larynx; *nerve supply,* upper cervical spinal nerves carried by hypoglossal. SYN musculus thyrohyoideus.

**thy·roid bru·it** (thī′royd brū-ē′) Vascular murmur heard over hyperactive thyroid glands.

**thy·roid col·lar** (thī′royd kol′ăr) Collar on a lead radiographic apron used to reduce radiation exposure to thyroid area of neck.

**thy·roid·ec·to·my** (thī′roy-dek′tŏ-mē) Removal of thyroid gland. [*thyroid* + G. *ektomē,* excision]

**thy·roid gland** (thī′royd gland) [TA] Endocrine (ductless) gland consisting of irregularly spheroid follicles, lying in front and to sides of upper part of trachea and lower part of larynx and of horseshoe shape, with two lateral lobes connected by a narrow central portion, the isthmus; secretes thyroid hormone and calcitonin.

**thy·roid·i·tis** (thī′roy-dī′tis) Inflammation of thyroid gland. [*thyroid* + G. *-itis,* inflammation]

**thy·ro·la·ryn·ge·al** (thī′rō-lă-rin′jē-ăl) Relating to thyroid gland or cartilage and larynx.

**thy·ro·lib·er·in** (thī′rō-lib′ĕr-in) Tripeptide hormone from hypothalamus, which stimulates anterior lobe of hypophysis to release thyrotropin. [*thyrotropin* + L. *libero,* to free, + *-in*]

**thy·ro·meg·a·ly** (thī′rō-meg′ă-lē) Enlargement of thyroid gland. [*thyro-* + G. *megas,* large]

**thy·ro·pal·a·tine** (thī′rō-pal′ă-tīn) Denoting the palatopharyngeus muscle.

**thy·rop·a·thy** (thī-rop′ă-thē) Disorder of thyroid gland. [*thyro-* + G. *pathos,* suffering]

**thy·ro·tox·ic cri·sis, thy·roid cri·sis** (thī′rō-tok′sik krī′sis, thī′royd) Exacerbation of symptoms of hyperthyroidism; marked by rapid pulse, nausea, diarrhea, fever, loss of weight, extreme nervousness, and sudden rise in metabolic rate; coma and death may occur. Also called thyroid storm.

**thy·ro·tox·i·co·sis** (thī′rō-tok′si-kō′sis) State produced by excessive quantities of endogenous or exogenous thyroid hormone. [*thyro-* + G. *toxikon,* poison, + *-osis,* condition]

**thy·rot·ro·pin** (thī′rō-trō′pin) Glycoprotein hormone produced by anterior lobe of hypophysis; also used as a diagnostic test to differentiate primary and secondary hypothyroidism. [fr. *thyro-* + G. *trophē,* nourishment; corrupted to *-tropin,* and reanalyzed as fr. G. *tropē,* a turning]

**thy·rox·ine, thy·rox·in** (thī-rok′sēn, -sin) The active iodine compound existing normally in the thyroid gland and extracted therefrom in crystalline form for therapeutic use; also prepared synthetically; used for the relief of congenital hypothyroidism, and myxedema.

**TIA** Abbreviation for transient ischemic attack.

**tic** (tik) Habitual, repeated contraction of some muscles, resulting in stereotyped individualized actions that can be voluntarily suppressed for only brief periods, e.g., clearing the throat, sniffing. [Fr.]

**tic dou·lou·reux** (tik dū-lū-ru′) SYN trigeminal neuralgia. [Fr. painful]

**tick·ling** (tik′ling) Denoting a peculiar itching or tingling sensation caused by excitation of surface nerves, as of the skin by light stroking.

**t.i.d.** Abbreviation for L. *ter in die,* three times a day.

**ti·dal air** (tī′dăl ār) SYN tidal volume.

**ti·dal vol·ume** (tī′dăl vol′yūm) Volume of air inspired or expired in a single breath during regular breathing. SYN tidal air.

st

**tide** (tīd) Alternate rise and fall, ebb and flow, or an increase or a decrease. [M.E., fr. O.E. *tīd*]

**time** (tīm) That relationship of events expressed by past, present, and future, and measured in units such as seconds, minutes, hours, days, months, years, or decades. [M.E., fr. O.E. *tīma*]

**tinc·ture (Tr)** (tingk′shŭr) An alcoholic or hydroalcoholic solution prepared from vegetable materials or chemical substances.

**tine** (tīn) 1. In dentistry, slender, pointed end of an explorer. 2. An instrument used to introduce antigen into skin; usually with several individual tines. [A.S. *tind,* a prong]

**tin·e·a** (tin′ē-ă) Fungal infection of keratin component of hair, skin, or nails.

**tin·e·a bar·bae** (tin′ē-ă bahr′bē) Fungal infection of beard, occurring as a follicular infection or as a granulomatous lesion.

**tin·e·a cap·i·tis** (tin′ē-ă kap′i-tis) Common form of fungal infection of scalp caused by various species of *Microsporum* and *Trichophyton* on or within hair shafts, occurring most commonly in children and characterized by irregularly placed and variously sized patches of apparent baldness because of hairs breaking off at the surface of the scalp, scaling, and black dots.

**tin·e·a cir·ci·na·ta** (tin′ē-ă sir-si-nā′tă) SYN tinea corporis.

**tin·e·a cor·po·ris** (tin′ē-ă kōr-pōr′is) A well-defined, scaling, macular eruption of dermatophytosis that frequently forms anular lesions and may appear on any part of the body.

**tin·e·a crur·is** (tin′ē-ă krūr′is) A form of tinea in the genitocrural region, inner side of thighs, perineal region, and groin. SYN eczema marginatum, jock itch.

**tin·e·a ker·i·on** (tin′ē-ă ker′ē-on) Inflammatory fungus infection of scalp and beard, marked by pustules and a boggy infiltration of surrounding parts.

**tin·e·a un·gui·um** (tin′ē-ă ŭng-gwī′ŭm) Ringworm of the nails due to a dermatophyte.

**tin·e·a ver·si·col·or** (tin′ē-ă vĕr′si-kŏ′lŏr) An eruption of tan or brown branny patches on the skin of the trunk, often appearing white, in contrast with hyperpigmented skin after exposure to the summer sun. SYN pityriasis versicolor.

**Ti·nel sign** (tē-nel′ sīn) Sensation of tingling, or of "pins and needles," felt at lesion site or more distally along course of a nerve when percussed; indicates partial lesion or early regeneration in nerve.

**tin·foil** (tin′foyl) 1. Base metal foil used as a separating material, as between cast and denture base material during flasking and curing procedures. 2. Tin rolled into extremely thin sheets.

**tin·foil sub·sti·tute** (tin′foyl sŭb′sti-tūt) A liquid material used in place of foil as a separating material (i.e., between cast and denture base material during flasking and curing procedures).

**tin·ni·tus** (tin′i-tŭs) Perception of a sound (e.g.,whistling, roaring) in the absence of an environmental stimulus.

**tint·ed den·ture base** (tint′ĕd den′chŭr bās) Dental appliance material that simulates coloring and shading of natural oral tissues.

**tip** (tip) 1. Point, more or less sharp. 2. Pointed third of the working end of an explorer, probe, or sickle scaler.

**tip of work·ing end** (tip wŏrk′ing end) A pointed working-end such as on a sickle scaler.

**tip pinch** (tip pinch) OCCUPATIONAL THERAPY pinch between the tips of the index finger and the thumb. SYN tip-to-tip pinch.

**tip·ping** (tip′ing) Tooth movement in which angulation of long axis of tooth is altered.

**tip-third of work·ing-end** (tip′thĭrd wŏrk′ing end) Portion of the working-end of a sickle kept in contact with tooth surface during instrumentation. SEE ALSO toe-third of working-end, leading-third of working-end.

**tip-to-tip pinch** (tip tip pinch) SYN tip pinch.

**tis·sue** (tish′ū) A collection of similar cells and intercellular substances surrounding them. Four basic kinds exist: epithelium; connective tissues including adipose tissue, blood, bone, and cartilage; muscle tissue; and nerve tissue. [Fr. *tissu,* woven, fr. L. *texo,* to weave]

**tis·sue-bear·ing a·re·a** (tish′ū-bār-ing ar′ē-ă) SYN denture foundation area.

**tis·sue dis·place·a·bil·i·ty** (tish′ū dis-plās′ă-bil′i-tē) Property of tissue that permits it to be moved from an initial or relaxed position or form. SYN compression of tissue.

**tis·sue mold·ing** (tish′ū mōld′ing) SYN border molding.

**tis·sue reg·is·tra·tion** (tish′ū rej′is-trā′shŭn) 1. Accurate registration of shape of tissues under any condition by means of a suitable material. 2. An impression.

**tis·sue res·pi·ra·tion** (tish′ū res′pir-ā′shŭn) Interchange of gases between blood and tissues. SYN internal respiration.

**tis·sue slough** (tish′ū slawf) External layer of tissue that loosens when exposed to extensive topical anesthetic, abrasive toothpaste, smokeless tobacco, or mouth rinses. SEE slough.

**tis·sue-trim·ming** (tish′yū-trim′ing) SYN border molding.

**ti·ta·ni·um** (tī-tā′nē-ŭm) A metallic element, used as an implant in dental work because of its uniquely high level of biocompatibility. [*Titans*, in G. myth., sons of Earth]

**ti·ta·ni·um al·loy** (tī-tā′nē-ŭm al′oy) A compound with elements other than titanium, often with aluminum to increase strength and decrease weight and with vanadium to prevent corrosion.

**ti·ta·ni·um di·ox·ide** (tī-tā′nē-ŭm dī-ok′sīd) Agent used in creams and powders to protect against external irritations and sun rays.

**ti·ter** (tī′tĕr) The standard of strength of a volumetric test solution. SYN titre. [Fr. *titre*, standard]

**tit·il·la·tion** (tit′i-lā′shŭn) The act or sensation of tickling. [L. *titillatio*, fr. *titillo*, pp. *-atus*, to tickle]

**ti·tra·tion** (tī-trā′shŭn) Volumetric analysis by addition of definite amounts of a test solution to a solution of the substance being assayed. [Fr. *titre*, standard]

**titre** [Br.] SYN titer.

**tit·u·ba·tion** (tit′yū-bā′shŭn) **1.** Tremor or shaking of head, of cerebellar origin. **2.** Staggering or stumbling in trying to walk. [L. *titubo*, pp. *-atus*, to stagger]

**TLC** Abbreviation for total lung capacity.

**T lym·pho·cyte** (lim′fŏ-sīt) Lymphocyte formed in bone marrow from which it migrates to thymic cortex to become an immunologically competent cell.

**TMD syndrome** (sin′drōm) Abbreviation for temporomandibular joint pain-dysfunction syndrome.

**TMJ** Abbreviation for temporomandibular joint dysfunction.

**TMJ syn·drome** (sin′drōm) SYN myofascial pain-dysfunction syndrome.

**TMP** Abbreviation for trimethoprim.

**TMP/SMX** Abbreviation for trimethoprim-sulfamethoxazole.

**to·bac·co** (tŏ-bak′ō) Herb of South American origin, *Nicotiana tabacum*, which has large ovate to lanceolate leaves; leaves contain 2–8% nicotine and are source of smoking tobacco, chewing tobacco, and snuff. Tobacco smoke contains nicotine, carbon monoxide (4%), nitric oxide, and numerous aromatic hydrocarbons and other substances known to be carcinogens.

**to·bac·co stain** (tŏ-bak′ō stān) Tenacious dark brown or black tooth discoloration that results from cigarette, pipe, or cigar smoking or the use of smokeless tobacco.

**α-to·coph·er·ol** (tŏ-kof′ĕr-ol) One of several forms of vitamin E. A light yellow, viscous, odorless, oily liquid that deteriorates on exposure to light, is obtained from wheat germ oil or by synthesis; an antioxidant retarding rancidity by interfering with autoxidation of fats. SYN vitamin E (1).

**toe** (tō) [TA] **1.** Rounded third of the working end of a curette. **2.** One of the digits of the feet. [A.S. *ta*]

**toe-drop** (tō′drop) Inability to dorsiflex the toes.

**toe of work·ing-end** (tō wŏrk′ing-end) Rounded working-end, as on a curette.

**toe-third of work·ing-end** (tō′thĭrd wŏrk′ing end) Portion of the working-end of a curette kept in contact with tooth surface during instrumentation.

**To·ga·vir·i·dae** (tō′gă-vir′i-dē) A family of viruses that includes the following genera: *Alphavirus*, which includes eastern equine encephalitis; western equine encephalitis; Venezuelan equine encephalitis; and the rubella virus (*Rubivirus*).

**toi·let** (toy-let′) In dentistry, cavity débridement, final step before placing a restoration in a tooth whereby cavity is cleaned and all debris removed. [Fr. *toilette*]

**tol·er·ance** (tol′ĕr-ăns) **1.** Ability to endure or be less responsive to a stimulus, especially over a period of continued exposure. **2.** Power of resisting the action of a poison or of taking a drug continuously or in large doses without harm. [L. *tolero*, pp. *-atus*, to endure]

**tol·er·ance dose** (tol′ĕr-ăns dōs) Largest dose of an agent that can be accepted without production of injurious symptoms.

**To·lo·sa-Hunt syn·drome** (tō-lō′sah-hŭnt′ sin′drōm) Cavernous sinus syndrome produced by an idiopathic granuloma.

**Tomes fi·bers** (tōmz fī′bĕrz) SYN dentinal fibers.

**Tomes gran·u·lar lay·er** (tōmz gran′yū-lăr lā′ĕr) Thin layer of dentin adjacent to cementum, appearing granular in ground sections.

**to·mo·graph** (tō′mŏ-graf) The radiographic equipment used in tomography. [G. *tomos*, a cutting (section), + *graphō*, to write]

**to·mog·ra·phy** (tŏ-mog′ră-fē) Making a radiographic image of a selected plane by means of reciprocal linear or curved motion of the x-ray tube and film cassette; images of all other planes are blurred ("out of focus") by being relatively displaced on the film. SYN planigraphy, planography, stratigraphy.

**tone** (tōn) **1.** Sound of distinct frequency. **2.** Character of the voice expressing an emotion.

st

**3.** Tension present in resting muscles. **4.** Firmness of tissues; normal functioning of all organs. **5.** To perform toning. [G. *tonos*, tone, or a tone]

**tongue** (tŭng) [TA] Mobile mass of muscular tissue covered with mucous membrane, occupying cavity of mouth and forming part of its floor, constituting also by its posterior portion anterior wall of pharynx; bears taste buds and assists in mastication, deglutition, and articulation of speech. See this page. SYN lingua. [A.S. *tunge*]

**tongue bone** (tŭng bōn) SYN hyoid bone.

**tongue crib** (tŭng krib) Appliance used to control visceral (infantile) swallowing and tongue thrusting and to encourage mature or somatic tongue posture and function.

**tongue phe·nom·e·non** (tŭng fĕ-nom´ĕ-non) SYN Schultze sign.

**tongue thrust** (tŭng thrŭst) Infantile pattern of suckle-swallow movement in which the

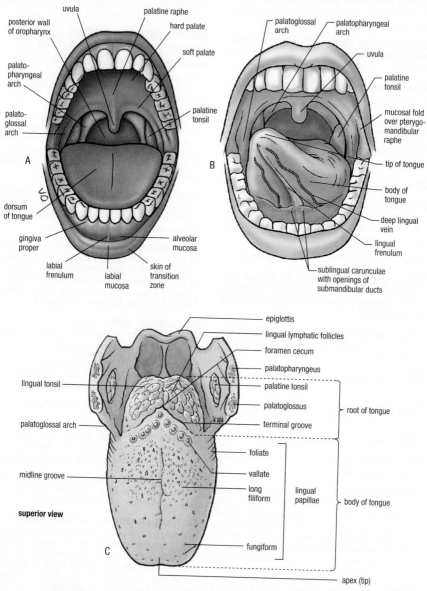

**tongue:** (A) oral cavity and dorsum of tongue; (B) inferior (dorsal) surface of tongue showing veins; (C) features of dorsum of tongue

tongue is placed between incisor teeth or alveolar ridges during initial stage of swallowing.

**ton·ic con·vul·sion** (ton'ik kŏn-vŭl'shŭn) Convulsion with sustained muscle contraction.

**ton·o·fi·bril** (ton'ō-fī'bril) One of a system of fibers found in the cytoplasm of epithelial cells.

**ton·sil** (ton'sil) **1.** Intramucosal collection of lymphocytes or aggregated lymphoid tissue closely associated with overlying epithelium, including pharyngeal tonsil (adenoid), palatine tonsil, and lingual tonsil, which collectively form a lymphoepithelial ring in pharynx. **2.** SYN palatine tonsil. **3.** An anatomic structure resembling palatine tonsil in form. [L. *tonsilla,* a stake, as a pl, the tonsils]

**ton·sil·la,** pl. **ton·sil·lae** (ton-sil'lă, -lē) [TA] SYN palatine tonsil.

**ton·sil·la lin·gua·lis** (ton-sil'lă ling-gwā'lis) [TA] SYN lingual tonsil.

**ton·sil·la pa·la·ti·na** (ton-sil'lă pal'ă-tī'nă) [TA] SYN palatine tonsil.

**ton·sil·la pha·ryn·ge·a·lis** (ton-sil'ă fă-rin'jē-ā'lis) [TA] SYN adenoid.

**ton·sil·lar, ton·sil·lar·y** (ton'si-lăr, -lar-ē) Relating to tonsils, especially palatine tonsil. SYN amygdaline (3).

**ton·sil·lar branch·es of glos·so·pha·ryn·ge·al nerve** (ton'si-lăr branch'ĕz glos'ō-fă-rin'jē-ăl nĕrv) [TA] Branches of glossopharyngeal nerve conducting sensory fibers from palatine tonsillar fossa.

**ton·sil·lar branch·es of less·er pal·a·tine nerves** (ton'si-lăr branch'ĕz les'ĕr pal'ă-tīn nĕrvz) [TA] Branches of the lesser palatine nerves that extend to the palatine tonsil and to its bed.

**ton·sil·lar branch of the fa·cial ar·te·ry** (ton'si-lăr branch fā'shăl ahr'tĕr-ē) [TA] Primary blood supply to palatine tonsil, with anastomoses with other tonsillar arteries.

**ton·sil·lar crypt** (ton'si-lăr kript) [TA] One of a variable number of deep recesses that extend into lingual, palatine, pharyngeal, and tubal tonsils from the free surface.

**ton·sil·lar fos·sa** (ton'si-lăr fos'ă) [TA] Depression between palatoglossal and palatopharyngeal arches occupied by palatine tonsil. SYN amygdaloid fossa, tonsillar sinus.

**ton·sil·lar fos·su·lae (pal·a·tine and pha·ryn·ge·al)** (ton'si-lăr fos'yū-lē pal'ă-tīn fă-rin'jē-ăl) [TA] Small pits at openings of tonsillar crypts onto external surface of tonsil.

**ton·sil·lar ring** (ton'si-lăr ring) SYN pharyngeal lymphatic ring.

**ton·sil·lar si·nus** (ton'si-lăr sī'nŭs) SYN tonsillar fossa.

**ton·sil·lec·to·my** (ton'si-lek'tŏ-mē) Removal of tonsil. [tonsil + G. *ektomē,* excision]

**ton·sil·li·tis** (ton'si-lī'tis) Inflammation of a tonsil. [tonsil + G. *-itis,* inflammation]

**ton·sil·lo·lin·gual sul·cus** (ton'si-lō-ling'gwăl sŭl'kŭs) Space between palatine tonsil and tongue.

▣**tooth,** pl. **teeth** (tūth, tēth) [TA] One of the hard conic structures set in alveoli of upper and lower jaws used in mastication and assisting in articulation; dermal structure composed of dentin and encased in cementum on anatomic root and enamel on anatomic crown. It consists of a root buried in the alveolus, a neck covered by gum, and a crown, the exposed portion. In the center, pulp cavity is filled with a connective tissue reticulum containing a jellylike substance (dental pulp) and blood vessels and nerves that enter through one or more apertures at the apex of the root. The 20 deciduous teeth or primary teeth appear between the 6th–9th and 24th months of life; these exfoliate and are replaced by 32 permanent teeth appearing between 5th–7th years and 17th–23rd years. There are four kinds of teeth: incisor, canine, premolar, and molar. See page 570. SYN dens (1) [TA]. SYN dens (1) [TA]. [A.S. *tōth*]

**tooth a·bra·sion** (tūth ă-brā'zhŭn) Loss or wearing away of tooth structure caused by abrasive characteristics of nonfood substances.

**tooth·ache** (tūth'āk) Pain in a tooth due to condition of pulp or periodontal ligament resulting from caries, infection, or trauma. SYN dentalgia, odontalgia, odontodynia.

**tooth-and-nail syn·drome** (tūth nāl sin'drōm) Hypodontia associated with absent or very small nails at birth.

**tooth ar·range·ment** (tūth ă-rānj'mĕnt) **1.** Placement of teeth on a denture base with definite objectives in mind. **2.** Setting of teeth on temporary bases.

**tooth a·vul·sion** (tūth ă-vŭl'shŭn) Traumatic separation of tooth from its alveolus. SYN tooth evulsion.

**tooth-borne** (tūth'bōrn) Term used to describe a prosthesis or part of a prosthesis that depends entirely on abutment teeth for support.

**tooth-borne base** (tūth'bōrn bās) Denture base restoring an edentulous area that has abutment teeth at each end for support; tissue that it covers is not used for support.

**tooth·brush** (tūth'brŭsh) A bristled or filamented home-care dental device intended to clean teeth, gums, and tongue.

**tooth·brush head** (tūth'brŭsh hed) That part of the implement composed of the tufts and the stock (extension of the handle to which tufts are attached).

▣**tooth bud** (tūth bŭd) Primordial structures from which a tooth is formed: enamel organ, dental papilla, and dental sac enclosing them. See page 570. SYN dental germ, tooth germ.

st

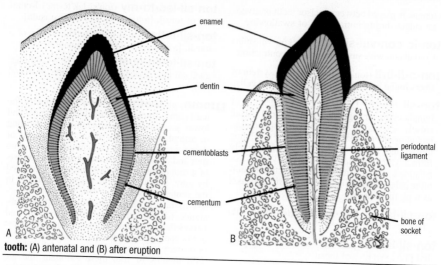

**tooth:** (A) antenatal and (B) after eruption

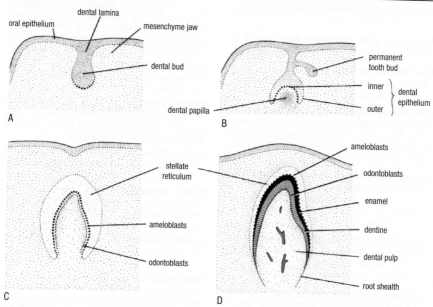

**tooth formation at successive stages of development:** (A) 8 weeks; (B) 10 weeks; (C) 3 months; (D) 6 months

**tooth ce·ment** (tūth sĕ-ment´) SEE cement (1). SYN cementum.

**tooth con·tour** (tūth kon´tūr) Outline or form of a tooth surface.

**tooth e·rup·tion** (tūth ĕ-rŭp´shŭn) SYN eruption (1).

**tooth e·vul·sion** (tūth ĕ-vŭl´shŭn) SYN tooth avulsion.

**tooth form** (tūth fōrm) Characteristics of the curves, lines, angles, and contours of various teeth that permit their identification and differentiation.

**tooth germ** (tūth jĕrm) SYN tooth bud.

**tooth im·pac·tion** (tūth im-pak´shŭn) SYN impacted tooth.

**tooth i·so·la·tion** (tūth ī´sŏ-lā´shŭn) In dentistry, separation of a tooth or group of teeth from oral tissues and saliva by use of a dental dam, cotton rolls, or other means to improve access, visibility, and control moisture contamination while restorative or operative dental procedures are performed.

**tooth li·ga·tion** (tūth lī-gā´shŭn) Binding together of teeth with wire for stabilization and immobilization after traumatic injury or orthognathic surgery, or during periodontal therapy.

**tooth mo·bil·i·ty** (tūth mō-bil´i-tē) Movement of a tooth due to lack of attachment and diminished supportive apparatus. SEE mobility.

**tooth num·ber·ing sys·tem** (tūth nŭm´bĕr-ing sis´tĕm) System used to identify and refer to permanent and primary dentition (i.e., Universal Numbering System, International Numbering System, Palmer Numbering System).

**tooth·pick** (tūth´pik) Small wood sliver or thin plastic device used to remove food particles from the interdental space.

**tooth plane** (tūth plān) Any imaginary plane of section of a tooth (e.g., axial, horizontal, or vertical).

**tooth pol·yp** (tūth pol´ip) SYN hyperplastic pulpitis.

**tooth pulp** (tūth pŭlp) SYN dental pulp.

**tooth sac** (tūth sak) Capsule that encloses the developing tooth.

**tooth sock·et** (tūth sok´ĕt) [TA] Socket in alveolar process of maxilla or mandible, into which each tooth fits and is suspended by means of periodontal ligament. SYN alveolus dentalis [TA], alveolus (1).

**tooth squeeze** (tūth skwēz) SYN barodontalgia.

**tooth trans·plan·ta·tion** (tūth trans´plan-tā´shŭn) Transfer of a tooth from one alveolus to another.

**tooth wear** (tūth wār) Loss of tooth structure due to friction or abrasion). SEE wear.

**to·phus**, pl. **to·phi** (tō´fŭs, -fī) A salivary calculus or tartar.

**top·i·cal** (top´i-kăl) Relating to a definite place or locality, anatomic or geographic; local. [G. topikos, fr. topos, place]

**top·i·cal ad·min·i·stra·tion** (top´i-kăl ad-min´i-strā´shŭn) SYN transdermal.

**top·i·cal an·es·the·si·a** (top´i-kăl an´es-thē´zē-ă) Superficial loss of sensation in conjunctiva, mucous membranes, or skin, produced by direct application of local anesthetic solutions, ointments, jellies, sprays, or solutions.

**topo-** Combining form meaning place, topical.

**to·pog·ra·phy** (tŏ-pog´ră-fē) ANATOMY the description of any part of the body, especially in relation to a definite and limited area of the surface. [topo- + G. graphē, a writing]

**Torn·waldt cyst** (tōrn´vahlt sist) Inflammation or obstruction of pharyngeal bursa with the formation of a lesion containing pus.

**torque** (tōrk) **1.** In dentistry, torsion force applied to a tooth to produce or maintain crown or root movement. **2.** A rotatory force. [L. torqueo, to twist]

**tor·sion** (tōr´shŭn) **1.** In dentistry, twisting or rotation of tooth part on its long axis. **2.** Twisting cut end of an artery to arrest hemorrhage. [L. torsio, fr. torqueo, to twist]

**tor·si·ver·sion, tor·so·ver·sion** (tōr´si-vĕr´zhŭn, tōr´sō-) Malposition of a tooth in which it is rotated on its long axis.

**tor·ti·col·lis** (tōr´ti-kol´is) Contraction, or shortening, of muscles of neck, chiefly those supplied by the accessory nerve (CN XI). [L. tortus, twisted, + collum, neck]

**to·rus**, pl. **to·ri** (tōr´ŭs, -ī) **1.** [TA] Rounded swelling, such as that caused by a contracting muscle. **2.** Geometric figure formed by revolution of a circle around the base of any of its arcs, such as the convex molding at the base of pillar. See this page. [L. swelling, knot, bulge]

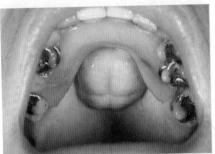

**torus palatinus:** a midline bony growth in hard palate, which is relatively common in adult patients, although size and lobulation vary widely; although alarming in appearance, it is generally harmless

**to·rus buc·cal·is** (tōr´ŭs bŭk-ā´lis) Longitudinal cheek fold opposite occlusal plane of teeth beginning at corner of mouth.

**to·rus man·di·bu·lar·is** (tōr´ŭs man-dib´yū-lā´ris) Bony protuberance on lingual aspect of lower jaw in canine-premolar region.

**tor·us pal·a·ti·nus** (tōr´ŭs pal´ă-tī´nŭs) Bony protuberance in midline of hard palate. SYN maxillary torus.

**to·tal lung ca·pac·i·ty (TLC)** (tō´tăl lŭng kă-pas´i-tē) The inspiratory capacity plus the functional residual capacity.

**to·tal par·en·ter·al nu·tri·tion (TPN)** (tō´tăl pă-ren´tĕr-ăl nū-trish´ŭn) Nutrition main-

st

tained entirely by central intravenous injection or other nongastrointestinal route.

**to·tal treat·ment plan** (tō'tăl trēt'měnt plan) Sequential outline of essential services and procedures that must be carried out by the dentist, the dental hygienist, and the patient to eliminate disease and restore the oral cavity.

**touch** (tŭch) **1.** Sense by which slight contact with skin or mucous membrane is appreciated. **2.** Digital examination. [Fr. *toucher*]

**Tou·rette syn·drome** (tūr-et' sin'drōm) Tic disorder appearing in childhood, characterized by multiple motor and vocal tics present for longer than 1 year. Coprolalia and echolalia rarely occur.

**tour·ni·quet** (tŭr'ni-kĕt) An instrument for temporarily arresting the flow of blood to or from a distal part by pressure applied with an encircling device. [Fr. fr. *tourner,* to turn]

**tox·e·mi·a** (tok-sē'mē-ă ) **1.** Clinical manifestations observed during some infectious diseases, assumed to be caused by toxins and other noxious substances elaborated by infectious agent. **2.** Clinical syndrome caused by toxic substances in blood. [G. *toxikon,* poison, + *haima,* blood]

**tox·ic** (tok'sik) Pertaining to a toxin. [G. *toxikon,* an arrow-poison]

**tox·ic·i·ty** (tok-sis'i-tē) State of being poisonous.

**tox·ic meg·a·co·lon** (tok'sik meg'ă-kō'lŏn) Acute nonobstructive dilation of the colon.

**toxico-** Combining form meaning poison, toxin.

**tox·i·coid** (tok'si-koyd) Having an action like that of a poison; temporarily poisonous. [*toxico-* + G. *eidos,* resemblance]

**tox·i·col·o·gist** (tok'si-kol'ŏ-jist) A specialist or expert in toxicology.

**tox·i·col·o·gy** (tok'si-kol'ŏ-jē) Science of poisons, including their source, chemical composition, action, tests, and antidotes. [*toxico-* + G. *logos,* study]

**tox·ic shock syn·drome (TSS)** (tok'sik shok sin'drōm) Infection with toxin-producing staphylococci, occurring most often in vagina of menstruating women using superabsorbent tampons but also prevalent in many soft tissue infections.

**tox·in** (tok'sin) Noxious or poisonous substance formed or elaborated either as an integral part of the cell or tissue (endotoxin), as an extracellular product (exotoxin), or as a combination, during metabolism and growth of some microorganisms and some higher plant and animal species. [G. *toxikon,* poison]

**tox·o·ca·ri·a·sis** (tok'sō-kă-rī'ă-sis) Infection with nematodes of the genus *Toxocara.*

**tox·oid** (tok'soyd) Toxin that has been treated (commonly with formaldehyde) to destroy its toxic property but retain its antigenicity, i.e., its capability of stimulating the production of antitoxin antibodies and thus of producing an active immunity. [*toxin* + G. *eidos,* resemblance]

**Tox·o·plas·ma gon·di·i** (tok'sō-plaz'mă gon'dē-ī) Abundant, widespread sporozoan species that may cause in utero infection. [G. *toxon,* bow or arc, + *plasma,* anything formed]

**tox·o·plas·mo·sis** (tok'sō-plaz-mō'sis) Disease caused by the protozoan parasite *Toxoplasma gondii,* which can produce various syndromes in humans. Prenatally acquired human infection can result in presence of abnormalities such as microcephalus or hydrocephalus at birth, development of jaundice with hepatosplenomegaly or meningoencephalitis in early childhood, or delayed appearance of ocular lesions such as chorioretinitis in later childhood.

**TPN** Abbreviation for total parenteral nutrition.

**Tr** Abbreviation for tincture; tragion; treatment.

**tra·bec·u·la,** pl. **tra·bec·u·lae** (tră-bek' yū-lă, -lē) [TA] Meshwork; one of the supporting bundles of fibers traversing substance of a structure, usually derived from the capsule or one of the fibrous septa. [L. dim. of *trabs,* a beam]

**tra·bec·u·lar bone** (tră-bek'yū-lăr bōn) SYN substantia spongiosa.

**trace** (trās) **1.** Evidence of former existence, influence, or action of an object, phenomenon, or event. **2.** Extremely small amount or barely discernible indication of something.

**trac·er** (trā'sĕr) **1.** A mechanical device with a marking point attached to one jaw and a graph plate or tracing plate attached to the other jaw; used to record direction and extent of mandibular movements. **2.** An element or compound containing atoms that can be distinguished from their normal counterparts by physical means (e.g., radioactivity assay or mass spectrography) and can thus be used to follow (trace) metabolism of normal substances. **3.** Colored or radioactive substance that can be injected in region of a tumor (e.g., melanoma, breast) to map lymph flow from tumor to its nearest nodal basin; used in sentinel node detection.

**tra·che·a,** pl. **tra·che·ae** (trā'kē-ă, -ē) [TA] Air tube extending from larynx into thorax to level of the fifth or sixth thoracic vertebra where it bifurcates into right and left bronchi. SYN windpipe. [G. *tracheia artēria,* rough artery]

**tra·che·al in·tu·ba·tion** (trā'kē-ăl in'tū-bā'shŭn) Passage of a tube through nose, mouth, or tracheotomy to maintain a patent airway.

**trach·e·lism, trach·e·lis·mus** (trăk′ĕ-lizm, -liz′mŭs) Bending the neck backward, such as sometimes ushers in an epileptic attack. [G. *trachēlismos*, a seizing by the throat]

**trach·e·los·chi·sis** (trak′ĕ-los′ki-sis) Congenital neck fissure. [*trachelo*- + G. *schisis*, fissure]

♻ **tracheo-, trache-** Combining forms denoting the trachea.

**tra·che·o·bron·chi·al** (trā′kē-ō-brong′kē-ăl) Relating to both trachea and bronchi, denoting especially a set of lymph nodes.

**tra·che·o·bron·chos·co·py** (trā′kē-ō-brong-kos′kŏ-pē) Inspection of the interior of the trachea and bronchi. [*tracheo*- + *bronchus*, + G. *skopeō*, to view]

**tra·che·o·e·so·pha·ge·al fold** (trā′kē-ō-ĕ-sof′ă-jē′ăl fōld) Longitudinal folds in respiratory diverticulum that fuse to form tracheoesophageal septum. SYN tracheoesophageal ridge.

**tra·che·o·e·so·pha·ge·al ridge** (trā′kē-ō-ĕ-sof′ă-jē′ăl rij) SYN tracheoesophageal fold.

**tra·che·o·la·ryn·ge·al** (trā′kē-ō-lă-rin′jē-ăl) Relating to the trachea and the larynx.

**tra·che·oph·o·ny** (trā′kē-of′ŏ-nē) Hollow voice sound heard in auscultation of the trachea. [*tracheo*- + G. *phōnē*, voice]

**tra·che·os·co·py** (trā′kē-os′kŏ-pē) Inspection of the interior of the trachea. [*tracheo*- + G. *skopeō*, to examine]

**tra·che·o·ste·no·sis** (trā′kē-ō-stĕ-nō′sis) Narrowing of the lumen of the trachea. [*tracheo*- + G. *stenōsis*, constriction]

**tra·che·os·to·my** (trā′kē-os′tŏ-mē) SYN tracheotomy. [*tracheo*- + G. *stoma*, mouth]

**tra·che·o·tome** (trā′kē-ō-tōm) A knife used to perform tracheotomy.

**tra·che·ot·o·my** (trā′kē-ot′ŏ-mē) The operation of creating an opening into the trachea, usually intended to be temporary. SYN tracheostomy. [*tracheo*- + G. *tomē*, incision]

**trac·ing** (trās′ing) In dentistry, line or lines, scribed on a table or plate by a pointed instrument, representing a record of mandibular movements; may be extraoral (made outside the oral cavity) or intraoral (made within the oral cavity).

**tract** (trakt) [TA] **1.** Elongated area; passage or pathway. **2.** Abnormal passage (e.g., a fistula or sinus communicating with an abscess cavity). [L. *tractus*, a drawing out]

**trac·tion** (trak′shŭn) Act of drawing or pulling, as by an elastic or spring force. [L. *tractio*, fr. *traho*, pp. *tractus*, to draw]

**trag·i·on (Tr)** (trāj′ē-on) A cephalometric point in the notch just above the tragus of the ear; it lies 1–2 mm below the spine of the helix, which can be palpated.

**tra·gus,** pl. **tra·gi** (trā′gŭs, -jī) A tonguelike projection of the cartilage of the auricle in front of the opening of the external acoustic meatus and continuous with the cartilage of this canal. SYN hircus (3). [G. *tragos*, goat, in allusion to the hairs growing on the part, like a goatee]

**trait** (trāt) **1.** A qualitative characteristic. **2.** Discrete attribute as contrasted with metric character. [Fr. from L. *tractus*, a drawing out, extension]

**tran·quil·iz·er** (trang′kwi-lī-zĕr) Drug that promotes tranquility by calming, and pacifying with minimal sedation.

**trans·am·i·nase** (tranz-am′i-nās) SYN aminotransferase.

**trans·am·i·na·tion** (tranz′am-i-nā′shŭn) The reaction between an amino acid and an α-keto acid through which the amino group is transferred from the former to the latter.

**tran·scrip·tase** (tran-skrip′tās) Polymerase associated with process of transcription; may be RNA or DNA dependent. [L. *transcribo*, pp. *transcriptum*, to copy, + *-ase*]

**trans·der·mal** (trans-dĕr′măl) Entering through the dermis or skin. SYN topical administration.

**trans·du·cer** (trans-dū′sĕr) A device that converts energy from one form to another.

**trans·fec·tion** (trans-fek′shŭn) A method of gene transfer using infection of a cell with nucleic acid (as from a retrovirus) resulting in subsequent viral replication in the transfected cell. [*trans*- + *infection*]

**trans·fer cop·ing** (trans′fĕr kōp′ing) In dentistry, metallic or acrylic resin or other covering or cap used to position a die in an impression.

**trans·for·ma·tion** (trans′fŏr-mā′shŭn) **1.** A change of one tissue into another, as in cartilage into bone. **2.** In metals, change in phase and physical properties in solid state caused by heat treatment. [L. *trans-formo*, pp. *-atus*, to transform]

**trans·fu·sion** (trans-fyū′zhŭn) Transfer of blood or blood component from one person (donor) to another person (recipient). [L. *trans-fundo*, pp. *-fusus*, to pour from one vessel to another]

**tran·si·ent** (trans′shĕnt, -sē-ĕnt) Short-lived; passing; not permanent. [L. *transeo*, pres. p. *transiens*, to cross over]

**tran·si·ent fa·cial pa·ral·y·sis** (trans′shĕnt fā′shăl păr-al′i-sis) Short-term loss of motor activity of a muscle innervated by the facial nerve because of injury or disease involv-

st

ing such nerve or muscle. A common cause is incorrect local anesthetic placement about the facial nerve that took place during an inferior alveolar nerve block.

**tran·si·ent is·che·mic at·tack (TIA)** (tran′shĕnt is-kē′mik ă-tak′) Sudden focal loss of neurologic function with complete recovery usually within 24 hours; caused by a brief period of inadequate perfusion in a portion of the territory of the carotid or vertebral basilar arteries.

**🔲trans·il·lu·mi·na·tion** (tranz′i-lū′mi-nā′shŭn) Method of examination by passage of light through tissues or a body cavity. See this page. [*trans-* + L. *illumino*, pp. *-atus*, to light up]

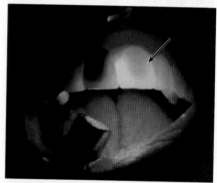

**transillumination:** light passing through an artificial crown; dark shadow (arrow) is remaining crown of natural tooth

**trans·il·lum·i·na·tion test** (tranz′i-lū′mi-nā′shŭn test) Dental assessment using transmitted light to produce a shadow of the root if the pulp is necrotic or has earlier been replaced by a filling material.

**tran·si·tion·al cell car·ci·no·ma** (tran-zish′ŭn-ăl sel kahr′si-nō′mă) A malignant neoplasm derived from transitional epithelium.

**tran·si·tio·nal den·ti·tion** (tran-zish′ŭn-ăl den-tish′ŭn) SYN mixed dentition.

**tran·si·tion·al den·ture** (tran-zish′ŭn-ăl den′chŭr) Partial denture that serves as a temporary prosthesis to which teeth will be added as more teeth are lost, and that will be replaced after postextraction tissue changes have occurred; may become an interim denture when all teeth have been removed from dental arch.

**trans·la·tion** (trans-lā′shŭn) In dentistry, movement of a tooth through alveolar bone without change in axial inclination.

**trans·lo·ca·tion** (trans′lō-kā′shŭn) 1. Transposition of two segments between nonhomologous chromosomes as a result of abnormal breakage and refusion of reciprocal segments. 2. Transport of a metabolite across a biomem-

brane. [*trans-* + L. *location*, placement, fr. *loco*, to place]

**trans·lu·cen·cy** (trans-lū′sĕn-sē) Characteristic of a substance that is partially able to allow light to pass through it.

**trans·mi·gra·tion** (trans′mī-grā′shŭn) Movement from one site to another; may entail crossing some usually limiting barrier, as in passage of blood cells through walls of vessels (diapedesis). [L. *transmigro*, pp. *-atus*, to remove from one place to another]

**trans·mis·si·ble** (trans-mis′i-bĕl) Capable of being transmitted (carried across) from one person to another.

**trans·mis·sion** (trans-mish′ŭn) 1. Conveyance of disease from one person to another. 2. Passage of a nerve impulse across an anatomic cleft. [L. *transmissio*, a sending across]

**trans·mu·co·sal de·liv·er·y** (trans-myū-kō′săl dĕ-liv′ĕr-ē) Drug delivery system wherein the drug traverses the intact mucosa.

**trans·par·ent den·tin** (trans-par′ĕnt den′tin) SYN sclerotic dentin.

**trans·plant** (trans-plant′, trans′plant) 1. To transfer from one part to another, as in grafting and transplantation. 2. The tissue or organ in grafting and transplantation. SEE ALSO graft. [*trans-* + L. *planto*, to plant]

**trans·port** (trans′pōrt) The movement or transference of biochemical substances in biologic systems. [L. *transporto*, to carry over, fr. *trans-* + *porto*, to carry]

**trans·pose** (trans-pōz′) To transfer one tissue or organ in place of another. [L. *trans-pono*, pp. *-positus*, to place across, transfer]

**trans·po·si·tion** (trans′pŏ-zish′ŭn) 1. Misplacement of teeth from normal sequence in the arch. 2. Removal from one place to another; metathesis. 3. Condition of being in wrong place or on wrong side of the body.

**trans·sep·tal fi·bers** (tran-sep′tăl fī′bĕrz) Type II collagen fibers running from tooth to tooth over crest of alveolus; constitute bulk of the interdental papilla.

**tran·su·date** (tran′sū-dāt) Any fluid (solvent and solute) that has passed through a presumably normal membrane, such as the capillary wall, as a result of imbalanced hydrostatic and osmotic forces. [*trans-* + L. *sudo*, pp. *-atus*, to sweat]

**tran·sude** (trans-yūd′) In general, to ooze or to pass a liquid gradually through a membrane.

**trans·verse** (trans-vĕrs′) [TA] Crosswise; lying across the long axis of the body or of a part. [L. *transversus*]

**trans·verse hor·i·zon·tal ax·is** (trans-věrs′ hōr′i-zon′tăl ak′sis) An imaginary line through both temporomandibular joints about which the mandible rotates in the sagittal plane during opening and closing of the mouth. SYN hinge axis, mandibular axis (1).

**trans·verse plane** (trans-věrs′ plān) [TA] Plane across body at right angles to coronal and sagittal planes; perpendicular to long axis of body or limbs, regardless of position of body or limb; in the anatomic position, they are horizontal; otherwise two terms not synonymous.

**trans·verse ridge** (trans-věrs′ rij) [TA] SYN crista transversalis.

**trans·verse sec·tion** (trans-věrs′ sek′ shŭn) A cross-section obtained by slicing, actually or through imaging techniques, the body or any part of the body structure, in a horizontal plane, i.e., a plane that intersects the longitudinal axis at a angle. SYN axial section.

**trans·ver·sion** (trans-věr′zhŭn) In dentistry, eruption of a tooth in a position normally occupied by another; transposition of a tooth.

**trans·ves·tism** (trans-ves′tizm) Practice of dressing or masquerading in the clothes of the opposite sex. [*trans-* + L. *vestio*, to dress]

**trau·ma**, pl. **trau·ma·ta, trau·mas** (traw′ mă, -mă-tă, -măz) An injury, physical or mental. See this page. [G. wound]

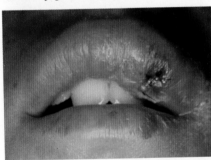

**trauma:** swollen ulcerated upper lip

**trau·ma from oc·clu·sion** (traw′mă ŏ-klū′zhŭn) Reversible lesion in periodontium caused by excessive movement of teeth.

**trau·mat·ic** (traw-mat′ik) Relating to or caused by trauma. [G. *traumatikos*]

**trau·mat·ic an·es·the·si·a** (traw-mat′ik an′es-thē′zē-ă) Loss of sensation resulting from nerve injury.

**trau·mat·ic brain in·ju·ry (TBI)** (traw-mat′ik brān in′jŭr-ē) An insult to the brain as the result of physical trauma or external force, not degenerative or congenital, which may cause a diminished or altered state of consciousness and may impair cognitive, behavioral, physical, or emotional functioning.

**trau·mat·ic fe·ver** (traw-mat′ik fē′vĕr) Elevation of temperature after an injury.

**trau·mat·ic neu·ro·ma** (traw-mat′ik nūr-ō′ mă) The nonneoplastic proliferative mass of Schwann cells and neurites that may develop at the proximal end of a severed or injured nerve. SYN amputation neuroma, false neuroma.

**trau·ma·tize** (traw′mă-tīz) To cause or inflict trauma. [G. *traumatizō*, to wound]

**trau·ma·to·gen·ic oc·clu·sion** (traw′mă-tō-jen′ik ŏ-klū′zhŭn) Malocclusion capable of hurting teeth or associated structures. Also called traumatic occlusion.

**trau·ma·to·ther·a·py** (traw′mă-tō-thār′ă-pē) Treatment of trauma or the result of injury.

**tra·verse** (tră-věrs′) In computed tomography, one complete linear movement of the gantry across the object being scanned.

**tray** (trā) A flat receptacle with raised edges.

**tray com·pound** (trā kom′pownd) Colloq. usage for impression compound used in an impression tray.

**Treach·er Col·lins syn·drome** (trěch′ĕr kol′inz sin′drōm) Mandibulofacial dysostosis characterized by bone abnormalities of structures formed from the first pharyngeal arch, including a large, fishlike mouth with dental abnormalities.

**treat** (trēt) To manage a defect or disease by medicinal, surgical, or other measures; to care for a patient surgically or medically. [Fr. *traiter*, fr. L. *tracto*, to drag, handle, perform]

**treat·ment (Tx, Tr)** (trēt′mĕnt) Medical or surgical management of a patient.

**treat·ment den·ture** (trēt′mĕnt den′chŭr) Dental prosthesis used to treat or condition tissues that are called on to support and retain a denture base.

**treat·ment plan** (trēt′mĕnt plan) Established sequence of dental therapy reached after diagnosis and case study.

**trem·a·tode, trem·a·toid** (trem′ă-tōd, -toyd) Common name for a fluke of the class Trematoda.

**trem·or** (trem′ŏr) 1. Repetitive, often regular, oscillatory movements caused by alternate, or synchronous, but irregular contraction of opposing muscle groups; usually involuntary. 2. Minute ocular movement occurring during fixation on an object. [L. a shaking]

**trench mouth** (trench mowth) SYN necrotizing ulcerative gingivitis.

**Tren·de·len·burg po·si·tion** (tren-del′ĕn-bŭrg pŏ-zish′ŭn) A supine position on the operating table, which is inclined at varying angles

st

so that the pelvis is higher than the head; used during and after operations in the pelvis or to treat shock.

**trep·a·na·tion** (trep′ă-nā′shŭn) SYN trephination.

**treph·i·na·tion** (tref′i-nā′shŭn) Removal of a circular piece of cranium by a trephine.

**tre·phine, tre·pan** (trē-fīn′, trĕ-pan′) **1.** A cylindric or crown saw used for the removal of a disc of bone, especially from the skull, or of other firm tissue. **2.** To remove a disc of bone or other tissue by means of a trephine. [contrived fr. L. *tres fines,* three ends]

**Trep·o·ne·ma** (trep′ō-nē′mă) A genus of anaerobic bacteria pathogenic and parasitic for humans and other animals, generally producing local lesions in tissues. [G. *trepō,* to turn, + *nēma,* thread]

**Trep·o·ne·ma pal·li·dum** (trep′ō-nē′mă pal′i-dŭm) Bacterial species that causes syphilis in humans.

**Tre·sil·i·an sign** (trē-sil′ē-ăn sīn) Reddish prominence at orifice of parotid duct, found in mumps.

**tre·sis** (trē′sis) SYN perforation.

**tret·i·no·in** (tret′i-nō′in) A keratolytic agent.

**tri·ad** (trī′ad) **1.** A collection of three things with something in common. **2.** The transverse tubule and the terminal cisternae on each side of it in skeletal muscle fibers. [G. *trias (triad-),* the number 3, fr. *treis,* three]

**tri·age** (trē′ahzh) **1.** Medical screening of patients to determine their relative priority for treatment. **2.** Separation of a large number of casualties, in military or civilian disaster medical care, into three groups: those who cannot be expected to survive even with treatment; those who will recover without treatment; and the highest priority, those who will not survive without treatment. [Fr. sorting]

**tri·al** (trī′ăl) A test or experiment, usually conducted under specific conditions.

**tri·al base** (trī′ăl bās) SYN baseplate. [M.E., fr. O.Fr. *trier,* to sort, distinguish]

**tri·al den·ture** (trī′ăl den′chŭr) Setup of artificial teeth fabricated so that it may be placed in the patient's mouth to verify esthetics, for making records, or any other operation deemed necessary before final completion of denture. SYN wax model denture.

**tri·an·gle** (trī′ang-gĕl) [TA] In anatomy and surgery, three-sided area with arbitrary or natural boundaries. [L. *triangulum,* fr. *tri-,* three, + *angulus,* angle]

**tri·an·gu·lar crest** (trī-ang′gyū-lăr krest) SYN crista triangularis.

**tri·an·gu·lar ridge** (trī-ang′gyū-lăr rij) [TA] SYN crista triangularis.

**tri·ceps,** pl. **tri·ceps, tri·cep·ses** (trī′seps, -ĕz) Three-headed; denoting especially two muscles. [L. fr. *tri-,* three, + *caput,* head]

**trich·al·gi·a** (trik-al′jē-ă) Pain produced by touching the hair; painful hair, as seen in atypical angina. [*trich-* + G. *algos,* pain]

**Trich·i·nel·la spi·ra·lis** (trik′i-nel′ă spī-rā′lis) The pork or trichina worm, a species of parasites that cause trichinosis, found in most regions of the world but more frequently in the Northern Hemisphere; transmission occurs as a result of ingesting raw or inadequately cooked meat (especially pork but now often associated with game animals such as bear or walrus).

**trich·i·no·sis** (trik-i-nō′sis) The disease resulting from ingestion of raw or inadequately cooked pork (or bear or walrus meat) that contains encysted larvae of the nematode parasite *Trichinella spiralis.* [*Trichinella* (trichina) + G. *-osis,* condition]

**tricho-** The hair; a hairlike structure. [G. *thrix (trich-)*]

**trich·o·ep·i·the·li·o·ma** (trik′ō-ep′i-thē′lē-ō′mă) Any of numerous small benign nodules, occurring mostly on the face, derived from basal cells of hair follicles enclosing small keratin cysts. SYN Brooke tumor. [*tricho-* + *epithelioma*]

**trich·o·es·the·si·a** (trik′ō-es-thē′zē-ă) Form of paresthesia in which there is a sensation as of a hair on the skin, on the mucous membrane of the mouth, or on the conjunctiva. [*tricho-* + G. *aisthēsis,* sensation]

**tri·choph·a·gy** (tri-kof′ă-jē) Habitual biting of one's hair. [*tricho-* + G. *phagein,* to eat]

**trich·o·phy·to·be·zo·ar** (trik′ō-fī′tō-bē′zōr) Mixed hair and food ball, consisting of vegetable fibers, seeds and skins of fruits, and animal hair matted together to form a ball in the stomach. [*tricho-* + G. *phyton,* plant, + *bezoar*]

**trich·o·rhi·no·pha·lan·ge·al syn·drome** (trik′ō-rī′nō-fă-lan′jē-ăl sin′drōm) Condition characterized by sparse fine hair, broad nose with a long philtrum, swollen middle phalanges with cone-shaped epiphyses, and growth retardation.

**trich·o·til·lo·ma·ni·a** (trik′ō-til′ō-mā′nē-ă) A compulsion to pull out one's own hair. [*tricho-* + G. *tillo,* pull out, + *mania,* insanity]

**trich·u·ri·a·sis** (trik′yū-rī′ă-sis) Infection with nematodes of the genus *Trichuris.* In humans, intestinal parasitization by *T. trichiura* is usually asymptomatic and not associated with peripheral eosinophilia.

**Tri·chu·ris** (tri-kyūr′is) A genus of aphasmid nematodes related to the trichina worm. [*tricho-* + G. *oura,* tail]

**tri·clo·san** (trī′klō-san) Biphenyl agent used in dentifrices.

**tri·co·no·dont** (trī-kŏ′nō-dont) Referring to a tooth having three cones or cusps in a linear arrangement; central one is largest. [*tri-* + G. *kōnos,* cone, + *odous,* tooth]

**tri·cus·pid, tri·cus·pi·dal, tri·cus·pi·date** (trī-kŭs′pid, -pi-dăl, -pi-dāt) **1.** In dentistry, having three tubercles or cusps, as second upper molar tooth (occasionally) and upper third molar (usually). **2.** In anatomy, having three points, prongs, or cusps, as the tricuspid valve of the heart.

**tri·cyc·lic an·ti·de·pres·sant (TCA)** (trī-sī′klik an′tē-dĕ-pres′ănt) Chemical group of antidepressants that share three-ringed nucleus.

**tri·dent** (trī′dent) SEE tridentate.

**tri·den·tate** (trī-den′tāt) Three-toothed; three-pronged. [*tri-* + L. *dentatus,* toothed]

**trid·y·mite** (trid′i-mīt) Form of silica used in dental casting investment. [fr. G. *tridymos,* threefold]

**tri·fa·cial** (trī-fā′shăl) Denoting trigeminal nerves. [*tri-* + L. *facies,* face]

**tri·fa·cial nerve** (trī-fā′shăl nĕrv) SYN trigeminal nerve [CN V].

**tri·fid** (trī′fid) Split into three parts. [L. *trifidus,* three-cleft]

**tri·fur·ca·ted root** (trī′fŭr-kā-tĕd rūt) Division of a tooth root structure into three sections.

**tri·fur·ca·tion** (trī′fŭr-kā′shŭn) **1.** Area where tooth roots divide into three distinct portions. **2.** A division into three branches. [*tri-* + L. *furca,* fork]

**tri·fur·ca·tion in·volve·ment** (trī′fŭr-kā′shŭn in-volv′mĕnt) Colloq. for dental decay or periodontal disease that affects the area of the tooth where the root separates into three parts. Maxillary molars have three roots and are most commonly affected.

**tri·gem·i·nal gan·gli·on** (trī-jĕm′i-năl gang′glē-ŏn) [TA] The large, flattened sensory ganglion of the trigeminal nerve lying close to the cavernous sinus along the medial part of the middle cranial fossa in the trigeminal cavity of the dura mater.

**tri·gem·i·nal nerve [CN V]** (trī-jem′i-năl nĕrv) [TA] Chief sensory nerve of face and motor nerve of muscles of mastication; its nuclei are in the mesencephalon and in the pons and medulla oblongata extending down into the cervical portion of the spinal cord. SYN fifth cranial nerve [CN V], nervus trigeminus [CN V], trifacial nerve.

**tri·gem·i·nal neu·ral·gi·a** (trī-jem′i-năl nūr-al′jē-ă) Severe, paroxysmal pain in one or more branches of trigeminal nerve; often induced by touching trigger points in or about the mouth. SYN facial neuralgia, tic douloureux.

**trig·ger point** (trig′ĕr poynt) Focus of hyper-irritability in tissue that, when palpated or otherwise stimulated, is locally tender and gives rise to referred pain.

**tri·gone** (trī′gōn) [TA] First three dominant cusps (protocone, paracone, and metacone), taken collectively, of an upper molar tooth. [L. *trigonum,* fr. G. *trigōnon,* triangle]

**tri·gon·id** (trī-gon′id) First three dominant cusps of a lower molar tooth.

**tri·l·o·gy of Fal·lot** (tril′ŏ-jē fah-lō′) A set of congenital defects including pulmonic stenosis, atrial septal defect, and right ventricular hypertrophy. SYN Fallot triad.

**tri·mes·ter** (trī′mes-tĕr) A period of 3 months. [L. *trimestris,* of 3-months′ duration]

**tri·meth·o·prim (TMP)** (trī-meth′ō-prim) An antimicrobial agent that potentiates effect of sulfonamides and sulfones.

**tri·meth·o·prim-sul·fa·meth·ox·a·zole (TMP/SMX)** (trī-meth′ō-prim sŭl′fă-meth-oks′ă-zōl) Drug combination consisting of a dihydrofolate reductase inhibitor and a sulfonamide antibacterial drug; drug combination is synergistic as the drugs interfere with two successive steps in formation/use of folic acid by microorganisms. Used to treat many infectious diseases.

**tri·plant im·plant** (trī′plant im′plant) Combination of three pin implants to form a single abutment to support or retain a dental prosthesis.

**tri·ple·gi·a** (trī-plē′jē-ă) **1.** Paralysis of an upper and a lower extremity and of the face. **2.** Paralysis of three limbs, both extremities on one side and one on the other. [*tri-* + G. *plēgē,* stroke]

**tris·mus** (triz′mŭs) Persistent contraction of masseter muscles due to failure of central inhibition; often initial manifestation of generalized tetanus. SYN ankylostoma, lockjaw. [L. fr. G. *trismos,* a creaking, rasping]

**tri·so·my** (trī′sō-mē) State of an individual or cell with an extra chromosome instead of normal pair of homologous chromosomes; in humans, the state of a cell containing 47 normal chromosomes. [*tri-* + (chromo)*some*]

**tri·so·my 8 syn·drome** (trī′sō-mē sin′drŏm) Full trisomy 8 is usually associated with early lethality, but most affected patients are mosaic with craniofacial dysmorphism; short, wide neck; narrow cylindric trunk; multiple joint and digital abnormalities; and deep creases of palms and soles.

**tri·so·my 13 syn·drome** (trī′sō-mē sin′drŏm) Chromosomal disorder usually fatal within 2 years; characterized by mental retardation, malformed ears, cleft lip or palate, micro-

st

phthalmia or coloboma, small mandible, polydactyly, cardiac defects, convulsions, renal anomalies, umbilical hernia, malrotation of intestines, and dermatoglyphic anomalies.

**tri·so·my 18 syn·drome** (trī′sō-mē sin′ drōm) Chromosomal disorder usually fatal within 2–3 years; characterized by mental retardation, abnormal skull shape, low-set and malformed ears, small mandible, cardiac defects, short sternum, diaphragmatic or inguinal hernia, ileal diverticulum, abnormal flexion of fingers, and dermatoglyphic anomalies.

**tri·so·my 20 syn·drome** (trī′sō-mē sin′ drōm) Chromosomal disorder characterized by profound mental retardation, coarse facies, macrostomia and macroglossia, minor anomalies of the ears, pigmentary dysplasia of skin, dorsal kyphoscoliosis, and other skeletal defects.

**tri·ta·no·pi·a** (trī′tă-nō′pē-ă) Deficient color perception in which there is an absence of blue-sensitive pigment in the retinal cones. [G. *tritos,* third, + *an-* priv. + *ōps,* eye]

**trit·ur·ate** (trit′yūr-āt, -ăt) 1. To accomplish trituration. 2. A triturated substance.

**trit·ur·a·tion** (trit′yūr-ā′shŭn) 1. Mixing dental amalgam in a mortar and pestle or with a mechanical device. 2. Reducing a drug to a fine powder and incorporating it thoroughly with sugar of milk by rubbing the two together in a mortar. [L. *trituratio,* fr. *trituro,* to thresh, fr. *tero,* pp. *tritus,* to rub]

**triv·i·al name** (triv′ē-ăl nām) A name of a chemical, no part of which is necessarily used in a systematic sense; i.e., it gives little or no indication as to chemical structure. Such names are common for drugs, hormones, proteins, and other biologicals, and are used by the general public. They may not be officially sanctioned, in contrast to nonproprietary names, but may be adopted as official nonproprietary names as a result of widespread usage.

**tro·che** (trō′kē) *Avoid the mispronunciation trōsh.* A small, discoid or rhombic body composed of solidifying paste containing an astringent, antiseptic, or demulcent drug, used for local treatment of mouth or throat. Troches are meant to dissolve in the mouth and are also called lozenges and pastilles. SYN lozenge, morsulus. [L. *trochiscus* fr. G. *trochiskos,* a little wheel, fr. *trochos,* a wheel]

**troch·le·a,** pl. **troch·le·ae** (trok′lē-ă, -ē) [TA] 1. Structure serving as a pulley. 2. Smooth articular surface of bone on which another glides. [L. pulley, fr. G. *trochileia,* a pulley, fr. *trechō,* to run]

**troch·le·ar nerve [CN IV]** (trok′lē-ăr nĕrv) [TA] Nerve that supplies superior oblique muscle of eye. SYN fourth cranial nerve [CN IV], nervus trochlearis [CN IV], pathetic nerve.

**troph·ic** (trō′fik) 1. Relating to or dependent on nutrition. 2. Resulting from interruption of nerve supply. [G. *trophē,* nourishment]

**troph·o·blast** (trō′fō-blast) Mesectodermal cell layer covering the blastocyst that erodes uterine mucosa and through which embryo receives nourishment from mother. [*tropho-* + G. *blastos,* germ]

**troph·o·derm** (trof′ō-dĕrm) The trophectoderm, or trophoblast, together with vascular mesodermal layer underlying it. [*tropho-* + G. *derma,* skin]

**troph·o·der·ma·to·neu·ro·sis** (trō′fō-dĕr′mă-tō-nūr-ō′sis) Trophic changes (e.g., dryness, thinness, increased susceptibility to infections) of a cutaneous area due to that area's innervation.

**troph·o·neu·ro·sis** (trō′fō-nūr-ō′sis) A trophic disorder, such as atrophy, hypertrophy, or a skin eruption, occurring as a consequence of disease or injury of nerves of the body part. [*tropho-* + G. *neuron,* nerve, + *-osis,* condition]

**trough** (trawf) 1. Long, narrow, shallow channel or depression. 2. Lowest point in variable measurement.

**Trous·seau sign** (trū-sō′ sīn) In latent tetany, occurrence of carpopedal spasm accompanied by paresthesia elicited when upper arm is compressed, as in use of a tourniquet or a blood pressure cuff.

**Trp** Abbreviation for tryptophan.

**true an·ky·lo·sis** (trū ang′ki-lō′sis) SYN synostosis.

**tru·sion** (trū′zhŭn) Displacement of a body, e.g., a tooth, from an initial position. [L. *trudo,* pp. *trusus,* to thrust]

**truth se·rum** (trūth sēr′ŭm) Colloquialism for a drug (e.g., amobarbital sodium, thiopental sodium) intravenously injected with scopolamine to elicit information from subject under its influence.

**try-in** (trī′in) Preliminary insertion of a complete denture wax-up (trial denture), of a partial denture casting, or of a finished restoration to determine fit, esthetics, and maxillomandibular relation.

**tryp·sin** (trip′sin) Proteolytic enzyme formed in small intestine from trypsinogen by action of enteropeptidase; serine proteinase that hydrolyzes peptides, amides, and esters, at bonds of carboxyl groups of L-arginyl or L-lysyl residues.

**tryp·tase** (trip′tās) A neutral protease released from mast cells during cellular activation and degranulation. [*trypt-,* fr. *trypsin,* fr. G. *tripsis,* a rubbing or grinding, + *-ase*]

**tryp·to·phan (Trp, W)** (trip′tŏ-fan) A nutritionally essential amino acid.

**TSS** Abbreviation for toxic shock syndrome.

**tube, tub·ing** (tūb, tūb´ing) [TA] *Avoid the redundant phrase hollow tube.* **1.** A hollow cylindric structure or canal. **2.** A hollow cylinder or pipe. [L. *tubus*]

**tube feed·ing** (tūb fēd´ing) Administering nutrition or other fluids by means of a tube inserted directly into the enteral tract. This method of administration is used when a patient is unable to swallow.

**tu·ber·cle** (tū´bĕr-kĕl) **1.** [TA] In dentistry, a small elevation arising on the surface of a tooth. **2.** [TA] A nodule, especially in an anatomic, not pathologic, sense. **3.** Circumscribed, rounded, solid elevation on skin, mucous membrane, surface of an organ, or bone surface, the last giving attachment to a muscle or ligament. **4.** A granulomatous lesion due to infection by *Mycobacterium tuberculosis*. [L. *tuberculum*, dim. of *tuber*, a knob, a swelling, a tumor]

**tu·ber·cle of tooth** (tū´bĕr-kĕl tūth) SYN dental tubercle.

**tu·ber·cle of up·per lip** (tū´bĕr-kĕl ŭp´ĕr lip) [TA] Slight projection on free edge of center of upper lip at lower extent of philtrum.

**tu·ber·cu·lid** (tū-bĕr´kyū-lid) Lesion of the skin or mucous membrane resulting from hypersensitivity to mycobacterial antigens disseminated from a distant site of active tuberculosis. [*tubercul-* + G. *-id*]

**tu·ber·cu·lin** (tū-bĕr´kyū-lin) A glycerin-broth culture of *Mycobacterium tuberculosis* evaporated to 1/10 volume at 100°C and filtered.

**tu·ber·cu·lin test** (tū-bĕr´kyū-lin test) A dermatologic procedure in which tuberculin or its purified protein derivative (PPD) is injected.

**tu·ber·cu·lin-·type hy·per·sen·si·tiv·i·ty** (tū-bĕr´kyū-lin-tīp hī´pĕr-sen´si-tiv´i-tē) SYN delayed hypersensitivity.

**tu·ber·cu·lo·sis (TB)** (tū-bĕr´kyū-lō´sis) A specific disease caused by infection with *Mycobacterium tuberculosis*, the tubercle bacillus, which can affect almost any tissue or organ of the body; most common site is in the lungs. [*tuberculo-* + G. *-osis*, condition]

**tu·ber·cu·lous spon·dy·li·tis** (tū-bĕr´kyū-lŭs spon´di-lī´tis) Tuberculous infection of the spine associated with a sharp angulation of the spine at the point of disease. SYN Pott disease.

**tu·ber·cu·lum im·par** (tū-bĕr´kyū-lŭm im´pahr) SYN median lingual swelling.

**tu·ber·os·i·ty** (tū´bĕr-os´i-tē) [TA] A large tubercle or rounded elevation, especially from bone surface.

**tu·ber·os·i·ty re·duc·tion** (tū´bĕr-os´i-tē rĕ-dŭk´shŭn) Surgical excision of excessive fibrous or bony tissue in area of maxillary tuberosity before making prosthetic appliances.

**tu·ber·ous scle·ro·sis** (tū´bĕr-ŭs skler-ō´sis) Phacomatosis characterized by the formation of multisystemic hamartomas producing seizures, mental retardation, and angiofibromas of the face. SYN Bourneville disease, epiloia.

**tube tooth** (tūb tūth) Artificial tooth constructed with a vertical, cylindric aperture extending from center of base up into tooth body into which a pin may be placed or cast to attach tooth to a denture base.

**tu·bo·cu·ra·rine chlo·ride** (tū´bō-kyūr-ahr´in klōr´īd) An alkaloid; used to produce muscular relaxation during surgical operations.

**tu·bu·lar vision** (tū´byū-lăr vizh´ŭn) A constriction of the visual field, as though one were looking through a hollow cylinder or tube. SYN tunnel vision.

**tu·bule** (tū´byūl) [TA] A small tube. [L. *tubulus*, dim. of *tubus*, tube]

**tu·bu·li·za·tion** (tū´byū-lī-zā´shŭn) Enclosing the joined ends of a divided nerve, after neurorrhaphy, in a cylinder of paraffin or of some slowly absorbable material to keep surrounding tissues from intruding and thereby preventing union.

**tu·bu·li·za·tion of nerve** (tū´byū-lī-zā´shŭn nĕrv) Enclosing the joined ends of a divided nerve, after neurorrhaphy, in a cylinder of paraffin or of some slowly absorbable material to keep surrounding tissues from pushing in and preventing union.

**tuft·ed floss** (tŭf´tĕd flaws) Combination of regular thin dental floss and a segment of a thicker, more yarnlike material. This tufted type is indicated for cleaning under crowns and bridgework, some types of orthodontic appliances, and where there are wide embrasures with missing interdental papillae.

**tug, tug·ging** (tŭg, tŭg´ing) A pulling or dragging movement or sensation.

**tu·me·fa·cient** (tū´mĕ-fā´shĕnt) Causing or tending to cause swelling. [L. *tume-facio*, to cause to swell, fr. *tumeo*, to swell]

**tu·mor** (tū´mŏr) *Avoid the jargonistic use of this word as a synonym of neoplasm.* **1.** Any swelling or tumefaction. **2.** One of the four signs of inflammation (the others are, calor, dolor, rubor) enunciated by Celsus. SYN tumour. [L. *tumor*, a swelling]

**tu·mor·i·ci·dal** (tū´mŏr-i-sī´dăl) Denoting an agent destructive to tumors. SYN tumouricidal. [*tumor* + L. *caedo*, to kill]

**tu·mor mark·er** (tū´mŏr mahr´kĕr) A substance released into the circulation by tumor tissue; its detection in the serum indicates the presence and specific type of tumor. SYN tumour marker, tumour marker.

**tu·mor sup·pres·sor gene** (tū′mŏr sŭ-pres′ŏr jēn) Gene that encodes a protein involved in controlling cellular growth. SYN tumour suppressor gene.

**tumour** [Br.] SYN tumor.

**tumouricidal** [Br.] SYN tumoricidal.

**tumour marker** [Br.] SYN tumor marker.

**tumour supressor gene** [Br.] SYN tumor suppressor gene.

**tung·sten car·bide** (tŭng′stĕn kahr′bīd) One of the hardest known materials, used as an abrasive and in manufacture of dental cutting instruments.

**tu·ni·ca in·ti·ma** (tū′ni-kă in′ti-mă) [TA] The innermost coat of a blood or lymphatic vessel; consists of endothelium, usually a thin fibroelastic subendothelial layer, and an inner elastic membrane of longitudinal fibers.

**tu·ni·ca me·di·a** (tū′ni-kă mē′dē-ă) [TA] The middle, usually muscular, coat of an artery or other tubular structure. SYN media (1).

**tun·ing** (tūn′ing) Adjusting the length of the stroke made by an electronically powered dental instrument.

**tun·nel** (tŭn′ĕl) An elongated passageway, usually open at both ends.

**tun·nel vi·sion** (tŭn′ĕl vizh′ŭn) SYN tubular vision.

**tur·bid·i·ty** (tŭr-bid′i-tē) The quality of being turbid, of losing transparency because of sediment or insoluble matter. [L. *turbiditas,* fr. *turbidus,* turbid]

**tur·gor** (tŭr′gŏr) Fullness. [L., fr. *turgeo,* to swell]

**tur·key gob·bler neck** (tŭr′kē gob′lĕr nek) Large skin folds hanging under the chin.

**Turn·er syn·drome** (tŭr′nĕr sin′drōm) A syndrome with chromosome count 45 and only one X chromosome; buccal and other cells usually test negative for sex chromatin; anomalies include dwarfism, webbed neck, valgus of elbows, pigeon chest, infantile sexual development, and amenorrhea. SYN XO syndrome.

**Turn·er tooth** (tŭr′nĕr tūth) Enamel hypoplasia involving a solitary permanent tooth; related to infection in the primary tooth that preceded it or to trauma during odontogenesis.

**tus·si·gen·ic** (tŭs′i-jen′ik) Causing cough. [L. *tussis,* cough, + *-gen,* producing]

**tus·sive frem·i·tus** (tŭs′iv frem′i-tŭs) Form of fremitus similar to vocal, produced by a cough.

**TWAR** (twahr) [Acronym derived from the laboratory designations of the first two isolates, TW-83 and AR-39] SYN *Chlamydia pneumoniae.*

**Tweed edge·wise treat·ment** (twēd ej′wīz trēt′mĕnt) SEE edgewise appliance.

**Tweed tri·an·gle** (twēd trī′ang-gĕl) Area defined by facial and dental landmarks on a lateral cephalometric film, using the Frankfurt horizontal plane as a base and intended for use as a guide in the evaluation and planning of orthodontic treatment.

**twelfth cra·ni·al nerve [CN XII]** (twelfth krā′nē-ăl nĕrv) SYN hypoglossal nerve [CN XII].

**twelfth-year mo·lar** (twelfth-yēr mō′lăr) Second permanent molar tooth.

**twin** (twin) **1.** One of two children born at a single birth. May be monozygotic or dizygotic. **2.** Double; growing in pairs. [A.S. *getwin,* double]

**twinge** (twinj) A sudden momentary sharp pain.

**twin·ning** (twin′ing) Production of equivalent structures by division; tendency of divided parts to assume symmetric relations. See this page.

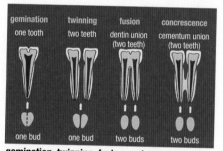

gemination, twinning, fusion, and concrescence

**twitch** (twich) **1.** To jerk spasmodically. **2.** Momentary spasmodic contraction of a muscle fiber. [A.S. *twiccian*]

**two-point con·tact** (tū′poynt kon′takt) Method of correct adaptation of a periodontal file to the tooth with the working-end on the calculus deposit and the lower shank resting against the tooth; provides additional stability and leverage needed when using a file.

**two-tone dis·clos·ing so·lu·tion** (tū′tōn dis-klōz′ing sŏ-lū′shŭn) Topically applied dye that stains older plaque blue and newer plaque red. SEE ALSO trifurcation.

**Tx** Abbreviation for treatment.

**tym·pan·ic** (tim-pan′ik) **1.** Relating to the tympanic cavity or membrane. **2.** Resonant.

**tym·pan·ic cav·i·ty** (tim-pan′ik kav′i-tē) [TA] An air chamber in the temporal bone, medial to the tympanic membrane, between the external acoustic meatus and the inner ear containing the ossicles. SYN cavity of middle ear.

**tym·pan·ic mem·brane** (tim-pan′ik mem′ brăn) [TA] A thin tense membrane forming the greater part of the lateral wall of the tympanic cavity and separating it from the external acoustic meatus. SYN eardrum. [L. *membrana tympani*]

**tym·pa·ni·tes** (timp′ă-nī′tēz) Swelling of the abdomen resulting from gas in intestinal or peritoneal cavity. [L. fr. G. *tympanitēs*, an edema in which the belly is stretched like a drum, *tympanon*]

**tym·pa·nit·ic** (tim′pă-nit′ik) **1.** Referring to tympanites. **2.** Denoting quality of sound elicited by percussing over inflated intestine or a large pulmonary cavity.

**tym·pa·no·hy·al** (tim′pă-nō-hī′ăl) Pertaining to the relationship between tympanic cavity and hyoid arch.

**tym·pa·no·hy·al bone** (tim′pă-nō-hī′ăl bōn) Small nodule of bone forming base of the cartilaginous styloid process of temporal bone at birth.

**tym·pa·no·man·dib·u·lar** (tim′pă-nō-man-dib′yū-lăr) Relating to the tympanic cavity and the mandible.

**tym·pa·no·mas·toid fis·sure** (tim′ pă-nō-mas′toyd fish′ŭr) [TA] A fissure that separates the tympanic portion from the mastoid portion of the temporal bone; it transmits the auricular branch of the vagus nerve. SYN auricular fissure.

**tym·pa·ny** (tim′pă-nē) Low-pitched, resonant, drumlike note obtained by percussing surface of a large air-containing space (e.g., distended abdomen).

**type** (tīp) Usual form, or a composite form, which all others of the class resemble more or less closely; model, denoting especially a disease or a symptom complex giving the stamp or characteristic to a class. [G. *typos*, a mark, a model]

**type A be·ha·vior, type A per·son·al· i·ty** (tīp bē-hāv′yŏr, pĕr′sŏn-al′i-tē) Behavior pattern characterized by aggressiveness, ambitiousness, restlessness, and a strong sense of time urgency. New research suggests that it is hostile behavior and associated with increased risk for coronary heart disease.

**type B be·ha·vior, type B per·son·al· i·ty** (tīp bē-hāv′yŏr, pĕr′sŏn-al′i-tē) Pattern of action characterized by absence or obverse of type A behavior characteristics.

**Type 1 di·a·be·tes** (tīp dī′ă-bē′tēz) Condition characterized by high blood glucose levels caused by a total lack of insulin. Occurs when body's immune system attacks the insulin-producing beta cells in the pancreas and destroys them. The pancreas then produces little or no insulin. Disorder develops most often in young people but can appear in adults. SYN juvenile-onset diabetes.

**Type 2 di·a·be·tes** (tīp dī-ă-bē′tēz) Condition characterized by high blood glucose levels caused by either a lack of insulin or body's inability to use insulin efficiently; develops most often in middle-aged and older adults but can appear in young people.

**ty·phoi·dal** (tī-foyd′ăl) Relating to or resembling typhoid fever.

**ty·phoid car·rier** (tī′foyd kar′ē-ĕr) A person carrying the pathogen for typhoid fever but not displaying any signs or symptoms; someone having the potential to spread the disease via bodily excretions. SEE ALSO carrier.

**ty·phoid fe·ver** (tī′foyd fē′vĕr) Acute infectious disease caused by *Salmonella typhi* characterized by a continued fever rising in a step-like curve the first week, severe physical and mental depression, an eruption of rose-colored spots on the chest and abdomen, tympanites, early onset constipation, diarrhea, and sometimes intestinal hemorrhage or perforation of the bowel. Sometimes called typhoid.

**ty·phus** (tī′fŭs) Group of acute infectious and contagious diseases, caused by rickettsiae that are transmitted by arthropods, occurring in two principal forms: epidemic typhus and endemic (murine) typhus. [G. *typhos*, smoke, stupor]

**typ·ic·al an·ti·psy·chot·ic a·gent** (tip′ĭ-kăl an′tē-sī-kot′ik ā′jĕnt) Functional category of older antipsychotic drugs thought to exert their action predominantly through dopaminergic blockade; now more generally called first-generation antipsychotics.

**ty·po·dont** (tīp′ō-dont) Model of upper and lower dental arches used in teaching dental treatment methods.

**TYR** Abbreviation for tyramine.

**Tyr** Abbreviation for tyrosine.

**ty·ra·mine (TYR)** (tī′ră-mēn, tir′ă-) Decarboxylated tyrosine, a sympathomimetic amine having an action in some respects resembling that of epinephrine; present in ergot, mistletoe, ripe cheese, beer, red wine, and putrefied animal matter.

**ty·ro·sine (Tyr)** (tī′rō-sēn) An α-amino acid present in most proteins.

**ty·ro·si·ne·mi·a** (tī′rō-si-nē′mē-ă) Inherited disorders of tyrosine metabolism associated with elevated blood concentration of tyrosine and enhanced urinary excretion of tyrosine and tyrosyl compounds. [*tyrosine* + G. *haima*, blood]

st

# U

**U** Abbreviation for uranium.

**🔲 ul·cer** (ŭl'sĕr) Lesion through skin or mucous membrane resulting from loss of tissue, usually with inflammation. SEE erosion. See this page and page A6. [L. *ulcus* (*ulcer-*), a sore, ulcer]

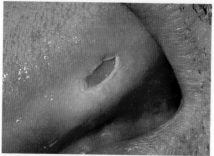

**traumatic ulcer: lateral lingual border of the tongue**

**ul·cer·at·ing gran·u·lo·ma of pu·den·da** (ŭl'sĕr-āt'ing gran'yū-lō'mă pū-den' dă) SYN granuloma inguinale.

**ul·cer·a·tion** (ŭl'sĕr-ā'shŭn) **1.** Formation of an ulcer. **2.** An ulcer or aggregation of ulcers.

**ul·cer·a·tive co·li·tis** (ŭl'sĕr-ă-tiv kō-lī'tis) Chronic disease of unknown cause characterized by ulceration of the colon and rectum, with rectal bleeding, mucosal crypt abscesses, inflammatory pseudopolyps, abdominal pain, and other symptoms.

**ul·cer·a·tive sto·ma·ti·tis** (ŭl'sĕr-ă-tiv stō'mă-tī'tis) SYN aphtha (2).

**ul·cer·o·mem·bra·nous gin·gi·vi·tis** (ŭl'sĕr-ō-mem'bră-nŭs jin'ji-vī'tis) SYN necrotizing ulcerative gingivitis.

**ul·na** (ŭl'nă, -nē) [TA] The medial and larger of the two bones of the forearm. SYN cubitus (2) [TA]. [L. elbow, arm, fr. G. *ōlenē*]

**ul·nar de·vi·a·tion** (ŭl'năr dē'vē-ā'shŭn) Movement of the wrist toward the little finger side of the forearm.

**♻ ulo-, ule-** **1.** Combining forms denoting scar, scarring. **2.** The gums. SEE ALSO gingivo-. **3.** Curly. [G. *oulē*]

**ULQ** Abbreviation for upper left quadrant (of mouth)

**ul·tra·cen·tri·fuge** (ŭl'tră-sen'tri-fyūzh) A high-speed centrifuge by means of which large molecules sediment at practicable rates.

**ul·tra·son·ic** (ŭl'tră-son'ik) Relating to energy waves similar to those of sound but of higher frequencies (above 20,000 Hz). [*ultra-* + L. *sonus*, sound]

**ul·tra·son·ic clean·ing** (ŭl'tră-son'ik

klēn'ing) **1.** In dentistry, use of a high-frequency vibrating point to remove deposits from tooth structure. **2.** Process of cleaning dentures by placing them in a special liquid in a container that generates high-frequency vibrations.

**ul·tra·son·ic scal·er** (ŭl'tră-son'ik skā'lĕr) SYN magnetostrictive ultrasonic device.

**ul·tra·son·o·gram** (ŭl'tră-sŏn'ŏ-gram) The image obtained by ultrasonography. SEE ALSO echogram. SYN sonogram.

**ul·tra·son·o·graph** (ŭl'tră-son'ŏ-graf) Computerized instrument used to create an image with ultrasound. SYN sonograph. [*ultra-* + L. *sonus*, sound, + G. *graphō*, to write]

**ul·tra·so·nog·ra·phy** (ŭl'tră-sŏ-nog'ră-fē) The location, measurement, or delineation of deep structures by measuring the reflection or transmission of high-frequency or ultrasonic waves. SYN echography, sonography. [*ultra-* + L. *sonus*, sound, + G. *graphō*, to write]

**ul·tra·sound** (ŭl'tră-sownd) Sound having a frequency greater than 30,000 Hz.

**U·lys·ses syn·drome** (yū-lis'ēz sin'drōm) Adverse effects of extensive diagnostic investigations conducted because of a false-positive result in routine laboratory screening.

**un·com·pen·sat·ed al·ka·lo·sis** (ŭn-kom'pĕn-sā'tĕd al'kă-lō'sis) Disorder in which the pH of body fluids is elevated because of lack of the compensatory mechanisms of compensated alkalosis.

**un·con·di·tion·ed re·sponse** (ŭn'kŏn-dish'ŭnd rĕ-spons') Response, such as salivation, which is a part of the animal or human behavior.

**un·con·scious** (ŭn-kon'shŭs) **1.** Not conscious. **2.** In psychoanalysis, the psychic structure comprising the drives and feelings of which one is unaware. SYN insensible (1).

**un·con·scious·ness** (ŭn-kon'shŭs-nĕs) An imprecise term for severely impaired awareness of self and surrounding environment; most often used as a synonym for coma.

**un·der·bite** (ŭn'dĕr-bīt) A nontechnical term applied to mandibular underdevelopment or to excessive maxillary development.

**un·der·cut** (ŭn'dĕr-kŭt) **1.** That portion of a tooth that lies between survey line (height of contour) and gingivae. **2.** Contour of a cross-section of a residual ridge or dental arch that would prevent insertion of a denture. **3.** Contour of a flasking stone that interlocks in such a way as to prevent separation of parts.

**un·der·cut gauge** (ŭn'dĕr-kŭt gāj) Device, used with a surveyor, to locate areas for placement of retentive components of clasps precisely when designing removable partial dentures.

**un·der·jet** (ŭn´dĕr-jet) Partial overlay of the maxillary and mandibular incisors; maxillary incisors are within the perimeter of the mandibular incisors. SEE ALSO underbite.

**un·der·nu·tri·tion** (ŭn´dĕr-nū-trish´ŭn) Malnutrition resulting from a reduced consumption of food.

**un·e·rup·ted** (un´ĕ-rŭp´tĕd) Condition of teeth that have not yet penetrated into oral cavity.

**un·e·rup·ted tooth** (ŭn´ĕ-rŭp´tĕd tūth) **1.** Tooth prior to emergence. **2.** Tooth unable to break out or emerge from dental alveolar tissues into oral cavity. See this page.

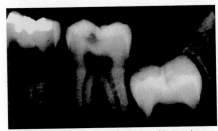

**unerupted 3rd molar:** crown is formed but roots are incomplete

**un·fill·ed seal·ant** (ŭn-fild´ sēl´ănt) Resin-based sealant material that does not contain filler particles; has a low viscosity that permits deeper penetration into the pits and fissures of a tooth. SEE ALSO sealant.

**u·ni·cus·pid, u·ni·cus·pi·date** (yū´ni-kŭs´pid, -pi-dāt) Having only one cusp, as a canine tooth.

**u·ni·lat·e·ral** (yū´ni-lat´ĕ-răl) Confined to one side only.

**un·in·ter·rupt·ed su·ture** (ŭn´in-tĕr-ŭp´tĕd sū´chŭr) SYN continuous suture.

**un·ion** (yūn´yŭn) **1.** Joining or amalgamation of two or more bodies. **2.** Structural adhesion or growing together of the edges of a wound. **3.** Healing of a fracture represented by the development of continuity between fractured fragments. [L. *unus*, one]

**u·nit** (yū´nit) *It is recommended that in handwritten material this word be written in full, because the abbreviation U is subject to frequent misinterpretation.* **1.** One; a single person or thing. **2.** A standard of measure, weight, or any other quality, by multiplication or fractions of which a scale or system is formed. **3.** A group of people or things considered as a whole because of mutual activities or functions. SEE ALSO international unit. [L. *unus*, one]

**Uni·ted States A·dopt·ed Names (USAN)** (yū-nī´tĕd stāts ă-dop´tĕd nāmz) Designation for nonproprietary names (for drugs) adopted by the USAN Council in cooperation with the manufacturers concerned.

**Uni·ted States Phar·ma·co·pei·a (USP)** (yū-nī´tĕd stāts fahr´mă-kō-pē´ă) SEE Pharmacopeia.

**Uni·ted States Pub·lic Health Ser·vice (USPHS)** (yū-nī´tĕd stāts pŭb´lik helth sĕr´vis) Bureau of the U.S. Department of Health and Human Services, served by a corps of medical officers presided over by the Surgeon General, concerned with scientific research, domestic and insular quarantine, administration of government hospitals, publication of sanitary reports, and statistics.

**unit of pen·i·cil·lin (in·ter·na·tion·al)** (yū´nit pen´i-sil´in in´tĕr-nash´ŏ-năl) Penicillin activity of 0.6 mcg of penicillin G.

**u·ni·ver·sal ap·pli·ance** (yū´ni-vĕr´săl ă-plī´ăns) Combination of edgewise and ribbon arch appliance techniques, affording precise control of individual teeth in all planes of space.

**u·ni·ver·sal cu·rette** (yū´ni-vĕr´săl kyūr-et´) Periodontal instrument used to remove calculus from crowns and roots of teeth designed to be used on all tooth surfaces. Working end has a rounded back, rounded toe, and two working cutting edges, and is semicircular in cross-section. One of the most frequently used and versatile periodontal débridement instruments.

**u·ni·ver·sal den·tal no·men·cla·ture** (yū´ni-vĕr´săl den´tăl nō´mĕn-klā-chŭr) **1.** A North American system of identifying teeth by assigning a sequential number to each permanent tooth beginning with upper right third molar (1) and continuing to upper left third molar (16), then continuing in the lower arch and finishing with the lower right third molar (32). **2.** System for deciduous teeth analogous to the permanent one using Arabic letters (A through T). SEE ALSO F.D.I. dental nomenclature, Palmer dental nomenclature.

**uni·ver·sal do·nor** (yū´ni-vĕr´săl dō´nŏr) In blood grouping, a person belonging to group O.

**u·ni·ver·sal in·stru·ment** (yū´ni-vĕr´săl in´strŭ-mĕnt) Tool or device that can be used on all dental surfaces.

**U·ni·ver·sal Pre·cau·tions** (yū´ni-vĕr´săl prē-kaw´shŭnz) (in full, Universal Blood and Body Fluid Precautions). A set of procedural directives and guidelines published in August 1987 by the U.S. Centers for Disease Control and Prevention (CDC) (as *Recommendations for Prevention of HIV Transmission in Health-Care Settings*) to prevent parenteral, mucous membrane, and nonintact skin exposures of health care workers to bloodborne pathogens.

**uv**

**u·ni·ver·sal re·cip·i·ent** (yū´ni-vĕr´săl rĕ-sip´ē-ĕnt) Patient with AB blood type who is able to receive a blood transfusion from any blood type in the ABO system.

**u·ni·ver·sal tooth cod·ing sys·tem** (yū´ni-vĕr´săl tūth kōd´ing sis´tĕm) A dental designation system in which the permanent teeth are numbered 1–32, beginning with the maxillary right third molar (No. 1) and ending with the mandibular right third molar (No. 32). The primary teeth have a similar designation, preceded by "D". The American Dental Association designation system is similar except the primary teeth are identified by the letters a–t.

**un·med·ul·lat·ed** (ŭn-med´yū-lāt´ĕd) SYN unmyelinated.

**un·mod·i·fied zinc ox·ide-eu·ge·nol ce·ment** (ŭn-mod´i-fīd zingk ok´sīd yū´jĕ-nol sĕ-ment´) SYN zinc oxide eugenol cement.

**un·my·e·li·nat·ed** (ŭn-mī´ĕ-li-nā-tĕd) Denoting nerve fibers (axons) lacking a myelin sheath. SYN amyelinated, amyelinic, unmedullated.

**un·of·fi·cial** (ŭn´ŏ-fish´ăl) Denoting a drug that is not listed in the United States Pharmacopeia or the National Formulary.

**un·op·er·a·ted cleft** (ŭn-op´ĕr-ā-tĕd kleft) Palatal gap that has not been surgically repaired.

**un·pair·ed work·ing-ends** (ŭn-pārd´ wŏrk´ing-endz) Double-ended instrument with dissimilar working-ends (e.g., explorer-probe combination). SEE ALSO paired working-end.

**un·sat·u·ra·ted chem·i·cal-va·por ster·il·iz·a·tion** (ŭn-sach´ŭr-ā-tĕd kem´i-kăl vā´pŏr ster´i-lī-zā´shŭn) Method of disinfection using vapor of a chemical solution in a closed, pressurized chamber.

**un·sat·ur·at·ed fat·ty ac·id** (ŭn-sach´ŭr-āt-ĕd fat´ē as´id) A fatty acid, the carbon chain of which possesses one or more double or triple bonds.

**un·sta·ble an·gi·na** (ŭn-stā´bĕl an´ji-nă) SYN acute coronary syndrome.

**un·strain·ed jaw re·la·tion** (ŭn-strānd´ jaw rĕ-lā´shŭn) SYN rest relation.

**un·strat·i·fied ep·i·the·li·um** (ŭn-strat´i-fīd ep´i-thē´lē-ŭm) Thin, membranous tissue that consists of a single layer of cells. SYN nonstratified epithelium.

**up·per left quad·rant (of mouth) (ULQ)** (ŭp´ĕr left kwah´drănt mowth) One of four areas in the oral cavity comprising (according to the numeration system of the American Dental Association) maxillary teeth 9 to 16.

**up·per right quad·rant (of mouth) (URQ)** (ŭp´ĕr rīt kwah´drănt mowth) One of four areas in the oral cavity comprising (according to the numeration system of the American Dental Association) maxillary teeth 1 to 8.

**up·reg·u·la·tion** (ŭp´reg´yū-lā´shŭn) Opposite of downregulation.

**up·reg·u·la·tion/down·reg·u·la·tion hy·poth·e·sis** (ŭp´reg-yū-lā´shŭn down´ reg-yū-lā´shŭn hī-poth´ĕ-sis) Theory of neurochemical basis of depression (an elaboration of the monoamine hypothesis) linking it to an increase in number (upregulation) of postsynaptic monoamine receptors, which are then effectively decreased in number (downregulation) as a result of antidepressant activity.

**up·right** (ŭp´rīt) Colloq. usage for moving a tooth into an erect position.

**u·ra·cil** (yūr´ă-sil) Pyrimidine (base) present in ribonucleic acid.

**uraemia** [Br.] SYN uremia.

**urano-, uranisco-** Combining forms denoting hard palate. [G. *ouranos*, sky vault, *ouraniskos*, roof of mouth (palate)]

**u·ra·nos·chi·sis, u·ra·nis·co·chasm** (yūr´ă-nos´ki-sis, -nis´kō-kazm) Cleft of hard palate. [*urano-* + G. *schisis*, fissure]

**u·ra·no·staph·y·lo·plas·ty, ura·no·staph·y·lor·rha·phy** (yūr´ă-nō-staf´i-lō-plas´tē, -ōr´ă-fē) Repair of a cleft of both hard and soft palates. [*urano-* + G. *staphylē*, uvula, + *plassō*, to form]

**u·ra·no·staph·y·los·chi·sis, u·ra·no·ve·los·chi·sis** (yūr´ă-nō-staf´i-los´ki-sis, -vĕ-los´ki-sis) Cleft of soft and hard palates. [*urano-* + G. *staphylē*, uvula, + *schisis*, fissure]

**u·re·a** (yūr-ē´ă) Chief end product of nitrogen metabolism in mammals. [G. *ouron*, urine]

**u·re·a frost, u·re·mic frost** (yūr-ē´ă frawst, -mik) Powdery deposits on the skin, especially face, due to excretion of nitrogenous compounds in sweat.

**u·re·a pe·rox·ide** (yūr-ē´ă pĕr-ok´sīd) White crystalline compound used in an aqueous solution as an oxidizing mouthwash.

**u·re·ase** (yūr´ē-ās) An enzyme used as an antitumor agent; it is present in intestinal bacteria.

**u·re·mi·a** (yūr-ē´mē-ă) **1.** Excess of urea and other nitrogenous waste in blood. **2.** Complex of symptoms due to severe persisting renal failure that can be relieved by dialysis. SYN uraemia. [G. *ouron*, urine, + *haima*, blood]

**u·re·mic breath** (yūr-ē´mik breth) Characteristic odor in patients with chronic renal failure, variously described as "fishy," "ammoniac," and "fetid," which is indicative of the systemic accumulation of volatile metabolites, usually excreted in urine; dimethylamine and trimethylamine have been identified and correlated with odor.

**u·re·ter·i·tis** (yūr-ē′tĕr-ī′tis) Inflammation of a ureter.

**u·re·thri·tis** (yūr′ē-thrī′tis) Inflammation of the urethra. [*ureth-* + G. *-itis,* inflammation]

**u·ric ac·id** (yūr′ik as′id) White crystals, poorly soluble, contained in solution in the urine of mammals.

**u·ri·dro·sis** (yūr′i-drō′sis) Excretion of urea or uric acid in sweat. [*uri-* + G. *hidrōs,* sweat]

**u·ri·nal·y·sis** (yūr′in-al′i-sis) Analysis of urine.

**u·ri·nar·y fever** (yūr′i-nar-ē fē′vĕr) Elevation of temperature, usually slight and transitory, following catheterization of the urethra, or the passage of blood clots, gravel, or a calculus.

**ur·i·nar·y tract** (yūr′i-nar-ē trakt) The passage from renal pelvis to the urinary meatus through the ureters, bladder, and urethra.

**u·ri·nary tract in·fec·tion (UTI)** (yūr′i-nar-ē trakt in-fek′shŭn) Microbial infection, usually bacterial, of any part of the urinary tract.

**u·rine** (yūr′in) The fluid and dissolved substances excreted by the kidney. [L. *urina;* G. *ouron*]

♻ **uro-** Combining form denoting urine. [G. *ouron*]

**u·ro·bi·lin** (yūr′ō-bī′lin) A uroporphyrin; an acyclic tetrapyrrole that is one of the natural breakdown products of heme. SYN urohematin.

**ur·o·cri·sis** (yūr′ō-krī′sis) Severe pain in any of the urinary organs or passages. [*uro-* + G. *krisis,* crisis]

**urohaematin** [Br.] SYN urohematin.

**u·ro·hem·a·tin** (yūr′ō-hē′mă-tin) SYN urobilin, urohaematin.

**ur·o·ki·nase** (yūr′ō-kī′nās) SYN plasminogen activator.

**ur·ol·o·gy** (yūr-ol′ŏ-jē) The medical specialty concerned with the study, diagnosis, and treatment of diseases of the genitourinary tract. [*uro-* + G. *logos,* study]

**ur·op·a·thy** (yūr-op′ă-thē) Any disorder involving the urinary tract. [*uro-* + G. *pathos,* suffering]

**URQ** Abbreviation for upper right quadrant (of mouth)

**ur·so·de·ox·y·chol·ic ac·id** (ŭr′sō-dē-oks′ē-kō′lik as′id) SYN ursodiol.

**ur·so·di·ol** (ŭr′sō-dī′ōl) A bile acid used to facilitate the dissolution of gallstones in patients; a potential alternative to cholecystectomy. SYN ursodeoxycholic acid.

**ur·ti·car·i·a** (ŭr′ti-kar′ē-ă) An eruption of itching wheals, colloquially called hives, usually of systemic origin; may be due to a state of hypersensitivity to foods or drugs, foci of infection, physical agents (heat, cold, light, friction), or psychic stimuli. [L. *urtica*]

**ur·ti·ca·tion** (ŭr′ti-kā′shŭn) Burning sensation resembling that produced by urticaria or resulting from nettle poisoning. [L. *urticatio*]

**USAN** Abbreviation for United States Adopted Names.

**USP** Abbreviation for United States Pharmacopeia.

**USPHS** Abbreviation for United States Public Health Service.

**USP u·nit** (yū′nit) Unit as defined and adopted by *United States Pharmacopeia.*

**UTI** Abbreviation for urinary tract infection.

**u·tri·cle** (yū′tri-kĕl) **1.** Small sac or pouch. **2.** A dilated portion of membranous labyrinth receiving ampullae of semicircular canals. [L. diminutive form of *uter,* leather bag]

**u·ve·i·tis,** pl. **u·ve·i·ti·des** (yū′vē-ī′tis, -it′i-dēz) Inflammation of the uveal tract: iris, ciliary body, and choroid. [*uvea* + G. *-itis,* inflammation]

**u·ve·o·pa·rot·id fe·ver** (yū′vē-ō-păr-ot′id fē′vĕr) Chronic enlargement of the parotid glands and inflammation of the uveal tract accompanied by a long-continued fever of low degree; a form of sarcoidosis. SYN Heerfordt disease.

**u·vu·la,** pl. **u·vu·lae** (yū′vyū-lă, -lē) [TA] An appendant fleshy mass. [Mod. L. dim. of L. *uva,* a grape, the uvula]

**u·vu·lec·to·my** (yū′vyū-lek′tŏ-mē) Excision of the uvula. [*uvula* + G. *ektomē,* excision]

**u·vu·li·tis** (yū′vyū-lī′tis) Inflammation of the uvula.

**u·vu·lop·to·sis, u·vu·lap·to·sis** (yū′vyū-lop-tō′sis, -lap-tō′sis) Relaxation or elongation of the uvula. [*uvulo-* + G. *ptōsis,* a falling]

**u·vu·lo·tome** (yū′vyū-lō-tōm) An instrument for cutting the uvula.

**u·vu·lot·o·my** (yū′vyū-lot′ŏ-mē) Any cutting operation on the uvula. [*uvulo-* + G. *tomē,* a cutting]

UV

# V

**V** Abbreviation for valine; volt.

**vac·ci·na·tion** (vak'si-nā'shŭn) The act of administering a vaccine.

**vac·cine** (vak-sēn') Originally, live vaccine (vaccinia, cowpox) virus inoculated in skin as prophylaxis against smallpox and obtained from skin of calves inoculated with seed virus. Usage has extended the meaning to include essentially any preparation intended for active immunologic prophylaxis. [L. *vaccinus,* relating to a cow, vacca]

**vac·u·ole** (vak'yū-ōl) 1. A minute space in any tissue. 2. A clear space in the substance of a cell. [Mod. L. *vacuolum,* dim. of L. *vacuum,* an empty space]

**vac·u·um** (vak'yūm) An empty space, one practically exhausted of air or gas. [L. ntr. of *vacuus,* empty]

**vac·u·um cast·ing** (vak'yūm kast'ing) Casting of a metal in the presence of a vacuum.

**vac·u·um head·ache** (vak'yūm hed'āk) Headache due to frontal sinus closure.

**vac·u·um in·vest·ing** (vak'yūm in-vest'ing) Investing of a pattern using a vacuum to remove trapped air from the investment material.

**va·go·glos·so·pha·ryn·ge·al** (vā'gō-glos'ō-fă-rin'jē-ăl) Relating to vagus and glossopharyngeal nerves.

**va·go·lyt·ic** (vā'gō-lit'ik) 1. Pertaining to or causing vagolysis. 2. A therapeutic or chemical agent that has inhibitory effects on the vagus nerve. 3. Denoting an agent having such effects.

**va·go·mi·met·ic** (vā'gō-mi-met'ik) Mimicking action of efferent fibers of vagus nerve.

**va·go·va·gal** (vā'gō-vā'găl) Pertaining to a process that uses both afferent and efferent vagal fibers.

**va·gus nerve [CN X]** (vā'gŭs nĕrv) [TA] Mixed nerve that arises from numerous small roots from side of medulla oblongata through retroolivary groove, between glossopharyngeal above and accessory below. SYN nervus vagus [CN X], tenth cranial nerve [CN X].

**Val** Abbreviation for valine.

**va·lence, va·len·cy** (vā'lĕns, -sē) The combining power of one atom of an element (or a radical), that of the hydrogen atom being the unit of comparison, determined by the number of electrons in the outer shell of the atom (v. electrons). [L. *valentia,* strength]

**val·id** (val'id) Effective; producing desired result; verifiably correct. [L. *valeo,* to be strong]

**val·i·da·tion** (val'i-dā'shŭn) Act or process of making valid.

**va·lid·i·ty** (vă-lid'i-tē) Index of how well a test or procedure in fact measures what it purports to measure; an objective index by which to describe how valid a test or procedure is.

**val·ine (Val, V)** (vā-lēn') A nutritionally essential amino acid.

**Val·leix points** (vahl'ā poynts) Various points in course of a nerve, pressure on which is painful in cases of neuralgia.

**val·ue** (val'yū) 1. Standard or quality denoting worth, utility, or merit; also, a thing or ideal that possesses value or is prized as desirable. 2. A precise quantity, measured or calculated. [M.E., fr. O.Fr., fr. L. *valeo,* to be of value]

**valve** (valv) [TA] 1. Fold of lining membrane of a canal or other hollow organ that serves to retard or prevent fluid reflux. 2. Any formation or reduplication of tissue, or flaplike structure, resembling or functioning as a valve. [L. *valva*]

**van Buch·em syn·drome** (vahn bū'kem sin'drōm) Osteosclerosing skeletal dysplasia, characterized by mandibular enlargement, thickening of diaphyses and calvaria, and increased serum alkaline phosphatase; autosomal recessive inheritance.

**van·co·my·cin** (van'kō-mī'sin) Antibiotic isolated from cultures of *Nocardia orientalis,* bactericidal against gram-positive organisms.

**va·por** (vā'pŏr) 1. Molecules in gaseous phase of a solid or liquid substance exposed to a gas. 2. Visible emanation of fine particles of a liquid. 3. Medicinal preparation to be administered by inhalation. SYN vapour. [L. steam]

**va·por·i·za·tion** (vā'pŏr-ī-zā'shŭn) 1. Change of a solid or liquid to a state of vapor. 2. The therapeutic application of a vapor.

**va·por·iz·er** (vā'pŏr-īz-ĕr) An apparatus for reducing medicated liquids to a state of vapor suitable for inhalation or application to accessible mucous membranes. SEE ALSO atomizer.

**vapour** [Br.] SYN vapor.

**Va·quez dis·ease** (vah-kā' di-zēz') SYN polycythemia vera.

**var·i·a·bil·i·ty** (var'ē-ă-bil'i-tē) The capability of being variable.

**var·i·a·ble** (var'ē-ă-bĕl) That which is inconstant, which can or does change, as contrasted with a constant. [L. *vario,* to vary, change, differ]

**var·i·ate** (var'ē-āt) Measurable quantity capable of taking on a number of values; may be binary, continuous, or discrete.

🔲**var·i·cel·la** (var'i-sel'ă) Acute contagious disease, usually occurring in children, caused by the Varicella-Zoster virus genus, *Varicellovirus*; marked by a sparse eruption of papules, which become vesicles and then pustules, like that of smallpox although less severe and varying in stages, usually with mild constitutional symptoms; incubation period is about 14–17 days. See page A12. SYN chickenpox. [Mod. L. dim. of *variola*]

**va·ri·o·la** (vă-rī'ō-lă) **1.** Species type of the genus *Orthopoxvirus* that causes human smallpox. **2.** Smallpox. [Med. L. dim of L. *varius, spotted*]

**var·ix**, pl. **va·ri·ces** (var'iks, -i-sēz) **1.** A dilated vein. **2.** An enlarged and tortuous vein, artery, or lymphatic vessel. [L. *varix* (*varic-*), a dilated vein]

**vas**, pl. **va·sa** (vas, vā'să) [TA] Duct or canal conveying any liquid (e.g., blood). [L. a vessel, dish]

**vas·cu·lar den·tin** (vas'kyū-lăr den'tin) SYN vasodentin.

**vas·cu·lar dis·eas·es** (vas'kyū-lăr di-zēz'ĕz) General term that refers to diseases that affect blood vessels.

**vas·cu·lar ring** (vas'kyū-lăr ring) Anomalous arteries congenitally encircling trachea and esophagus.

**vas·cu·li·tis** (vas'kyū-lī'tis) SYN angiitis.

**va·so·ac·tive in·tes·ti·nal pol·y·pep·tide (VIP)** (vā'sō-ak'tiv in-tes'ti-năl pol'ē-pep'tīd) Polypeptide hormone secreted most commonly by non-β islet cell tumors of the pancreas; excess production causes copious watery diarrhea and fecal electrolyte loss.

**va·so·con·stric·tion** (vā'sō-kŏn-strik'shŭn) Narrowing of blood vessels.

**va·so·con·stric·tive** (vā'sō-kŏn-strik'tiv) **1.** Causing narrowing of the blood vessels. **2.** SYN vasoconstrictor (1).

**va·so·con·stric·tor** (vā'sō-kŏn-strik'tŏr) **1.** An agent that narrows blood vessels. SYN vasoconstrictive (2). **2.** A nerve, stimulation of which causes vascular constriction.

**va·so·den·tin** (vā'sō-den'tin) Dentin in which primitive capillaries have remained uncalcified and so are wide enough to give passage to formed blood elements. SYN vascular dentin.

**va·so·de·pres·sion** (vā'sō-dĕ-presh'ŭn) Reduction of tone in blood vessels with vasodilation and resulting in lowered blood pressure.

**va·so·de·pres·sor** (vā'sō-dĕ-pres'ŏr) **1.** Producing vasodepression. **2.** An agent that produces vasodepression.

**va·so·di·la·tion** (vā'sō-dī-lā'shŭn) Widening of the lumen of blood vessels.

**va·so·di·la·tive** (vā'sō-dī-lā'tiv) **1.** Causing dilation of the blood vessels. **2.** SYN vasodilator (1).

**va·so·di·la·tor** (vā'sō-dī'lā-tŏr) **1.** An agent that causes dilation of blood vessels. SYN vasodilative (2). **2.** A nerve, stimulation of which results in dilation of the blood vessels.

**va·so·gen·ic shock** (vā'sō-jen'ik shok) Shock resulting from depressed activity of higher vasomotor centers in brainstem and medulla, producing vasodilation without loss of fluid so that container is disproportionately large. In oligemic shock, blood volume is reduced; in both, return of venous blood is inadequate.

**va·so·in·hib·i·tor** (vā'sō-in-hib'i-tŏr) Agent that restricts or prevents functioning of vasomotor nerves.

**va·so·mo·tor** (vā'sō-mō'tŏr) **1.** Causing dilation or constriction of the blood vessels. **2.** Denoting nerves that have this action.

**va·so·mo·tor a·tax·i·a** (vā'sō-mō'tŏr ă-tak'sē-ă) Form of autonomic ataxia causing irregularity in peripheral circulation, marked by alternations of pallor and suffusion, due to spasm of the smaller blood vessels.

**va·so·pres·sin (VP)** (vā'sō-pres'in) Nonapeptide neurohypophysial hormone related to oxytocin and vasotocin. [*vaso*- + L. *premo*, pp. *pressum*, to press down, + *-in*]

**va·so·pres·sor** (vā'sō-pres'ŏr) Agent producing vasoconstriction and a rise in blood pressure, usually understood to be systemic arterial pressure unless otherwise specified.

**va·so·stim·u·lant** (vā'sō-stim'yū-lănt) Agent that excites vasomotor action.

**vault** (vawlt) A part resembling an arched roof or dome: e.g., the pharyngeal vault or fornix, the nonmuscular upper part of the nasopharynx; the palatine vault, arch of the plate; or vault of the vagina, fornix of vagina. [thr. O. Fr., fr. L. *volvo*, pp. *volutus*, to turn round]

**V-bends** (bendz) V-shaped arcs incorporated in an archwire, usually placed mesially or distally to canines (cuspids) and used as a "dead" area of wire through which torquing bends may be placed.

**VC** Abbreviation for vital capacity.

**VDRL test** (test) A flocculation test for syphilis, developed by the Venereal Disease Research Laboratory of the U.S. Public Health Service.

**vec·tor** (vek'tŏr) **1.** An invertebrate animal (e.g., tick, mite, mosquito, bloodsucking fly) capable of transmitting an infectious agent among vertebrates. **2.** Anything (e.g., velocity, mechanical force, electromotive force) having magnitude and direction. **3.** SYN recombinant vector. [L. *vector,* a carrier]

**uv**

**ve·gan** (vē′găn) Strict vegetarian; i.e., one who consumes no animal or dairy products.

**veg·e·tar·i·an** (vej′ĕ-tar′ē-ăn) One whose diet is restricted to foods of vegetable origin, excluding primarily animal meats. Cf. vegan.

**veg·e·ta·tive bac·te·ri·a** (vej′ĕ-tā-tiv bak-tēr′ē-ă) The growing form of bacteria.

**ve·hi·cle** (vē′i-kĕl) **1.** An excipient or a menstruum; a substance, usually without therapeutic action, used as a medium to give bulk for the administration of medicines. **2.** An inanimate substance by or on which an infectious agent passes from an infected to a susceptible host. [L. *vehiculum,* a conveyance, fr. *veho,* to carry]

**veil** (vāl) **1.** SYN velum (1). **2.** SYN caul (1). [L. *velum*]

**vein** (vān) [TA] Blood vessel carrying blood toward the heart; postnatally, all veins except the pulmonary carry dark unoxygenated blood. [L. *vena*]

**vel·o·car·di·o·fa·cial syn·drome** (vē′lō-kahr′dē-ō-fā′shăl sin′drōm) Disorder with hypernasal speech, dysmorphic facial features (long midface, cylindric nose, downward turned corners of mouth), and cardiac abnormalities.

**ve·loc·i·ty** (vĕ-los′i-tē) Rate and direction of movement. [L. *velocitas,* fr. *velox (veloc-),* quick, swift]

**vel·o·pha·ryn·ge·al seal** (vē′lō-fă-rin′jē-ăl sēl) Closure between oral and nasopharyngeal cavities.

**ve·lum,** pl. **ve·la** (vē′lŭm, -lă) **1.** Any structure resembling a veil or curtain. SYN veil (1), velamen. **2.** SYN caul (1). **3.** SYN greater omentum. **4.** Any serous membrane or membranous envelope or covering. [L. veil, sail]

**ve·lum pa·la·ti·num** (vē′lŭm pal′ă-tī′nŭm) SYN soft palate.

**ve·nec·ta·si·a** (vē′nek-tā′zē-ă) SYN phlebectasia.

◼**ve·neer** (vĕ-nēr′) **1.** In dentistry, a layer of tooth-colored material, usually porcelain or composite resin, attached to and covering surface of a metal crown or natural tooth structure. **2.** A thin surface layer laid over a base of common material. See this page. [Fr. *fournir,* to furnish]

◼**ve·neer crown** (vĕn-ēr′ krown) Metal tooth crown with a thin layer of porcelain covering all or part of its surface. See this page. SYN porcelain fused to metal crown, porcelain veneer crown, veneered metal crown, ceramo metal crown.

**ve·neer·ed met·al crown** (vĕn-ērd′ me′tăl krown) SYN veneer crown.

**ve·ne·re·al dis·ease** (vĕ-nēr′ē-ăl di-zēz′) SYN sexually transmitted disease.

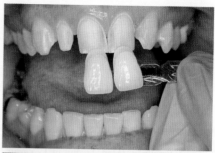
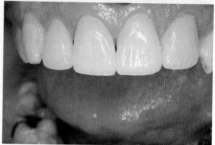

**veneers:** (A) teeth prepared for indirect veneers; (B) veneers cemented in place

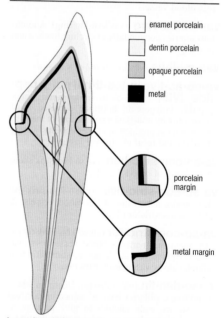

enamel porcelain

dentin porcelain

opaque porcelain

metal

porcelain margin

metal margin

**layers in construction of ceramometal crown**

**ven·i·punc·ture** (ven′i-pŭngk′shŭr) The puncture of a vein, usually to withdraw blood.

**ve·nog·ra·phy** (vē-nog′ră-fē) Radiographic demonstration of a vein, after the injection of contrast medium. [*veno-* + G. *graphō,* to write]

**ve·nous** (vē′nŭs) Relating to a vein or veins. [L. *venosus*]

**ve·nous blood** (vē′nŭs blŭd) Blood that has passed through capillaries of various tissues, except the lungs, and is found in veins, right chambers of heart, and pulmonary arteries; usually dark red due to lower oxygen content.

**ve·nous pulse** (vē′nŭs pŭls) A pulsation occurring in the veins.

**ve·nous re·turn** (vē′nŭs rē-tŭrn′) Amount of blood per unit of time returning to heart through great veins and coronary sinus.

**ven·ti·late** (ven′ti-lāt) To aerate, or oxygenate, blood in the pulmonary capillaries. SYN air (2). [L. *ventilo*, pp. *-atus*, to fan, fr. *ventus*, the wind]

**ven·ti·la·tion** (ven′ti-lā′shŭn) 1. Replacement of air or other gas in a space by fresh air or gas. 2. Movement of gas(es) into and out of the lungs. SYN respiration (2).

**ven·ti·la·tion me·ter** (ven′ti-lā′shŭn mē′tĕr) Meter used to measure tidal and minute ventilatory volumes.

**ven·til·a·tor** (ven′til-ā-tŏr) SYN respirator. [L. *ventilo*, to fan, fr. *ventus*, wind, + *-ator*, agent suffix]

**vent·plant** (vent′plant) An endosteal implant, usually made of titanium, used to provide support and fixation for a dental prosthesis by transmucosal projections; also used to designate a family of implants.

**ven·trad** (ven′trad) Toward the ventral aspect; opposed to dorsad. [L. *venter*, belly, + *ad*, to]

**ven·tral** (ven′trăl) [TA] 1. Pertaining to the belly or to any venter. 2. SYN anterior. [L. *ventralis*]

**ven·tri·cle** (ven′tri-kĕl) [TA] A normal cavity, as of the brain or heart. [L. *ventriculus*, dim. of *venter*, belly]

**ven·tric·u·lar dys·func·tion** (ven-trik′yū-lăr dis-fŭngk′shŭn) Abnormal pumping function of the cardiac ventricles.

**ven·tric·u·lar fib·ril·la·tion** (ven-trik′yū-lăr fib′ri-lā′shŭn) Coarse or fine, rapid, fibrillary movements of the ventricular muscle that replace the normal contraction.

**ven·tric·u·lar pre·load** (ven-trik′yū-lăr prē′lōd) The pressure stretching the ventricular walls at the onset of ventricular contraction. SYN preload (2).

**ven·tric·u·lar sep·tal de·fect (VSD)** (ven-trik′yū-lăr sep′tăl dē′fekt) *Avoid the incorrect form ventriculoseptal.* Congenital defect in septum between cardiac ventricles, usually resulting from failure of spiral aorticopulmonary septum to close interventricular foramen.

**ven·tric·u·li·tis** (ven-trik′yū-lī′tis) Inflammation of the ventricles of the brain. [*ventricle* + G. *-itis*, inflammation]

**ven·tric·u·lo·a·tri·al shunt** (ven-trik′yū-lō-ā′trē-ăl shŭnt) Surgical procedure for hydrocephalus. SYN ventriculoatriostomy.

**ven·tric·u·lo·a·tri·os·to·my** (ven-trik′yū-lō-ā′trē-os′tŏ-mē) SYN ventriculoatrial shunt.

**ven·ule** (ven′yūl) [TA] Venous radicle continuous with a capillary.

**VEP** Abbreviation for visual evoked potential.

**ver·mi·cide** (vĕr′mi-sīd) An agent that kills intestinal parasitic worms. [*vermi-* + L. *caedo*, to kill]

**ver·mil·ion bor·der** (vĕr-mil′yŏn bōr′dĕr) Junction between skin aspect of the lip and vermilion zone. Cf. vermilion zone.

**ver·mil·i·o·nec·to·my** (vĕr-mil′yŏn-ek′tŏ-mē) Excision of vermilion border of lip. [*vermilion* border + G. *ektomē*, cutting out]

**ver·mil·ion zone, ver·mil·ion tran·si·tion·al zone** (vĕr-mil′yŏn zōn, tran-zish′ŭn-ăl) The red margin of the upper and lower lip that commences at the exterior edge of the intraoral labial mucosa (''moist line'') and extends outward, terminating at the extraoral labial cutaneous junction; a thinly keratinized type of stratified squamous epithelium deeply penetrated by well-vascularized dermal papillae which show through the translucent epidermis to impart the typical red appearance of the lips.

**Ver·net syn·drome** (ver-nā′ sin′drōm) Syndrome characterized by paralysis of motor components of glossopharyngeal, vagus, and accessory cranial nerves as they lie in posterior fossa; most commonly due to head injury.

**ver·nix** (vĕr′niks) SYN dental varnish. [Mod. L.]

**ver·ru·ca,** pl. **ver·ru·cae** (vĕr-ū′kă, -kē) Flesh-colored growth characterized by circumscribed hypertrophy of papillae of corium, with thickening of malpighian, granular, and keratin epidermal layers, caused by human papillomavirus; also applied to epidermal verrucous tumors of nonviral etiology. SYN wart. [L.]

**ver·ru·ca vul·ga·ris** (vĕr-ū′kă vŭl-gā′ris) An epidermal keratotic papilloma that occurs frequently in young people due to localized infection by human papillomavirus. See this page.

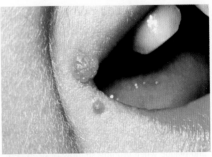

**verruca vulgaris**

**UV**

**ver·ru·cous** (vĕr-ū´kŭs) Denotes anything having a wartlike appearance. SEE ALSO verruca. [L. *verruca,* wart, + *-ous* adj. suffix]

**ver·ru·cous car·ci·no·ma** (vĕr-ū´kŭs kahr´si-nō´mă) Malignant tumor of the oral epithelium that has a papillary appearance.

**ver·sive sei·zure** (vĕr´siv sē´zhŭr) Seizure characterized by sustained, forced conjugate ocular and cephalic and/or truncal deviation.

**ver·te·bra** (vĕr´tĕ-bră) [TA] *Avoid the mispronunciation verte'bra.* One of the segments of vertebral column; in humans, there are usually 33 vertebrae. [L. joint, fr. *verto,* to turn]

**ver·ti·cal** (vĕr´ti-kăl) [TA] **1.** Relating to the vertex, or crown of the head. **2.** Perpendicular. **3.** Denoting any plane or line that passes longitudinally through the body in the anatomic position.

**ver·ti·cal ax·is** (vĕr´ti-kăl aks´is) In dentistry, line around which working side condyle rotates in horizontal plane during mandibular movement.

**ver·ti·cal di·men·sion** (vĕr´ti-kăl di-men´shŭn) Measurement of face between any two arbitrarily selected points that are conveniently located, one above and one below the mouth, usually in the midline.

**ver·ti·cal e·las·tic** (vĕr´ti-kăl ĕ-las´tik) Pliable material used in a direction perpendicular to occlusal plane, connecting one arch wire to the other, and often used to improve intercuspation.

**ver·ti·cal os·te·ot·o·my** (vĕr´ti-kăl os´tē-ot´ŏ-mē) Oral surgical procedure similar to sliding oblique osteotomy.

**ver·ti·cal o·ver·lap** (vĕr´ti-kăl ō´vĕr-lap) **1.** Extension of upper teeth over lower teeth in a vertical direction when opposing posterior teeth are in contact in centric occlusion. **2.** Distance that teeth lap over their antagonists vertically, especially for distance that the upper incisal edges drop below lower ones, but may also describe vertical relations of opposing cusps. **3.** Relationship of maxillary to mandibular incisors when incisal edges pass each other in centric occlusion. SYN overbite.

**ver·ti·cal stroke ac·tion** (vĕr´ti-kăl strōk ak´shŭn) Instrumentation strokes parallel to long axis of tooth involving a pulling action; used on the mesial and distal surfaces of posterior teeth.

**ver·ti·cal tech·nique** (vĕr´ti-kăl tek-nēk´) Using the working-end of an electronically powered instrument in a manner similar to that of a calibrated periodontal probe, with the point directed toward the junctional epithelium. Instrument tip is in a vertical orientation to the long axis of the tooth; used to remove calculus and plaque when probing shallow or deep periodontal pockets with instruments.

**ver·ti·cal trans·mis·sion** (vĕr´ti-kăl trans-mish´ŭn) **1.** Passing a virus by means of the genetic apparatus of a cell in which the viral genome is integrated. **2.** For infectious agents in general, transmission of an agent from an individual to its offspring.

**ver·ti·go** (vĕr´ti-gō) **1.** A sensation of spinning or whirling motion; implies a definite sensation of rotation of the subject or of objects about the subject. **2.** Imprecisely used to describe dizziness. [L. *vertigo* (*vertigin-*), dizziness, fr. *verto,* to turn]

**ves·i·cant** (ves´i-kănt) An agent that produces a vesicle.

**ves·i·ca·tion** (ves´i-kā´shŭn) SYN vesiculation.

**ves·i·cle** (ves´i-kĕl) **1.** [TA] Small bladder or bladderlike structure. **2.** A small circumscribed skin elevation containing fluid. **3.** Small sac containing liquid or gas. See this page. [L. *vesicula,* a blister, dim. of *vesica,* bladder]

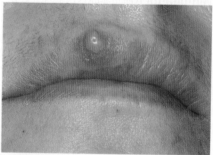

**vesicle:** manifestation of recurrent herpes simplex infection

**ves·i·cos·to·my** (ves´i-kos´tŏ-mē) SYN cystostomy. [*vesico-* + G. *stoma,* mouth]

**ve·sic·u·la·tion** (vĕ-sik´yū-lā´shŭn) **1.** The formation of vesicles. SYN blistering, vesication. **2.** SYN inflation.

**ve·sic·u·lo·bron·chi·al** (vĕ-sik´yū-lō-brong´kē-ăl) Denoting an auscultatory sound that has both vesicular and bronchial qualities.

**ve·sic·u·lo·tu·bu·lar** (vĕ-sik´yū-lō-tū´byū-lăr) Denoting an auscultatory sound having both vesicular and tubular qualities.

**ve·sic·u·lo·tym·pan·ic** (vĕ-sik´yū-lō-tim-pan´ik) Denoting a percussion sound having both vesicular and tympanic qualities.

**ve·sic·u·lo·tym·pa·nit·ic res·o·nance** (vĕ-sik´yū-lō-tim´pă-nit´ik rez´ŏ-năns) Peculiar, partly tympanitic, partly vesicular sound, obtained on percussion in cases of pulmonary emphysema. SYN bandbox resonance.

**ves·sel** (ves´ĕl) [TA] Structure conveying or containing a fluid.

**ves·tib·u·lar** (ves-tib′yū-lăr) Relating to a vestibule, especially of the ear.

**ves·ti·bu·lar ap·pa·ra·tus** (ves-tib′yū-lăr ap′ă-rat′ŭs) Receptor organ of vestibular portion of eighth cranial nerve consisting of three semicircular canals and the otolith, located within petrous portion of temporal bone of cranium.

**ves·tib·u·lar a·que·duct** (ves-tib′yū-lăr ahk′wĕ-dŭkt) [TA] Bony canal running from vestibule and opening on posterior surface of petrous portion of temporal bone, giving passage to endolymphatic duct and a small vein.

**ves·tib·u·lar a·re·a** (ves-tib′yū-lăr ar′ē-ă) [TA] Part of floor of the fourth ventricle lateral to sulcus limitans [TA] and medial to the restiform body [TA] that overlies vestibular nuclei and portions of cochlear nuclei.

**ves·tib·u·lar lab·y·rinth** (ves-tib′yū-lăr lab′i-rinth) [TA] Portion of membranous labyrinth concerned with sense of equilibration. SYN vestibular organ.

**ves·tib·u·lar lip of spi·ral lim·bus** (ves-tib′yū-lăr lip spīr′ăl lim′bŭs) [TA] The upper, short periosteal extension of the limbus laminae spiralis osseae that provides the central attachment for the tectorial membrane. SYN lamina dentata.

**ves·tib·u·lar nerve** (ves-tib′yū-lăr nĕrv) [TA] Portion of vestibulocochlear nerve [CN VIII] peripheral to vestibular root. SYN vestibular part of vestibulocochlear nerve.

**ves·tib·u·lar neu·ro·ni·tis** (ves-tib′yū-lăr nūr′ō-nī′tis) Paroxysmal attack of severe vertigo, not accompanied by deafness or tinnitus, which affects young to middle-aged adults, often following nonspecific upper respiratory infection.

**ves·tib·u·lar or·gan** (ves-tib′yū-lăr ōr′găn) SYN vestibular labyrinth.

**ves·tib·u·lar part of ves·tib·u·lo·co·chle·ar nerve** (ves-tib′yū-lăr pahrt ves-tib′yū-lō-kok′lē-ăr nĕrv) SYN vestibular nerve.

**ves·tib·u·lar screen** (ves-tib′yū-lăr skrēn) Screen made of acrylic resin that covers labial or buccal surfaces of one or both dental arches; used to stimulate tooth movement by using perioral muscle force.

**ves·tib·u·lar sur·face of coch·le·ar duct** (ves-tib′yū-lăr sŭr′făs kok′lē-ăr dŭkt) [TA] Membrane separating cochlear duct from vestibular canal; consists of squamous epithelial cells with microvilli toward ductus, a basement membrane, and thin layer of connective tissue toward scala.

**ves·tib·u·lar sur·face of tooth** (ves-tib′yū-lăr sŭr′făs tūth) [TA] Tooth surface that faces buccal or labial mucosa of vestibule of

mouth; opposite lingual tooth surface. SYN facial surface of tooth, facies facialis dentis, facies vestibularis dentis.

**ves·ti·bule** (ves′ti-byūl) [TA] **1.** Small cavity or a space at entrance of a canal. **2.** Specifically, central, somewhat ovoid, cavity of osseous labyrinth communicating with semicircular canals posteriorly and cochlea anteriorly. [L. *vestibulum*]

**ves·ti·bule of lar·ynx** (ves′ti-byūl lar′ ingks) [TA] Upper part of laryngeal cavity from superior aperture to vestibular folds or rima vestibuli, bounded anteriorly by epiglottis, laterally by mucosa overlying quadrangular membranes and posteriorly by mucosa overlying arytenoid cartilages and arytenoideus muscle.

**ves·tib·u·lo·cer·e·bel·lar a·tax·i·a** (ves-tib′yū-lō-ser′ĕ-bel′ăr ă-tak′sē-ă) Ataxia due to central vestibular system disease or its cerebellar components, manifested clinically by unsteady gait, nystagmus, and incoordination of arm and leg movements.

**ves·tib·u·lo·co·chle·ar** (ves-tib′yū-lō-kok′ lē-ăr) Relating to vestibule and cochlea of ear.

**ves·tib·u·lo·co·chle·ar nerve [CN VIII]** (ves-tib′yū-lō-kok′lē-ăr nĕrv) [TA] Composite sensory nerve innervating receptor cells of membranous labyrinth. SYN eighth cranial nerve [CN VIII], eighth nerve, nervus acusticus [CN VIII], nervus octavus [CN VIII], nervus statoacusticus [CN VIII], nervus vestibulocochlearis [CN VIII], octavus.

**ves·tib·u·lo·co·chle·ar organ** (ves-tib′yū-lō-kok′lē-ăr ōr′găn) [TA] Organ comprising external, middle, and internal ear; end organs of vestibular and auditory systems.

**ves·tib·u·lo·co·chle·ar vein** (ves-tib′yū-lō-kok′lē-ăr vān) [TA] Companion vein of vestibulocochlear artery, a tributary vein of the cochlear canaliculus.

**ves·tib·u·lop·a·thy** (ves-tib′yū-lōp′ă-thē) Any abnormality of vestibular apparatus.

**ves·tib·u·lo·plas·ty** (ves-tib′yū-lō-plas-tē) Any of a series of surgical procedures designed to restore alveolar ridge height by lowering muscles attaching to buccal, labial, and lingual jaw aspects. [*vestibulo-* + G. *plassō*, to form]

**ves·tib·u·lo·spi·nal re·flex** (ves-tib′yū-lō-spī′năl rē′fleks) Effect of vestibular stimulation on body posture.

**Vet·er·ans Ad·min·is·tra·tion hos·pi·tal** (vet′ĕr-ănz ăd-min′i-strā′shŭn hos′pi-tăl) Hospital operated at federal government expense and administered by the U.S. Veterans Administration for care of veterans, their dependents, and other retired military personnel.

**vi·a·ble** (vī′ă-bĕl) Capable of living; denoting

**uv**

a fetus sufficiently developed to live outside of uterus. [Fr. fr. *vie*, life, fr. L. *vita*]

**vi·bes·ate** (vī′bĕ-sāt) Mixture of polvinate and malrosinol in organic solvent and a propellant; used as a topical spray for wounds.

**vi·brat·ing line** (vī′brāt-ing līn) Imaginary line across posterior part of palate; division between movable and immovable tissues.

**Vick·ers hard·ness test** (vik′ĕrz hahrd′ nĕs test) Common dental assessment to determine the hardness of materials using a diamond point to produce a square impression. SEE ALSO Brinell hardness test.

**vi·dar·a·bine** (vī-dar′ă-bēn) Purine nucleoside used to treat herpes simplex infections.

**view box** (vyū boks) Backlit framed surface on wall or table used for examination of dental radiographs.

**vig·a·bat·rin** (vī-ga′bă-trin) An antiepileptic agent.

**vil·lus,** pl. **vil·li** (vil′ŭs, -ī) *Do not confuse this word with the adjective villous.* **1.** Projection surface, especially from a mucous membrane. **2.** An elongated dermal papilla projecting into an intraepidermal vesicle or cleft.

**Vin·cent an·gi·na** (van[h]-sawn[h]′ an′ji-nă) Ulcerative infection of oral soft tissues including tonsils and pharynx caused by fusiform and spirochetal organisms; usually associated with necrotizing ulcerative gingivitis; may progress to noma. Death from suffocation or sepsis may result.

**Vin·cent ba·cil·lus** (van[h]-sawn[h]′ bă-sil′ŭs) SYN *Fusobacterium nucleatum.*

**Vin·cent gin·gi·vi·tis** (van[h]-sawn[h]′ jin′ji-vī′tis) SYN necrotizing ulcerative gingivitis.

**Vin·cent in·fec·tion** (van[h]-sawn[h]′ in-fek′shŭn) SYN necrotizing ulcerative gingivitis.

**Vin·cent spi·ril·lum** (van[h]-sawn[h]′ spī-ril′ŭm) Spirochete found in association with Vincent bacillus.

**vin·e·gar** (vin′ĕ-găr) Impure dilute acetic acid, made from wine, cider, malt, etc. SYN acetum. [Fr. *vinaigre,* fr. *vin,* wine, + *aigre,* sour]

**VIP** Abbreviation for vasoactive intestinal polypeptide.

**VIP·o·ma** (vi-pō′mă) Endocrine tumor, usually originating in pancreas, which produces a *v*asoactive *i*ntestinal *p*olypeptide believed to cause profound cardiovascular and electrolyte changes with vasodilatory hypotension, watery diarrhea, hypokalemia, and dehydration. [*v*asoactive *i*ntestinal *p*olypeptide + G. *-ōma,* tumor]

**viraemia** SYN viremia.

**vi·ral hep·a·ti·tis** (vī′răl hep′ă-tī′tis) Hepatitis caused by various immunologically unrelated viruses: hepatitis A virus, hepatitis B virus, hepatitis C virus, hepatitis D virus, hepatitis E virus, and hepatitis G virus.

**vi·ral hep·a·ti·tis an·ti·bod·ies** (vī′răl hep′ă-tī′tis an′ti-bod-ēz) Immunoglobulins induced in a patient who is exposed to a hepatitis-causing virus.

**vi·ral hep·a·ti·tis an·ti·gens** (vī′răl hep′ ă-tī′tis an′ti-jĕnz) Immunogenic components of hepatitis viruses.

**vi·ral hep·a·ti·tis, type A** (vī′răl hep′ă-tī′tis tīp) A viral disease with a short (15–50 days) incubation period caused by hepatitis A virus, often transmitted by fecal-oral route.

**vi·ral hep·a·ti·tis, type B** (vī′răl hep′ă-tī′tis tīp) A viral disease with a long incubation period (usually 50–160 days), caused by a hepatitis B virus, usually transmitted by injection of infected blood or blood derivatives or by use of contaminated needles, lancets, or other instruments or by sexual transmission. SYN infectious hepatitis, short-incubation hepatitis.

**vi·ral hep·a·ti·tis, type C** (vī′răl hep′ă-tī′tis tīp) Principal cause of non-A, non-B posttransfusion hepatitis caused by an RNA virus; high percentage of patients develop chronic liver disease leading to cirrhosis.

**vi·ral hep·a·ti·tis, type D** (vī′răl hep′ă-tī′tis tīp) Acute or chronic hepatitis caused by a satellite virus, the hepatitis delta virus; chronic type appears to be more severe than other types of viral hepatitis.

**vi·ral hep·a·ti·tis type E** (vī′răl hep′ă-tī′ tis tīp) Hepatitis caused by a nonenveloped, single-stranded, positive-sense RNA virus unrelated to other forms of hepatitis. Principal cause of enterically transmitted, waterborne, epidemic NANB hepatitis occurring primarily in Asia, Africa, and South America.

**vi·ral shed·ding** (vī′răl shed′ing) Presence of virus in body secretions, in excretions, or in body surface lesions with potential for disease transmission and infection. SYN virus shedding.

**vi·re·mi·a** (vī-rē′mē-ă) The presence of a virus in the bloodstream. SYN viraemia.

**vi·ri·dans strep·to·coc·ci** (vir′i-danz strep-tō-kok′sī) A name applied not to a distinct species but rather to the group of α-hemolytic streptococci as a whole; have been isolated from the mouth and intestines of humans, the intestines of horses, the milk and feces of cows, milk products, and the sputum and lungs. SYN *Streptococcus viridans.*

**vi·ri·on** (vī′rē-on) The complete virus particle that is structurally intact and infectious.

**vi·rol·o·gy** (vī-rol′ŏ-jē) The study of viruses and of viral disease. [*virus* + G. *logos,* study]

**vi·ro·ther·a·py** (vī′rō-thār′ă-pē) Treatment of malignancies using engineered viruses to target cancerous cells.

**vir·u·lence** (vir′yū-lĕns) The disease-evoking power of a pathogen. [L. *virulentia*, fr. *virulentus*, poisonous]

**vi·rus**, pl. **vi·rus·es** (vī′rŭs, -ĕz) 1. Formerly, the specific agent of an infectious disease. 2. Term for a group of infectious agents, which, with few exceptions, are capable of passing through fine filters that retain most bacteria, are usually not visible through the light microscope, lack independent metabolism, and are incapable of growth or reproduction apart from living cells. 3. Relating to or caused by a virus, as a viral disease. [L. poison]

**vis·cer·a** (vis′ĕr-ă) Plural of viscus.

**vis·cer·al swal·low** (vis′ĕr-ăl swahl′ō) Immature swallowing pattern of an infant or older person with tongue thrust.

**vis·cer·o·cra·ni·um** (vis′ĕr-ō-krā′nē-ŭm) [TA] That part of the cranium derived from embryonic pharyngeal arches. SYN facial skeleton, jaw skeleton. [*viscero- + cranium*]

**vis·cer·o·gen·ic re·flex** (vis′ĕr-ō-jen′ik rē′fleks) Any of a number of reflexes (e.g., headache, cough, disturbed pulse), caused by disordered visceral conditions.

**vis·cer·o·mo·tor, vis·cer·i·mo·tor** (vis′ĕr-ō-mō′tŏr, vis′ĕr-i-) Relating to or controlling visceral movement; denoting autonomic nerves innervating viscera, especially intestines.

**vis·cer·o·mo·tor re·flex** (vis′ĕr-ō-mō′tŏr rē′fleks) Contraction of muscles of the thorax or abdomen in response to a stimulus from one of the viscera therein.

**vis·cer·o·skel·e·ton** (vis′ĕr-ō-skel′ĕ-tŏn) 1. Any bony formation in an organ. 2. Bony framework protecting viscera (e.g., ribs and sternum, pelvic bones, and anterior portion of the cranium).

**vis·cos·i·ty** (vis-kos′i-tē) In general, the resistance to flow or alteration of shape by any substance as a result of molecular cohesion. [L. *viscositas*, fr. *viscosus*, viscous]

**vis·cus**, pl. **vis·cer·a** (vis′kŭs, -ĕr-ă) An organ of the digestive, respiratory, urogenital, and endocrine systems as well as the spleen, the heart, and great vessels; hollow and multilayered walled organs. [L. the soft parts]

**vis·i·ble-light cure** (viz′i-bĕl-līt′ kyūr) Polymerization induced by visible light; does not start setting until the light is activated, thereby allowing longer working time for adapting the dressing material.

**vis·ion** (vizh′ŭn) The act of seeing. [L. *visio*, fr. *video*, pp. *visus*, to see]

**vis·u·al a·cu·ity** (vizh′ū-ăl ă-kyū′i-tē) Sharpness or clarity of vision, measured as the ability to distinguish letters or other images of various sizes at a fixed distance, usually with a Snellen chart. Normal rating by such means is 20/20 vision.

**vis·u·al au·ra** (vizh′ū-ăl awr′ă) Epileptic aura characterized by visual illusions or hallucinations, formed or unformed.

**vis·u·al e·val·u·a·tion** (vizh′ū-ăl ĕ-val′yū-ā′shŭn) Examination of a cutting edge to evaluate sharpness accomplished by holding the working-end under a strong light source. A dull cutting edge reflects light because it is rounded and thick and reflected light appears as a bright line running along the edge of the face. A sharp cutting edge is more of a line—with no thickness—and so does not reflect light.

**vis·u·al e·voked po·ten·tial (VEP)** (vizh′ū-ăl ē-vōkt′ pŏ-ten′shăl) Voltage fluctuations that may be recorded from occipital area of scalp due to retinal stimulation by a light flashing at quarter-second intervals.

**vis·u·al pur·ple** (vizh′ū-ăl pŭr′pĕl) SYN rhodopsin.

**vis·u·o·au·di·tor·y** (vizh′yū-ō-aw′di-tōr′ē) Relating to both vision and hearing; denoting nerves connecting centers for these senses.

**vis·u·og·no·sis** (vizh′ū-og-nō′sis) Recognition and understanding of visual impressions. [L. *visus*, vision, + G. *gnōsis*, knowledge]

**vi·tal** (vī′tăl) Relating to life. [L. *vitalis*, fr. *vita*, life]

**vi·tal bleach·ing** (vī′tăl blēch′ing) Bleaching of teeth to remove stains or lighten the color; usually done with peroxides.

**vi·tal ca·pa·ci·ty (VC)** (vī′tăl kă-pas′i-tē) The greatest volume of air that can be exhaled from the lungs after a maximum inspiration. SYN respiratory capacity.

**vi·tal·i·ty test** (vī-tal′i-tē test) Group of thermal and electrical assessments of dental pulp health. SYN pulp test.

**vi·ta·lom·e·ter** (vī′tă-lom′ĕ-tĕr) Electrical device for determining vitality of tooth pulp.

**vit·al pulp** (vī′tăl pŭlp) Pulp composed of viable tissue, either normal or diseased, responds to electric stimuli and to heat and cold.

**vi·tal signs (VS)** (vīt′ăl sīnz) Clinical determination of temperature, pulse rate, rate of breathing, and level of blood pressure.

**vi·tal sta·tis·tics** (vī′tăl stă-tis′tiks) Systematically tabulated information concerning births, marriages, divorces, separations, and deaths.

**vi·tal tooth** (vī′tăl tūth) Tooth with a living pulp.

UV

**vi·ta·min** (vīt′ă-min) One of a group of organic substances, present in minute amounts in natural foodstuffs, which are essential to normal metabolism; insufficient amounts in the diet may cause deficiency diseases. [L. *vita,* life, + *amine*]

**vi·ta·min A** (vīt′ă-min) **1.** Any β-ionone derivative, except provitamin A carotenoids, possessing qualitatively the biologic activity of retinol; deficiency interferes with production and resynthesis of rhodopsin, thereby causing night blindness. **2.** Retinol, original vitamin A.

**vi·ta·min A2** (vī′tă-min) SYN dehydroretinol.

**vi·ta·min A1 ac·id** (vīt′ă-min as′id) SYN retinoic acid.

**vi·ta·min B** (vī′tă-min) Group of water-soluble substances originally considered as one vitamin.

**vi·ta·min B1** (vī′tă-min) SYN thiamin.

**vi·ta·min B2** (vī′tă-min) SYN riboflavin.

**vi·ta·min B6** (vī′tă-min) Pyridoxine and related compounds (e.g., pyridoxal; pyridoxamine).

**vi·ta·min B12** (vī′tă-min) Generic descriptor for compounds exhibiting biologic activity of cyanocobalamin.

**vi·ta·min Bc con·ju·gase** (vī′tă-min kon′jŭ-gās) Enzyme catalyzing hydrolysis of the pteroylpolyglutamic acids to pteroylmonoglutamic acid, with consequent increase in vitamin activity; obsolete term for folic acid.

**vi·ta·min B com·plex** (vī′tă-min kom′pleks) Pharmaceutic term applied to drug products containing a mixture of the B vitamins, usually B1, B2, B3, B5, and B6.

**vi·ta·min B12 with in·trin·sic fac·tor con·cen·trate** (vī′tă-min in-trin′sik fak′tŏr kon′sĕn-trāt) Combination of vitamin B12 with suitable preparations of mucosa of the stomach or intestine of domestic animals used for food by humans.

**vi·ta·min C** (vīt′ă-min) SYN ascorbic acid.

**vi·ta·min C test** (vī′tă-min test) SYN capillary fragility test.

**vi·ta·min C u·nit (in·ter·na·tion·al)** (vī′tă-min yū′nit in′tĕr-nash′ŏ-năl) Vitamin C activity of 0.05 mg of the standard crystalline levoascorbic acid.

**vi·ta·min D** (vī′tă-min) Generic descriptor for all steroids exhibiting biologic activity of ergocalciferol or cholecalciferol, the antirachitic vitamins popularly called "sun-ray vitamins." They promote the proper use of calcium and phosphorus, thereby producing growth, together with proper bone and tooth formation, in young children.

**vi·ta·min D2** (vī′tă-min) SYN ergocalciferol.

**vi·ta·min D milk** (vī′tă-min milk) Cow's milk to which vitamin D has been added, to contain 400 USP units of vitamin D per quart.

**vi·ta·min D–re·sis·tant rick·ets** (vī′tă-min rĕ-zis′tănt rik′ĕts) Metabolic disorder characterized by renal tubular defects in phosphate transport and bone abnormalities resulting in hypophosphatemic rickets or osteomalacia.

**vi·ta·min D u·nit (in·ter·na·tion·al)** (vī′tă-min yū′nit in′tĕr-nash′ŏ-năl) Antirachitic activity contained in 0.025 mcg of a preparation of crystalline vitamin D3.

**vi·ta·min E** (vī′tă-min) **1.** SYN alpha-tocopherol. **2.** Generic descriptor of tocol and tocotrienol derivatives possessing the biologic activity of α-tocopherol; contained in various oils (e.g., wheat germ, cotton seed, palm, rice) and whole grain cereals where it constitutes the nonsaponifiable fraction.

**vi·ta·min E u·nit** (vī′tă-min yū′nit) Potency usually expressed in terms of weight of pure α-tocopherol.

**vi·ta·min F** (vī′tă-min) Term sometimes applied to the essential unsaturated fatty acids: linoleic, linolenic, and arachidonic acids.

**vi·ta·min K** (vī′tă-min) Generic descriptor for compounds with the biologic activity of phylloquinone; fat-soluble, thermostable compounds found in alfalfa, pork, liver, fish meal, and vegetable oils.

**vit·a·min K1, vit·a·min K1(20)** (vī′tă-min) SYN phylloquinone.

**vi·ta·min K3** (vī′tă-min) SYN menadione.

**vi·ta·min K4** (vī′tă-min) SYN menadiol diacetate.

**vi·ta·min K5** (vī′tă-min) An antihemorrhagic vitamin.

**vi·ta·min K u·nit** (vī′tă-min yū′nit) SEE Dam unit.

**vi·ta·min P** (vī′tă-min) Mixture of plant bioflavonoids (especially citrus fruits); reduces permeability and fragility of capillaries and is useful in treatment of some cases of purpura that are resistant to vitamin C therapy.

**vi·ta·min U** (vī′tă-min) Term given to a factor in fresh cabbage juice that encourages healing of peptic ulcers.

**vit·i·a·tion** (vish′ē-ā′shŭn) Change that impairs use or reduces efficiency. [L. *vitiatio* fr. *vitio,* pp. *vitiatus,* to corrupt, fr. *vitium,* vice]

**vit·i·li·go,** pl. **vit·i·lig·i·nes** (vit′i-lī′gō, -lij′nēz) The appearance on otherwise normal skin of nonpigmented white patches of varied sizes; hair in the affected areas is usually white. Epidermal melanocytes are completely lost in depigmented areas by an autoimmune process. [L. a skin eruption, fr. *vitium,* blemish, vice]

**vit·re·o·den·tin** (vit′rē-ō-den′tin) Dentin of a particularly brittle quality character.

**vit·ri·fi·ca·tion** (vit′ri-fi-kā′shŭn) Conversion of dental porcelain (frit) to a glassy substance by heat and fusion. [L. *vitrium,* glassy, + *facio,* to make]

**vit·ri·ol** (vit′rē-ol) Any of the various salts of sulfuric acid.

**V-MI** Abbreviation for Volpe-Manhold Index.

**vo·cal frem·i·tus** (vō′kăl frem′i-tŭs) Vibration in the chest wall, felt on palpation, produced by the spoken voice. [L. *fremitus vocalis*]

**vo·cal res·o·nance (VR)** (vō′kăl rez′ŏ-năns) Voice sounds as heard on auscultation of the chest.

**voice** (voys) The sound made by air passing out through the larynx and upper respiratory tract, the vocal folds being approximated.

**void** (voyd) To evacuate urine or feces.

**vol·a·tile** (vol′ă-til) 1. Tending to evaporate rapidly. 2. Tending toward violence, explosiveness, or rapid change. [L. *volatilis,* fr. *volo,* to fly]

**vol·a·tile an·es·thet·ic** (vol′ă-til an′es-thet′ik) Liquid anesthetic that volatilizes to a vapor at room temperature and, when inhaled, is capable of producing general anesthesia.

**vol·a·tile oil** (vol′ă-til oyl) A substance of oily consistency and feel, derived from a plant and containing the principles to which the odor and taste of the plant are due (essential oil). SYN ethereal oil.

**Volk·mann chei·li·tis** (fōlk′mahn kī-lī′tis) SYN cheilitis glandularis.

**Vol·pe-Man·hold In·dex (V-MI)** (vōl′pē man′hōld in′deks) Assessment tool for comparing the amount of dental calculus in different patients.

**volt (v, V)** (vōlt) The unit of electromotive force; the electromotive force that will produce a current of 1 ampere in a circuit that has a resistance of 1 ohm.

**volt·age** (vōl′tăj) Electromotive force, pressure, or potential expressed in volts.

**vol·ume** (vol′yūm) Space occupied by matter,

expressed usually in cubic millimeters, cubic centimeters, liters, and other measures. [L. *volumen,* something rolled up, scroll, fr. *volvo,* to roll]

**vol·un·tar·y** (vol′ŭn-tar-ē) Relating or acting in obedience to the will; not obligatory. [L. *voluntarius,* fr. *voluntas,* will, fr. *volo,* to wish]

**vol·un·tar·y mut·ism** (vol′ŭn-tar-ē myū′tizm) SYN elective mutism.

**vo·mer** (vō′mĕr) [TA] A trapezoidal bone forming the inferior and posterior portion of the nasal septum. [L. ploughshare]

**vom·it** (vom′it) 1. To eject matter from the stomach through the mouth. 2. Vomitus; the matter so ejected. SYN vomitus (2). [L. *vomo,* pp. *vomitus,* to vomit]

**vom·it·ing** (vom′it-ing) Ejection of matter from stomach in retrograde fashion through the esophagus and mouth. SYN emesis (1), vomitus (1).

**vom·it·ing re·flex** (vom′it-ing rē′fleks) Vomiting elicited by a variety of stimuli, especially one applied to region of fauces. SYN pharyngeal reflex (2).

**vom·it·u·ri·tion** (vom′i-tyūr-ish′ŭn) SYN retching.

**vom·i·tus** (vom′i-tŭs) 1. SYN vomiting. 2. SYN vomit (2). [L. a vomiting, vomit]

**von Grae·fe syn·drome II** (von grā′fĕ sin′drōm) SYN Moebius syndrome.

**von Spee curve** (fahn shpē kŭrv) SYN curve of Spee.

**von Wil·le·brand dis·ease** (fahn vil′ĕ-brahnt di-zēz′) Hemorrhagic diathesis characterized by tendency to bleed primarily from mucous membranes (i.e., oral), prolonged bleeding time, normal platelet count, normal clot retraction, partial and variable deficiency of factor VIIIR.

**VP** Abbreviation for vasopressin.

**VR** Abbreviation for vocal resonance.

**VS** Abbreviation for vital signs.

**VSD** Abbreviation for ventricular septal defect.

**vul·ner·a·bil·i·ty** (vŭl′nĕr-ă-bil′i-tē) Weakness of susceptibility to damage. [L. *vulnerabilis,* susceptible to injury, fr. *vulnero,* to wound, fr. *vulnus,* wound]

**UV**

# W

**W** Abbreviation for tryptophan; watt.

**Wa·chen·dorf mem·brane** (vahk´en-dŏrf mem´brān) **1.** SYN pupillary membrane. **2.** SYN cell membrane.

**wad·ding** (wahd´ing) Carded cotton or wool in sheets, used for surgical dressing.

**wad·dling gait** (wahd´ling gāt) Rolling ambulation in which weight-bearing hip is not stabilized; it bulges outward with each step, opposite side of pelvis drops, resulting in alternating lateral trunk movements; due to gluteus medius muscle weakness, and seen with muscular dystrophies, among other disorders.

**walk·er** (wawk´ĕr) A light, portable framework used for support and assistance in walking by a person with a gait impairment for which a cane or crutches are inadequate.

**walk·ing stroke** (wawk´ing strōk) Movement of a calibrated probe around the perimeter of the base of a sulcus or pocket.

**walk·ing stroke ac·tion** (wawk´ing strōk ak´shŭn) A combination push-pull motion used with a light grasp during exploration of teeth and root surfaces.

**wall** (wawl) [TA] An investing part enclosing a cavity such as the thorax, abdomen or any hollow unit, or that covers a cell or any anatomic unit. [L. *vallum*]

**W-arch** (ahrch) Fixed maxillary expansion device attached to lingual part of molars, with either bilateral or unilateral extension arms.

**war·fa·rin** (wōr´fă-rin) Anticoagulant with same actions as dicumarol.

**warn·ing** (wōrn´ing) Strong cautionary advice about possible dangers or contraindications in health-care-related activity or pharmacy.

**wart** (wōrt) SYN verruca.

**wash·ed field tech·nique** (wawsht fēld tek-nēk´) Cutting cavity preparations in teeth by using a constant irrigant that is immediately suctioned from the mouth with a vacuum device.

**waste man·age·ment** (wāst man´ăj-mĕnt) Administration of activities that provide safe collection, transport, processing, recycling or disposal of potentially hazardous waste products (i.e. needles, tissue specimens).

**wast·ing** (wāst´ing) **1.** SYN emaciation. **2.** Denoting a disease characterized by emaciation.

**wa·ter** (waw´tĕr) **1.** A clear, odorless, tasteless liquid, solidifying at 0°C (32°F) and boiling at 100°C (212°F), present in all animal and vegetable tissues and dissolves more substances than any other liquid. **2.** Euphemism for urine. [A.S. *waeter*]

**wa·ter-cool·ed in·stru·ment tip** (waw´tĕr-kūld in´strŭ-mĕnt tip) Sonic or ultrasonic instrument tip cooled by a constant stream of water provided near the point of the instrument tip.

**wa·ter di·u·re·sis** (waw´tĕr dī´yūr-ē´sis) Excretion of urine after drinking water; results from reduced secretion of antidiuretic hormone of neurohypophysis in response to the lowered osmotic blood pressure.

**Wa·ter·house-Frid·er·ich·sen syn·drome** (waw´tĕr-hows frē´der-ik-sen sin´drŏm) Condition occurring mainly in children younger than 10 years of age, characterized by vomiting, diarrhea, extensive purpura, cyanosis, tonic-clonic convulsions, and circulatory collapse.

**wa·ter·shed** (waw´tĕr-shed) **1.** Area of marginal blood flow at the extreme periphery of a vascular bed. **2.** Slopes in the abdominal cavity, formed by projections of the lumbar vertebrae and the pelvic brim.

**wa·ter·shed in·farc·tion** (waw´tĕr-shed in-fahrk´shŭn) Infarction in a region of the cerebral cortex, the spinal cord, or a peripheral nerve where the distributions of nutrient arteries meet or overlap.

**Wat·son-Crick he·lix** (waht´sŏn-krik´ hē´liks) Helical structure assumed by two strands of deoxyribonucleic acid, held together throughout their length by hydrogen bonds between bases on opposite strands, referred to as Watson-Crick base pairing.

**watt (W)** (waht) The SI unit of electrical power.

**wave** (wāv) **1.** Movement of particles in an elastic body, whether solid or fluid, which produces a progression of alternate elevations and depressions, or rarefactions and condensations. **2.** The elevation of the pulse, felt by the finger or represented in the curved line of the sphygmograph. [A.S. *wafian*, to fluctuate]

**wave·length** (wāv´length) The distance from one point on a wave (frequently shaped like a sine curve) to the next point in the same phase; i.e., from peak to peak or from trough to trough.

**wax** (waks) **1.** A substance, plastic at room temperature, secreted by bees for building honeycomb cells. See this page. SYN cera. **2.** Any substance with physical properties similar to those of beeswax, of animal, vegetable, or mineral origin (e.g., oils, lipids, or fats that are solids at room temperature). See page 597. [A.S. *weax*]

**wax-bite reg·is·tra·tion** (waks´bīt rej´is-trā´shŭn) A record, made in wax, of the occlusal relationship of the maxilla and the mandible.

**wax ex·pan·sion** (waks eks-pan´shŭn) In dentistry, a method of expanding wax patterns

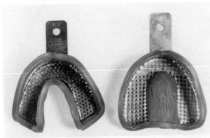

**beading or periphery wax**

to compensate for shrinkage of gold during casting process.

**wax·ing, wax·ing-up** (waks'ing, -ŭp') Contouring a pattern in wax, generally applied to shaping in wax of contours of a trial denture or a crown prior to casting in metal.

**wax mod·el den·ture** (waks mod'ĕl den' chŭr) SYN trial denture.

**wax pat·tern** (waks pat'ĕrn) Casting wax molded or carved to replicate a restoration to replace missing tooth structure or to produce a metal framework for a removable prosthesis.

**wax·y cast** (waks'ē kast) Form of urinary cast consisting of homogeneous proteinaceous material that has a high refractive index, in contrast to the low refractive index of hyaline casts; waxy casts probably represents an advanced stage of the disintegrative process that results in coarsely and finely granular casts and are usually indicative of advanced renal disease.

**WBC** Abbreviation for white blood cell.

**wean·ing** (wēn'ing) **1.** Transition of the human infant from breast-feeding or bottle nursing and commencement of nourishment with other food. **2.** Gradual withdrawal of a patient from dependency on a life-support system or other form of therapy. **3.** Gradual elimination of physical or psychological dependence on a harmful or otherwise inappropriate substance or activity.

**wear** (wār) Wasting or deterioration caused by friction.

**We·ber syn·drome** (web'ĕr sin'drōm) Midbrain tegmentum lesion characterized by ipsilateral oculomotor nerve paresis and contralateral paralysis of the extremities, face, and tongue.

**We·del·staedt chis·el** (wād'ĕl-stāt chiz' ĕl) Tool with slightly curved blade aligned with long axis of shank.

**wedge** (wej) A solid body having the shape of an acute-angled triangular prism. [A.S. *weeg*]

**weight** (wāt) **1.** In scientific usage, product of the force of gravity, defined internationally as 9.80665 m/s², times the mass of the body. **2.** In common usage, apparent mass of a body when measured in air by comparison to standard masses of prescribed composition, the effects of the buoyancy of air being ignored. **3.** A piece of material, usually metal, of known mass, used as a comparison object in weighing. [A.S. *gewiht*]

**well·ness** (wel'nĕs) A philosophy of life and personal hygiene that views health as not merely the absence of illness but the full realization of one's physical and mental potential, as achieved through positive attitudes, fitness training, a diet low in fat and high in fiber, and the avoidance of unhealthful practices (smoking, drug and alcohol abuse, overeating).

**Wer·nic·ke-Kor·sa·koff syn·drome** (ver'ni-kĕ-kōr'sĕ-kof sin'drōm) The coexistence of Wernicke and Korsakoff syndromes.

**Wer·nic·ke syn·drome** (ver'ni-kĕ sin' drōm) Common condition in patients with long-term alcoholism, resulting largely from thiamin deficiency and characterized by disturbances in ocular motility, pupillary alterations, nystagmus, and ataxia with tremors.

**Wes·tern blot, Wes·tern blot·ting** (wes' tĕrn blot, blot'ing) SYN Western blot analysis.

**West·ern blot a·nal·y·sis** (wes'tĕrn blot ă-nal'i-sis) A procedure in which proteins separated by electrophoresis in polyacrylamide gels are transferred (blotted) onto nitrocellulose or nylon membranes and identified by specific complexing with antibodies that are either pre- or posttagged with a labeled secondary protein. SYN Western blot, Western blotting.

**West Nile vi·rus** (west nīl vī'rŭs) Mosquito-borne virus; human infection is usually subclinical but can lead to fatal encephalitis, particularly in old people.

**wet gang·rene** (wet gang-grēn') Ischemic necrosis of an extremity with bacterial infection, producing cellulitis adjacent to the necrotic areas. SYN moist gangrene.

**Whar·ton duct** (wōr'tŏn dŭkt) SYN submandibular duct.

**wheal** (wēl) Circumscribed, evanescent papule or irregular plaque or dermal edema, appearing as an urticarial lesion, slightly reddened, often changing in size and shape and extending to adjacent areas, and usually accompanied by intense itching; produced by intradermal injection or test, or by exposure to allergenic substances in susceptible people. [A.S. *hwēle*]

**wheat germ** (wēt jĕrm) Embryo of wheat; contains thiamin, riboflavin, and other vitamins.

**wheat germ oil** (wēt jĕrm oyl) Oil obtained by expression from germ of the wheat seed, one of the richest sources of natural vitamin E; used as a nutritional supplement.

**WX**

**wheeze** (wēz) **1.** To breathe noisily and with difficulty. **2.** A whistling, squeaking, musical, or puffing sound made on exhalation by air passing through fauces, glottis, or narrowed tracheobronchial airways. [A.S. *hwēsan*]

**whe·wel·lite** (wē′wel-īt) A monohydrate of calcium oxalate; found in renal calculi.

**whe·wel·lite cal·cu·lus** (wē′wel-īt kal′kyū-lŭs) Dental calculus in which the crystalloid component is calcium oxalate monohydrate.

**whis·key** (wis′kē) An alcoholic liquid obtained by the distillation of the fermented mash of wholly or partly malted cereal grains (e.g., barley, corn, rye, and wheat). [Gael, *usquebaugh,* water of life]

**white blood cell (WBC)** (wīt blŭd sel) SYN leukocyte.

**white cor·pus·cle** (wīt kōr′pŭs-ĕl) Any type of leukocyte.

**white hair·y tongue** (wīt hār′ē tŭng) Lingual disorder characterized by elongation of the filiform papillae. SYN lingua alba, lingua villosa alba.

**whit·en·ing** (wīt′ĕn-ing) Lightening of teeth to a whiter color by use of dental bleaching materials. See this page.

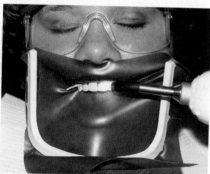

office-applied vital tooth whitening using light to enhance the effects of the whitening agent

**white sponge ne·vus** (wīt spŭnj nē′vŭs) Disorder of oral cavity characterized by soft, white or opalescent, thickened, and corrugated folds of mucous membrane; other mucosal sites are occasionally involved simultaneously. See this page and page A10. SYN oral epithelial nevus.

**white spot le·sion** (wīt spot lē′zhŭn) First sign of demineralization of the enamel surface of a tooth; produces a chalky white appearance.

**whit·ing** (wīt′ing) Chalk ($CaCO_3$) used to polish metal or plastic appliances.

**whit·low** (wit′lō) Purulent infection through a perionychial fold causing an abscess of the

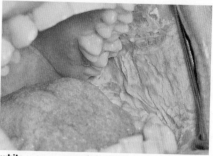

white sponge nevus: buccal mucosa

bulbous distal end of a finger. SEE ALSO herpetic whitlow. [M.E. *whitflawe*]

**WHO** Abbreviation for World Health Organization.

**whoop** (hūp, wūp) The loud sonorous inspiration in pertussis with which the paroxysm of coughing terminates, due to spasm of the larynx.

**whoop·ing cough** (hūp′ing kawf, wūp′) SYN pertussis.

**whorl** (wŏrl) Turn of the spiral cochlea of the ear.

**whorl·ed e·nam·el** (wŏrld ĕ-nam′ĕl) Enamel in which rods assume a twisting course.

**will** (wil) A legal document expressing the writer's wishes for the disposal of personal property after death. [M.E., fr. O.E. *willa*]

**Wil·liams syn·drome** (wil′yăms sin′drōm) Disorder characterized by distinctive facies with shallow supraorbital ridges, medial eyebrow flare, stellate patterning of the irises, small nose with anteverted nares, and loquacious personality.

**Wil·son dis·ease** (wil′sŏn di-zēz′) Disorder of copper metabolism, characterized by cirrhosis, basal ganglia degeneration, neurologic manifestations, and deposition of green or golden brown pigmentation in the periphery of the cornea. [S.A.K. *Wilson*]

**win·dow** (win′dō) **1.** SYN fenestra. **2.** Any opening in space or time, particularly a critical interval within which a given event must, or cannot, occur. **3.** In computed tomography, range of CT numbers (expressed in Hounsfield units) across which all shades of the gray scale are distributed in a given image so as to emphasize slight differences in x-ray absorption coefficients between tissues of similar density (e.g., mediastinal soft tissues).

**win·dow pe·ri·od** (win′dō pēr′ē-ŏd) **1.** Critical time interval. **2.** Time between infection with a bloodborne virus and the appearance of specific laboratory evidence of infection in a specimen of blood obtained from the asymptomatic host for the purpose of diagnostic screening, or in blood or blood products donated by the host.

**wind·pipe** (wind′pīp) SYN trachea.

**wing** (wing) [TA] Any flattened, laterally projecting process. SYN ala. [Fr. Middle English *winge, wenge,* from Old Norse *vaenger,* wing]

**wink re·flex** (wingk rē′fleks) General term for reflex closure of eyelids caused by any stimulus.

**wire** (wīr) A slender, pliable rod or thread of metal, used in dentistry and surgery.

**wire arch** (wīr ahrch) Wire conforming to the dental arch; used to restore normal curve to a denture.

**wire splint** (wīr splint) 1. Device for stabilizing teeth loosened by trauma or by a periodontal condition in maxilla or mandible. 2. Device for reducing and stabilizing maxillary or mandibular fractures; applied to both jaws, with its two components connected by intermaxillary wires or rubber bands.

**wir·ing** (wīr′ing) Fastening together the ends of a broken bone by wire sutures.

**wir·y** (wīr′ē) 1. Resembling or having the hard, threadlike feel of wire. 2. Denoting a small, fine, incompressible pulse.

**wis·dom tooth** (wiz′dŏm tūth) SYN third molar tooth.

**Wiss·ler syn·drome** (vis′ler sin′drōm) High intermittent fever; irregularly recurring macular and maculopapular eruption of the face, chest, and limbs; leukocytosis; arthralgia; occasionally eosinophilia and raised erythrocyte sedimentation rate; occurs in children and adolescents, with varying duration.

**with·draw·al** (with-draw′ăl) 1. Act of removal or retreat. 2. Psychological and/or physical syndrome caused by abrupt cessation of use of a drug in a habituated person. 3. Therapeutic process of discontinuing a drug to avoid the symptoms of withdrawal.

**with·draw·al syn·drome** (with-draw′ăl sin′drōm) Development of a substance-specific syndrome that follows cessation of, or reduction in, intake of a psychoactive substance that the person previously used regularly; e.g., clinical syndrome of disorientation, perceptual disturbance, and psychomotor agitation following cessation of chronic use of excessive quantities of alcohol is termed alcohol withdrawal syndrome.

**WN** Abbreviation for well-nourished.

**wolff·i·an bod·y** (vōlf′ē-ăn bod′ē) SYN mesonephros.

**Wolff law** (vōlf law) 1. Every change in the

form and the function of a bone is followed by changes in the bone's internal architecture and secondary alterations in its external conformation; these changes usually represent responses to alterations in weight-bearing stresses. 2. Bone forms in areas of stress and is resorbed in areas of nonstress.

**Wo·lin·el·la** (wō′li-nel′ă) Genus of gramnegative, microaerophilic bacteria isolated from gingival sulcus and root canal infections in humans. Type species is *W. succinogenes.*

**work con·di·tion·ing** (wŏrk kŏn-dish′ŏn-ing) 1. A treatment program focused on functional requirements of a job or employment setting, incorporating the basic components of physical conditioning such as strength, endurance, flexibility, and coordination. 2. A component of an industrial therapy program that serves as a precursor to a work hardening program; it is undertaken after acute care or basic rehabilitation treatment has been completed.

**work hard·en·ing** (wŏrk hahr′dĕn-ing) A multidisciplinary progam where actual work tasks are performed to rehabilitate an injured worker. The focus of therapy is to stimulate a regular work routine where therapy is regimented as a precursor to return to work. SEE ALSO work conditioning.

**work·ing con·tacts** (wŏrk′ing kon′takts) Points of contact of artificial or natural teeth on side of occlusion toward which mandible has deviated.

**work·ing cut·ting edge** (wŏrk′ing kŭt′ing ej) Cutting edge used for periodontal débridement. Universal curettes have two working cutting edges per working-end; area-specific curettes have only one.

**work·ing-end** (wŏrk′ing end) The part of an instrument used to perform a task or procedure. See this page.

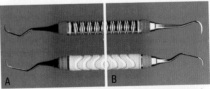

**unpaired and paired working-ends:** (A) instrument with unpaired dissimilar working-ends; (B) instrument with paired, mirror image working-ends

**work·ing oc·clu·sal sur·faces** (wŏrk′ing ŏ-klū′zăl sŭr′făs-ĕz) Dental areas on which mastication can occur.

**work·ing path** (wŏrk′ing path) Trajectory of ipsilateral condyle during lateral jaw movement.

**work·ing side** (wŏrk′ing sīd) In dentistry,

lateral segment of a dentition toward which mandible is moved during occlusal function.

**work·ing side con·dyle** (wŏrk´ing sīd kon´dīl) In dentistry, mandibular condyle on the side toward which mandible moves in a lateral excursion.

**work·ing stroke** (wŏrk´ing strōk) Scaling or root planing action of a dental instrument.

**work sim·pli·fi·ca·tion** (wŏrk sim´pli-fi-kā´shŭn) Application to clinical procedures of time-and-motion studies, analysis of dental instruments and other equipment, and use of body mechanics to smooth patient's therapy.

**World Health Or·ga·ni·za·tion (WHO)** (wŏrld helth ōr´găn-ĭ-zā´shŭn) Branch of the United Nations having as its aim "the attainment of all peoples of the highest possible level of health" (Article 1, UN Charter).

**World Health Or·gan·i·za·tion probe** (wŏrld helth ōr´găn-ĭ-zā´shŭn prōb) Periodontal probe developed by the World Health Organization and used with the Periodontal Screening and Recording (PSR) System for periodontal assessment. The WHO probe has a colored band (called the reference marking) located 3.5–5.5 mm from the probe tip. This colored reference marking is used when performing a PSR screening examination on dental patients.

**wound** (wūnd) 1. Trauma to any body tissues, especially caused by physical means and with interruption of continuity. 2. A surgical incision. 3. To inflict with a wound. [O.E. *wund*]

**wo·ven bone** (wō´vĕn bōn) Bony tissue characteristic of the embryonal skeleton, in which the collagen fibers of the matrix are arranged

irregularly in the form of interlacing networks. SYN nonlamellar bone, reticulated bone.

**wrist** (rist) [TA] The proximal segment of the hand consisting of the carpal bones and the associated soft parts. [A.S. wrist joint, ankle joint]

**wrist clo·nus re·flex** (rist klō´nŭs rē´fleks) Sustained clonic movement of the hand induced by sudden extension of the wrist.

**wrist-drop** (rist´drop) Paralysis of extensors of wrist and fingers; most often caused by radial nerve lesion.

**wrist mo·tion ac·ti·va·tion** (rist mō´shŭn ak´ti-vā´shŭn) Rotating the hand and wrist as a unit to provide power for an instrumentation stroke.

**writ·ing** (rīt´ing) 1. The act of forming letters to produce a visible and intelligible body of coherent language. 2. The product of such activity.

**writ·ing hand** (rīt´ing hand) SYN dominant hand.

**wrought wire** (rawt wīr) Wire formed by drawing a cast structure through a die into a desired shape and size; used in dentistry for partial denture clasps and orthodontic appliances.

**wrought-wire clasp** (rawt-wīr´ klasp) Fitting on a removable partial denture made of an alloy drawn or worked into a wire and formed appropriately.

**Wy·burn-Ma·son syn·drome** (wī´bŭrn-mā´sŏn sin´drōm) Combination of findings include arteriovenous malformation on the cerebral cortex, arteriovenous malformation of the retina and intracranial optic pathway, and facial nevus, usually occurs in people with mental retardation.

# X

**X** Abbreviation for crossbite.

**xan·the·las·ma pal·pe·bra·rum** (zan′thĕ-laz′mă pal′pē-brā′rŭm) Soft, yellow-orange plaques on eyelids or medial canthus, most common form of xanthoma; may be associated with low-density lipoproteins, especially in younger adults. SYN xanthoma palpebrarum.

**xan·thene** (zan′thēn) Basic structure of many natural products, drugs, dyes (e.g., fluorescein, pyronin, eosins), indicators, pesticides, and antibiotics.

**xan·thi·nu·ri·a, xan·thi·u·ri·a, xan·thur·i·a** (zan′thi-nyū′rē-ă, -thē-yūr′ē-ă, -thyūr′ē-ă) **1.** Excretion of abnormally large amounts of xanthine in the urine. **2.** A disorder characterized by urinary excretion of xanthine in place of uric acid, hypouricemia, and occasionally the formation of renal xanthine stones. [*xanthine* + G. *ouron*, urine]

**xan·tho·dont** (zan′thō-dont) Someone who has yellow teeth. [*xantho-* + G. *odous*, tooth]

**xan·tho·gran·u·lo·ma** (zan′thō-gran′yū-lō′mă) An infiltration of retroperitoneal tissue by lipid macrophages, occurring most commonly in women.

**xan·tho·ma** (zan-thō′mă) Yellow nodule or plaque, especially dermatologic, composed of lipid-laden histiocytes. [G. *xantho-*, blond + G. *-oma*, tumor]

**xan·tho·ma di·a·be·ti·co·rum** (zan-thō′mă dī-ă-bet-i-kō′rŭm) Eruptive xanthoma associated with severe diabetes.

**xan·tho·ma pal·pe·bra·rum** (zan-thō′mă pal′pē-brā′rŭm) SYN xanthelasma palpebrarum.

**xan·tho·ma pla·num** (zan-thō′mă plā′nŭm) Form of xanthoma marked by the occurrence of yellow, flat bands or minimally palpable rectangular plates in the corium.

**xan·tho·ma·to·sis** (zan′thō-mă-tō′sis) Widespread xanthomas, especially on elbows and knees, which sometimes affect mucous membranes and may be associated with metabolic disturbances.

**xan·tho·sis** (zan-thō′sis) A yellowish discoloration of degenerating tissues, especially seen in malignant neoplasms. [*xantho-* + G. *-osis*, condition]

**X chro·mo·some, Y chro·mo·some** (krō′mŏ-sōm) SEE sex chromosomes.

♻ **xeno-** *This combining form is correctly pronounced zĕn″ō, not zē′nō.* Strange; consisting of foreign material; parasitic. [G. *xenos*, guest, host, stranger, foreign]

**xen·o·bi·ot·ic** (zen′ō-bī-ot′ik) Pharmacologically, endocrinologically, or toxicologically active substance not endogenously produced and therefore foreign to an organism. [*xeno-* + G. *bios*, life + *-ic*]

**xen·o·graft** (zen′ō-graft, zē′nō-graft) A graft transferred from an animal of one species to one of another species. SYN heterograft, heterologous graft.

**xen·o·pho·bi·a** (zen′ō-fō′bē-ă) Morbid fear of strangers or foreigners. [*xeno-* + G. *phobos*, fear]

♻ **xero-** *Avoid misspelling this combining form zero-.* Combining form denoting dry. [G. *xeros*]

**xe·ro·chi·li·a** (zēr′ō-kī′lē-ă) Dryness of the lips. [*xero-* + G. *cheilos*, lip]

**xe·ro·der·ma, xe·ro·der·mi·a** (zēr′ō-dĕr′mă, -mē-ă) Mild form of ichthyosis characterized by excessive dryness of skin due to slight thickening of horny layer and diminished water content of stratum corneum due to decreased perspiration or exposure to wind, or low humidity; associated with aging, atopic dermatitis, and vitamin A deficiency. [*xero-* + G. *derma*, skin]

**xe·ro·der·ma pig·men·to·sum** (zēr′ō-dĕr′mă pig′men-tō′sŭm) Eruption of exposed skin occurring in childhood and characterized by photosensitivity with severe sunburn in infancy and the development of numerous pigmented spots resembling freckles, larger atrophic lesions eventually resulting in glossy white thinning of the skin surrounded by telangiectases, and multiple solar keratoses that undergo malignant change at an early age.

**xe·ro·gen·ic** (zēr′ō-jen′ik) Denotes that which causes dry mouth.

**xe·rog·ra·phy** (zē-rog′ră-fē) SYN xeroradiography.

**xe·ro·ma** (zēr-ō′mă) SYN xerophthalmia.

**xe·ro·pha·gi·a, xe·roph·a·gy** (zē′rō-fā′jē-ă, zēr-of′ă-jē) Consumption of dry foodstuffs; subsistence on a dry diet. [*xero-* + G. *phagō*, to eat]

**xe·roph·thal·mi·a** (zēr′of-thal′mē-ă) Excessive dryness of the conjunctiva and cornea, which lose their luster and become keratinized; may be due to local disease or to a systemic deficiency of vitamin A. SYN xeroma. [*xero-* + G. *ophthalmos*, eye]

**xe·ro·ra·di·og·ra·phy** (zē′rō-rā′dē-og′ră-fē) Radiography using a specially coated charged plate instead of x-ray film, developing with a dry powder rather than liquid chemicals, and transferring the powder image onto paper for a permanent record; edge enhancement is inherent. SYN xerography.

**xe·ro·sto·mi·a** (zēr'ō-stō'mē-ă) Dryness of the mouth, having a varied etiology, resulting from diminished or arrested salivary secretion, or asialism. See this page. [*xero-* + G. *stoma,* mouth]

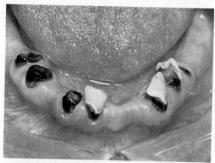

**rampant caries associated with xerostomia**

**X-link·ed** (lingkt) Pertaining to genes borne on the X chromosome.

**X-link·ed ich·thy·o·sis** (lingkt ik'thē-ō-sis) Form of skin disorder with onset at birth or in early infancy and affecting males; characterized by scaling predominantly on the scalp, neck, and trunk that progresses centripetally; palms and soles are spared; histologic manifestations are hyperkeratosis, a granular layer in the epidermis, and normal epidermal cell turnover; X-linked recessive inheritance.

**XO syn·drome** (sin'drōm) SYN Turner syndrome.

**x-ray** (rā) **1.** Ionizing electromagnetic radiation emitted from a highly evacuated tube, resulting from excitation of inner orbital electrons by bombardment of the target anode with a stream of electrons from a heated cathode. **2.** Ionizing electromagnetic radiation produced by the excitation of the inner orbital electrons of an atom by other processes, such as nuclear delay and its sequelae. **3.** SYN radiograph.

**x-ray beam** (rā bēm) Emission of electromagnetic radiation or particles from the x-ray tube. SEE ALSO x-ray.

**x-ray tube** (rā tūb) Vacuum tube containing electrodes that are directed onto a metal target to produce an x-ray. SEE ALSO x-ray.

**XS** Abbreviation for excess.

**xy·li·tol** (zī'li-tol) An optically inactive sugar alcohol; often used as a sugar substitute in diabetic diets; synthesis of xylitol from L-xylulose is blocked in patients with idiopathic pentosuria.

**xy·lol** (zī'lol) A volatile liquid obtained from coal tar; used as a solvent, in the manufacture of chemicals and synthetic fibers, and in histology as a clearing agent. SYN dimethylbenzene.

**xy·lose** (zī'lōs) An aldopentose, isomeric with ribose, obtained by fermentation or hydrolysis of carbohydrate.

**xy·lu·lose** (zī'lyū-lōs) A 2-ketopentose that appears in urine in patients with essential pentosuria; it is also an intermediate in the glucuronate pathway.

**xy·lu·lose re·duc·tase** (zīl'yū-lōs rĕ-dŭk'tās) Enzyme that reversibly converts xylulose to xylitol using either NADH (D-xylulose reductase) or NADPH (L-xylulose reductase); a deficiency of the L form is seen in patients with essential pentosuria.

# Y

**Y** Symbol for yttrium.

**yawn** (yawn) **1.** To gape. **2.** An involuntary opening of the mouth, usually accompanied by inspiration; it may be a sign of drowsiness or of vital depression, as after hemorrhage, but is often caused by suggestion. [A.S. *gānian*]

**yaws** (yawz) Infectious disease caused by *Treponema pertenue* and characterized by development of crusted granulomatous ulcers on extremities; may involve bone, but, unlike syphilis, does not affect central nervous or cardiovascular pathology systems. [of Caribbean origin; similar to Calinago word yaya, the disease]

**Y-ax·is** (aks´is) Cephalometric indicator of vertical and horizontal coordinates of mandibular growth expressed in degrees of inferior facial angle formed by intersection of the sella-gnathion plane with the Frankfurt horizontal plane.

**Yb** Symbol for ytterbium.

**yeast** (yēst) A general term denoting true fungi that are widely distributed in substrates that contain sugars (e.g., fruits), and in soil, animal excreta, and vegetative parts of plants. Because of their ability to ferment carbohydrates, some yeasts are important in brewing and baking industries. [A.S. *gyst*]

**Yer·sin·i·a** (yĕr-sin´ē-ă) Genus of motile and nonmotile, non-spore-forming bacteria containing gram-negative, unencapsulated, ovoid to rod-shaped cells; parasitic on humans and other animals; type species is *Y. pestis.* [A. J. E. *Yersin,* Swiss bacteriologist, 1862–1943]

**Yer·sin·i·a en·ter·o·co·li·ti·ca** (yĕr-sin´ ē-ă en´tĕr-ō-kō-lit´i-kă) A bacterial species that causes yersiniosis in humans; found in feces and lymph nodes of sick and healthy animals, including humans, and in material contaminated with feces.

**Yer·sin·i·a pseu·do·tu·ber·cu·lo·sis** (yĕr-sin´ē-ă sū´dō-tū-bĕr´kyū-lō´sis) Bacterial species causing pseudotuberculosis in birds, rodents, and, rarely, in humans.

**yer·sin·i·o·sis** (yĕr-sin´ē-ō´sis) A common human infectious disease caused by *Yersinia enterocolitica* marked by diarrhea, enteritis, pseudoappendicitis, ileitis, erythema nodosum, and sometimes septicemia or acute arthritis.

**yin-yang** (yin´yang) In ancient Chinese thought, concept of two complementary and opposing influences, Yin and Yang, which underpin and control all nature. The aim of Chinese medicine is to keep them in proper balance.

**Y-link·ed in·her·i·tance** (lingkt in-her´i-tăns) The pattern of inheritance that may result from a mutant gene located on a Y chromosome.

**Y-link·ed lo·cus** (lingkt lō´kŭs) Any (haploid) locus that in normal karyotypes is borne on the Y chromosome.

**yo·gurt, yo·ghurt** (yō´gŭrt) Fermented, partially evaporated, whole milk prepared by maintaining it at 50°C for 12 hours after addition of a mixed culture of *Lactobacillus bulgaricus, L. acidophilus,* and *Streptococcus lactis;* consumed as a food. [Turkish]

**yo·him·bine** (yō-him´bēn) An alkaloid, active principle of yohimbé, bark of *Corynanthe yohimbi;* it produces a competitive blockade, of limited duration, of adrenergic α-receptors; has also been used for its alleged aphrodisiac properties.

**yoke** (yōk) [TA] SYN jugum (1). [A.S. *geoc*]

**yolk** (yōk) One of the types of nutritive material stored in the oocyte (ovum) for the nutrition of the embryo; particularly abundant and conspicuous in birds' eggs. [A.S. *geolca; geolu,* yellow]

**Young mod·u·lus** (yŭng mod´yū-lŭs) A type of modulus of elasticity that specifies the force applied to a body in one direction, per unit cross-sectional area of the body perpendicular to that direction, divided by the fractional change in length of the body in that direction.

**yt·ter·bi·um (Yb)** (i-tĕr´bē-ŭm) A metallic element of the lanthanide group; used in cisternography and in brain scans.

**yt·tri·um (Y)** (it´rē-ŭm) A metallic element used in lasers.

yz

# Z

**ZDV** Abbreviation for zidovudine.

**ze·lo·typ·i·a** (zē′lō-tip′ē-ă) Excessive zeal, carried to the point of morbidity, in the advocacy of any cause. [G. *zēlotypia*; rivalry, envy, fr. *zēlos*, zeal, + *typtō*, to strike]

**ze·ro** (zēr′ō) *The JCAHO directs that a zero always be inserted before a decimal point when no other digit appears there (e.g., 0.5 mg, not .5 mg) and that a zero never be inserted after a decimal point when no other digit appears there (e.g., 5 mg, not 5.0 mg).* **1.** The figure 0, indicating the absence of magnitude, or nothing. **2.** In thermometry, point from which figures on scale start in one or the other direction; in Celsius and Réaumur scales, zero indicates freezing point for distilled water; in the Fahrenheit scale, it is 32° below freezing point of water. [Sp. fr. Ar. *sifr*, cipher]

**ze·ro de·gree teeth** (zēr′ō dě-grē′ tēth) Prosthetic teeth having no cusp angles in relation to the horizontal.

**zi·do·vu·dine (ZDV)** (zī-dō′vyū-dēn) A thymidine analogue that is an inhibitor of in vitro replication of HIV virus; also used in pharmacotherapeutic management of AIDS.

**zig·zag plas·ty** (zig′zag plast′ē) SYN Z-plasty.

**zinc** (zingk) A metallic element and essential bioelement; many salts are used in medicine; a cofactor in many proteins. [Ger. *Zink*]

**zinc ox·ide** (zingk ok′sīd) Used as a protective in ointment and as a dusting powder; also used in paint as a substitute for lead carbonate.

**zinc ox·ide and eu·ge·nol** (zingk ok′sīd yū′jě-nol) Compound used as a base material beneath metallic dental restorations and as a temporary filling material or impression material; setting and hardening result from complex reactions between the two ingredients.

**zinc ox·ide eu·ge·nol ce·ment (ZOE)** (zink oks′īd yū′jě-nol sě-ment′) A dental fixative made by mixing zinc oxide and eugenol commonly used to cement restorations in place temporarily. SYN unmodified zinc oxide-eugenol cement.

**zinc ox·y·phos·phate ce·ment** (zingk ok′sē-fos′fāt sě-ment′) SYN zinc phosphate cement.

**zinc phos·phate ce·ment** (zingk fos′fāt sě-ment′) Powder, containing primarily zinc oxide mixed with a liquid containing orthophosphoric acid to form a hard crystalline mass on standing, used in dentistry as a luting agent for cast metal restorations and orthodontic bands, and as a temporary restorative material, or a base under restorations, particularly in deep cavities. See page 605. SYN zinc oxyphosphate cement.

**zinc pol·y·car·bo·nate ce·ment** (zingk pol′ē-kahr′bŏ-nāt sě-ment′) SYN polycarboxylate cement.

**zir·co·ni·um (Zr)** (zǐr-kō′nē-ŭm) A metallic element, widely distributed in nature, but never great in quantity in any one place. [*zircon*, a mineral, fr. Ar. *zarkūn*, cinnabar, Pers, *zargun*, goldlike]

**ZOE** Abbreviation for zinc oxide eugenol cement.

**Zol·lin·ger-El·li·son syn·drome** (zol′in-jĕr-el′i-sŏn sin′drōm) Peptic ulceration with gastric hypersecretion and non-beta cell tumor of the pancreatic islets, sometimes associated with familial polyendocrine adenomatosis.

**zol·pi·dem** (zol′pi-děm) A sedative/hypnotic drug useful for treating anxiety and resembling benzodiazepines in its pharmacology but differing somewhat in chemical structure. Unlike benzodiazepines, zolpidem lacks prominent anticonvulsant properties, and less tolerance may develop with its use.

**zone** (zōn) [TA] A segment; any encircling or beltlike structure, either external or internal, longitudinal or transverse. [L. *zona*]

**zon·og·ra·phy** (zō-nog′ră-fē) A form of tomography with a relatively thick plane of focus; especially used in renal radiography. [*zone* + G. *graphō*, to write]

**zos·ter** (zos′tĕr) SYN herpes zoster. [G. *zōstēr*, a girdle]

**Z-plas·ty** (plas′tē) Surgery to elongate a contracted scar or to rotate tension 90 degrees; the middle line of a Z-shaped incision is made along the line of greatest tension or contraction, and triangular flaps are raised on opposite sides of the two ends and transposed. SYN zigzag plasty.

**Zr** Symbol for zirconium.

**Zsig·mon·dy den·tal no·men·cla·ture** (tsig′mawn-dē den′tăl nō′měn-klā-chŭr) SYN Palmer dental nomenclature.

**Z-tract in·jec·tion** (trakt in-jek′shŭn) Technique in which skin and subcutaneous tissue are displaced laterally before inserting the needle intramuscularly; used to prevent leakage along track of the needle and consequent tissue irritation. See page 605.

**zwei·back** (zwī′bak) Sweetened bread that has been baked twice, preferred for infant feeding during teething. [Ger. twice-baked]

**zy·go·ma** (zī-gō′mă) **1.** SYN zygomatic bone. **2.** SYN zygomatic arch. [G. a bar, bolt, the os jugale, fr. *zygon*, yoke]

**zy·go·mat·ic arch** (zī′gō-mat′ik ahrch) [TA] Arch formed by temporal process of zygomatic bone that joins zygomatic process of tem-

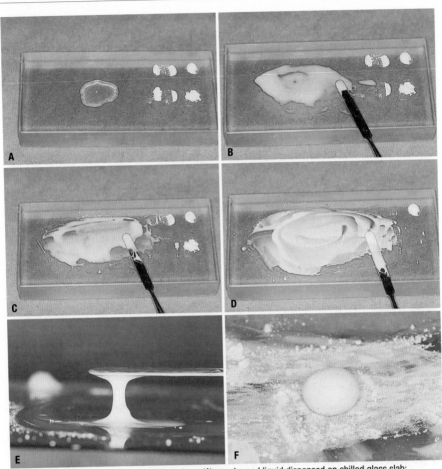

**cement:** mixing process for zinc-phosphate type; (A) powder and liquid dispensed on chilled glass slab; (B) first increment mixed with liquid; (C, D) increments added to mixture gradually, using entire glass slab; (E) as mixed for luting, cement produces 1" "string"; (F) mixture for base can be rolled into a ball

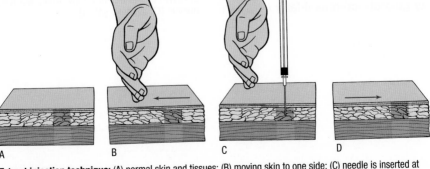

**Z-tract injection technique:** (A) normal skin and tissues; (B) moving skin to one side; (C) needle is inserted at 90-degree angle, to aspirate for blood; (D) once needle is withdrawn, displaced tissue is allowed to return to its normal position, preventing solution from escaping from muscle tissue

poral bone. SYN arcus zygomaticus, cheek bone (2), malar arch, zygoma (2).

**zy·go·mat·ic bone** (zī´gō-mat´ik bōn) [TA] Quadrilateral bone that forms prominence of cheek, lateral wall and margin of orbit, and anterior two thirds of zygomatic arch; it articulates with the frontal, sphenoid, temporal, and maxillary bones. SYN cheek bone (1), mala (2), malar bone, zygoma (1).

**zy·go·mat·ic nerve** (zī´gō-mat´ik nĕrv) [TA] Branch of maxillary nerve [CN V2] in inferior orbital fissure through which it passes; gives rise to two sensory branches, the zygomaticotemporal and zygomaticofacial, which supply skin of temporal and zygomatic regions and is continued as communicating branch of the lacrimal nerve with the zygomatic nerve. SYN temporomandibular nerve.

**zy·go·mat·i·co·au·ric·u·lar** (zī´gō-mat´i-kō-aw-rik´yū-lăr) Relating to zygomatic bone and auricle.

**zy·go·mat·i·co·au·ric·u·lar in·dex** (zī´gō-mat´i-kō-awr-ik´yū-lăr in´deks) Ratio between zygomatic and auricular diameters of the cranium or head.

**zy·go·ma·ti·co·au·ri·cu·lar·is** (zī´gō-măt´i-kō-awr-ik´yū-lar´is) Facial muscle of external ear; *origin*, epicranial aponeurosis, *insertion*, cartilage of auricle; *action*, draws pinna of ear upward and forward; *nerve supply*, facial. Considered by some to be the anterior part of the temporoparietalis muscle.

**zy·go·mat·i·co·fa·cial** (zī´gō-mat´i-kō-fā´shăl) Relating to zygomatic bone and face.

**zy·go·mat·i·co·fa·cial for·a·men** (zī´gō-mat´i-kō-fā´shăl fōr-ā´mĕn) [TA] Opening on the lateral surface of the zygomatic bone below the orbital margin that transmits the zygomaticofacial nerve.

**zy·go·mat·i·co·fron·tal** (zī´gō-mat´i-kō-frŏn´tăl) Relating to zygomatic and frontal bones.

**zy·go·mat·i·co·max·il·lar·y** (zī´gō-mat´i-

kō-mak´si-lar-ē) Relating to zygomatic bone and maxilla.

**zy·go·mat·i·co·max·il·lar·y su·ture** (zī´gō-mat´i-kō-mak´si-lar-ē sū´chŭr) [TA] Articulation of the zygomatic bone with the zygomatic process of the maxilla.

**zy·go·mat·i·co·or·bi·tal** (zī´gō-mat´i-kō-ōr´bi-tăl) Relating to zygomatic bone and orbit.

**zy·go·mat·i·co·or·bi·tal ar·te·ry** (zī´gō-mat´i-kō-ōr´bi-tăl ahr´tĕr-ē) [TA] *Origin*, superficial temporal, sometimes middle temporal; *distribution*, orbicularis oculi muscle and portions of the orbit; *anastomoses*, lacrimal and palpebral branches of ophthalmic.

**zy·go·mat·i·co·or·bi·tal for·a·men** (zī´gō-mat´i-kō-ōr´bi-tăl fōr-ā´mĕn) [TA] Common opening on orbital surface of zygomatic bone of canals transmitting zygomaticofacial and zygomaticotemporal nerves; sometimes each of these canals has a separate opening on orbital surface.

**zy·go·mat·ic pro·cess of max·il·la** (zī´gō-mat´ik pro´ses mak-sil´ă) [TA] Rough projection from maxilla that articulates with zygomatic bone. SYN malar process.

**zy·go·mat·ic pro·cess of tem·po·ral bone** (zī´gō-mat´ik pro´ses tem´pŏr-ăl bōn) [TA] Anterior process that articulates with temporal process of zygomatic bone to form zygomatic arch.

**zy·go·mat·ic re·gion** (zī´gō-mat´ik rē´jŏn) [TA] Area of the face outlined by zygomatic bone; prominence above the cheek.

**zy·go·max·il·lar·y** (zī´gō-mak´si-lar-ē) Relating to zygomatic bone and maxilla.

**zy·gos·i·ty** (zī-gos´i-tē) Nature of the zygotes from which individuals are derived; e.g., whether by separation of the division of one zygote, in which case they will be genetically identical, or from two separate zygotes.

**zy·gote** (zī´gōt) **1.** Diploid cell resulting from union of a sperm and a secondary oocyte. **2.** Early embryo that develops from a fertilized oocyte. [G. *zygōtos,* yoked]

# Contents to the Appendices

**Units of Measure**

Weights and Measures ..................................................................... APP 2

**Affixes and Abbreviations**

Medical/Dental Prefixes, Suffixes, and Combining Forms ....................... APP 6

Common Medical/Dental Abbreviations and Acronyms .......................... APP 12

Common Abbreviations Used in Medication Orders ............................. APP 21

Common Abbreviations Not to Be Used in Medication Orders ................. APP 22

**Reference Values**

Laboratory Reference Range Values .................................................. APP 24

**Dental/Periodontal Classifications and Charting**

Classifications of Periodontal Diseases and Conditions .......................... APP 34

Caries Classification .................................................................... APP 37

Classifications of Furcation Involvement ........................................... APP 38

Dental and Periodontal Charting ..................................................... APP 40

Documenting Gingival Margin Level ................................................ APP 43

Periodontal Screening and Recording (PSR) System .............................. APP 44

Tooth Numbering Systems ............................................................. APP 47

**Infection Control**

Guidelines for Infection Control in Dental Health Care Settings ............... APP 49

Infection Control for the Dental Office: A Checklist ............................. APP 60

**Dental Imaging**

Panoramic Radiograph .................................................................. APP 62

Paralleling Technique ................................................................... APP 64

Guidelines for Prescribing Dental Radiographs .................................... APP 68

Automatic Film Processing Errors .................................................... APP 70

Film Handling Errors ................................................................... APP 71

Intraoral Projection and Technique Errors .......................................... APP 72

Panoramic Patient Positioning Errors ................................................ APP 73

Panoramic Procedural Errors .......................................................... APP 75

**Professional Information**

Professional Organizations ............................................................. APP 76

# Weights and Measures

## Scale of the Metric System and International System of Units (SI)

| Prefix | Symbol | Power |
|---|---|---|
| yotta- | Y | $10^{24}$ |
| zetta- | Z | $10^{21}$ |
| exa- | E | $10^{18}$ |
| peta- | P | $10^{15}$ |
| tera- | T | $10^{12}$ |
| giga- | G | $10^{9}$ |
| mega- | M | $10^{6}$ |
| kilo- | k | $10^{3}$ |
| hecto- | h | $10^{2}$ |
| deca- | da | $10^{1}$ |
| base unit | — | 1 |
| deci- | d | $10^{-1}$ |
| centi- | c | $10^{-2}$ |
| milli- | m | $10^{-3}$ |
| micro- | mc | $10^{-6}$ |
| nano- | n | $10^{-9}$ |
| pico- | p | $10^{-12}$ |
| femto- | f | $10^{-15}$ |
| atto- | a | $10^{-18}$ |
| zepto- | z | $10^{-21}$ |
| yocto- | y | $10^{-24}$ |

## SI Base Units

| Quantity | Name | Symbol |
|---|---|---|
| length | meter | m |
| mass* | kilogram[†] | kg |
| time | second | s |
| electric current | ampere | A |
| thermodynamic temperature | kelvin[‡] | K |
| luminous intensity | candela | cd |
| amount of substance | mole | mol |

*In commercial and everyday use, *weight* usually means *mass* (e.g., when speaking of a person's weight, the quantity referred to is *mass*).

[†]For historical reasons, *kilogram* is the only base unit with a prefix. Multiples and submultiples of the kilogram are formed by attaching the appropriate prefix to the stem -*gram* (e.g., *milligram*) and the appropriate prefix symbol to the symbol *g* (e.g., *mg*).

[‡]The degree Celsius (°C) is still widely accepted usage for expressing temperature and temperature intervals. Celsius (formerly centigrade) *temperature* is converted to Kelvin (K) thermodynamic temperature by adding 273.16 to the Celsius scale. For *temperature interval*, 1°C equals K.

## Some SI-Derived Units Expressed in Terms of Base Units

| Quantity | Name | Symbol |
|---|---|---|
| area | square meter | $m^2$ |
| volume* | cubic meter | $m^3$ |
| specific volume | cubic meter per kilogram | m3/kg |
| speed, velocity | meter per second | m/s |
| acceleration | meter per second squared | $m/s^2$ |
| mass density | kilogram per cubic meter | $kg/m^3$ |
| concentration | mole per cubic meter | $mol/m^3$ |
| luminance candela | per square meter | $cd/m^2$ |

*Liter (L, l). $10^{-3}$ m3 is used as a special name for the cubic decimeter.

## Some SI-Derived Units with Special Names

| Quantity | Name | Symbol | Expression |
|---|---|---|---|
| frequency | hertz | Hz | $s^{-1}$ |
| force | newton | N | $m\ kg\ s^{-2}$ |
| pressure, stress | pascal | Pa | $m^{-1}\ kg\ s^{-2}$ |
| energy | joule | J | $m^2\ kg\ s^{-2}$ |
| power | watt | W | $m^2\ kg\ s^{-3}$ |
| quantity of electricity, electric charge | coulomb | C | $s\ A$ |
| electric potential, electromotive force | volt | V | $m2\ kg\ s^{-3}A^{-1}$ |
| capacitance | farad | F | $m^{-2}\ kg^{-1}\ s^4A^{-2}$ |
| electrical resistance | ohm | $\Omega$ | $m^2\ kg^{-2}\ A^{-2}$ |
| electrical conductance | siemens | S | $m^{-2}kg\ s^{-2}A^{-1}$ |
| magnetic flux | weber | Wb | $m^2\ kg\ s^{-2}A^{-1}$ |
| magnetic flux density | tesla | T | $kg\ s^{-2}A^{-1}$ |
| activity of radionuclide | becquerel* | Bq | $s^{-1}$ |
| absorbed dose of radiation | gray† | Gy | $m^2\ s^{-2}$ |
| exposure (x and $\gamma$ radiation) | coulomb per kilogram‡ | C kg | $kg^{-1}\ s\ A$ |

*Replacing the curie (Ci), $3.7 \times 10^{10}$ $s^{-1}$. †Replacing the rad, $10^{-2}$ J $kg^{-1}$. ‡Replacing the roentgen (R), $2.58 \times 10^{-4}$ C $kg^{-1}$.

## Measures of Length

| Micrometers | Millimeters | Centimeters | Meters | Kilometers | Miles | Yards | Feet | Inches |
|---|---|---|---|---|---|---|---|---|
| 1 | 0.001 | $10^{-4}$ | | | | | | 0.000039 |
| $10^3$ | 1 | $10^{-1}$ | | | | | .00328 | 0.03937 |
| $10^4$ | 10 | 1 | 0.01 | 0.0109 | | | .03281 | 0.3937 |
| 254,000 | 25.4 | 2.54 | 0.0254 | | | 0.0278 | .0833 | 1 |
| | 304.8 | 30.48 | 0.3048 | | | 0.333 | 1 | 12 |
| $10^6$ | $10^3$ | $10^2$ | 1 | 0.001 | 0.0006213 | 1.0936 | 3.2808 | 39.37 |
| 914,400 | 914.40 | 91.44 | 0.9144 | 0.009 | 0.0005681 | 1 | 3 | 36 |
| $10^9$ | $10^6$ | $10^5$ | $10^3$ | 1 | 0.6215 | 1093.6121 | 3280.8 | |
| | | | 1609.0 | 1.609 | 1 | 1760.0 | 5280.0 | |

To convert:

Millimeters to inches: divide by 25.4
Inches to millimeters: multiply by 25.4

Centimeters to feet: divide by 30.7
Feet to centimeters: multiply by 30.7

Meters to yards: multiply by 1.09375
Yards to meters: multiply by 0.9143

Kilometers to miles: multiply by 0.625
Miles to kilometers: multiply by 1.6

## Measures of Mass (Weight)

| Avoirdupois Weights | | | | Metric Equivalents | | |
|---|---|---|---|---|---|---|
| Grains | Drams | Ounces | Pounds | Milligrams | Grams | Kilograms |
| 1 | 0.0366 | 0.0023 | 0.00014 | 64.8 | 0.0648 | 0.000065 |
| 27.34 | 1 | 0.0625 | 0.0039 | | 1.772 | 0.001772 |
| 437.5 | 16 | 1 | 0.0625 | | 28.350 | 0.028350 |
| 7,000 | 256 | 16 | 1 | | 453.5924 | 0.453592 |
| 0.0154 | | | | 1 | 0.001 | |
| 15.4324 | 0.5648 | 0.0353 | 0.002205 | 1000 | 1 | 0.001 |
| 15,432.358 | 564.32 | 35.27 | 2.2046 | | 1000 | 1 |

To convert (approximately):

Kilograms to pounds: multiply by 2.2
Pounds to kilograms: multiply by 0.454

Grams to ounces: multiply by 0.03527
Ounces to grams: multiply by 28.35

| Apothecaries' Weights | | | | | Metric Equivalents | | |
|---|---|---|---|---|---|---|---|
| Grains | Scruples | Drams | Ounces | Pounds | Milligrams | Grams | Kilograms |
| 1 | 0.05 | 0.0167 | 0.0021 | 0.00017 | 64.8 | 0.0648 | 0.000065 |
| 20 | 1 | 0.333 | 0.042 | 0.0035 | | 1.296 | 0.001296 |
| 60 | 3 | 1 | 0.125 | 0.0104 | | 3.888 | 0.000389 |
| 480 | 24 | 8 | 1 | 0.0833 | | 31.103 | 0.031103 |
| 5,760 | 288 | 96 | 12 | 1 | | 373.2417 | 0.373242 |
| 0.0154 | | | | | 1 | 0.001 | |
| 15.4324 | | 0.2572 | 0.0322 | 0.0027 | 1000 | 1 | 0.001 |
| 15,432.358 | | 257.2 | 32.15 | 2.6792 | | 1000 | 1 |

## Measures of Capacity

| | Apothecaries' Measures | | | | Metric Equivalents | | |
|---|---|---|---|---|---|---|---|
| Minims | Fluid Drams | Fluid Ounces | Pints | Quarts | Gallons | Liters | Milliliters |
| 1 | 0.0167 | 0.002 | 0.00013 | | | 0.0006 | 0.06161 |
| 60 | 1 | 0.125 | 0.0078 | 0.0039 | | 0.0037 | 3.6967 |
| 480 | 8 | 1 | 0.0625 | 0.0312 | 0.0078 | 0.0296 | 29.5737 |
| 7,680 | 128 | 16 | 1 | 0.5 | 0.125 | 0.4732 | 473.166 |
| 15,360 | 256 | 32 | 2 | 1 | 0.25 | 0.9464 | 946.358 |
| 61,440 | 1024 | 128 | 8 | 4 | 1 | 3.7854 | 3785.434 |
| 16,230 | 270.52 | 33.8418 | 2.1134 | 1.0567 | 0.2642 | 1 | 1000 |
| 16.23 | 0.2705 | 0.0338 | 0.00212 | 0.00106 | 0.000265 | 0.001 | 1 |

To convert (approximately):

1 British imperial gallon = 1.201 U.S. gallon    Liters to gallons: multiply by 0.264
1 U.S. gallon = 0.8327 British imperial gallon    Gallons to liters: multiply by 3.788

Liters to pints: multiply by 2.1
Pints to liters: multiply by 0.4732

## Approximate Household Measures and Weights*

| Teaspoons | Tablespoons | Cups or Glasses† | Drams | Fluid Ounces | Milliliters | Grams |
|---|---|---|---|---|---|---|
| 1 | | | 1 | 0.125 | 5 | 5 |
| 3 | 1 | | 4 | 0.50 | 15 | 15 |
| 48 | 16‡ | 1 | 64 | 8 | 237 | 240 |

*A drop is a measure of uncertain quantity, depending on the nature of the liquid as well as the shape of the container and of the opening from which the liquid falls. One drop of water is roughly equivalent to 1 minim.

†"Tumbler or glass" generally means 8 fluid ounces.

‡For dry measure, 12 tablespoons equal 1 cup.

# Medical/Dental Prefixes, Suffixes, and Combining Forms

**a-** not, without, less

**ab-** from, away from, off

**abs-** from, away from, off

**acantho-** thorn

**ad-** increase, adherence, motion toward, very

**-ad** toward, in the direction of, -ward

**adeno-** gland

**adip-** fat

**adipo-** fat

**-agogue,** promoter, stimulator

**-al** pertaining to

**alb-** white

**albo-** white

**alge-** pain

**algesi-** pain

**algio-** pain

**algo-** pain

**allo-** other, different

**ambi-** around, on (both) sides, on all sides, both

**amyl-** starch, polysaccharide

**amylo-** starch, polysaccharide

**an-** not, without, -less

**ana-** up, toward, apart

**andro-** male

**angi-** vessel

**angio-** vessel

**ankylo-** crooked

**ante-** before

**anthraco-** coal, carbon

**anti-** 1 against, opposing, 2 curative, 3 antibody

**apo-** separated from, derived from

**aque-** water

**aqueo-** water

**-ar** pertaining to

**-arche** beginning

**arteri-** artery

**arterio-** artery

**arthr-** joint, articulation

**arthro-** joint, articulation

**-ary** pertaining to

**-ase** an enzyme

**-ate** a salt or ester of an ''-ic'' acid

**athero-** pasty, fatty

**atto-** one quintillionth $(10^{-18})$

**audi-** hearing

**audio-** hearing

**aur-** ear

**auri-** ear

**auro-** ear

**aut-** self, same

**auto-** self, same

**bacteri-** bacteria

**bacterio-** bacteria

**bi-** twice, double

**bio-** life

**blasto-** budding by cells or tissue

**brachi-** arm

**brachio-** arm

**brachy-** short

**bronch-** bronchus

**bronchi-** bronchus

**broncho-** bronchus

**carcin-** cancer

**carcino-** cancer

**cardi-** 1 heart, 2 esophageal opening of stomach

**cardio-** 1 heart, 2 esophageal opening of stomach

**carpo-** wrist

**caud-** tail, lower part of body

**caudo-** tail, lower part of body

**-cele** hernia, swelling

**celio-** abdomen

**-centesis** surgical puncture

**centi-** one hundredth $(10^{-2})$

**cephal-** the head

**cephalo-** the head

**cervic-** 1 neck, 2 uterine cervix

**cervico-** 1 neck, 2 uterine cervix

**cheil-** lip

**cheilo-** lip

**chem-** 1 chemistry, 2 drug

**chemo-** 1 chemistry, 2 drug

**chir-** hand

**chiro-** hand

**chlor-** 1 green, 2 chlorine

**chloro-** 1 green, 2 chlorine

**chol-** bile

**chondrio-** 1 cartilage, 2 granular, 3 gritty

**chondro-** 1 cartilage, 2 granular, 3 gritty

**chrom-** color

**chromat-** color

**chromo-** color

**chron-** time

**chrono-** time

**-cidal** killing, destroying

**-cide** killing, destroying

**cis-** on this side, on the near side
**-clast** breaker
**-clysis** washing
**co-** with, together, in association, very, complete
**col-** with, together, in association, very, complete
**com-** with, together, in association, very, complete
**con-** with, together, in association, very, complete
**conio-** dust
**cor-** with, together, in association, very, complete
**cost-** rib
**costo-** rib
**crani-** cranium
**cranio-** cranium
**-crine** secretion
**cry-** cold
**cryo-** cold
**crypt-** hidden
**crypto-** hidden
**culdo-** cul-de-sac
**cyan-** 1 blue, 2 cyanide
**cyano-** 1 blue, 2 cyanide
**cycl-** 1 circle, cycle, 2 ciliary body
**cyst-** 1 bladder, 2 cyst, 3 cystic duct
**cysti-** 1 bladder, 2 cyst, 3 cystic duct
**cysto-** 1 bladder, 2 cyst, 3 cystic duct
**cyt-** cell
**-cyte** cell
**cyto-** cell
**dacry-** tears
**dacryo-** tears
**dactyl-** finger, toe
**dactylo-** finger, toe
**de-** away from, cessation
**deca-** ten
**deci-** one tenth ($10^{-1}$)
**deka-** ten
**dent-** tooth
**denti-** tooth
**derm-** skin
**derma-** skin
**dermat-** skin
**dermato-** skin
**dermo-** skin
**dextr-** right, toward or on the right side
**dextro-** right, toward or on the right side
**di-** separation, taking apart, reversal, not, un-
**dif-** separation, taking apart, reversal, not, un-
**dipso-** thirst

**dir-** separation, taking apart, reversal, not, un-
**dis-** separation, taking apart, reversal, not, un-
**duo-** two
**duodeno-** duodenum
**-dynia** pain
**dynamo-** force, energy
**dys-** bad, difficult
**ect-** outer, on the outside
**-ectasia** dilatation, stretching
**-ectasis** dilatation, stretching
**ecto-** outer, on the outside
**-ectomy** excision
**-emphraxis** obstruction
**encephal-** brain
**encephalo-** brain
**end-** within, inner
**endo-** within, inner
**enter-** intestine
**entero-** intestine
**ent-** inner, within
**ento-** inner, within
**epi-** upon, following, subsequent to
**ergo-** work
**erythr-** red, redness
**erythro-** red, redness
**eso-** inward
**esthesio-** sensation, perception
**eu-** good, well
**ex-** out of, from, away from
**exo-** exterior, external, outward
**extra-** outside of, without
**ferri-** ferric ion ($Fe^{3+}$)
**ferro-** 1 metallic iron, 2 ferrous ion ($Fe^{2+}$)
**fibr-** fiber
**fibro-** fiber
**-form** in the form or shape of
**galact-** milk
**galacto-** milk
**gastr-** 1 stomach, 2 belly
**gastro-** 1 stomach, 2 belly
**-gen** 1 producing, coming to be, 2 precursor
**gen-** 1 producing, coming to be, 2 precursor
**giga-** one billion ($10^9$)
**gingiv-** gums
**gingivo-** gums
**gloss-** tongue
**glosso-** tongue
**gluco-** glucose
**glyco-** sugars
**gnath-** jaw
**gnatho-** jaw

**gonio-** angle
**-gram** a recording
**granul-** granular, granule
**granulo-** granular, granule
**-graph** recording instrument
**hecto-** one hundred ($10^{10}$)
**hem-** blood
**hema-** blood
**hemat-** blood
**hemato-** blood
**hemi-** one half
**hemo-** blood
**hepat-** liver
**hepatico-** liver
**hepato-** liver
**hept-** seven
**hepta-** seven
**hidr-** sweat
**hidro-** sweat
**hist-** tissue
**histio-** tissue
**histo-** tissue
**homeo-** same, constant
**hydr-** water, hydrogen
**hydro-** water, hydrogen
**hyper-** excessive, above normal
**hypo-** beneath, diminution, deficiency, the
   lowest
**-ia** a condition
**-iasis** condition, state
**-ic** pertaining to
**-ics** organized knowledge, practice,
   treatment
**ileo-** ileum
**ilio-** ilium
**in-** 1 in, 2 not
**-in** chemical suffix
**-ine** chemical suffix
**infra-** below
**inter-** between, among
**intra-** within
**intro-** within
**irid-** iris
**irido-** iris
**ischi-** ischium
**ischio-** ischium
**-ism** 1 condition, disease, 2 practice,
   doctrine
**-ismus** spasm, contraction
**iso-** 1 equal, like, 2 isomer, 3 sameness
**-ite** the nature of, resembling
**-ites** -y, -like
**-itides** plural of -itis

**-itis** inflammation
**kal-** potassium
**kali-** potassium
**karyo-** nucleus
**kerat-** cornea
**kerato-** cornea
**kilo-** one thousand ($10^{3}$)
**kin-** movement
**kine-** movement
**kinesi-** motion
**kinesio-** motion
**kineso-** motion
**kino-** movement
**labio-** lip
**lacrim-** tears
**lacrimo-** tears
**laparo-** abdomen, abdominal wall
**laryng-** larynx
**laryngo-** larynx
**lateri-** lateral, to one side, side
**latero-** lateral, to one side, side
**-lepsis** seizure
**-lepsy** seizure
**lepto-** light, slender, thin, frail
**leuk-** white
**leuko-** white
**linguo-** tongue
**lip-** fat, lipid
**lipo-** fat, lipid
**lith-** stone, calculus, calcification
**litho-** stone, calculus, calcification
**-log** speech, words
**log-** speech, words
**logo-** speech, words
**-logy** 1 study of, 2 collecting
**lymph-** lymph
**lympho-** lymph
**lys-** lysis, dissolution
**lyso-** lysis, dissolution
**macr-** large, long
**macro-** large, long
**mal-** bad, deficient
**-malacia** softening
**masto-** breast
**meg-** large, oversize
**mega-** 1 large, oversize, 2 one million ($10^{6}$)
**megal-** large
**megalo-** large
**-megaly,** enlargement
**melan-** black
**melano-** black
**mening-** meninges
**meningo-** meninges

**ment-** chin
**mento-** chin
**-mer** member of a series
**mes-** 1 middle, mean, intermediate,
  2 attaching membrane
**meso-** 1 middle, mean, intermediate,
  2 attaching membrane
**meta-** 1 after, behind, 2 joint action,
  sharing
**-meter** measurement, measuring device
**micr-** small, microscopic
**micro-** 1 small, microscopic, 2 one
  millionth ($10^{-6}$)
**milli-** one thousandth ($10^{-3}$)
**mon-** single
**mono-** single
**morph-** form, shape, structure
**morpho-** form, shape, structure
**my-** muscle
**myo-** muscle
**myel-** 1 bone marrow, 2 spinal cord
**myelo-** 1 bone marrow, 2 spinal cord
**myx-** mucus
**myxo-** mucus
**nano-** 1 dwarf, 2 one billionth ($10^{-9}$)
**nas-** nose
**naso-** nose
**natr-** sodium
**natri-** sodium
**necr-** death, necrosis
**necro-** death, necrosis
**neo-** new
**nephr-** kidney
**nephro-** kidney
**neur-** nerve, nervous system
**neuri-** nerve, nervous system
**neuro-** nerve, nervous system
**norm-** normal
**normo-** normal
**octo-** eight
**odont-** tooth
**odonto-** tooth
**odyn-** pain
**odyno-** pain
**-oid** resemblance to
**olig-** few, little
**oligo-** few, little
**-oma** tumor, neoplasm
**-omata** plural of -oma
**oncho-** onco
**onco-** tumor, bulk, volume
**-one** ketone (–CO– group)
**onych-** fingernail, toenail

**onycho-** fingernail, toenail
**or-** mouth
**ori-** mouth
**oro-** mouth
**-ose** sugar
**-oses** plural of -osis
**-osis** process, condition, state
**ossi-** bone
**osseo-** bony
**ost-** bone
**oste-** bone
**osteo-** bone
**oxa-** oxygen
**oxo-** oxygen
**oxy-** 1 sharp, acid, 2 acute, shrill, quick,
  3 oxygen
**pachy-** thick
**pan-** all, entire
**pant-** all, entire
**panto-** all, entire
**para-** 1 abnormal, 2 involvement of two
  like parts
**pari-** equal
**path-** disease
**patho-** disease
**-pathy** disease
**ped-** 1 child, 2 foot
**pedi-** 1 child, 2 foot
**pedo-** 1 child, 2 foot
**-penia** deficiency
**penta-** five
**per-** through, thoroughly, intensely
**peri-** around, about
**-pexy** fixation, usually surgical
**-phage** eating, devouring
**-phagia** eating, devouring
**phago-** eating, devouring
**-phagy** eating, devouring
**phako-** lens
**phanero-** visible, evident
**pharmaco-** drugs, medicine
**pharyng-** pharynx
**pharyngo-** pharynx
**phil-** 1 attraction, 2 chemical affinity
**-philia** 1 attraction, 2 chemical affinity
**philo-** 1 attraction, 2 chemical affinity
**phleb-** vein
**phlebo-** vein
**-phobia** fear
**phon-** sound, speech
**phono-** sound, speech
**phor-** carrying, bearing
**phoro-** carrying, bearing

**phos-** light
**phot-** light
**photo-** light
**phreno-** 1 diaphragm, 2 mind, 3 phrenic
**-phylaxis** protection
**physi-** 1 physical, 2 natural
**physio-** 1 physical, 2 natural
**physo-** 1 swelling, inflation, 2 air, gas
**phyt-** plants
**phyto-** plants
**pico-** one trillionth ($10^{-12}$)
**plan-** flat
**plani-** flat
**plano-** flat
**-plasia** formation
**plasma-** plasma
**plasmat-** plasma
**plasmato-** plasma
**plasmo-** plasma
**platy-** wide, flat
**-plegia** paralysis
**pleo-** more
**plesio-** near, similar
**pleur-** rib, side, pleura
**pleura-** rib, side, pleura
**pleuro-** rib, side, pleura
**pluri-** several, more
**-pnea** breath, respiration
**pneo-** breath, respiration
**pneum-** 1 air, gas, 2 lung, 3 breathing
**pneuma-** 1 air, gas, 2 lung, 3 breathing
**pneumat-** 1 air, gas, 2 lung, 3 breathing
**pneumato-** 1 air, gas, 2 lung, 3 breathing
**pod-** foot, foot-shaped
**-pod** foot, foot-shaped
**podo-** foot, foot-shaped
**-poiesis** production
**poikilo-** irregular, variable
**poly-** 1 multiplicity, 2 polymer
**post-** after, behind, posterior
**pre-** anterior, before
**pro-** 1 before, forward, 2 precursor
**prot-** first
**proto-** first
**pseud-** false
**pseudo-** false
**-ptosis** sagging, falling
**pykn-** dense, compact
**pykno-** dense, compact
**pyo-** suppuration, pus
**pyreto-** fever
**pyro-** fire, heat, fever
**quadr-** four

**quadri-** four
**radio-** 1 radiation, x-ray, 2 radius
**re-** again, backward
**reno-** kidney
**retro-** backward, behind
**rhin-** nose
**rhino-** nose
**-rrhagia** discharge
**-rrhaphy** surgical suturing
**-rrhea** flow
**-rrhexis** rupture
**salping-** tube
**salpingo-** tube
**sarco-** flesh, muscle
**schisto-** split, cleft
**schiz-** split, cleft, division
**schizo-** split, cleft, division
**scler-** hardness (induration), sclerosis, ocular sclera
**sclero-** hardness (induration), sclerosis, ocular sclera
**scolio-** crooked
**-scope** instrument for viewing
**-scopy** viewing
**scot-** shadow, darkness
**scoto-** shadow, darkness
**semi-** one half, partly
**sept-** 1 seven, 2 septum, 3 sepsis, infection
**septi-** seven
**septo-** 1 seven, 2 septum, 3 sepsis, infection
**sial-** saliva, salivary gland
**sialo-** saliva, salivary gland
**sider-** iron
**sidero-** iron
**sin-** sinus
**sino-** sinus
**sinu-** sinus
**sito-** food, grain
**somat-** body, bodily
**somato-** body, bodily
**somatico-** body, bodily
**somno-** sleep
**son-** 1 sound, 2 ultrasound
**sono-** 1 sound, 2 ultrasound
**spasmo-** spasm
**spermo-** semen, spermatozoa
**sperma-** semen, spermatozoa
**sphygmo-** pulse
**spir-** breathing
**spiro-** breathing
**splanchn-** viscera
**splanchni-** viscera

**splanchno-** viscera
**splen-** spleen
**spleno-** spleen
**staphyl-** grape, bunch of grapes, staphylococci
**staphylo-** grape, bunch of grapes, staphylococci
**-stasis** stopping
**-stat** arresting change or movement
**steno-** narrowness, constriction
**stereo-** solid
**stheno-** strength, force, power
**stom-** mouth
**stoma-** mouth
**stomat-** mouth
**stomato-** mouth
**sub-** beneath, less than normal, inferior
**super-** in excess, above, superior, in the upper part
**supra-** above
**sy-** together
**syl-** together
**sym-** together
**syn-** together
**sys-** together
**tachy-** rapid
**tel-** distant
**tele-** distant
**ten-** tendon
**tendin-** tendon
**teno-** tendon
**tenont-** tendon
**tenonto-** tendon
**tera-** one quadrillion ($10^{15}$)
**tetra-** four
**therm-** heat
**thermo-** heat
**thorac-** chest, thorax
**thoracico-** chest, thorax

**thoraco-** chest, thorax
**thromb-** blood clot
**thrombo-** blood clot
**-tome 1** cutting instrument, **2** segment, section
**-tomy** cutting operation
**tono-** tone, tension, pressure
**top-** place, topical
**topo-** place, topical
**tox-** toxin, poison
**toxi-** toxin, poison
**toxico-** toxin, poison
**toxo-** toxin, poison
**trache-** trachea
**tracheo-** trachea
**trans-** across, through, beyond
**tri-** three
**trich-** hair
**trichi-** hair
**-trichia** hair
**tricho-** hair
**tris-** three
**-trophic** food, nutrition
**tropho-** food, nutrition
**-trophy** food, nutrition
**-tropia** turning
**-tropic** turning toward, affinity
**ultra-** beyond
**uni-** one, single
**vas-** duct, blood vessel
**vasculo-** blood vessel
**vaso-** duct, blood vessel
**vesico-** urinary bladder, vesicle
**xanth-** yellow, yellowish
**xantho-** yellow, yellowish
**xero-** dry
**zo-** **1** animal, **2** life
**zoo-** **1** animal, **2** life
**zym-** fermentation, enzymes
**zymo-** fermentation, enzymes

# Common Medical/Dental Abbreviations and Acronyms

**a** (specific) absorption (coefficient) (USUALLY ITALIC); (total) acidity; area; (systemic) arterial (blood) (SUBSCRIPT); asymmetric; atto

**A** absorbance

**Å** angstrom; Ångström unit

**aa** [G.] ana of each (USED in prescriptions)

**AA** amino acid; aminoacyl

**Ab** antibody

**ABG** arterial blood gas

**ABO** blood group system

**a.c.** [L.] *ante cibum,* before a meal

**AC** acetate; acromioclavicular; air conduction; alternating current; atriocarotid

**ACE** angiotension converting enzyme

**ACEI** angiotensin converting enzyme inhibitor

**ACh, Ach** acetylcholine

**ACTH** adrenocorticotropic hormone (corticotropin)

**ad lib.** [L.] *ad libitum,* freely, as desired

**ADH** antidiuretic hormone

**ADHD** attention deficit hyperactivity disorder

**ADLs** activities of daily living

**ADR** adverse drug reaction

**AED** automated external defibrillator

**AFB** acid fast bacillus

**Ag (or AG)** amalgam restoration, silver alloy amalgam; antigen; [L.] *argentum,* silver

**A:G R** albumin globulin ratio

**AIDS** acquired immunodeficiency syndrome

**Al** aluminum

**ALL** acute lymphocytic leukemia

**ALS** advanced life support; amyotrophic lateral sclerosis; antilymphocyte serum

**ALT** alanine aminotransferase

**Am** americium

**AML** acute myelogenous leukemia

**ANOVA** analysis of variance

**ANS** autonomic nervous system

**ANUG** acute necrotizing ulcerative gingivitis

**AP** anteroposterior

**APAP** acetaminophen

**ARDS** adult *or* acute respiratory distress syndrome

**ARF** acute renal failure; acute rheumatic fever

**As** arsenic

**ASA** acetylsalicylic acid (aspirin)

**ASCP** American Society of Clinical Pathologists

**AST** aspartate aminotransferase

**at. wt.** atomic weight

**ATL** adult T cell leukemia; adult T cell lymphoma

**atm** (standard) atmosphere

**ATP** adenosine 5′ triphosphate

**ATPase** adenosine triphosphatase

**ATPD** ambient temperature and pressure, dry

**ATPS** ambient temperature and pressure, saturated (with water vapor)

**Au** [L.] *aurum,* gold

**AUC** area under the curve

**AV** arteriovenous

**A-V** arteriovenous; atrioventricular

**AVM** arteriovenousmalformation

**AVN** atrioventricular node

**AW** atomic weight

**ax.** axis

**AZT** azidothymidine (zidovudine)

**B** barometric (pressure) (SUBSCRIPT); boron

**B or Bucc** buccal surface (caries or restoration)

**Ba** barium

**BBB** blood brain barrier; bundle branch block

**BBT** basal body temperature

**BCG** bacille bilié de Calmette Guérin (vaccine)

**Be** beryllium

**Bi** bismuth

**b.i.d.** [L.] *bis in die,* twice a day

**BMD** bone mineral density

**BMI** body mass index

**BP** blood pressure; boiling point; *British Pharmacopoeia*

**BPH** Bachelor of Public Health, benign prostatic hyperplasia

**Bq** becquerel (SI unit of radionuclide activity)

**Br** bromine

**BS, BSc** Bachelor of Science (Baccalaureus Scientiae)

**BSA** body surface area

**BSN** Bachelor of Science in Nursing

**BT** bleeding time

**BTPS** body temperature, ambient pressure, saturated (with water vapor)

**BTU** British thermal unit

**BTX** botulinum toxin

**BUN** blood urea nitrogen

**BUS** Bartholin glands, urethra, Skene glands

**Bx** biopsy

**c** calorie (small); capillary (blood); centi

**C** calorie (large); carbon; Celsius; centigrade; clearance (rate, renal) c;

compliance; concentration; cylindric (lens); cytidine

**c** [L.] *cum,* with

**C&S** culture and sensitivity

**C.C.** chief complaint

**c/o** complains of

**ca.** [L.] *circa,* about, approximately

**Ca** calcium; cathodal; cathode

**CA** cancer; carcinoma; cardiac arrest; chronologic age; contrast angiography; croup associated (virus); cytosine arabinoside

**CABG** coronary artery bypass graft

**CAD** coronary artery disease

**cal** calorie (small)

**Cal** calorie (large)

**CAM** complementary and alternative medicine

**CAO** conscious, alert, oriented

**cap** capsule

**CAPD** continuous ambulatory peritoneal dialysis

**CAT** computerized axial tomography (obsolete)

**CBC** complete blood (cell) count

◊**cc, c.c.** cubic centimeter

**CCU** coronary care unit; critical care unit

**Cd** cadmium

**CD** compact disc

**CDA** Certified Dental Assistant

**CDC** (U.S.) Centers for Disease Control and Prevention

**CDP** cytidine 5′ diphosphate

**Ce** cerium

**CEU** continuing education unit

**Cf** californium

**CF** complement fixation; cystic fibrosis; coupling factor

**CGA** catabolite gene activator

**cGMP** cyclic guanosine monophosphate

**cgs, CGS** centimeter-gramsecond (system, unit)

**ChB** Bachelor of Surgery (Chirurgiae Baccalaureus)

**ChD, Chir Doct** Doctor of Surgery (Chirurgiae Doctor)

**CHF** congestive heart failure

**CHO** carbohydrate

**Ci** curie

**CI** color index; *Colour Index*; confidence interval

**CJD** Creutzfeldt-Jakob disease

**CK** creatine kinase

**Cl** chlorine

**CL** cardiolipin

**CLA(ASCP)** Clinical Laboratory Assistant (American Society of Clinical Pathologists)

**CLIA** Clinical Laboratory Improvement Amendments

**CLL** chronic lymphocytic leukemia

**cm** centimeter

**Cm** curium

**CMA** Certified Medical Assistant

**CME** continuing medical education

**CMI** cell mediated immunity

**CML** chronic myelogenous leukemia

**CMO** Chief Medical Officer

**CMT** Certified Medical Transcriptionist

**CMV** controlled mechanical ventilation; cytomegalovirus

**CNS** central nervous system

**Co** cobalt

**Comp** composite resin restoration

**COPD** chronic obstructive pulmonary disease

**COS** Chief of Staff

**CPK** creatine phosphokinase

**CPR** cardiopulmonary resuscitation

**cps** cycles per second

**CPT** *Current Procedural Terminology*

**Cr** chromium; creatinine

**CR** Chief Resident; conditioned reflex; crown rump (length)

**CRD** chronic respiratory disease

**CRNA** Certified Registered Nurse Anesthetist

**CRNP** Certified Registered Nurse Practitioner

**CRP** cross reacting protein

**CRT** Certified Respiratory Therapist

**Cs** cesium

**CSF** cerebrospinal fluid; colony-stimulating factor

**CT** computed tomography

**Cu** [L.] *cuprum,* copper

**CV** cardiovascular

**CVA** cerebral vascular (cerebrovascular) accident, costovertebral angle

**CVP** central venous pressure

**CVS** cardiovascular system; chorionic villus sampling

**CXR** chest x-ray

**Δ** delta; change; heat

**d** deci-; day

*d* dextrorotatory

**D-** prefix indicating that a molecule is sterically analogous to D glyceraldehyde

**da** deca

**Da** dalton

**DA** developmental age

**db, dB** decibel

**DC** Dental Corps; Doctor of Chiropractic; direct current

◊**D/C** discharge; discontinue

**DCh** Doctor of Surgery (Doctor Chirurgiae)

---

The forbidden symbol (◊) appears opposite abbreviations prohibited by the Joint Commission on Accreditation of Healthcare Organizations (JCAHO).

**DDS** Doctor of Dental Surgery

**def** decayed, extracted, or filled (deciduous teeth)

**DEF** decayed, extracted, or filled (permanent teeth)

**DEXA** dual energy x-ray absorptiometry

**df** decayed and filled (deciduous teeth)

**DF** decayed and filled (permanent teeth)

**DH** Dental Hygienist

**DIC** disseminated intravascular coagulation

**DIF** direct immunofluorescence

**DJD** degenerative joint disease

**dk** deca-, deka-

**DKA** diabetic ketoacidosis

**dL** deciliter

**dM** decimorgan

**DM** diabetes mellitus

**DMD** Doctor of Dental Medicine; Duchenne muscular dystrophy

**DME** Director of Medical Education

**dmf** decayed, missing, or filled (deciduous teeth)

**DMF** decayed, missing, or filled (permanent teeth)

**DMSO** dimethyl sulfoxide

**DMT** *N,N* dimethyltryptamine

**DMV** Doctor of Veterinary Medicine

**DNR** do not resuscitate

**DO** disto-occlusal surfaces (caries or restoration); Doctor of Osteopathy

**DOA** dead on arrival

**DOB** date of birth

**DP** Doctor of Pharmacy; Doctor of Podiatry

**DPH** Doctor of Public Health; Doctor of Public Hygiene

**DPharm** Doctor of Pharmacy

**DPM** Doctor of Physical Medicine; Doctor of Podiatric Medicine

**dr** dram

**Dr Med** Doctor of Medicine

**DRG** diagnosis-related group

**DrPH** Doctor of Public Health; Doctor of Public Hygiene

**DRVVT** dilute Russell viper venom test

**D-S** Doerfler Stewart (test)

**DSA** digital subtraction angiography

**DSc** Doctor of Science

**DSD** dry sterile dressing

**DVM** Doctor of Veterinary Medicine

**DVT** deep vein thrombosis

**Dx** diagnosis

**EB** Epstein Barr (virus)

**EBV** Epstein Barr virus

**ECF** extended care facility; extracellular fluid

**ECG** electrocardiogram

**ECM** erythema chronicum migrans

**ECMO** extracorporeal membrane oxygenation

**ECS** electrocerebral silence

**ECT** electroconvulsive therapy

**ED** eating disorder; effective dose; emergency department; erectile dysfunction

**EEG** electroencephalogram

**EENT** eye, ear, nose, and throat

**EIA** enzyme immunoassay

**EKG** [German] *Elektrokardiogramme*, electrocardiogram

**ELISA** enzyme-linked immunosorbent assay

**EMF** electromotive force

**EMG** electromyogram; exomphalos, macroglossia, and gigantism (syndrome)

**EMS** eosinophilia-myalgia syndrome

**EMT** Emergency Medical Technician

**ENT** ear, nose, and throat

**EPO** erythropoietin

**ER** endoplasmic reticulum; emergency room

**Er** erbium

**ERBF** effective renal blood flow

**ERPF** effective renal plasma flow

**ERT** estrogen replacement therapy

**Es** einsteinium

**ESEP** extreme somatosensory evoked potential

**ESR** electron spin resonance; erythrocyte sedimentation rate

**ESRD** end stage renal disease

**ESWL** extracorporeal shock-wave lithotripsy

**EtOH** ethyl alcohol

**Eu** europium

**ev, eV** electron volt

**F** Fahrenheit; faraday (constant); fertility (factor); field (of vision); fluorine; force; fractional (concentration); free (energy)

**f** femto-; (respiratory) frequency

**FAAN** Fellow of the American Academy of Nursing

**FAAP** Fellow of the American Academy of Pediatrics

**FACA** Fellow of the American College of Anesthesiology

**FACAL** Fellow of the American College of Allergy

**FACC** Fellow of the American College of Cardiologists

**FACD** Fellow of the American College of Dentists

**FACFP** Fellow of the American College of Family Physicians

**FACO** Fellow of the American College of Otolaryngology

**FACOG** Fellow of the American College of Obstetricians and Gynecologists

**FACOS** Fellow of the American College of Orthopaedic Surgeons

**FACP** Fellow of the American College of Physicians

**FACR** Fellow of the American College of Radiology

**FACS** Fellow of the American College of Surgeons

**FAMA** Fellow of the American Medical Association

**FB** foreign body

**FBS** fasting blood sugar

**FDA** (U.S.) Food and Drug Administration

**Fe** [L.] *ferrum,* iron

**FEF** forced expiratory flow

**FET** forced expiratory time

**FEV** forced expiratory volume

**FF** filtration fraction

**FFD** focus film distance

**FIA** fluorescent immunoassay

**FISH** fluorescent in situ hybridization

**Fm** fermium

**FNA** fine-needle aspiration

**FPD** Fixed Partial Denture

**fps, FPS** foot pound second (system, unit)

**Fr** francium; French (gauge, scale)

**FRC** functional residual capacity (of lungs)

**French** (catheter gauge)

**FTA-ABS** fluorescent treponemal antibody absorption (test)

**F/U** follow-up

**FUO** fever of unknown origin

**FVC** forced vital capacity

**Fx** fracture

**G** giga; glucose; gravitation (newtonian constant of); guanosine (or guanylic acid) residues in polynucleotides

**g** gram

**Ga** gallium

**GABA** γ-aminobutyric acid

**GABHS** group-A β-hemolytic *Streptococcus*

**Gal** galactose

**GC** gonococcus, gonorrhea

**Gd** gadolinium

**Ge** germanium

**GERD** gastroesophageal reflux disease

**GFR** glomerular filtration rate

**GGT** γ-glutamyl transferase

**GH-RH** growth hormone releasing hormone

**GI** gastrointestinal; Gingival Index

**GIC** glass ionomer cement

**GLC** gas liquid chromatography

**GMO** General Medical Officer

**GMS** Gomori (or Grocott) methenamine silver (stain)

**GN** Graduate Nurse

**GOT** glutamic oxaloacetic transaminase (aspartate aminotransferase)

**GPI** Gingival Periodontal Index

**gr** grain

**GSW** gunshot wound

**gt.** [L.] *gutta,* a drop

**gtt.** [L.] *guttae,* drops

**GTT** glucose tolerance test

**GU** genitourinary

**GVHD** graft versus host disease

**Gy** gray (unit of absorbed dose of ionizing radiation)

**H** henry; hydrogen; hyperopia; hyperopic

**h** Planck constant

**H & E** hematoxylin and eosin

**H & H** hematocrit and hemoglobin

**H⁺** hydrogen ion

**HAART** highly active anti-retroviral therapy

**HAV** hepatitis A virus

**Hb** hemoglobin

**HbA** adult hemoglobin

**HB^cAg** Hepatitis B core antigen

**HB^e** Hepatitis B early antigen

**HB^cAb** Hepatitis B early antibody

**Hb^eAg** Hepatitis B early antigen

**Hbg** hemoglobin

**HBIG** hepatitis B immune globulin

**HBO** hyperbaric oxygen

**HB^sAb** hepatitis B surface antibody

**HBsAg** hepatitis B surface antigen

**HBV** hepatitis B virus

**HCFA** Health Care Financing Administration

**HCl** hydrochloric acid; hydrochloride

**Hct** hematocrit

**HCV** Hepatitis C virus

**h. d.** [L.] *hora decubitus,* at bedtime

**HDL** high-density lipoprotein

**Hg** [L.] *hydrargyrum,* mercury

**Hgb** hemoglobin

**HGE** human granulocytic ehrlichiosis

**HGH** human (pituitary) growth hormone

**HGSIL** high-grade squamous intraepithelial lesion

**HIPAA** Health Insurance Portability and Accountability Act

**HIV** human immunodeficiency virus

**HLA** human lymphocyte antigen, human leukocyte antigen

**HMG** CoA 3 hydroxy 3 methylglutaryl coenzyme A
**HMO** Health Maintenance Organization
**h/o** history of
**HPF** high power field
**HPI** history of present illness
**HPV** human papillomavirus
**⃠h. s., HS [L.]** *hora somni,* at bedtime
**HSV** herpes simplex virus
**5-HT** 5-hydroxytryptamine (serotonin)
**Ht** hyperopia, total
**HTLV** human T cell lymphocytotrophic virus; human T cell lymphoma/leukemia virus
**HTN** hypertension
**Hx** (medical) history
**Hz** hertz
**¹²⁵I** iodine 125
**¹³¹I** iodine 131
**¹²³I** iodine 123 (radioisotope)
**I & D** incision and drainage
**I & O** (fluid) intake and output
**IADLs** instrumental activities of daily living
**IBD** inflammatory bowel disease
**IBS** irritable bowel syndrome
**IBW** ideal body weight
**ICD** *International Classification of Diseases of the World Health Organization*; implantable cardioverterdefibrillator
**ICDA** *International Classification of Diseases, Adapted for Use in the United States*
**ICP** intracranial pressure
**ICU** intensive care unit
**ID** infective dose
**IDU** idoxuridine; injecting/injection drug user

**IF** initiation factor; intrinsic factor
**IFN** interferon
**Ig** immunoglobulin
**IGF** insulinlike growth factor
**IL** interleukin
**ILA** insulinlike activity
**IM** internal medicine; intramuscular(ly); infectious mononucleosis
**IMS** Indian Medical Service
**IND** investigational new drug
**INR** international normalized ratio
**IOML** infraorbitomeatal line
**IP** interphalangeal; intraperitoneal(ly)
**IPAP** inspiratory positive airway pressure
**IQ** intelligence quotient
**IRB** institutional review board
**IU** International Unit
**IV** intravenous, intravenously; intraventricular
**IVDA** intravenous drug abuse(r)
**IVP** intravenous pyelogram
**J** flux (density)
**J** joule
**K [Mod. L.]** *kalium,* potassium; kelvin
**k** kilo
**kat** katal
**kb** kilobase
**kc** kilocycle
**kcal** kilocalorie
**kDa** kilodalton
**kg** kilogram
**KOH** potassium hydroxide
**KS** Kaposi sarcoma
**kv** kilovolt
**kVp** kilovolt peak
**l, L** liter (use of CAPITAL letter preferred)
**L or Ling** lingual surface (caries or restoration)

**LD** lethal dose
**LDL** low-density lipoprotein
**LE** lupus erythematosus
**LGV** lymphogranuloma venereum
**LP** lumbar puncture
**LPN** Licensed Practical Nurse
**⃠µ** mu; micro; heavy chain class corresponding to IgM
**⃠µCi** microcurie
**⃠µg** microgram
**⃠µl,µL** microliter
**⃠µm** micrometer
**µµ** micromicro
**m** mass; meter; milliminim; molar
**m- *meta***
**M** mega, meg; molar; moles (per liter); morgan; myopic; myopia
**M** molar; moles (per liter)
**m** moles (per liter)
**mA** milliampere
**MA** Master of Arts (Magister Artium); Medical Assistant; mental age
**MAb** monoclonal antibody
**MAC** *Mycobacterium avium* complex
**MAI** *Mycobacterium aviumintracellulare*
**MAO** monoamine oxidase
**MAOI** monoamine oxidase inhibitor
**mA-S** milliampere second
**MBC** maximum breathing capacity
**MC** Medical Corps
**mCi** millicurie
**mcm** millimicron
**MD [L.]** *Medicinae Doctor,* Doctor of Medicine
**Med Tech** Medical Technician; Medical Technologist
**MEDLARS** Medical Literature Analysis and Retrieval System
**meq, mEq** milliequivalent

---

The forbidden symbol (⃠) appears opposite abbreviations prohibited by the Joint Commission on Accreditation of Healthcare Organizations (JCAHO).

**MEV** million electron volts ($10^6$ ev)

**mg** milligram

**Mg** magnesium

**MHC** major histocompatibility complex

**MHz** megahertz

**MI** mitral insufficiency; myocardial infarction

**ml, mL** milliliter

**MLC** mixed lymphocyte culture (test)

**MLD** minimal lethal dose

**mm** millimeter

**mmHg** millimeters of mercury (torr)

**mmol** millimole

**MMPI** Minnesota Multiphasic Personality Inventory (test)

**MMR** measles-mumps-rubella (vaccine)

**Mn** manganese

**Mo** molybdenum

**MO** mesio-occlusal surfaces (caries or restoration); Medical Officer; mineral oil

**MOC** Medical Officer on Call

**MOD** Medical Officer of the Day

**mol** mole

**mol wt** molecular weight

**MOM** Milk of Magnesia

**MOPP** Mustargen (mechlorethamine hydrocholoride), Oncovin (vincristine sulfate), procarbazine hydrochloride, and prednisone

**MPD** maximal permissible dose

**MPH** Master of Public Health

**MRCP** Member of the Royal College of Physicians

**MRCS** Member of the Royal College of Surgeons

**MRI** magnetic resonance imaging

**mRNA** messenger RNA

**MRSA** methicillin-resistant *Staphylococcus aureus*

**MS** Master of Science

⃠**MS** multiple sclerosis; magnesium sulfate; morphine sulfate

**msec** millisecond

**m/sec** meters per second

**MSG** monosodium glutamate

**MSM** men who have sex with men

**MSN** Master of Science in Nursing

**MT** Medical Technologist; Medical Transcriptionist; Monitor Technician

**mtDNA** mitochondrial DNA

**MUGA** multiple gated acquisition (imaging)

**mV** millivolt

**Mv** mendelevium

**MVA** motor vehicle accident

**MW** molecular weight

***v*** nu; kinematic viscosity

**n** index of refraction; nano

**N** newton; nitrogen; normal (concentration)

ɴ normal (SMALL caps)

**Na** [Modern L.] *natrium*, sodium

ɴᴀ *Nomina Anatomica*

**NAD** nicotinamide adenine dinucleotide; no apparent (or acute) distress

**NCV** nerve conduction velocity

**Nd** neodymium

**Nd:YAG** neodymium: yttriumaluminum- garnet [laser]

**NDA** New Drug Application

**Ne** neon

**NE** norepinephrine; not examined

**NF** National Formulary

**ng** nanogram

**NGF** nerve growth factor (antigen)

**Ni** nickel

**NIH** National Institutes of Health

**NK** natural killer (cell)

**NKA** no known allergies

**NLM** National Library of Medicine

**nm** nanometer

**NP** Nurse Practitioner

**NPO** [L.] *nihil per os*, nothing by mouth

**NS** normal saline

**NSAID** nonsteroidal antiinflammatory drug

**NSR** normal sinus rhythm

**NUG** necrotizing ulcerative gingivitis

**Ω** omega; ohm

***o-*** *ortho*

**O** [L.] *oculus*, eye; opening (in formulas for electrical reactions); oxygen

**OB** obstetrics

**OB/GYN** obstetrics (and) gynecology

**OC** oral contraceptive

**Occ** occlusal surfaces (caries or restoration)

**OCD** obsessive compulsive disorder

**OD** Doctor of Optometry; Officer of the Day; overdose

⃠**OD** [L.] *oculus dexter*, right eye

**ODD** oculodentodigital (dysplasia, syndrome)

**Oe** oersted (centimeter gram second unit of magnetic field strength)

**OFD** orofaciodigital (dysostosis, syndrome)

**OML** orbitomeatal line

**OMM** ophthalmomandibulomelic (dysplasia, syndrome)

**OP** osmotic pressure; outpatient

**OPV** oral poliovirus vaccine

**OR** operating room

---

The forbidden symbol (⃠) appears opposite abbreviations prohibited by the Joint Commission on Accreditation of Healthcare Organizations (JCAHO).

**ORIF** open reduction and internal fixation
**Os** osmium
**OSA** obstructive sleep apnea
**OSHA** Occupational Safety and Health Administration
**OT** occupational therapy; Koch old tuberculin
**OTC** over the counter (nonprescription) drug
✑**OU** [L.] *oculus uterque*, each eye (both eyes)
**oz** ounce
**p** pico; pupil
*p-* para
**P** partial (pressure); peta; phosphorus, phosphoric (residue); plasma (concentration); pressure; para (obstetric history)
$^{32}$**P** phosphorus-32
**PA** Physician Assistant; posteroanterior
**Pa** pascal
**PA** Physician's Assistant; posteroanterior; pulmonary artery
**Pb** [L.] *plumbum*, lead
**p.c.** [L.] *post cibum*, after a meal
**PCB** polychlorinated biphenyl
**Pco2** partial pressure of carbon dioxide
**PCP** phencyclidine; plasma cell pneumonia (Pneumocystic carinii pneumonia); primary care provider
**PCR** polymerase chain reaction
**PCWP** pulmonary capillary wedge pressure
**Pd** palladium
**PDA** patent ductus arteriosus; posterior descending artery
**PDGF** platelet derived growth factor
**PDR** *Physicians' Desk Reference*

**PEEP** positive end expiratory pressure
**PEG** polyethylene glycol
**PET** positron emission tomography
**PFM** porcelain fused to metal (crown)
**pg** picogram
**PG** prostaglandin
**PGA** prostaglandin A
**PGB** prostaglandin B
**PGE** prostaglandin E
**PGF** prostaglandin F
**pH** hydrogen ion concentration; p (power) of $[H+]_{10}$
**Pharm D** Doctor of Pharmacy *(Pharmaciae Doctor)*
**PhD** Doctor of Philosophy *(Philosophiae Doctor)*
**PhD** [L.] *Philosophiae Doctor*, Doctor of Philosophy
**PhG** [L.] *Pharmacopoeia Germanica*, German Pharmacopeia
**PhG** Graduate in Pharmacy
**PHN** Public Health Nurse; postherpetic neuralgia
**PICC** peripherally inserted central catheter
**PK** pyruvate kinase
**PKU** phenylketonuria
**pm** picometer
**Pm** promethium
**PM** post mortem
**PMI** point of maximum intensity
**PMN** polymorphonuclear (leukocyte)
**PN** Practical Nurse
**PND** paroxysmal nocturnal dyspnea; postnasal drip
**PO** [L.] *per os,* by mouth
**PPD** purified protein derivative (of tuberculin)
**ppm** parts per million
**PPV** positive pressure ventilation

**p.r.n. PRN,** [L.] *pro re nata,* as needed
**psi** pounds per square inch
**PSV** pressure-supported ventilation
**PT** physical therapy; prothrombin time
**Pt** platinum
**PTH** parathyroid hormone
**PTT** partial thromboplastin time
**PVC** premature ventricular contraction
**PVL** plasma viral load
**PVP** polyvinylpyrrolidone (povidone)
**q** [L.] *quisque*, every
**Q** coulomb; volume of blood flow
**Qco$_2$** microliters CO2 given off per milligram of dryweight of tissue per hour
✑**q.d.** [L.] *quaque die*, every day
**q.i.d.** [L.] *quater in die*, four times a day
**QNS** quantity not sufficient
✑**q.o.d.** every other day
**q.s.** [L.] *quantum satis*, as much as is enough; [L.] *quantum sufficiat*, as much as may suffice; quantity sufficient
**r** racemic; roentgen
**RA** rheumatoid arthritis
**RAD** reactive airways disease
**rbc** red blood cell; red blood (cell) count
**RBC** red blood cell; red blood (cell) count
**RBF** renal blood flow
**RCM** right costal margin
**RCT** root canal treatment
**RD** reaction of degeneration; reaction of denervation; Registered Dietitian
**RDA** recommended daily allowance

---

The forbidden symbol (✑) appears opposite abbreviations prohibited by the Joint Commission on Accreditation of Healthcare Organizations (JCAHO).

**RDH** Registered Dental Hygienist

**RDS** respiratory distress syndrome

**RE** right ear; right eye

**rem** roentgen equivalent, man

**REM** rapid eye movement (sleep); reticular erythematous mucinosis

**rep** roentgen equivalent, physical

**RF** release factor; rheumatoid factor

**Rh** Rhesus (Rh blood group); rhodium

**RIA** radioimmunoassay

**RN** Registered Nurse

**RNA** Registered Nurse Anesthetist; ribonucleic acid

**RNC** Registered Nurse, Certified

**RNP** Registered Nurse Practitioner

**R/O** rule out

**ROM** range of motion

**ROS** review of systems

**RP** Registered Pharmacist

**RPD** Removable Partial Denture

**RPh** Registered Pharmacist

**rpm** revolutions per minute

**RPR** rapid plasma reagin (test)

**RQ** respiratory quotient

**RT** Radiologic Technologist; Registered Technologist; Respiratory Therapist

**RVEF** right ventricular ejection fraction

**RVH** right ventricular hypertrophy

**σ** sigma; reflection coefficient; standard deviation; 1 millisecond (0.001 sec)

**s** [L.] *semis*, half; steady state (SUBSCRIPT); [L.] *sinister*, left

**s** sine, without

**s/s** signs and symptoms

**S** [L.] *sinister*, left; saturation of hemoglobin (percentage of) (followed by subscript $o_2$ **or** $co_2$); siemens; spheric; spheric (lens); sulfur; Svedberg (unit)

**SA** sinuatrial

**S-A** sinuatrial

**SAD** seasonal affective disorder

**S and P** Scale and Polish (periodontics)

**SARS** severe acute respiratory syndrome

**SBE** subacute bacterial endocarditis

**sc** subcutaneous(ly)

**ScD** Doctor of Science

**SCID** severe combined immunodeficiency

**SD** standard deviation; streptodornase

**SGOT** serum glutamicoxaloacetic transaminase (aspartate aminotransferase)

**SGPT** serum glutamic-pyruvic transaminase (alanine aminotransferase)

**SH** serum hepatitis

**SI** [French] *Système International d'Unités;* International System of Units

**SID** source-to-image (-receptor) distance

**SIDS** sudden infant death syndrome

**sig.** [L.] *signa*, affix a label, inscribe

**SIRD** source-to-imagereceptor distance

**SL** sublingual(ly)

**SLE** systemic lupus erythematosus

**Sn** [L.] *stannum*, tin

**SN** Student Nurse

**SOB** short(ness) of breath

**sol.** solution

**soln.** solution

**SP** Speech Pathologist

**sp. gr.** specific gravity

**sp.** species

**SPF** sun protection (or protective) factor

**spp.** species (plural)

**SQ** subcutaneous

**ssp.** subspecies

**SSRI** selective serotonin reuptake inhibitor

**stat; STAT** [L.] *statim*, immediately, at once

**STD** sexually transmitted disease

**STEL** short-term exposure limit

**STI** sexually transmitted infection

**STM** short-term memory

**STPD** standard temperature (0° C) and pressure (760 mmHg absolute), dry

**STS** serologic test for syphilis

**Sv, SV** sievert (unit)

**SVT** supraventricular tachycardia

**t** metric ton

**t** temperature (Celsius); tritium

**T** temperature, absolute (Kelvin); tension (intraocular); tera; tesla; tetanus (toxoid); tidal (volume) (SUBSCRIPT); tocopherol; transverse (tubule); tritium; tumor (antigen)

**T** absolute temperature (Kelvin)

**T & C** type and crossmatch

**Ta** tantalum

**TA** *Terminologia Anatomica*

**tab** tablet

**TB** tuberculosis

**TBV** total blood volume

**Tc** technetium

**$^{99m}$Tc** technetium 99m

**TCA** tricarboxylic acid; trichloracetic acid

**TEN** toxic epidermal necrolysis

**TFCI** transient focal cerebral ischemia

**THC** tetrahydrocannabinol
**Ti** titanium
**TIA** transient ischemic attack
**TIBC** total iron-binding capacity
**t.i.d.** [L.] *ter in die*, three times a day
**tinct.** tincture
◌**t.i.w.** three times a week
**Tl** thallium
**TMJ** temporomandibular joint
**TNF** tumor necrosis factor
**TNM** tumor, node, metastasis (tumor staging)
**t-PA, TPA** tissue plasminogen activator
**TPHA** *Treponema pallidum* hemagglutination (test)
**TPI** *Treponema pallidum* immobilization (test)
**TPN** total parenteral nutrition
**TPR** temperature, pulse, and respirations

**tr.** tincture
**TSH** thyroid stimulating hormone
**TSS** toxic shock syndrome
**TTP** thrombotic thrombocytopenic purpura
**TU** toxic unit, toxin unit
**Tx** treatment
**Tyr** tyrosine (and its radicals) ◌**U** unit
**URI** upper respiratory infection
**US** ultrasound
**USAN** United States Adopted Names (Council)
**USP** *United States Pharmacopeia*
**USPHS** United States Public Health Service
**UTI** urinary tract infection
**VDRL** Venereal Disease Research Laboratory (test)
**VHDL** very high density lipoprotein

**VLDL** very low density lipoprotein
**Vmax** maximal velocity
**VN** Visiting Nurse, Vocational Nurse
**VO** vocal order
**VS** vital signs; volumetric solution
**VT** tidal volume
**VZIG** varicella-zoster immune globulin
**W** watt; [German] *Wolfram*, tungsten
**WD** well-developed
**WDLL** well-differentiated lymphocytic (or lymphatic) lymphoma
**WHO** World Health Organization
**WN** well nourished
**Y** yttrium
**YAG** yttrium-aluminumgarnet (laser)
**Yb** ytterbium
**Zn** zinc
**Zr** zirconium

---

The forbidden symbol (◌) appears opposite abbreviations prohibited by the Joint Commission on Accreditation of Healthcare Organizations (JCAHO).

# Common Abbreviations Used in Medication Orders

| | | | |
|---|---|---|---|
| a or a. | before | om | on morning |
| a.c. | before meals | on | on night |
| ad lib | as desired | oz | ounce |
| alt. h. | alternate hours | p or p. | after, per |
| am | in the morning; before noon | p.c. | after meals |
| | | PO | by mouth |
| aq. | water | pm | afternoon, evening |
| bid | twice a day | prn | as needed, according to necessity |
| c̄ | with | | |
| cap., caps. | capsule | q | each, every |
| dil. | dilute | qh | every hour |
| dist. | distilled | qid, Qqds | four times a day |
| DS | double strength | q1h | every 1 hour |
| EC | enteric coated | q2h | every 2 hours |
| elix. | elixir | q3h | every 3 hours |
| ext. | external, extract | q4h | every 4 hours |
| fl, fld | fluid | q6h | every 6 hours |
| g | gram | q8h | every 8 hours |
| gr | grain | q12h | every 12 hours |
| gtt | drop | qs | as much as needed, quantity, sufficient |
| H | hypodermic | | |
| h, hr | hour | qt | quart |
| IM | intramuscular | R. or PR | rectally, per rectum |
| inj. | injection | Rx | take, prescription |
| IV | intravenous | S, Sig | give the following directions |
| IVP | IV push | s̄ | without |
| IVPB | IV piggyback | sid | once daily |
| kg | kilogram | sol. or soln. | solution |
| L | liter | SQ | subcutaneous |
| lb | pound | stat. | immediately, at once |
| liq. | liquid | tab. | tablet |
| mcg, mg | microgram | tbsp, T | tablespoon |
| mEq | milliequivalent | tds, tid | three times a day |
| mg | milligram | tinct., tr | tincture |
| mL | milliliter | tsp, t | teaspoon |
| noct. | night | ung. | ointment |

Modified from Craven RF, Hirnle CJ, eds. *Fundamentals of Nursing: Human Health and Function*. Philadelphia: Lippincott Williams & Wilkins, 2000.

# Common Abbreviations Not to Be Used in Medication Orders

The Joint Commission on Accreditation of Healthcare Organizations' list of dangerous abbreviations, acronyms, and symbols not to be used was originally created in 2004 and updated May 2005.

Joint Commission on Accreditation of Healthcare Organizations (JCAHO): *www.jcaho.org*

As of May 2005, the survey and scoring of this requirement applies to all orders and all medication-related documentation that is handwritten (including free-text computer entry) or on preprinted forms.

## Official "Do Not Use" List

| Abbreviation | Potential Problem | Preferred Term |
|---|---|---|
| U (for unit) | Mistaken as 0 (zero), 4 (four), or cc. | Write "unit." |
| IU (for international unit) | Mistaken as IV (intravenous) or 10 (ten) | Write "international unit." |
| Q.D., QD, q.d., qd (daily), Q.O.D., QOD, q.o.d, qod (every other day) | Mistaken for each other. Period after the Q mistaken for "I" and the "O" mistaken for "I." | Write "daily." Write "every other day." |
| Trailing zero (X.0 mg), lack of leading zero (.X mg) | Decimal point is missed. | Never write a zero by itself after a decimal point (X mg)*. Always use a zero before a decimal point (0.X mg). |
| MS, MSO4 and MgSO4 | Can mean morphine sulfate or magnesium sulfate. Confused for one another. | Write "morphine sulfate." Write "magnesium sulfate." |

**An abbreviation on the "do not use" list should not be used in any of its forms—upper or lower case, with or without periods. For example, if Q.D. is on your list, you cannot use QD or qd. Any of those variations may be confusing and could be misinterpreted.**

* Exception: a "trailing zero" may be used only where required to demonstrate the level of precision of the value being reported, such as for laboratory results, imaging studies that report size of lesions, or catheter/tube sizes. It may not be used in medication orders or other medication-related documentation.

# Additional Abbreviations, Acronyms, and Symbols

Organizations may consider adding any or all of these to their own list of abbreviations not to use. The following items will be reviewed annually by JCAHO for possible future inclusion on the official "do not use" list.

| Abbreviation | Potential Problem | Preferred Term |
|---|---|---|
| > (greater than)<br>< (less than) | Mistaken for 7 (seven) or the letter "L."<br>Confused for one another. | Write "greater than" or "less than." |
| Abbreviations for drug names | Misinterpreted due to similar abbreviations for multiple drugs. | Write drug names in full. |
| Apothecary units | Unfamiliar to many practitioners.<br>Confused with metric units. | Use metric units. |
| @ | Mistaken for 2 (two). | Write "at." |
| cc (for cubic centimeter) | Mistaken for U (units) when poorly written. | Write "ml" or "milliliters." |
| μg (for microgram) | Mistaken for mg (milligrams), resulting in one thousand-fold overdose. | Write "mcg" or "micrograms." |

# Laboratory Reference Range Values

Show-Hong Duh, PhD, DABCC, Department of Pathology,
University of Maryland School of Medicine
Janine Denis Cook, PhD, Department of Medical and Research Technology,
University of Maryland School of Medicine

Reference range values are for apparently healthy people and often overlap significantly with values for those who are sick. Actual values may vary significantly due to differences in assay methodologies and standardization. Institutions may also set up their own reference ranges based on the particular populations that they serve, thus regional differences may occur. Consequently, values reported by individual laboratories may differ from those listed in this appendix.

All values are given in conventional and SI units. However, in cases where SI units have not been widely accepted, conventional units are used. In case of the heterogenous nature of the materials measured or uncertainty about the exact molecular weight of the compounds, SI measurements cannot be used so that mass per volume remains as the unit of concentration.

## Abbreviations:

**ACD,** acid-citrate-dextrose; **AMP,** adenosine monophosphate; **CEA,** carcinoembryonic antigen; **CHF,** congestive heart failure; **Cit,** citrate; **Cl,** chlorine; **CNS,** central nervous system; **CSF,** cerebrospinal fluid; **cyclic AMP,** adenosine 3′,5′-cyclic phosphate; **EDTA,** ethylenediaminetetraacetic acid; **Hb,** hemoglobin; **HDL,** high-density lipoprotein; **Hep,** heparin; **LDL-C,** low-density lipoprotein-cholesterol; **MB,** myoglobin; **NaCit,** sodium citrate; **NAPA,** N-acetylprocainomide; **Ox,** oxalate; **RBC,** red blood cell(s); **RIA,** radioimmunoassay; **SD,** standard deviation; **WBC,** white blood cell(s)

## References:

Burtis CA, Ashwood ER. eds. Tietz textbook of clinical chemistry, 3rd ed. Philadelphia; WB Saunders, 1998.

Children's Hospital, St. Louis, The Department of Clinical Laboratories, High Density Lipoprotein Lipid Panel: Cholesterol, HDL, Cholesterol, LDL (calculated), Cholesterol, Total, Triglycerides, Parathyroid Hormone (PTH).

Clinical chemistry laboratory: Reference range values in clinical chemistry. Professional services manual. Baltimore, Department of Pathology, University of Maryland Medical System, 1999.

Harmening DM, ed. Hematologic values in chemical hematology and fundamentals of hemostasis, 2nd ed. Philadelphia: FA Davis, 1992.

Laboratory Corporation of America. Available at: http://www.labcorp.com/datasets/labcorp/html/chapter/mono/he005000.htm. Accessed September 7, 2010.

National cholesterol education program: Report of the expert panel on detection, evaluation, and treatment of high blood cholesterol in adults. *Arch Intern Med* 1988;148:36–69.

Triglyceride, high density lipoprotein and coronary heart disease. National Institute of Health Consensus Statement, NIH Consensus Development Conference, 1992;10(2).

University of Texas Health Center at San Antonio. Neonatal Bilirubin.

University of Texas Medical Branch. Erythrocyte Sedimentation Rate, Wintrobe. Available at: http://www.utmb.edu/lsg/hem/Sedimentation_Rate.htm. Accessed September 15, 2010.

University of Virginia Children's Medical Center. Therapy Review: Warfarin (Coumadin®). *Pediatric Pharmacotherapy*. January 1995;1(5):386.

Wafarin Therapy in Children Who Require Long-Term Total Parenteral Nutrition. *Pediatrics* [electronic article]. November 2003;112(5):386. Available at: http://pediatrics.aappublications.org/cgi/content/full/112/5/e386. Accessed September 15, 2010.

| Tests | Conventional Units | SI Units |
|---|---|---|
| Acetaminophen, serum or plasma (Hep or EDTA) | | |
| Therapeutic | 10–30 mcg/mL | 66–199 mcmol/L |
| Toxic | >200 mcg/mL | >1324 mcmol/L |
| Acetone | | |
| Serum | | |
| Qualitative | Negative | Negative |
| Quantitative | 0.3–2.0 mg/dL | 0.05–0.34 mmol/L |
| Urine | | |
| Qualitative | Negative | Negative |
| *Alanine aminotransferase (ALT, SGPT), serum | | |
| Male | 13–40 U/L (37°C) | 0.22–0.68 mckat/L (37°C) |
| Female | 10–28 U/L (37°C) | 0.17–0.48 mckat/L (37°C) |
| Albumin | | |
| Serum | | |
| Adult | 3.5–5.2 g/dL | 35–52 g/L |
| >60 y | 3.2–4.6 g/dL | 32–46 g/L |
| | Avg. of 0.3 g/dL higher in patients in upright position | Avg. of 3 g/L higher in patients in upright position |
| Urine | | |
| Qualitative | Negative | Negative |
| Quantitative | 50–80 mg/24 h | 50–80 mg/24 h |
| CSF | 10–30 mg/dL | 100–300 mg/L |
| *Amylase | | |
| Serum | 27–131 U/L | 0.46–2.23 mckat/L |
| Urine | 1–17 U/h | 0.017–0.29 mckat/h |
| *Aspartate aminotransferase (AST, SGOT), serum | 10–59 U/L (37°C) | 0.17–1.00 −2 to +3 kat/L (37°C) |
| Bicarbonate, serum (venous) | 22–29 mEq/L | 22–29 mmol/L |
| †*Bilirubin | | |
| Bilirubin, direct | | |
| Birth–death | 0.0–0.4 mg/dL | |
| Bilirubin, total | | |
| Birth–1 day | 1.0–6.0 mg/dL | |
| 1–2 days | 6.0–7.5 mg/dL | |
| 2–5 days | 4.0–13.5 mg/dL | |
| 5 days–death | 0.2–1.2 mg/dL | |
| Total bilirubin, neonatal | | |
| Birth–1 day | 1.0–6.0 mg/dL | |
| 1–2 days | 6.0–7.5 mg/dL | |
| 2–5 days | 4.0–13.5 mg/dL | |
| 5 days–1 month | 0.0–1.8 mg/dL | |
| 1 month–death | 0.0–1.8 mg/dL | |
| Bone marrow, differential cell count | | |
| Adult | | |
| Undifferentiated cells | 0–1% | 0–0.01 |
| Myeloblast | 0–2% | 0–0.02 |
| Promyelocyte | 0–4% | 0–0.04 |
| Myelocytes | | |
| Neutrophilic | 5–20% | 0.05–0.20 |
| Eosinophilic | 0–3% | 0–0.03 |
| Basophilic | 0–1% | 0–0.01 |

*(continued)*

Test values dependent on laboratory methods used
† Bilirubin data—Source: University of Texas Health Center at San Antonio

| Tests | Conventional Units | | SI Units |
|---|---|---|---|
| Bone marrow, differential cell count *(continued from previous page)* | | | |
| Metamyeolocytes and bands | | | |
| Neutrophilic | 5–35% | | 0.05–0.35 |
| Eosinophilic | 0–5% | | 0–0.05 |
| Basophilic | 0–1% | | 0–0.01 |
| Segmented neutrophils | 5–15% | | 0.05–0.15 |
| Pronormoblast | 0–1.5% | | 0–0.015 |
| Basophilic normoblast | 0–5% | | 0–0.05 |
| Polychromatophilic normoblast | 5–30% | | 0.05–0.30 |
| Orthochromatic normoblast | 5–10% | | 0.05–0.10 |
| Lymphocytes | 10–20% | | 0.10–0.20 |
| Plasma cells | 0–2% | | 0–0.02 |
| Monocytes | 0–5% | | 0–0.05 |
| Calcium, serum | 8.6–10.0 mg/dL (Slightly higher in children) | | 2.15–2.50 mmol/L (Slightly higher in children) |
| Calcium, ionized, serum | 4.64–5.28 mg/dL | | 1.16–1.32 mmol/L |
| Calcium, urine | | | |
| Low calcium diet | 50–150 mg/24 h | | 1.25–3.75 mmol/24 h |
| Usual diet; trough | 100–300 mg/24 h | | 2.50–7.50 mmol/24 h |
| Carbon dioxide, total, serum/plasma (Hep) | 22–28 mmol/L | | 22–28 mmol/L |
| Carbon dioxide ($PCO_2$), blood, arterial | Male 35–48 mmHg Female 32–45 mmHg | | 4.66–6.38 kPa 4.26–5.99 kPa |
| Carbon monoxide as carboxyhemoglobin (HbCO), whole blood (EDTA) | | | |
| Nonsmokers | 0.5–1.5% total Hb | | 0.005–0.015 HbCO fraction |
| Smokers | | | |
| 1–2 packs/d | 4–5% total Hb | | 0.04–0.05 HbCO fraction |
| >2 packs/d | 8–9% total Hb | | 0.08–0.09 HbCO fraction |
| Toxic | >20% total Hb | | >0.20 HbCO fraction |
| Lethal | >50% total Hb | | >0.5 HbCO fraction |
| *Cell counts, adult | | | |
| Erythrocytes | | | |
| Male | $4.7–6.1 \times 10^6$/mcL | | $4.7–6.1 \times 10^{12}$/L |
| Female | $4.2–5.4 \times 10^6$/mcL | | $4.2–5.4 \times 10^{12}$/L |
| Leukocytes | | | |
| Total | $4.8–10.8 \times 10^3$/mcL | | $4.8–10.8 \times 10^6$/L |
| Differential | Percentage | Absolute | Absolute (SI) |
| Myelocytes | 0 | 0/mcL | 0/L |
| Neutrophils | | | |
| Band | 3–5 | 150–400/mcL | $150–400 \times 10^6$/L |
| Segmented | 54–62 | 3000–5800/mcL | $3000–5800 \times 10^6$/L |
| Lymphocytes | 20.5–51.1 | $1.2–3.4 \times 10^3$/mcL | $1.2–3.4 \times 10^9$/L |
| Monocytes | 1.7–9.3 | $0.11–0.59 \times 10^3$/mcL | $0.11–0.59 \times 10^9$/L |
| Granulocytes | 42.2–75.2 | $1.4–6.5 \times 10^3$/mcL | $1.4–6.5 \times 10^9$/L |
| Eosinophils | | $0–0.7 \times 10^3$/mcL | $0–0.7 \times 10^9$/L |
| Basophils | | $0–0.2 \times 10^3$/mcL | $0–0.2 \times 10^9$/L |
| Platelets | 130–400 | $\times 10^3$/mcL | $130–400 \times 10^9$/L |
| Reticulocytes | 0.5–1.5% RBCs | | 0.005–0.015 of RBCs |
| | 24,000–84,000/mcL | | $24–84 \times 10^9$/L |
| Cells, CSF | 0–10 leukocytes/mm³ 0 RBC/mm³ | | 0–10 leukocytes/mm³ 0 RBC/mm³ |

* Test values dependent on laboratory methods used.

| Tests | Conventional Units | SI Units |
|---|---|---|
| **Chloride** | | |
| Serum or plasma (Hep) | 98–107 mmol/L | 98–107 mmol/L |
| Sweat | | |
| Normal | 5–35 mmol/L | 5–35 mmol/L |
| Cystic fibrosis | 60–200 mmol/L | 60–200 mmol/L |
| Urine, 24 h (vary greatly with Cl intake) | | |
| Infant | 2–10 mmol/24 h | 2–10 mmol/24 h |
| Child | 15–40 mmol/24 h | 15–40 mmol/24 h |
| Adult | 110–250 mmol/24 h | 110–250 mmol/24 h |
| **Cholesterol, serum** | | |
| Adult desirable | <200 mg/dL | <5.2 mmol/L |
| borderline | 200–239 mg/dL | 5.2–6.2 mmol/L |
| high-risk | ≥240 mg/dL | ≥6.2 mmol/L |
| **Coagulation tests** | 80–120% of normal | 0.8–1.2 of normal |
| Antithrombin III (synthetic substrate) | | |
| Bleeding time (Duke) | 0–6 min | 0–6 min |
| Bleeding time (Ivy) | 1–6 min | 1–6 min |
| Bleeding time (template) | 2.3–9.5 min | 2.3–9.5 min |
| Clot retraction, qualitative | 50–100% in 2 h | 0.5–1.0/2 h |
| Coagulation time (Lee-White) | 5–15 min (glass tubes) | 5–15 min (glass tubes) |
| | 19–60 min (siliconized tubes) | 19–60 min (siliconized tubes) |
| Cold hemolysin test (Donath-Landsteiner) | No hemolysis | No hemolysis |
| **Complement components** | 75–160 U/mL | 75–160 kU/L |
| Total hemolytic complement activity, plasma (EDTA) | | |
| Total complement decay rate (functional), plasma (EDTA) | 10–20% | Fraction decay rate: 0.10–0.20 |
| | Deficiency: >50% | >0.50 |
| C1q, serum | 14.9–22.1 mg/dL | 149–221 mg/L |
| C1r, serum | 2.5–10.0 mg/dL | 25–100 mg/L |
| C1s (C1 esterase), serum | 5.0–10.0 mg/dL | 50–100 mg/L |
| C2, serum | 1.6–3.6 mg/dL | 16–36 mg/L |
| C3, serum | 90–180 mg/dL | 0.9–1.8 g/L |
| C4, serum | 10–40 mg/dL | 0.1–0.4 g/L |
| C5, serum | 5.5–11.3 mg/dL | 55–113 mg/L |
| C6, serum | 17.9–23.9 mg/dL | 179–239 mg/L |
| C7, serum | 2.7–7.4 mg/dL | 27–74 mg/L |
| C8, serum | 4.9–10.6 mg/dL | 49–106 mg/L |
| C9, serum | 3.3–9.5 mg/dL | 33–95 mg/L |
| **Corpuscular values of erythrocytes** (values are for adults; in children, values vary with age) | | |
| Mean corpuscular hemoglobin (MCH) | 27–31 pg | 0.42–0.48 fmol |
| Mean corpuscular hemoglobin concentration (MCHC) | 33–37 g/dL | 330–370 g/L |
| Mean corpuscular volume (MCV) | Male 80–94 mcm$^3$ | 80–94 fL |
| | Female 81–99 mcm$^3$ | 81–99 fL |
| *[†]Creatine kinase (CK), serum | | |
| Male | 15–105 U/L (30°C) | 0.26–1.79 mckat/L (30°C) |
| Female | 10–80 U/L (30°C) | 0.17–1.36 mckat/L (30°C) |
| Note: Strenuous exercise or intramuscular injections may elevate transient CK levels. | | |

* Test values dependent on laboratory methods.
[†] Test values dependent on patient's race.

| Tests | Conventional Units | SI Units |
|---|---|---|
| Ethanol (alcohol), whole blood (Ox) or serum | | |
|   Depression of CNS | >100 mg/dL | >21.7 mmol/L |
|   Fatalities reported | >400 mg/dL | >86.8 mmol/L |
| α-Fetoprotein (AFP), serum | <15 ng/mL | <15 mcg/L |
| ††Fat, fecal, F, 72 h | | |
|   Infant, breast-fed | <1 g/d | |
|   Pediatrics (0–6 y) | <2 g/d | |
|   Adult | <7 g/d | |
|   Adult (fat-free diet) | <4 g/d | |
| §Fatty acids, total, serum | 190–240 mg/dL | 7–15 mmol/L |
|   Nonesterified, serum | 8–25 mg/dL | 0.28–0.89 mmol/L |
| Ferritin, serum | 20–150 ng/mL | 20–250 mcg/L |
|   Male | | |
|   Female | 10–120 ng/mL | 10–120 mcg/L |
|   Ferritin values of <20 ng/mL (20 mcg/L) have been reported to be generally associated with depleted iron stores. | | |
| Fluoride | | |
|   Plasma (Hep) | 0.01–0.2 mcg/mL | 0.5–10.5 mcmol/L |
|   Urine | 0.2–3.2 mcg/mL | 10.5–168 mcmol/L |
|   Urine, occupational exposure | <8 mcg/mL | <421 mcmol/L |
| Glucose (fasting) | | |
|   Blood | 65–95 mg/dL | 3.5–5.3 mmol/L |
|   Plasma or serum | 74–106 mg/dL | 4.1–5.9 mmol/L |
|   Glucose, 2 h postprandial, serum | <120 mg/dL | <6.7 mmol/L |
| Glucose, urine | | |
|   Quantitative | <500 mg/24 h | <2.8 mmol/24 h |
|   Qualitative | Negative | Negative |
| Glucose, CSF | 40–70 mg/dL | 2.2–3.9 mmol/L |
| Glycated hemoglobin (Hemoglobin A1c), whole blood (EDTA) | 4.2%–5.9% | 0.042–0.059 |
| HDL-lipid panel | | |
|   Cholesterol, HDL | >40 mg/dL | |
|   Cholesterol, LDL (calculated) | | |
|     optimal | <100 mg/dL | |
|     near optimal | 100–129 mg/dL | |
|     borderline high | 130–159 mg/dL | |
|     high | >160 mg/dL | |
|   Cholesterol, total | | |
|     0–1 year | 50–120 mg/dL | |
|     1–2 years | 70–190 mg/dL | |
|     2–16 years | 120–220 mg/dL | |
|     >16 years | 0–199 mg/dL | |
|     desirable | <200 mg/dL | |
|     borderline | 200–239 mg/dL | |
|     high | >240 mg/dL | |

*(continued)*

†† Reference values vary from laboratory to laboratory, but are generally found within the range of 5–7 g/d. It should be noted that children, especially infants, cannot ingest the 100 g/d of fat that is suggested for the test. Therefore, a fat retention coefficient is determined by measuring the difference between ingested fat and fecal fat, and expressing that difference as a percentage. The figure, called the fat retention coefficient, is 95% or greater in healthy children and adults. A low value indicates steatorrhea. http://www.labcorp.com/datasets/labcorp/html/chapter/mono/sc008000.htm

§ "Fatty acids" include a mixture of different aliphatic acids of varying molecular weight; a mean molecular weight of 284 D has been assumed.

| Tests | Conventional Units | SI Units |
|---|---|---|
| HDL-lipid panel *(continued from previous page)* | | |
| ¶Tryglycerides | | |
|    desirable | <150 mg/dL | |
|    borderline high | 150–199 mg/dL | |
|    high | >200 mg/dL | |
| Hematocrit | | |
|    Males | 42–52% | 0.42–0.52 |
|    Females | 37–47% | 0.37–0.47 |
|    Newborn | 53–65% | 0.53–0.65 |
|    Children (varies with age) | 30–43% | 0.30–0.43 |
| Hemoglobin (Hb) | | |
|    Males | 14.0–18.0 g/dL | 2.17–2.79 mmol/L |
|    Females | 12.0–16.0 g/dL | 1.86–2.48 mmol/L |
|    Newborn | 17.0–23.0 g/dL | 2.64–3.57 mmol/L |
|    Children (varies with age) | 11.2–16.5 g/dL | 1.74–2.56 mmol/L |
| Hemoglobin, fetal | ≥1 y old: <2% of total Hb | ≥1 y old: <0.02% of total Hb |
| Hemoglobin, plasma | <3 mg/dL | <0.47 mcmol/L |
| Immunoglobulins, serum | | |
|    IgG | 700–1600 mg/dL | 7–16 g/L |
|    IgA | 70–400 mg/dL | 0.7–4.0 g/L |
|    IgM | 40–230 mg/dL | 0.4–2.3 g/L |
|    IgD | 0–8 mg/dL | 0–80 mg/L |
|    IgE | 3–423 IU/mL | 3–423 kIU/L |
| Immunoglobulin G (IgC), CSF | 0.5–6.1 mg/dL | 0.5–6.1 g/L |
| Insulin, plasma (fasting) | 2–25 mcU/mL | 13–174 pmol/L |
| *Iron, serum | | |
|    Males | 65–175 mcg/dL | 11.6–31.3 mcmol/L |
|    Females | 50–170 mcg/dL | 9.0–30.4 mcmol/L |
| Iron binding capacity, serum, total (TIBC) | 250–425 mcg/dL | 44.8–71.6 mcmol/L |
| Iron saturation, serum | | |
|    Male | 20–50% | 0.2–0.5 |
|    Female | 15–50% | 0.15–0.5 |
| LDL-cholesterol (LDL-C), serum or plasma (EDTA) | | |
|    Adult desirable | <130 mg/dL | <.2 mmol/L |
|    borderline | 130–159 mg/dL | 3.37–4.12 mmol/L |
|    high risk | ≥160 mg/dL | ≥4.13 mmol/L |
| Lead, | | |
|    Whole blood (Hep) | <25 mcg/dL | <0.48 mcmol/L |
|    Urine, 24 h | <80 mcg/d | <0.39 mcmol/d |
| Lidocaine, serum or plasma (Hep or EDTA); 45 min after bolus dose | | |
| Therapeutic | 1.5–6.0 mcg/mL | 6.4–26 mcmol/L |
| Toxic | | |
|    CNS, cardiovascular depression | 6–8 mcg/mL | 26–34.2 mcmol/L |
|    Seizures, obtundation, decreased cardiac output | >8 mcg/mL >34.2 mcmol/L | |
| *Lipase, serum | 23–300 U/L (37°C) | 0.39–5.1 mckat/L (37°C) |

¶ If the triglyceride value is >400 mg/dL, the LDL calculation is invalid. http://webserver01.bjc.org/slch/pro/Professional.htm? http://webserver01.bjc.org/labtestguide/Lab%20Test%20Guidebook/slchlabsiteonline.htm.
* Test values dependent on laboratory methods used.

| Tests | Conventional Units | SI Units |
|---|---|---|
| Magnesium | | |
|   Serum | 1.3–2.1 mEq/L | 0.65–1.07 mmol/L |
| | 1.6–2.6 mg/dL | 16–26 mg/L |
|   Urine | 6.0–10.0 mEq/24 h | 3.0–5.0 mmol/24 h |
| Mercury | | |
|   Whole blood (EDTA) | 0.6–59 mcg/L | <0.29 mcmol/L |
|   Urine, 24 h | <20 mcg/d | <0.1 mcmol/d |
|   Toxic | >150 mcg/d | >0.75 mcmol/d |
| Methemoglobin | 0.06–0.24 g/dL or | 9.3–37.2 mcmol/L or |
|       (hemoglobin), whole blood | 0.78 ± 0.37% of total Hb (SD) | mass fraction of total Hb: |
|       (EDTA, Hep or ACD) | | 0.008 ± 0.0037 (SD) |
| Occult blood, feces, random | Negative (<2 mL blood/150 g stool/d) | Negative (<13.3 mL blood/kg stool/d) |
|   Qualitative, urine, random | Negative | Negative |
| Osmolality | | |
|   Serum | 275–295 mOsm/kg serum water | 275–295 mmol/kg serum water |
|   Urine | 50–1200 mOsm/kg water | 50–1200 mmol/kg water |
|   Ratio, urine:serum | 1.0–3.0 | 1.0–3.0 |
| | 3.0–4.7 after 12 h fluid restriction | 3.0–4.7 after 12 h fluid restriction |
| Osmotic fragility of erythrocytes | Begins in 0.45–0.39% NaCl | Begins in 77–67 mmol/L NaCl |
| | Complete in 0.33–0.30% NaCl | Complete in 56–51 mmol/L NaCl |
| Oxygen, blood | | |
|   Capacity | 16–24 vol% (varies with hemoglobin) | 7.14–10.7 mmol/L (varies with hemoglobin) |
|   Content | | |
|     Arterial | 15–23 vol% | 6.69–10.3 mmo |
|     Venous | 10–16 vol% | 4.46–7.14 mmol/L |
|   Saturation | | |
|     Arterial and capillary | 95–98% of capacity | 0.95–0.98 of capacity |
|     Venous | 60–85% of capacity | 0.60–0.85 of capacity |
|   Tension | | |
|     $pO_2$ arterial and capillary | 83–108 mmHg | 11.1–14.4 kPa |
|     Venous | 35–45 mmHg | 4.6–6.0 kPa |
| P50, blood | 25–29 mmHg (adjusted to pH 7.4) | 3.33–3.86 kPa |
| Partial thromboplastin time activated (APTT) | <35 sec | <35 sec |
| *Phosphatase, acid, prostatic, serum radioimmunoassay | <3.0 ng/mL | <3.0 mcg/L |
| *Phosphatase, alkaline, total, serum | 38–126 U/L (37°C) | 0.65–2.14 mckat/L |
| Phosphate, inorganic, serum | | |
|   Adults | 2.7–4.5 mg/dL | 0.87–1.45 mmol/L |
|   Children | 4.5–5.5 mg/dL | 1.45–1.78 mmol/L |
| Phospholipids, serum | 125–275 mg/dL | 1.25–2.75 g/L |
| Phosphorus, urine | 0.4–1.3 g/24 h | 12.9–42 mmol/24 h |
| Potassium, plasma (Hep) | | |
|   Males | 3.5–4.5 mEq/L | 3.5–4.5 mmol/L |
|   Females | 3.4–4.4 mEq/L | 3.4–4.4 mmol/L |

(continued)

*Test values dependent on laboratory methods used.

| Tests | Conventional Units | SI Units |
|---|---|---|
| Potassium | | |
|   Serum | | |
|     Premature | | |
|       Cord | 5.0–10.2 mEq/L | 5.0–10.2 mmol/L |
|       48 h | 3.0–6.0 mEq/L | 3.0–6.0 mmol/L |
|     Newborn, cord | 5.6–12.0 mEq/L | 5.6–12.0 mmol/L |
|     Newborn | 3.7–5.9 mEq/L | 3.7–5.9 mmol/L |
|     Infant | 4.1–5.3 mEq/L | 4.1–5.3 mmol/L |
|     Child | 3.4–4.7 mEq/L | 3.4–4.7 mmol/L |
|     Adult | 3.5–5.1 mEq/L | 3.5–5.1 mmol/L |
|   Urine, 24 h | 25–125 mEq/d, varies with diet | 25–125 mmol/d; varies with diet |
|   CSF | 70% of plasma level or 2.5–3.2 mEq/L; rises with plasma hyperosmolality | 0.70 of plasma level or 2.5–3.2 mmol/L; rises with plasma hyperosmolality |
| *Prostate-specific antigen (PSA), serum | | |
|   Male | <4.0 ng/mL | <4.0 mcg/L |
| *Protein, serum | | |
|   Total | 6.4–8.3 g/dL | 64–83 g/L |
|   Albumin | 3.9–5.1 g/dL | 39–51 g/L |
|   Globulin | | |
|     $\alpha^1$ | 0.2–0.4 g/dL | 2–4 g/L |
|     $\alpha^2$ | 0.4–0.8 g/dL | 4–8 g/L |
|     $\beta$ | 0.5–1.0 g/dL | 5–10 g/L |
|     $\gamma$ | 0.6–1.3 g/dL | 6–13 g/L |
|   Urine | | |
|     Qualitative | Negative | Negative |
|     Quantitative | 50–80 mg/24 h (at rest) | Same |
|   CSF, total | 8–32 mg/dL | 80–320 mg/dL |
| †Sedimentation rate, erythrocyte | | |
|   Westergren | | |
|       Male: 0–50 y | 0–15 mm/h | |
|       Male: >50 y | 0–20 mm/h | |
|       Female: 0–50 y | 0–20 mm/h | |
|       Female: >50 y | 0–30 mm/h | |
|   Wintrobe | | |
|       Males | <10 mm/h | |
|       Females | <20 mm/h | |
|       Critical value | >75 mm/h | |
| Sodium | | |
|   Serum or plasma (Hep) | | |
|     Premature | | |
|       Cord | 116–140 mEq/L | 116–140 mmol/L |
|       48 h | 128–148 mEq/L | 128–148 mmol/L |
|     Newborn, cord | 126–166 mEq/L | 126–166 mmol/L |
|     Newborn | 133–146 mEq/L | 133–146 mmol/L |
|     Infant | 139–146 mEq/L | 139–146 mmol/L |
|     Child | 138–145 mEq/L | 138–145 mmol/L |
|     Adult | 136–145 mEq/L | 136–145 mmol/L |
|   Urine, 24 h | 40–220 mEq/d (diet dependent) | 40–220 mmol/d (diet dependent) |
|   Sweat | | |
|     Normal | 10–40 mEq/L | 10–40 mmol/L |
|     Cystic fibrosis | 70–190 mEq/L | 70–190 mmol/L |
| Specific gravity, urine | 1.002–1.030 | 1.002–1.030 |

*(continued)*

*Test values dependent on laboratory methods used.
†http://www.labcorp.com/datasets/labcorp/html/chapter/mono/he005000.htm

| Tests | Conventional Units | SI Units |
|-------|-------------------|----------|
| *Thyroid-stimulating hormone (TSH), serum | 0.4–4.2 mcU/mL | 0.4–4.2 mU/L |
| Thyroxine serum | 5–12 mcg/dL (varies with age, higher in children and pregnant women) | 65–155 nmol/L (varies with age, higher in children and pregnant women) |
| *Thyroxine, free, serum | 0.8–2.7 ng/dL | 10.3–35 pmol/L |
| Thyroxine binding globulin (TBG), serum | 1.2–3.0 mg/dL | 12–30 mg/L |
| Triglycerides, serum, fasting<br>Desirable<br>Borderline high<br>Hypertriglyceridemia | <250 mg/dL<br>250–500 mg/dL<br>>500 mg/dL | <2.83 mmol/L<br>2.83–5.67 mmol/L<br>>5.65 mmol/L |
| Urea nitrogen, serum | 6–20 mg/dL | 2.1–7.1 mmol urea/L |
| Urea nitrogen:creatinine ratio, serum | 12:1 to 20:1 | 48–80 urea:creatinine mole ratio |
| *Uric acid<br>Serum, enzymatic<br>Male<br>Female<br>Child<br>Urine | <br><br>4.5–8.0 mg/dL<br>2.5–6.2 mg/dL<br>2.0–5.5 mg/dL<br>250–750 mg/24 h (with normal diet) | <br><br>0.27–0.47 mmol/L<br>0.15–0.37 mmol/L<br>0.12–0.32 mmol/L<br>1.48–4.43 mmol/24 h (with normal diet) |
| Viscosity, serum | 1.00–1.24 cP | 1.00–1.24 cP |
| Vitamin A, serum | 30–80 mcg/dL | 1.05–2.8 mcmol/L |
| Vitamin B12, serum | 110–800 pg/mL | 81–590 pmol/L |
| Vitamin E, serum<br>Normal<br>Therapeutic | <br>5–18 mcg/mL<br>30–50 mcg/mL | <br>12–42 mcmol/L<br>69.6–116 mcmol/L |
| Zinc, serum | 70–120 mcg/dL | 10.7–18.4 mcmol/L |

*Test values dependent on laboratory methods used.

# Classifications of Periodontal Diseases and Conditions

## I. Gingival Diseases

A. Dental plaque-induced gingival diseases*

   1. Gingivitis associated with dental plaque only
     a. Without other local contributing factors
     b. With local contributing factors

   2. Gingival diseases modified by systemic factors
     a. Associated with the endocrine system
       1) Puberty-associated gingivitis
       2) Menstrual cycle-associated gingivitis
       3) Pregnancy-associated
         a) Gingivitis
         b) Pyogenic granuloma
       4) Diabetes mellitus-associated gingivitis
     b. Associated with blood dyscrasias
       1) Leukemia-associated gingivitis
       2) Other

   3. Gingival diseases modified by medications
     a. Drug-influenced gingival diseases
       1) Drug-influenced gingival enlargements
       2) Drug-influenced gingivitis
         a) Oral contraceptive associated gingivitis
         b) Other

   4. Gingival diseases modified by malnutrition
     a. Ascorbic acid-deficiency gingivitis
     b. Other

B. Non-plaque-induced gingival lesions

   1. Gingival diseases of specific bacterial origin
     a. *Neisseria gonorrhea*-associated lesions
     b. *Treponema palladium*-associated lesions
     c. Streptococcal species-associated lesions
     d. Other

   2. Gingival diseases of viral origin
     a. Herpesvirus infections
       1) Primary herpetic gingivostomatitis
       2) Recurrent oral herpes
       3) Varicella zoster infections
     b. Other

   3. Gingival diseases of fungal origin
     a. *Candida*-species infections
       1) Generalized gingival candidosis
     b. Linear gingival erythema
     c. Histoplasmosis
     d. Other

   4. Gingival lesions of genetic origin
     a. Hereditary gingival fibromatosis
     b. Other

   5. Gingival manifestations of systemic conditions
     a. Mucocutaneous disorders
       1) Lichen planus
       2) Pemphigoid
       3) Pemphigus vulgaris
       4) Erythema multiforme
       5) Lupus erythematosus
       6) Drug-induced
       7) Other

b. Allergic reactions
  1) Dental restorative materials
    a) Mercury
    b) Nickel
    c) Acrylic
    d) Other
  2) Reactions attributable to
    a) Toothpastes/ dentifrices
    b) Mouthrinses/ mouthwashes
    c) Chewing gum additives
    d) Foods and additives
  3) Other

6. Traumatic lesions (factitious, iatrogenic, accidental)
  a. Chemical injury
  b. Physical injury
  c. Thermal injury

7. Foreign body reactions

8. Not otherwise specified (NOS)

## II. Chronic Periodontitis**

A. Localized
B. Generalized

## III. Aggressive Periodontitis**

A. Localized
B. Generalized

## IV. Periodontitis as a Manifestation of Systemic Diseases

A. Associated with hematological disorders
  1. Acquired neutropenia
  2. Leukemias
  3. Other

B. Associated with genetic disorders
  1. Familial and cyclic neutropenia
  2. Down syndrome
  3. Leukocyte adhesion deficiency syndromes
  4. Papillon-Lefèvre syndrome
  5. Chediak-Higashi syndrome
  6. Histiocytosis syndromes
  7. Glycogen storage disease
  8. Infantile genetic agranulocytosis
  9. Cohen syndrome
  10. Ehlers-Danlos syndrome (Types IV and VIII)
  11. Hypophosphatasia
  12. Other

C. Not otherwise specified (NOS)

## V. Necrotizing Periodontal Diseases

A. Necrotizing ulcerative gingivitis (NUG)
B. Necrotizing ulcerative periodontitis (NUP)

## VI. Abscesses of the Periodontium

A. Gingival abscess
B. Periodontal abscess
C. Pericoronal abscess

## VII. Periodontitis Associated with Endodontic Lesions

A. Combined periodontic-endodontic lesions

## VIII. Developmental or Acquired Deformities and Conditions

A. Localized tooth-related factor that modify or predispose to plaqueinduced gingival diseases or periodontitis
  1. Tooth anatomic factors
  2. Dental restorations/ appliances
  3. Root fractures
  4. Cervical root resorption and cemental tears

B. Mucogingival deformities and conditions around teeth
  1. Gingival/soft tissue recession
    a. Facial or lingual surfaces
    b. Interproximal (papillary)
  2. Lack of keratinized gingiva
  3. Decreased vestibular depth
  4. Aberrant frenum/muscle position
  5. Gingival excess
    a. Pseudopocket
    b. Inconsistent gingival margin
    c. Excessive gingival display
    d. Gingival enlargement
  6. Abnormal color

C. Mucogingival deformities and conditions on edentulous ridges
   1. Vertical and/or horizontal ridge deficiency
   2. Lack of gingiva/keratinized tissue
   3. Gingival/soft tissue enlargement
   4. Aberrant frenum/muscle position
   5. Decreased vestibular depth
   6. Abnormal color

D. Occlusal trauma
   1. Primary occlusal trauma
   2. Secondary occlusal trauma

---

*Can occur on a periodontium with no attachment loss or on a periodontium with attachment loss that is not progressing.
** Can be further classified on the basis of extent and severity.

From 1999 International Workshop for a Classification of Periodontal Diseases and Conditions. Papers. Oak Brook, Illinois, October 30–November 2, 1999. *Ann Periodontol.* 1999; 4(1): 2–3.

# Caries Classification

| Classification Location | Appearance | Method of Examination |
|---|---|---|
| **Class I**<br>Cavities in pits of fissures<br>• Occlusal surfaces of premolars and molars<br>• Buccal and lingual surfaces of molars (pit and fissure)<br>• Lingual surfaces of maxillary incisors | | Direct or indirect visual<br>Exploration<br>Radiographs are not diagnostic |
| **Class II**<br>Cavities in proximal surfaces of premolars and molars | | Early caries: by radiograph only<br>Moderate caries not broken through from proximal to occlusal:<br>• Visual by color changes in tooth and loss of translucency<br>• Exploration from proximal<br>Extensive caries involving occlusal: direct visual |
| **Class III**<br>Cavities in proximal surfaces of incisors and canines that do not involve the incisal angle | | Early caries: by radiograph or transillumination<br>Moderate caries not broken through to lingual or facial:<br>• Visual by tooth color change<br>• Exploration<br>• Radiograph<br>Extensive caries: direct visual |
| **Class IV**<br>Cavities in proximal surfaces of incisors or canines that involve the incisal angle | | Visual<br>Transillumination |
| **Class V**<br>Cavities in the cervical 1/3 of facial or lingual surfaces (not pit or fissure) | | Direct visual: dry surface for vision<br>Exploration to distinguish demineralization: whether rough or hard and unbroken<br>Areas may be sensitive to touch |
| **Class VI**<br>Cavities on incisal edges of anterior teeth and cusp tips of posterior teeth | | Direct visual<br>May be discolored |

Adapted from Wilkins EM. *Clinical Practice of the Dental Hygienist*, 9th ed. Baltimore: Lippincott Williams & Wilkins, 2005.

# Classifications of Furcation Involvement

Furcation involvement should be recorded on a periodontal chart using a scale that quantifies the severity (or extent) of the furcation invasion. Below is a common furcation-rating scale, including charting symbols.

| Class | Description | Symbol |
|---|---|---|
| **Class I**<br><br>JE<br>bone level | The concavity—just above the furcation entrance—on the root trunk can be felt with the probe tip; however, the furcation probe cannot enter the furcation area. | ∧ |
| **Class II**<br><br>JE<br>bone level<br>facial view | The probe is able to partially enter the furcation—extending approximately one third of the width of the tooth—but it is not able to pass completely through the furcation. | △ |
| **Class III**<br><br>bone level<br>facial view | In *mandibular molars,* the probe passes completely through the furcation between the mesial and distal roots.<br>In *maxillary molars,* the probe passes between the mesiobuccal and distobuccal roots and touches the palatal root. | ▲ |
| **Class IV**<br><br>JE<br>bone level<br>facial view | Same as a class III furcation involvement except that the entrance to the furcation is visible clinically owing to tissue recession. | ◆ |

## Documenting Furcation Involvement

On this sample periodontal chart, all four classes of furcation involvement are represented. Tooth 2 has a class IV furcation involvement on the facial aspect. Tooth 3 has a class I furcation involvement on the facial aspect between the mesiobuccal and distobuccal roots. On the lingual aspect, tooth 2 has a class III furcation involvement between the distobuccal and palatal roots and a class II furcation involvement between the mesiobuccal and palatal roots.

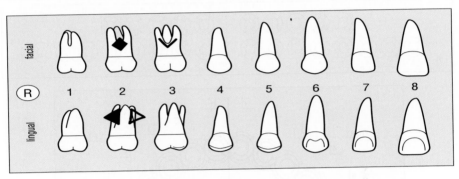

Adapted from Wilkins EM. *Clinical Practice of the Dental Hygienist,* 9th ed. Baltimore: Lippincott Williams & Wilkins, 2005.

# Dental & Periodontal Charting

## Geometric Charting

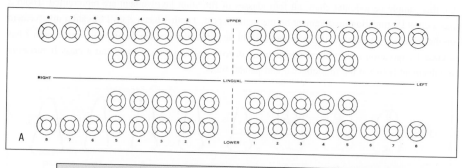

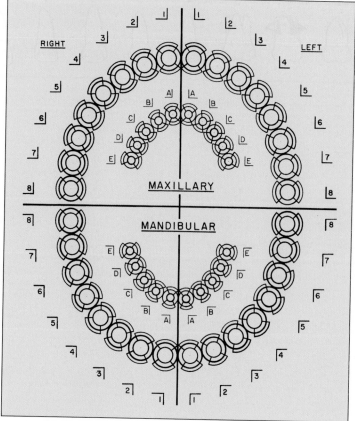

(A) Linear format with primary teeth between the permanent teeth. (B) Permanent teeth in arch format with primary teeth inside.

In this example, teeth are numbered according to the Palmer system (by quadrant, either 1–8 or A–E). Each tooth includes two circles. The inner circle represents the occlusal surface, and the outer circle, divided into four parts, represents the mesial, facial, distal, and lingual.

From Wilkins EM. *Clinical Practice of the Dental Hygienist,* 9th ed. Baltimore: Lippincott Williams & Wilkins, 2005.

# Combined dental and periodontal charting

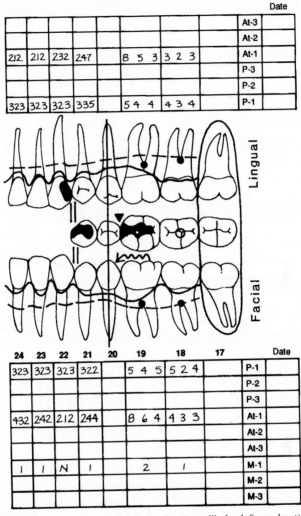

| | | | | | | | | | Date | |
|---|---|---|---|---|---|---|---|---|---|---|
| | | | | | | | | At-3 | |
| | | | | | | | | At-2 | |
| 212 | 212 | 232 | 247 | | 8 5 3 | 3 2 3 | | At-1 | |
| | | | | | | | | P-3 | |
| | | | | | | | | P-2 | |
| 323 | 323 | 323 | 335 | | 5 4 4 | 4 3 4 | | P-1 | |

Lingual

Facial

| 24 | 23 | 22 | 21 | 20 | 19 | 18 | 17 | Date | |
|---|---|---|---|---|---|---|---|---|---|
| 323 | 323 | 323 | 322 | | 5 4 5 | 5 2 4 | | P-1 | |
| | | | | | | | | P-2 | |
| | | | | | | | | P-3 | |
| 432 | 242 | 212 | 244 | | 8 6 4 | 4 3 3 | | At-1 | |
| | | | | | | | | At-2 | |
| | | | | | | | | At-3 | |
| I | I | N | I | | 2 | I | | M-1 | |
| | | | | | | | | M-2 | |
| | | | | | | | | M-3 | |

Section of a combined dental and periodontal charting (mandibular left quadrant). In this example, teeth are numbered according to the Universal (or ADA) system. Dental caries and restorations are marked on the anatomic crowns and/or roots. The gingival margin is clearly drawn to show areas of recession. Boxes at the apices of each tooth provide spaces for probing depths and clinical attachment level recordings, as well as for mobility notations.

From Wilkins EM. *Clinical Practice of the Dental Hygienist*, 9th ed. Baltimore: Lippincott Williams & Wilkins, 2005.

# Periodontal charting

| 1 | 2 | 3 | 4 | 5 | 6 | 7 | 8 | 9 | 10 | 11 | 12 | 13 | 14 | 15 | 16 | Maxilla |
|---|---|---|---|---|---|---|---|---|----|----|----|----|----|----|----|---------|
|  |  |  |  |  | I | I |  |  |  |  |  | I |  |  | I | Mobility (I, II, III) |
| + | + |  | + | + | + | + |  |  | + | + | + | + | + | + | + | Bleeding/Purulence (+) |
|  |  |  |  |  |  |  |  |  |  |  |  |  |  |  |  | Attachment Level (CEJ to BP) |
| 646 | 635 |  | 325 | 536 | 525 | 435 | 433 | 334 | 425 | 435 | 536 | 626 | 638 | 846 | 746 | Probing Depth (FGM to BP) |
|  |  |  |  |  |  |  |  |  |  |  |  |  |  |  |  | Facial |
|  |  |  |  |  |  |  |  |  |  |  |  |  |  |  |  | Palatal |
| + | + |  | + | + | + | + | + | + | + | + | + | + | + | + | + | Bleeding/Purulence (+) |
|  |  |  |  |  |  |  |  |  |  |  |  |  |  |  |  | Attachment Level (CEJ to BP) |
| 636 | 525 |  | 335 | 526 | 536 | 425 | 443 | 324 | 424 | 525 | 535 | 626 | 627 | 827 | 736 | Probing Depth (FGM to BP) |
|  |  |  |  |  |  |  |  |  |  |  |  |  |  |  |  | F/P Plaque |
|  | ✓ |  | ✓ | ✓ |  |  |  | ✓ | ✓ |  |  |  | ✓ | ✓ | ✓ | Supragingival Calculus |
| ✓ | ✓ |  | ✓ | ✓ | ✓ | ✓ | ✓ | ✓ | ✓ | ✓ | ✓ | ✓ | ✓ | ✓ | ✓ | Subgingival Calculus |
|  |  |  | 4 |  |  |  | 3 |  |  |  |  | 4 |  |  |  | PSR Code |

Right / Left

| 32 | 31 | 30 | 29 | 28 | 27 | 26 | 25 | 24 | 23 | 22 | 21 | 20 | 19 | 18 | 17 | Mandible |
|----|----|----|----|----|----|----|----|----|----|----|----|----|----|----|----|----------|
|  |  |  |  |  | I |  | I | I |  |  |  |  |  |  |  | Mobility (I, II, III) |
| + |  | + | + | + | + |  | + |  |  | + | + | + |  | + | + | Bleeding/Purulence (+) |
|  |  |  |  |  |  |  |  |  |  |  |  |  |  |  |  | Attachment Level (CEJ to BP) |
| 546 | 736 | 626 | 635 | 535 | 534 | 324 | 423 | 323 | 324 | 324 | 434 | 435 | 536 | 746 | 635 | Probing Depth (FGM to BP) |
|  |  |  |  |  |  |  |  |  |  |  |  |  |  |  |  | Lingual |
|  |  |  |  |  |  |  |  |  |  |  |  |  |  |  |  | Facial |
| + | + | + | + | + |  | + | + | + |  | + |  | + |  | + | + | Bleeding/Purulence (+) |
|  |  |  |  |  |  |  |  |  |  |  |  |  |  |  |  | Attachment Level (CEJ to BP) |
| 546 | 736 | 625 | 535 | 635 | 534 | 324 | 423 | 323 | 324 | 324 | 434 | 435 | 526 | 736 | 625 | Probing Depth (FGM to BP) |
|  |  |  |  |  |  |  |  |  |  |  |  |  |  |  |  | L/F Plaque |
|  |  |  |  | ✓ | ✓ | ✓ | ✓ | ✓ |  |  | ✓ | ✓ |  |  |  | Supragingival Calculus |
| ✓ | ✓ | ✓ | ✓ | ✓ | ✓ | ✓ | ✓ | ✓ | ✓ | ✓ | ✓ | ✓ | ✓ | ✓ | ✓ | Subgingival Calculus |
|  |  |  | 4 |  |  |  | 3 |  |  |  |  | 4 |  |  |  | PSR Code |

In this example, teeth are numbered according to the Universal (or ADA) system.

From Nield-Gehrig JS, Willmann DE. *Foundations of Periodontics for the Dental Hygienist.* Baltimore: Lippincott Williams & Wilkins, 2003.

# Documenting Gingival Margin Level

Most periodontal charts include rows of boxes that are used to record the gingival margin level on the facial and lingual aspects of teeth. Customarily, the following notations indicate the gingival margin level on a periodontal chart:

- A zero (0) indicates that the gingiva is at the cemento-enamel junction (CEJ; normal level of gingival margin)
- A negative ( − ) number indicates that the gingiva significantly covers the CEJ
- A positive ( + ) number indicates gingival recession

## SAMPLE PERIODONTAL CHART WITH GINGIVAL MARGIN LEVELS

On the sample periodontal chart shown below, the gingival margin level is charted in the row of boxes labeled "GM to CEJ"–gingival margin to cemento-enamel junction. In addition, the level of the gingival margin may be drawn across the teeth on a periodontal chart.

In this example chart, the level of the gingival margin is significantly coronal to the CEJ on teeth 22, 23 and 24. The gingival margin level is normal for teeth 20 and 21. Recession is present on teeth 18 and 19.

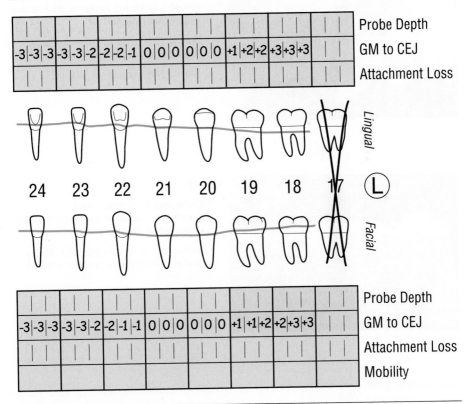

Adapted from Nield-Gehrig JS. *Fundamentals of Periodontal Instrumentation & Advanced Root Instrumentation,* 5th ed. Baltimore: Lippincott Williams & Wilkins, 2004.

# Periodontal Screening and Recording (PSR) System

## Criteria for Assigning PSR Codes

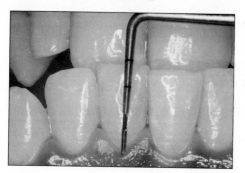

### Code 0

- Color-coded reference mark is completely visible in the deepest sulcus or pocket of the sextant.

- No calculus or defective margins on restorations are present.

- Gingival tissues are healthy with no bleeding evident on gentle probing.

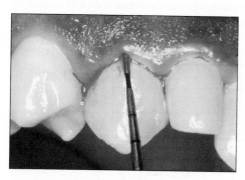

### Code 1

- Color-coded reference mark is completely visible in the deepest sulcus or pocket of the sextant.

- No calculus or defective margins on restorations are present.

- Bleeding IS present on probing.

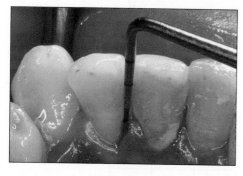

### Code 2

- Color-coded reference mark is completely visible in the deepest sulcus or pocket of the sextant.

- Supragingival or subgingival calculus and/or defective margins are detected.

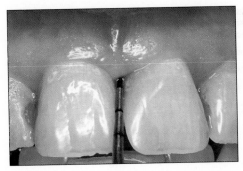

### Code 3

- Color-coded reference mark is partially visible in the deepest sulcus or pocket of the sextant.

- This code indicates a probing depth between 3.5 and 5.5 mm.

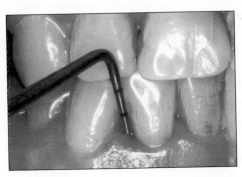

### Code 4

- Color-coded reference mark is not visible in the deepest sulcus or pocket in the sextant.

- This code indicates a probing depth of greater than 5.5 mm.

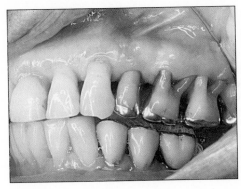

### Code *

The * symbol is added to the code of a sextant exhibiting any of the following abnormalities:

- furcation involvement

- mobility

- mucogingival problems

- recession extending into the colored area of the probe

Pictured here is an example of a sextant that has teeth with furcation involvement. Therefore, the symbol should be recorded next to the sextant code.

| Implications of PSR Codes | |
|---|---|
| Code | Further Clinical Documentation |
| Code 0, 1, or 2 in all sextants | No further documentation needed |
| Code 3 in one sextant | Comprehensive periodontal assessment of sextant with 3 code |
| Code 3 in two or more sextants | Comprehensive periodontal assessment of entire mouth |
| Code 4 in one or more sextants | Comprehensive periodontal assessment of entire mouth |

## Documenting PSR Codes

For a PSR completed on May 14, 2004, the PSR box chart would look like the chart shown below.

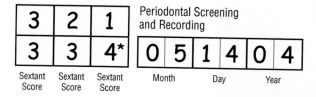

On this sample PSR chart, the following codes have been entered:

- Maxillary right posteriors = Code 3

- Maxillary anterior sextant = Code 2

- Maxillary left posteriors = Code 1

- Mandibular right posteriors = Code 3

- Mandibular anterior sextant = Code 3

- Mandibular left posteriors = Code 4 plus the * symbol to indicate one of the following problems: furcation involvement, mobility, mucogingival problems, or recession extending into the colored area of the probe.

Adapted from Nield-Gehrig JS. *Fundamentals of Periodontal Instrumentation & Advanced Root Instrumentation,* 5th ed. Baltimore: Lippincott Williams & Wilkins, 2004.

# Tooth Numbering Systems

The three tooth designation systems in general use are the Universal, adopted by the American Dental Association; the F.D.I. (or International), adopted by the Fédération Dentaire Internationale; and the Palmer.

## Universal or ADA System

### Permanent Teeth

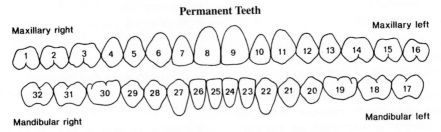

Maxillary right  Maxillary left

Mandibular right  Mandibular left

### Primary Teeth

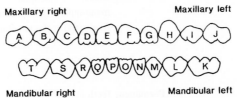

Maxillary right  Maxillary left

Mandibular right  Mandibular left

### Permanent Teeth

Start with the right maxillary third molar (number 1) and follow around the arch to the left maxillary third molar (16); descend to the left mandibular third molar (17); and follow around to the right mandibular third molar (32).

### Primary or Deciduous Teeth

Use continuous upper case letters A through T in the same sequence as for permanent teeth: right maxillary second molar (A) around to the left maxillary second molar (J); descend to the left mandibular second molar (K); and around to the right mandibular second molar (T).

## International or F.D.I. System

### Permanent Teeth

| Q-1 Maxillary right | | | | | | | | Q-2 Maxillary left | | | | | | | |
|---|---|---|---|---|---|---|---|---|---|---|---|---|---|---|---|
| 18 | 17 | 16 | 15 | 14 | 13 | 12 | 11 | 21 | 22 | 23 | 24 | 25 | 26 | 27 | 28 |
| 48 | 47 | 46 | 45 | 44 | 43 | 42 | 41 | 31 | 32 | 33 | 34 | 35 | 36 | 37 | 38 |
| Mandibular right Q-4 | | | | | | | | Mandibular left Q-3 | | | | | | | |

### Primary Teeth

| Q-5 Maxillary right | | | | | Q-6 Maxillary left | | | | |
|---|---|---|---|---|---|---|---|---|---|
| 55 | 54 | 53 | 52 | 51 | 61 | 62 | 63 | 64 | 65 |
| 85 | 84 | 83 | 82 | 81 | 71 | 72 | 73 | 74 | 75 |
| Mandibular right Q-8 | | | | | Mandibular left Q-7 | | | | |

## Permanent Teeth

Each tooth is numbered by the quadrant (1 to 4) and by the tooth within the quadrant (1 to 8).

*Quadrant Numbers*
1 = Maxillary right
2 = Maxillary left
3 = Mandibular left
4 = Mandibular right

*Tooth Numbers Within Each Quadrant.* Start with number 1 at the midline (central incisor) to number 8, third molar.

*Designation.* The digits are pronounced separately. For example, "two-five" (25) is the maxillary left second premolar, and "four-two" (42) is the mandibular right lateral incisor.

## Primary or Deciduous Teeth

Each tooth is numbered by quadrant (5 to 8) to continue with the permanent quadrant numbers. The teeth are numbered within each quadrant (1 to 5).

*Quadrant Numbers*
5 = Maxillary right
6 = Maxillary left
7 = Mandibular left
8 = Mandibular right

*Tooth Numbers Within Each Quadrant.* Number 1 is the central incisor, and number 5 is the second primary molar.

*Designation.* The digits are pronounced separately. For example, "eight-three" (83) is the mandibular right primary canine, and "six-five" (65) is the maxillary left second primary molar.

# Palmer System

### Permanent Teeth

**Maxillary right**                                                         **Maxillary left**

| 8 | 7 | 6 | 5 | 4 | 3 | 2 | 1 | 1 | 2 | 3 | 4 | 5 | 6 | 7 | 8 |
| 8 | 7 | 6 | 5 | 4 | 3 | 2 | 1 | 1 | 2 | 3 | 4 | 5 | 6 | 7 | 8 |

**Mandibular right**                                                        **Mandibular left**

### Primary Teeth

**Maxillary right**                          **Maxillary left**

| E | D | C | B | A | A | B | C | D | E |
| E | D | C | B | A | A | B | C | D | E |

**Mandibular right**                         **Mandibular left**

## Permanent Teeth

With number 1 for each central incisor, the teeth in each quadrant are numbered to 8, the third molar. To identify individual teeth, horizontal and vertical lines are drawn to indicate the quadrant. For example, the left maxillary first premolar is ⌊4, the right mandibular first and second molars are 76⌉. An entire quadrant may be represented by the use of the letter Q, for example, the maxillary right quadrant is Q⌋.

## Primary or Deciduous Teeth

Upper case letters A through E are used instead of the numbers. Examples are the mandibular left canine ⌈C and the maxillary right first primary molar D⌋.

Adapted from Wilkins EM. *Clinical Practice of the Dental Hygienist,* 9th ed. Baltimore: Lippincott Williams & Wilkins, 2005.

# Guidelines for Infection Control in Dental Health Care Settings

## Categories

These recommendations are designed to prevent or reduce potential for disease transmission from patient to dental health care personnel (DHCP), from DHCP to patient, and from patient to patient. Each recommendation is categorized on the basis of existing scientific data, theoretical rationale, and applicability. Rankings are based on the system used by CDC and the Healthcare Infection Control Practices Advisory Committee (HICPAC) to categorize recommendations:

*Category IA.* Strongly recommended for implementation and strongly supported by well-designed experimental, clinical, or epidemiologic studies.

*Category IB.* Strongly recommended for implementation and supported by experimental, clinical, or epidemiologic studies and a strong theoretical rationale.

*Category IC.* Required for implementation as mandated by federal or state regulation or standard. When IC is used, a second rating can be included to provide the basis of existing scientific data, theoretical rationale, and applicability. Because of state differences, the reader should not assume that the absence of a IC implies the absence of state regulations.

*Category II.* Suggested for implementation and supported by suggestive clinical or epidemiologic studies or a theoretical rationale.

*Unresolved issue.* No recommendation. Insufficient evidence or no consensus regarding efficacy exists.

## I. Preventing Transmission of Bloodborne Pathogens

### A. Hepatitis B Virus (HBV) Vaccination

1. Offer the HBV vaccination series to all DHCP with potential occupational exposure to blood or other potentially infectious material (IA, IC).
2. Always follow U.S. Public Health Service/CDC recommendations for hepatitis B vaccination, serologic testing, follow-up, and booster dosing (IA, IC).
3. Test DHCP for anti-HBs 1–2 months after completion of the 3-dose vaccination series (IA, IC).
4. DHCP should complete a second 3-dose vaccine series or be evaluated to determine if they are HBsAg-positive if no antibody response occurs to the primary vaccine series (IA, IC).
5. Retest for anti-HBs at the completion of the second vaccine series. If no response to the second 3-dose series occurs, nonresponders should be tested for HBsAg (IC).
6. Counsel nonresponders to vaccination who are HBsAg-negative regarding their susceptibility to HBV infection and precautions to take (IA, IC).
7. Provide employees appropriate education regarding the risks of HBV transmission and the availability of the vaccine. Employees who decline the vaccination should sign a declination form to be kept on file with the employer (IC).

### B. Preventing Exposures to Blood and Other Potentially Infectious Materials (OPIM)

1. General recommendations
   a. Use standard precautions (OSHA's bloodborne pathogen standard retains the term "universal precautions") for all patient encounters (IA, IC).
   b. Consider sharp items (e.g., needles, scalers, burs, lab knives, and wires) that are contaminated with patient blood and saliva as potentially infective and establish engineering controls and work practices to prevent injuries (IB, IC).
   c. Implement a written, comprehensive program designed to minimize and manage DHCP exposures to blood and body fluids (IB, IC).

2. Engineering and work-practice controls

    a. Identify, evaluate, and select devices with engineered safety features at least annually and as they become available on the market (e.g., safer anesthetic syringes, blunt suture needle, retractable scalpel, or needleless IV systems) (IC).

    b. Place used disposable syringes and needles, scalpel blades, and other sharp items in appropriate puncture-resistant containers located as close as feasible to the area in which the items are used (IA, IC).

    c. Do not recap used needles by using both hands or any other technique that involves directing the point of a needle toward any part of the body. Do not bend, break, or remove needles before disposal (IA, IC).

    d. Use either a one-handed scoop technique or a mechanical device designed for holding the needle cap when recapping needles (e.g., between multiple injections and before removing from a nondisposable aspirating syringe) (IA, IC).

3. Postexposure management and prophylaxis

    a. Follow CDC recommendations after percutaneous, mucous membrane, or nonintact skin exposure to blood or other potentially infectious material (IA, IC).

## II. Hand Hygiene

### A. General Considerations

1. Perform hand hygiene with either a nonantimicrobial or antimicrobial soap and water when hands are visibly dirty or contaminated with blood or other potentially infectious material. If hands are not visibly soiled, an alcohol-based hand rub can also be used. Follow the manufacturer's instructions (IA).

2. Indications for hand hygiene include:

    a. when hands are visibly soiled (IA, IC);

    b. after barehanded touching of inanimate objects likely to be contaminated by blood, saliva, or respiratory secretions (IA, IC);

    c. before and after treating each patient (IB);

    d. before donning gloves (IB); and

    e. immediately after removing gloves (IB, IC).

3. For oral surgical procedures, perform surgical hand antisepsis before donning sterile surgeon's gloves. Follow the manufacturer's instructions by using either an antimicrobial soap and water, or soap and water followed by drying hands and application of an alcohol-based surgical hand-scrub product with persistent activity (IB).

4. Store liquid hand-care products in either disposable closed containers or closed containers that can be washed and dried before refilling. Do not add soap or lotion to (i.e., top off) a partially empty dispenser (IA).

### B. Special Considerations for Hand Hygiene and Glove Use

1. Use hand lotions to prevent skin dryness associated with handwashing (IA).

2. Consider the compatibility of lotion and antiseptic products and the effect of petroleum or other oil emollients on the integrity of gloves during product selection and glove use (IB).

3. Keep fingernails short with smooth, filed edges to allow thorough cleaning and prevent glove tears (II).

4. Do not wear artificial fingernails or extenders when having direct contact with patients at high risk (e.g., those in intensive care units or operating rooms) (IA).

5. Use of artificial fingernails is usually not recommended (II).

6. Do not wear hand or nail jewelry if it makes donning gloves more difficult or compromises the fit and integrity of the glove (II).

## III. Personal Protective Equipment (PPE)

### A. Masks, Protective Eyewear, and Face Shields

1. Wear a surgical mask and eye protection with solid side shields or a face shield to protect mucous membranes of the eyes, nose, and mouth during procedures likely to generate splashing or spattering of blood or other body fluids (IB, IC).
2. Change masks between patients or during patient treatment if the mask becomes wet (IB).
3. Clean with soap and water, or if visibly soiled, clean and disinfect reusable facial protective equipment (e.g., clinician and patient protective eyewear or face shields) between patients (II).

### B. Protective Clothing

1. Wear protective clothing (e.g., reusable or disposable gown, laboratory coat, or uniform) that covers personal clothing and skin (e.g., forearms) likely to be soiled with blood, saliva, or OPIM (IB, IC).
2. Change protective clothing if visibly soiled (134); change immediately or as soon as feasible if penetrated by blood or other potentially infectious fluids (IB, IC).
3. Remove barrier protection, including gloves, mask, eyewear, and gown, before departing work area (e.g., dental patient care, instrument processing, or laboratory areas) (IC).

### C. Gloves

1. Wear medical gloves when a potential exists for contacting blood, saliva, OPIM, or mucous membranes (IB, IC).
2. Wear a new pair of medical gloves for each patient, remove them promptly after use, and wash hands immediately to avoid transfer of microorganisms to other patients or environments (IB).
3. Remove gloves that are torn, cut, or punctured as soon as feasible and wash hands before regloving (IB, IC).
4. Do not wash surgeon's or patient examination gloves before use or wash, disinfect, or sterilize gloves for reuse (IB, IC).
5. Ensure that appropriate gloves in the correct size are readily accessible (IC).
6. Use appropriate gloves (e.g., puncture- and chemical-resistant utility gloves) when cleaning instruments and performing housekeeping tasks involving contact with blood or OPIM (IB, IC).
7. Consult with glove manufacturers regarding the chemical compatibility of glove material and dental materials used (II).

### D. Sterile Surgeon's Gloves and Double Gloving During Oral Surgical Procedures

1. Wear sterile surgeon's gloves when performing oral surgical procedures (IB).
2. No recommendation is offered regarding the effectiveness of wearing two pairs of gloves to prevent disease transmission during oral surgical procedures. The majority of studies among HCP and DHCP have demonstrated a lower frequency of inner glove perforation and visible blood on the surgeon's hands when double gloves are worn; however, the effectiveness of wearing two pairs of gloves in preventing disease transmission has not been demonstrated (Unresolved issue).

## IV. Contact Dermatitis and Latex Hypersensitivity

### A. General Recommendations

1. Educate DHCP regarding the signs, symptoms, and diagnoses of skin reactions associated with frequent hand hygiene and glove use (IB).
2. Screen all patients for latex allergy (e.g., take health history and refer for medical consultation when latex allergy is suspected) (IB).
3. Ensure a latex-safe environment for patients and DHCP with latex allergy (IB).
4. Have emergency treatment kits with latex-free products available at all times (II).

# V. Sterilization and Disinfection of Patient-Care Items

## A. General Recommendations

1. Use only FDA-cleared medical devices for sterilization and follow the manufacturer's instructions for correct use (IB).
2. Clean and heat-sterilize critical dental instruments before each use (IA).
3. Clean and heat-sterilize semicritical items before each use (IB).
4. Allow packages to dry in the sterilizer before they are handled to avoid contamination (IB).
5. Use of heat-stable semicritical alternatives is encouraged (IB).
6. Reprocess heat-sensitive critical and semi-critical instruments by using FDA-cleared sterilant/high-level disinfectants or an FDA-cleared low-temperature sterilization method (e.g., ethylene oxide). Follow manufacturer's instructions for use of chemical sterilants/high-level disinfectants (IB).
7. Single-use disposable instruments are acceptable alternatives if they are used only once and disposed of correctly (IB, IC).
8. Do not use liquid chemical sterilants/high-level disinfectants for environmental surface disinfection or as holding solutions (IB, IC).
9. Ensure that noncritical patient-care items are barrier-protected or cleaned, or if visibly soiled, cleaned and disinfected after each use with an EPA-registered hospital disinfectant. If visibly contaminated with blood, use an EPA-registered hospital disinfectant with a tuberculocidal claim (i.e., intermediate level) (IB).
10. Inform DHCP of all OSHA guidelines for exposure to chemical agents used for disinfection and sterilization. Using this report, identify areas and tasks that have potential for exposure (IC).

## B. Instrument Processing Area

1. Designate a central processing area. Divide the instrument processing area, physically or, at a minimum, spatially, into distinct areas for 1) receiving, cleaning, and decontamination; 2) preparation and packaging; 3) sterilization; and 4) storage. Do not store instruments in an area where contaminated instruments are held or cleaned (II).
2. Train DHCP to employ work practices that prevent contamination of clean areas (II).

## C. Receiving, Cleaning, and Decontamination Work Area

1. Minimize handling of loose contaminated instruments during transport to the instrument processing area. Use work-practice controls (e.g., carry instruments in a covered container) to minimize exposure potential (II). Clean all visible blood and other contamination from dental instruments and devices before sterilization or disinfection procedures (IA).
2. Use automated cleaning equipment (e.g., ultrasonic cleaner or washer-disinfector) to remove debris to improve cleaning effectiveness and decrease worker exposure to blood (IB).
3. Use work-practice controls that minimize contact with sharp instruments if manual cleaning is necessary (e.g., long-handled brush) (IC).
4. Wear puncture- and chemical-resistant/heavy-duty utility gloves for instrument cleaning and decontamination procedures (IB).
5. Wear appropriate PPE (e.g., mask, protective eyewear, and gown) when splashing or spraying is anticipated during cleaning (IC).

## D. Preparation and Packaging

1. Use an internal chemical indicator in each package. If the internal indicator cannot be seen from outside the package, also use an external indicator (II).
2. Use a container system or wrapping compatible with the type of sterilization process used and that has received FDA clearance (IB).
3. Before sterilization of critical and semicritical instruments, inspect instruments for cleanliness, then wrap or place them in containers designed to maintain sterility during storage (e.g., cassettes and organizing trays) (IA).

### E. Sterilization of Unwrapped Instruments

1. Clean and dry instruments before the unwrapped sterilization cycle (IB).

2. Use mechanical and chemical indicators for each unwrapped sterilization cycle (i.e., place an internal chemical indicator among the instruments or items to be sterilized) (IB).

3. Allow unwrapped instruments to dry and cool in the sterilizer before they are handled to avoid contamination and thermal injury (II).

4. Semicritical instruments that will be used immediately or within a short time can be sterilized unwrapped on a tray or in a container system, provided that the instruments are handled aseptically during removal from the sterilizer and transport to the point of use (II).

5. Critical instruments intended for immediate reuse can be sterilized unwrapped if the instruments are maintained sterile during removal from the sterilizer and transport to the point of use (e.g., transported in a sterile covered container) (IB).

6. Do not sterilize implantable devices unwrapped (IB).

7. Do not store critical instruments unwrapped (IB).

### F. Sterilization Monitoring

1. Use mechanical, chemical, and biological monitors according to the manufacturer's instructions to ensure the effectiveness of the sterilization process (IB).

2. Monitor each load with mechanical (e.g., time, temperature, and pressure) and chemical indicators (II).

3. Place a chemical indicator on the inside of each package. If the internal indicator is not visible from the outside, also place an exterior chemical indicator on the package (II).

4. Place items/packages correctly and loosely into the sterilizer so as not to impede penetration of the sterilant (IB).

5. Do not use instrument packs if mechanical or chemical indicators indicate inadequate processing (IB).

6. Monitor sterilizers at least weekly by using a biological indicator with a matching control (i.e., biological indicator and control from same lot number) (IB).

7. Use a biological indicator for every sterilizer load that contains an implantable device. Verify results before using the implantable device, whenever possible (IB).

8. The following are recommended in the case of a positive spore test:

   a. Remove the sterilizer from service and review sterilization procedures (e.g., work practices and use of mechanical and chemical indicators) to determine whether operator error could be responsible (II).

   b. Retest the sterilizer by using biological, mechanical, and chemical indicators after correcting any identified procedural problems (II).

   c. If the repeat spore test is negative, and mechanical and chemical indicators are within normal limits, put the sterilizer back in service (II).

9. The following are recommended if the repeat spore test is positive:

   a. Do not use the sterilizer until it has been inspected or repaired or the exact reason for the positive test has been determined (II).

   b. Recall, to the extent possible, and reprocess all items processed since the last negative spore test (II).

   c. Before placing the sterilizer back in service, rechallenge the sterilizer with biological indicator tests in three consecutive empty chamber sterilization cycles after the cause of the sterilizer failure has been determined and corrected (II).

10. Maintain sterilization records (i.e., mechanical, chemical, and biological) in compliance with state and local regulations (IB).

**G. Storage Area for Sterilized Items and Clean Dental Supplies**

1. Implement practices on the basis of date- or event-related shelf-life for storage of wrapped, sterilized instruments and devices (IB).

2. Even for event-related packaging, at a minimum, place the date of sterilization, and if multiple sterilizers are used in the facility, the sterilizer used, on the outside of the packaging material to facilitate the retrieval of processed items in the event of a sterilization failure (IB).

3. Examine wrapped packages of sterilized instruments before opening them to ensure the barrier wrap has not been compromised during storage (II).

4. Reclean, repack, and resterilize any instrument package that has been compromised (II).

5. Store sterile items and dental supplies in covered or closed cabinets, if possible (II).

## VI. Environmental Infection Control

### A. General Recommendations

1. Follow the manufacturers' instructions for correct use of cleaning and EPA-registered hospital disinfecting products (IB, IC).

2. Do not use liquid chemical sterilants/high-level disinfectants for disinfection of environmental surfaces (clinical contact or housekeeping) (IB, IC).

3. Use PPE, as appropriate, when cleaning and disinfecting environmental surfaces. Such equipment might include gloves (e.g., puncture- and chemical-resistant utility), protective clothing (e.g., gown, jacket, or lab coat), protective eyewear/face shield, and mask (IC).

### B. Clinical Contact Surfaces

1. Use surface barriers to protect clinical contact surfaces, particularly those that are difficult to clean (e.g., switches on dental chairs) and change surface barriers between patients (II).

2. Clean and disinfect clinical contact surfaces that are not barrier-protected, by using an EPA-registered hospital disinfectant with a low- (i.e., HIV and HBV label claims) to intermediate-level (i.e., tuberculocidal claim) activity after each patient. Use an intermediate-level disinfectant if visibly contaminated with blood (IB).

### C. Housekeeping Surfaces

1. Clean housekeeping surfaces (e.g., floors, walls, and sinks) with a detergent and water or an EPA-registered hospital disinfectant/detergent on a routine basis, depending on the nature of the surface and type and degree of contamination, and as appropriate, based on the location in the facility, and when visibly soiled (IB).

2. Clean mops and cloths after use and allow to dry before reuse; or use single-use, disposable mop heads or cloths (II).

3. Prepare fresh cleaning or EPA-registered disinfecting solutions daily and as instructed by the manufacturer (II).

4. Clean walls, blinds, and window curtains in patient-care areas when they are visibly dusty or soiled (II).

### D. Spills of Blood and Body Substances

1. Clean spills of blood or OPIM and decontaminate surface with an EPA-registered hospital disinfectant with low- (i.e., HBV and HIV label claims) to intermediate-level (i.e., tuberculocidal claim) activity, depending on size of spill and surface porosity (IB, IC).

### E. Carpet and Cloth Furnishings

1. Avoid using carpeting and cloth-upholstered furnishings in dental operatories, laboratories, and instrument processing areas (II).

### F. Regulated Medical Waste

1. General Recommendations

   a. Develop a medical waste management program. Disposal of regulated medical waste must follow federal, state, and local regulations (IC).

b. Ensure that DHCP who handle and dispose of regulated medical waste are trained in appropriate handling and disposal methods and informed of the possible health and safety hazards (IC).

2. Management of Regulated Medical Waste in Dental Health-Care Facilities
   a. Use a color-coded or labeled container that prevents leakage (e.g., biohazard bag) to contain nonsharp regulated medical waste (IC).
   b. Place sharp items (e.g., needles, scalpel blades, orthodontic bands, broken metal instruments, and burs) in an appropriate sharps container (e.g., puncture resistant, color-coded, and leakproof). Close container immediately before removal or replacement to prevent spillage or protrusion of contents during handling, storage, transport, or shipping (IC).
   c. Pour blood, suctioned fluids or other liquid waste carefully into a drain connected to a sanitary sewer system, if local sewage discharge requirements are met and the state has declared this an acceptable method of disposal. Wear appropriate PPE while performing this task (IC).

## VII. Dental Unit Waterlines, Biofilm, and Water Quality
### A. General Recommendations
1. Use water that meets EPA regulatory standards for drinking water (i.e., <500 CFU/mL of heterotrophic water bacteria) for routine dental treatment output water (IB, IC).
2. Consult with the dental unit manufacturer for appropriate methods and equipment to maintain the recommended quality of dental water (II).
3. Follow recommendations for monitoring water quality provided by the manufacturer of the unit or waterline treatment product (II).
4. Discharge water and air for a minimum of 20–30 seconds after each patient, from any device connected to the dental water system that enters the patient's mouth (e.g., handpieces, ultrasonic scalers, and air/water syringes) (II).
5. Consult with the dental unit manufacturer on the need for periodic maintenance of antiretraction mechanisms (IB).

### B. Boil-Water Advisories
1. The following apply while a boil-water advisory is in effect:
   a. Do not deliver water from the public water system to the patient through the dental operative unit, ultrasonic scaler, or other dental equipment that uses the public water system (IB, IC).
   b. Do not use water from the public water system for dental treatment, patient rinsing, or handwashing (IB, IC).
   c. For handwashing, use antimicrobial-containing products that do not require water for use (e.g., alcohol-based hand rubs). If hands are visibly contaminated, use bottled water, if available, and soap for handwashing or an antiseptic towelette (IB, IC).
2. The following apply when the boil-water advisory is cancelled:
   a. Follow guidance given by the local water utility regarding adequate flushing of waterlines. If no guidance is provided, flush dental waterlines and faucets for 1–5 minutes before using for patient care (IC).
   b. Disinfect dental waterlines as recommended by the dental unit manufacturer (II).

## VIII. Special Considerations
### A. Dental Handpieces and Other Devices Attached to Air and Waterlines
1. Clean and heat-sterilize handpieces and other intraoral instruments that can be removed from the air and waterlines of dental units between patients (IB, IC).
2. Follow the manufacturer's instructions for cleaning, lubrication, and sterilization of handpieces and other intraoral instruments that can be removed from the air and waterlines of dental units (IB).

3. Do not surface-disinfect, use liquid chemical sterilants, or use ethylene oxide on handpieces and other intraoral instruments that can be removed from the air and waterlines of dental units (IC).

4. Do not advise patients to close their lips tightly around the tip of the saliva ejector to evacuate oral fluids (II).

## B. Dental Radiology

1. Wear gloves when exposing radiographs and handling contaminated film packets. Use other PPE (e.g., protective eyewear, mask, and gown) as appropriate if spattering of blood or other body fluids is likely (IA, IC).

2. Use heat-tolerant or disposable intraoral devices whenever possible (e.g., film-holding and positioning devices). Clean and heat-sterilize heat-tolerant devices between patients. At a minimum, high-level disinfect semicritical heat-sensitive devices, according to manufacturer's instructions (IB).

3. Transport and handle exposed radiographs in an aseptic manner to prevent contamination of developing equipment (II).

4. The following apply for digital radiography sensors:

    a. Use FDA-cleared barriers (IB).

    b. Clean and heat-sterilize, or high-level disinfect, between patients, barrier-protected semicritical items. If the item cannot tolerate these procedures then, at a minimum, protect with an FDA-cleared barrier and clean and disinfect with an EPA-registered hospital disinfectant with intermediate-level (i.e., tuberculocidal claim) activity, between patients. Consult with the manufacturer for methods of disinfection and sterilization of digital radiology sensors and for protection of associated computer hardware (IB).

## C. Aseptic Technique for Parenteral Medications

1. Do not administer medication from a syringe to multiple patients, even if the needle on the syringe is changed (IA).

2. Use single-dose vials for parenteral medications when possible (II).

3. Do not combine the leftover contents of single-use vials for later use (IA).

4. The following apply if multidose vials are used:

    a. Cleanse the access diaphragm with 70% alcohol before inserting a device into the vial (IA).

    b. Use a sterile device to access a multiple-dose vial and avoid touching the access diaphragm. Both the needle and syringe used to access the multidose vial should be sterile. Do not reuse a syringe even if the needle is changed (IA).

    c. Keep multidose vials away from the immediate patient treatment area to prevent inadvertent contamination by spray or spatter (II).

    d. Discard the multidose vial if sterility is compromised (IA).

5. Use fluid infusion and administration sets (i.e., IV bags, tubings and connections) for one patient only and dispose of appropriately (IB).

## D. Single-Use (Disposable) Devices

1. Use single-use devices for one patient only and dispose of them appropriately (IC).

## E. Preprocedural Mouth Rinses

1. No recommendation is offered regarding use of preprocedural antimicrobial mouth rinses to prevent clinical infections among DHCP or patients. Although studies have demonstrated that a preprocedural antimicrobial rinse (e.g., chlorhexidine gluconate, essential oils, or povidone-iodine) can reduce the level of oral microorganisms in aerosols and spatter generated during routine dental procedures and can decrease the number of microorganisms introduced in the patient's bloodstream during invasive dental procedures, the scientific evidence is inconclusive that using these rinses prevents clinical infections among DHCP or patients (Unresolved issue).

**F. Oral Surgical Procedures**

1. The following apply when performing oral surgical procedures:
   a. Perform surgical hand antisepsis by using an antimicrobial product (e.g., antimicrobial soap and water, or soap and water followed by alcohol-based hand scrub with persistent activity) before donning sterile surgeon's gloves (IB).
   b. Use sterile surgeon's gloves (IB).
   c. Use sterile saline or sterile water as a coolant/irrigatant when performing oral surgical procedures. Use devices specifically designed for delivering sterile irrigating fluids (e.g., bulb syringe, single-use disposable products, and sterilizable tubing) (IB).

**G. Handling of Biopsy Specimens**

1. During transport, place biopsy specimens in a sturdy, leakproof container labeled with the biohazard symbol (IC).
2. If a biopsy specimen container is visibly contaminated, clean and disinfect the outside of a container or place it in an impervious bag labeled with the biohazard symbol (IC).

**H. Handling of Extracted Teeth**

1. Dispose of extracted teeth as regulated medical waste unless returned to the patient (IC).
2. Do not dispose of extracted teeth containing amalgam in regulated medical waste intended for incineration (II).
3. Clean and place extracted teeth in a leakproof container, labeled with the biohazard symbol, and maintain hydration for transport to educational institutions or a dental laboratory (IC).
4. Heat-sterilize teeth that do not contain amalgam before they are used for educational purposes (IB).

**I. Dental Laboratory**

1. Use PPE when handling items received in the laboratory until they have been decontaminated (IA, IC).
2. Before they are handled in the laboratory, clean, disinfect, and rinse all dental prostheses and prosthodontic materials (e.g., impressions, bite registrations, occlusal rims, and extracted teeth) by using an EPA-registered hospital disinfectant having at least an intermediate-level (i.e., tuberculocidal claim) activity (IB).
3. Consult with manufacturers regarding the stability of specific materials (e.g., impression materials) relative to disinfection procedures (II).
4. Include specific information regarding disinfection techniques used (e.g., solution used and duration), when laboratory cases are sent off-site and on their return (II).
5. Clean and heat-sterilize heat-tolerant items used in the mouth (e.g., metal impression trays and face-bow forks) (IB).
6. Follow manufacturers' instructions for cleaning and sterilizing or disinfecting items that become contaminated but do not normally contact the patient (e.g., burs, polishing points, rag wheels, articulators, case pans, and lathes). If manufacturer instructions are unavailable, clean and heat-sterilize heat-tolerant items or clean and disinfect with an EPA-registered hospital disinfectant with low- (i.e., HIV, HBV effectiveness claim) to intermediate-level (i.e., tuberculocidal claim) activity, depending on the degree of contamination (II).

**J. Laser/Electrosurgery Plumes/Surgical Smoke**

1. No recommendation is offered regarding practices to reduce DHCP exposure to laser plumes/surgical smoke when using lasers in dental practice. Practices to reduce HCP exposure to laser plumes/surgical smoke have been suggested, including use of a) standard precautions (e.g., high-filtration surgical masks and possibly full face shields); b) central room suction units with in-line filters to collect particulate matter from minimal plumes; and c) dedicated mechanical smoke exhaust systems with a high-efficiency filter to remove substantial amounts of laser-plume particles. The effect of the exposure (e.g., disease

transmission or adverse respiratory effects) on DHCP from dental applications of lasers has not been adequately evaluated (Unresolved issue).

### K. *Mycobacterium tuberculosis*

1. General Recommendations

   a. Educate all DHCP regarding the recognition of signs, symptoms, and transmission of TB (IB).

   b. Conduct a baseline tuberculin skin test (TST), preferably by using a two-step test, for all DHCP who might have contact with persons with suspected or confirmed active TB, regardless of the risk classification of the setting (IB).

   c. Assess each patient for a history of TB as well as symptoms indicative of TB and document on the medical history form (IB).

   d. Follow CDC recommendations for 1) developing, maintaining, and implementing a written TB infection-control plan; 2) managing a patient with suspected or active TB; 3) completing a community risk-assessment to guide employee TSTs and follow-up; and 4) managing DHCP with TB disease (IB).

2. The following apply for patients known or suspected to have active TB:

   a. Evaluate the patient away from other patients and DHCP. When not being evaluated, the patient should wear a surgical mask or be instructed to cover mouth and nose when coughing or sneezing (IB).

   b. Defer elective dental treatment until the patient is noninfectious (IB).

   c. Refer patients requiring urgent dental treatment to a previously identified facility with TB engineering controls and a respiratory protection program (IB).

### L. Creutzfeldt-Jakob Disease (CJD) and Other Prion Diseases

1. No recommendation is offered regarding use of special precautions in addition to standard precautions when treating known CJD or vCJD patients. Potential infectivity of oral tissues in CJD or vCJD patients is an unresolved issue. Scientific data indicate the risk, if any, of sporadic CJD transmission during dental and oral surgical procedures is low to nil. Until additional information exists regarding the transmissibility of CJD or vCJD during dental procedures, special precautions in addition to standard precautions might be indicated when treating known CJD or vCJD patients.

## Infection-Control Internet Resources

**Advisory Committee on Immunization Practices**
http://www.cdc.gov/vaccines/recs/acip/default.htm

**American Dental Association**
http://www.ada.org

**American Institute of Architects Academy of Architecture for Health**
http://www.aahaia.org

**American Society of Heating, Refrigeration, Air-conditioning Engineers**
http://www.ashrae.org

**Association for Professionals in Infection Control and Epidemiology, Inc.**
http://www.apic.org

**CDC, Division of Healthcare Quality Promotion**
http://www.cdc.gov/ncidod/hip

**CDC, Division of Oral Health, Infection Control**
http://www.cdc.gov/OralHealth/infectioncontrol/index.htm

**CDC,** *Morbidity and Mortality Weekly Report*
http://www.cdc.gov/mmwr

**CDC, NIOSH**
http://www.cdc.gov/niosh/homepage.html

**CDC Recommends, Prevention Guidelines System**
http://wonder.cdc.gov/wonder/prevguid/topics.html

**EPA, Antimicrobial Chemicals**
http://www.epa.gov/oppad001/chemregindex.htm

**FDA**
http://www.fda.gov

**Immunization Action Coalition**
http://www.immunize.org

**Infectious Diseases Society of America**
http://www.idsociety.org/PG/toc.htm

**OSHA, Dentistry, Bloodborne Pathogens**
http://www.osha.gov/SLTC/bloodbornepathogens/index.html

**Organization for Safety, Asepsis and Prevention**
http://www.osap.org

**Society for Healthcare Epidemiology of America**
http://www.shea-online.org

Adapted from Centers for Disease Control and Prevention. Guidelines for Infection Control in Dental Health-Care Settings–2003. MMWR 2003;52 (No. RR-17). Available at: http://www.cdc.gov/mmwr/preview/mmwrhtml/rr5217a1.htm.

# Infection Control for the Dental Office: a Checklist

## Immunization

- Health care workers should have appropriate immunizations such as that for hepatitis B virus.

## Before Patient Treatment

- Obtain a thorough medical history.
- Disinfect prostheses and appliances received from the laboratory.
- Place disposable coverings to prevent contamination of surfaces, and/or disinfect surfaces after treatment.
- Set out supplies and instruments needed for the procedure.
- Flush waterlines before connecting handpieces, air/water syringes, or ultrasonic scalers.

## During Patient Treatment

- Treat all patients as potentially infectious.
- Use protective attire and barrier techniques when contact with body fluids or mucous membranes is anticipated.
    - Wear gloves.
    - Wear a mask.
    - Wear protective eyewear.
    - Wear a uniform, laboratory coat, or gown.
- Disinfect film packets before taking them into the darkroom.
- Open intraorally contaminated x-ray film packets in the darkroom with disposable gloves without touching the films.
- Use aseptic technique to retrieve additional items.
- Minimize formation of droplets, spatters, and aerosols.
- Use a rubber dam to isolate the tooth/teeth and field when appropriate.
- Use high-volume vacuum evacuation.
- Protect hands.
    - Wash hands before gloving and after gloves are removed.
    - Change gloves between each patient.
    - Discard gloves that are torn, cut, or punctured.
    - Avoid hand injuries.
- Avoid injury with sharp instruments and needles.
    - Handle sharp items carefully.
    - Do not bend or break disposable needles.
    - If needles are not recapped, place them in a separate field. If recapping is necessary, use a method that protects hands from injury, such as a holder for the cap.
    - Place sharp items in appropriate containers.
    - Remove burs from handpieces when not in use.

## After Patient Treatment

- Wear heavy-duty rubber gloves.
- Clean instruments thoroughly.
- Heat-sterilize instruments.
    - Sterilize instruments that penetrate soft tissue or bone.
    - Sterilize all instruments that come in contact with oral mucous membranes and body fluids, and all instruments that have been contaminated by secretions of patients. Otherwise, use appropriate chemical sterilization.

-Wrap instruments for sterilization to maintain sterility until use. Do not reuse single-use wraps.

-Monitor the sterilizer with biological monitors.

-Clean handpieces, dental units, and ultrasonic scalers.

-Flush handpieces, dental units, ultrasonic scalers, and air/water syringes between patients.

-Clean and sterilize air/water syringes or use disposable tips.

-Clean and sterilize ultrasonic scalers if possible; otherwise, disinfect them appropriately.

-Clean and sterilize handpieces.

-Process single-use water delivery systems according to the manufacturer's directions.

- Handle sharp instruments with caution.

-Place disposable needles, scalpels, and other sharp items intact into puncture-resistant containers before disposal.

- Replace any disposable surface covers on environmental surfaces.
- Decontaminate environmental surfaces.

-Wipe work surfaces with absorbent toweling to remove debris, and dispose of this toweling appropriately.

-Disinfect with suitable chemical disinfectant.

-Change protective coverings on light handles, the x-ray unit head, and other items.

- Decontaminate supplies and materials.

-Rinse and disinfect impressions, bite registrations, and appliances to be sent to the laboratory.

- Communicate the infection control program to the dental laboratory.
- Dispense a small amount of pumice in a disposable container for individual use on each lab case and discard any excess.
- Remove contaminated wastes appropriately.

-Pour blood, suctioned fluids, and other liquid waste into a drain connected to a sanitary sewer system.

-Place solid waste contaminated with blood or saliva in sealed, sturdy, impervious, red bags labeled ''biohazard'' (with the biohazard symbol affixed to the bag) and dispose of according to local government regulations.

- Remove gloves and wash hands.

## Daily

- Flush cleansing solution through evacuation lines, and clean or replace the unit's solid waste filter traps.
- Flush waterlines for 2–3 minutes after periods of nonuse if waterlines were not drained.
- If in-line water filters are used, change daily.
- For in-line check valves, change daily or as directed by the manufacturer.

## Overnight

- If possible, drain waterlines for dry storage periods of nonuse (overnight, weekends).

## Weekly

- Clean and disinfect the main evacuation trap.
- Clean and disinfect inside and outside of drawers and cabinets.
- Perform weekly disinfection procedures on waterlines as directed by the manufacturer.

Adapted from Cottone JA, Terezhalmy GT, Molinari JA, *Practical Infection Control in Dentistry,* 3rd ed. Baltimore: Lippincott Williams & Wilkins, 2001.

# Panoramic Radiograph

## Panoramic Radiograph Zones

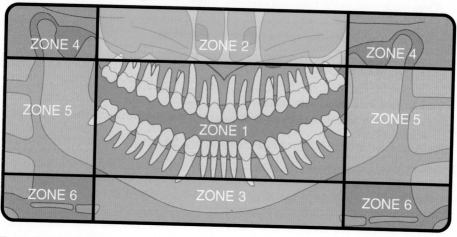

**Zone 1:** Dentition
The teeth should be separated and arranged with an upward curve posteriorly, producing a smile-like arrangement.

**Zone 2:** Nose and Sinus
The inferior turbinates should be within the nasal fossa, and the hard palate shadows above the root apices.

**Zone 3:** Mandibular Body
The inferior cortex of the mandibular body should be smooth and uninterrupted.

**Zone 4:** TMJ
The condyles are centered in this zone and are equal in size and position bilaterally.

**Zone 5:** Ramus-Spine
The ramus should be equal in width bilaterally, and the spine should not be superimposed on the ramus.

**Zone 6:** Hyoid
The hyoid bone should remain in this zone.

In a properly positioned patient, structures are projected onto the image with specific interrelation-ships to each other to form a pattern one can recognize as an error-free exposure.

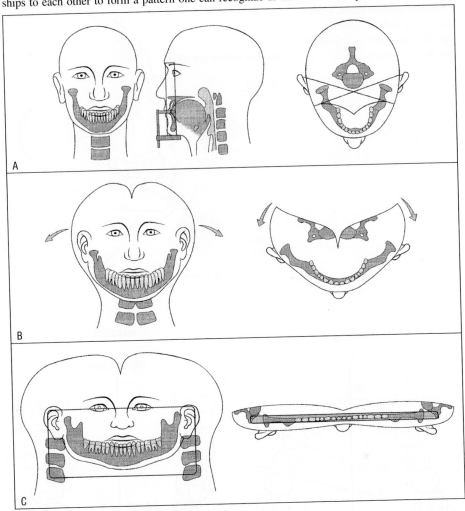

**Correct panoramic projection of anatomical structures:** (A) note the relation of anterior teeth and biteblock groove to the image layer and the path of the rotation center; (B) the unfolding of anatomical structures in three dimensions, much like opening a book with the cover toward you; (C) the relative position of key anatomical structures within the panoramic image (left) and within the image layer (right).

Adapted from Langland OE, Langlais RP, Preece JW. *Principles of Dental Imaging,* 2nd ed. Baltimore: Lippincott Williams & Wilkins, 2002.

# Paralleling Technique

**Vertical angulation of BID:**
note the difference between
positive and negative angulation
of the x-ray beam.

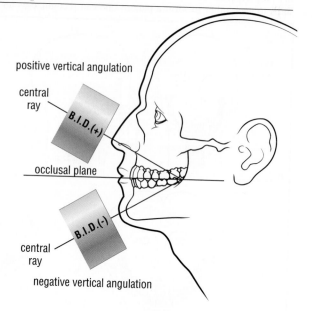

positive vertical angulation

central
ray

B.I.D.(+)

occlusal plane

B.I.D.(-)

central
ray

negative vertical angulation

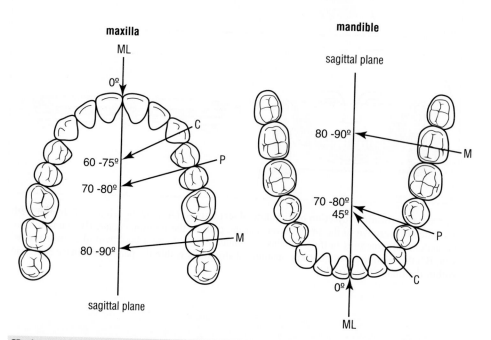

**maxilla**

ML

0º

C

60 -75º

P

70 -80º

M

80 -90º

sagittal plane

**mandible**

sagittal plane

80 -90º

M

70 -80º
45º

P

0º

C

ML

**Horizontal angulation of BID:** to position the horizontal angulation of the BID correctly, the central ray of the beam should be directed at an angle to the sagittal plane, as specified by the anatomical region; C = canine, M = molar, ML = midline, P = premolar.

# Maxillary

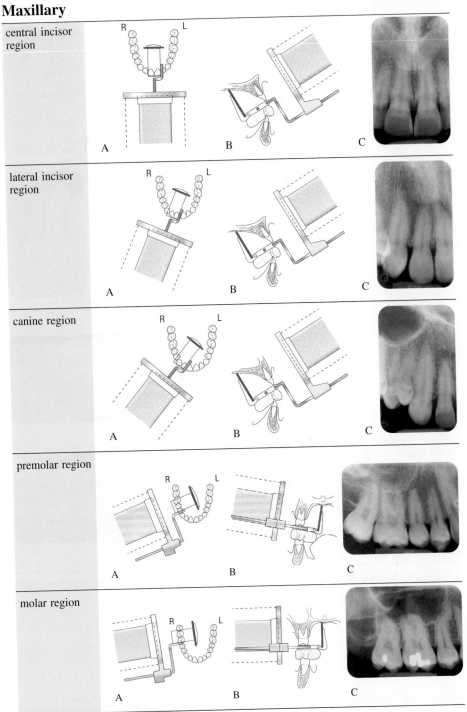

central incisor region

lateral incisor region

canine region

premolar region

molar region

A = horizontal film and BID placement; B = vertical film and BID placement; C = resultant radiograph.

# Mandibular

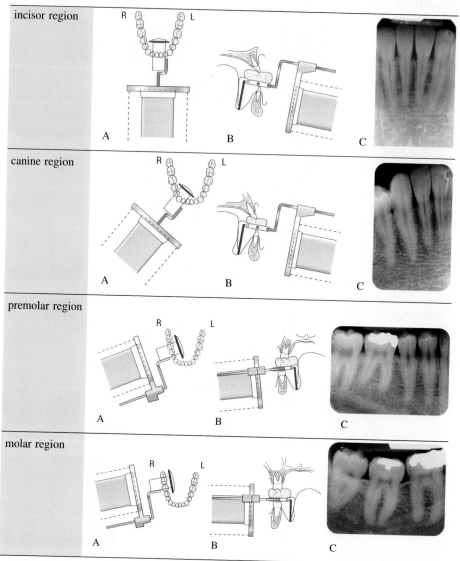

incisor region

A    B    C

canine region

A    B    C

premolar region

A    B    C

molar region

A    B    C

A = horizontal film and BID placement; B = vertical film and BID placement; C = resultant radiograph.

# Bitewing

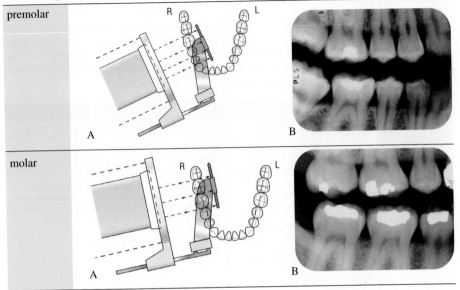

A = horizontal film and BID placement; B = resultant radiograph.

Adapted from Langland OE, Langlais RP, Preece JW. *Principles of Dental Imaging,* 2nd ed. Baltimore: Lippincott Williams & Wilkins, 2002.

# Guidelines for Prescribing Dental Radiographs

The recommendations in this chart are subject to clinical judgment and may not apply to every patient. They are to be used by dentists only after reviewing the patient's health history and completing a clinical examination. Because every precaution should be taken to minimize radiation exposure, protective thyroid collars and aprons should be used whenever possible. This practice is strongly recommended for children, women of childbearing age, and pregnant women.

| Type of Encounter | Patient Age and Dental Developmental Stage | | | | |
|---|---|---|---|---|---|
| | Child with Primary Dentition (prior to eruption of first permanent tooth) | Child with Transitional Dentition (after eruption of first permanent tooth) | Adolescent with Permanent Dentition (prior to eruption of third molars) | Adult, Dentate or Partially Edentulous | Adult, Edentulous |
| **New patient\*** being evaluated for dental diseases and dental development | Individualized radiographic exam consisting of selected periapical/occlusal views and/or posterior bitewings if proximal surfaces cannot be visualized or probed. Patients without evidence of disease and with open proximal contacts may not require a radiographic exam at this time. | Individualized radiographic exam consisting of posterior bitewings with panoramic exam or posterior bitewings and selected periapical images. | Individualized radiographic exam consisting of posterior bitewings with panoramic exam or posterior bitewings and selected periapical images. A full mouth intraoral radiographic exam is preferred when the patient has clinical evidence of generalized dental disease or a history of extensive dental treatment. | | Individualized radiographic exam, based on clinical signs and symptoms. |
| **Recall patient\*** with clinical caries or at increased risk for caries\*\* | Posterior bitewing exam at 6–12 month intervals if proximal surfaces cannot be examined visually or with a probe. | | | Posterior bitewing exam at 6–18 month intervals. | Not applicable |
| **Recall patient\*** with no clinical caries and not at increased risk for caries\*\* | Posterior bitewing exam at 12–24 month intervals if proximal surfaces cannot be examined visually or with a probe. | | Posterior bitewing exam at 18–36 month intervals. | Posterior bitewing exam at 24–36 month intervals. | Not applicable |
| **Recall patient\*** with periodontal disease | Clinical judgment as to the need for and type of radiographic images for the evaluation of periodontal disease. Imaging may consist of, but is not limited to, selected bitewing and/or periapical images of areas where periodontal disease (other than nonspecific gingivitis) can be identified clinically. | | | | Not applicable |
| **Patient** for monitoring of growth and development | Clinical judgment as to need for and type of radiographic images for evaluation and/or monitoring of dentofacial growth and development. | | Clinical judgment as to need for and type of radiographic images for evaluation and/or monitoring of dentofacial growth and development. Panoramic or periapical exam to assess developing third molars. | Usually not indicated | |

| | Patient Age and Dental Developmental Stage | | | | |
|---|---|---|---|---|---|
| Type of Encounter | Child with Primary Dentition (prior to eruption of first permanent tooth) | Child with Transitional Dentition (after eruption of first permanent tooth) | Adolescent with Permanent Dentition (prior to eruption of third molars) | Adult, Dentate or Partially Edentulous | Adult, Edentulous |
| **Patient** with other circumstances including, but not limited to, proposed or existing implants, pathology, restorative/ endodontic needs, treated periodontal disease and caries remineralization | Clinical judgment as to need for and type of radiographic images for evaluation and/or monitoring in these circumstances. | | | | |

**\*Clinical situations for which radiographs may be indicated include but are not limited to:**

**A. Positive Historical Findings**
1. Previous periodontal or endodontic treatment
2. History of pain or trauma
3. Familial history of dental anomalies
4. Postoperative evaluation of healing
5. Remineralization monitoring
6. Presence of implants or evaluation for implant placement

**B. Positive Clinical Signs/Symptoms**
1. Clinical evidence of periodontal disease
2. Large or deep restorations
3. Deep carious lesions
4. Malposed or clinically impacted teeth
5. Swelling
6. Evidence of dental/facial trauma
7. Mobility of teeth

8. Sinus tract ("fistula")
9. Clinically suspected sinus pathology
10. Growth abnormalities
11. Oral involvement in known or suspected systemic disease
12. Positive neurologic findings in the head and neck
13. Evidence of foreign objects
14. Pain and/or dysfunction of the temporomandibular joint
15. Facial asymmetry
16. Abutment teeth for fixed or removable partial prosthesis
17. Unexplained bleeding
18. Unexplained sensitivity of teeth
19. Unusual eruption, spacing, or migration of teeth
20. Unusual tooth morphology, calcification, or color
21. Unexplained absence of teeth
22. Clinical erosion

**\*\*Factors increasing risk for caries may include but are not limited to:**

1. High level of caries experience or demineralization
2. History of recurrent caries
3. High titers of cariogenic bacteria
4. Existing restoration(s) of poor quality
5. Poor oral hygiene
6. Inadequate fluoride exposure
7. Prolonged nursing (bottle or breast)
8. Frequent high sucrose content in diet
9. Poor family dental health

10. Developmental or acquired enamel defects
11. Developmental or acquired disability
12. Xerostomia
13. Genetic abnormality of teeth
14. Many multisurface restorations
15. Chemo/radiation therapy
16. Eating disorders
17. Drug/alcohol abuse
18. Irregular dental care

From American Dental Association, United States Food & Drug Administration. *The Selection of Patients for Dental Radiograph Examinations.* Revised 2004.

# Automatic Film Processing Errors

| Condition | Cause |
| --- | --- |
| Low-density (light) films | Solution temperature too low<br>Exhausted developer (underreplenishment)<br>Improper agitation or massaging action of rollers<br>Processing too fast (higher temperature and/or faster roller speed) |
| High-density (dark) films | Solutions overheated<br>Light leaks in the processor cover<br>Too much replenishment |
| Wet or tacky films | Dryer & developer temperatures too low<br>Dryer thermostatic control or heater inoperative<br>Dryer air circulation inadequate (high humidity in dryer section)<br>Wrong chemistry and/or film<br>Processing too fast (higher temperature and/or faster roller speed) |
| Film discoloration (brown) | Contamination of fixer by the developer solution |
| Film discoloration (greenish yellow) | Fixer solution exhausted (underreplenishment)<br>Processing too fast (higher temperature and/or faster roller speed)<br>Wrong type of film for the processor solution |
| Fogged films (unwanted density) | Incorrect or defective safelight filter or bulb<br>Light leaks in the darkroom<br>Developer temperature too high<br>Improper storage of films |
| Streaking (uneven density) | Underreplenishment<br>Rollers encrusted with chemical deposits<br>Dirty wash water<br>Film not hardened properly by chemicals |
| Surface marks | Foreign materials or irregularities on the surface of the rollers<br>Rough handling of the film before processing |
| Films chalky or dirty | No wash water or dirty wash water<br>Fixer contaminated |
| Jams or failure of film to transport | Chemicals contaminated or diluted<br>Chemical temperature too high<br>Films excessively soft and not adequately hardened; when enough gelatin lubricates the rollers, films will jam up with one another<br>Dirty rollers<br>Racks not seated properly<br>Dirty wash water<br>Incorrect dryer temperature<br>Hesitation in drive assembly, causing film to pause in transit<br>Film not tracking through the processor in straight line (improper feeding of films)<br>Bent film corners as leading edge |

Adapted from Langland OE, Langlais RP, Preece JW. *Principles of Dental Imaging*, 2nd ed. Baltimore: Lippincott Williams & Wilkins, 2002.

# Film Handling Errors

| Error | Cause |
|---|---|
| Black pressure marks on film | Teeth marks on film (especially pediatric occlusal film) |
| Black bend lines on films | From bending film to reduce patient discomfort |
| Black marks on film | Saliva contamination of black protective paper covering film; caused by failure to blot film packet with paper towel |
| Black "lightning- or tree-like" marks on film | Static electricity; removing film too rapidly from packet or box in air with dry humidity |
| Torn emulsion and scratches on film | Careless handling of film during processing when emulsion is soft and swollen |
| Dust and powder artifacts | Film contact with dust, grit, or glove powder before processing |
| White ball-point pen marks | Writing on front of film packet with ball-point pen |
| Fogged film (unwanted density): | |
|    Light fog | Light leaks in the darkroom |
| | Improper safelight; check bulb wattage, distance, and filter-film compatibility |
| | Turning overhead (white) light on too soon; be certain films have cleared in fixer first |
|    Radiation fog | Improper storage; insufficient protection of film next to x-ray machine |
|    Processing (chemical fog) | Developer temperatures too high |
| | Over-strength developer (check manufacturer's instructions) |
| | Prolonged development for temperature |
| | Contaminated developer (clean tank routinely) |
|    Deterioration of film | Temperature of storage area too high (store in refrigerator) |
| | Humidity of storage area too high (store in refrigerator) |
| | Strong fumes (ammonia, paint) |

Adapted from Langland OE, Langlais RP, Preece JW. *Principles of Dental Imaging,* 2nd ed. Baltimore: Lippincott Williams & Wilkins, 2002.

# Intraoral Projection and Technique Errors

| Error | Cause |
| --- | --- |
| Radiopaque artifacts on radiograph | Leaving dental appliance in mouth and/or eyeglasses or jewelry on the patient |
| Blurred image on radiograph | Movement of film, patient, or tubehead during exposure |
| Apical ends of teeth cut off | Film placed too close to the teeth in the maxillary arch in paralleling technique |
|  | Too flat a vertical angulation, which causes elongation |
| All of specific region not showing | Faulty film placement (center the film over the area of interest) |
| Herringbone effect or ping-pong ball and light density | Printed back side of film placed toward beam of radiation (film reversed) |
| Black dot in apical area | Manufacturer's identifying depression on film placed toward apical area of the teeth (place "dot in slot"—XCP instrument) |
| Double images of radiographs | Film exposed twice to radiation; "use film cup" |
| "Phalangioma" (patient's finger in image) | In holding the film (bisecting angle technique), the finger is placed between the film and the teeth |
| Tongue image | Placing the film on top of the tongue |
| Overlapping of teeth | Plane of the film is not parallel to the lingual surface of the teeth |
|  | Incorrect horizontal angulation of the cone (BID) |
| Foreshortening of image | Bisecting technique: vertical angulation of cone (BID) too steep |
|  | Paralleling technique: film not parallel with long axes of the teeth |
|  | Paralleling technique: long cone (BID) is not positioned correctly |
| Elongation of image | Bisecting technique: vertical angulation of cone (BID) is too flat |
|  | Paralleling technique: film is not positioned parallel to the long axes of the teeth |
|  | Paralleling technique: long cone (BID) not positioned correctly |
| Dimensional distortion of image | Inherent error in bisecting angle technique produces elongation of palatal roots and foreshortening of buccal roots of molars in the same view |
| Image distorted severely | Film is bent as patient bites on the film-holder or biteblock |
| Partial image "cone-cut" | Cone (BID) of radiation not covering the area of interest |
| Crowns of teeth not showing | Not enough film ($\frac{1}{8}$") showing below or above the crowns of the teeth |
|  | Vertical angulation too steep |

Adapted from Langland OE, Langlais RP, Preece JW. *Principles of Dental Imaging*, 2nd ed. Baltimore: Lippincott Williams & Wilkins, 2002.

# Panoramic Patient Positioning Errors

| Error and Cause | Identifying Features | Correction |
|---|---|---|
| Patient too far forward | Narrow blurred anterior teeth with pseudospace<br>Superimposition of spine on ramus<br>Bicuspid overlap bilaterally | Use incisal bite guide<br>Line up incisal edge of teeth with notch<br>Edentulous patients should bite about 5 mm behind notch |
| Patient too far back | Wide, blurred anterior teeth<br>Ghosting of rami; spread-out turbinates, ears, and nose in image; condyles off lateral edges of film | Use incisal bite guide<br>Line up incisal edge of teeth with notch |
| Chin tipped too low | Excessive curving of the occlusal plane<br>Loss of image of the roots of the lower anterior teeth<br>Narrowing of the intercondylar distance and loss of head of the condyles at the top of the film | Tip chin down, but ala-tragus line should not exceed $-5$ to $-7$ degrees downward<br>Use chin rest |
| Chin raised too high | Flattening or reverse curvature of occlusal plane<br>Loss of image of the roots of the upper anterior teeth<br>Lengthening of intercondylar distance and loss of head of the condyles at the edges of the film<br>Hard palate shadow wider and superimposed on the apices of the maxillary teeth | Tip chin down $-5$ to $-7$ degrees<br>Use chin rest |
| Head twisted | Unequal right-left magnification, particularly teeth and ramus<br>Severe overlap of contact points and blurring | Line up patient's midline with middle of incisal bite guide<br>Close side guide |
| Head tilted | Mandible appears tilted on film<br>Unequal distance between mandible and chin rest at a given point on the right and left sides<br>One condyle is higher and larger than the other | Position the chin firmly on both sides of the chin rest<br>Close side guide |
| Slumped position | Ghost image of cervical spine superimposed on the anterior region | Stand-up machines: have the patient step forward or place feet on markers<br>All machines: be certain the patient is sitting or standing erect |
| Chin not on the chin rest | Sinus not visible on the film<br>Tops of condyles are cut off<br>Excessive distance between inferior border of the mandible and the lower edge of the film | Position the chin on the chin rest |
| Bite guide not used | Incisal and occlusal surfaces of the upper and lower teeth overlapped | Use bite guide<br>Compensate for missing anterior teeth with cotton rolls |
| Tongue not on palate | Relative radiolucency obscuring apices of the maxillary teeth (palatoglossal air space) | Place the tongue firmly against the palate<br>Ask the patient to swallow, or to suck on his or her tongue |
| Lips open | Relative radiolucency on the coronal portion of the upper and lower teeth | Close lips |

| Error and Cause | Identifying Features | Correction |
|---|---|---|
| Patient movement | Wavy outline of the cortex of the interior border of the mandible | Ask the patient to hold still and not swallow |
| | Blurring of the image above wavy cortical outline | Explain the function of the machine to avoid startling the patient |
| | | Be certain the patient's clothing will not interfere |
| Prostheses | Evidence of prostheses in the image | Remove all complete and partial dentures, eyeglasses, and jewelry |
| | Acrylic denture teeth and bases do not show | |

Adapted from Langland OE, Langlais RP, Preece JW. *Principles of Dental Imaging,* 2nd ed. Baltimore: Lippincott Williams & Wilkins, 2002.

# Panoramic Procedural Errors

| Error and Cause | Identifying Features | Correction |
|---|---|---|
| Not starting at "home base" | A portion of the film is blank<br>A portion of the anatomy is lost at the edge of the film | Align the machine and/or cassette with starting point |
| Cassette resistance | One or several dark vertical bands on the film; these represent areas of overexposure as the casette is stopped, but radiation continues to be emitted until the end of the cycle | Be certain to remove thickly padded items of clothing<br>In stocky patients with a short neck, the cassette may need to be raised slightly above the ideal position |
| Paper or lint in screen | Radiopacity of unusual shape and location<br>Foreign object prevents complete exposure of film by fluorescent screen | Periodic inspection and cleaning of the screen |
| "Fingernail" artifact | Crescent-shaped radiolucency | Avoid rough handling of the film when removing from the box or cassette |
| Static electricity | Lightning-like radiolucency; dot-like radiolucencies<br>Starburst and other patterns, such as tree-shaped objects | Dry air in the darkroom can be humidified with a humidifier or large bowl of water<br>Avoid rapidly pulling the film from envelopetype cassettes or full box of film |
| White-light exposure | A portion of film appears overexposed | Avoid smoking near film<br>Check other sources of light leaks in the darkroom (i.e., unsafe safelight or radio)<br>Check integrity of cassette |
| Double exposure | Two images on the same film | Always place exposed films in the same location and where they may not be mistaken for unexposed films |
| Underexposed | Film too light | Increase kV and/or mA depending on the machine<br>Place film between screens, not to one side only<br>Check developer solution |
| Overexposed | Film too dark | Decrease kV and/or mA depending on the machine |
| No name | Patient's name or identification number not on film | Use film imprinter, special labeling tape, or special pen |

Adapted from Langland OE, Langlais RP, Preece JW. *Principles of Dental Imaging,* 2nd ed. Baltimore: Lippincott Williams & Wilkins, 2002.

# Professional Organizations

This directory, by no means exhaustive, lists professional organizations in the U.S. and some other English-speaking countries. Each country's name is followed by its country code for international calling. City codes or other area codes are listed with individual telephone numbers.

## Australia (61)

Academy of Australian and New Zealand
  Prosthodontists
Dr. Ian Lander, Secretary/Treasurer
Suite 15, Gateway Building
Andrea Lane
Booragoon WA 6154
08 9316 2811
08 9316 2813 (fax)
ianita@bigpond.net.au
www.aanzp.com.au

Australasian Academy of Paediatric
  Dentistry
Children's Dentistry
Angle House
7 Whitehorse Road
Balwyn VIC 31303
3 9817 3222
3 9817 3122 (fax)
mala@drmala.com.au
www.aapd.org.au

Australasian Osseointegration Society
Dr. Stan Stewart, Federal Secretary
13 Filipi Drive
St. Albans Park VIC 3219
03 5248 6641
www.aos.org.au

Australian Dental Association
75 Lithgow Street
St. Leonards NSW 2065
02 9906 4412
02 9906 4917 (fax)
adainc@ada.org.au
www.adad.org.au

Australian and New Zealand Academy of
  Endodontists
Dr. Mark Evans, Secretary/Treasurer
517 St. Kilda Road
Melbourne VIC 3004
03 9866 4528
03 9820 3102 (fax)
evansm@netspace.net.au
www.ada.org.au/_ANZAE.asp

Australian and New Zealand Society for
  Paediatric Dentistry
Dr. John Winters, Federal President
Suite 7, 38 Meadowvale Avenue
South Perth WA 6151
08 9367 9277
08 9367 9244 (fax)
drwinters@kidsdentist.com.au
www.anzspd.org.au

Australian and New Zealand Academy of
  Periodontists
Dr. Scott Parsons, Honorary Secretary
  ANZAP
Suite 15, McKay Gardens Professional
  Centre
Mackay Gardens TURNER ACT 2612
61 2 6247 6534
61 2 6247 0190 (fax)
capitalperio@bigpond.com
www.perio.org.au

Australian and New Zealand Association of
  Oral & Maxillofacial Surgeons
PO Box 576
Crows Nest NSW 1585
02 9431 8620
02 9431 8677 (fax)
anzaoms@apcaust.com.au
www.anzaoms.org

Australian Prosthodontic Society Inc.
Dr. A. Lidums, President
195 North Terrace
Adelaide SA 5000
(08) 8223 3531
(08) 8232 7772 (fax)
alidums@senet.com.au
www.ada.org.au/_APS.asp

Australian Society for Dental
   Anaesthesiology
Dr. A. Viljoen, President
Unit 2, Brindabella Specialist Centre
Cnr. Hinderman Drive & Palmer Street
Garran ACT 2605
02 6281 7666
02 6281 7667 (fax)
andrejv@bigpond.com
www.ada.org.au/_ASDA.asp

Australian Society of Endodontology
Dr. Glen Weston, Federal Secretary/
   Treasurer
573 Old Cleveland Road
South Perth QLD 4152
7 3395 2299
glenweston@internode.on.net
www.ada.org.au/Societies/ASE/_Home.asp

Australian Society of Forensic Dentistry
Dr. Russell Lain, Secretary
Oral Surgery Department
United Dental Hospital of Sydney
2 Chalmers Street
Surry Hills NSW 2010
(02) 9293 3293
r_lain@s054.aone.net.au
www.uq.edu.au/asfd

Australian Society of Implant Dentistry
Dr. David Rosenwax, Secretary
30 Portland Street
Dover Heights NSW 2030
02 93718407
02 93718542 (fax)
drosenwax@bigpond.com
www.asid.org.au

Australian Society of Orthodontists Inc.
PO Box 576
Crows Nest NSW 1585
02 9431 8666
02 9431 8677 (fax)
www.aso.org.au

Australian Society of Periodontology
Dr. B. James, President
69 Thuringowa Drive
Kirwan QLD 4817
07 4723 6560
07 4723 6562 (fax)
brianejames@bigpond.com
www.ada.org.au/_ASP.asp

Dental Hygienists'Association of Australia
PO Box 10030
Gouger Street
Adelaide SA 5000
08 8177 0196
0409 011 516 (mobile)
dhaainc@primus.com.au
www.dhaa.asn.au

Royal Australasian College of Dental
   Surgeons
Level 6, 64 Castlereagh Street
Sydney NSW 2000
2 9232 3800
2 9221 8108 (fax)
registrar@racds.org
www.racds.org

## Bermuda (1)

The Bermuda Dental Association
PO Box 3059
Hamilton HMNX
(441) 236-9375
(441) 292-4577 (fax)
bdadental@ibl.bm
www.bermudadental.bm

## Canada (1)

The Canadian Academy of Periodontology
#105-1815 Alta Vista Drive
Ottawa, ON K1G 3Y6
(613) 523-9800
(613) 523-1968 (fax)
central-office@cap-acp.ca

Canadian Association of Oral &
  Maxillofacial Surgeons
174 Colonnade Road
Unit 25
Ottawa, ON K2E 7J5
(613) 721-1816
(613) 721-3581 (fax)
info@caoms.com
www.caoms.com

Canadian Association of Orthodontists
2175 Sheppard Avenue East
Suite 310
Toronto, ON M2J 1W8
(416) 491-3186
(416) 491-1670 (fax)
cao@taylorenterprises.com
www.cao-aco.org

Canadian Dental Association
1815 Alta Vista Drive
Ottawa, ON KIG 3Y6
(613) 523-1770
reception@cda-adc.ca
www.cda-adc.ca

Canadian Dental Hygienists Association
96 Centerpointe Drive
Ottawa, ON K2G 6B1
(613) 224-5515
(613) 224-7283 (fax)
info@cdha.ca
www.cdha.ca

## Egypt (20)

Egyptian Dental Association
84 Mathaf El-Manyal Street
PO Box 11451
Cairo
02 365 8568
02 318 9143 (fax)
eda@internetegypt.com
www.eda-egypt.org

Egyptian Orthodontic Society
Faculty of Dentistry
University of Alexandria
Alexandria 21521
info@egortho.org
www.egortho.org

## India (91)

Indian Dental Association
Dr. V. M. Veerabahu
83, Dewan Bahadur Road
R. S. Puram, Coimbatore 641002
Ansari Nagar
New Dehli 110 020
(0422) 2553684/2450838
idatrustcbe@eth.net
www.dentalhealthindia.com

## Ireland (353)

Irish Dental Association Ltd.
Unit 2, Leopardstown Office Park
Sandyford
Dublin 18
353 1 2950072
353 1 2950092 (fax)
www.dentist.ie

## New Zealand (64)

New Zealand Dental Association
3 St. Marks Road
PO Box 28 084
Remuera, Auckland, 1136
09 524 2778
09 520 5256 (fax)
nzdainfo@nzda.org.nz
www.nzda.org.nz

New Zealand Dental
  Hygienists'Association
PO Box 36 529
Merivale
Christchurch
member@nzdha.co.nz

Academy of Australian and New Zealand
  Prosthodontists
(*see under* Australia)

Australian and New Zealand Academy of
  Endodontists
(*see under* Australia)

Australian and New Zealand Association of
Oral & Maxillofacial Surgeons
(*see under* Australia)

Australian and New Zealand Academy of
Periodontists
(*see under* Australia)

Australian and New Zealand Society for
Paediatric Dentistry
(*see under* Australia)

## Pakistan (92)

Pakistan Dental Association
Flat #3, 20 Floor, 31-c Zamzama
Commercial Lane-2, phase V, D.H.A.
Karachi
21-5823196, 21-5873075
21-5379393 (fax)
info@pda.org.pk
www.pda.org.pk

## Singapore (65)

Singapore Dental Association
2 College Road
Singapore 169850
223 9343
224 7967 (fax)
www.sda.org.sg

## South Africa (27)

Health Professions Council of South Africa
PO Box 205, Pretoria, 0001
553 Vermeulen Street
Arcadia
Pretoria
(012) 338 9300, (012) 338 6680
(012) 328 5120, (012) 325 2074 (fax)
hpcsa@hpcsa.co.za
www.hpcsa.co.za/about-us/contact-us.html

Dental Therapy and Oral Hygiene
The Registrar
Health Professions Council of South Africa
Professional Board for Dental Therapy and
Oral Hygiene
PO Box 25
Pretoria, 0001
012 338 9339
emmanuelc@hpcsa.co.za

Medical and Dental Professions
The Registrar
Health Professions Council of South Africa
Professional Board for Dental Therapy and
Oral Hygiene
PO Box 25
Pretoria, 0001
012 338 9325
daniek@hpcsa.co.za

## United Kingdom (44)

The British Association of Dental Nurses
11 Pharos Street
Fleetwood FY7 6BG
01253 778631
01253 773266 (fax)
admin@badn.org.uk
www.badn.org.uk

British Association of Oral and
Maxillofacial Surgeons
Royal College of Surgeons of England
35-43 Lincoln's Inn Fields
London WC2A 3PN
020 7405 8074
020 7430 9997 (fax)
office@baoms.org.uk
www.baoms.org.uk

British Dental Association
64 Wimpole Street
London WIG 8YS
020 7935 0875
020 7487 5232 (fax)
enquiries@bda.org
www.bda-dentistry.org.uk

British Dental Hygienists' Association
Mobbs Miller House
Ardington Road
Northampton
NN1 5LP
0870 2430752
enquiries@bdha.org.uk

The British Orthodontic Society
BOS Office
12 Bridewell Place
London EC4V 6AP
020 7353 8680
020 7353 8682 (fax)
ann.wright@bos.org.uk
www.bos.org.uk

British Society of Periodontology
44 Pool Road
Hartley Wintney
Hook
Hampshire RG27 8RD
01252 843598

The Commonwealth Dental Association
3 Rodney House
12/13 Pembridge Crescent
London W11 3DY
20 7229 3931
20 7681 2758 (fax)
www.cdauk.com

European Association for Cranio-
  Maxillofacial Surgery
PO Box 85
Midhurst GU29 9WS
West Sussex
1730 810951
1790 812042 (fax)
secretariat@eacmfs.org
www.eurofaces.com

European Orthodontic Society
Flat 20
49 Hallam Street
London W1W 6JN
20 7935 2795
20 7323 0410 (fax)
eoslondon@aol.com
www.eoseurope.org

Orthodontic National Group
11 Rutland Close
Copmanthorpe
York YO2 3SS
(01904) 725614
www.orthodontic-ong.co.uk

## United States (1)

Academy of Gp Orthodontics
9701 Wesley Street, Suite 202
Greenville, TX 75402-3745
(800) 634-2027
(888) 634-2028 (fax)
www.academygportho.com

American Academy of Gnathologic
  Orthopedics
2651 Oak Grove Road
Walnut Creek, CA 94598
(800) 510-2246
aago@astound.net
www.aago.com

American Academy of Periodontology
737 N. Michigan Avenue, Suite 800
Chicago, IL 60611-6660
(312) 787-5518
(312) 787-3670 (fax)
www.perio.org

The American Association for Functional
  Orthodontics
106 South Kent Street
Winchester, VA 22601
(540) 662-2200
(540) 665-8910 (fax)
aafo@verizon.net
www.aafo.org

American Association of Oral and
  Maxillofacial Surgeons
9700 West Bryn Mawr Avenue
Rosemont, IL 60018-5701
(847) 678-6200
(847) 678-6286 (fax)
www.aaoms.org

American Association of Orthodontists
401 N. Lindbergh Boulevard
St. Louis, MO 63141
(314) 993-1700
(314) 997-1745 (fax)
info@aaortho.org
www.braces.org

American Dental Assistants Association
35 E. Wacker Drive, Suite 1730
Chicago, IL 60601
(312) 541-1550
(312) 541-1496 (fax)
srobles@adaa1.com
www.dentalassistant.org

American Dental Association
211 E. Chicago Avenue
Chicago, IL 60611
(312) 440-2500
www.ada.org

American Dental Education Association
1400 K Street, NW, Suite 1100
Washington, DC 20005
(202) 289-7201
(202) 289-7204 (fax)
www.adea.org

American Dental Hygienists' Association
444 N. Michigan Avenue, Suite 3400
Chicago, IL 60611
(312) 440-8900
member.services@adha.net
www.adha.org

The American Orthodontic Society
11884 Greenville Avenue, Suite 112
Dallas, TX 75243
(800) 448-1601
aos@orthodontics.com
www.orthodontics.com

American Student Dental Association
211 E. Chicago Avenue, Suite 1160
Chicago, IL 60611-2687
(312) 440-2795
(312) 440-2820 (fax)
ASDA@ASDAnet.org

College of Diplomats of the American
   Board of Orthodontics
3260 Upper Bottom Road
St. Charles, MO 63303
(636) 922-5551
(636) 244-1650 (fax)
www.cdabo.org

Hispanic Dental Association
1224 Centre West, Suite 400B
Springfield, IL 62704
(217) 793-0035
(217) 793-0041 (fax)
HispanicDental@hdassoc.org
www.hdassoc.org

Holistic Dental Association
PO Box 151444
San Diego, CA 92175
info@holisticdental.org

International Academy of Periodontology
Boston University
100 E. Newton Street
Boston, MA 02118
(617) 638-4758
(617) 638-4799
bujiap@bu.edu
www.perioiap.org

International Association for Dental
   Research & American Association for
   Dental Research
1619 Duke Street
Alexandria, VA 22314-3406
(703) 548-0066
(703) 548-1883 (fax)
research@iadr.org
www.dentalresearch.org

International Association of Oral and
   Maxillofacial Surgeons
17 W220 22nd Street, Suite 420
Oakbrook Terrace, IL 60181
(630) 833-0945
(630) 833-1382 (fax)
info@iaoms.org
www.iaoms.org

International Association for Orthodontics
750 North Lincoln Memorial Drive, Suite
422
Milwaukee, WI 53202
(414) 272-2757
(414) 272-2754 (fax)
worldheadquarters@iaortho.org
www.iaortho.org

National Dental Association
3517 16th Street, NW
Washington, DC 20010
(202) 588-1697
(202) 588-1244 (fax)
admin@ndaonline.org
www.ndaonline.org

National Dental Hygienists' Association
PO Box 22463
Tampa, FL 33622
(800) 234-1096
forNDHA@aol.com
www.ndhaonline.org

World Federation of Orthodontists
401 North Lindbergh Boulevard
St. Louis, MO 63141
(314) 993-1700
(314) 993-5208 (fax)
www.wfo.org